AF248528

Congenital Heart Disease in Pediatric and Adult Patients

Ali Dabbagh • Antonio Hernandez Conte
Lorraine Lubin

Editors

Congenital Heart Disease in Pediatric and Adult Patients

Anesthetic and Perioperative Management

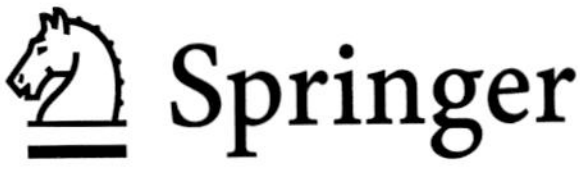

Editors
Ali Dabbagh, MD
Cardiac Anesthesiology Department
Anesthesiology Research Center
Shahid Beheshti University of
Medical Sciences
Tehran
Iran

Lorraine Lubin, MD
Department of Anesthesiology
Cedars-Sinai Medical Center
Los Angeles, CA
USA

Antonio Hernandez Conte, MD, MBA
Kaiser Permanente Los Angeles Medical
Center
Division of Cardiac Anesthesiology
Los Angeles, CA
USA

ISBN 978-3-319-44689-9   ISBN 978-3-319-44691-2   (eBook)
DOI 10.1007/978-3-319-44691-2

Library of Congress Control Number: 2017933707

Printed on acid-free paper

This Springer imprint is published by Springer Nature
The registered company is Springer International Publishing AG
The registered company address is: Gewerbestrasse 11, 6330 Cham, Switzerland

Foreword

Teach What You Practice!

There is an old educational aphorism, which has been used by educators for centuries: *Practice what you preach.* All too often teachers are somewhat distant from the educational frontlines. Although their opinions may be scientifically or evidence based, their edicts are not practical to clinicians treating complex patients in the real world (e.g., those with congenital heart disease). Rather, what the trainee (student, resident, or fellow) requires is an authoritative book edited and written by experts who manage these patients full time. They utilize evidence-based medicine to add to their clinical exposure and synthesize for the student an approach that "works." It is as if you are taking a master class with a master clinician whose "pearls" will make you a better doctor. Certainly, Drs. Ali Dabbagh, Antonio Hernandez Conte, and Lorraine Lubin represent an exemplary international composite of this type of physician. These are clinician-educators, who on a daily if not hourly basis interact with the patients with congenital heart disease.

From my own personal experience as a resident and cardiac anesthesia fellow, I desired to have a practical book that gave me a rapid overview of this field and allowed me to put my clinical observations in perspective. The editors have achieved just that. First, in 44 chapters, they take the reader from basic science to preoperative decision-making, monitoring and lesion-based intraoperative care, and finally care in the ICU setting. Second, the book is uniform in its presentation, showing the handiwork of the editors. This is the book you want available at 3 am in the morning when you called to manage the care of a patient undergoing an emergency surgical procedure or are facing a complex clinical dilemma in the ICU. Third, importantly, with the spectacular surgical results currently obtainable, pediatric patients are now living a productive life as adults. This means that many clinicians in nonacademic medical centers will be confronted by this reality. Thus, another group of physicians will benefit from the editors' and contributors' practical insights.

In this day of worldwide medical missions, the last chapter of this book deserves special mention. The coverage of *Pediatric Cardiac Anesthesia and Surgery in Developing Countries* is most likely unique to this book. This chapter will serve as an exceptional guide for use in settings where resources are limited.

In summary, the editors and contributors have skillfully fulfilled their mission as both *teachers* and *preachers*!

Paul Barash, MD
Professor of Anesthesiology
Yale University, School of Medicine
New Haven, CT, USA

Introduction

Congenital cardiac disease encompasses a wide range of disorders that are usually diagnosed in the early infancy. The cardiac pathology may be life-threatening and require immediate intervention and/or surgery, or it may be less severe and allow for a series of interventions over the course of the patient's early childhood and into adulthood. In *Congenital Heart Disease in Pediatric and Adult Patients: Anesthetic and Perioperative Management*, we have collaborated with a vast array of leading cardiac clinicians from around the world who manage this patient population on a daily basis in order to highlight the subtle and not so subtle nuances. Their expertise allows for a practical approach in the management of a complex series of problems and issues.

Congenital Heart Disease in Pediatric and Adult Patients: Anesthetic and Perioperative Management is organized into six major sections. Each section describes a particular facet unique to this subspecialty and is designed to allow the clinician managing this patient population to rapidly become oriented with the specific pathologies and care issues.

Part I focuses upon the history of pediatric anesthesia as well as embryology and pediatric physiology and pharmacology.

Part II entails the technical requirements for diagnostic methods and for monitoring patients undergoing congenital corrective surgery.

Part III focuses upon the preoperative evaluation and considerations unique to patients with congenital heart disease.

Part IV describes in great detail the intraoperative care of patients with congenital heart disease with specific chapters on each of the congenital anomalies.

Part V expounds upon postoperative care of patients with congenital heart disease.

Part VI of the book addresses emerging trends and clinical care outside of the traditional operating room that is creating the new field of "hybrid" procedures for congenital issues. Also, the final chapter in this section discusses pediatric cardiac surgery in emerging countries.

We believe that *Congenital Heart Disease in Pediatric and Adult Patients: Anesthetic and Perioperative Management* will allow the reader to gain a general and detailed knowledge base to optimally care for both pediatric and adult patients who undergo congenital heart surgery in the twenty-first century, both containing basic information and practical day-to-day data.

The editors would like to acknowledge the kind cooperation of all our contributors who have done their great work in preparing the chapters. Also, the kind cooperation and friendly patients of Springer authorities, especially Mr. Grant Weston and Mr. André Tournois, are highly acknowledged.

Tehran, Iran
Los Angeles, CA, USA
Los Angeles, CA, USA

Ali Dabbagh, MD
Antonio Hernandez Conte, MD, MBA
Lorraine Lubin, MD

Contents

Contributors

Mohammad-Amin Abdollahifar, PhD Department of Anatomy, School of Medicine, Shahid Beheshti University of Medical Sciences, Tehran, Iran

Iki Adachi, MD Division of Congenital Heart Surgery, Mechanical Circulatory Support, Texas Children's Hospital, Mechanical Circulatory Support, Baylor College of Medicine, Houston, TX, USA

Felice Eugenio Agrò, MD Anesthesia, Intensive Care and Pain Management Department, University School of Medicine Campus Bio-Medico of Rome, Rome, Italy

Abdullah Amini, PhD Department of Anatomy, School of Medicine, Shahid Beheshti University of Medical Sciences, Tehran, Iran

Gerald A. Bushman, MD Children's Hospital Los Angeles, Anesthesia Critical Care Medicine, Keck School of Medicine, Los Angeles, CA, USA

Marcelo Cardarelli, MD, MPH Pediatric and Congenital Cardiac Surgeon, Inova Children Hospital, Falls Church, VA, USA

William Novick Global Cardiac Alliance, Memphis, TN, USA

Alessandro Centonze, MD Department of Anesthesiology, Intensive Care and Pain Management, Campus Bio-Medico University Hospital of Rome, Rome, Italy

Renzo Cifuentes, MD Novick Cardiac Alliance, Universidad de Guayaquil, Guayaquil, Ecuador

Antonio Hernandez Conte, MD, MBA Division of Cardiac Anesthesiology, Kaiser Permanente Los Angeles Medical Center, Los Angeles, CA, USA

Cedars-Sinai Medical Center, Los Angeles, CA, USA

Ali Dabbagh, MD Cardiac Anesthesiology Department, Anesthesiology Research Center, Shahid Beheshti University of Medical Sciences, Tehran, Iran

Filip De Somer, PhD University Hospital Gent, Heart Center 5IE-K12, Gent, Belgium

Elham Hashemi Dehkordi, MD Pediatric Endocrinology, Child Growth and Development Research Center, Isfahan University of Medical Sciences, Isfahan, Iran

Edmo Atique Gabriel, MD, PhD Cardiac Surgeon, Coordinator and Professor of Medicine of União das Faculdades dos Grandes Lagos (Unilago), São José do Rio Preto, São Paulo, Brazil

Sthefano Atique Gabriel, MD, PhD Vascular and Endovascular Surgeon, Fellowship of Advanced Aortic Surgery at Ospedale San Raffaele, Milan, Italy

Ruchira Garg, MD Cedars-Sinai Medical Center, Los Angeles, CA, USA

Mahmoud Ghasemi, MD Pediatric Department, Kermanshah University of Medical Sciences, Kermanshah, Iran

Dheeraj Kumar Goswami, MD Anesthesiology and Pediatric Critical Care, Johns Hopkins Hospital, Baltimore, MD, USA

Majid Haghjoo, MD Department of Cardiac Electrophysiology, Rajaie Cardiovascular Medical and Research Center, Iran University of Medical Sciences, Tehran, Iran

Mahin Hashemipour, MD Pediatric Endocrinology. Endocrine and Metabolism Research Center, Isfahan University of Medical Sciences, Isfahan, Iran

Alireza Imani, PhD Department of Physiology, School of Medicine, Tehran University of Medical Sciences, Tehran, Iran

Mohammadrafie Khorgami, MD Department of Cardiac Electrophysiology, Rajaie Cardiovascular Medical and Research Center, Iran University of Medical Sciences, Tehran, Iran

Lorraine Lubin, MD Cedars Sinai Medical Center, Department of Anesthesiology, Los Angeles, CA, USA

Stacey Marr, MSc, RN, NP William Novick Global Cardiac Alliance, Memphis, TN, USA

Ali Mazaheri, MD Pediatric Department, Lorestan University of Medical Sciences, Lorestan, Iran

Marion McRae, MScN Cedars-Sinai Medical Center, Los Angeles, CA, USA

David Geffen School of Medicine, UCLA, Los Angeles, CA, USA

Evelyn Carolina Monico, MD Pediatric Anesthesia, Texas Children's Hospital, Baylor College of Medicine, Houston, TX, USA

Neda Mostofizadeh, MD Pediatric Endocrinology, Child Growth and Development Research Center, Isfahan University of Medical Sciences, Isfahan, Iran

Pablo Motta, MD Baylor College of Medicine, Texas Children's Hospital, Division of Pediatric Cardiovascular Anesthesiology, Houston, TX, USA

Yamile Muñoz, MD Cardiovascular and Thoracic Anesthesia, Novick Cardiac Alliance, Clínica Cardio VID, Medellín, Colombia

Pooja Nawathe, MD Cedars-Sinai Medical Center, Los Angeles, CA, USA

William M. Novick, MD Surgery and International Child Health, University of Tennessee Health Science Center, Memphis, TN, USA

William Novick Global Cardiac Alliance, Memphis, TN, USA

Antonio Perez-Ferrer, MD Department of Pediatric Anesthesiology and Intensive Care, La Paz University Hospital, Madrid, Spain

Alistair Phillips, MD, FACC, FACS Congenital Heart Program, the Heart Institute, Division of Congenital Heart Surgery, Division of Cardiothoracic Surgery, Department of Surgery, Cedars-Sinai Medical Center, Los Angeles, CA, USA

Zoel Augusto Quiñónez, MD Baylor College of Medicine, Texas Children's Hospital, Division of Pediatric Cardiovascular Anesthesiology, Houston, TX, USA

Shahzad G. Raja, BSc, MBBS, MRCS, FRCS(C-Th) Department of Cardiac Surgery, Harefield Hospital, London, UK

Samira Rajaei, MD, PhD Department of Immunology, School of Medicine, Tehran University of Medical Science, Tehran, Iran

Michael A. E. Ramsay, MD, FRCA Department of Anesthesiology and Pain Management, Baylor Research Institute, Baylor University Medical Center and Baylor Research Institute, Dallas, TX, USA

Sri O. Rao, MD Novick Cardiac Alliance, Memphis, TN, USA

Noushin Rostampour, MD Pediatric Department, Shahrekord University of Medical Sciences, Shahrekord, Iran

Mohammad Ali Saghafi, MD Anesthesiology Research Center, Cardiac Anesthesiology Department, Shahid Beheshti University of Medical Sciences, Tehran, Iran

Jose E. Santoro, MD Yale University School of Medicine, Yale New Haven Children's Hospital, New Haven, USA

Jamie Wingate Sinton, MD Anesthesiology Department, Baylor College of Medicine & Texas Children's Hospital, Houston, TX, USA

Fahimeh Soheilipour, MD Minimally Invasive Surgery Research Center, Iran University of Medical Sciences, Tehran, Iran

Zahra Talebi, PharmD Anesthesiology Research Center, Shahid Beheshti University of Medical Sciences, Tehran, Iran

Ramin Baghaei Tehrani, MD Pediatric Cardiac Surgery Department, Modarres Hospital, Shahid Beheshti University of Medical Sciences, Tehran, Iran

Premal M. Trivedi, MD Baylor College of Medicine, Texas Children's Hospital, Division of Pediatric Cardiovascular Anesthesiology, Houston, TX, USA

David Freed Vener, MD Department of Anesthesia and Pediatrics, Baylor College of Medicine and Texas Children's Hospital, Houston, TX, USA

Marialuisa Vennari, MD Department of Anesthesiology, Intensive Care and Pain Management, Campus Bio-Medico University Hospital of Rome, Rome, Italy

Robert Wong, MD Cedars-Sinai Medical Center, Los Angeles, CA, USA

Ian Gavin Wright, MB ChB FCA(SA) Department of Anaesthesiology, Intensive Care and Pain Management, Harefield Hospital, London, UK

Part I
History, Embryology, Physiology and Pharmacology

Chapter 1
History of Pediatric Anesthesia and Pediatric Cardiac-Congenital Surgery

Antonio Hernandez Conte

Pediatric surgery has a long history that dates back to the early twentieth century. In the early 1900s, pediatric medicine and surgery were undistinguishable from general adult surgical care, therefore, adult and pediatric patients were treated in a similar manner. Whereas in contemporary medicine, pediatric surgery is a completely separate specialty with different training pathways compared to a surgeon treating adult patients. It was soon discovered that the mortality rates in the younger population were extraordinarily high and that if improved results were expected, the pediatric patient would need a separate treatment approach.

Pediatric patients have traditionally been defined as patients under the age of 18; however, as will be discussed in later chapters, this age demarcation has once again become less defined as patients who manifested congenital heart disease grow into adulthood and require additional cardiologic or cardiac surgical interventions. Pediatric cardiac and congenital surgery focuses upon the surgical correction of major anomalies pertaining to the heart and surround vascular structures. As the subspecialty of pediatric surgery evolved in the mid-1900s, pediatric surgical care becomes more commonly based at children's specialty hospitals throughout Europe and the United States. In the period of less than 50 years, the initial development and evolution of medical and technical advances led by key scientists and physicians focusing upon care of the pediatric patient allowed the fields of pediatric surgery, pediatric cardiac/congenital surgery, and pediatric anesthesia to become a mainstay of modern-day medicine.

A. Hernandez Conte, MD, MBA
Division of Cardiac Anesthesiology, Kaiser Permanente Los Angeles Medical Center, Los Angeles, CA, USA

Cedars-Sinai Medical Center, Los Angeles, CA, USA
e-mail: sedated@bellsouth.net; antonio.conte@kp.org

© Springer International Publishing Switzerland 2017
A. Dabbagh et al. (eds.), *Congenital Heart Disease in Pediatric and Adult Patients*, DOI 10.1007/978-3-319-44691-2_1

The Birth of Pediatrics and "Children's Hospitals" in the United States

The status of pediatric care in the 1800s and early 1900s was profoundly different than current standards. As mentioned earlier, pediatric patients were in essence treated in a manner similar to adults. Some examples of prevailing treatments and trends included lack of understanding of intravenous therapy, and fluid balance was based on adult models. Additionally, blood transfusions were not utilized, and appendicitis was the fourth common cause of death in children. The most common surgical procedures in children were abscess drainage, appendectomies, tumors, and hernia repairs. There was 90 % mortality for colostomies and intussusceptions. With the concomitant medical and surgical advances that had begun in the mid-1930s and continued thereafter in each decade, pediatric care was finally becoming entrenched in newly formed children's hospitals.

Dr. Abraham Jacobi is considered to be the father of pediatrics in the United States and offered the first lectures on pediatric disease in 1860. Generally speaking, adult medicine focused upon organ issues or technology. Dr. Jacobi believed that children warranted a broader approach with respect to child health and well-being and not just disease states. In 1880, Dr. Jacobi along with a few other physicians founded the American Medical Association's section on the diseases of children. They stressed the need for more children's hospitals and for the expansion of pediatric content in medical school curricula. By 1900, ten schools of medicine had full-time pediatricians.

In the pre-1850s, US hospitals generally had no place for children outside of the maternity ward. Childhood illnesses were therefore most often handled at home. When families sought medical care outside of their home, children were treated as tiny adults. This view lead to high infant and children mortality rates who had been admitted to hospitals, due to improper medical care. Dr. Francis West Lewis visits the Great Ormond Street Hospital for Sick Children in London. At the time this was the leading institution in the world for not only pediatric care but also the education of practitioners in the field. Dr. Lewis was inspired to bring what he saw in London to the United States. Lewis and his colleague Dr. Hewson Bache begin to work on what has now become the Children's Hospital of Philadelphia.

In 1850, the Children's Hospital of Pennsylvania (CHOP) in Philadelphia opened its doors. By 1871, CHOP was performing its first pediatric surgeries, and in 1871 the first pediatric-centered medical training program was established. Surgical clinics were created to train surgeons who were now working at the few emerging children's hospitals across the country. As early as the 1870s, physicians at the Children's Hospital of Philadelphia, for example, pressured the lay trustees who managed the hospital to increase patient turnover and accept more acutely ill children, especially orthopedic surgical patients who had something to offer physician education and on whom new surgical techniques and therapies could be tried. This new emphasis on the medical needs of patients and the experimental needs of doctors and nurses conflicted with the social welfare role children's hospitals saw themselves as performing.

The Children's Hospital in Boston was the second such specialty hospital in the United States and admitted its first patient in 1869. By the 1920s and 1930s, The Children's Hospital in Boston was becoming a major center for advanced care of the pediatric patient while also performing novel and innovative procedures for the first time. Advancements at The Children's Hospital in Boston have continued, and notable accomplishments include the first correction of hypoplastic left heart syndrome (1983) and the first pediatric open-heart transplant (1986).

Surgical Pioneers in Pediatric Surgery

William E. Ladd is often referred to as the *father* of pediatric surgery. A Harvard-educated physician, Dr. Ladd's career path was dramatically altered after being dispatched by U.S President Lowell to treat the approximately 9000 victims who were innocent bystanders at the accidental collision of two ships in the Halifax Harbour in Nova Scotia in 1917. The explosion was the most powerful nonnuclear explosion that had ever occurred in history, and 4 % of the population of Halifax was killed instantly. Dr. Ladd was sent on one of the first trains deployed to the accident site in Nova Scotia, and his experiences in Halifax had a profound effect upon him. After returning to Boston, Dr. Ladd devoted himself entirely to the surgical care of infants and children. Dr. Ladd recognized that children needed a very gentle and thorough physical evaluation, and surgeons needed to rely upon their own senses. Additionally, adult surgical instruments were not suitable for children, and he began to develop appropriately sized instruments.

In 1918, Dr. Ladd became an instructor in surgery at Harvard Medical School, and by 1927, he was named the chief of surgery. In 1931, Dr. Ladd became a full Harvard Medical School Professor, and in 1941, he published the seminal textbook entitled *Abdominal Surgery of Infancy and Childhood*. As quoted by Donald Watson, "Dr. Ladd brought the diagnosis and management of surgical lesions of infancy and childhood into new perspective." Indeed Dr. Ladd's pioneer efforts truly initiated pediatric surgery as a separate discipline in the Western Hemisphere." Physicians who trained under Dr. Ladd in Boston perpetuated the specialty and achieved their own independent successes to further cement and validate the emerging specialty. These physicians included Drs. Robert E. Gross, Theodore Jewett, Earle Wrenn, Donald Rooney, C. Everett Koop, and Monford Custer—all of them continued to advance the field of pediatric surgery in the twentieth century.

Origins of Pediatric Anesthesiology

The subspecialty of pediatric anesthesia has significantly evolved since its origin in Jefferson, Georgia, when Dr. Crawford Long administered the first documented ether anesthetic to an 8-year-old boy for a toe amputation on July 3, 1842. From the very beginning, it was clear that children were at higher risk than adults for anesthesia-related complications and death because of differences in their physiology, anatomy, and functional development. The progression of pediatric anesthesia as a subspecialty arose from the evolution of pediatric surgery. The history of pediatric anesthesia is intertwined with Dr. Ladd's advances in pediatric surgery and his work in creating the subspecialty Children's Hospital of Boston.

Prior to World War II, two anesthesiologists played a pivotal role in establishing pediatric anesthesia's role as an important necessity for successful surgery in pediatric patients. Dr. Charles H. Robson from Toronto's Hospital for Sick Children was perhaps the first pediatric anesthesiologist. Dr. Robson's practice of administering open-drop ether and cyclopropane and his use of tracheal intubations in children in the 1930s demonstrated early clinical applications of his research in pediatric anesthesia. Dr. Philip Ayer working in England during the same period contributed to the development of the "T-piece" as part of the breathing circuit. Post-World War II, a group of six anesthesiologists around the world played key roles in further refining the role of the pediatric anesthesiologist. In Boston, Dr. Robert M. Smith's invention of the precordial stethoscope was groundbreaking, and in Philadelphia Dr. Margo van Deming developed tools to determine anesthetic blood levels in infants. Dr. Digby Leigh, based out of Montreal and Los Angeles, and Dr. Jackson Rees further refined pediatric breathing apparatus. Meanwhile in New York City, Dr. Virginia Apgar developed infant scoring systems to determine neonatal well-being immediately after birth. Finally, Dr. Smith's first pediatric anesthesia textbook is among the pioneering influences that helped shape the early phases of pediatric anesthesia.

The aforementioned events coincided with the elevation of anesthesiology to a specialty rank distinct and equal to surgery and medicine, with its own specialty board (established in 1937) and training programs. By 1941, the American Board of Medical Specialties (ABMS) approved the American Board of Anesthesiology (ABA) as a separate primary board. In the 1960s and 1970s, pediatric anesthesia entered into its first explosive period of growth fueled by translational discoveries in human biology, including fundamental understandings of the transition from fetal to postnatal circulation. Research on homeostatic fluid regulation, electrolytes, metabolism, temperature regulation, monitoring of blood gases, mechanical ventilation, and cardiopulmonary resuscitation helped in developed neonatal and pediatric care that previously did not exist.

The 1980s and 1990s were transformative years that witnessed the establishment of pediatric anesthesia as a formal subspecialty fellowship training programs implemented across the United States. In 1997, the American Council on Graduate Medical Education recognized pediatric anesthesia as subspecialty, and pediatric anesthesiology falls under its purview. In 2012, the ABMS approved the ABA's time-limited pediatric anesthesiology subspecialty certificate for physician credentialing.

Developments Leading to Pediatric Heart and Congenital Surgery

The development of pediatric cardiac and congenital surgery arose from the confluence of multiple events. At the very basis of the field was the initial descriptive study of pediatric cardiac defects—many of which were acquired from birth or deemed to be *congenital*. In the early 1600s, a group of anatomists published vastly descriptive accounts of the pediatric cardiac anatomy and vasculature. Dr. Lee Harvey published *De Motu Cordis*, an account of the pulmonary and systemic circulations. In 1671, Niels Stenson of Copenhagen described the cardiac pathology of a stillborn fetus with multiple congenital anomalies including the cardiac lesion, which is now recognized as tetralogy of Fallot. Dr. Stenson correctly described the physiologic consequences of the anatomic malformation. More than 100 years later, Dr. Edwardo Sandifort, for the first time, described the clinical symptoms of a young child whom he called "blue boy." Because the child had appeared normal at birth, he suspected that the condition was acquired, but when he died at twelve and one-half years of age, it was apparent, at postmortem study, that this was a congenital defect, which included a patent foramen ovale, a small pulmonary artery with a blocked pulmonary valve, and a ventricular communication between the two ventricles. In 1888, the anatomic lesion, now called tetralogy of Fallot, was named for Etienne-Louis Fallot who stated that 75 % of patients with cyanotic heart disease would have either pulmonary stenosis or atresia, an overriding aorta, a ventricular septal defect, and right ventricular hypertrophy; his assertions were validated by autopsy findings.

Clinicians who advanced the study of pediatric cardiology began to manifest their findings by the early 1800s. In 1819, Rene Laennec developed the stethoscope, and this allowed physicians to begin to relate murmurs heard by auscultation and correlate them to pathologic findings found at autopsy. In the 1850s, Thomas Peacock noted the characteristic radiation of the murmur of pulmonary stenosis. In 1858, he published a book that contained beautiful illustrations of various congenital malformations, including descriptions of ventricular septal defects, pulmonary stenosis, and transposition of the aorta and pulmonary artery. By 1874, Henri Roger described a loud murmur accompanied by a thrill to be pathognomonic of a communication between the two ventricles that was compatible with a long life. Gibson described the murmur as well as the pathophysiology of patent ductus arteriosus in 1898.

In 1930, Helen Taussig was placed in charge of the cardiac clinic at the Harriet Lane Home for Invalid Children in Baltimore, Maryland, and had a fluoroscope installed. Helen Taussig learned to utilize the fluoroscope so that she might learn more about congenital malformations of the heart. Using both electrocardiogram and fluoroscopy, Taussig was able to correlate physical findings with the pathology noted at autopsy. Dr. Taussig's descriptions of anatomic lesions corroborated with fluoroscopy led to the final crucial knowledge needed to provide surgeons with conclusive evidence that would warrant a surgical approach. In 1938, Dr. Robert Gross ligated the patent ductus of a patient, and thus the discipline of pediatric cardiology and cardiac surgery was born.

A few physicians recognized that infants with tetralogy of Fallot were often pink until the ductus arteriosus closed. Dr. Taussig hypothesized that if a patent ductus could be ligated, then why not surgically construct a ductus. Taussig initially approached Dr. Gross to attempt such a procedure but he declined; however, she found another surgeon, Alfred Blalock, to possibly consider such an operation. Blalock had already performed anastomoses between the left subclavian artery and pulmonary artery in his attempt to learn more about pulmonary artery hypertension. In November 1944, Blalock anastomosed the left subclavian artery to the pulmonary artery; this positively impacted the life of a severely cyanotic child with tetralogy of Fallot. The Blalock-Taussig operation, as it was named, soon had worldwide recognition. The following year, Crayfoord and Nylin from Stockholm, Sweden, successfully repaired a coarctation of the aorta with an end-to-end anastomosis. All of these surgical procedures were performed on the beating heart. To repair intracardiac lesions, cardiopulmonary bypass was necessary. In 1955, Walt Lillehei and colleagues in Minneapolis reported the results in 32 patients with ventricular septal defect, tetralogy of Fallot, and atrioventricular communis defects using a human cross-circulation technique.

The arrival of a mechanical cardiopulmonary bypass device was not an overnight event, and it took a long series of events to occur prior to the arrival of the "heart-lung" machine to be invented. An Austrian-German physiologist, Maximilian von Frey, developed an early prototype of a heart-lung machine in 1885 at the University of Leipzig. However, the utilization of this machine was not feasible before the discovery of heparin in 1916 which was necessary to prevent clotting of the mechanical components within the device. A Soviet scientist Sergei Brukhonenko developed a heart-lung machine for total body perfusion in 1926 which was used in experiments with canines. Dr. Clarence Dennis led the team that conducted the first known operation involving open cardiotomy with temporary mechanical takeover of both heart and lung functions in 1951 at the University of Minnesota Hospital; the patient did not survive due to an unexpected complex congenital heart defect. This followed 4 years of laboratory experimentation with dogs with a unit called the *Iron Heart*. A team of scientists at Birmingham University (including Eric Charles, a chemical engineer) were among the pioneers of this technology. Another member of the team was Dr. Russell M. Nelson, who performed the first open-heart surgery in Utah.

The first successful mechanical support of left ventricular function was performed in July 3, 1952, by Forest Dewey Dodrill using a machine, the Dodrill-GMR, codeveloped with General Motors. The machine was later used to support right ventricular function. The first successful open-heart procedure on a human utilizing the heart-lung machine was performed by John Gibbon in 1953 at Thomas Jefferson University Hospital in Philadelphia. He repaired an atrial septal defect in an 18-year-old woman. Dr. Gibbon's cardiopulmonary bypass machine was further developed into a reliable instrument by a surgical team led by John W. Kirklin at the Mayo Clinic in Rochester, Minnesota, in the mid-1950s (Fig. 1.1).

Future Directions

As a medical specialty, pediatric cardiology and pediatric heart/congenital surgery have always required a team—pathologists, physiologists, cardiologists, surgeons, intensivists, interventionalists, and anesthesiologists—each playing a critical and pivotal role in the treatment of children with cardiac congenital disease. In the twenty-first century, geneticists, molecular biologists, and other basic scientists are contributing their innovative discoveries to this broad multidisciplinary team to

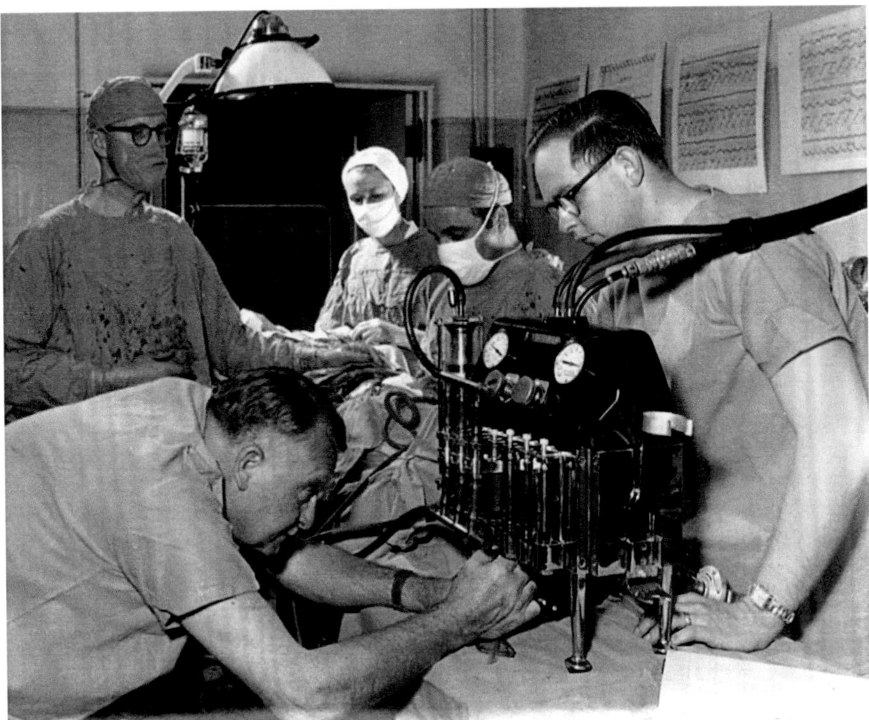

Fig. 1.1 The Dodrill-GMR heart pump (Dr Dodrill is in scrub cap and mask on the left. Used with permission from Dr. William S. Stoney. Adapted from Stoney WS. Historical perspectives in cardiology. Circulation 2009;119:2844–53)

ensure an exciting future for pediatric cardiology and the children yet to be born. The amalgamation of specialties with seeming divergent interests is now allowing the formation of "hybridized" environments where multidisciplinary teams create new procedures combining elements of traditional open-heart surgery with minimally invasive techniques. New techniques in DNA sequencing will allow early recognition of genetic disorders predisposing individuals to congenital cardiac disease. Minimally invasive techniques will continue to play a larger role in the repair of congenital lesions either in utero or post-delivery in the neonatal period. The traditional "operating room" of the twenty-first century will continue to evolve and transform into a complex array of medical and surgical specialists working alongside with basic scientists in a state-of-the-art environment to allow translational endeavors to flourish.

Chapter 2
Cardiovascular System Embryology and Development

Ali Dabbagh, Abdollah Amini, Mohammad-Amin Abdollahifar, and Mohammad Ali Saghafi

Establishing Cardiac Crescent

The first organ which is formed and began to function during the embryonic periods is the heart. In fact, when the embryo could no more support its nutritional requirements just by the *simple diffusion from the placenta*, the heart appears as a new organ.

From epiblast, the primitive streak comes out; however, the primitive streak, in turn, gives origin to mesoderm. Myocardial progenitor cells come out of anterior splanchnic mesoderm. As described by Abu-Issa and Kirby, these myocardial progenitor cells start their development process through four "sequential but at times, overlapping" stages (Abu-Issa and Kirby 2007; Lin et al. 2012):

1. Cardiogenic *mesoderm* specification
2. Bilateral *establishment* of heart fields
3. Composition and configuration of *heart field*
4. Differentiation of cardiomyocyte and formation of *heart tube*

The heart as noted is one of the organs originating from anterior splanchnic mesoderm. Also, parts of the endoderm are involved in the development of the heart; these endodermal parts are enveloped by mesoderm to form the endodermal portions of the heart (Lin et al. 2012).

A. Dabbagh, MD (⊠) • M.A. Saghafi, MD
Cardiac Anesthesiology Department, Anesthesiology Research Center,
Shahid Beheshti University of Medical Sciences, Tehran, Iran
e-mail: alidabbagh@yahoo.com; alidabbagh@sbmu.ac.ir

A. Amini, PhD • M.-A. Abdollahifar, PhD
Department of Anatomical and Biological Sciences, School of Medicine, Shahid Beheshti
University of Medical Sciences, Tehran, Iran

© Springer International Publishing Switzerland 2017
A. Dabbagh et al. (eds.), *Congenital Heart Disease in Pediatric and Adult Patients*, DOI 10.1007/978-3-319-44691-2_2

The cardiac progenitor cells develop locally into the splanchnic layers of the lateral mesoderm on both left and right sides of the embryo to form bilateral blood islands in splanchnic mesoderm, leading to *cardiogenic mesoderm specification.* Also, blood islands appear bilaterally in this mesoderm, which will later form blood cells and two dorsal aortae (Gittenberger-de Groot et al. 2005).

In the next stage, after the development of the cardiac progenitor cells in the lateral mesoderm, two "lateral mesodermal islands" or "lateral cardiogenic plates" are created. These two lateral islands fuse together in the midline to form the *cardiac crescent* which has the following features (Yutzey and Kirby 2002; Lockhart et al. 2011):

- It has an "arch-shaped" or "bow-shaped" or "horseshoe-shaped" feature in the caudal part of the embryo.
- It constitutes the so-called primary heart field or first heart field (PHF or FHF), in days 16–18.
- Then, PHF gives rise to some of the main structure of the mature heart: atria, left ventricle, atrioventricular (AV) canal, and most part of the right ventricle (Fig. 2.1).

PHF has two poles with the following order in migration and looping:

- A cephalad pole will later constitute the bulbus cordis and aortic roots (i.e., the outflow tract).
- The caudal pole, which is also known as the sinus venosus, will later constitute the ventricles and the ends of those major veins that bring the venous blood to the heart; also, some segments of the atria are made from the caudal pole (Lin et al. 2012).

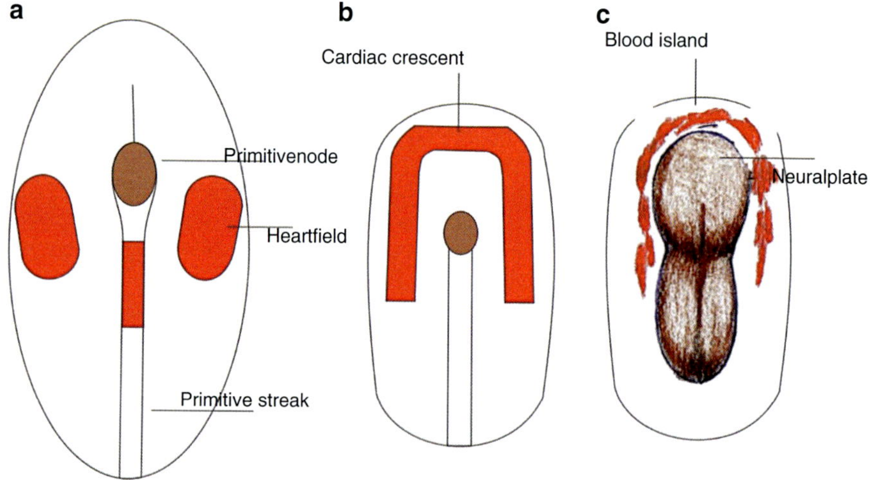

Fig. 2.1 Early development of the heart; (**a–c**) Dorsal view of an embryo. Hemangioblasts reside in the splanchnic mesoderm in front of the neural plate and on each side of the embryo

While the cardiovascular system forms in about the middle of the third week, this primary heart tube has rhythmic peristalsis activity by the end of the third week. After rightward looping of the primary heart tube, these two poles of the primary heart tube are changed accordingly:

- Anterior specification: ventricular segments
- Posterior specification: atrial segments

During later stages of the cardiac development, another important part named *secondary heart field* (SHF) is created with the following characteristics (Moorman et al. 2003; Verzi et al. 2005; Restivo et al. 2006; Watanabe and Buckingham 2010; Xin et al. 2013; Calkoen et al. 2016):

- SHF is "a second cellular pool."
- It is derived from the *ventral pharyngeal splanchnic mesoderm.*
- SHF is located medial and anterior to the cardiac crescent (i.e., medial and anterior to PHF and dorsal to the primary heart tube).
- Its main function is to give cellular origin to "the arterial and venous side of the heart."
- SHF, during days 20 and 21, primarily gives origin to the conotruncal region of the heart, which includes mainly the following segments in the mature heart: other primordial parts of the right ventricle, the interventricular septum (IVS), and endothelial and myocardial components of *the outflow tract* (i.e., conotruncus).
- Another major function of the SHF is laterality of cardiac constituents.

Clinical Note
Some of the most common congenital heart disorders due to conotruncal defects are:

- Persistent truncus arteriosus
- Tetralogy of Fallot
- Double-outlet right ventricle
- Pulmonary atresia
- Pulmonary stenosis (Restivo et al. 2006)

Formation of the Heart Tube

The heart arises from a common mesodermal pool of progenitor cells, which is part of the cardiopharyngeal region. During the early phases of cardiac development, some parts of the primary cardiogenic area are anterior to the neural tubes; however, due to the very rapid growth of brain vesicles, there is a cephalad movement of the oropharyngeal membrane, which in turn pushes the heart into the more caudal parts; then, the heart comes to an inner position to be part of the future thorax. From another point of view, the oropharyngeal region becomes compressed in between the brain, the yolk, and the heart (Soukup et al. 2013; Diogo et al. 2015).

The process of body folding involves both cephalocaudal and lateral folding of the embryonic plate. As the embryonic plates fold laterally, the endocardial tubes fuse with each other to form a heart tube; by this process, the heart tube is gradually formed (Yutzey and Kirby 2002; Abu-Issa and Kirby 2007).

Usually, *looping of the heart tube* which is discussed in the next paragraphs is considered as the primary visible sign for asymmetry during embryo development. However, formation of the atrioventricular canal is structurally asymmetric associated with left-sided bulging (Moorman et al. 2003).

Therefore, the heart tube is composed of three distinct layers (Yutzey and Kirby 2002; Lockhart et al. 2011):

1. The inner endothelial cover, i.e., *endocardium* (which lines the inner layer of the heart tube).
2. The outer myocardial layer, i.e., *myocardium*; the endocardium and myocardium are separated by an acellular space which is rich in extracellular matrix (ECM); this thick ECM, also named *cardiac jelly*, is secreted by myocardium and is rich in a number of specific molecules including hyaluronic acid, hyaluronan, fibronectin, fibrillin, proteoglycans, and collagens which have important roles in heart development, especially for proper development of endocardial cushion of the atrioventricular junctions.
3. The epicardium (visceral pericardium) is derived from mesodermal cells that arise from splanchnic mesoderm on the surface of the septum transversum and sinus venous which migrate onto the outer surface of the myocardium.

During later developmental phases, the heart tube become swelled and progressively invaginates into the pericardial cavity. At first, it is attached to the dorsal wall of the body through the dorsal mesocardium which is a fold of the mesodermal tissue (Moorman et al. 2003; Lin et al. 2012). However, the central portion of dorsal mesocardium degenerates and forms the transverse pericardial sinus, which is located between the left and the right sides of the pericardial cavity (Fig. 2.2).

The heart is now attached only at its caudal and cranial parts in the pericardial cavity by blood vessels; i.e., the ventricular loop of the heart has gained both "inlet and outlet components." The inflow to the heart is initially supplied by three pairs of drainage veins into the tubular heart through vitelline veins (return poorly oxygenated blood from the umbilical vesicle), umbilical veins (carry well-oxygenated blood from the chorion), and common cardinal veins (return poorly blood with low oxygen from the embryo body) (Moorman et al. 2003; Lin et al. 2012). On the other side, the outlet supports the cardiac outflow tract; it means that the left and right dorsal aortae make the outflow of the heart vessels, which in turn leads to arteries emerging from the aortic sac and then going to pharyngeal arcs. In the area of the arches, the dorsal aortae are arranged as paired vessels, but caudal parts of the dorsal aorta join together to form a single aorta (thoracic aorta and abdominal aorta).

However, with improvements in heart development, the heart loop is completed and expands; the dorsal mesocardium breaks up, except in the most caudal segment

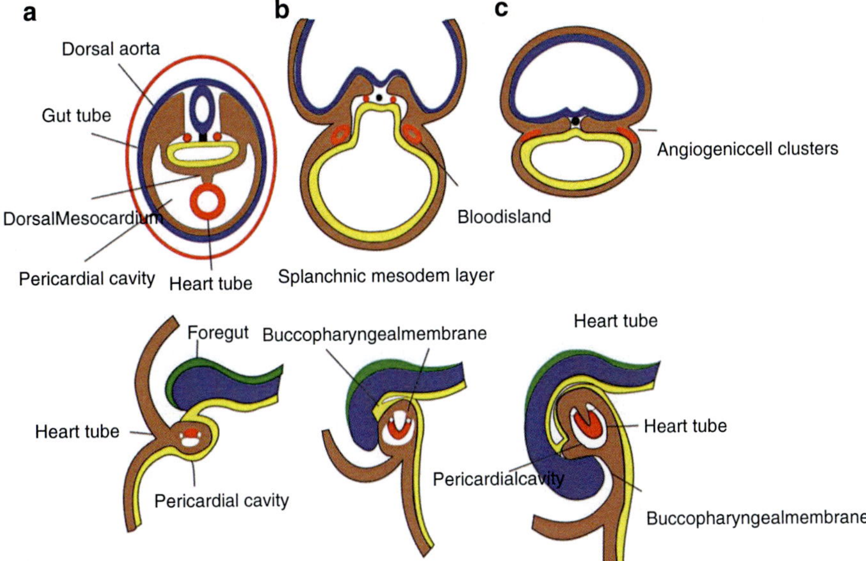

Fig. 2.2 Transverse sections and longitudinal section through embryo at different stages of heart tube formation; (**a**) 17 days, (**b**) 18 days, (**c**) 22 days

which plays the role of venous pole for the heart; this dorsal mesenchymal part has a central role in some major events of heart development like pulmonary vein development and atrioventricular mesenchymal complex formation.

The Looping of Cardiac Tissue

The primitive heart tube begins to elongate on day 23; however, signaling pathway guaranteeing right-sided looping is initiated earlier. It means that the looping process is signaled during gastrulation; as mentioned earlier, *looping of the heart tube* is the primary visible sign for asymmetry during embryo development. The process of cardiac loop is completed by day 28 (Yutzey and Kirby 2002; Moorman et al. 2003; Jacobs et al. 2007).

As the primitive heart tube elongates in both cranial and caudal parts, the dorsal mesocardium is detached from the developing left ventricle, leading to liberation of the heart tube. The heart tube bends rightward after its liberation (Moorman et al. 2003).

Then, in the process of looping, the *cephalic part* of the heart tube bends in three directions:

- Ventral
- Caudal
- To the right

However, the *caudal part* itself bends again and extends in these three directions:

- Dorsal
- Cranial
- To the left

As mentioned before, these processes of bending are completed by day 28 and lead finally to the *cardiac loop*.

Over the next 5 weeks, a series of "strictures" and "bulged areas" are created in the primitive heart tube. Through the bulged regions, the following structures come out:

- Bulbus cordis (which includes truncus arteriosus, conus arteriosus, and conus cordis)
- Ventricle
- Atrium
- Sinus venosus

The resultant "ventricular loop" has two main components:

- The inlet gives origin to the sinus venosus, which starts at the caudal end and consists of left and right sinus horns; these right and left horns are partially confluent; also, the common cardinal veins drain into the sinus venosus (Yutzey and Kirby 2002).
- The outlet consists of the conus and truncus, and the arterial system (including aorta and pharyngeal arcs) originates from the outflow tract SHF which is the origin of the outflow tract myocardium which comes out of the ventricular outlet (Restivo et al. 2006; Watanabe and Buckingham 2010).

There are two other chambers that are cranial to the sinus venosus; these are:

- *The primitive atrium* which will form the common atrium (also known as primitive atrium); this primitive atrium will form the left and the right atria.
- *The primitive ventricle* which will form the left ventricle; however, the primitive ventricle is separated from the next expansion (i.e., the bulbus cordis) by the bulboventricular sulcus; the latter segment will form much of the right ventricle.

Conotruncal segment The distal outflow tract of the right and left ventricles has the same origin. The *conotruncal segment* is the cranial-most segment of the ventricles and forms the following parts:

- *Outflow tract*: the distal outflow region each of the left and right ventricles.
- *Conus cordis* (*or conus arteriosus*): after creating the outflow tract, the conotruncal segment is further subdivided into the conus cordis (or conus arteriosus) and the truncus arteriosus; conus cordis will be eventually incorporated into the corresponding right and left ventricles.
- *Truncus arteriosus*: this is the third part of the conotruncal segment and splits into two parts to form the pulmonary artery and the ascending aorta; however, the most cranial end of the truncus arteriosus is connected to a dilated expansion called *the aortic sac* (Fig. 2.3).

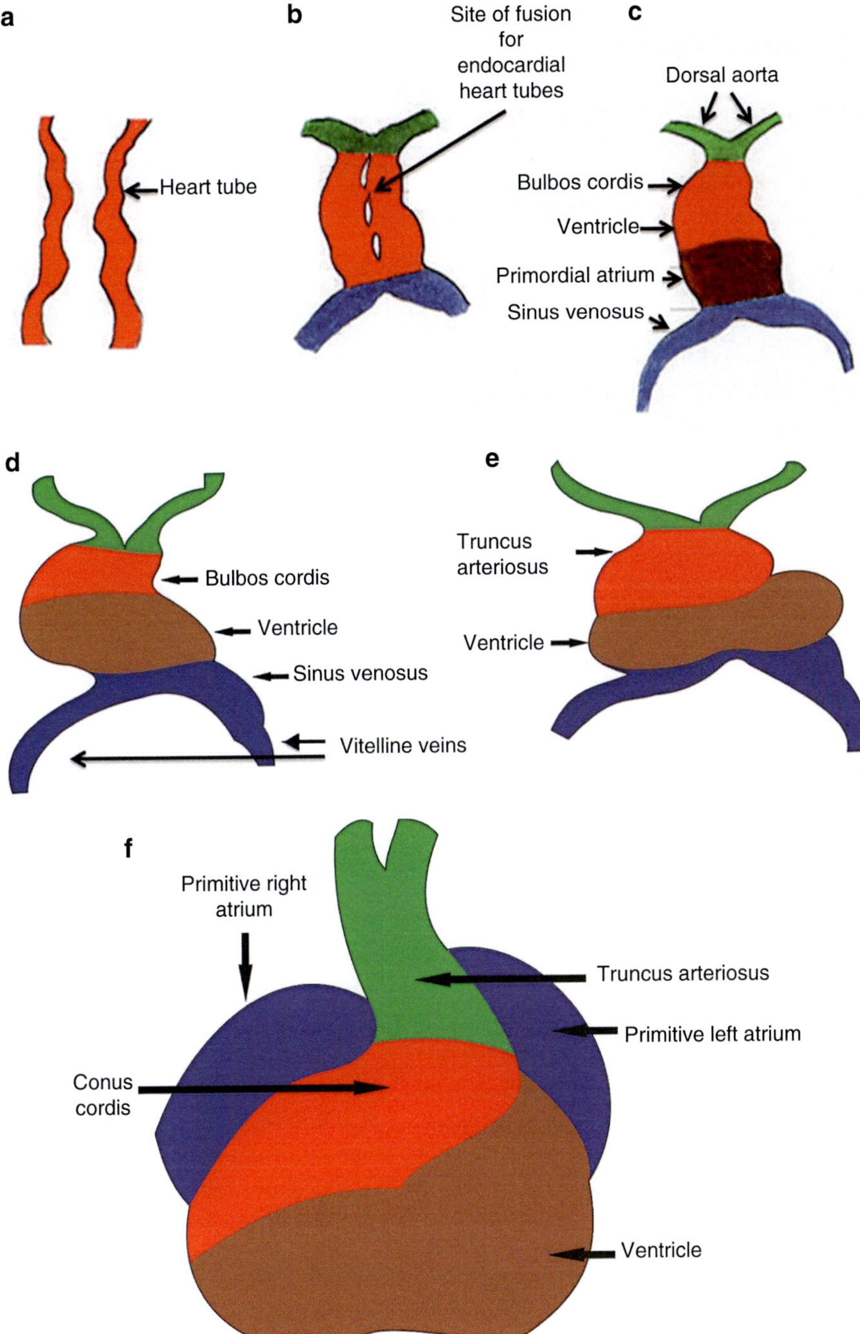

Fig. 2.3 Developing of the cardiac loop. (**a**) 18 days. (**b**) 22 days. (**c**) 23 days. (**d**) 24 days. (**e**) 28 days. (**f**) 35 days

The aortic sac is continuous with the first aortic arch and, eventually, with the other four aortic arches. The aortic arches form major arteries that transport blood to the head and also to the trunk. On the other hand, the sinus venosus receives blood from the common cardinal vein, the umbilical vein, and the vitelline vein which bring the blood back to the heart from the chorion, the umbilical vesicle, and the embryo, respectively.

Clinical Note

In the case of abnormal looping, there may be:

- Random looping
- Anterior looping
- Leftward looping

In clinic, abnormal looping could be seen in the following clinical syndromes:

- Abnormal atrial situs (situs inversus or isomerism)
- Dextrocardia
- Ventricular inversion

We never see heterotaxia patterns in ventricles; heterotaxia is exclusively seen in the atria of the heart (Gittenberger-de Groot et al. 2005; Jacobs et al. 2007).

The Formation of the Sinus Venosus

At the end of the fourth week, the heart contracts synchronously that led to moving of the blood in one direction. During this time the venous blood from right and left sinus horns enters to the sinus venosus. Usually three important veins enter to the right and left horns including (1) embryo via the common cardinal veins, (2) developing placenta via the umbilical veins, and (3) umbilical vesicle via the vitelline vein. The primordial atrium receives blood from the sinus venosus under the control of sinoatrial valves. The blood then enters into the primordial ventricle through the atrioventricular canal. Simultaneously, with the contraction of the ventricle, the blood is pumped via the bulbus cordis and truncus arteriosus and enters into the aortic sac. The blood then distributes to the embryo, umbilical vesicle, and placenta through the dorsal aortas. Initially, the opening between the atrium and the sinus is big. Soon, however, the sinus entrance shifts to the right side. This shift is affected primarily by left-to-right shunts of blood, which take place in the venous system during the fourth and fifth weeks of development (Fig. 2.4).

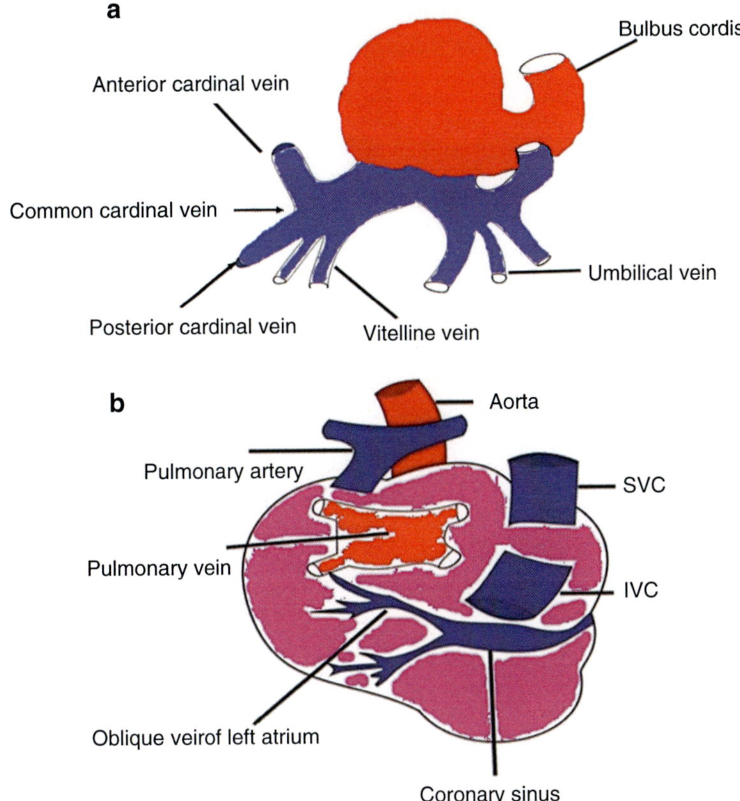

Fig. 2.4 Different stages of development in "sinus venosus"; (**a**) 24 days, (**b**) 35 days

The Next Steps in Differentiation: Atrial Development

Blood flow from left to right causes enlargement of the right sinus and right-sided veins. The right horn is the main confluence between the original sinus venosus and the atrium; this right horn develops gradually into the right atrium and makes the smooth part of the right atrial wall. Now, the sinoatrial orifice is edged on each side by a valvular fold; these folds will create *the right and the left venous valves.* After a while, the dorsocranial parts of these valves fuse together; the result is formation of a ridge called *septum spurium* (Fig. 2.5a).

In the next stage, the right sinus horn is merged into the atrial wall; however, the left venous valve and the septum spurium fuse with the atrial septum. Meanwhile, all of the superior parts of the right venous valve are drawn back, but the inferior parts are changed into two parts: the inferior vena cava valve and the coronary sinus valve (Fig. 2.5b).

										A. Dabbagh et al.

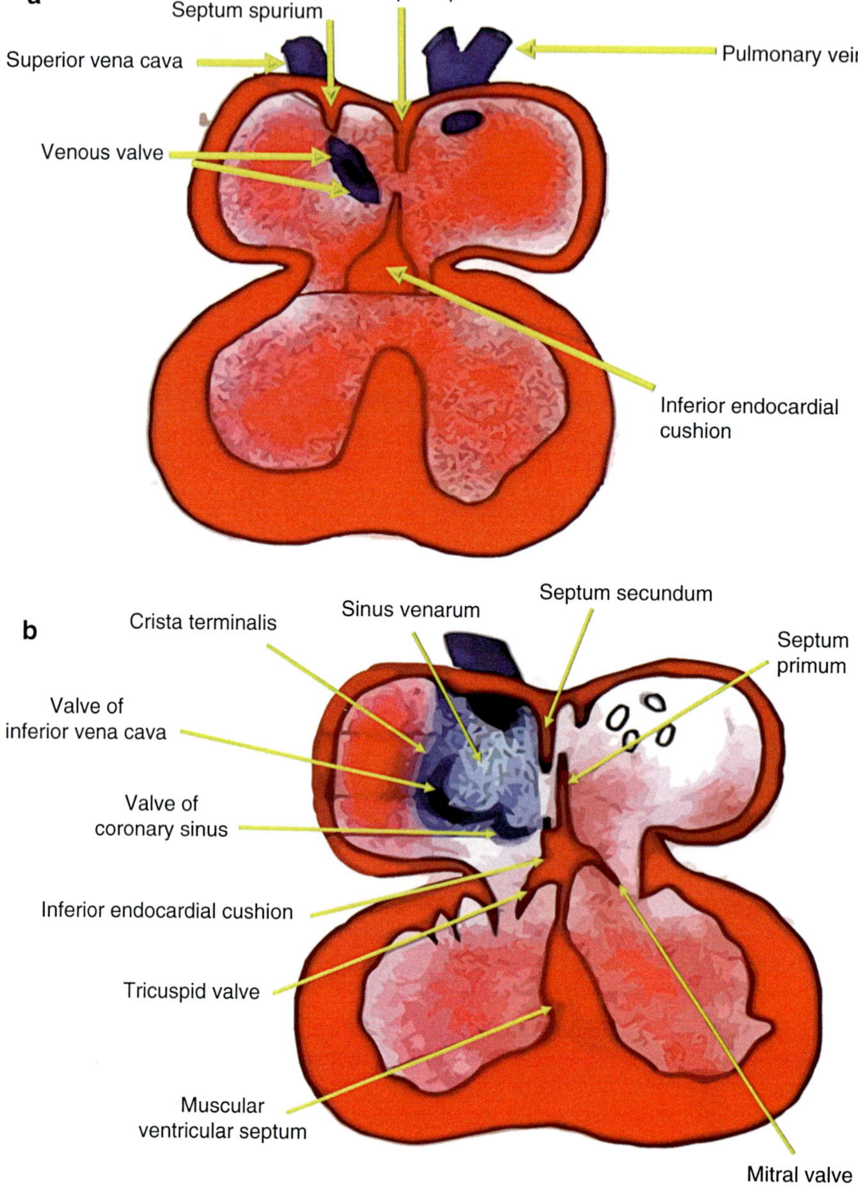

Fig. 2.5 Coronal sections of the heart at the atrioventricular canal level; (**a**) 5 weeks, (**b**) fetal stage

As mentioned in the previous segments, during development of the heart, the heart segments are arranged from cephalad to caudal as the order (Fig. 2.3d):

- Vitelline veins
- Primitive atrium

- Sinus venosus
- Ventricle
- Conotruncal segment (including outflow tract, bulbus cordis, and truncus arteriosus)

However, the sinus venosus is located between vitelline veins (cephalad) and primitive atrium chamber (caudad). In fact, the sinus venosus persists until adulthood, when the sinus venosus forms the smooth-walled parts of the right atrium; in the mature heart, this smooth part of the right atrium is called *sinus venarum* or *venarum sinus*, which composes the main parts of the posterior atrial wall and the majority of the interatrial septum and the lateral wall of right atrium; in the adult heart, sinus venarum surrounds the openings of the venae cavae and the coronary sinus (Taylor and Taylor 1997; Ho et al. 2002).

There is a junction between the sinus venosus and the primary atrium which is called *crista terminalis* (Fig. 2.5b); in the mature heart, crista terminalis is a fibromuscular ridge at the posterolateral region of the right atrium. Crista terminalis is the anatomical margin between the anterior wall of the right atrium (i.e., the trabeculated-walled right atrium which contains pectinate muscles and the right atrial appendage) and the posterior wall of the right atrium (i.e., the smooth-walled parts of the right atrium also named sinus venarum) (Freedom et al. 2005).

> **Clinical Note**
> Crista terminalis functions as the anterior pathway for typical atrial fibrillation or atrial flutter. Also, in some patients, crista terminalis mimics the right atrium masses in echocardiographic exams especially in patients with supraventricular arrhythmias in which a suspicious mass in the right atrium is of utmost importance and needs vigilance for differential diagnosis; sophisticated transesophageal echocardiography and/or cardiac computed tomography/magnetic resonance imaging are needed to rule out the differential diagnosis (Ellis et al. 2000; Gaudio et al. 2004; Akcay et al. 2007; Salustri et al. 2010; Na et al. 2011; Siddiqui et al. 2013; Nakanishi et al. 2015).

The primary atrium starts to be formed at about 2 weeks of gestation. As the primitive atrium enlarges, it partially envelops the bulbus cordis; meanwhile, the right atrium and the left atrium are created out of the primary atrium mainly due to the growth of the septum primum:

- The primitive right atrium is created out of the primitive atrium by fusion of the right sinus horn; as mentioned above, the right atrium is consisted of two main parts, the trabeculated right atrial appendages which give origin to pectinate muscle and the smooth-walled sinus venarum originating from the right horn of the sinus venosus; the pectinate muscles cover the entire wall of the right atrial appendage (Ho et al. 2002).

- The primitive left atrium expands according to the following order: first of all, an outgrowth of the posterior left atrial wall develops in the left side of the septum primum to the primary pulmonary vein (Fig. 2.5a); this primitive pulmonary vein connects with the veins of the developing lung buds; however, during the next expansion, the pulmonary vein and its branches are merged into the left atrium, making the large part of smooth wall of adult left atrium. In the left atrium, there is not such a structure like crista terminalis; so, the mouth of the appendage plays the differentiation role between rough and smooth parts of the left atrium. Only one vein opens initially into the left atrium; however, in the mature heart, four pulmonary veins drain into the left atrium. The left atrial wall is smooth in the majority of its segments; but, a few parts are rough; meanwhile, much less amount of pectinate muscle is seen in the left atrium compared to the right atrium. In complied heart, the left atrium originates from the appendage of the trabeculated atrial wall, and its roof is adjacent to the aorta and pulmonary artery with its trabeculated surface. On the other hand, the smooth-walled portion covers the majority of left atrial surface, initiates from the pulmonary vein component, and is continued up to the body and the vestibule of the left atrium; also, the smooth wall includes the superior and posterior walls of the left atrium (Fig. 2.5a, b) (Ho et al. 2002).

The Primordial Heart Septation

After cardiac looping, the heart, composed of inner endocardial lining and outer myocardial cells, is septated into four main independent regions, which eventually conform the typical anatomy of the future heart chambers and extracardiac arterial system (Lin et al. 2012):

- The atrium
- The atrioventricular canal (also contains *endocardial cushions*)
- The ventricle
- The outflow tract (also contains *endocardial cushions*)

Septation is a critical transitional stage event in heart development, since during septation, the heart is changed from a *single chamber peristaltic tube* to a *four-chambered pump with unidirectional valves* and specific cardiac routes for blood circulation; also, we should note that in normal developmental sequence of the heart, cardiac looping is an essential prerequisite for septation; so we will have the following three stages as the logical and subsequent stages which constitute cardiac development:

- Cardiac looping
- Septation
- Chamber formation

Also, septation, though a single stage in cardiac development, takes place at three different anatomic levels that any defect in each of these levels results in specific lesions; these levels are (Gittenberger-de Groot et al. 2005):

- The atrium
- The ventricle
- The arterial pole

However, myocytes participating in chamber formation are not materially involved in septation (Lamers and Moorman 2002; Lin et al. 2012).

Human heart septation starts at the fourth week and is accomplished by the end of the seventh week and involves two main phases which are composed of sequential events:

- During the *first phase*, two actively growing tissue masses (known as ridges) advance toward each other, until they fuse and make a septum (Fig. 2.6a, b). This septum primarily divides the heart lumen *into two main single canals* (Fig. 2.6a). Similar septum may also be actively shaped by a single mass of growing tissue which will develop till it launches into the opposite side of the lumen (Fig. 2.6c). Synthesis of extracellular matrices and cell proliferation play a main role in the formation of such tissue masses.
- The *endocardial cushions* develop into the conotruncal and atrioventricular parts; *endocardial cushions* are local tissue swellings, made of accumulated "cardiac jelly"; in fact, cardiac jelly is abundant masses of extracellular matrix incorporated between the endocardium and the myocardium (Lin et al. 2012). Cardiac jelly is acellular at first; however, after formation of AV cushions, there is an epithelial-to-mesenchymal transition (EMT) of the endocardial cells which cover the cushions (Lockhart et al. 2011).
- However, *endocardial cushions* when created participate in the formation of membranous parts of atrial and ventricular septa, the atrioventricular canals, the atrioventricular (AV) valves, and the aortic and pulmonary valves. But, we

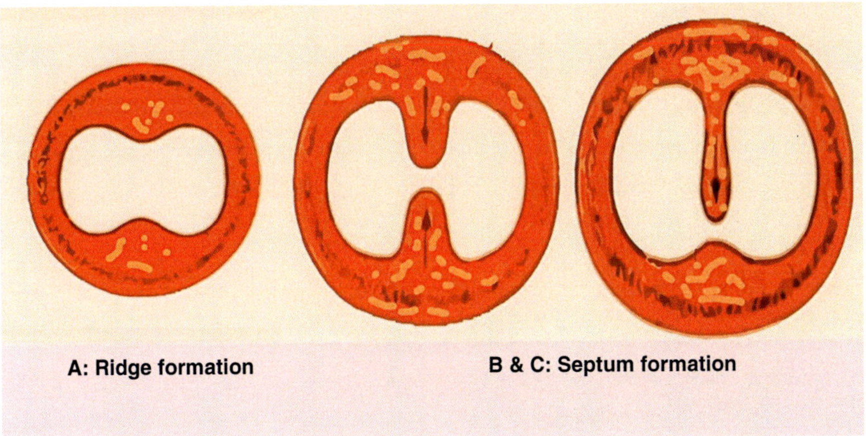

Fig. 2.6 (**a**) Ridge formation by two actively growing masses; (**b**) septation and septum formation by two actively growing masses that close to each other until they fuse and make a septum; (**c**) septation by a single actively growing mass

should remember that endocardium cushions usually do not participate in *true* septum formation. Instead, endocardial cushions take part in septation process in a different way. Their mechanism is that a thin strip of mass tissue in the walls of the atria and ventricles grows and spreads around to well expand the surrounding tissue, until it makes a thin ridge between two contralateral parts; each of these contralateral thin ridges grows on either side until they reach each other and eventually fuse to form a septum. However, this septation mechanism usually does not completely divide the original lumen; but, it leaves a thin link between the two contralateral parts; while later on, the thin canal is endorsed and secondarily supported by proliferation of neighboring tissues. This mechanism of septation separates the ventricles and atria *partially* (Fig. 2.6a–c). At times, due to this mechanism or other similar mechanisms, some of the cardiac structures are created that are known as *classic septum* while they are not real septum and are in fact *folds* or *layers* of the myocardial tissue that engulf some adipose tissue in between (Anderson et al. 2003a).

Whatever the mechanism of septation, the process of septum formation and cardiac *chambering* is not completed until three major subsequent events will happen which eventually will lead into the typical "four-chambered heart":

- Creation of the primitive atrial septum (PAS)
- Creation of the atrioventricular (AV) cushions which also gives origin into tricuspid valve apparatus and mitral valve apparatus
- Creation of the interventricular septum (IVS)

These three major events are discussed in the next paragraphs.

Septum development in the common atrium   Creation of the primitive atrial septum (PAS)

The septation process in the common atrium starts at the beginning of the fifth week and includes the following steps (McCarthy et al. 2003; Gittenberger-de Groot et al. 2005; Sukernik and Bennett-Guerrero 2007; Asrress et al. 2015; Calkoen et al. 2016):

- A sickle-formed crest derived from the roof of the common atrium grows toward the middle of the heart lumen; this crest makes the first part of the structure called *septum primum.*
- The caudal end of this septum primum develops toward the fused endocardial cushion which is located in the atrioventricular canal.
- In this stage, there is a gap between two parts of the common atrium which is called the *ostium primum* and allows blood flow between the two parts of the common atrium (i.e., interatrial flow).
- The septum primum is fenestrated spontaneously in its superior regions by apoptosis to create *ostium secundum*; these fenestrations appear in order to create right-to-left shunt in the fetal circulation which allows flow of oxygenated blood

coming from the umbilical vein to the other organs of fetal body; in this way, the superior part of the septum primum will be obliterated, though it will be completed by *septum secundum.*

- A crescent muscular mass of the ventrocranial common atrial wall originates from the right atrium and grows downward on the right side of the septum primum; this infolding will produce the superior segment of the future interatrial septum; this structure is called *septum secundum* and it will cover the main part of the *ostium secundum*; this muscular *septum secundum* develops during the fifth and sixth weeks of gestation.
- So, we see that the future interatrial septum is the result of two merging septa: *septum primum* and *septum secundum.*
- The left venous valve and the septum spurium merge with the right side of the septum secundum.
- Meanwhile, the pulmonary veins will be relocated from the right atrium to the dorsal wall of the left atrium.
- The defect in the septum secundum is called the *fossa ovalis* which is usually compensated by *septum primum.*
- There is a defect in the borders of septum primum and septum secundum called the *foramen ovale*, an obliquely elongated cleft in the interatrial septum which is open as long as fetal circulation persists; after birth, transition of circulation from fetal circulation to normal circulation leads to increased pressure in the left cardiac chambers and closure of the foramen ovale, at first physiologically and after a while, anatomically.
- The *sinus venosus* is the part of the tissue separating right pulmonary veins from the SVC from the posterior and inferior aspects of the free wall of the right atrium; *coronary sinus septum* is the part of the myocardial tissue separating the coronary sinus from the left atrium (Geva et al. 2014).

The communication between the endocardial cushions and the lower edge septum primum named the foramen primum or the ostium primum. The ostium primum, as a shunt, helps the oxygenated blood to cross from the left to the right atrium. In the next growth, expansions of the lower and higher endocardia cushions develop toward the rim of the septum primum and block the ostium primum.

Genetic factors related to the development of interatrial septum: a set of genetic studies have shown that atrial septal defects and defects in the conduction system are closely related to NKX2.5 mutations. The other genes that play a main role in the heart development are GATA4 gene. The product of this gene and its interaction with other gene products including TBX5 play an important role in cardiac development. Mutations in this gene alter the transcriptional activity of GATA4 and result in ASD, VSD, and pulmonary valvular stenosis (Gourdie et al. 1999; Gourdie et al. 2003; Christoffels et al. 2004; Moorman et al. 2005; Tomita-Mitchell et al. 2007; Remme et al. 2009; Moskowitz et al. 2011; Xin et al. 2013; Stefanovic and Christoffels 2015).

Clinical Notes

- ASD is discussed in detail in Chap. 19; however, some of its developmental notes are discussed here in brief.
- If the pulling-down process of septum primum and septum secundum is deficient, a type of defect occurs in the interatrial septum known as ASD secundum or ostium secundum ASD (*ASD II*) which is *the most common type of ASD*.
- If the ostium primum is not closed by septum primum coming from the underlying AV cushions, primary atrial septal defect (*ASD I*) occurs which is often in combination with varying degrees of abnormalities in AV cushions, namely, AVSD which is discussed in Chap. 18—AV Septal Defects.
- In a minority of newborns, fetal circulation persists, leading to a clinical status called persistent fetal circulation (PFC) which is discussed in detail in Chap. 3—Cardiac Physiology; however, PFC leads to increased pressure in the right side over the left side which is the main etiology for persistence of the foramen ovale, a disease known as *persistent foramen ovale (PFO)* which is discussed under the interatrial defects.
- The last major type of interatrial defects is called *sinus venosus atrial septal defect*, which is due to abnormal attachment of venae cavae (often the superior vena cava) leading to atrial septal defect which is usually associated with anomalous attachment of pulmonary veins; this defect is often discussed under anomalous pulmonary venous drainage (Kerut et al. 2001; Sukernik et al. 2001; Oliver et al. 2002; McCarthy et al. 2003; Van Praagh et al. 2003; Sukernik and Bennett-Guerrero 2007; John et al. 2011; Briggs et al. 2012).

Septum development in the atrioventricular canal Creation of the atrioventricular cushions associated with tricuspid and mitral valves

At the fifth week of gestation, the superior and inferior endocardial cushions are going to be created, so they gradually appear over the primitive left ventricle. Then, an endocardial mass is produced on the ventral and dorsal parts of atrioventricular (AV) canal, and at the same time, this mass is penetrated by mesenchymal cells. In this way, the AV endocardial cushions are made close to each other, while in the next stage, they merge together and are separated to form the left and the right AV canals; these AV canals could discriminate incompletely the primordial ventricle from the primordial atrium.

However, specialized parts of extracellular matrix or cardiac jelly play a crucial role in the development of endocardial cushion; this is why the effect of specific molecules including hyaluronic acid, hyaluronan, fibronectin, fibrillin, proteoglycans, and collagens in cardiac jelly is a leading role (Lockhart et al. 2011; Ray and Niswander 2012; Lalani and Belmont 2014).

The cells that constitute the endocardial cushion tissues are primarily endocardial in origin; however, these endothelial cells migrate into the inner layers of the heart tube to create the primitive mesodermal tissue of this tube which is located in the crux of the heart. This critical process in formation of cardiac cushions is called *endothelial-to-mesenchymal transition of endothelial cells* in cardiac cushions (Zhang et al. 2014; Davey and Rychik 2016).

There is a detailed list of cellular and molecular factors which play their role in the development of cardiac cushions, and any impairment in their role may lead to endocardial cushion defects; these factors include but are not limited to the following:

- Transforming growth factors and proteins (like bone morphogenetic protein, BMP)
- Intercellular signaling molecules and enzymes
- Extracellular matrices
- Transcription factors and mutations in their related genes, like *GATA4* transcription factor, *TGF beta*, *FOG* factor, *Smad4*, Zic family member 3 (*Zic3*), *NK2* homeobox 5 (Nkx2.5), and T-box protein 5 (Tbx5)
- Mutations in genes such as *CYSTEINE-RICH PROTEIN WITH EGF-LIKE DOMAINS* (*CRELD1*, a cell adhesion molecule) (Yamagishi et al. 2009; Lockhart et al. 2011; Moskowitz et al. 2011; Ray and Niswander 2012; Garside et al. 2013; Liu et al. 2013; Paffett-Lugassy et al. 2013; Xin et al. 2013; Lalani and Belmont 2014; Kathiriya et al. 2015; Stefanovic and Christoffels 2015; Gordon and Gordon 2016)

Atrioventricular Valves

For the creation of the atrioventricular (AV) valves, the following steps happen:

- The AV valves are produced in a process called *endothelial-to-mesenchymal transition of endothelial cells* in cardiac cushions through the following subsequent stages.
- The endocardial cushions are the "progenitors" of the AV valves.
- The embryologic cells that constitute the endocardial cushions are endothelial cells migrating into the inner layer of the heart tube; this migration creates the primary mesodermal tissue of the heart tube which is located in the heart crux.
- Afterward, the AV endocardial cushions merge.
- Then the mesenchymal tissue proliferates locally and surrounds the orifice of the AV canals.
- In the next stage, the blood flow dips out the tissue on the ventricular surface of the mesenchymal proliferations, which leads to more final form of the valves.
- However, there is still persistence of the *valve links* to the ventricular wall by muscular cords; in the last stage, the muscular cords are changed to a dense connective tissue, followed by obliteration of muscular part of the cords.

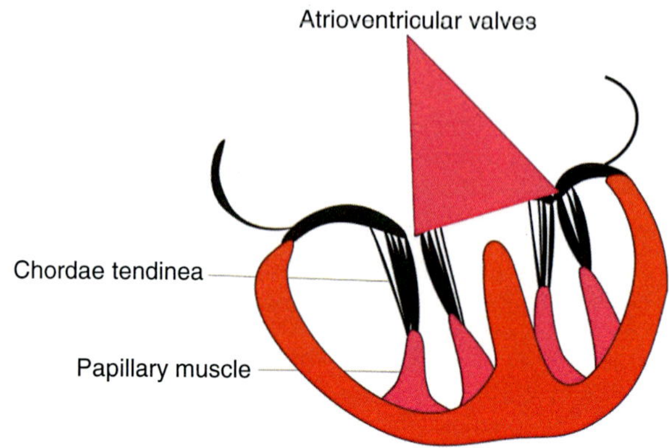

Fig. 2.7 Development of the atrioventricular valves and chordae tendineae

- Now the valves include the connective tissue endorsed by endocardium, which are attached by chordae tendineae to the papillary muscles (Fig. 2.7).
- And now we have two final valves: the *two-leaflet* valve in the left atrioventricular canal which is bicuspid, known as the *mitral valve*, and *three-leaflet* valve in the right atrioventricular canal known as the *tricuspid valve* (Gaussin et al. 2005; Zhang et al. 2014; Davey and Rychik 2016).

Many cellular and molecular factors play their role in the normal development of AV cushions; any impairment in their process leads to impaired endocardial cushion development; some of these factors are presented here:

- Transforming growth factors and proteins (like bone morphogenetic protein, BMP)
- Intercellular signaling molecules and enzymes
- Transcription factors and mutations in their related genes, like GATA4 transcription factor, TGF beta, FOG factor, Smad4, Zic family member 3 (Zic3), NK2 homeobox 5 (Nkx2.5), and T-box protein 5 (Tbx5)
- Extracellular matrices (Yamagishi et al. 2009; Moskowitz et al. 2011; Ray and Niswander 2012; Garside et al. 2013; Liu et al. 2013; Kathiriya et al. 2015; Stefanovic and Christoffels 2015)

Clinical Note
If normal development of the endocardial cushions is impaired, the resulting defects would be seen as *defects in the septum* (at the crux of the heart) and, also, impairment in normal development of the AV valves, a clinical state known as atrioventricular septal defect "AVSD." However, these abnormalities in the septum and the AV valves do not have a constant spectrum with varying degrees; so, there are different phenotypes seen in patients with AVSD; detailed discussion on this disease could be found in Chap. 18—AV Septal Defects.

Septum development in the ventricles Creation of the interventricular septum (IVS)

At the beginning of the fifth week, the primeval ventricles start to expand and create the apical portions of the future ventricles from the primary heart tube. The interventricular septum (IVS) sulcus is the externally separating margin of right and left ventricles, while the internal separator of right and left ventricle is the bulboventricular flange which is part of the primitive ventricle and leads to the development of the muscular part of IVS. Development of the primeval ventricles is one of the main steps in the development of IVS. There are two main parts in IVS:

- The muscular IVS developed from the bulboventricular flange.
- The membranous IVS connects the upper margin of the bulboventricular flange to the anterior and posterior endocardial cushions.

However, there are a number of following sequential events leading to the development of IVS:

- The *first* sign of division in primordial ventricle is the creation of muscular IVS which is a median ridge in the ventricle floor adjacent to its apex; the edge of muscular IVS is concave and free.
- During early stage of development, IVS achieves its height by expansion of the ventricles on each side.
- Afterward, IVS myoblasts start active proliferation, resulting in increased size.
- The next step is conus septum completion, which happens as a result of tissue extension, starting from the inferior part of endocardial cushion alongside top of the muscular IVS; these parts of tissue finally merge with the neighboring portion of the conus septum.
- And the final step is closure of the opening above the muscular IVS; when the interventricular foramen closes completely, the membranous part of the IVS is formed.
- Three sources of tissue take part in the closure of the interventricular opening and formation of the membranous IVS: the *left* bulbar ridge, the *right* bulbar ridge, and the endocardial cushions.

The *primary ventricular septum* or *primary ventricular fold* is produced following the trabeculation of the ventral part of the muscular IVS. However, there is a smooth part on the dorsal wall of IVS, named the *inlet septum*; this nomenclature is used because it is located nearby the AV canals. The *moderator band* or *septomarginal trabecula* is located on the right wall of muscular IVS, between the primary trabeculated fold and the inlet septum. This structure is a firm connection between the muscular septum and the anterior papillary muscle. When the right ventricular chamber expands, the moderator band is formed nearby the AV canal and dorsal muscular IVS. Eventually, a large part of the mature right ventricular chamber is formed by this expansion. However, if this anatomic area expands incompletely, the developing tricuspid part of the atrioventricular canal remains attached to the interventricular foramen, leading to tricuspid atresia and/ or other tricuspid valve anomalies (Lamers and Moorman 2002; Gittenberger-de Groot et al. 2005; Togi et al. 2006; Lin et al. 2012; Poelmann et al. 2014).

Failure or gaps in the development of IVS leads to different forms of VSD; a detailed discussion on VSD is found in Chap. 19.

Septum Development in the Truncus Arteriosus and Conus Cordis

There is a paired ridge, composed of two cushions, which appears in opposing sites of the truncus. These two ridges are located as follows:

- On the *right side* of superior wall: the right swelling lies on the superior truncus.
- On the *left side* of the inferior wall: the left swelling lies on the inferior truncus.

During the fourth week of gestation, *the right-sided swelling* located on the superior site of truncus progresses distally and toward the left. Meanwhile, *the left-sided swelling* located on inferior truncus develops distally to the right. Henceforward, these swellings grow toward the aortic arch, while at the same time, they turn around each other. During this turning movement, they foreshadow the spiral pathway of the upcoming septum (Webb et al. 2003; Anderson et al. 2010).

These swellings deal with a spiral twist of about 180°. Some of the neural crest cells are transferred from the embryonic pharynx and pharyngeal arches to arrive in these edges. The streaming of the blood from the ventricles is one of the main factors that may play a major role in the spiral orientation of the bulbar and truncal edges (Webb et al. 2003; Anderson et al. 2012).

Anyway, this model of development results in the formation of a spiral *aortico-pulmonary septum* when the edges merge. However, after these edges are completely merged, they make the *aorticopulmonary septum*, separating the truncus into two parts: an *aortic channel* and a *pulmonary channel* (Fig. 2.8) (Steding and Seidl 1981; Webb et al. 2003; Okamoto et al. 2010).

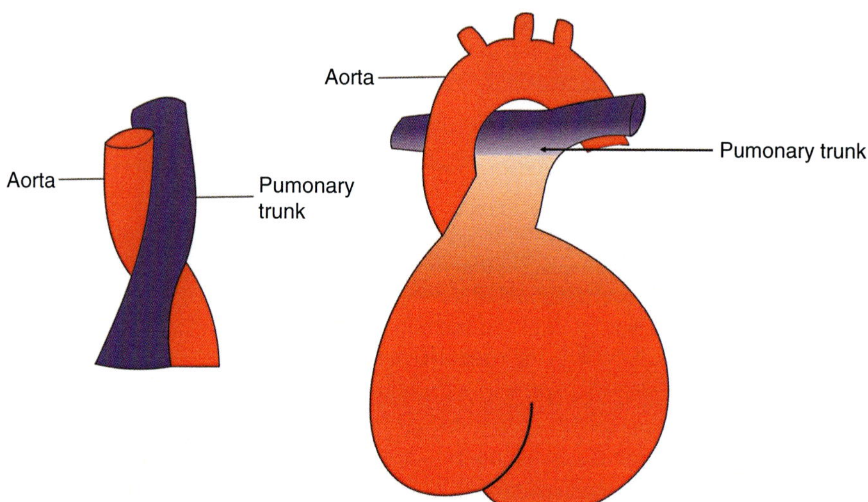

Fig. 2.8 Septation of the heart outflow tract and complete the ventricular separation. Formation of the conotruncal ridge; conotruncal ridge fuses with the other compartment to complete the interventricular septum

During the fifth week of gestation, ridges from the subendocardial tissue are formed in the *common outflow tract*. The spiral orientation of these ridges results in a spiral *aorticopulmonary septum* during fusion of these ridges. This is the septum that divides the outflow tract into two channels, the pulmonary trunk and the aorta. The second heart field (SHF) plays a crucial role in the development of the outflow tract. Any impairment in SHF or neural crest results in major defects in growth and development of the conotruncal region (Steding and Seidl 1981; Webb et al. 2003; Restivo et al. 2006).

Semilunar Valve Formation

When conotruncal septa are formed, two other cushions are developed which oppose each other in the outflow tract; they are called "the intercalated cushion in the distal conal fragment"; the new cushions, after being remodeled, make two main *outflow tract* cushions. These two cushions together with the lateral intercalated cushions are excavated; the final result of this process is creating cavities at the origin of the future pulmonary artery and ascending aorta. The primordial deviations from these cavities and the intervening tissues are *valvular sinuses* and *semilunar valves*. A set of studies in mice show that semilunar valve leaflets originate mainly from endocardial cushion tissue, associated somewhat with neural crest cells and epicardial cells. The development of semilunar valves in human is completed up to the ninth week (Fig. 2.9) (Anderson et al. 2003b; Hinton and Yutzey 2011; Goenezen et al. 2012; Lin et al. 2012; Sherif 2014; van Geemen et al. 2016).

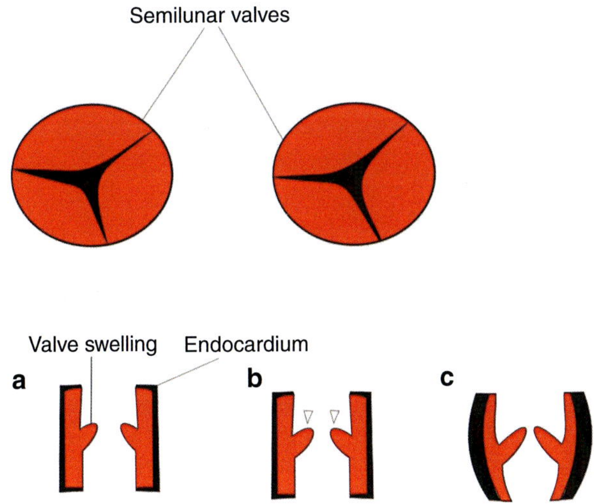

Fig. 2.9 Development of semilunar valves at weeks 6 (**a**), 7 (**b**), and 9 (**c**). The superior surface is hollowed to form the valves

Development of the Cardiac Conducting System in the Heart

The cardiac conducting system (CCS) is composed of several integral components in a delicate hierarchy which is the mainstay for effective mechanical contractions of the heart chambers (Desplantez et al. 2007; Dun and Boyden 2008; Atkinson et al. 2011).

- The sinoatrial (SA) node which is the main *excitatory and impulse generating* location in the heart, generating the regular and rhythmic leading impulses of the heart; they have the most rapid intrinsic rate for impulse generation all over the cardiac cells.
- Specialized conduction system known as *conductive cells* which is mainly composed of the atrioventricular conduction pathways, atrioventricular (AV) node, His bundle, and its right and left branches; finally, there are the Purkinje fiber cells or the Purkinje fiber network which is distributed over all parts of the ventricles and conducts the electrical impulse effectively and rapidly over the ventricles (Fig. 2.10).

Development of the sinoatrial (SA) node During the very early phases of heart development, while there is no conduction system development, all of the epithelioid myocytes are electrically active; however, more sophisticated studies have shown that pacemaking area cells have been evolved as a primitive area in the primary sinus venosus and atrium well before the heart begins; these cells are developed and start signaling toward the outflow tract of the developing heart well before any other part of the CCS is developed; their impulses are spread over the heart through gap junctions and connexin proteins (Jalife et al. 1999; Mikawa and Hurtado 2007).

The pacemaker cells changing later to SA node are placed in the caudal portion of the left heart tube at the beginning of their development. At first, the primitive atrium plays the main role of pacemaker in the heart, but in the next phases of development, this role is transferred to sinus venosus. Later, during the fourth week, SA node develops. It is located in the right wall of the sinus venous during early phases of development; however, in the next couple of weeks, its gradual development leads to its merge with the right atrial wall. In the normal heart, SA node lies in the cephalic portion of the posterior wall of right atrium just near the orifice of SVC. During its normal function, SA node has a complex architecture leading to heterogeneous electrical activity. Also, pacemaking cells, especially in SA node, have a number of specific specifications:

- Higher rate of spontaneous beating
- Faster activation of the funny current (I_f)
- Greater density of the funny current (Mikawa and Hurtado 2007)

Development of AV node During the next phases of CCS development, the cells derived from left wall of sinus venous form the atrioventricular node and bundle; these cells are usually placed in the inferior part of interatrial septum and anterior to

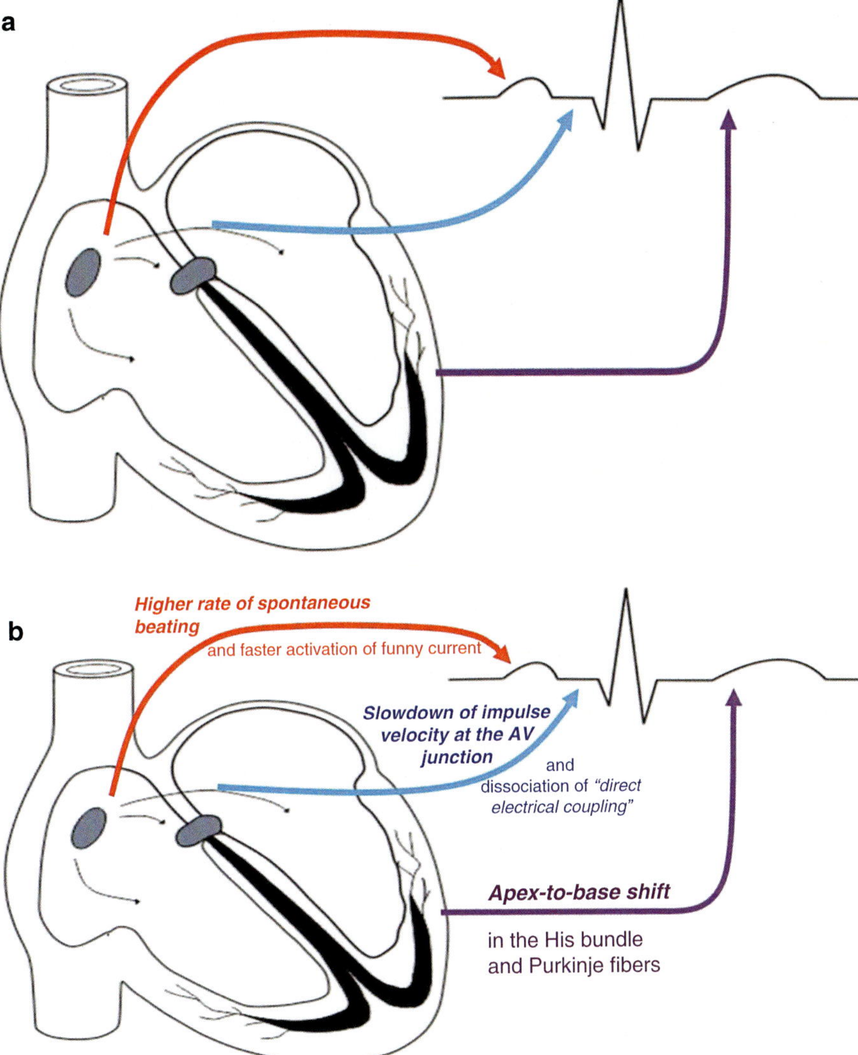

Fig. 2.10 Cardiac conductive system and its elements; in the left, see the relationship of normal electrocardiography with the elements of the system. (**a**) Relationship of each anatomical segment with electrocardiograph; (**b**) the embryologic "role definition" for each of the electrical segments of the heart during its development (Modified from Dabbagh (2014). Published with kind permission from © Springer, 2014. All Rights Reserved)

the coronary sinus foramen. The AV node lies just superior to the endocardial cushions. Development of AV node is a multiple step mechanism. The first theory is that AV node cells are in fact a subpopulation of the primary myocardial cells which their differentiation into "normal" mature myocardial cells is restrained, leading to AV node cells with slow conducive properties; however, additional cellular and molecular theories (including signaling mechanism) are proposed for AV node development; these are beyond the scope of this chapter (Christoffels et al. 2004; Moorman et al. 2005; Mikawa and Hurtado 2007).

During the development of AV node, there are three basic changes in differentiation of the impulse propagation pattern of the CCS; these changes occur during looping of the heart tube and ensure productive and successful pumping of the blood in the four-chambered heart; they are mainly the result of the following three major developmental steps:

1. *Significant slowdown of impulse velocity at the AV junction*: this impulse slowdown is synchronized with morphologic cleavage between atrial and ventricular chambers; also, this time delay in combination with development of AV cushions leads to production of an effective peristaltic wave in myocardial contraction; the final result will be augmented pumping efficiency of the developing heart.
2. The second step is *dissociation of direct electrical coupling* between atrial syncytium and ventricular syncytium due to the creation of the interventricular septum.
3. *Shift in the electrical direction of the impulse*: when septation occurs in the ventricular chambers, there is a very clear and specific change in the process of impulse generation and propagation and that is a dramatic shift in the electrical direction of the impulse from *base-to-apex* model to *apex-to-base* model (Mikawa and Hurtado 2007).

Development of bundle branches and His bundles During the next developmental phases, the AV node bundle fibers pass through the atrium to the ventricles and divide into the right and left bundle branches, distributing over the ventricular myocardial tissue. The growth of the AV node is simultaneous with the formation of the bundle of His, a specialized conducting fiber, connecting the bundle branches to the Purkinje fibers in the peripheral ventricular conduction system. His bundles distribute into the left and the right ventricles by the moderator band.

Development of Purkinje fibers Development of the Purkinje fibers is from the "working myocytes" as a result of interactions between contractile myocytes with endocardial cells and arterial cells, leading to the development of *subendocardial* and *intramyocardial* Purkinje cells, respectively; also, coronary arteries have a very essential role in differentiation of Purkinje cells; endothelin signaling is another main factor that promotes transdifferentiation process of the Purkinje fiber (Gourdie et al. 1999, 2003; Gassanov et al. 2004; Mikawa and Hurtado 2007; Hua et al. 2014).

The CCS has a pivotal role in the function of the heart; any developmental defects leading to abnormalities in the CCS lead to life-threatening cardiac arrhythmias (Wu et al. 2014). Also, the repair of congenital heart defects, especially in patients with ventricular septal defects, is associated with a great risk of damage during surgical correction in all of these conducting structures (Racker 2004).

Atrioventricular (AV) Valve Anomalies

Abnormalities in AV valve development significantly contribute to errors in the remodeling process that leads to formation of valve leaflets, chordae tendineae, and papillary muscles; they originate from endocardial cushion and ventricular myocardium. Partitioning of truncus arteriosus and conus arteriosus in the fifth week of embryologic development is associated with the spiral development and twisting migration of neural crest cells; the final result as mentioned before is the development of the structures known later as "outflow tracts" and "great arteries" (Anderson et al. 2003b; Restivo et al. 2006).

In the *pulmonary tract* system, the related conus known as *pulmonary conus* takes part in the formation of the infundibulum which is the anatomic structure between pulmonary valve and the AV valves on one side and the muscular infundibulum on the other side. In the *outflow tract* of the systemic circulation, the sub-aortic conus is obliterated leading to the development of the aortic valve surrounded by fibrous continuity of the AV valves (Hinton and Yutzey 2011).

Till now, the main pathogenesis mechanism of AV valve atresia (leading to complete obliteration of the orifice of each valve) is not well known. When the AV septum is not formed, the wedging and remodeling of valves are impaired, and consequently, alignment of the AV canals with their appropriate ventricles fails. It seems to be the underlying mechanism leading to single inlet for the ventricle: ventricular inflow from both atria.

Likewise, in *double-outlet right ventricle (DORV)*, there may be double outlets for a ventricle, due to malalignment of the outflow tract; in other words, the affected ventricle has both the aorta and the pulmonary artery. In this disease, the aortic and pulmonary outflow tracts link to the right ventricle, associated in almost all cases with a ventricular septal defect, leading to arterial blood flow leaving the right ventricle while the blood is a mixture of high oxygenated and poor oxygenated blood. In these patients, the ductus arteriosus links the pulmonary trunk and aorta to each other. Impairment in biventricular circulation leading to a univentricular heart function leads to left ventricle-driven circulation and enlargement of the left ventricle and hypoplastic right ventricle; ductus arteriosus should remain open. Usually this condition leads to cardiac failure unless treated. This disease is discussed more in Chap. 30—Double Outlet Right Ventricle (Anderson et al. 2001, 2003b; Mahle et al. 2008).

Stenosis of Cardiac Semilunar Valves

Stenosis of the semilunar valve is defined as stenosis of either the aortic valve or the pulmonary valve. These conditions are discussed in Chap. 24, Right-Sided Obstructive Lesions, and Chap. 26, Congenital Aortic Valve Anomalies. Congenital valvular stenosis is due to abnormal cavitation and remodeling within the distal conal cushion tissue responsible for forming the aortic semilunar valves, leading to different congenital diseases of the aortic valve.

Cardiac Outflow Tract Septation Anomalies

Truncus arteriosus Cardiac neural crest cells are multipotent migratory cells that contribute to the cardiac outflow tract formation and the pharyngeal arch arteries. Today we know that a great number of many of the outflow tract septation malformations are in association with abnormal development of neural crest cells; as a result, the conotruncal septa do not form at all, leading to *persistent truncus arteriosus*. This abnormality will inevitably embrace a defect in ventricular septation, leading to mixing of the blood during departure from two ventricles, i.e., in the common outflow tract; however, the result of this mixing is mainly a left-to-right shunt leading to pulmonary hypertension (Fig. 2.11). If not treated, the child usually dies within the first 2 years of life. This defect is usually corrected surgically, by fixing the VSD and implanting a valved prosthetic shunt connecting the right ventricle and the pulmonary arteries.

Transposition of the great vessels In about 5 per 10,000 live-born infants, the conotruncal septa develop but without the usual spiral pattern, leading to transposition of the great vessels, in which the left ventricle empties into the pulmonary circulation and the right ventricle empties into the systemic circulation. Inversion of the great vessels is often fatal unless the ductus arteriosus remains patent or is accompanied by intrinsic ASD or VSD or by surgically introduced atrial defects aiming to establish an interatrial communication and hence allowing the deoxygenated systemic and the newly oxygenated pulmonary blood to mix. Inversion can be surgically modified with a favorable prognosis. Nevertheless, it is the main cause of death in infants with cyanotic heart disease younger than 1 year old. A full discussion of the disease is presented in Chap. 21—Transposition of Great Vessels.

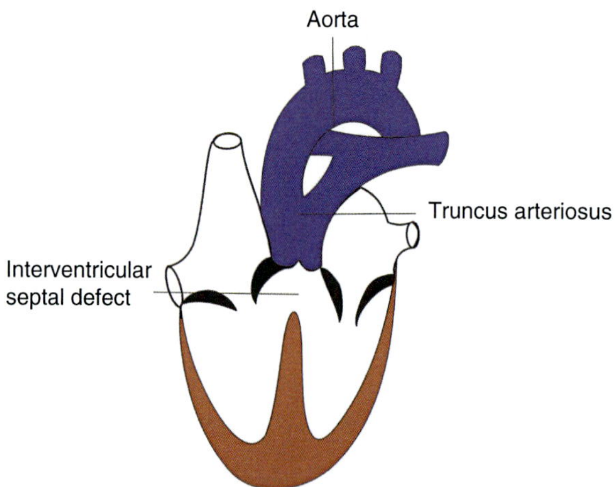

Fig. 2.11 The outflow cardiac tract septation defects

Tetralogy of Fallot (TOF) TOF is a syndrome described by Danish Niels Stensen in 1671, then reported by Eduard Sandifort in 1777, and the exact anatomy of TOF illustrated by William Hunter from St George's Hospital Medical School, London, in 1784. It was in 1888 that Etienne-Louis Arthur Fallot described L'anatomie pathologique de la maladie bleu; in 1924, the term "tetralogy of Fallot" was created for the first time by Canadian Maude Abbott (Berry 2006; Evans 2008; Van Praagh 2009). The term *tetralogy* refers to four classic malformations, demonstrated as a graphic in Fig. 2.12, and includes:

- Pulmonary stenosis
- Ventricular septal defect
- Rightward displacement of the aorta (usually known as overriding of the aorta)
- Right ventricular hypertrophy

The main etiologic mechanism is uneven separation of the outflow tract which results to overriding of the aorta and also malalignment of the muscular outlet septum regarding right and left ventricles; these defects lead to increased filling pressures in the right ventricle, with resultant right ventricular hypertrophy. TOF is among the common cyanotic congenital heart diseases and is generally corrected surgically, including release of the pulmonary trunk obstruction, repair of ventricular septal defect, and, at the same time, correction of overriding; a few years later a considerable number of patients refer for correction of the pulmonary insufficiency which is a sequel of pulmonary stenosis repair. TOF is presented in detail in Chap. 20 (Therrien et al. 2005; Apitz et al. 2009; Starr 2010).

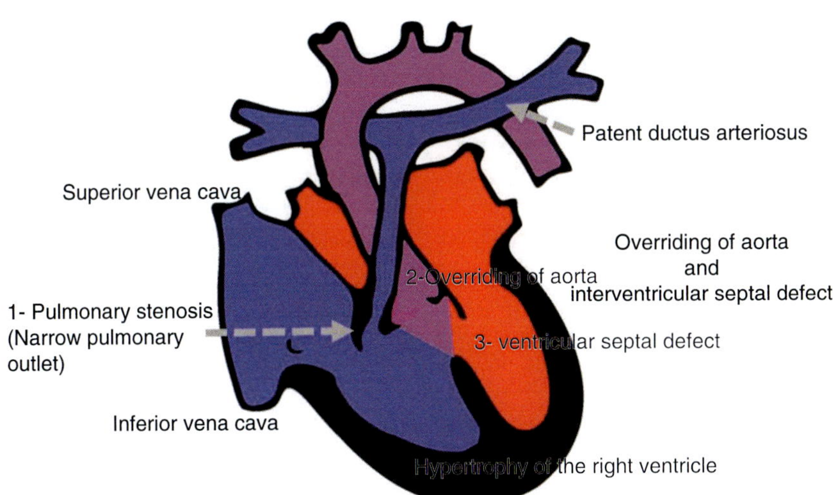

Fig. 2.12 Tetralogy of Fallot: (1) pulmonary stenosis, (2) overriding of aorta, (3) interventricular septal defect, and (4) hypertrophy of the right ventricle

Vascular Formation

Two main mechanisms are involved in the development of blood vessels:

1. *Vasculogenesis*, a process producing vessels through the process of angioblast coalescence; this mechanism is responsible for the production of the two main vessels, the dorsal aorta and cardinal veins (Williams et al. 2010; Charpentier et al. 2015).
2. *Angiogenesis*, new buds emerge from the preexisting vessels, and in this way, new vessels are created; this is the mechanism responsible for the development of all body vessels except for dorsal aorta and cardinal veins; however, vascular endothelial growth factor (VEGF) and other growth factors play a crucial role throughout this mechanism (Charpentier and Conlon 2014).

Arterial System

Development of Aortic Arches

The *aortic arches* are a series of paired developing vascular organs in the embryological development; in addition, they are also known as *pharyngeal arch arteries* or *branchial arches*, and they give origin to a number of important vascular structures.

The creation of aortic arches begins between 22nd and 24th days of development. At first a pair of arches is formed; then, following the folding of body, the endocardial tubes move toward the future thorax; meanwhile, the cranial ends of the attached aortae are drawn into a dorsoventral loop. This leads to the location of the first aortic arch pair into the condensed mesenchyme of the first pharyngeal arches in each side of the developing pharynx.

The arterial lumen of the aortic arch arises from the ventral part of the aortic sac, which is an enlargement at the cranial part of the truncus arteriosus. They are linked to the right and left dorsal aortae. Aortic arches are located ventral to the dorsal aorta. The dorsal aortae persist as discrete vessels in the aortic arches area; however, in the fourth week of gestation, they merge together throughout the fourth thoracic segment to the fourth lumbar segment to make a dorsal aorta in midline. Development of aorta occurs during the third week of development, in relation with development of the endocardial tube. During days 26–29, through the process of angiogenesis and vasculogenesis, the second, third, fourth, and sixth arches grow inside their related pharyngeal arches; then, they are incorporated with EPCs that are transferred from the inclosing mesoderm. Also, neural crest mesenchymal cells in the pharyngeal arches play a main role in the usual growth of the arch arteries; here the neural crest cells do not have a direct relationship with the endothelium of these vessels (Kau et al. 2007).

Development of Arterial Tree from Aortic Arches

During 28th to 32nd days of embryonic development, the blood departs the heart via the outflow tract and comes back to the heart through the extrapericardial aortic sac. There is a very important connection between the *aortic sac* and *bilateral dorsal aortae*; this connection is developed through third, fourth, and sixth pharyngeal arch arteries, which run in their corresponding pharyngeal arches and then separate in the dorsal region; finally, they merge with the paired dorsal aortae. Later, during the course of development, the *aortic sac* obliterates and is no more recognized (days 37–42). A summary of the organs created during the embryologic period from the aortic arches is discussed here *for each aortic arch* based on related extensive studies; also, a very brief summary is presented in Table 2.1 (Graham 2003; Kau et al. 2007; Strilic et al. 2009; Kellenberger 2010; Mirilas 2011; Lammert and Axnick 2012; Stojanovska et al. 2012; Bamforth et al. 2013; Neufeld et al. 2014; Rana et al. 2014; Gupta et al. 2015, 2016; Menshawi et al. 2015; Plein et al. 2015).

The first aortic arches As the future arches are going to be formed, the first two arches go to remission and go to their earlier states. Later, as the second arch develops, the first arch degenerates absolutely (except a small remnant which makes a part of the maxillary arteries).

The second aortic arches By day 26, the second aortic arch grows in the second pharyngeal arches and joins the dorsal aortae to the aortic sac; however, the second arch degenerates at the time that the sixth arch is developed; just a small part of the second arch remains which makes the stapedial artery, providing future blood supply to the stapes bone in the developing ear.

Table 2.1 Embryologic aortic arch pairs (Kau et al. 2007; Rana et al. 2014)

Aortic arch pair	Originated arteries
First pair	Maxillary and external carotid arteries
Second pair	Stapedial arteries
Third pair (carotid arch)	Internal carotid artery also, proximal parts of the third pair constitute the common carotid arteries
Fourth pair	*Right arch*: constitutes the proximal right subclavian artery until the origin of right internal mammary branch *Left arch*: originates the aortic arch between the left common carotid artery and left subclavian artery (ductus arteriosus)
Fifth pair	Rudimentary vessels
Sixth pair	*Right arch*: constitutes the right pulmonary artery *Left arch*: the main and left pulmonary artery and ductus arteriosus
Seventh pairs	*Right arch*: constitutes part of the right subclavian artery; in addition, the right fourth arch and the right dorsal aorta contribute information of the right subclavian artery *Left arch*: the left subclavian artery

The third and fourth aortic arches During regression of the first arch on day 25, the third and fourth aortic arches are formed; the aortic arch is made of the joint venture of left fourth aortic arch with the merged dorsal aorta and a small part of the aortic sac; this combination is converted to *ascending aorta* or to *aortic arch* and *the most cranial part of the descending aorta*. When the dorsal aortic segments are merged, they lead to caudal parts of the descending aorta at the fourth thoracic level.

During these developmental processes, the fourth arch is much more profuse and protuberant than the third and sixth arterial arches.

The *third aortic arch* is attached to the dorsal aortae at its cranial part; this attachment has an "end-to-side" fashion, leading to the development of *internal carotid arteries* as cranial extensions of this attachment.

There is another part of dorsal aorta located between the third and the fourth aortic arches, known as *carotid duct*; this arterial segment is narrower than caudal segments of the dorsal aorta.

In the next stage of the arterial system development, the dorsal aorta disappears on either side by day 35; these aortic parts join the third and the fourth arch arteries. Therefore, the third aortic arches drain totally into the cranial parts of the dorsal aortae which perfuse the head.

The arteries derived from the third arch include:

- Right common carotid artery
- Left common carotid artery
- Proximal part of the right and left internal carotid arteries

The distal part of each *internal carotid artery* is developed from the cranial part of the ipsilateral dorsal aorta, and the right and left external carotid arteries develop from the common carotids.

The fifth aortic arches The fifth pair is *not* involved in these developmental stages; as a matter of fact, some authors have even questioned its presence or at least claimed that no specific role is attributable to this arch in the development of congenital heart diseases; however, others have defined some role (Bamforth et al. 2013; Gupta et al. 2015, 2016).

The sixth aortic arches It is formed on day 29 while the second arch degenerates simultaneously; the proximal end of the aortic sac gives rise to the right and left sixth arches which are asymmetrical in the next developmental phases. The right sixth arch loses its distal connection with the right dorsal aorta by the end of the eighth week; in comparison, the left sixth arch does not disappear and its distal part forms the *ductus arteriosus*. This duct lets the blood transfer from the pulmonary trunk into the descending aorta during gestation. After birth, this duct is closed and is transformed later to ligamentum arteriosum, a rudimentary joint between the pulmonary trunk and aorta.

The uneven growth of the right and left sixth arches has another consequence: *asymmetry between left and right recurrent laryngeal nerves*, which are branches of the vagus nerves. The laryngeal nerves rise initially under the level of the sixth arch; then, they pass under the right and left sixth arches. Recurrent laryngeal nerves innervate intrinsic muscles of the laryngeal system. Throughout development, the larynx moves cranially in relation to aortic arch; however, the left recurrent laryngeal nerve is trapped below the left sixth arch and remains circled under the developing ligamentum arteriosum. In contrast to the left recurrent nerve, the right recurrent laryngeal nerve is entrapped below the fourth arch which is changed later to the right subclavian artery due to the degeneration of the distal portion of the right sixth aortic arch and also no further development in the fifth arch.

Finally, during these phases, *sprouts of pulmonary trunk* emerge as the following order: sprouts of the pulmonary trunk could be visible at the caudal segment of the sixth aortic arch. The embryonic pulmonary arteries grow in the splanchnopleuric mesoderm; they initially join the fourth aortic arch; then, they create a new and secondary link with the sixth arch before missing their link with the fourth aortic arches. In fact, the pulmonary arteries join the sixth arch arteries and in the next stages, to the pulmonary trunk; however, pulmonary artery buds are not near each other in this stage; instead, the lumen of the aortic sac is insinuated between them; at this time, the right primary pulmonary artery is more laterally located compared to the left primary pulmonary artery. The distal part of the pulmonary arteries in the lung tissue anastomoses with the existing vasculature in the mesenchymal tissue surrounding the bronchial sprouts.

The seventh aortic arches The seventh pair of dorsal intersegmental aortae meets and joins; left and right *subclavian arteries* originate at the caudal point of their convergence; then, they vegetate toward the sprouts of the corresponding upper limb. The *right subclavian* artery which will supply the upper limbs has a triple-based origin:

1. The right seventh intersegmental artery
2. A short segment of the right dorsal aorta
3. The right fourth arch

The brachiocephalic arteries are derived by the modification of the joint area of the aortic sac and the right fourth arch. The *left subclavian artery* provides blood to left upper limb; it is developed progressively from the ascending aorta (Menshawi et al. 2015).

By the seventh week, the right dorsal aorta is disconnected from the merged "right sixth arch and midline dorsal aorta"; however, preserving its connection to the right fourth arch. In addition, the right dorsal aorta obtains a branch named the right seventh cervical intersegmental artery, which grows into the right upper limb sprout area.

Also, at the dorsal aspect of the dorsal aortae, a number of small intersegmental arteries sprout at regular distances; they run toward the developing spinal cord to support blood supply to the future spinal cord.

Fate of the Vitelline and Umbilical Arteries

The umbilical vesicle (yolk sac), allantois, and chorion are supplied by the unpaired ventral branches of the dorsal aorta. The three vitelline arteries perfuse the embryologic segments as they pass to the vesicle and later the primitive gut by the following order:

Celiac arterial trunk is the most superior of the three abdominal vitelline arteries and supplies the *foregut*. During its course, celiac trunk initially joins the dorsal aorta at the seventh cervical level; later, this connection continues down to the 12th thoracic level. The branches of celiac artery vascularize the abdominal part of the foregut, the abdominal esophagus up to the descending segment of the duodenum, and also the liver, pancreas, gallbladder, and spleen. The branch perfusing the spleen develops within the mesoderm of the dorsal mesogastrium. Dorsal mesogastrium is the portion of the dorsal mesentery that suspends the stomach (Cavdar et al. 1997; Yi et al. 2008; Stimec et al. 2011).

Superior mesenteric artery (SMA) is the second abdominal vitelline artery which supplies the *midgut*. At the beginning of its course, SMA joins the dorsal aorta at the second thoracic level. This connection moves later to the first lumbar level. This artery supplies the developing midgut, including the *part of intestine extending from descending segment of the duodenum to transverse colon near the left colic flexure* (Rouwet et al. 2000; Bhatnagar et al. 2013).

Inferior mesenteric artery (IMA) is the third and final segment of abdominal vitelline artery which supplies the *hindgut*. IMA initially joins the dorsal aorta at the 12th thoracic level and later ends at the third lumbar level supplying *distal portion of transverse colon, descending colon, sigmoid colon, and the superior rectum* (Moonen et al. 2012; Bhatnagar et al. 2013).

Blood supply to the inferior end of the anorectal canal comes from the branches of the iliac arteries. Two umbilical arteries pass from the connecting stalk (primordial umbilical cord) and locate along sides with vessels in the chorion, the embryonic part of the placenta. The umbilical arteries carry poorly oxygenated blood to the placenta. Proximal parts of the umbilical arteries form the *internal iliac* and *superior vesical* arteries. However, after birth, distal parts of umbilical artery obliterate and become the medial umbilical ligaments.

Dorsal Aorta Gives Rise to Lateral Branches

Lateral branches of the descending aorta supply the suprarenal glands, gonads, and kidneys. However, these three organs and their arteries have different developmental pathway.

The suprarenal glands originate in the posterior body wall between the sixth and 12th thoracic segments; they are supplied by a pair of lateral aortic branches that arise at an upper lumbar level. Also, some branches from the renal artery and inferior phrenic artery supply the suprarenal glands, but the suprarenal arteries developing from these aortic branches remain the major supply to the glands (Dutta 2010; Sato 2013).

The presumptive gonads become vascularized by *gonadal arteries* which arise initially at the tenth thoracic level. The gonads descend during development, but the origin of the gonadal arteries becomes stable at the third or fourth lumbar segments. The gonadal arteries elongate, as the gonads (especially the testes) descend further; there are many retroperitoneal anastomoses of the gonadal veins in fetal period, and afterward, left side anastomoses are much more common in both sexes (Raz 2004; Szpinda et al. 2005; Hen et al. 2014; Alfahad and Scott 2015).

In contrast, *the definitive kidneys* arise in the sacral region and move upward to a lumbar position just below the suprarenal glands. As they migrate, they are vascularized by a sequence of transient aortic side streams that originate at higher levels. These arteries do not elongate for following the ascending kidneys; in contrast, they degenerate. The definitive renal arteries develop from final pair of arteries in the upper lumbar region. Sometimes, a more inferior pair of renal arteries remains as accessory renal arteries (Alfahad and Scott 2015).

Intersegmental Branches

At the beginning of the fourth week, the vasculogenesis process leads to the rise of small sprouts in the posterolateral segments; these primitive sprouts are located alongside the cervical somites extending through to the sacral somites; they grow up and at the same time join to dorsal aorta. In *lumbar* and *thoracic* segments, the dorsal branch derived from each of these intersegmental vessels vascularizes toward the growing neural tube and also the epimeres (i.e., the dorsal portion of each somite which gives origin to dorsal muscles that are innervated from the related spinal somite). In addition, the dorsal skin is supplied by the cutaneous branches of these arteries (Gans and Northcutt 1983; Northcutt and Gans 1983; Technau and Scholz 2003).

Besides, these intersegmental vessels vascularize the hypomeres; i.e., hypomeric muscles and related skin are supplied by the ventral branches of intersegmental vessel (hypomeric muscles are those muscles derived from a hypomere and are also innervated by an anterior ramus of the related spinal nerve; also, hypomere is the lateral plate of the mesoderm which grows up to form the ventral body parts) (Finnegan 1961a, b; Technau and Scholz 2003).

The *ventral intersegmental arteries* in the *thoracic* segments are transformed to intercostal arteries and cutaneous branches, while in the *sacral* and *lumbar* regions, they are developed to lateral sacral and lumbar arteries.

A small branch, the median sacral artery, arises from the dorsal aorta in the area of common iliac artery bifurcation.

In *cervical* regions, the branches derived from intersegmental arteries link together and create a new complex form of vascularization. Some paired vertebral arteries rise from longitudinal branches that anastomose together in order to form a longitudinal vessel, while in back, they secondarily miss their intersegmental links to the aorta. The anastomoses of intersegmental arteries cause to the development of some arteries such as ascending cervical, deep cervical, internal thoracic, superior intercostal, and inferior and superior epigastric arteries (Adameyko and Fried 2016).

Formation of Limb Arteries

During the development of the limb buds, the arteries derived from seven cervical and five lumbar intersegmental arteries grow into the limb buds to provide blood to them; this primitive perfusion system works through an axial artery, which develops alongside the central axis of each limb. In the upper limb, the axial artery gives origin to the following arteries:

- Brachial artery
- Anterior interosseous artery of the forearm
- Deep palmar arch of the hand
- Radial, ulnar, and median arteries

In the lower limb, in contrast to the upper limb, the axial artery degenerates; so, the external arteries supply the blood flow of the lower limb, finally leading to these main arteries (Funke and Kuhn 1998):

- The small sciatic artery which provides the blood for the sciatic nerve in the posterior thigh.
- A branch of the popliteal artery.
- A segment of the peroneal artery in the foreleg.
- All additional arteries of the lower limb are derived from the external iliac artery.

The Formation of Coronary Arteries

Coronary arteries originate from two different segments:

1. The proepicardial cells
2. The epicardial cells

Vascular development in the myocardial tissue follows the initial development of cardiac loop. The primary coronary beds are formed in the trabeculations of the myocardial tissue, while the underling myocardial cells lead to some degrees of epicardial cell change in the form of "epithelial-to-mesenchymal transition," in such a way that the newly formed mesenchymal cells penetrate the *endothelial* and *smooth muscle* cells located in the walls of coronary arteries. The endothelial plexus located in the subepicardial layer is connected to the endothelial sprouts which are located in the walls of the aortic sinuses.

On the other hand, the neural crest cells help smooth muscle cells alongside the proximal division of coronary arteries. The endothelial sprouts of coronary arteries develop some forms of vascular ring which is peritruncal; then, they penetrate and merge into the aortic wall. In fact, coronary arteries attach to the aorta following the development of endothelial cells in such a way that coronary arteries penetrate into the aorta. However, there are only two sprouts of coronary arteries which can produce their lumen and orifices: these are the left and the right coronary arteries. This is one of the main differences between coronary arteries and cardiac veins: coronary arteries are perfused from the systemic circulation through the root of aorta; however, coronary sinuses are the specific site for cardiac veins to connect general circulation. Coronary arteries are perfused in the third trimester. Chapter 34 deals in detail with coronary artery anomalies (Song et al. 2015; Perez-Pomares et al. 2016) (Fig. 2.13).

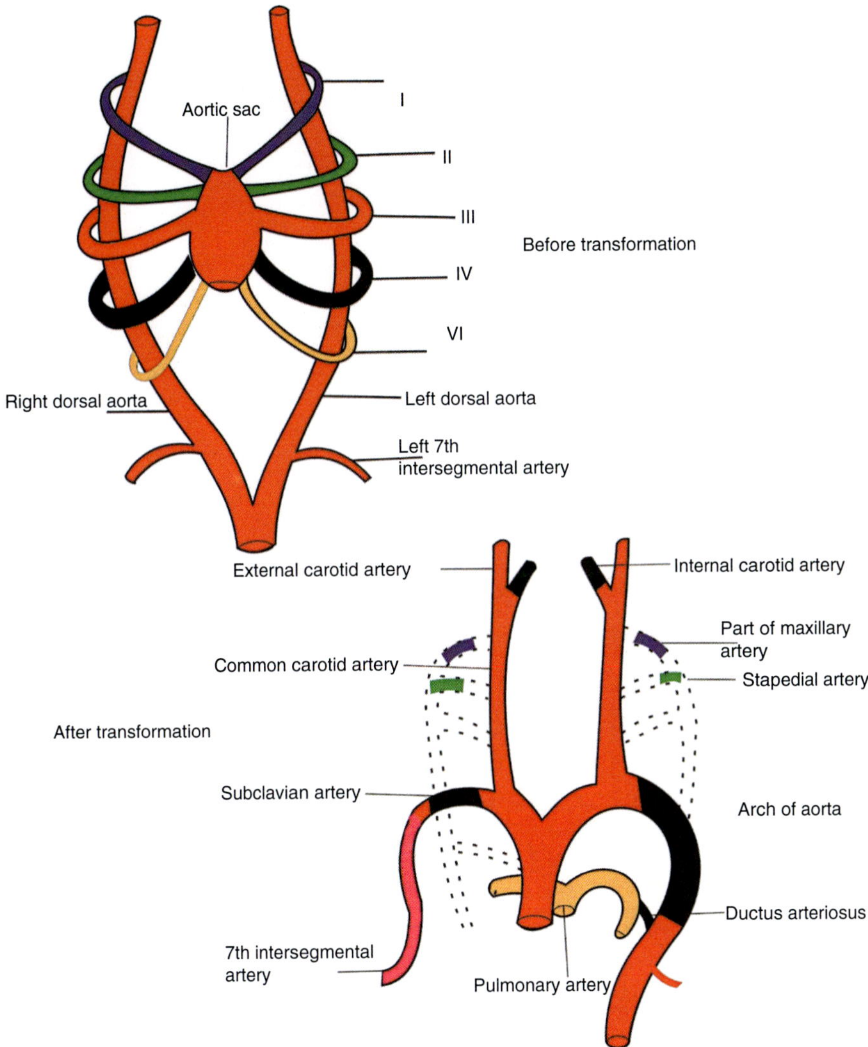

Fig. 2.13 Schematic drawings of the aortic arches and dorsal aorta before transformation into the definitive vascular pattern and after transformation

The Formation of Venous System

During the early 2nd month, three main veins can be found in each side of the body: vitelline vein, umbilical vein, and cardinal vein; these veins are discussed here (Fig. 2.14):

1. *Vitelline veins* or omphalomesenteric veins transfer blood from yolk sac to the sinus venosus. The vitelline veins make a plexus around the duodenal part of the small intestine; afterward, they arrive in sinus venosus after crossing septum transversum. After trespassing the septum transversum, they are invaded by the liver cords growing into the septum; this will lead to interruption of venous courses. In the final stage, hepatic sinusoids are formed as a wide vascular network. Blood transfer from the left side to the right side of the liver leads to formation of an expanded right vitelline vein. In the next developmental phases, the right hepatocardiac channel gives origin to the hepatocardiac segment of IVC; but the proximal portion of the left vitelline vein gradually disappears.

   The set of arteries around the duodenum anastomose and grow as a single vessel: *portal vein*. A small bud of artery grows from the right vitelline vein and creates the superior mesenteric vein. Later on, the distal part of left vitelline vein degenerates.

2. *Umbilical veins* originate from the chorionic villi and transfer highly oxygenated blood from the placenta to the embryo body. During the early stages, a pair of veins, i.e., the umbilical veins, passes from both sides of the liver, to connect in later stages to sinusoids of the liver. At this time, the proximal portion of each

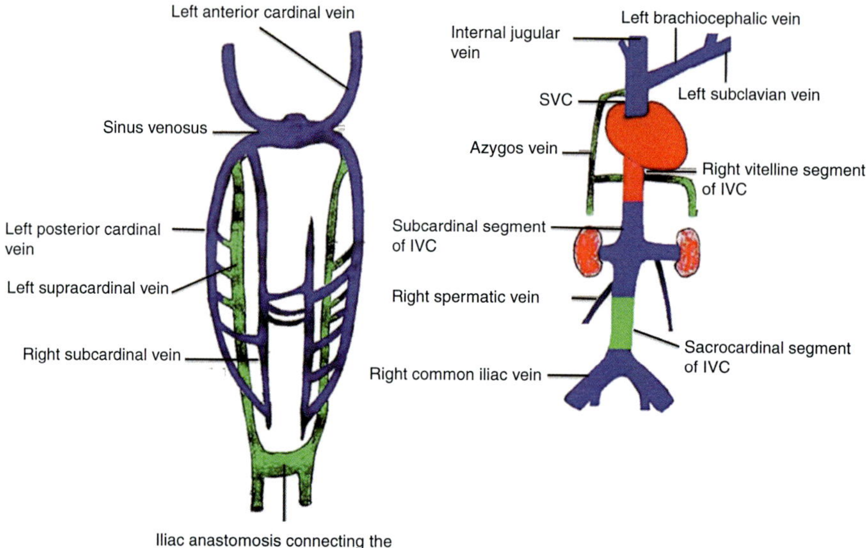

Fig. 2.14 Illustrations of the primordial veins; initially, three systems of veins are present: the umbilical veins from the chorion, the vitelline veins from the yolk sac, and the cardinal veins from the body of the embryo

umbilical vein and the remnants of the right umbilical vein begin to disappear. Therefore, the left vein is the only vein that transfers blood from the placenta to the liver. With increased blood flow through the placenta, a direct connection, named ductus venosus, is created between the right hepatocardiac channel and the left umbilical veins. Ductus venosus bypasses the sinusoidal plexus in the liver. However, obliteration of the left umbilical vein leads to ligamentum venosum and obliteration of ductus venosus leads to ligamentum teres.

3. *Cardinal veins* drain the whole embryo body. In the embryonic period, cardinal veins are the early main veins draining the cephalic portion of the embryo. Anterior and posterior cardinal veins are derived from this early venous system; the anterior cardinal vein drains the *cephalic* segment of the embryo, while the posterior cardinal vein drains other segments of embryo. These anterior and posterior veins connect together before arriving into the sinus horn, making the *short common cardinal* vein. Throughout the 2nd embryologic month, a considerable number of veins are created including:

- The sacrocardinal veins which drain the lower limbs
- The subcardinal veins which drain the left and right kidneys
- The supracardinal veins which drain the body wall

The anastomosis between the left and right veins leads to development of *vena cava system*, transferring the blood from the left side to the right side.

Inferior vena cava (IVC) development The development of IVC occurs during the fourth to eighth gestation weeks. Creation of IVC has many different stages with many developmental complexities, involving all the anatomic venous segments originating from different venous parts (Spentzouris et al. 2014). It was in 1793 that IVC anomalies were first described by Abernethy in a 10-month-old baby with concomitant polysplenia and dextrocardia (Petik 2015).

IVC has four distinct segments (Spentzouris et al. 2014; Petik 2015; Smillie et al. 2015):

Hepatic IVC: vitelline vein is the origin of the hepatic IVC.
Suprarenal IVC is originated from right subcardinal vein.
Renal IVC is created after anastomosis between right subcardinal and right supracardinal veins.
Infrarenal IVC: embryologic development of infrahepatic IVC is the neatly ordered sequence of regression and formation between three paired embryonic veins:

- *Subcardinal* veins
- *Supracardinal* veins
- *Posterior cardinal* veins

The anterior cardinal veins anastomose together and form the *left brachiocephalic* vein. This will lead to an important event in the future: *the venous blood drains from the left side of the head and the left upper limbs to the right venous side.* Also, the right common cardinal vein and the proximal part of the right anterior cardinal vein join to make the *superior vena cava.*

The end part of the *left posterior cardinal* vein enters the left brachiocephalic vein; this venous segment is preserved as a small vessel named the *left superior intercostal vein*; venous blood from the second and third intercostal spaces drains into these vessels.

The *left renal vein* is formed by the anastomosis between the subcardinal veins. After that, the left subcardinal vein gradually disappears; only remnants of its distal portion remain which are named the *left gonadal vein*. Therefore, the right subcardinal vein remains as a main drainage channel which forms the *renal segment of the inferior vena cava*.

The sacrocardinal veins merge together and make the *left common iliac veins*. The right sacrocardinal vein forms the *sacrocardinal portion of the inferior vena cava*.

When the renal and hepatic parts of inferior vena cava anastomose together, the formation of hepatic, renal, and sacrocardinal segments is completed.

After degeneration of the posterior cardinal veins, the supracardinal veins take the main role in body wall venous drainage. The *azygos vein* is formed after merging of these veins:

- The fourth to 11th right intercostal veins
- The right supracardinal vein
- Part of the posterior cardinal vein

However, the left fourth to seventh intercostal veins merge and create the *hemiazygos vein* which is drained into the left supracardinal vein; later on, the hemiazygos vein drains into the azygos vein. One should always consider that during the fetal life and later on until adulthood, there are many anatomical variations of the azygos and hemiazygos veins (Krakowiak-Sarnowska et al. 2003; Keskin et al. 2013; Piciucchi et al. 2014).

The Formation of Lymphatic System

The development of the lymphatic system starts around the end of the sixth week, i.e., 2 weeks after recognition of the primordial cardiovascular system. The growth pattern of the lymphatic vessels is much similar to blood vessels. In the final fate of the lymphatic system, there are some connections with the venous system. The early lymphatic capillaries connect with each other to make a lymphatic network (Park et al. 2015).

Development of Lymph Sacs and Lymphatic Ducts

At the end of the embryonic period, there are six primary lymph sacs that include:

- Two jugular lymph sacs which are located near the junction of the subclavian veins with the anterior cardinal veins which will be the future internal jugular veins

- Two iliac lymph sacs close to the junction of the iliac veins with the posterior cardinal veins
- One retroperitoneal lymph sac which is located in the root of the mesentery, located on the posterior abdominal wall
- One cisterna chili located dorsal to the retroperitoneal lymph sac

In earlier phases, lymphatic vessels create some connections with the lymph sacs and pass along the main veins, in such a way that they create these connections:

- From the jugular lymph sacs to the head, neck, and upper limbs.
- From the iliac lymph sacs to the lower trunk and lower limbs.
- From the retroperitoneal lymph sac and the chyle cistern to the primordial gut; the cistern connects two large channels (right and left thoracic ducts) which are connected to the jugular lymph sacs; later on, between these channels, large anastomosis develops.

The Development of Thoracic Duct

The thoracic duct develops from different parts including:

- The caudal part of the right thoracic duct
- The anastomosis between the left and right thoracic ducts
- The cranial part of the left thoracic duct

Therefore, there are various variations in the origin, course, and insertion of the adult thoracic duct. The right lymphatic duct is created after merging of the right thoracic duct in its cranial part. Both the thoracic duct and the right lymphatic duct join with the venous system at the venous angle which is located between the internal jugular vein and the subclavian vein (Butler et al. 2009; Park et al. 2015).

Circulation Before and After Birth

Fetal Circulation

Prior to birth, the umbilical vein transfers the blood from placenta to the fetus while 80 % of its content is oxygen saturated; when the blood reaches the liver, it goes directly through the ductus venosus into the *inferior vena cava* (IVC) in a phenomenon called "short-circuiting the liver." A small amount of this blood arrives to the liver sinusoids; then, it is combined with the blood coming from the portal circulation. The flow of the umbilical blood via the liver sinusoids is regulated by the sphincter of the ductus venosus, located near the entry of the umbilical vein. The sphincter of ductus venosus closes as soon as the first uterine contraction occurs in order to increase venous entry as much as possible and avoid unexpected overloading of the heart.

The blood coming from the *placenta* is well oxygenated; it comes from the maternal circulation, going through placenta to the umbilical veins and ductus venosus; there, the deoxygenated blood coming from the lower limbs is mixed with the oxygenated blood; from here, the mixed, though still oxygenated, blood is transferred through IVC, going finally to the right atrium.

From this point, part of *oxygenated blood* trespasses the foramen ovale to go from the right atrium to the *left atrium*, then the left ventricle and aorta to perfuse systemic organs, including brain and heart muscles, which are the first organs receiving well-oxygenated blood coming from the placenta.

In addition, the remaining oxygenated blood coming from IVC goes through the right atrium to the right ventricle and goes to the *pulmonary trunk* perfusing the lungs and then returning through pulmonary veins to the left atrium, left ventricle, and descending aorta to go to the to the umbilical artery. However, part of the blood goes through the *pulmonary trunk* to the ductus arteriosus and aorta to flow into the systemic circulation.

Superior vena cava (SVC) drains the desaturated blood coming from the arms and head; then, in the left atrium, this blood is combined with the desaturated blood coming from the lungs. Afterward, the blood goes into the left ventricle and ascending aorta.

In fetal life, because of high resistance of pulmonary vessels, the majority of blood directly goes from the ductus arteriosus to the descending aorta and does not pass through pulmonary vessels. In the descending aorta, the blood is combined with the blood coming from the proximal aorta. Finally, the desaturated blood goes through the descending aorta and then two umbilical arteries toward the placenta to leave fetal circulation.

As a brief, mixture of the saturated and desaturated blood takes places in the following locations:

1. In the *liver*, a small amount of the desaturated blood coming from the portal system mixes the saturated blood.
2. In *IVC*, the deoxygenated blood returned from the organs such as the lower limbs, kidneys, and pelvis is added to the saturated blood.
3. In the *right atrium*, the desaturated blood returned from the upper and lower limbs and the head is added to the saturated blood.
4. In the *left atrium*, the blood returned from the lungs is added to the saturated blood.
5. At the junction of the *ductus arteriosus* with the descending aorta, the desaturated blood coming from the pulmonary trunk is added to "now relatively saturated blood" which finally enters the descending aorta.

Circulatory Alterations After Birth

The events in circulation after birth are discussed in detail in Chap. 3—Pediatric Cardiovascular Physiology. In summary, the fetal circulation shift to a neonatal circulation pattern is an adaptive change in order to tolerate the new "out of the uterus" environment; the final goal is achieving a *biventricular parallel circulation pattern instead of the series circulation of the fetus*; here, these steps are discussed in brief (Rabi et al. 2006; Gao and Raj 2010; Katheria and Leone 2012; Noori et al. 2012; Rabe et al. 2012; Duley and Batey 2013; Galinsky et al. 2013; McDonald et al. 2013; Azhibekov et al. 2014; van Vonderen et al. 2014a, b; Baik et al. 2015; van Vonderen and Te Pas 2015; Yigit et al. 2015):

1. The establishment of the first inspiratory effort leads to inflation of the lungs and commencement of gas exchange; the result is increased oxygen pressure in the pulmonary vascular bed and the alveoli, which is among the earliest initiatives for transition of circulation; as a result, *pulmonary vascular resistance* (PVR) drops suddenly in the first 10 min after birth.
2. Placental vessels are clamped; abrupt increase in systemic vascular resistance (SVR) happens.
3. Foramen ovale is closed due to increased pressure in the left atrial chamber over the right atrial chamber; the mechanism of closure is anatomic relationship between septum primum and septum secundum; however, very shortly afterward, the ductus arteriosus is closed, preventing flow between pulmonary artery and the aorta; this is an essential "shift" in body circulation from a "series circulation" to a "parallel circulation."
4. Complete anatomical closure of the foramen ovale and ductus arteriosus occurs later; often, the foramen ovale is closed physiologically first and then anatomically during a few days, with a minority having only physiologic closure of the foramen ovale even in adulthood; however, the ductus arteriosus is closed during the first 48–72 h after birth.
5. The umbilical vein stops its venous flow at birth.
6. Portal venous system pressure increases, leading to redirection of flow through the hepatic veins.
7. *β-receptors* are not as much frequent in the newborn heart; but, they increase in myocardium after birth.
8. This transitional circulation needs a minimum of 5 min during the first stages of life, resulting in the "normal postnatal oxygen saturation" state.
9. Blood pressure in the early postnatal period depends on a number of factors, mainly cardiac output (CO) and systemic vascular resistance (SVR); in addition, these factors affect blood pressure: neonatal asphyxia, drugs transferred from the mother like antihypertensive agents or some anesthetics, term infants vs preterm infants, vaginal delivery compared to cesarean section, and gender (female vs male neonates).
10. Cardiac output considered as left and right heart output assumes the "normal" pattern after birth; in fact, in the fetal circulation, the main load of cardiac output is on the right heart; however, just after birth, i.e., in the postnatal period, while the transition from series circulation to parallel circulation ensues, left ventricle and right ventricle cardiac output equalizes and the dominancy of right ventricle output (RVO) disappears, and at the same time, left ventricle output (LVO) and left ventricle stroke volume (SV) increase; also, cardiac output increases in the early postnatal 2–5 h, while after that, due to closure of ductus arteriosus, cardiac output gradually drops to a bit lower level to become stable.
11. If any pathology impairs this process, the transition from fetal to neonatal circulation does not occur correctly, leading to *persistence of fetal circulation*.

12. Increased PVR due to hypoxia, acidosis, and hypercarbia, history of diabetes in mother during pregnancy, intrauterine inflammation due to infection or other reasons, increased pressure in the right atrium over the left atrium leading to impaired closure of foramen ovale, or patency of ductus arteriosus are among the main etiologies for *persistence of fetal circulation.*

Angiomas

Abnormal and unnecessary growth of small capillary networks is named a capillary hemangioma. On the other side, accumulating and germinating bundle of large venous sinuses is a cavernous hemangioma. Infantile hemangiomas are the most common vascular tumors in childhood. These tumors develop rapidly and cause an uncontrolled growing mass composed of endothelial cells, lumen obstruction, multilayered basement membranes, and fibrous tissue. Their only risk is when they are located on critical anatomical points like the skull or vertebral canal or in the airways (Marler and Mulliken 2005).

Genetic basis linked with developmental syndromes or chromosomal abnormalities has been proposed for some hemangiomas. For example:

- *5q31-33* of chromosomal region has close link with some hemangioma, containing genes such as *FGF4, PDGFβ*, and *FMS-RELATED TYROSINE KINASE*, coding the molecules essential in blood vessel growth.
- Dysregulation of the *TIE/ANG* signaling pathways.
- Mutations of *VEGFR2*.
- Multiple hemangioblastomas are related with *von Hippel-Lindau disease*, with mutations in a gene at chromosome *3p25-26*.
- Excessive angiogenesis may be due to great levels of vascular endothelial growth factor (*VEGF*) and hypoxia inducible factor 1-alpha (*HIF1α*) secretion by stromal tumor cells.

Abnormalities of the Ductus Arteriosus

The ductus arteriosus which is located in the right side of the aortic arch grows toward the right side either in front or behind the esophagus and trachea, making ligamentum arteriosum after its postnatal closure.

If it passes from behind of the esophagus, it can lead to a constriction of the esophagus and trachea with clinical dysphagia and/or dyspnea.

When the right and left fourth aortic arches are disappeared and the distal right of dorsal aorta persists, a disease state known as interrupted aortic arch happens. After birth, the aorta supplies the upper body, upper limbs, and head, but the pulmonary artery (contains blood with poorly oxygenated) supplies the lower body and limbs through a patent ductus arteriosus. Detailed discussion about interrupted aortic arch could be found in Chap. 27.

Aortic Coarctation

Coarctation of the aorta (CoA) is one of the common congenital defects, more common in males than females. CoA may occur as a separated abnormality or in association with various other injuries, usually bicuspid aortic valve (BAV) and ventricular septal defect. The disease is discussed in Chap. 24.

CoA is often defined as a restricted aortic segment encompassing localized medial thickening, with some enfolding of the medial and overlaid neointimal tissue.

The underlying mechanism for aortic coarctation is still controversial, although the deformity may be initiated by genetic factors or by teratogens.

There are two main potential etiologies proposed as the causative mechanism for CoA, namely, "ductal theory or ductus tissue theory" and "hemodynamic theory or flow theory" described as follows:

- *Hemodynamic theory or flow theory*: more widely accepted, this theory known as *Rudolph theory* states that during the fetal period, the development of the aortic arch (including the length and the diameter of the arch) depends on *the amount of blood flow which passes through the arch*; if this blood flow is impaired, it leads to a narrowed and/or hypoplastic aortic arch. This phenomenon explains three main features of CoA: (1) the *posterior shelf*, (2) the *intracardiac defects* which are concomitant embryologic lesions, (3) *tubular hypoplasia* which is often a concomitant lesion of CoA, and (4) the right-sided obstructive lesions which are very rarely associated with CoA.
- *Ductal theory or ductus tissue theory*: this theory is also known as *Skodaic hypothesis* which assumes "abnormal distribution or aberrant migration" of smooth muscle cells (SMC) from the ductus arteriosus to the adjacent aortic tissue as the etiology of CoA; in other words, the ectopic ductal tissue in the aortic isthmus causes CoA and aortic constriction, usually in the isthmus of the aorta (i.e., the junction of aorta with ductus arteriosus) (Krediet 1965; Gillman and Burton 1966; Hutchins 1971; Heymann and Rudolph 1972; Rudolph et al. 1972; Shinebourne and Elseed 1974; Moore and Hutchins 1978; Ho and Anderson 1979; Momma et al. 1982; Van Meurs-Van Woezik and Krediet 1982; Russell et al. 1991; Jimenez et al. 1999; Liberman et al. 2004; Carroll et al. 2006; Kenny and Hijazi 2011).

CoA occurs in three forms:

- Juxtaductal location which is close to the ductus arteriosus, which is more common than other forms.
- Preductal CoA, i.e., proximal location which is upstream of the ductus; usually, collateral circulation does not develop, since the ductus arteriosus connects most of the oxygen- and nutrient-enriched blood from the placenta to the lower portion of the body (Fig. 2.15).
- Postductal CoA, i.e., distal location which is downstream of ductus; postductal CoA is asymptomatic in some newborn infants, since other arteries including subclavian, internal thoracic, transverse cervical, suprascapular, superior epigastric, intercostal, and lumbar arteries create collateral circulation throughout the embryonic and fetal period (Fig. 2.15).

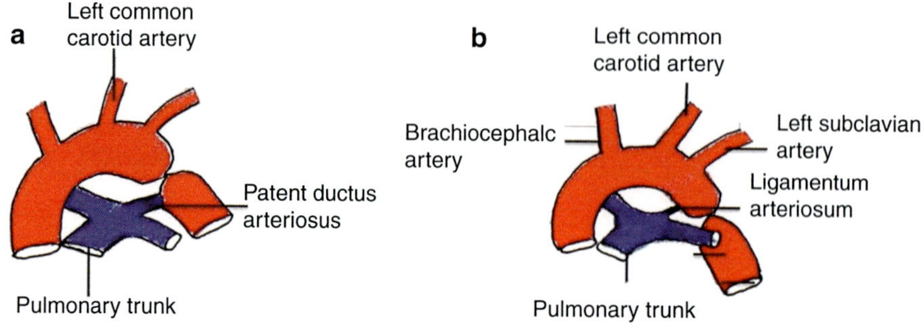

Fig. 2.15 Coarctation of the aorta: (**a**) preductal type, (**b**) postductal type

When the ductus is closed after birth, the infants suffering from CoA are imposed with many abnormalities. In this disease the upper part of the body and head are well perfused but the lower part is somewhat ischemic. CoA repair may be done by surgery, stenting, or balloon dilation angioplasty with different outcomes and chance of recurring stenosis. More detailed discussion on this topic is found in Chap. 24 of this book.

Alagille syndrome refers to genetic problems that result in various symptoms in different parts of the body, including the liver, kidney, heart, and other systems of the body such as paucity of bile ducts and arterial stenosis. Abnormalities related to the disorder generally become apparent in early childhood or infancy.

Vena Cava Anomalies

The anomalies of venae cavae are categorized under two main classes: IVC anomalies and SVC anomalies.

IVC Anomalies

Inferior vena cava (IVC) anomalies were first described in 1793 by Abernethy in a 10-month-old baby who had polysplenia and dextrocardia (Petik 2015).

Embryologic development of IVC is the neatly ordered sequence of regression and formation between three paired embryonic veins (Fig. 2.14):

- Subcardinal veins
- Supracardinal veins
- Postcardinal veins

As mentioned in the previous pages, under IVC development, these events occur between the fourth and eighth gestational weeks, in a multistage process; so, embryologic development of IVC is a potential process for many developmental malformations. Since the development of cross-sectional imaging, congenital anomalies of the IVC and its side streams have been encountered much more frequently, and in a large number of affected patients, these anomalies have been symptom-free.

Congenital anomalies of IVC are diverse, and at least 14 types of anomalies have been reported till now; among these 14, the most important ones are these four types (Srivastava et al. 2005; Dutta 2010):

- Double IVC, also known as duplication of IVC
- Left IVC or left-sided IVC
- Retroaortic left renal vein
- Circumaortic left renal vein

Among the other lesions are interrupted IVC, other left renal vein anomalies, gonadal vein anomalies, and preduodenal portal vein (Malaki et al. 2012; G et al. 2014; Hagans et al. 2014; Spentzouris et al. 2014; Petik 2015).

Persistent left IVC is usually the result of two events which happen together: *regression of the right supracardinal veins plus persistence of the left supracardinal veins.*

The typical form of persistent left IVC is that it will merge with the left renal vein then crosses to the other side, reaching the right renal vein, anterior to the aorta; this crossover from left to right is almost always at the level of renal veins. The final result is a normal right-sided IVC which is located in prerenal position (Bass et al. 2000; Malaki et al. 2012; Petik 2015).

There may be two forms of azygos continuation of IVC:

- Left IVC and absent infrarenal IVC with azygos continuation of IVC
- Left IVC and absent infrarenal IVC with azygos and hemiazygos continuation

Double IVC is a rare anomaly; its etiology is failure of regression in the caudal part of the left supracardinal veins, leading to persistence of *both supracardinal veins* and creation of an abnormal left IVC accompanied with right IVC; hence, there will be two IVCs. Significant asymmetry between the sizes of right and left IVCs is possible. The venous blood arriving left IVC will ultimately drain into one of the following veins:

- Right IVC via the left renal vein
- Hemiazygos vein rising from thoracic part of the supracardinal system (Bass et al. 2000; Malaki et al. 2012)

SVC Anomalies

Left Superior Vena Cava

In some patients, the left anterior cardinal vein remains, leading to preserved connection between the anterior cardinal vein and the left sinus venosus. Its incidence in general population is about 0.3–0.5 %. If left SVC persists, the blood coming

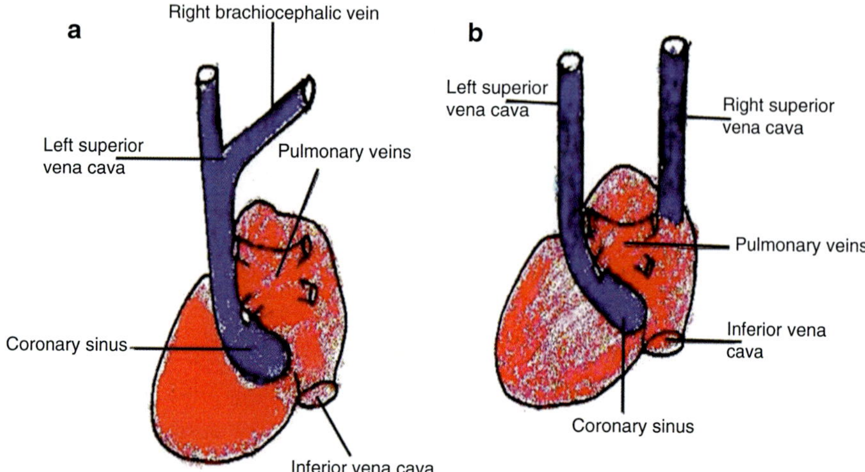

Fig. 2.16 Left SVC: (**a**) double SVC, (**b**) single left SVC

from the left side of the head, neck, and the upper extremity is emptied through the abnormal left SVC into the coronary sinus. This anomaly is presented either as a steady left (double) SVC or a single left SVC. A single left SVC is seen if the left anterior cardinal vein persists while at the same time, the right one is eliminated. In this situation, the left anterior cardinal vein leads to a superior vena cava draining the blood from the entire head and neck, both upper extremities, and the azygos system, then directing all this venous blood into the coronary sinus and right atrium. However, when double and left SVC are present, left SVC drains directly into the left atrium; this condition is seen more commonly in heterotaxy cases (Fig. 2.16). In about 65 % of all left SVC cases, the left brachiocephalic vein is either very small or does not exist at all.

Lymphatic System Anomalies

Lymphedema may result from lymphatic hypoplasia. Primary lymphedemas also known as lymphatic obstruction are swellings of the lymphatic vasculature and a major hereditary congenital disorder of the lymphatic system which is induced by hypoplasia of the lymphatic system. This condition usually is accompanied with other abnormalities. There are a number of genes involved in development of lymphedema (Dellinger et al. 2008; Stoll et al. 2013; Sabine and Petrova 2014; Yang and Oliver 2014; Park et al. 2015):

- FOXC2 gene
- The transcription factors related to the Forkhead family
- SOX18 gene mutations and SRY-related transcription factor
- Ang2, Nrp2, Net, Podoplanin, and Syk

The most severe swellings usually take place in the legs, but, for lymphedema related to *Turner syndrome*, the lymphatic ducts are obstructed in the neck region and upper trunk; however, this clinical feature may also be the result of lymph-filled cyst development (known as cystic hygromas). These cysts may withdraw if drainage of lymphatic recovers during subsequent stages of development.

Milroy disease is associated with impaired function of the lymphatic system; so, it is a primary lymphedema syndrome due to mutations in the VEGFR3 gene.

References

Abu-Issa R, Kirby ML. Heart field: from mesoderm to heart tube. Annu Rev Cell Dev Biol. 2007;23:45–68.

Adameyko I, Fried K. The nervous system orchestrates and integrates craniofacial development: a review. Front Physiol. 2016;7:49.

Akcay M, Bilen ES, Bilge M, Durmaz T, Kurt M. Prominent crista terminalis: as an anatomic structure leading to atrial arrhythmias and mimicking right atrial mass. J Am Soc Echocardiogr Off Publ Am Soc Echocardiogr. 2007;20:197.e199–110.

Alfahad A, Scott P. Testicular arteries originating from accessory renal arteries. J Vasc Interv Radiol. 2015;26:205.

Anderson RH, Chaudhry B, Mohun TJ, Bamforth SD, Hoyland D, Phillips HM, Webb S, Moorman AF, Brown NA, Henderson DJ. Normal and abnormal development of the intrapericardial arterial trunks in humans and mice. Cardiovasc Res. 2012;95:108–15.

Anderson RH, Cook A, Brown NA, Henderson DJ, Chaudhry B, Mohun T. Development of the outflow tracts with reference to aortopulmonary windows and aortoventricular tunnels. Cardiol Young. 2010;20 Suppl 3:92–9.

Anderson RH, McCarthy K, Cook AC. Continuing medical education. Double outlet right ventricle. Cardiol Young. 2001;11:329–44.

Anderson RH, Webb S, Brown NA, Lamers W, Moorman A. Development of the heart: (2) Septation of the atriums and ventricles. Heart. 2003a;89:949–58.

Anderson RH, Webb S, Brown NA, Lamers W, Moorman A. Development of the heart: (3) formation of the ventricular outflow tracts, arterial valves, and intrapericardial arterial trunks. Heart. 2003b;89:1110–8.

Apitz C, Webb GD, Redington AN. Tetralogy of Fallot. Lancet. 2009;374:1462–71.

Asrress KN, Marciniak M, Marciniak A, Rajani R, Clapp B. Patent foramen ovale: the current state of play. Heart. 2015;101:1916–25.

Atkinson A, Inada S, Li J, Tellez JO, Yanni J, Sleiman R, Allah EA, Anderson RH, Zhang H, Boyett MR, Dobrzynski H. Anatomical and molecular mapping of the left and right ventricular His-Purkinje conduction networks. J Mol Cell Cardiol. 2011;51:689–701.

Azhibekov T, Noori S, Soleymani S, Seri I. Transitional cardiovascular physiology and comprehensive hemodynamic monitoring in the neonate: relevance to research and clinical care. Semin Fetal Neonatal Med. 2014;19:45–53.

Baik N, Urlesberger B, Schwaberger B, Freidl T, Schmolzer GM, Pichler G. Cardiocirculatory monitoring during immediate fetal-to-neonatal transition: a systematic qualitative review of the literature. Neonatology. 2015;107:100–7.

Bamforth SD, Chaudhry B, Bennett M, Wilson R, Mohun TJ, Van Mierop LH, Henderson DJ, Anderson RH. Clarification of the identity of the mammalian fifth pharyngeal arch artery. Clin Anat (New York, NY). 2013;26:173–82.

Bass JE, Redwine MD, Kramer LA, Huynh PT, Harris Jr JH. Spectrum of congenital anomalies of the inferior vena cava: cross-sectional imaging findings. Radiographics. 2000;20:639–52.

Berry D. History of cardiology: Etienne-Louis Fallot, MD. Circulation. 2006;114:f152.

Bhatnagar S, Rajesh S, Jain VK, Patidar Y, Mukund A, Arora A. Celiacomesenteric trunk: a short report. Surg Radiol Anat. 2013;35:979–81.

Briggs LE, Kakarla J, Wessels A. The pathogenesis of atrial and atrioventricular septal defects with special emphasis on the role of the dorsal mesenchymal protrusion. Differentiation Res Biol Divers. 2012;84:117–30.

Butler MG, Isogai S, Weinstein BM. Lymphatic development. Birth Defects Res C Embryo Today. 2009;87:222–31.

Calkoen EE, Hazekamp MG, Blom NA, Elders BB, Gittenberger-de Groot AC, Haak MC, Bartelings MM, Roest AA, Jongbloed MR. Atrioventricular septal defect: from embryonic development to long-term follow-up. Int J Cardiol. 2016;202:784–95.

Carroll SJ, Ferris A, Chen J, Liberman L. Efficacy of prostaglandin E1 in relieving obstruction in coarctation of a persistent fifth aortic arch without opening the ductus arteriosus. Pediatr Cardiol. 2006;27:766–8.

Cavdar S, Sehirli U, Pekin B. Celiacomesenteric trunk. Clin Anat (New York, NY). 1997;10:231–4.

Charpentier MS, Conlon FL. Cellular and molecular mechanisms underlying blood vessel lumen formation. BioEssays News Rev Mol Cell Dev Biol. 2014;36:251–9.

Charpentier MS, Tandon P, Trincot CE, Koutleva EK, Conlon FL. A distinct mechanism of vascular lumen formation in Xenopus requires EGFL7. PLoS One. 2015;10:e0116086.

Christoffels VM, Hoogaars WM, Tessari A, Clout DE, Moorman AF, Campione M. T-box transcription factor Tbx2 represses differentiation and formation of the cardiac chambers. Dev Dyn Off Publ Am Assoc Anatomists. 2004;229:763–70.

Dabbagh A. Cardiac physiology. In: Dabbagh A, Esmailian F, Aranki SF, editors. Postoperative critical care for cardiac surgical patients. Berlin: Springer; 2014. p. 1–39.

Davey BT, Rychik J. The natural history of atrioventricular valve regurgitation throughout fetal life in patients with atrioventricular canal defects. Pediatr Cardiol. 2016;37:50–4.

Dellinger MT, Thome K, Bernas MJ, Erickson RP, Witte MH. Novel FOXC2 missense mutation identified in patient with lymphedema-distichiasis syndrome and review. Lymphology. 2008;41:98–102.

Desplantez T, Dupont E, Severs NJ, Weingart R. Gap junction channels and cardiac impulse propagation. J Membr Biol. 2007;218:13–28.

Diogo R, Kelly RG, Christiaen L, Levine M, Ziermann JM, Molnar JL, Noden DM, Tzahor E. A new heart for a new head in vertebrate cardiopharyngeal evolution. Nature. 2015;520:466–73.

Duley L, Batey N. Optimal timing of umbilical cord clamping for term and preterm babies. Early Hum Dev. 2013;89:4.

Dun W, Boyden PA. The Purkinje cell; 2008 style. J Mol Cell Cardiol. 2008;45:617–24.

Dutta S. Suprarenal gland-arterial supply: an embryological basis and applied importance. Rom J Morphol Embryol Revue roumaine de morphologie et embryologie. 2010;51:137–40.

Ellis WS, SippensGroenewegen A, Auslander DM, Lesh MD. The role of the crista terminalis in atrial flutter and fibrillation: a computer modeling study. Ann Biomed Eng. 2000;28:742–54.

Evans WN. "Tetralogy of Fallot" and Etienne-Louis Arthur Fallot. Pediatr Cardiol. 2008;29:637–40.

Finnegan CV. An analysis of the postgastrula differentiation of the hypomere. I. The influence of tissue mass and of endoderm in Ambystoma punctatum. J Embryol Exp Morphol. 1961a;9:294–309.

Finnegan CV. An analysis of the postgastrula differentiation of the hypomere. II. The influence of endoderm and tissue mass in Taricha torosa. J Embryol Exp Morphol. 1961b;9:609–17.

Freedom RM, Jaeggi ET, Lim JS, Anderson RH. Hearts with isomerism of the right atrial appendages – one of the worst forms of disease in 2005. Cardiol Young. 2005;15:554–67.

Funke C, Kuhn HJ. The morphogenesis of the arteries of the pelvic extremity. A comparative study of mammals with special reference to the tree shrew Tupaia belangeri (Tupaiidae, Scandentia, Mammalia). Adv Anat Embryol Cell Biol. 1998;144:1–97.

Galinsky R, Hooper SB, Wallace MJ, Westover AJ, Black MJ, Moss TJ, Polglase GR. Intrauterine inflammation alters cardiopulmonary and cerebral haemodynamics at birth in preterm lambs. J Physiol. 2013;591:2127–37.

Gans C, Northcutt RG. Neural crest and the origin of vertebrates: a new head. Science (New York, NY). 1983;220:268–73.

Gao Y, Raj JU. Regulation of the pulmonary circulation in the fetus and newborn. Physiol Rev. 2010;90:1291–335.

Garside VC, Chang AC, Karsan A, Hoodless PA. Co-ordinating Notch, BMP, and TGF-beta signaling during heart valve development. Cell Mol Life Sci. 2013;70:2899–917.

Gassanov N, Er F, Zagidullin N, Hoppe UC. Endothelin induces differentiation of ANP-EGFP expressing embryonic stem cells towards a pacemaker phenotype. FASEB J Off Publ Fed Am Soc Exp Biol. 2004;18:1710–2.

Gaudio C, Di Michele S, Cera M, Nguyen BL, Pannarale G, Alessandri N. Prominent crista terminalis mimicking a right atrial mixoma: cardiac magnetic resonance aspects. Eur Rev Med Pharmacol Sci. 2004;8:165–8.

Gaussin V, Morley GE, Cox L, Zwijsen A, Vance KM, Emile L, Tian Y, Liu J, Hong C, Myers D, Conway SJ, Depre C, Mishina Y, Behringer RR, Hanks MC, Schneider MD, Huylebroeck D, Fishman GI, Burch JB, Vatner SF. Alk3/Bmpr1a receptor is required for development of the atrioventricular canal into valves and annulus fibrosus. Circ Res. 2005;97:219–26.

Geva T, Martins JD, Wald RM. Atrial septal defects. Lancet. 2014;383:1921–32.

Gillman RG, Burton AC. Constriction of the neonatal aorta by raised oxygen tension. Circ Res. 1966;19:755–65.

Gittenberger-de Groot AC, Bartelings MM, Deruiter MC, Poelmann RE. Basics of cardiac development for the understanding of congenital heart malformations. Pediatr Res. 2005;57:169–76.

Goenezen S, Rennie MY, Rugonyi S. Biomechanics of early cardiac development. Biomech Model Mechanobiol. 2012;11:1187–204.

Gordon NK, Gordon R. The organelle of differentiation in embryos: the cell state splitter. Theor Biol Med Model. 2016;13:11.

Gourdie RG, Kubalak S, Mikawa T. Conducting the embryonic heart: orchestrating development of specialized cardiac tissues. Trends Cardiovasc Med. 1999;9:18–26.

Gourdie RG, Harris BS, Bond J, Justus C, Hewett KW, O'Brien TX, Thompson RP, Sedmera D. Development of the cardiac pacemaking and conduction system. Birth Defects Res C Embryo Today. 2003;69:46–57.

Graham A. Development of the pharyngeal arches. Am J Med Genet A. 2003;119a:251–6.

Gupta SK, Bamforth SD, Anderson RH. How frequent is the fifth arch artery? Cardiol Young. 2015;25:628–46.

Gupta SK, Gulati GS, Anderson RH. Clarifying the anatomy of the fifth arch artery. Ann Pediatr Cardiol. 2016;9:62–7.

Hagans I, Markelov A, Makadia M. Unique venocaval anomalies: case of duplicate superior vena cava and interrupted inferior vena cava. J Radiol Case Rep. 2014;8:20–6.

Hen G, Friedman-Einat M, Sela-Donenfeld D. Primordial germ cells in the dorsal mesentery of the chicken embryo demonstrate left-right asymmetry and polarized distribution of the EMA1 epitope. J Anat. 2014;224:556–63.

Heymann MA, Rudolph AM. Effects of congenital heart disease on fetal and neonatal circulations. Prog Cardiovasc Dis. 1972;15:115–43.

Hinton RB, Yutzey KE. Heart valve structure and function in development and disease. Annu Rev Physiol. 2011;73:29–46.

Ho SY, Anderson RH. Coarctation, tubular hypoplasia, and the ductus arteriosus. Histological study of 35 specimens. Br Heart J. 1979;41:268–74.

Ho SY, Anderson RH, Sanchez-Quintana D. Atrial structure and fibres: morphologic bases of atrial conduction. Cardiovasc Res. 2002;54:325–36.

Hua LL, Vedantham V, Barnes RM, Hu J, Robinson AS, Bressan M, Srivastava D, Black BL. Specification of the mouse cardiac conduction system in the absence of Endothelin signaling. Dev Biol. 2014;393:245–54.

Hutchins GM. Coarctation of the aorta explained as a branch-point of the ductus arteriosus. Am J Pathol. 1971;63:203–14.

Jacobs JP, Anderson RH, Weinberg PM, Walters 3rd HL, Tchervenkov CI, Del Duca D, Franklin RC, Aiello VD, Beland MJ, Colan SD, Gaynor JW, Krogmann ON, Kurosawa H, Maruszewski

B, Stellin G, Elliott MJ. The nomenclature, definition and classification of cardiac structures in the setting of heterotaxy. Cardiol Young. 2007;17 Suppl 2:1–28.

Jalife J, Morley GE, Vaidya D. Connexins and impulse propagation in the mouse heart. J Cardiovasc Electrophysiol. 1999;10:1649–63.

Jimenez M, Daret D, Choussat A, Bonnet J. Immunohistological and ultrastructural analysis of the intimal thickening in coarctation of human aorta. Cardiovasc Res. 1999;41:737–45.

John J, Abrol S, Sadiq A, Shani J. Mixed atrial septal defect coexisting ostium secundum and sinus venosus atrial septal defect. J Am Coll Cardiol. 2011;58:e9.

Katheria A, Leone T. Altered transitional circulation in infants of diabetic mothers with strict antenatal obstetric management: a functional echocardiography study. J Perinatol. 2012;32: 508–13.

Kathiriya IS, Nora EP, Bruneau BG. Investigating the transcriptional control of cardiovascular development. Circ Res. 2015;116:700–14.

Kau T, Sinzig M, Gasser J, Lesnik G, Rabitsch E, Celedin S, Eicher W, Illiasch H, Hausegger KA. Aortic development and anomalies. Semin Intervent Radiol. 2007;24:141–52.

Kellenberger CJ. Aortic arch malformations. Pediatr Radiol. 2010;40:876–84.

Kenny D, Hijazi ZM. Coarctation of the aorta: from fetal life to adulthood. Cardiol J. 2011;18:487–95.

Kerut EK, Norfleet WT, Plotnick GD, Giles TD. Patent foramen ovale: a review of associated conditions and the impact of physiological size. J Am Coll Cardiol. 2001;38:613–23.

Keskin S, Keskin Z, Sekmenli N. The independent right and left azygos veins with hemiazygos absence: a rare case presentation. Case Rep Vasc Med. 2013;2013:282416.

Krakowiak-Sarnowska E, Wisniewski M, Szpinda M, Krakowiak H. Variability of the azygos vein system in human foetuses. Folia Morphol. 2003;62:427–30.

Krediet P. An hypothesis of the development of coarctation in man. Acta Morphol Neerl Scand. 1965;6:207–12.

Lalani SR, Belmont JW. Genetic basis of congenital cardiovascular malformations. Eur J Med Genet. 2014;57:402–13.

Lamers WH, Moorman AF. Cardiac septation: a late contribution of the embryonic primary myocardium to heart morphogenesis. Circ Res. 2002;91:93–103.

Lammert E, Axnick J. Vascular lumen formation. Cold Spring Harb Perspect Med. 2012;2: a006619.

Latha GA, Kagali NA, Kagali NA, M S. Preduodenal portal vein in adult with polysplenia syndrome revisited with a case report. Indian J Surg. 2014;76:137–42.

Liberman L, Gersony WM, Flynn PA, Lamberti JJ, Cooper RS, Stare TJ. Effectiveness of prostaglandin E1 in relieving obstruction in coarctation of the aorta without opening the ductus arteriosus. Pediatr Cardiol. 2004;25:49–52.

Lin CJ, Lin CY, Chen CH, Zhou B, Chang CP. Partitioning the heart: mechanisms of cardiac septation and valve development. Development. 2012;139:3277–99.

Liu Y, Lu X, Xiang FL, Lu M, Feng Q. Nitric oxide synthase-3 promotes embryonic development of atrioventricular valves. PLoS One. 2013;8:e77611.

Lockhart M, Wirrig E, Phelps A, Wessels A. Extracellular matrix and heart development. Birth Defects Res A Clin Mol Teratol. 2011;91:535–50.

Mahle WT, Martinez R, Silverman N, Cohen MS, Anderson RH. Anatomy, echocardiography, and surgical approach to double outlet right ventricle. Cardiol Young. 2008;18 Suppl 3:39–51.

Malaki M, Willis AP, Jones RG. Congenital anomalies of the inferior vena cava. Clin Radiol. 2012;67:165–71.

Marler JJ, Mulliken JB. Current management of hemangiomas and vascular malformations. Clin Plast Surg. 2005;32:99–116, ix.

McCarthy K, Ho S, Anderson R. Defining the morphologic phenotypes of atrial septal defects and interatrial communications. Images Paediatr Cardiol. 2003;5:1–24.

McDonald SJ, Middleton P, Dowswell T, Morris PS. Effect of timing of umbilical cord clamping of term infants on maternal and neonatal outcomes. Cochrane Database Syst Rev. 2013;7:CD004074.

Menshawi K, Mohr JP, Gutierrez J. A functional perspective on the embryology and anatomy of the cerebral blood supply. J Stroke. 2015;17:144–58.

Mikawa T, Hurtado R. Development of the cardiac conduction system. Semin Cell Dev Biol. 2007;18:90–100.

Mirilas P. Lateral congenital anomalies of the pharyngeal apparatus: part I. Normal developmental anatomy (embryogenesis) for the surgeon. Am Surg. 2011;77:1230–42.

Momma K, Takao A, Ando M. Angiocardiographic study of coarctation of the aorta–morphology and morphogenesis. Jpn Circ J. 1982;46:174–83.

Moonen RM, Kessels CG, Zimmermann LJ, Villamor E. Mesenteric artery reactivity and small intestine morphology in a chicken model of hypoxia-induced fetal growth restriction. J Physiol Pharmacol Off J Polish Physiol Soc. 2012;63:601–12.

Moore GW, Hutchins GM. Association of interrupted aortic arch with malformations producing reduced blood flow to the fourth aortic arches. Am J Cardiol. 1978;42:467–72.

Moorman A, Webb S, Brown NA, Lamers W, Anderson RH. Development of the heart: (1) formation of the cardiac chambers and arterial trunks. Heart. 2003;89:806–14.

Moorman AF, Christoffels VM, Anderson RH. Anatomic substrates for cardiac conduction. Heart Rhythm. 2005;2:875–86.

Moskowitz IP, Wang J, Peterson MA, Pu WT, Mackinnon AC, Oxburgh L, Chu GC, Sarkar M, Berul C, Smoot L, Robertson EJ, Schwartz R, Seidman JG, Seidman CE. Transcription factor genes Smad4 and Gata4 cooperatively regulate cardiac valve development. [corrected]. Proc Natl Acad Sci U S A. 2011;108:4006–11.

Na JO, Kim EJ, Mun SJ, Choi EH, Mun JH, Lee HR, Kim YK, Yong HS. Prominent crista terminalis in patients with embolic events. J Cardiovasc Ultrasound. 2011;19:156–8.

Nakanishi T, Fukuzawa K, Yoshida A, Itoh M, Imamura K, Fujiwara R, Suzuki A, Yamashita S, Matsumoto A, Konishi H, Ichibori H, Hirata K. Crista terminalis as the anterior pathway of typical atrial flutter: insights from entrainment map with 3D intracardiac ultrasound. Pacing Clin Electrophysiol. 2015;38:608–16.

Neufeld S, Planas-Paz L, Lammert E. Blood and lymphatic vascular tube formation in mouse. Semin Cell Dev Biol. 2014;31:115–23.

Noori S, Wlodaver A, Gottipati V, McCoy M, Schultz D, Escobedo M. Transitional changes in cardiac and cerebral hemodynamics in term neonates at birth. J Pediatr. 2012;160:943–8.

Northcutt RG, Gans C. The genesis of neural crest and epidermal placodes: a reinterpretation of vertebrate origins. Q Rev Biol. 1983;58:1–28.

Okamoto N, Akimoto N, Hidaka N, Shoji S, Sumida H. Formal genesis of the outflow tracts of the heart revisited: previous works in the light of recent observations. Congenit Anom. 2010;50:141–58.

Oliver JM, Gallego P, Gonzalez A, Dominguez FJ, Aroca A, Mesa JM. Sinus venosus syndrome: atrial septal defect or anomalous venous connection? A multiplane transoesophageal approach. Heart. 2002;88:634–8.

Paffett-Lugassy N, Singh R, Nevis KR, Guner-Ataman B, O'Loughlin E, Jahangiri L, Harvey RP, Burns CG, Burns CE. Heart field origin of great vessel precursors relies on nkx2.5-mediated vasculogenesis. Nat Cell Biol. 2013;15:1362–9.

Park SJ, Park SY, Choi H. Aberrent thoracic duct cyst in postrior mediastinum. Korean J Thorac Cardiovasc Surg. 2015;48:225–7.

Perez-Pomares JM, de la Pompa JL, Franco D, Henderson D, Ho SY, Houyel L, Kelly RG, Sedmera D, Sheppard M, Sperling S, Thiene G, van den Hoff M, Basso C. Congenital coronary artery anomalies: a bridge from embryology to anatomy and pathophysiology-a position statement of the development, anatomy, and pathology ESC Working Group. Cardiovasc Res. 2016;109:204–16.

Petik B. Inferior vena cava anomalies and variations: imaging and rare clinical findings. Insights Imaging. 2015;6:631–9.

Piciucchi S, Barone D, Sanna S, Dubini A, Goodman LR, Oboldi D, Bertocco M, Ciccotosto C, Gavelli G, Carloni A, Poletti V. The azygos vein pathway: an overview from anatomical variations to pathological changes. Insights Imaging. 2014;5:619–28.

Plein A, Fantin A, Ruhrberg C. Neural crest cells in cardiovascular development. Curr Top Dev Biol. 2015;111:183–200.

Poelmann RE, Gittenberger-de Groot AC, Vicente-Steijn R, Wisse LJ, Bartelings MM, Everts S, Hoppenbrouwers T, Kruithof BP, Jensen B, de Bruin PW, Hirasawa T, Kuratani S, Vonk F, van de Put JM, de Bakker MA, Richardson MK. Evolution and development of ventricular septation in the amniote heart. PLoS One. 2014;9:e106569.

Rabe H, Diaz-Rossello JL, Duley L, Dowswell T. Effect of timing of umbilical cord clamping and other strategies to influence placental transfusion at preterm birth on maternal and infant outcomes. Cochrane Database Syst Rev. 2012;8:CD003248.

Rabi Y, Yee W, Chen SY, Singhal N. Oxygen saturation trends immediately after birth. J Pediatr. 2006;148:590–4.

Racker DK. The AV junction region of the heart: a comprehensive study correlating gross anatomy and direct three-dimensional analysis. Part II. Morphology and cytoarchitecture. Am J Physiol Heart Circ Physiol. 2004;286:H1853–71.

Rana MS, Sizarov A, Christoffels VM, Moorman AF. Development of the human aortic arch system captured in an interactive three-dimensional reference model. Am J Med Genet A. 2014;164a:1372–83.

Ray HJ, Niswander L. Mechanisms of tissue fusion during development. Development. 2012;139:1701–11.

Raz E. Guidance of primordial germ cell migration. Curr Opin Cell Biol. 2004;16:169–73.

Remme CA, Verkerk AO, Hoogaars WM, Aanhaanen WT, Scicluna BP, Annink C, van den Hoff MJ, Wilde AA, van Veen TA, Veldkamp MW, de Bakker JM, Christoffels VM, Bezzina CR. The cardiac sodium channel displays differential distribution in the conduction system and transmural heterogeneity in the murine ventricular myocardium. Basic Res Cardiol. 2009;104:511–22.

Restivo A, Piacentini G, Placidi S, Saffirio C, Marino B. Cardiac outflow tract: a review of some embryogenetic aspects of the conotruncal region of the heart. Anat Rec A Discov Mol Cell Evol Biol. 2006;288:936–43.

Rouwet EV, De Mey JG, Slaaf DW, Heineman E, Ramsay G, Le Noble FA. Development of vasomotor responses in fetal mesenteric arteries. Am J Physiol Heart Circ Physiol. 2000;279:H1097–105.

Rudolph AM, Heymann MA, Spitznas U. Hemodynamic considerations in the development of narrowing of the aorta. Am J Cardiol. 1972;30:514–25.

Russell GA, Berry PJ, Watterson K, Dhasmana JP, Wisheart JD. Patterns of ductal tissue in coarctation of the aorta in the first three months of life. J Thorac Cardiovasc Surg. 1991;102:596–601.

Sabine A, Petrova TV. Interplay of mechanotransduction, FOXC2, connexins, and calcineurin signaling in lymphatic valve formation. Adv Anat Embryol Cell Biol. 2014;214:67–80.

Salustri A, Bakir S, Sana A, Lange P, Al Mahmeed WA. Prominent crista terminalis mimicking a right atrial mass: case report. Cardiovasc Ultrasound. 2010;8:47.

Sato Y. Dorsal aorta formation: separate origins, lateral-to-medial migration, and remodeling. Dev Growth Differ. 2013;55:113–29.

Sherif HM. Heterogeneity in the segmental development of the aortic tree: impact on management of genetically triggered aortic aneurysms. Aorta (Stamford). 2014;2:186–95.

Shinebourne EA, Elseed AM. Relation between fetal flow patterns, coarctation of the aorta, and pulmonary blood flow. Br Heart J. 1974;36:492–8.

Siddiqui AU, Daimi SR, Gandhi KR, Siddiqui AT, Trivedi S, Sinha MB, Rathore M. Crista terminalis, musculi pectinati, and taenia sagittalis: anatomical observations and applied significance. ISRN Anat. 2013;2013:803853.

Smillie RP, Shetty M, Boyer AC, Madrazo B, Jafri SZ. Imaging evaluation of the inferior vena cava. Radiographics. 2015;35:578–92.

Song G, Ren W, Tang L, Hou Y, Zhou K. Coronary artery fistula from the left circumflex to coronary sinus in infant: case report with literature review. Int J Cardiol. 2015;188:37–9.

Soukup V, Horacek I, Cerny R. Development and evolution of the vertebrate primary mouth. J Anat. 2013;222:79–99.

Spentzouris G, Zandian A, Cesmebasi A, Kinsella CR, Muhleman M, Mirzayan N, Shirak M, Tubbs RS, Shaffer K, Loukas M. The clinical anatomy of the inferior vena cava: a review of common congenital anomalies and considerations for clinicians. Clin Anat (New York, NY). 2014;27:1234–43.

Srivastava A, Singh KJ, Suri A, Vijjan V, Dubey D. Inferior vena cava in urology: importance of developmental abnormalities in clinical practice. Scientific World Journal. 2005;5: 558–63.

Starr JP. Tetralogy of fallot: yesterday and today. World J Surg. 2010;34:658–68.

Steding G, Seidl W. Contribution to the development of the heart, Part II: morphogenesis of congenital heart diseases. Thorac Cardiovasc Surg. 1981;29:1–16.

Stefanovic S, Christoffels VM. GATA-dependent transcriptional and epigenetic control of cardiac lineage specification and differentiation. Cell Mol Life Sci. 2015;72:3871–81.

Stimec BV, Terraz S, Fasel JH. The third time is the charm–anastomosis between the celiac trunk and the left colic artery. Clin Anat (New York, NY). 2011;24:258–61.

Stojanovska J, Cascade PN, Chong S, Quint LE, Sundaram B. Embryology and imaging review of aortic arch anomalies. J Thorac Imaging. 2012;27:73–84.

Stoll SJ, Bartsch S, Kroll J. HOXC9 regulates formation of parachordal lymphangioplasts and the thoracic duct in zebrafish via stabilin 2. PLoS One. 2013;8:e58311.

Strilic B, Kucera T, Eglinger J, Hughes MR, McNagny KM, Tsukita S, Dejana E, Ferrara N, Lammert E. The molecular basis of vascular lumen formation in the developing mouse aorta. Dev Cell. 2009;17:505–15.

Sukernik MR, Bennett-Guerrero E. The incidental finding of a patent foramen ovale during cardiac surgery: should it always be repaired? A core review. Anesth Analg. 2007;105:602–10.

Sukernik MR, Mets B, Bennett-Guerrero E. Patent foramen ovale and its significance in the perioperative period. Anesth Analg. 2001;93:1137–46.

Szpinda M, Frackiewicz P, Flisinski P, Wisniewski M, Krakowiak-Sarnowska E. The retroperitoneal anastomoses of the gonadal veins in human foetuses. Folia Morphol (Warsz). 2005;64:72–7.

Taylor JR, Taylor AJ. The relationship between the sinus node and the right atrial appendage. Can J Cardiol. 1997;13:85–92.

Technau U, Scholz CB. Origin and evolution of endoderm and mesoderm. Int J Dev Biol. 2003;47:531–9.

Therrien J, Provost Y, Merchant N, Williams W, Colman J, Webb G. Optimal timing for pulmonary valve replacement in adults after tetralogy of Fallot repair. Am J Cardiol. 2005;95:779–82.

Togi K, Yoshida Y, Matsumae H, Nakashima Y, Kita T, Tanaka M. Essential role of Hand2 in interventricular septum formation and trabeculation during cardiac development. Biochem Biophys Res Commun. 2006;343:144–51.

Tomita-Mitchell A, Maslen CL, Morris CD, Garg V, Goldmuntz E. GATA4 sequence variants in patients with congenital heart disease. J Med Genet. 2007;44:779–83.

van Geemen D, Soares AL, Oomen PJ, Driessen-Mol A, Janssen-van den Broek MW, van den Bogaerdt AJ, Bogers AJ, Goumans MJ, Baaijens FP, Bouten CV. Age-dependent changes in geometry, tissue composition and mechanical properties of fetal to adult cryopreserved human heart valves. PLoS One. 2016;11:e0149020.

Van Meurs-Van Woezik H, Krediet P. Changes after birth in the tunica media and in the internal diameter of the aortic isthmus in normal newborns. J Anat. 1982;134:573–81.

Van Praagh R. The first Stella van Praagh memorial lecture: the history and anatomy of tetralogy of Fallot. Semin Thorac Cardiovasc Surg Pediatr Card Surg Annu. 2009;19–38.

Van Praagh S, Geva T, Lock JE, Nido PJ, Vance MS, Van Praagh R. Biatrial or left atrial drainage of the right superior vena cava: anatomic, morphogenetic, and surgical considerations–report of three new cases and literature review. Pediatr Cardiol. 2003;24:350–63.

van Vonderen JJ, Roest AA, Siew ML, Blom NA, van Lith JM, Walther FJ, Hooper SB, te Pas AB. Noninvasive measurements of hemodynamic transition directly after birth. Pediatr Res. 2014a;75:448–52.

van Vonderen JJ, Roest AA, Siew ML, Walther FJ, Hooper SB, te Pas AB. Measuring physiological changes during the transition to life after birth. Neonatology. 2014b;105:230–42.

van Vonderen JJ, Te Pas AB. The first breaths of life: imaging studies of the human infant during neonatal transition. Paediatr Respir Rev. 2015;16:143–6.

Verzi MP, McCulley DJ, De Val S, Dodou E, Black BL. The right ventricle, outflow tract, and ventricular septum comprise a restricted expression domain within the secondary/anterior heart field. Dev Biol. 2005;287:134–45.

Watanabe Y, Buckingham M. The formation of the embryonic mouse heart: heart fields and myocardial cell lineages. Ann N Y Acad Sci. 2010;1188:15–24.

Webb S, Qayyum SR, Anderson RH, Lamers WH, Richardson MK. Septation and separation within the outflow tract of the developing heart. J Anat. 2003;202:327–42.

Williams C, Kim SH, Ni TT, Mitchell L, Ro H, Penn JS, Baldwin SH, Solnica-Krezel L, Zhong TP. Hedgehog signaling induces arterial endothelial cell formation by repressing venous cell fate. Dev Biol. 2010;341:196–204.

Wu M, Peng S, Zhao Y. Inducible gene deletion in the entire cardiac conduction system using Hcn4-CreERT2 BAC transgenic mice. Genesis (New York, NY : 2000). 2014;52:134–40.

Xin M, Olson EN, Bassel-Duby R. Mending broken hearts: cardiac development as a basis for adult heart regeneration and repair. Nat Rev Mol Cell Biol. 2013;14:529–41.

Yamagishi T, Ando K, Nakamura H. Roles of TGFbeta and BMP during valvulo-septal endocardial cushion formation. Anat Sci Int. 2009;84:77–87.

Yang Y, Oliver G. Transcriptional control of lymphatic endothelial cell type specification. Adv Anat Embryol Cell Biol. 2014;214:5–22.

Yi SQ, Terayama H, Naito M, Hirai S, Alimujang S, Yi N, Tanaka S, Itoh M. Absence of the celiac trunk: case report and review of the literature. Clin Anat (New York, NY). 2008;21:283–6.

Yigit M, Kowalski W, Hutchon D, Pekkan K. Transition from fetal to neonatal circulation: modeling the effect of umbilical cord clamping. J Biomech. 2015;48(9):1662–70.

Yutzey KE, Kirby ML. Wherefore heart thou? Embryonic origins of cardiogenic mesoderm. Dev Dyn Off Publ Am Assoc Anatomists. 2002;223:307–20.

Zhang H, von Gise A, Liu Q, Hu T, Tian X, He L, Pu W, Huang X, He L, Cai CL, Camargo FD, Pu WT, Zhou B. Yap1 is required for endothelial to mesenchymal transition of the atrioventricular cushion. J Biol Chem. 2014;289:18681–92.

Chapter 3
Pediatric Cardiovascular Physiology

Ali Dabbagh, Alireza Imani, and Samira Rajaei

Evolutional Transition in Cardiac Physiology

The physiologic change from fetal to neonatal circulation constitutes two main items which have a number of main impacts: lack of lung ventilation in fetus and "series" model of circulation. A number of these are discussed here more; however, some of the other developmental changes, especially those related to contractile processes, are discussed in the next parts of this chapter.

Fetal Circulation

Fetal circulation and its developmental changes:

- The lungs are not ventilated in the fetus; so, pulmonary vessels are nearly collapsed having a very high vascular resistance, leading to only about 10 % of the cardiac output through the lungs.

A. Dabbagh, MD (✉)
Cardiac Anesthesiology Department, Anesthesiology Research Center,
Shahid Beheshti University of Medical Sciences, Tehran, Iran
e-mail: alidabbagh@yahoo.com; alidabbagh@sbmu.ac.ir

A. Imani, PhD
Department of Physiology, School of Medicine, Tehran University of Medical Science,
Tehran, Iran
e-mail: aimani@tums.ac.ir

S. Rajaei, MD, PhD
Department of Immunology, School of Medicine, Tehran University of Medical Science,
Tehran, Iran
e-mail: samirarajaei@tums.ac.ir

- The placental vessels have a very low resistance leading to a highly perfused vascular bed in the fetal circulation.
- The main gas exchange is through the placental vessels.
- The blood circulation does not follow two parallel circuits; instead one circulation pathway exists and the blood flows through a "series" circuit to perfuse all the organs; complete mixing occurs through the ductus arteriosus, foramen ovale, umbilical vessels, and placental vessels.
- The right and left ventricles (RV and LV) are connected through foramen ovale, and so, there is not a significant pressure difference between the two chambers; the right ventricle has a greater workload (about two thirds of the heart workload is tolerated by RV and one third by LV).
- The blood inside the superior vena cava (SVC) is deoxygenated, passes the right atrium to the right ventricle, and then goes through the ductus arteriosus to the descending aorta; deoxygenated blood does not go to the pulmonary vascular system due to its high resistance.
- The oxygenated blood comes from the placenta to the inferior vena cava (IVC) and then goes through the foramen ovale, left atrium, and left ventricle to the ascending aorta to perfuse the whole body organs.
- Finally, when assessing the fetal circulation as a whole, there are three main shunts in the fetal circulation:

   1. *Ductus venosus*: the oxygenated blood passes from the umbilical vein to the inferior vena cava.
   2. *Foramen ovale*: the blood from the right atrium through the foramen ovale enters into the left atrium.
   3. *Ductus arteriosus*: the blood from pulmonary artery (due to the high resistance) passes through the ductus arteriosus to the aorta and then returned to the placenta for oxygenation through the umbilical arteries (Hines 2013; Azhibekov et al. 2014; van Vonderen and Te Pas 2015).

Changes in Circulation at Birth

The fetal circulation should be changed to a neonatal circulation pattern in order to adapt the new environment out of the uterus; this is an obligatory change which is achieved through a number of sequential events in the circulation; these events are well ordered and delicately arranged, one after the other, to achieve the goal of "transition" and achieving a "biventricular parallel circulation pattern" instead of the series circulation in the fetus. The main bulk of our knowledge regarding this human neonatal transition is based on human fetal data from studies performed in 1970s; however, animal studies have been added to them; a summary of these studies is presented here as the following transitional physiologic steps (Rabi et al. 2006, 2012; Gao and Raj 2010; Katheria and Leone 2012; Noori et al. 2012; Duley and Batey 2013; Galinsky et al. 2013; McDonald et al. 2013; Azhibekov et al. 2014;

van Vonderen et al. 2014a, b; Baik et al. 2015; van Vonderen and Te Pas 2015; Yigit et al. 2015):

1. Lungs are inflated and gas exchange starts, with resultant increase in oxygen pressure of the pulmonary vascular bed and the alveoli; this would be one of the very crucial and among the earliest initiatives for transition of circulation; so, as a result, *pulmonary vascular resistance* (PVR) drops suddenly and significantly during the first 10 min after birth which will result in a rapid surge in pulmonary blood flow.

2. Placental vessels are occluded after cord clamp leading to abrupt increase in systemic vascular resistance (SVR); this is probably due to thermal and mechanical stimulation and an alteration in oxygen tension; in addition, the contraction of the smooth muscles in the wall of umbilical arteries causes their closure, which usually occurs a few minutes after birth, though the real destruction of the lumen by fibrous proliferation may happen 2–3 months later; the distal portion of umbilical artery forms the medial umbilical ligaments and the proximal portion of umbilical artery stay open, making the superior vesical arteries; however, just following the closure of the umbilical arteries, the ductus venosus and umbilical veins are also closed; this is why blood could enter from the placenta to the newborn circulation for a short time interval after birth. Following obliteration, the ligamentum teres hepatis is formed from the umbilical vein.

3. With the increased pressure in the left atrial chamber over the right atrial chamber, the foramen ovale is closed and also, in a very short time, ductus arteriosus is closed; closure of ductus arteriosus leads to flow reversal in the ductus, which prevents any further flow between the pulmonary artery and the aorta; this is an essential "shift" in body circulation: in other words, the circulation changes from a "series circulation" to a "parallel circulation."

4. The complete anatomical closure of the *foramen ovale* and *ductus arteriosus* is not abrupt; in fact, the *foramen ovale* is closed physiologically first, and then, it will be closed anatomically during a few days; however, there are a minority of "normal" children in whom the foramen ovale is not closed anatomically even till adulthood, leading to the potential opening of the foramen ovale in case of increased pulmonary vascular resistance and the possibility of right-to-left embolization; on the other hand, the ductus arteriosus is closed during the first 48–72 h after birth; on the other hand, *ductus arteriosus* is closed directly after birth due to contraction of the neighboring muscles; here, bradykinin (a substance released from the lungs after early inflation) plays the main role in contraction and closure of ductus. It is estimated that the anatomical obliteration of ductus arteriosus by proliferation of its intima takes about 1–3 months. In the adult period, the ligamentum arteriosum is formed by the obliteration of ductus arteriosus.

5. Venous flow from the umbilical vein stops at the time of birth; also, the muscular contraction causes the ductus venosus to be closed; the ligamentum venosum is formed after closure of the ductus venosus.

6. Pressure in the portal venous system increases, which leads to redirect flow through the hepatic veins.

7. Throughout this transitional period, there is a marked increase in blood levels of stress hormones including catecholamines and activation of renin-angiotensin-aldosterone level.

8. *β-receptors* are not as much frequent in the newborn heart as the adult heart; however, after birth, a number of factors lead to increased levels of β-receptors in myocardium; the effect of thyroid hormone is of great importance.

9. In normal newborn, at least the first 5 min of life is needed to pass the transitional circulation and to reach the "normal postnatal oxygen saturation" state according to the following order:

   - Just in the first min of life, blood oxygen saturation is about "60–70 %."
   - During the first 5 min of life, blood oxygen saturation increases to "80–90 %."
   - And finally, in the first 10 min of life, blood oxygen saturation increases to more than 90 %.

   The above trend in oxygen saturation demonstrates the "normal shift" from fetal to neonatal circulation; all these saturation levels are a somewhat lower after cesarean delivery compared with normal vaginal delivery. There are some controversies regarding the effect of delayed umbilical cord clamping on the neonatal physiology and the transition from fetal to neonatal physiologic status; currently, the available evidence is toward delayed cord clamping since it would improve the neonatal hemodynamics and blood volume accompanied with "sustained placental respiration" (Rabi et al. 2006; Noori et al. 2012; Azhibekov et al. 2014).

10. Blood pressure in the early postnatal period depends on cardiac output (CO) and systemic vascular resistance (SVR); meanwhile, in the neonatal period, these factors affect blood pressure:

    - Neonatal asphyxia decreases blood pressure.
    - Some drugs decrease blood pressure (like antihypertensive drugs used in mothers or mothers receiving some anesthetic drugs for cesarean delivery).
    - Blood pressure is higher in preterm infants compared to term infants.
    - Blood pressure is higher in neonates after vaginal delivery compared to cesarean section.
    - Blood pressure is higher in female neonates compared to male ones (Baik et al. 2015).

11. Cardiac output considered as the left and right heart output assumes the "normal" pattern after birth; in fact, in the fetal circulation, the main load of cardiac output is on the right heart; however, just after birth, i.e., in the postnatal period, while the transition from series circulation to parallel circulation ensues, the left ventricle and right ventricle cardiac output equalize and the dominancy of the right ventricle output (RVO) disappears, and, at the same time, the left ventricle output (LVO) and left ventricle stroke volume (SV) increase; also, cardiac output increases in the early postnatal 2–5 h, while after

that, due to closure of ductus arteriosus, cardiac output gradually drops to a bit lower levels to become stable (van Vonderen et al. 2014a; Baik et al. 2015).

12. There are a number of associated problems which could affect the process of transition from fetal to neonatal circulation and, hence, cause some delay or even impairment in the process of normal transition leading to *persistence of fetal circulation*; among them, the following could be mentioned:

- Any kind of impairment in pulmonary circulation which could increase the pulmonary vascular resistance (PVR); hypoxia, acidosis, and hypercarbia may lead to pulmonary vasoconstriction and increased PVR.
- Increased pressure in the right atrium over the left atrium could lead to reopening of the foramen ovale which would severely exacerbate the right-to-left shunt and aggravate the unwanted phenomenon of "persistence of fetal circulation"; if closure of the ductus arteriosus also does not happen, persistence of fetal circulation goes much more worse, which may mandate surgical intervention in order to treat persistence of fetal circulation.
- History of diabetes in mother during pregnancy.
- Intrauterine inflammation due to infection or other reasons.

Myocardial Electromechanical Function

To produce lifelong cardiac output, the heart needs to initiate electrical activity, to disseminate it in a well-designed and sequential manner to all parts of the heart and to produce cardiac output as "projectile" stroke volume in each beat. However, if we want to analyze the physiologic job of the heart, we will have the three following steps as the main cardiac tasks which, when integrated together, produce the function of the heart; for these tasks to be done, specialized cells are arranged in a delicate manner (Xin et al. 2013):

- Electrical function (due to action potential) of the heart mainly though pacemaker cells and Purkinje fibers (these are specialized cardiomyocytes that we call them together as the conductive cells; they generate and conduct the electrical impulse).
- Excitation-contraction coupling (ECC) is the intermediary step between electrical and mechanical activities of the myocardium, which is done by a complex of cellular systems inside the myocardial syncytia.
- Mechanical (contractile) function of the myocardium which is performed after a series of sub-functions between contractile proteins which initiate, modulate, and terminate each cardiac contraction and relaxation, i.e., systole and diastole; the contractile function is the role of atrial and ventricular cardiomyocytes, which form the cardiac muscular segment; however, they are supported by integration of connective tissue and cardiac fibroblasts.

These physiologic jobs are done mainly through two important cardiac syncytia:

1. *Atrial syncytium* which is composed of the myocardial tissue of left and right atria, plus the interatrial septum and sinoatrial node (SA node)

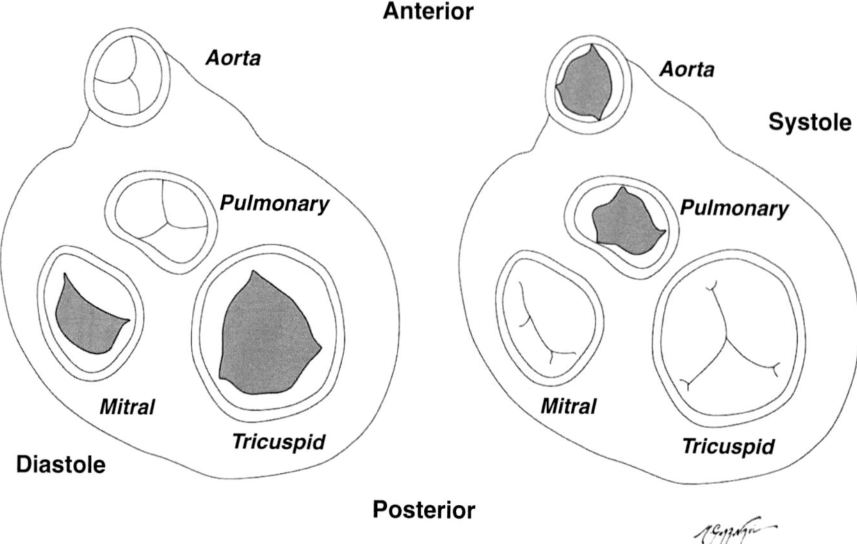

Fig. 3.1 The apex of the heart when viewed from above in systole and diastole; note the position of the valves and their relationships (Modified from Dabbagh (2014). Published with kind permission from © Springer, 2014. All Rights Reserved)

2. *Ventricular syncytium* which is composed of the myocardial tissue of left and right ventricles, the interventricular septum and atrioventricular node (AV node), atrioventricular bundle, and the other conducting structures distal to AV bundle

On the other hand, the function of the heart is performed in two time domain: systole and diastole. In systole, the contractile function of the ventricular syncytium causes blood pumping during an ejection process which is associated with blood pumping out of the ventricles; aortic and pulmonary valves are open and mitral and tricuspid valves are closed. On the other hand, in diastole, the ventricles expand in an active process leading to return of blood from atria to related ventricles; mitral and tricuspid valves are open, while aortic and pulmonary valves are closed (Fig. 3.1).

Let's discuss here the three main myocardial jobs in more detail (i.e., electrical function, ECC, and contractile function).

Electrical Function of the Myocardium: Action Potential

The electrical part of cardiac function is done through a well-organized and highly specialized *electrical network*; this network has two main cell types (Fig. 3.2):

"Impulse-generating cells" which have excitatory function and produce impulse; these cells mainly compose the *sinoatrial (SA) node*.

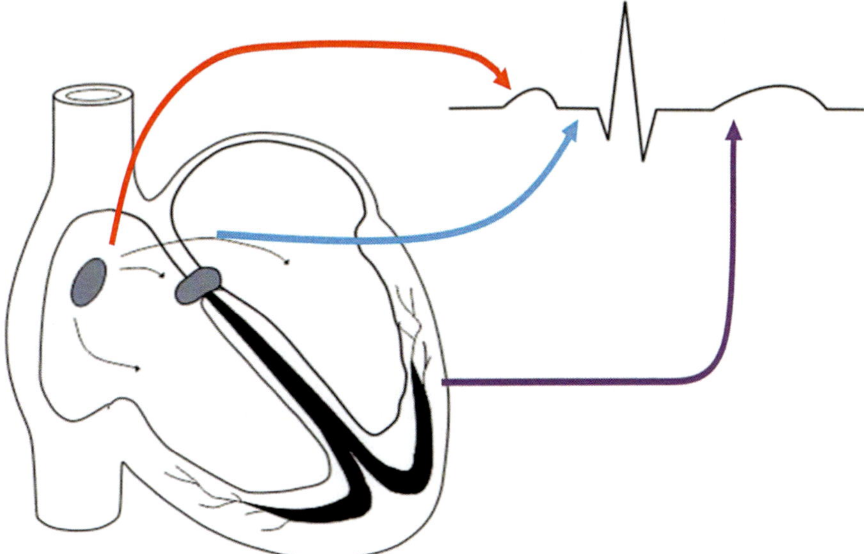

Fig. 3.2 Cardiac conductive system and its elements; in left, see the relationship of normal electrocardiography with the elements of the system (Modified from Dabbagh (2014). Published with kind permission from © Springer, 2014. All Rights Reserved)

The SA node lies in the cephalic portion of the posterior wall of the right atrium just near to the orifice of SVC. The SA node has a complex architecture leading to heterogeneous electrical activity throughout the SA node. Also, pacemaking cells, especially in the SA node, have a number of specific specifications:

- Higher rate of spontaneous beating
- Faster activation of the funny current (I_f) which is described later
- Greater density of the funny current (Mikawa and Hurtado 2007)

"Conductive cells" which are a well-defined network for conduction of the impulse and is composed of:

- The atrioventricular (AV) conduction pathways.
- The atrioventricular (AV) node which lies just superior to the endocardial cushions, in the inferior part of the interatrial septum and anterior to the coronary sinus foramen.
- The *His bundle*.
- The right and left branches of His bundle.
- The network of *Purkinje fiber cells* also known as *Purkinje fiber network*; the Purkinje fiber network is an extension of the His bundle distributed all over the ventricular tissue, in such a way to propagate and to conduct the electrical impulse throughout the ventricles as fast as possible (Desplantez et al. 2007; Dun and Boyden 2008; Atkinson et al. 2011).

Action Potential in Cardiac Cells

Certain ions, ion currents over both sides of the myocardial cell membrane and the cell membrane itself (including its integral structures like membrane channels, receptors, and enzymes), and, also, a number of internal cell structures work together to produce the electrical activity of myocardial cells. Electrical activity achieved as a result of different ion currents (Na^+, K^+, and Ca^{2+}) and activation of certain receptors or enzymes can alter this activity. In fact, the ion currents have the main role, and other factors like sympathetic and parasympathetic effects do not exert roles in generation of action potential; if we denervate the heart of an animal in lab, action potential and impulse generation would not be stopped but can affect the generation and shape of the action potentials.

Generation of action potential is essential for producing mechanical activity in the muscular wall of atria and ventricles, depolarization for contraction and repolarization for relaxation. For this, the action of the heart is called electromechanical activity.

Generally, there are two types of action potential in the heart: fast response action potential in the myocardium and Purkinje system and slow response action potential in nodal cells. Myocardial action potential consists of five sequential phases: phase 0 to phase 4. These phases compose together the electrical wave of myocardial cells known as action potential, "AP", which are described here in Table 3.1 and Fig. 3.3.

Cardiac Automaticity and Its Mechanism(s)

How does the pacemaker activity in the cardiac cells happens? For answering this question, we should look for the main difference between "myocardial cells" and "pacemaker cells" regarding action potential.

Action potential (AP) in cardiac pacemaker cells Although the main mechanisms in AP of cardiac pacemaker cells are similar to those in myocardial cells, there are a number of differences:

1. *Resting membrane potential* in pacemaker cells is higher than myocardial cells; i.e., while resting potential is about −90 to −80 in myocardial cell population, it is about −60 to −50 in cardiac pacemaker cells; one of the main mechanisms for this upper level of resting potential in pacemaker cells is Na^+ influx during repolarization known as the funny current abbreviated as $I(f)$ (DiFrancesco and Noble 2012; Papaioannou et al. 2013; Weisbrod et al. 2013).
2. There are two main Ca^{2+} channels in the heart tissue: T (transient) type Ca^{2+} channels (abbreviated as I_{CaT}) and L (long-lasting) type Ca^{2+} channels (abbreviated as I_{CaL}); both I_{CaT} and I_{CaL} are categorized under voltage-gated Ca^{2+} channels (VGCC) and have their role in impulse generation (i.e., SA node) and atrioventricular impulse conduction (i.e., AV node); though I_{CaT} typically diminishes in the normal adult heart, they have an active role in the final segments of repolarization and play their role in combination with I(f) to produce prepotential steep which is in fact the "pacemaker potential"; I_{CaT} has two isoforms in

Table 3.1 Action potential in myocardial cells

Phase	Event in action potential	Ion current	Electrical status (mV)
Phase 0	Rapid upstroke: *Depolarizaton*	Na^+ influx	Starts from -90 to -80 and goes up to about +10 to +15
Phase 1	Very short and initial *repolarization* which is "Incomplete repolarization"	K^+ outflux	Starts from +10 to + 15 and decreases to about +5
Phase 2	Initiation of contraction due to Ca^{2+} influx; this phase is also titled *"Plateau"* Usually determines the *action potential duration* and also, the *refractory period*	Ca^{2+} influx due to opening of slow (L) type Ca^{2+} channels; also, K^+ outflux	Starts from + 5 and has a nearly steady level; maximum drop to 0
Phase 3	*Final Repolarization*	Huge K^+ outflux	Starts from about "0" Ends at -80 to -90
Phase 4	Resting potential *i.e.* no active potential)	K^+ influx and outflux	Stays at -80 to -90

cardiac tissue: Ca(V)3.1 and Ca(V)3.2; also, Ca(V)1.3 is the main isomer of I_{CaL} in the heart; Mesirca et al. expressed that severe forms of congenital bradycardia and atrioventricular block in pediatric patients are associated with functional loss of Ca(V)3.1 isomer of I_{CaT} receptors; however, all types of VGCC, Ca(v)1.2, mediate excitation-contraction coupling which is a crucial process in contractile function and discussed later in the chapter (Sobie et al. 2006; Ono and Iijima 2010; Mesirca et al. 2014, 2015).

3. In cardiac pacemaker cells, the slope of AP in phase 4 is not as flat as myocardial cells; instead it is upward, known as *prepotential steep phase*, and is mainly due to three main factors:

- Funny current: I(f)
- Ca^{2+} influx by I_{CaT}
- K^+ efflux by potassium channel (I_K)

4. On the other hand, the main role of I_{CaL} is in phase 0; in fact, in pacemaker cells (SA node and AV node), I_{CaL} exerts its main role in phase 0, and "Ca^{2+} influx" in pacemaker cells replaces "Na^+ influx" of myocardial cells.

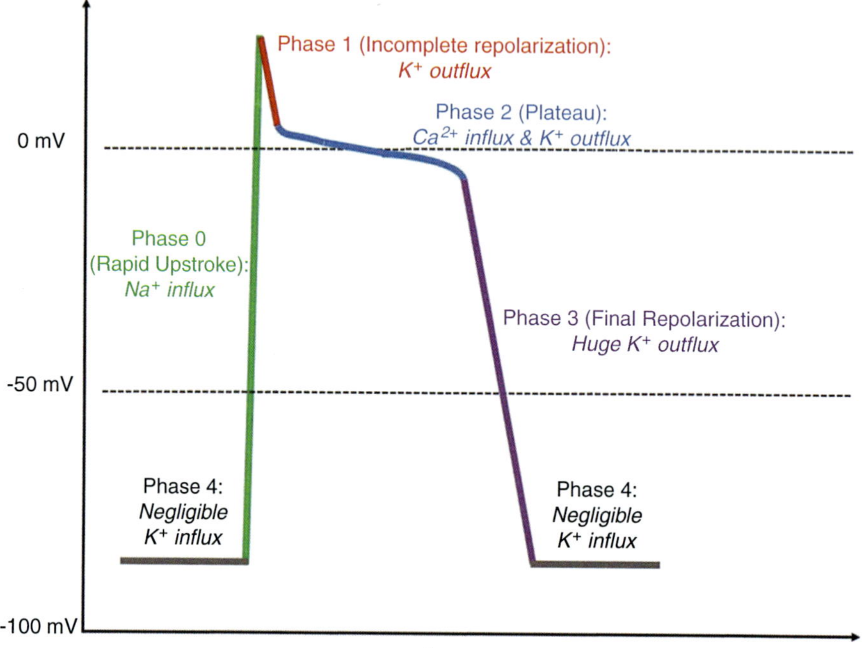

Fig. 3.3 Progress of action potential phases (Marcotti et al. 2004; Parham et al. 2006; Wolf and Berul 2008; Amanfu and Saucerman 2011; Marionneau and Abriel 2015)

5. Phase 1 (i.e., short-term repolarization) is nearly deleted or, better to say, integrated in phases 2 and 3.
6. Both phase 2 and phase 3 are merged to create a downhill in repolarization; so, there is no sensible plateau; instead, we see phases 1, 2, and 3 as a single repolarization phase which is terminated by phase 4. A summary of these phases is demonstrated in Table 3.2; Figs. 3.4 and 3.5.

There is another important concept in action potential of many cells including myocardial cells and that is "refractory period" which is the time interval during which there is no response to new impulse or the response could be sluggish: *absolute* refractory period or *relative* refractory period, respectively. Though described as one of the basic properties of currents alongside the cell membrane, some studies strongly believe that post-repolarization refractoriness plays a protective role against "reentrant" mechanisms of arrhythmias, especially in preventing atrial fibrillation.

In all cells having refractory period, the time interval for refractoriness is proportional to the time duration of action potential, and it is primarily dependent on the duration of phase 2 "plateau," so:

- In atrial cells, the refractory period is usually shorter (about 0.15 s).
- In ventricular cells it is about 0.25–0.3 s.

Table 3.2 Action potential in cardiac pacemaker cells

Term (Phase)	Event in action potential	Ion current	Electrical status (mV)	Difference with myocardial AP
Phase 0	Rapid upstroke	Ca^{2+} influx by I_{CaL}	Start from threshold level (-40) and goes up to about 0 to +5	**Shorter duration than cardiomyocyte**
Phase 1	Nearly *deleted & Integrated* in phases 2 & 3			
Phase 2	No sensible "*Plateau*": merged with phase 3 as a "Single Repolarization phase"			
Phase 3	Main *repolarization* wave	K^+ efflux	Starts from about "0 to +5"; ends at -50 to -60	Merged with phase 2 as a single "Repolarization phase"
Phase 4	Resting potential (prepotential)	I(f): Funny current Ca^{2+} influx by I_{CaT} K^+ efflux by I_K	Potential level increases from -50 or -60 to threshold level (-40)	Slope of AP is upward

- In pacemaker cells the refractory period is about 0.3 s, while the refractory period continues up to the middle of prepotential steep phase (Veenhuyzen et al. 2004; Coronel et al. 2012).

What is the underlying mechanism for automaticity of pacemaker cells? Three theories are proposed: *M-clock* theory, *Ca^{2+} clock* theory, and *coupled clock* theory, described here in brief:

M-clock theory This theory, known as membrane clock (or just briefly *M-clock*), implicates that ion channels and ion transporters located on myocardial cell membrane, their inward and outward currents, and their associated channels (i.e., mainly L-type Ca^{2+} channels, K^+ outflux channels, Na^+/Ca^{2+} exchanger "NCX," Na^+/K^+ ATPase, and funny currents) are the main generators of action potentials needed for pacemaker activity; this theory involves mainly the role of sarcolemma-related structures.

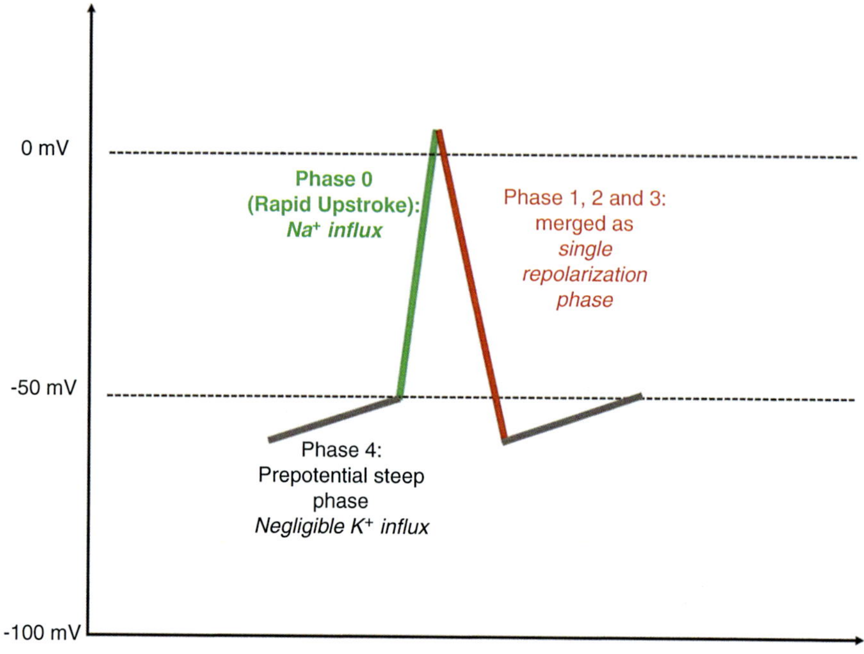

Fig. 3.4 Action potential (AP) in cardiac pacemaker cells

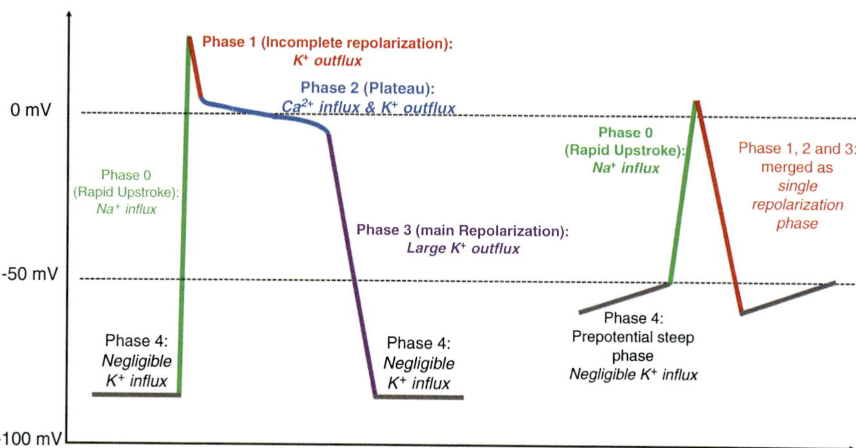

Fig. 3.5 The difference between action potential phases in normal and pacemaker cells

Ca^{2+} clock theory This theory implies that Ca^{2+} is restored in the sarcoplasmic reticulum, the related Ca^{2+} pumps (sarcoplasmic/endoplasmic Ca^{2+} ATPase, "SERCA"), Ca^{2+} channels including ryanodine receptor family (*RYRs*), and some members of the protein kinase family oscillate rhythmically and periodically to produce the pacemaker automaticity.

Coupled clock theory Though none of the two above theories are frankly dominant over the other theories, both cooperate to produce the pacemaker function in the heart having important role in impulse generation; however, their cooperation with other proteins like protein kinase A (PKA) or Ca^{2+}/calmodulin-dependent protein kinase II (CaMK II) is the basis for the model known as "coupled clock theory" being the most recent proposed theory for impulse generation and automaticity in the heart especially in SA node; this theory implicates the wide interactions between cell membrane-related mechanisms and intracellular mechanisms leading to impulse generation (Maltsev et al. 2006, 2014; Sobie et al. 2006; Maltsev and Lakatta 2007, 2012; Mangoni and Nargeot 2008; Lakatta et al. 2010; Yaniv et al. 2012, 2015).

Excitation-Contraction Coupling: ECC

ECC is the "linkage" phenomenon which translates the electrical activities of the heart to the mechanical activities; hence, it is the "electromechanical interface." Nearly 50 years ago, this concept was proposed, and since then, a great bulk of researches have been done on this topic (Quinn et al. 2014). The terminal and eventual goal in ECC is the process of Ca2+ cycling leading to rhythmic initiation and termination of myocardial contraction. ECC has three main parts:

Ca^{2+}
Functioning organelles of ECC
ECC-modulating mechanisms

Calcium Homeostasis

Calcium homeostasis should be discussed at first since Ca^{2+} homeostasis has a central role in ECC. As a matter of fact, Ca^{2+} homeostasis is one of the most important cellular processes in all cells including myocardial cells. Intracellular Ca^{2+} is not only a second messenger, but in myocytes, it has other roles; the *dual-phase pattern of Ca^{2+} cycling* (i.e., Ca^{2+} release and Ca^{2+} reuptake) is the basis for lifelong contraction and relaxation of the heart; needless to say, many intracellular proteins are involved in Ca^{2+} homeostasis; on the other hand, many intracellular interactions of the heart are dependent on Ca^{2+} homeostasis, including:

- Electrical function (with Ca^{2+} influx and efflux as integral parts of action potential)
- Mechanical activities (with Ca^{2+} surge in systole and Ca^{2+} reuptake in diastole)
- Cell energetics, especially inside the mitochondria
- Buffering capacity of the cells for stress control
- Apoptosis and cell death-dependent mechanisms

The sarcoplasmic reticulum (SR) is the main source of intracellular Ca^{2+} storage; however, in "pediatric heart" the amount of Ca^{2+} in SR is not as abundant as the SR of adult heart; so, the myocardium of the neonates, infants, and children is highly dependent on extracellular levels of Ca^{2+} for functioning normally, especially when considering the fact that the calcium transport system in the myocardium of infants and children is immature. These unique features of Ca^{2+} homeostasis in pediatric heart is among the main causes for reduced myocardial in this age group compared to the normal healthy adult (Bers 2002; Maier et al. 2005; Gustafsson and Gottlieb 2009; Asp et al. 2013).

The excitation-contraction coupling (ECC) involves a number of ongoing and interrelated events to act as a machine to promote cardiac function. The following steps occurring in sequential cascade constitute the ECC:

1. I_{CaL} or dihydropyridine receptor (DHPR) opens for initial primary Ca^{2+} influx, (Ca^{2+} trigger) from extracellular fluid (ECF).
2. The primary "Ca^{2+} trigger" causes release of huge Ca^{2+} amounts from the junctional sarcoplasmic reticulum through ryanodine receptor-2 and other intracellular calcium reservoirs; in fact, this small primary amount of Ca^{2+} sparks the release of next huge amounts of Ca^{2+}; this phenomenon is called *calcium-induced calcium release* (CICR); among many interesting features of CICR is that in some pathologies, CICR instability contributes to cardiac arrhythmias (Fabiato and Fabiato 1977, 1978; Fabiato 1983; Bers 2002).
3. CIRC causes huge Ca^{2+} release; then, Ca^{2+} interacts with contractile elements of the myocardial cells, starting myocardial contraction.
4. Immediately afterward, Ca^{2+} recycling from the cytosol back to the sarcoplasmic reticulum (SR) happens; this process is the main mechanism for Ca^{2+} reuptake and is done mainly by an ATP-dependent protein called sarco-/endoplasmic reticulum Ca^{2+} transport ATPase (abbreviated as SERCA) functioning as a pump to recollect Ca^{2+}; more than ten isoforms of SERCA have been recognized in different tissues; however, the primary isoform recognized in myocardial cells is SERCA2a; however, SERCA2a activity is not limitless and is modulated by another protein called phospholamban (PLB); PLB blocks SERCA2a through biochemical and structural transitions of its molecule (Sobie et al. 2006; Williams et al. 2010).
5. Besides SERCA2a, the remainder of Ca^{2+} is returned to ECF by NCX.

So, these three main proteins interact together in handling of Ca^{2+} homeostasis:

First: SERCA2a mediates Ca^{2+} reuptake and starts myocardial relaxation; in *diastolic dysfunction*, SERCA2a is one of the most important therapeutic targets which is the goal for novel therapies aimed to augment SERCA2a or phosphorylation of PLB (i.e., inactivation of PLB; also see next paragraph) (Shareef et al. 2014). In one study, Pavlovic et al. demonstrated that the "PLB/SERCA ratio was significantly reduced in atrial myocardial tissue of pediatric patients with volume overload" (Pavlovic et al. 2005).

Second: PLB modulates SERCA2a activity and so stops myocardial relaxation and, indirectly, stops diastole; also, PLB determines cardiac response to beta-1 adrenergic stimulation. When cardiac muscle is stimulated through β-1 receptor, increased cAMP ensues leading to increased activity of protein kinase

A (PKA); increased phosphorylation of PLB on serine-16 as the result of increased PKA activity results in relieving PLB inhibitory effect on SERCA2a activity; the final outcome of this story is increased Ca^{2+} pumping to the SR and accelerated reuptake of Ca^{2+} from cytosol; the physiologic picture of this cascade would be speeding up the myocardial relaxation and shortening diastole; augmented PLB phosphorylation could be a potential future therapy for diastolic dysfunction (Frank et al. 2003; Asp et al. 2013; Espinoza-Fonseca et al. 2015).

Third: Sarcolipin (SLN) is another cytosol protein that regulates Ca^{2+} homeostasis mainly in atrial myocytes somewhat similar to PLB in ventricular myocytes; though SLN and PLB are not the same regarding their structure, function, and anatomic site of action, their final function is to inhibit SERCA2a activity in order to terminate SERCA2a role in Ca^{2+} reuptake; decreased SLN in atrial myocytes is associated with augmented activity of SERCA2a in atrial myocytes and SR Ca^{2+} overload which is associated with atrial fibrillation and atrial remodeling (Bhupathy et al. 2007; Periasamy et al. 2008; Xie et al. 2012).

- There are a number of congenital heart diseases titled under "conotruncal defects" resulting from altered neural crest migration which include tetralogy of Fallot (TOF), transposition of great arteries, persistent truncus arteriosus, double-outlet right ventricle, interrupted aortic arch, and other anomalies of aortic arch; in these congenital cardiac anomalies, neural crest impairment leads to important defects in SR, especially impaired RYR-2, impaired ECC, and defective I_{CaL}; also, in some of these anomalies (mainly in TOF), impaired function of PLB and SLN is seen as a prominent defect in the myocardial cytosol (Vittorini et al. 2007).
- Other proteins like calmodulin (*cal*cium-*mod*ulated prote*in*) and calsequestrin are discussed here.
- There is another protein named calmodulin-dependent protein kinase II (CaMK II) which also could control and modulate SERCA2a (i.e., somewhat similar to PLB) (Tables 3.3 and 3.4).

Functioning Organelles of ECC

Functioning organelles of ECC are cell membrane, thick and thin filaments, T tubules, and sarcoplasmic reticulum:

1. The myocardial cell membrane or sarcolemma is the main player for both parts of ECC, i.e., the electrical phase of ECC (which includes creation of different phases of action potential) and the mechanical phase of ECC (which is primarily through Ca^{2+} trigger).
2. Thick and thin filaments.
3. Transverse tubules (T tubules).
4. Sarcoplasmic reticulum (SR), being divided to longitudinal SR (LSR) and junctional SR (JSR), acts as the main intracellular Ca^{2+} reservoir which releases and reuptakes Ca^{2+} per needed into and out of the cytosol; RyR-2 and SERCA are the main Ca^{2+} releasing and reuptaking pump located on JSR, respectively.

ECC-Modulating Mechanisms

There are a number of modulators which balance the different interactions in ECC (Yang et al. 2011; Asghari et al. 2014; Brunet et al. 2015; Motloch et al. 2016):

- PKC modulates ECC.
- All types of VGCC, Ca(v)1.2, mediate ECC.
- There are a number of uncoupling proteins (UCPs), mainly located in the inner membrane of cardiac mitochondria; they belong to a superfamily of mitochondrial ion transporters, and they modulate intracellular Ca2+; so, they modulate ECC by modulating mitochondrial Ca2+ uptake.
- The micro-architecture of the myocardial tissue has many aspects which have modulating role on ECC which are under further assessments.

Table 3.3 A summary of ECC

	Event	Protein or channel in-charge	The main phenomenon	Result
1.	Initial Ca^{2+} influx (Ca^{2+} entry to the cell)	I_{CaL} DHPR	DHPR channel opens	Triggers CICR (opening of RyR-2)
2.	Ca^{2+} release (CICR) due to opening of RyR-2	RyR-2	Channel opens and huge Ca^{2+} is released from SR	Starts myocardial contraction
3.	Ca^{2+} recycling, from cytosol back to SR, i.e., Ca^{2+} reuptake and Ca^{2+} efflux	SERCA2a (mainly) and NCX	Recollection of Ca^{2+} from cytosol	Starts myocardial relaxation
4.	Modulation of SERCA2a	PLB	Stopping Ca^{2+} reuptake by SERCA2a	Stops myocardial relaxation; the next contraction could now start

Table 3.4 A summary of the composing aspects of ECC and their related items

1.	Functioning organelles of ECC	Cell membrane
		Thick and thin filaments
		T tubules
		Sarcoplasmic reticulum
2.	Calcium ion (Ca2+)	Ca^{2+} influx to the cardiomyocytes (by L-type Ca^{2+} channels in *systole*)
		Ca^{2+} release inside the cell (by RyR in systole)
		Ca^{2+} efflux from the cardiomyocytes (by NCX in diastole)
		Ca^{2+} reuptake from the cell (by SERCA in diastole)
3.	Controllers of ECC	Ryanodine receptor (RyR) family
		Dihydropyridine receptor (DHPR)
		Calmodulin

Mechanical (Contractile) Function of the Myocardium

The contractile function of the myocardium is the specific duty performed by two syncytia: *atrial* and *ventricular*. These two syncytia are composed of a huge number of units called sarcomere. Each sarcomere is defined as a specialized part of the myocardial muscle located between two Z lines; the main ingredients of sarcomere are:

Contractile proteins which are responsible for myocardial contraction (actin and myosin) and the backbone (such as titin); these are arranged in a delicate structure between two Z lines and are discussed later.

Regulatory proteins which control the cyclic contraction-relaxation phases; these are mainly troponin, tropomyosin, tropomodulin, and myosin-binding protein C, which activate and modulate sarcomere functions. The contractile elements of the myocardium could be divided as shown in Table 3.5.

Inside each of the sarcomere, actin and myosin interactions lead to "Ca^{2+}-triggered crossbridges" between actin and myosin leading to contraction; this contraction is the third stage after electrochemical action potential translated via "ECC" pathway to contraction; so, the more crossbridges, the more contractile force. After each contraction, troponin I (TnI) detaches actin and myosin from each other; hence crossbridge sites (active sites) are disappeared. Crossbridges need great amounts of fuel supplied as sarcomere ATP reservoirs; both attachment and separation of crossbridges are energy consuming. This is the basis for cardiac systolic contraction and diastolic relaxation.

Although there are many similarities in the function and structure of the contractile tissue between healthy adult heart and the pediatric hearth, we should always keep in mind that the texture of the myocardium in pediatric heart is organized in such a way that only about 50 % of the tissue is composed of contractile elements, while the rest 50 % of the tissue is composed of noncontractile elements, including mitochondria and large nuclei. This unique structural feature has a number of specificities:

1. In the pediatric myocardium, the percentage of contractile mass in the total mass of myocardium is less than the adult myocardium; on the other hand, decreased contractile mass leads to decreased compliance of the ventricular muscle (compared to the adult healthy heart); this is one of the main reasons why the myocardial contractile reserve is significantly reduced compared to the healthy adult myocardium.

Table 3.5 Categories of myocardial filaments

	Contractile proteins	Modulatory proteins
Thick filament	Myosin Titin	Myosin-binding protein C (MBPC)
Thin filament	Actin	Tropomyosin Troponin (TnC, TnT, TnI) Tropomodulin

2. Due to decreased compliance of the LV, the filling pressures (compared with adult healthy myocardium) are higher, and preload augmentation is limited to just 1–7 mmHg.
3. The neonatal myocardium is hence highly dependent on the resting tone of β-adrenergic stimulation; in clinical practice, we see very high sensitivity of the neonatal myocardium to even low doses of β-blockers, and on the other side, the response to β-agonists is not so much exaggerated as adult healthy myocardium.

Here, we first describe the main ingredients of each sarcomere, and then we will describe their assembly including Z disc (Z line), M band, I band, and A band and how thin and thick filaments are integrated in the framework of these structures in sarcomere.

Thick Filament

Thick filament Thick filament is composed mainly of two contractile proteins (myosin and titin) and one modulatory protein (myosin-binding protein C or briefly MBPC).

Myosin has a structured framework. First of all, the 15 nanometer myosin rods are composed of the following elements:

- One myosin heavy chain (1 MHC)
- Two myosin light chains (2 MLCs)

Then, one MHC plus two MLCs compose a single myosin strand (MS); so, we will have:

$$1\,MHC + 2\,MLCs = MS$$

Afterward, two MSs woven together produce one myosin molecule (MM); in other words, each MM is composed of two MSs:

$$1\,MM = 2\,MS = 2\,MHCs + 4\,MLCs$$

However, each MM resembles a "golf club" which has two functional domains: the four MLCs in the *head region* and the *tail region* of MM which is like the handle of the golf club (Fig. 3.1). Ca^{2+} trigger causes the head of MM to cross bridge with actin leading contractions. Also, TnI inhibits the crossbridges at the end of each interaction to detach actin from myosin head.

About 300 MMs collectively form together in a parallel fashion forming myosin rod (MR) which resembles "a bundle of golf clubs" collected together while their heads protrude out of the bundle and their bodies and handles are attached together (Fig. 3.6).

Titin is the most frequent filament after actin and myosin; "the largest protein known to date," titin is a very giant filament extending from each side of the Z line

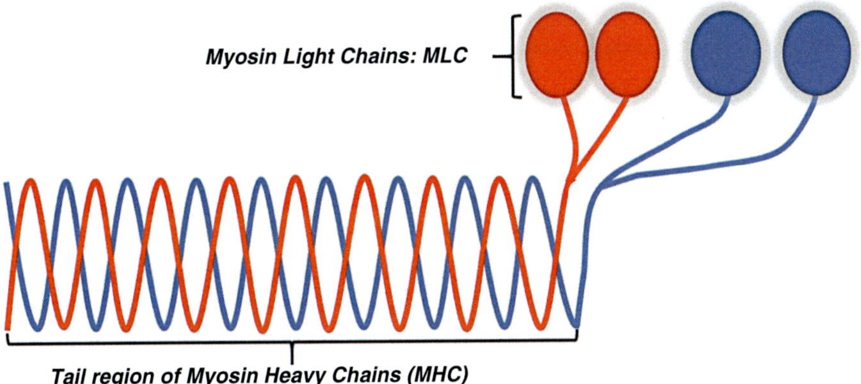

Fig. 3.6 Schematic presentation of a myosin molecule

toward the M line; it has been simply named as the "bidirectional molecular spring" of the cardiac sarcomere; in other words, during diastole, the extensible properties of titin help myocardial tissue to preserve its primary configuration, returning to the primary size of the heart; in this way, titin acts as a "passive force generator" in diastole; on the other hand, titin plays its role in restoration of sarcomere length when it is shorter than its slack length. Besides, titin has attachments with actin-myosin crossbridge sites through myosin-binding protein C (MBPC). This is why titin has a very strategic role in cardiac sarcomere to keep it stable during contraction and relaxation (Pyle and Solaro 2004; Solaro 2005; Kobirumaki-Shimozawa et al. 2014).

Titin has a specific structure which helps create its elastic role. Functionally speaking, titin has two segments:

- The extensible segment anchored to each side of the Z line located in the I band domain; this is the N terminal of titin.
- The non-extensible segment located in the A band; the end of C terminal is bound to the thick filament.

On the other hand, if we want to explain titin based on a structural classification of the molecule, it has two parts:

- Immunoglobulin-like segment.
- PEVK segment abbreviated for the four amino acids: proline (P), glutamate (E), valine (V), and lysine (K); these amino acids compose about 75 % of the PEVK segment.

The role of titin in "fine-tune passive myocardial stiffness" and "diastolic function and diastolic force generation" is highly dependent on phosphorylation of titin molecule by calcium-/calmodulin-dependent protein kinase II delta (CaMKIIδ); those regions of titin located in "I band" are important in phosphorylation mechanisms. Impairment in CaMKII-dependent phosphorylation of titin is considered as a major etiology for diastolic dysfunction. Mutations in those genes related to titin are often considered as the etiologic factor for dilated cardiomyopathy, since titin disruption ends to impairment of structure of the heart and its elasticity (LeWinter et al. 2007; Nishikawa et al. 2012; Hamdani et al. 2013a, b; Hidalgo et al. 2013; Kotter et al. 2013; Rain et al. 2014; McNally et al. 2015; Zile et al. 2015).

Titin stiffness could lead to RV diastolic dysfunction in pulmonary hypertension patients, of course in association with factors like reduced phosphorylation of cTnI and altered phosphorylation of Ca2+ (Rain et al. 2014).

Also, in heart failure patients, impaired phosphorylation of the thick filament protein myosin-binding protein C (cMyBP-C) has a main role especially in patients with diagnosis of familial hypertrophic cardiomyopathy due to mutations in MYBPC3 (Kuster et al. 2012).

Thin Filament

Thin filament is composed of actin (mainly in the form of filamentous actin "F actin"), tropomyosin (TM), and troponin complex (Tc); if we want to compare the number of molecules for each protein in the thin filament, then we will have one F actin, two TM, and two Tc in each imaginary unit of thin filament.

Actin Actin is made of F actin; so, F actin is the backbone of the thin filament, while TM is located in the groove of F actin strand; however, Tc is located at defined and regular intervals along F actin. Each molecule of F actin is composed of 13 subunits called globular actin "G actin," which twist to form a 360 degree turn in F actin strand. In cardiac sarcomere, F actin is alpha subtype.

Tropomyosin (TM) Tropomyosin is a *right-handed helical coiled coil* and inhibitory protein located on F actin. Two adjacent TM molecules attach together and turn round each other; then, this coiled filament (composed of two turned TM molecules) twists once more while being attached to actin filament; so, it is termed "the prototype coiled coil" protein. Each TM molecule is in contact with seven subsequent G actin molecules; so their molecular ratio is "Tm 1:G actin 7." The end of one TM molecule is attached to the head of the next TM molecule; this attachment, called head-to-tail overlap of TM, has about eight amino acids. This head-to-tail interaction of each two subsequent TM molecules is of the most determining factors modulating the function of thin filament. Of course, recent studies have demonstrated that this description is somewhat a simplified picture of the real structure of TM (Kobayashi et al. 2008; Nevzorov and Levitsky 2011).

TM is under the control of two parts of troponin complex: troponin T (TnT) and troponin I (TnI); in cardiac muscle, Ca^{2+} attachment to troponin C (TnC) causes TM to be detached from the actin-myosin crossbridge site; this is exactly the point which is inhibited by TM; in other words, Ca^{2+} inhibits TM; then, this "inhibition" exposes the "crossbridge site" to myosin molecule; this is exactly the myosin binding site on actin molecule known as *crossbridge site* or active site; in this process, when TM is pushed far from crossbridge sites, myosin crossbridge finds the opportunity to directly attach

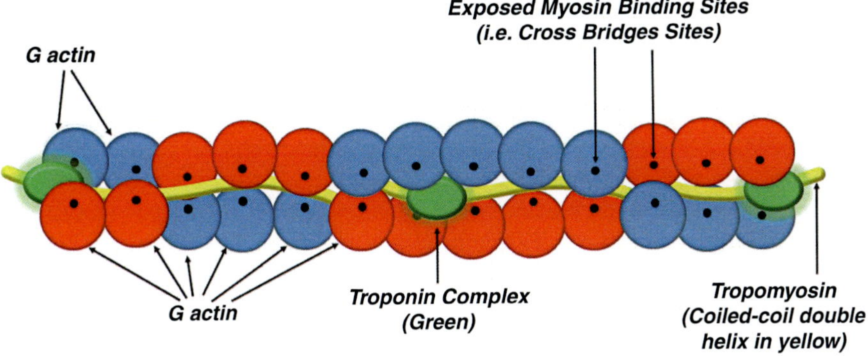

Fig. 3.7 Schematic presentation of a thin filament (also see Fig. 3.8a): each helix of F actin contains two strands of G actin each containing 13 G actin molecules (*blue* and *red globes*) and myosin binding sites which expose actin for crossbridging with myosin and located on each G actin (demonstrated as a *black dot*); troponin complex (*green knobs*) and tropomyosin double-strand coiled coils as (*yellow threads*)

to this critical point, i.e., the crossbridge; and these interactions lead to sarcomere contraction. At the end of the contraction, when Ca^{2+} concentration in sarcomere falls, troponin I (TnI) augments the role of TM, in such a way that again TM becomes closer to crossbridge sites, attaches to crossbridge, and pushes myosin away from crossbridge; the final outcome is inhibition of contraction. In this process, the two most important modulators for sensitivity of sarcomere filaments to Ca^{2+} are the sarcomere length (i.e., Frank-Starling relationship) and the role of protein phosphorylation in sarcomere which causes posttranslational modification of these proteins; the reader can find detailed discussion in a number of reviews published in the last years (Hitchcock-DeGregori 2008; Kobayashi et al. 2008; Jagatheesan et al. 2010; Bai et al. 2013).

There are two specific inherited diseases involving impaired function of TM in Ca^{2+} attachment: dilated cardiomyopathy (DCM) and hypertrophic cardiomyopathy (HCM); both are due to "missense mutations" in genes coding TM. In summary, in DCM, the mutation causes decreased sensitivity of TM to Ca^{2+} binding, while in HCM, the mutation ends to increased sensitivity of TM to Ca^{2+} (Bai et al. 2013; Redwood and Robinson 2013; Kalyva et al. 2014) (Fig. 3.7).

Troponin complex (Tn) Troponin complex is composed of three subsegments: troponin C (TnC), troponin I (TnI), and troponin T (TnT); TnI inhibits the crossbridge by inhibiting the actin-myosin-TM interactions, while TnC activates muscle contraction by "inhibiting the inhibitory role of TnI"; TnT is the modulator for troponin activity. Troponin complex is not just a simple attachment of three proteins; instead, the conformational interactions between these three components are mandatory for the activity of troponin complex.

Troponin C (TnC) This protein acts as a "Ca^{2+} sensor" which senses and regulates the sequential events involved in initiation and control of contraction inside the sarcomere. The shape of TnC is much similar a dumbbell; two heads of the dumbbell are the N terminus and the C terminus of TnC molecule.

There are two Ca^{2+} binding sites (CBS) on C terminus (CBS III and CBS IV); Ca^{2+} is attached firmly to both of them; so none of them is involved in controlling Ca^{2+}-dependent muscular contractions; however, these two Ca^{2+} binding sites (i.e., CBS III and IV) are attached to TnC and TnI. On the other hand, there are two other Ca^{2+} binding sites on the N terminus of TnC: CBS I and CBS II; however, CBS I cannot attach to Ca^{2+} firmly, while *CBS II* is the only and most important CBS that attaches to Ca^{2+} and performs the regulatory and modification roles of TnC in muscle contraction. Attachment of Ca^{2+} to CBS II on N terminus of TnC causes structural and functional changes in both "actin-TM" complex and troponin complex; these changes cause activation of the thin filament. TnC mutations are involved in both HCM and DCM (Marston and Redwood 2003; Kobayashi et al. 2008; Kekenes-Huskey et al. 2012; Craig et al. 2014; Kalyva et al. 2014; Kobirumaki-Shimozawa et al. 2014; Shi et al. 2015).

Troponin I (TnI) This part of troponin has an inhibitory role; not only TnI alone inhibits actin, but also, when combined with TM, the TnI-TM complex acts as a potent inhibitor of actin-myosin interaction and so prevents generation of forceful contractions. Some genetic disorders in TnI cause hypertrophic cardiomyopathy (HCM) or restrictive cardiomyopathy (RCM) because of impairment in inhibitory effects of TnI in diastole. The interested reader is addressed to detailed references for TnI (Chang et al. 2008; Kobayashi et al. 2008; Ohtsuki and Morimoto 2008; Solaro et al. 2008; 2013).

Troponin T (TnT) TnT is an integrating component of thin filament and connects TM to troponin complex. TnT attaches to the "head-to-tail" segment of two subsequent TM segments on one hand and to the Z disc on the other hand; this protein has a cooperative role in thin filament activation through its modulatory role on TM activity. To explain more, the inhibition of TnI would be relieved without any need of Ca^{2+} if there was no TnT; but in the presence of TnT, Ca^{2+} is mandatory for TnC activity in order to lift the inhibitory role of TnI. TnT is composed of two subfragments: TnT1 (N terminal) and TnT2 (C terminal). TnT1 binds strongly to tropomyosin, while TnT2 has the important role in Ca^{2+} regulation; the function of TnT on Ca^{2+} regulation would be impaired without TnT2. The majority of the mutations leading to DCM are related to TnT though TnI and TnC also have mutations leading to DCM. Also, some mutations in TnT lead to HCM (Chang et al. 2008; Kobayashi et al. 2008; Ohtsuki and Morimoto 2008).

A main functional part of interactions between these proteins is the crossbridging phenomenon, a basic phenomenon with its integral role in myocardial contraction, which is based on continuous interactions between the thick and thin filaments.

Z Disc, I Band, A Band, and M Line

Z disc, I band, A band, and M line (the following components are demonstrated in Fig. 3.8a, b): Sarcomeres are cylindrical repeating units; the margin of each sarcomere is Z disc or Z line.

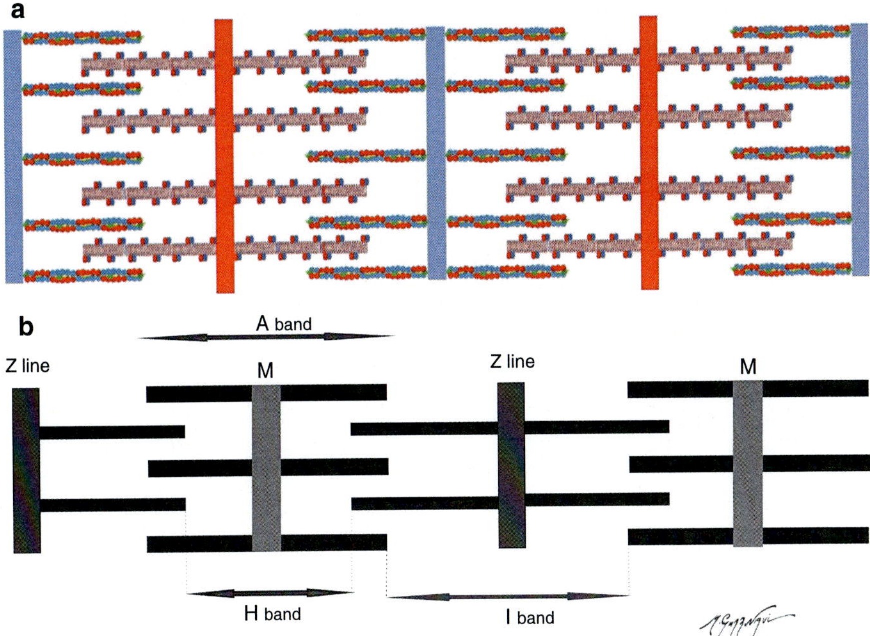

Fig. 3.8 (**a**) Schematic presentation of microscopic structure of a sarcomere from a wide view (also, see Fig. 3.7). (**b**) Schematic presentation of microscopic structure of a sarcomere (compare each part with its compared part in Section A) (Figure **b** is modified from Dabbagh (2014). Published with kind permission from © Springer, 2014. All Rights Reserved)

Z in Z discs stands for Zuckung, a German name meaning twitch; Z discs are three-dimensional structures about 100 nm (0.1 μ) composing the margins of each sarcomere; in fact, Z discs are the border of two neighboring sarcomeres, and they divide the sarcomeres from each other. However, each Z disc is a complex of many proteins including those located at Z disc and those attached to Z disc.

Functionally, Z discs have the main following roles:

- Producing mechanical stability in each contraction and relaxation, since Z discs are the anchoring site of many sarcomere proteins and, also, thin filament and titin
- Transmission and transduction of signal between two adjacent sarcomeres

Each Z disc is surrounded in each side by *I band*, which is the dark band adjacent to the Z disc; in fact each I band spans thin filaments of the two adjacent sarcomeres with Z disc located in its center.

There is a pivotal band for the thick filaments called *M band*; these bands are in the *M*iddle of the sarcomere, so *M* band. *Both Z discs and M bands are transversally oriented multi-protein scaffolds* (Stehle et al. 2009). On either side of each M band, thick filaments compose the "A band." In fact, A band is the band on each side of the M band which is the region of thick filaments; the lateral border of A band contains the terminal segment of the thin filaments which, together with thick filaments, slide into each other during contraction and come out during relaxation (Tskhovrebova and Trinick 2010).

One A band in the middle plus two "half I bands" in each side compose the span of one sarcomere which is between two Z discs.

On the other side, the specific segment of the A band located in the center of A band which is devoid of thin filaments is called "H band" (Solaro 2005; Kobayashi et al. 2008).

In summary, the attachment of filaments of sarcomeres is as follows (Stehle et al. 2009):

- *Thick filaments* are anchored just at its midpoint to the M line; then, each thick filament spans in each of the two lateral sides toward the Z discs; however, it does not attach Z disc.
- *Thin filaments* are attached and anchored to Z lines and extend from Z line toward the midpoint of the sarcomere, i.e., the M line; again, thin filaments do not attach to M line.
- *Titin*, the huge protein of the thick filament, is attached on one side to Z disc and on the other side to M band; so, titin is spread *all along the sarcomere* from the Z disc on one hand to the M band of the sarcomere on the other hand; also, there is alpha actinin, a specific protein located in Z line, connecting thin filament with titin (Anderson and Granzier 2012).

Novel Therapeutic Agents Against Heart Failure

Based on the protein molecules and the protein architecture involved in myocardial contraction, a wide array of novel therapeutic agents are under assay which is briefed here:

Omecamtiv mecarbil, a *myosin activator* agent, enables myosin to be attached much more "firmly" to actin to produce more forceful myocardial contraction; this drug acts directly on sarcomere, without any perturbation in myocardial Ca^{2+} homeostasis inside the cell; in fact, omecamtiv mecarbil increases the rate of actin-dependent release of phosphate, resulting in increased actin-attached myosin heads, causing increased number of active, force-generating myosin heads during systole and also increased effectiveness of myosin crossbridge formation and duration; so, systolic ejection time increases without any unwanted effects on the left ventricular filling pressure or any unwanted increase in myocardial contraction velocity; the drug seems to be a good pharmacologic agent for systolic heart failure; however, it is not yet available for clinical use (Cleland et al. 2011; Malik and Morgan 2011; Teerlink et al. 2011; Aronson and Krum 2012; Garg and Frishman 2013).

Istaroxime has a dual function; first, it inhibits sarcolemmal Na+/K+ ATPase to increase intracellular Na+ concentration and to decrease Ca^{2+} efflux through NCX, increasing intracellular Ca^{2+} concentration; second, istaroxime stimulates SERCA2a to augment lusitropic properties of the myocardium and decreases the chance for arrhythmias; it also protects the heart through stabilization of SERCA2a (George et al. 2014; Ahmad et al. 2015).

In diastole, Ca^{2+} overload happens which is either due to decreased rate of Ca^{2+} reuptake or increased sensitivity of myocardium to Ca^{2+}. Novel therapies have been proposed to treat diastolic dysfunction through augmentation of SERCA2a or partial inhibition of PLB (Kawase and Hajjar 2008; Teerlink et al. 2009; Kawamura et al. 2010; Asp et al. 2013).

Control Mechanisms of Cardiac Function

Autonomic Control of the Heart

The autonomic nervous system (ANS) as a portion of the peripheral nervous system continuously controls cardiovascular functions.

The ANS, on the other hand, is regulated by other centers such as the brain stem and hypothalamus.

The sympathetic and parasympathetic systems are the main component of ANS.

The preganglionic nerves of sympathetic system originate from T1-L2 segment of the spinal cord and enter the sympathetic chain ganglia located along the side of the viscera column (i.e., paravertebral ganglia). Postganglionic fibers of the cardiac sympathetic originate from the stellate ganglia and extend to different parts of the heart (SA and AV nodes, atria, and ventricles).

The long preganglionic nerves of cardiac parasympathetic system originate in the dorsal motor nucleus of the tenth cranial nerves (left and right vagi) or in the nucleus ambiguous. The short postganglionic nerves lie on epicardial surface and within the atrial and ventricular walls. There is no equal vagi distribution to different cardiac structures, because the vagi mainly affect SA and AV nodes and there is a slight distribution for atria and ventricles.

In the newborn heart, the number of α-adrenergic receptors is reduced; this is among the factors that limit the function of the left ventricle; also, the level of the circulating catecholamines increases dramatically to compensate for the limited function of the heart, an important fact that should be considered when anesthetizing a child or newborn especially for cardiac procedures; it is logic to avoid suppressing the sympathetic tone of the body in order to prevent decreased cardiac output.

Since the right and left sides of the embryonic structures are the sites for developing the SA and AV nodes, respectively, the SA node receives its ANS branches mainly from the right vagus and right stellate ganglion, and the AV node takes its branches mostly from the left vagus and left stellate ganglion. Sympathetic β-receptors are epicardial and parasympathetic muscarinic receptors are endocardial (Gordan et al. 2015).

Sympathetic and Parasympathetic Receptors

There are different subtypes of α- (α_{1A}, α_{1B}, and α_{1D}) and β (β_1 and β_2)-sympathetic (or adrenergic) receptors in the heart.

Although, the number of α_1-receptors is less than β-receptors, activation of α_1-receptors leads to increased ventricular contraction, sensitivity of contractile myofilaments to calcium ions, and cardiac hypertrophy. Activation of the α_1-receptor as a $G_{q/11}$-coupled receptor by stimulating phospholipase-C (PLC) leads to enhanced intracellular inositol triphosphate (IP3) and diacylglycerol (DAG) concentration.

The β_1-adrenergic receptors are expressed on the different portions of the heart such as the SA node, AV node, and atrial and ventricular cardiomyocytes. The activation of β_1-receptors increases heart rate and augments myocardial contractility by increasing of the intracellular calcium concentrations through calcium currents from extracellular fluid, and the sarcoplasmic reticulum (SR) stores and enhances the AV node conduction velocity. The β_1-adrenoceptor is a G_s-protein-coupled receptor, and activation of α_s (as a subunit of G-protein) by stimulation of adenylyl cyclase increases the cAMP production and raises protein kinase A (PKA) activity. Although, the number of the β_2-receptors subtype is less than the β_1-receptor, the effects of both subtypes are similar to each other.

The M_2 subtype of muscarinic receptors is dominant receptor for parasympathetic nervous system in the heart. This receptor is coupled to the Gi-protein, and activation of α_i by inhibition of adenylyl cyclase reduces cAMP production and lessens PKA activity. In addition, the $\beta\gamma$ portion of Gi-protein activates acetylcholine-sensitive potassium channels (I_{KAch}) and creates hyperpolarization (Thomas 2011).

Functions of the ANS in the Heart

The ANS has a prominent effect on the different features of the heart due to its capacity to modify heart rate (chronotropy), contractility (inotropy), conduction velocity (dromotropy), rate of relaxation (lusitropy), and degree of excitability (bathmotropy).

Chronotropy changes are created via changes in steepness of pacemaker potential in SA node; inotropy is regulated by modulation of myocardial force generation through different mechanisms; dromotropy is altered by changes in the speed of impulse conduction in the AV node; lusitropy is controlled by the manners that return the heart muscle to its initial relaxed condition after each muscle contraction, and bathmotropy is modified by changes in the threshold of heart excitation. The different effects of the β_1- and M_2 receptor activation on the heart has been summarized in Table 3.6 (Myslivecek and Trojan 2003).

Table 3.6 Myocardial receptors characterized by their properties

Receptor type	Inotropy	Chronotropy	Dromotropy	Lusitropy	Bathmotropy
β_1	+	+	+	+	+
M_2	–	–	–	–	–

Inotropic Effects of the β_1- and M_2 Receptor Activation

Intracellular rise of free Ca^{2+} concentration is a fundamental factor for initiating myocardial contraction, and for this, two important Ca^{2+} sources play a part: (1) extracellular fluid (ECF) and (2) sarcoplasmic reticulum (SR). Nearly, 20 % of needed Ca^{2+} is provided from ECF and the remaining (80 %) from SR. During the plateau phase of the action potential, Ca^{2+} enters the muscle fiber from ECF via L-type Ca^{2+} channels for generating the great release of Ca^{2+} from the SR through ryanodine channel in the CICR phenomenon described earlier in this chapter.

There are many reasons for positive inotropic effect of β_1-adrenoceptor stimulation by released catecholamines from postganglionic neuron of sympathetic system (norepinephrine) and the adrenal gland (epinephrine):

1. Increase in the PKA activity via phosphorylation of L-type Ca^{2+} channel leads to increase in the Ca^{2+} influx.
2. Increase in the Ca^{2+} influx leads to a greater release of Ca^{2+} from the SR, and this action reinforces the intracellular concentration of Ca^{2+}.
3. Catecholamines provide further Ca^{2+} stores in the SR for next contraction by increase in activity of SERCA and further Ca^{2+} pumping into the SR at the end of previous contraction. In addition, enhanced Ca^{2+} influx through L-type Ca^{2+} channels leads to increase in Ca^{2+} availability for more storage in the SR.
4. Sensitivity of troponin C for Ca^{2+} is increased, and this action facilitates the sliding of actin and myosin filaments for contraction achievement.

As mentioned earlier, stimulation of the vagus nerve has a slight direct effect on myocardial contractility due to poor distribution of parasympathetic on the atria and ventricles. On the other hand, severe stimulation of the vagus nerve has a significant inhibitory effect on myocardial contractility mainly by reducing heart rate.

Chronotropic Effects of the β_1- and M_2 Receptor Activation

Activation of Gs-protein-coupled β_1-adrenoceptor by pharmaceutical agents like epinephrine and norepinephrine enhances the heart rate through two mechanisms:

1. By increasing I_F (I_h) and I_{Ca} in the SA node which leads to increase in steepness of pacemaker potential of action potential
2. By increasing I_{Ca}, which causes more negative threshold of the action potential

Both of the above mechanisms accelerate the generation of the next action potential and shorten the interval between two consecutive action potentials.

On the other hand, in contrary to β_1-adrenoceptor, activation of Gi-protein-coupled M_2 receptor by acetylcholine (Ach) slows the pacemaker activity of the SA node through three mechanisms, leading to decreased heart rate:

1. Acetylcholine decreases the steepness of pacemaker potential by reducing I_F and I_{Ca}.
2. Activated $\beta\gamma$ portion of Gi-protein opens acetylcholine-sensitive potassium channels (I_{KAch}) and increases outward potassium current; this effect produces "a hyperpolarization state" in the SA node.
3. Reduction of I_{Ca} changes the threshold of action potential to more positive level.

All these three mechanisms decrease the speed of action potential generation, finally reducing heart rate (Chemla et al. 2000).

Lusitropic Effects of the β_1-Receptor Activation

Catecholamines enhance cardiac relaxation by stimulation of β_1-adrenoceptor. After binding of catecholamines to these receptors, protein kinase A (PKA) is activated. This activated enzyme can phosphorylate some proteins in the cardiomyocytes such as *phospholamban* which is a regulator of ion transport and a major substrate for PKA. Phospholamban reduces the uptake of Ca^{2+} into the sarcoplasmic reticulum by inhibiting SERCA and this effect creates delay for starting myocardial relaxation after each contraction. Phosphorylation of phospholamban by PKA declines the inhibitory effect of phospholamban on SERCA and leads to an increase in reuptake of Ca^{2+} into the SERCA (as described earlier in this chapter). Finally, reduction of intracellular Ca^{2+} level creates the earlier relaxation.

Phosphorylation of the troponin I is another action of PKA in order to augment myocardial relaxation; this effect reduces affinity of troponin C for Ca^{2+} binding and provides relaxation condition for cardiomyocytes.

Developmental Changes in Fetal Cardiac Contractile System

In this section, a number of developmental changes in cardiovascular system are discussed. Of course, in the first sections of this chapter, "evolutional transition in cardiac physiology" is discussed in detail and is not repeated here.

Developmental Changes in Cardiac Ca^{2+} Homeostasis

- Ca^{2+} homeostasis is not as fast in embryonic age as the adult heart; however, it develops to increase its speed regarding Ca^{2+} transport after the mid-embryonic stage.
- Development of SERCA2a activity starts to develop during embryonic stages.
- In embryonic and neonatal heart, mitochondrial Ca^{2+} transport is not as active as adult cardiac cells.

- Ca²⁺ transport through the sarcolemma and the SR of neonatal myocytes is immature; *this is mainly due to deficient or incomplete T tubules and also scant and small SR*; also, Ca²⁺ content of the SR is not enough; as far as myocardial tissue development goes on, these structures develop and also Ca²⁺ content increases to normal levels (Nakanishi et al. 1988; Wetzel et al. 1991; Mahony 1996). In clinical practice, two very important facts are seen:

  1. Myocardial contractility in neonates and infants is highly dependent on extracellular Ca²⁺ stores, since intracellular Ca²⁺ stores are negligible.
  2. Volatile anesthetics suppress myocardial contractility in neonates and children much more than adults, a finding which supports immature SR and limited intracellular Ca²⁺ stores in this patient population, especially regarding the degree of maturity of NCX; however, some believe that Ca²⁺ influx channels – not immature SR – are the main mechanism responsible for the effects of volatile agents (Frank et al. 1994; Seckin et al. 2001; Prakash et al. 2002; Park et al. 2007).

- CICR is not a dominant phenomenon in embryonic heart Ca²⁺ homeostasis; however, it develops as a cellular mechanism as far as the heart changes from an embryonic heart to a mature type heart.
- The compliance of myocardium is less in neonates and infants than older children and adults; in fact, ventricles in neonates and infants are more stiff and do not relax during diastole as much as adult ventricles; this stiffness in part is related to decreased concentration of SERCA2a, RyR, and NCX.
- Also, diastolic relaxation in embryonic heart is not as fast as the adult heart; this delay is not only due to decreased speed of Ca²⁺ kinetics in cytosol but also due to incomplete development of diastole (Kawamura et al. 2010).
- L-type Ca²⁺ channels have a unique model for their development which dominates their role in the heart; so, as age increases, their developmental course changes and improvement in their function happens (Qu et al. 2011).

Developmental Changes in Cardiac Action Potential

- Resting membrane potential in neonates is less dependent on K⁺ current, though this process changes with increasing age which develops to become as in the adult heart (Chen et al. 1991).

Developmental Changes in Mechanical Force Production and Contractile Function

- The fetal heart has "low specific force"; as gestation goes on, the force production property of the heart increases and force development is augmented; also, the rate of force development and the rate of relaxation are both slow in the fetal heart; however, this rate increases as much as the embryonic heart develops (Marston and Redwood 2003; Schwan and Campbell 2015; Racca et al. 2016).

- The myofibrils of the cardiac muscle elongate and also their width increases as the age of the embryo increases.
- M line and Z band are among the very early appearing structures of the cardiomyocyte; they are apparent about day 52 in the fetal period (Schwan and Campbell 2015; Racca et al. 2016).
- β-myosin is among those structures and proteins which is seen so much early in cardiac muscle cells (Marston and Redwood 2003).
- Cardiac troponin I (TnI) increases progressively while at the same time slow skeletal TnI decreases (Sasse et al. 1993; Schwan and Campbell 2015).
- All these changes during gestation of the cardiac myocytes lead to improvements and development of the contractile function; so, these developmental changes are the basis for improved force production as the embryonic heart develops; however, the trend of maturation continues after birth and during childhood and adolescence to lead to the final cardiac structure seen in the adult heart with the contractile properties of the adult heart.

Developmental Changes in Myocardial Function

The myocardium of an infant has a relatively fixed volume. The main reason is in the texture of an infant; the myocardium has about 50 % connective tissue with just the remaining 50 % being contractile tissue. So, the reserve of the heart is really limited and the cardiac output in an infant is highly dependent on heart rate. If preload increases, there is not much significant difference in cardiac output due to limited cardiac tolerance for diastolic filling pressures: a small increase in diastolic volume load leads to large increase in diastolic filling pressures. This is why the least amount of parasympathetic over activity is poorly tolerated in a borderline heart of an infant with underlying cardiac disease. Also, the cardiovascular system of an infant keeps increased heart rate up to 6 years old to compensate for this phenomenon.

Cardiac Cycle and Cardiac Work

Normal Cardiac Cycle

Cardiac pathologies cause different grades of impairment in the normal physiology of the heart, leading to altered cardiac work. So, we aim to move toward normal condition as much as possible; it means that we want to have a heart as much normal as possible with its pumping activity in an appropriate manner and also with proper timing and force; in other words, our treatment goal is to make cardiac work as much as possible normal. For this purpose, in diseased heart, we need the "cardiac cycle" to be as much as possible normal.

So, we should have normal function in the following items:

- *Diastole*: with proper timing and normal filling pressures, over-pressurized chambers are in contradiction with normal work; a major part of normal diastole is having normal pressures in the pulmonary vasculature.
- *Systole*: appropriate amount of blood with appropriate force and timing should be propelled out of the cardiac chambers in systole.

Systole and diastole are divided more into four stages which are organized one after another in a cycle called cardiac cycle:

Phase 1 – "Diastolic filling" with "mitral and tricuspid" valves are open and "aortic and pulmonary" valves are closed; so, ventricular cavities gradually fill; the following forces are the main determinants of ventricular cavity filling in diastole:

- Diastolic compliance of the ventricles which is very low especially in neonates and younger children
- The difference between pressure in atrial and ventricular cavities (i.e., atrial-ventricular pressure gradient)
- The atrial kick force (atrial contraction)

Phase 2 – "Isovolumic systole": no change in volume of the ventricle, instead, continued rise in ventricular pressure; during the very early stages of this phase, the atrioventricular (AV) valves are closed; however, the aortic and pulmonary valves are opened just at the late milliseconds of this stage, i.e., when intracavity pressure increases above a critical level; this is the start of the next phase.

Phase 3 – "Systolic ejection" is accompanied with blood ejection from the left ventricle to the aorta and the right ventricle to the pulmonary artery; the systemic and pulmonary vascular beds are perfused thereof; ventricles are emptied and decompressed after ejection.

Phase 4 – "Isovolumic relaxation": both ventricles relax and their dimensions increase; due to the falling pressure of the ventricular cavity, the aortic and pulmonary valves are closed; meanwhile, due to the same reason, mitral and tricuspid valves open. Now, the cardiac cycle starts a new cycle from phase 1 and this goes on (Tanaka et al. 1993; Gibson and Francis 2003; Carlsson et al. 2012; Chatterjee 2012; Mitchell and Wang 2014) (Table 3.7).

Cardiac Work

Cardiac work Cardiac work implies the product of myocardial performance and is the algebraic sum of two different items: First is the "external work" which is equivalent to the total myocardial energy used for ejecting blood out of the ventricles to the systemic and pulmonary vascular bed. The second parameter is the

Table 3.7 The sequence of phases in normal cardiac cycle

	Name of the phase	Intracavitary pressure	Intracavitary volume	State of the valves
1.	Diastolic filling	Gradually ↑	Gradually ↑	AV valves open; aortic and pulmonary closed
2.	Isovolumic systole	Increases up to a critical level	No change: ↔	AV valves closed; aortic and pulmonary valves *just* open
3.	Systolic ejection	Blood ejection causes sudden drop	Suddenly decreases	AV valves closed; aortic and pulmonary valves completely open
4.	Isovolumic relaxation	Gradually ↓	Starts filling	AV valves open; aortic and pulmonary valves closed

"internal work" which is the total energy needed by myocardial tissue to maintain cell energetic, myocardial integrity and homeostasis of cardiomyocytes. For calculating the external work, we use the product of *stroke work* multiplied by *ventricular cavity pressure*. However, we usually calculate the external work by calculating the area under curve of pressure-volume loop of left ventricle (i.e., LV pressure-volume AUC). The main myocardial need for energy reserve and its oxygen consumption is for used for external work; however, myocardial ischemia would jeopardize mainly the external work. There are a number of clinical indices for assessment of cardiac work. Since we could not measure the cellular energetic easily in clinical practice, we use a number of indices which are discussed here. These are stroke volume, cardiac output, and ejection fraction.

Stroke volume Each "stroke volume" is the amount of blood ejected from the heart in each cardiac beat. Stroke volume (SV) is the result of "end-diastolic volume (EDV) minus end-systolic volume (ESV)" or simply "SV = EDV-ESV." According to this equation, both EDV and ESV could affect SV. However, which factors could affect EDV and ESV?

- EDV depends directly at two factors:

  1. *Venous return* is the returned blood to the ventricles from veins, i.e., from inferior and superior vena cava (IVC and SVC) to RV and from pulmonary veins to LV.
  2. Diastolic time of ventricular filling or simply "filling time" which is the time in diastole that blood accumulates in ventricles; the longer the filling time, the more would be SV.

- ESV depends on three factors:

  1. *Preload* is the amount of ventricular stretching; the more stretch in ventricle, the more contractile force; this is discussed more in the section of "Frank-Starling relationship"; the relationship between preload and ESV is a converse relationship.

2. *Contractility* is the contractile force of the myocardium; this factor has a converse relationship with ESV, i.e., the more contractility, the less volume would remain in the ventricle; however, there are a multitude of factors affecting contractility which are discussed later.
3. *Afterload* is the resistance against the pumping action of ventricles; there is a direct relationship between ESV and afterload; for LV, afterload is mainly the systemic vascular resistance (SVR) which is about 90% of LV afterload; however, pulmonary vascular resistance (PVR) produces about 50% of RV afterload, and the RV wall stress is responsible for the other half of RV afterload.

Cardiac output Abbreviated as CO is the amount of blood which is pumped out of the heart during a 1 min interval; so, CO is the product of SV multiplied by heart rate; so, "cardiac output (ml/min) = stroke volume (ml/beat) × heart rate (beat/min)" or simply: $CO = HR \times SV$.

Ejection fraction Another important variable is ejection fraction or more commonly known as "EF.". EF is calculated based on this equation: $EF = SV/EDV$. (In this formula, EDV stands for end-diastolic volume.) Usually EF is expressed in percentage. Normal EF is usually between 55–70%, though more than 50% is considered normal for EF and consider patients having EF > 50% as good LV performance. EF is directly a very determining index of cardiac function and global clinical outcome. Patients with EF < 30% are often considered as very high risk cases impressing the global outcome.

Among the above three main factors (i.e., SV, ESV, and EDV), the cardiac work is much related to EDV and less to the other two factors; this is due to the length-tension concept of sarcomere which affects the cardiac contractility, cardiac work, and cardiac output more than the others. To understand this latter fact, we have to discuss Frank-Starling relationship in the next paragraph (Germano et al. 1995; Ababneh et al. 2000; Rozanski et al. 2000; Sharir et al. 2006; Lomsky et al. 2008; Mahadevan et al. 2008) (Tables 3.8, 3.9, 3.10, and 3.11).

Frank-Starling Relationship

For the first time, it was in 1895 that Otto Frank, the German physician and physiologist, described the relationship between length and activation of cardiac muscle fibers; the experiment was completed two decades later by Ernest Henry Starling, an English physiologist, and was named "length-dependent activation or LDA" or more commonly the "Frank-Starling relationship." Frank and Starling, in their animal model, demonstrated that increased blood accumulation in each ventricle during diastole will result in proportional increase in the amount of output from the same ventricle during systole (Markwalder and Starling 1914; Patterson et al. 1914; Cingolani et al. 2013; Neves et al. 2015).

Table 3.8 The main pressures in the cardiovascular system

	Variable
1.	Heart rate (HR)
2.	Central venous pressure (CVP)
3.	Right atrial pressure (RAP)
4.	Right ventricular pressure (RVP)
5.	Pulmonary artery pressure (PAP)
6.	Pulmonary artery wedge pressure (PAWP); pulmonary capillary wedge pressure (PCWP)
7.	Left atrial pressure (LAP)
8.	Left ventricular end-systolic pressure (LVESP)
9.	Left ventricular end-diastolic pressure (LVEDP)
10.	Aortic pressure

Parts are modified from Dabbagh (2014). Published with kind permission from © Springer, 2014. All Rights Reserved (National High Blood Pressure Education Program Working Group on High Blood Pressure in Children and Adolescents 2004; Dionne et al. 2012)

Table 3.9 Calculation formulas of main physiologic variables in the cardiovascular system

	Variable	Formula
1.	Cardiac output (CO)	$CO = SV \times HR$
2.	Cardiac index (CI)	$CI = CO/BSA$
3.	Stroke volume (SV)	$SV = (CO \times 1000)/HR$
4.	Mean arterial pressure (MAP)	$MAP = (2DBP + SBP)/3$
5.	Systemic vascular resistance (SVR)	$SVR = [(MAP\text{-}CVP) \times 80]/CO$
6.	Pulmonary vascular resistance (PVR)	$PVR = [(PAP\text{-}PAWP) \times 80]/CO$

Parts are modified from Dabbagh (2014). Published with kind permission from © Springer, 2014. All Rights Reserved (Brzezinski 1990; Dionne et al. 2012; Bonafide et al. 2013)
HR heart rate (beats/minute), *BSA* body surface area (m$_2$), *DBP* diastolic blood pressure, *SBP* systolic blood pressure

This property of cardiac muscle and cardiac fibers is preserved even when they are removed out of the body. So, cardiac muscle has a wide range of adaptation against cardiac work; in fact, preload and afterload changes are tolerated and appropriately responded due to this internal property. Under different physiologic states, cardiac muscle acts appropriately for different physiologic states from deep sleep to severe exercise, so the mechanism is named length-dependent activation (Bollensdorff et al. 2011; Neves et al. 2015).

The basis for Frank-Starling property of the heart has been explained at different levels: from the cellular level of cardiomyocytes to the neurohormonal control mechanisms of the heart. Based on Frank-Starling relationship, there is an *optimal interaction length* for sarcomere; in human sarcomere, the "optimal length" is about 2.2 μ for the sarcomere which causes the best interaction between actin and myosin (Solaro 2007; Neves et al. 2015).

Table 3.10 Normal range of blood pressure in *boys* with especial focus on "The Fourth Report on the Diagnosis, Evaluation, and Treatment of High Blood Pressure in Children and Adolescents" of the "National High Blood Pressure Education Program Working Group on High Blood Pressure in Children and Adolescents"

Age (year)	DBP mmHg		SBP mmHg		MAP mmHg	
	50% DBP	95% DBP	50% SBP	95% SBP	50% MAP	95% MAP
1	34–39	54–58	80–89	98–106	49–55	69–75
2	39–44	59–63	84–92	101–110	54–60	73–79
3	44–48	63–67	86–95	104–112	58–64	77–82
4	47–52	66–71	88–97	106–115	61–67	79–86
5	50–55	69–74	90–98	108–116	63–69	82–88
6	53–57	72–76	91–100	109–117	66–71	84–90
7	55–59	74–78	92–101	110–119	67–73	86–92
8	56–61	75–80	94–102	111–120	69–75	87–93
9	57–62	76–81	95–104	113–121	70–76	88–94
10	58–63	77–82	97–106	115–123	71–77	90–96
11	59–63	78–82	99–107	117–125	72–78	91–97
12	59–64	78–83	101–110	119–127	73–79	92–98
13	60–64	79–83	104–112	121–130	75–80	93–99
14	60–65	80–84	106–115	124–132	76–82	95–100
15	61–66	81–85	109–117	126–135	77–83	96–102
16	63–67	82–87	111–120	129–137	79–85	98–104
17	65–70	84–89	114–122	131–140	81–87	100–106

McLain (1976); Blumenthal et al. (1977); Horan and Sinaiko (1987); Feld and Springate (1988); Brzezinski (1990); Zubrow et al. (1995); Bartosh and Aronson (1999); Dionne et al. (2012); Bonafide et al. (2013); Heys et al. (2013); Shieh et al. (2013); Bassareo and Mercuro (2014); Ingelfinger (2014); Shah et al. (2015)

Each sarcomere has the internal property of length-dependent activation, i.e., if diastolic length of a contractile segment of cardiomyocyte (i.e., sarcomere) increases, then the generated force of the sarcomere during systole increases proportionally; however, this trend has a plateau. Whenever the plateau is reached, the sarcomere would produce less force during its contractions, hence, length-dependent activation. One of the proposed cellular explanations for this finding is that when the sarcomere length is more than the optimal length, the heads of actin and myosin go far from each other; then, their physiologic function impairs and less contraction is produced. On the other side of the spectrum, sudden decrease in diastolic length of sarcomere results in suppression of force generation, again with a plateau after a time period (Solaro 2007; Ribaric and Kordas 2012; Neves et al. 2015).

Though more than 100 years has passed from the findings of Frank and Starling, the exact underlying mechanisms are not fully elucidated yet, especially in the diastolic counterpart of Frank-Starling relationship (Campbell 2011; Neves et al. 2015). Today, we know that a number of different molecular mechanisms cooperate and interact together in each cardiac sarcomere to produce "strain-dependent activation," but all of

Table 3.11 Normal range of blood pressure in *girls* with especial focus on "The Fourth Report on the Diagnosis, Evaluation, and Treatment of High Blood Pressure in Children and Adolescents" of the "National High Blood Pressure Education Program Working Group on High Blood Pressure in Children and Adolescents"

Age (year)	DBP mmHg		SBP mmHg		MAP mmHg	
	50 % DBP	95 % DBP	50 % SBP	95 % SBP	50 % MAP	95 % MAP
1	38–42	56–60	83–90	100–107	53–58	71–76
2	43–47	61–65	85–91	102–109	57–62	75–80
3	47–51	65–69	86–93	104–110	60–66	78–83
4	50–54	68–72	88–94	105–112	63–67	80–85
5	52–56	70–74	89–96	106–114	64–69	82–87
6	54–58	72–76	91–98	108–115	66–71	84–89
7	55–59	73–77	92–101	110–119	67–73	85–91
8	57–60	75–78	94–102	111–120	69–74	87–92
9	58–61	76–79	95–104	113–121	70–75	88–93
10	59–62	77–80	97–106	115–123	72–77	90–94
11	60–63	78–81	99–107	117–125	73–78	91–96
12	61–64	79–82	102–109	119–126	75–79	92–97
13	62–65	80–83	104–110	121–128	76–80	94–98
14	63–66	81–84	106–112	123–129	77–81	95–99
15	64–67	82–85	107–113	124–131	78–82	96–100
16	64–68	82–86	108–114	125–132	79–83	96–101
17	64–68	82–86	108–115	125–132	81–84	96–101

McLain (1976); Blumenthal et al. (1977); Horan and Sinaiko (1987); Feld and Springate (1988); Brzezinski (1990); Zubrow et al. (1995); Bartosh and Aronson (1999); Dionne et al. (2012); Heys et al. (2013); Bassareo and Mercuro (2014); Ingelfinger (2014); Shah et al. (2015)

the fact is not discovered. At cellular and subcellular levels, a number of mechanisms have been proposed; some are more important over the others; however, more studies are underway:

- If diastolic tension increases, the number of crossbridges will increase; in turn, the overlap status of the cardiac myofilaments improves, which is in favor of more effective contractions; it could be translated that the inter-digitations of actin and myosin in diastole become more effective in production of systolic contractions (de Tombe and Ter Keurs 2015).
- With increasing length of sarcomere, the contractile force is increased in response to each level of Ca^{2+} concentration; so, the increased contractile force is the result of improved response to Ca^{2+} (Fuchs and Smith 2001; Cingolani et al. 2013; Goldhaber and Philipson 2013).
- Other proposed mechanisms are not related to "interfilament spacing" or the interaction of actin and myosin; based on these mechanisms, stretch induces some "structural rearrangements" in the thin and thick filaments of the myocardium which result in myofilament length-dependent activation and titin strain (Ait-Mou et al. 2016).

Cardiac Reflexes

Baroreceptor Reflex (or Carotid Sinus Reflex)

Baroreceptor reflex (or carotid sinus reflex) is among the most important reflexes in the cardiovascular system, affecting the hemodynamics on a beat-to-beat pattern. The discovery of different parts of this reflex is the result of the work of many scientists on this reflex and *chemoreceptor reflex*. These scientists include (but are not limited to) Claude Bernard in 1852; Heinrich Ewald Hering in 1921 and at the same time Jean-François Heymans and his son, Corneille, and De Castro in 1925; Edgar Douglas Adrian in 1932; Corneille Heymans in 1938; and Cowley and Arthur C. Guyton during the last decades (Trippodo et al. 1977; Zimmer 2004; De Castro 2009; Estanol et al. 2011). Baroreceptor reflex has a number of main components:

- *Importance*: control of blood pressure in the normal range especially for perfusion of vital organs
- *Stimulus*: severe increase or severe drop in blood pressure out of the normal values
- *Response and Physiologic Effect*: compensation for abnormal blood pressure through sympathetic or parasympathetic stimulation leading to modulation of vascular bed tone (decreased vascular tone and, hence, drop in blood pressure and bradycardia in case of sudden hypertension; increased vascular tone and, hence, rise in blood pressure and tachycardia in case of sudden hypotension). In this way, the baroreceptor reflex leads to regulation of blood pressure and systemic vascular tone, especially if it is highly elevated or there is a severe drop in blood pressure; however, many chronic cardiovascular diseases including chronic hypertension, heart failure, prolonged atherosclerosis, or other systemic diseases like chronic renal disorders, diabetes mellitus, or other chronic diseases impair the reflex partially or totally.
- *Neural pathway of the reflex*
- *Afferent limb*: carotid artery body and aortic arch

    - The receptors of the reflex are circumferential and longitudinal stretch receptors, located in carotid sinus and aortic arch; these receptors respond to increased blood pressure and then generate impulses.
    - The impulse goes from carotid sinus through the ninth cranial verve and from the aortic arch through the tenth cranial nerve.
    - Then, the impulses go from these two locations to the *nucleus solitarius*, which is the CNS center which processes the input and creates response.

- *CNS processing*

    Nucleus solitarius is located in the cardio-regulatory and vasomotor centers of the medulla.

    Nucleus solitarius is composed of two individual segments: first segment is the lateral and rostral segment also called the "pressor center," and the second segment is the central and caudal segment also named the "depressor" center.

In these two segments of *nucleus solitarius*, the afferent signals from carotid body and aortic arch are integrated with the limbic and hypothalamic inputs; finally, after these neural interactions, the efferent limb of the reflex is created.

- *Efferent limb*

When the response of the reflex should be toward decreasing blood pressure, decreased sympathetic tone is the main efferent response, which is mainly done through suppression and inhibition of sympathetic pathways; the result is *hypotension* and *bradycardia*; also, systemic vascular tone decreases which leads to dilatation of blood vessel and systemic vasodilation.

Increased tone of *parasympathetic* system is mainly through the vagus nerve and leads to bradycardia and depression of myocardial contractility.

Finally, blood pressure returns to its normal limits and the triggering of baroreceptors turns off.

However, in the event of hypotension, the above steps work in the opposite direction to augment systemic vascular tone, to augment myocardial contractility, and to increase heart rate, i.e., the other limb of the reflex would work (Vasquez et al. 1997; Pilowsky and Goodchild 2002; Campagna and Carter 2003; Kashihara 2009).

Bainbridge Reflex

Bainbridge reflex was first described in 1915 by Francis Bainbridge (British physiologist, 1874–1921).

- What did Francis Bainbridge discovered first? He infused "saline or blood into the jugular vein of the anesthetized dog" and observed *reflex tachycardia*. So, atrial reflex is another name for this reflex.
- *Stimulus*: dilation of the main systemic veins, left and right atrium.
- *Response*: increased heart rate in response to dilation of "the main systemic veins, left and right atrium."
- *Physiologic effect*: dilation of the right atrium causes activation of its neural pathway; then the signal is processed in CNS, and the response to this afferent impulse is increased sympathetic tone; in turn, increased sympathetic tone leads to increased contractility and tachycardia; finally, increased contractility and tachycardia helps the heart to become empty of the "extra load"; if we want to summarize the Bainbridge reflex, we can simply say: "Bainbridge reflex causes hypervolemia-induced tachycardia."
- *Importance*: Bainbridge reflex plays an important role in controlling heart rate and other hemodynamic variables; also, Bainbridge reflex is in contrary to the effects of the "carotid baroreceptor reflex."

- *Neural pathway* of the reflex:

  Afferent limb: the sympathetic neural pathways; the reflex is sensed in the atrial type B mechanoreceptors located in atrial tissue, just located at the junction of venae cavae and right atrial tissue and the junction of pulmonary veins and left atrial tissue; this in turn will send impulse through the vagus nerve (tenth cranial nerve) to CNS.
  Efferent limb: increased sympathetic drive through CNS to induce tachycardia.

- How is reflex blocked? If the patient is premedicated with atropine or in animal models, it is blocked by "bilateral vagotomy, or combined cholinergic and beta-adrenergic blockades" (Vatner and Zimpfer 1981; Boettcher et al. 1982; Hakumaki 1987; Hajdu et al. 1991; Barbieri et al. 2002; Crystal and Salem 2012; Cui et al. 2013).

Bezold-Jarisch Reflex

Bezold-Jarisch reflex (BJR) is known as "cardioinhibitory" reflex.

- *Who described the reflex first?*: BJR was described first by *von Bezold* and *Hirt* in 1867; *Adolf Jarisch* and *Richter* performed complementary studies in the late 1930s. They described the reflex briefly, especially its triad of "bradycardia, hypotension, and peripheral vasodilation" which is usually accompanied with *hypopnea* or *apnea*. Also, coronary artery vasodilation has been mentioned among the items of the reflex. Interestingly, Bezold and Hirt discovered the reflex during their investigations related to the effects of *veratridine* on the heart (Chandler and McDougal 2014).
- *Importance*: BJR has some cardioprotective effects; in some myocardial stress states like the acute phase of myocardial ischemia, infarction, or reperfusion syndrome, especially in the posterior or inferior myocardial walls, BJR is activated to do its protective effects (Shah and Waxman 2013).
- *Stimulus*: myocardial stressors like ischemia/reperfusion or infarction.
- *Response and physiologic effect*: *parasympathetic* overactivity is the main underlying phenomenon in BJR, associated with some degrees of *sympathetic* inhibition.
- *Neural pathway* of the reflex
- *Afferent limb*

  Mechanical stimuli (like volume or pressure overload) or chemical stimuli (like metabolites of myocardial ischemia or some chemicals) trigger some specific receptors inside the heart and located in left ventricle wall, atrial walls, atrial-caval junctions, and some other chambers of the heart.
  This trigger starts the pathway of the reflex.
  The afferent fibers are mainly non-myelinated C fibers, and 75 % of these afferent fibers are distributed over all chambers of the heart; on the other side, 25 % of the afferent fibers are myelinated and are located on the atrial walls and the atrial-caval junctions.

- *CNS processing*

  The role of the afferent fibers is to inhibit *medullary vasomotor center*, located in the medulla oblongata.

- *Efferent limb*

  When the inhibitory message reaches the medulla, two distinct effects go out of the *medullary vasomotor center*: bradycardia and suppression of the sympathetic output. Also, there is another indirect effect: decreased sympathetic output suppresses the peripheral vascular tone leading to peripheral vasodilation; systemic hypotension is the final result (Robertson et al. 1985; Hakumaki 1987; Meyrelles et al. 1997; Campagna and Carter 2003; Kashihara et al. 2004; Salo et al. 2007; Kashihara 2009; Iwase et al. 2014).

Chemoreceptor Reflex

Chemoreceptor reflex is the reflex in which changes in partial pressure of arterial oxygen and CO2 leads to respiratory control; this process is mainly through two pathways: chemoreceptor activation primarily leads to increased drive for ventilatory response and secondarily to increased sympathetic output which is associated with increased blood pressure.

Importance Both peripheral and central chemoreceptors affect and modulate the sympathetic system powerfully; so, they have great impacts in both health and disease; for example, they have contribution in generation of some diseases like heart failure, hypertension, and obstructive sleep apnea (Schultz et al. 2015; Lopez-Barneo et al. 2016).

Stimulus Decreased arterial pressure of oxygen triggers peripheral chemoreceptors in aortic arch and carotid bodies, while increased arterial pressure of CO2 (hypercarbia) triggers central chemoreceptors in brainstem.

  Neural pathway of the reflex

- *Afferent limb*:

  - There are two main chemoreceptors: peripheral chemoreceptors and central chemoreceptors; peripheral chemoreceptors respond to hypoxia; decreased pressure of oxygen in arterial blood below 80 mmHg triggers *peripheral chemoreceptors*, which are located in carotid body and aortic arch; the set point for hypoxic sensing by the carotid body is mediated in each individual by hypoxia-inducible factor-1 (HIF-1) and HIF-2 (Prabhakar and Semenza 2016). On the other hand, *central chemoreceptors* are located in brainstem and are triggered by hypercarbia (increased CO2 pressure or decreased pH of the blood).
  - Afferent nerves are the ninth (glossopharyngeal) and tenth (vagus) cranial nerves.
  - These nerves send the impulses to the medulla.

- *CNS processing*: rostral ventrolateral medulla is the main central location for processing the inputs from chemoreceptors.
- *Efferent limb*: sympathetic pathway is the main efferent limb; however, if hypoxia and hypercarbia persist, *parasympathetic* pathway is activated.

Response and physiologic effect The response would be increased sympathetic tone to compensate for hypoxia and hypercarbia, but in the cases of unresolved hypoxia and hypercarbia, the response of the reflex would be altered as *parasympathetic* stimulation which will be presented as bradycardia and coronary vasodilation (both through activation of the vagus nerve) in order to decrease oxygen demands (Schultz and Sun 2000; Kara et al. 2003; Schultz and Li 2007; Ding et al. 2011; Schultz 2011; Campanucci et al. 2012; Schultz et al. 2012; Schultz and Marcus 2012; Lopez-Barneo et al. 2016).

Valsalva Maneuver

Valsalva maneuver is the name for a cardiac reflex starting with a forced expiration against a "closed glottis."

Who described the reflex first? The "Valsalva maneuver" was first described by Valsalva in 1704.

Neural Pathway

- *Afferent limb*: baroreceptors of the arterial system
- *CNS processing*: medulla
- *Efferent limb*: sympathetic pathway

Response and physiologic effect Due to forced expiration against closed glottis, intrathoracic pressure increases suddenly with resultant increased central venous pressure (CVP) which subsequently leads to decreased venous return. The result is decreased cardiac output and a drop in blood pressure. However, baroreceptors of the arterial system will sense this blood pressure drop and will start firing the triggering signals for sympathetic stimulation leading to tachycardia.

Whenever the glottis is opened and venous return resumes, cardiac output and blood pressure are normalized, and this will lead to baroreceptor inhibition and "normal heart rate."

Importance We usually see a "sequence of rapid changes in preload and afterload stress" during Valsalva maneuver which is used for some clinical therapeutic and diagnostic implications, for example, for assessment of the interatrial shunts during echocardiography exam (like patent foramen ovale exam), for assessment of the treatment in supraventricular arrhythmias, or for assessment of the murmurs in hypertrophic cardiomyopathy, atrial septal defect, mitral valve prolapse, pulmonary stenosis, aortic stenosis, and tricuspid regurgitation (Sharpey-Schafer 1955; Porth et al. 1984; Nagappan et al. 2002; Zuber et al. 2008; Smith 2012; Wang et al. 2013).

Cushing Reflex

Cushing reflex – This reflex is among the cardiovascular reflexes that aim to protect the brain. Cushing reflex is very well known with its triad.

Who described the reflex first? Cushing reflex was introduced in 1901–1902 by Harvey Cushing (1869–1939).

Importance response and physiologic effect The Cushing reflex is an alarm for abnormal increase in intracranial pressure (ICP); in other words, Cushing reflex is an important sign for impaired cerebral perfusion status and potential cerebral ischemia. Also, sudden and inadvertent intravenous epinephrine administration could elicit the reflex. The reflex is usually seen in clinic as the following triad:

- Bradycardia
- Hypertension (increased systolic blood pressure and wide pulse pressure)
- Respiratory depression (respiratory irregularity ending to bradypnea and apnea)

Often an abrupt increase in ICP is due to increased production of cerebrospinal fluid (CSF), decreased CSF reabsorption, or a mass effect in the CNS; in a considerable number of the patients, these could be associated with cerebral herniation and death.

Stimulus Increase in ICP; (often) leading to cerebral ischemia

Neural Pathway

Afferent limb Increased ICP causes impaired CNS perfusion leading to ischemia of the brain which is sensed by perfusion receptors of the brain; these inputs activate the sympathetic pathway.

CNS processing Medulla sends the orders to the sympathetic system.

Efferent limb Sympathetic pathway is activated in an attempt to compensate for reduced cerebral perfusion; alpha-1 adrenergic stimulation is one of the main targets of sympathetic activation which leads to widespread arteriolar vasoconstriction. The resulting clinical picture is increased heart rate, blood pressure, and myocardial contractility; however, hypertension is sensed by baroreceptors located in the aortic arch and carotid sinus, and then, reflex bradycardia happens. Finally, increased blood pressure affects the respiratory pattern leading to irregularity in respiration. In this way, the triad of Cushing reflex is completed: hypertension, bradycardia, and respiratory depression (Grady and Blaumanis 1988; Dickinson 1990; Ayling 2002; Fodstad et al. 2006; Molnar et al. 2008; Wan et al. 2008; Robbins et al. 2016).

Oculocardiac Reflex

Oculocardiac reflex also known as trigeminal cardiac reflex (TCR) is triggered by traction on the extraocular muscles (especially rectus medialis), or it may be elicited by painful stimulation of the eyeball or some other structures of the face. Aging decreases the frequency of occurrence of the reflex. Also, the reflex is somewhat prevented by anticholinergic pretreatment like atropine. The pathway of this reflex is composed of:

- *Afferent limb*: ophthalmic division of the fifth cranial nerve (trigeminal nerve); the other branches of the trigeminal nerve (maxillary and mandibular branches) might also be involved; the impulses go to CNS via the Gasserian ganglion.
- *CNS processing*: sensory nucleus of the trigeminal nerve goes through internuncial fibers to the reticular formation and then to the motor nucleus of the vagus nerve.
- *Efferent limb*: tenth cranial nerve (vagus nerve) causing sinus bradycardia as the final clinical presentation of the reflex; at times, junctional rhythms, asystole, other arrhythmias, atrioventricular blocks, or even hypotension may be seen (Arasho et al. 2009; Tsai and Heitz 2012; Bhargava et al. 2014; Meuwly et al. 2015).

References

Ababneh AA, Sciacca RR, Kim B, Bergmann SR. Normal limits for left ventricular ejection fraction and volumes estimated with gated myocardial perfusion imaging in patients with normal exercise test results: influence of tracer, gender, and acquisition camera. J Nucl Cardiol. 2000; 7:661–8.

Ahmad S, Ahmad A, Hendry-Hofer TB, Loader JE, Claycomb WC, Mozziconacci O, Schoneich C, Reisdorph N, Powell RL, Chandler JD, Day BJ, Veress LA, White CW. Sarcoendoplasmic reticulum ca(2+) ATPase. A critical target in chlorine inhalation-induced cardiotoxicity. Am J Respir Cell Mol Biol. 2015;52:492–502.

Ait-Mou Y, Hsu K, Farman GP, Kumar M, Greaser ML, Irving TC, de Tombe PP. Titin strain contributes to the Frank-Starling law of the heart by structural rearrangements of both thin- and thick-filament proteins. Proc Natl Acad Sci U S A. 2016;113:2306–11.

Amanfu RK, Saucerman JJ. Cardiac models in drug discovery and development: a review. Crit Rev Biomed Eng. 2011;39:379–95.

Anderson BR, Granzier HL. Titin-based tension in the cardiac sarcomere: molecular origin and physiological adaptations. Prog Biophys Mol Biol. 2012;110:204–17.

Arasho B, Sandu N, Spiriev T, Prabhakar H, Schaller B. Management of the trigeminocardiac reflex: facts and own experience. Neurol India. 2009;57:375–80.

Aronson D, Krum H. Novel therapies in acute and chronic heart failure. Pharmacol Ther. 2012;135:1–17.

Asghari P, Scriven DR, Sanatani S, Gandhi SK, Campbell AI, Moore ED. Nonuniform and variable arrangements of ryanodine receptors within mammalian ventricular couplons. Circ Res. 2014;115:252–62.

Asp ML, Martindale JJ, Heinis FI, Wang W, Metzger JM. Calcium mishandling in diastolic dysfunction: mechanisms and potential therapies. Biochim Biophys Acta. 2013;1833:895–900.

Atkinson A, Inada S, Li J, Tellez JO, Yanni J, Sleiman R, Allah EA, Anderson RH, Zhang H, Boyett MR, Dobrzynski H. Anatomical and molecular mapping of the left and right ventricular His-Purkinje conduction networks. J Mol Cell Cardiol. 2011;51:689–701.

Ayling J. Managing head injuries. Emerg Med Serv. 2002;31:42.

Azhibekov T, Noori S, Soleymani S, Seri I. Transitional cardiovascular physiology and comprehensive hemodynamic monitoring in the neonate: relevance to research and clinical care. Semin Fetal Neonatal Med. 2014;19:45–53.

Bai F, Wang L, Kawai M. A study of tropomyosin's role in cardiac function and disease using thin-filament reconstituted myocardium. J Muscle Res Cell Motil. 2013;34:295–310.

Baik N, Urlesberger B, Schwaberger B, Freidl T, Schmolzer GM, Pichler G. Cardiocirculatory monitoring during immediate fetal-to-neonatal transition: a systematic qualitative review of the literature. Neonatology. 2015;107:100–7.

Barbieri R, Triedman JK, Saul JP. Heart rate control and mechanical cardiopulmonary coupling to assess central volume: a systems analysis. Am J Physiol Regul Integr Comp Physiol. 2002;283:R1210–20.

Bartosh SM, Aronson AJ. Childhood hypertension. An update on etiology, diagnosis, and treatment. Pediatr Clin North Am. 1999;46:235–52.

Bassareo PP, Mercuro G. Pediatric hypertension: an update on a burning problem. World J Cardiol. 2014;6:253–9.

Bers DM. Cardiac excitation-contraction coupling. Nature. 2002;415:198–205.

Bhargava D, Thomas S, Chakravorty N, Dutt A. Trigeminocardiac reflex: a reappraisal with relevance to maxillofacial surgery. J Maxillofac Oral Surg. 2014;13:373–7.

Bhupathy P, Babu GJ, Periasamy M. Sarcolipin and phospholamban as regulators of cardiac sarcoplasmic reticulum Ca2+ ATPase. J Mol Cell Cardiol. 2007;42:903–11.

Blumenthal S, Epps RP, Heavenrich R, Lauer RM, Lieberman E, Mirkin B, Mitchell SC, Boyar Naito V, O'Hare D, McFate Smith W, Tarazi RC, Upson D. Report of the task force on blood pressure control in children. Pediatrics. 1977;59:I-II, 797–820.

Boettcher DH, Zimpfer M, Vatner SF. Phylogenesis of the Bainbridge reflex. Am J Physiol. 1982;242:R244–6.

Bollensdorff C, Lookin O, Kohl P. Assessment of contractility in intact ventricular cardiomyocytes using the dimensionless 'Frank-Starling Gain' index. Pflugers Arch. 2011;462:39–48.

Bonafide CP, Brady PW, Keren R, Conway PH, Marsolo K, Daymont C. Development of heart and respiratory rate percentile curves for hospitalized children. Pediatrics. 2013;131:e1150–7.

Brunet S, Emrick MA, Sadilek M, Scheuer T, Catterall WA. Phosphorylation sites in the Hook domain of CaVbeta subunits differentially modulate CaV1.2 channel function. J Mol Cell Cardiol. 2015;87:248–56.

Brzezinski WA. Blood pressure. In: Walker HK, Hall WD, Hurst JW, editors. Clinical methods: the history, physical, and laboratory examinations. Boston: Butterworth Publishers, a division of Reed Publishing; 1990.

Campagna JA, Carter C. Clinical relevance of the Bezold-Jarisch reflex. Anesthesiology. 2003;98:1250–60.

Campanucci VA, Dookhoo L, Vollmer C, Nurse CA. Modulation of the carotid body sensory discharge by NO: an up-dated hypothesis. Respir Physiol Neurobiol. 2012;184:149–57.

Campbell KS. Impact of myocyte strain on cardiac myofilament activation. Pflugers Arch. 2011;462:3–14.

Carlsson M, Andersson R, Bloch KM, Steding-Ehrenborg K, Mosen H, Stahlberg F, Ekmehag B, Arheden H. Cardiac output and cardiac index measured with cardiovascular magnetic resonance in healthy subjects, elite athletes and patients with congestive heart failure. J Cardiovasc Magn Reson. 2012;14:51.

Chandler CM, McDougal OM. Medicinal history of North American. Phytochem Rev. 2014;13:671–94.

Chang AN, Parvatiyar MS, Potter JD. Troponin and cardiomyopathy. Biochem Biophys Res Commun. 2008;369:74–81.

Chatterjee K. Pathophysiology of systolic and diastolic heart failure. Med Clin North Am. 2012;96:891–9.

Chemla D, Coirault C, Hebert JL, Lecarpentier Y. Mechanics of relaxation of the human heart. News Physiol Sci. 2000;15:78–83.

Chen F, Wetzel GT, Friedman WF, Klitzner TS. Single-channel recording of inwardly rectifying potassium currents in developing myocardium. J Mol Cell Cardiol. 1991;23:259–67.

Cingolani HE, Perez NG, Cingolani OH, Ennis IL. The Anrep effect: 100 years later. Am J Physiol Heart Circ Physiol. 2013;304:H175–82.

Cleland JG, Teerlink JR, Senior R, Nifontov EM, Mc Murray JJ, Lang CC, Tsyrlin VA, Greenberg BH, Mayet J, Francis DP, Shaburishvili T, Monaghan M, Saltzberg M, Neyses L, Wasserman SM, Lee JH, Saikali KG, Clarke CP, Goldman JH, Wolff AA, Malik FI. The effects of the cardiac myosin activator, omecamtiv mecarbil, on cardiac function in systolic heart failure: a double-blind, placebo-controlled, crossover, dose-ranging phase 2 trial. Lancet. 2011;378:676–83.

Coronel R, Janse MJ, Opthof T, Wilde AA, Taggart P. Postrepolarization refractoriness in acute ischemia and after antiarrhythmic drug administration: action potential duration is not always an index of the refractory period. Heart Rhythm. 2012;9:977–82.

Craig R, Lee KH, Mun JY, Torre I, Luther PK. Structure, sarcomeric organization, and thin filament binding of cardiac myosin-binding protein-C. Pflugers Arch. 2014;466:425–31.

Crystal GJ, Salem MR. The Bainbridge and the "reverse" Bainbridge reflexes: history, physiology, and clinical relevance. Anesth Analg. 2012;114:520–32.

Cui J, Gao Z, Blaha C, Herr MD, Mast J, Sinoway LI. Distension of central great vein decreases sympathetic outflow in humans. Am J Physiol Heart Circ Physiol. 2013;305:H378–85.

Dabbagh A. Cardiac physiology. In: Dabbagh A, Esmailian F, Aranki SF, editors. Postoperative critical care for cardiac surgical patients. Berlin: Springer; 2014. p. 1–39.

De Castro F. The discovery of sensory nature of the carotid bodies – invited article. Adv Exp Med Biol. 2009;648:1–18.

de Tombe PP, Ter Keurs HE. Cardiac muscle mechanics: Sarcomere length matters. J Mol Cell Cardiol. 2015;91:148–50.

Desplantez T, Dupont E, Severs NJ, Weingart R. Gap junction channels and cardiac impulse propagation. J Membr Biol. 2007;218:13–28.

Dickinson CJ. Reappraisal of the Cushing reflex: the most powerful neural blood pressure stabilizing system. Clin Sci (Lond). 1990;79:543–50.

DiFrancesco D, Noble D. The funny current has a major pacemaking role in the sinus node. Heart Rhythm. 2012;9:299–301.

Ding Y, Li YL, Schultz HD. Role of blood flow in carotid body chemoreflex function in heart failure. J Physiol. 2011;589:245–58.

Dionne JM, Abitbol CL, Flynn JT. Hypertension in infancy: diagnosis, management and outcome. Pediatric Nephrol (Berlin, Germany). 2012;27:17–32.

Duley L, Batey N. Optimal timing of umbilical cord clamping for term and preterm babies. Early Hum Dev. 2013;89:4.

Dun W, Boyden PA. The Purkinje cell; 2008 style. J Mol Cell Cardiol. 2008;45:617–24.

Espinoza-Fonseca LM, Autry JM, Ramirez-Salinas GL, Thomas DD. Atomic-level mechanisms for phospholamban regulation of the calcium pump. Biophys J. 2015;108:1697–708.

Estanol B, Porras-Betancourt M, Padilla-Leyva MA, Senties-Madrid H. A brief history of the baroreceptor reflex: from Claude Bernard to Arthur C. Guyton. Illustrated with some classical experiments. Arch Cardiol Mex. 2011;81:330–6.

Fabiato A. Calcium-induced release of calcium from the cardiac sarcoplasmic reticulum. Am J Physiol. 1983;245:C1–14.

Fabiato A, Fabiato F. Calcium release from the sarcoplasmic reticulum. Circ Res. 1977;40:119–29.

Fabiato A, Fabiato F. Calcium-induced release of calcium from the sarcoplasmic reticulum of skinned cells from adult human, dog, cat, rabbit, rat, and frog hearts and from fetal and newborn rat ventricles. Ann N Y Acad Sci. 1978;307:491–522.

Feld LG, Springate JE. Hypertension in children. Curr Probl Pediatr. 1988;18:317–73.

Fodstad H, Kelly PJ, Buchfelder M. History of the cushing reflex. Neurosurgery. 2006;59:1132–7; discussion 1137.

Frank JS, Mottino G, Chen F, Peri V, Holland P, Tuana BS. Subcellular distribution of dystrophin in isolated adult and neonatal cardiac myocytes. Am J Physiol. 1994;267:C1707–16.

Frank KF, Bolck B, Erdmann E, Schwinger RH. Sarcoplasmic reticulum Ca2 + –ATPase modulates cardiac contraction and relaxation. Cardiovasc Res. 2003;57:20–7.

Fuchs F, Smith SH. Calcium, cross-bridges, and the Frank-Starling relationship. News Physiol Sci. 2001;16:5–10.

Galinsky R, Hooper SB, Wallace MJ, Westover AJ, Black MJ, Moss TJ, Polglase GR. Intrauterine inflammation alters cardiopulmonary and cerebral haemodynamics at birth in preterm lambs. J Physiol. 2013;591:2127–37.

Gao Y, Raj JU. Regulation of the pulmonary circulation in the fetus and newborn. Physiol Rev. 2010;90:1291–335.

Garg V, Frishman WH. A new approach to inotropic therapy in the treatment of heart failure: cardiac myosin activators in treatment of HF. Cardiol Rev. 2013;21:155–9.

George M, Rajaram M, Shanmugam E, VijayaKumar TM. Novel drug targets in clinical development for heart failure. Eur J Clin Pharmacol. 2014;70:765–74.

Germano G, Kiat H, Kavanagh PB, Moriel M, Mazzanti M, Su HT, Van Train KF, Berman DS. Automatic quantification of ejection fraction from gated myocardial perfusion SPECT. J Nucl Med. 1995;36:2138–47.

Gibson DG, Francis DP. Clinical assessment of left ventricular diastolic function. Heart. 2003;89:231–8.

Goldhaber JI, Philipson KD. Cardiac sodium-calcium exchange and efficient excitation-contraction coupling: implications for heart disease. Adv Exp Med Biol. 2013;961:355–64.

Gordan R, Gwathmey JK, Xie LH. Autonomic and endocrine control of cardiovascular function. World J Cardiol. 2015;7:204–14.

Grady PA, Blaumanis OR. Physiologic parameters of the Cushing reflex. Surg Neurol. 1988;29: 454–61.

Gustafsson AB, Gottlieb RA. Autophagy in ischemic heart disease. Circ Res. 2009;104:150–8.

Hajdu MA, Cornish KG, Tan W, Panzenbeck MJ, Zucker IH. The interaction of the Bainbridge and Bezold-Jarisch reflexes in the conscious dog. Basic Res Cardiol. 1991;86:175–85.

Hakumaki MO. Seventy years of the Bainbridge reflex. Acta Physiol Scand. 1987;130:177–85.

Hamdani N, Franssen C, Lourenco A, Falcao-Pires I, Fontoura D, Leite S, Plettig L, Lopez B, Ottenheijm CA, Becher PM, Gonzalez A, Tschope C, Diez J, Linke WA, Leite-Moreira AF, Paulus WJ. Myocardial titin hypophosphorylation importantly contributes to heart failure with preserved ejection fraction in a rat metabolic risk model. Circ Heart Fail. 2013a;6:1239–49.

Hamdani N, Krysiak J, Kreusser MM, Neef S, Dos Remedios CG, Maier LS, Kruger M, Backs J, Linke WA. Crucial role for Ca2(+)/calmodulin-dependent protein kinase-II in regulating diastolic stress of normal and failing hearts via titin phosphorylation. Circ Res. 2013b;112:664–74.

Heys M, Lin SL, Lam TH, Leung GM, Schooling CM. Lifetime growth and blood pressure in adolescence: Hong Kong's "Children of 1997" birth cohort. Pediatrics. 2013;131:e62–72.

Hidalgo CG, Chung CS, Saripalli C, Methawasin M, Hutchinson KR, Tsaprailis G, Labeit S, Mattiazzi A, Granzier HL. The multifunctional Ca(2+)/calmodulin-dependent protein kinase II delta (CaMKII delta) phosphorylates cardiac titin's spring elements. J Mol Cell Cardiol. 2013;54:90–7.

Hines MH. Neonatal cardiovascular physiology. Semin Pediatr Surg. 2013;22:174–8.

Hitchcock-DeGregori SE. Tropomyosin: function follows structure. Adv Exp Med Biol. 2008;644:60–72.

Horan MJ, Sinaiko AR. Synopsis of the report of the second task force on blood pressure control in children. Hypertension. 1987;10:115–21.

Ingelfinger JR. Clinical practice. The child or adolescent with elevated blood pressure. N Engl J Med. 2014;370:2316–25.

Iwase S, Nishimura N, Mano T. Role of sympathetic nerve activity in the process of fainting. Front Physiol. 2014;5:343.

Jagatheesan G, Rajan S, Wieczorek DF. Investigations into tropomyosin function using mouse models. J Mol Cell Cardiol. 2010;48:893–8.

Kalyva A, Parthenakis FI, Marketou ME, Kontaraki JE, Vardas PE. Biochemical characterisation of Troponin C mutations causing hypertrophic and dilated cardiomyopathies. J Muscle Res Cell Motil. 2014;35:161–78.

Kara T, Narkiewicz K, Somers VK. Chemoreflexes – physiology and clinical implications. Acta Physiol Scand. 2003;177:377–84.

Kashihara K. Roles of arterial baroreceptor reflex during bezold-jarisch reflex. Curr Cardiol Rev. 2009;5:263–7.

Kashihara K, Kawada T, Li M, Sugimachi M, Sunagawa K. Bezold-Jarisch reflex blunts arterial baroreflex via the shift of neural arc toward lower sympathetic nerve activity. Jpn J Physiol. 2004;54:395–404.

Katheria A, Leone T. Altered transitional circulation in infants of diabetic mothers with strict antenatal obstetric management: a functional echocardiography study. J Perinatol. 2012;32:508–13.

Kawamura Y, Ishiwata T, Takizawa M, Ishida H, Asano Y, Nonoyama S. Fetal and neonatal development of Ca2+ transients and functional sarcoplasmic reticulum in beating mouse hearts. Circ J. 2010;74:1442–50.

Kawase Y, Hajjar RJ. The cardiac sarcoplasmic/endoplasmic reticulum calcium ATPase: a potent target for cardiovascular diseases. Nat Clin Pract Cardiovasc Med. 2008;5:554–65.

Kekenes-Huskey PM, Lindert S, McCammon JA. Molecular basis of calcium-sensitizing and desensitizing mutations of the human cardiac troponin C regulatory domain: a multi-scale simulation study. PLoS Comput Biol. 2012;8:e1002777.

Kobayashi T, Jin L, de Tombe PP. Cardiac thin filament regulation. Pflugers Arch. 2008;457: 37–46.

Kobirumaki-Shimozawa F, Inoue T, Shintani SA, Oyama K, Terui T, Minamisawa S, Ishiwata S, Fukuda N. Cardiac thin filament regulation and the Frank-Starling mechanism. J Physiol Sci. 2014;64:221–32.

Kotter S, Gout L, Von Frieling-Salewsky M, Muller AE, Helling S, Marcus K, Dos Remedios C, Linke WA, Kruger M. Differential changes in titin domain phosphorylation increase myofilament stiffness in failing human hearts. Cardiovasc Res. 2013;99:648–56.

Kuster DW, Bawazeer AC, Zaremba R, Goebel M, Boontje NM, van der Velden J. Cardiac myosin binding protein C phosphorylation in cardiac disease. J Muscle Res Cell Motil. 2012;33: 43–52.

Lakatta EG, Maltsev VA, Vinogradova TM. A coupled SYSTEM of intracellular Ca2+ clocks and surface membrane voltage clocks controls the timekeeping mechanism of the heart's pacemaker. Circ Res. 2010;106:659–73.

LeWinter MM, Wu Y, Labeit S, Granzier H. Cardiac titin: structure, functions and role in disease. Clin Chim Acta. 2007;375:1–9.

Lomsky M, Johansson L, Gjertsson P, Bjork J, Edenbrandt L. Normal limits for left ventricular ejection fraction and volumes determined by gated single photon emission computed tomography – a comparison between two quantification methods. Clin Physiol Funct Imaging. 2008;28: 169–73.

Lopez-Barneo J, Ortega-Saenz P, Gonzalez-Rodriguez P, Fernandez-Aguera MC, Macias D, Pardal R, Gao L. Oxygen-sensing by arterial chemoreceptors: mechanisms and medical translation. Mol Aspects Med. 2016;47–48:90–108.

Mahadevan G, Davis RC, Frenneaux MP, Hobbs FD, Lip GY, Sanderson JE, Davies MK. Left ventricular ejection fraction: are the revised cut-off points for defining systolic dysfunction sufficiently evidence based? Heart. 2008;94:426–8.

Mahony L. Calcium homeostasis and control of contractility in the developing heart. Semin Perinatol. 1996;20:510–9.

Maier LS, Wahl-Schott C, Horn W, Weichert S, Pagel C, Wagner S, Dybkova N, Muller OJ, Nabauer M, Franz WM, Pieske B. Increased SR Ca2+ cycling contributes to improved contractile performance in SERCA2a-overexpressing transgenic rats. Cardiovasc Res. 2005;67: 636–46.

Malik FI, Morgan BP. Cardiac myosin activation part 1: from concept to clinic. J Mol Cell Cardiol. 2011;51:454–61.

Maltsev VA, Lakatta EG. Cardiac pacemaker cell failure with preserved I(f), I(CaL), and I(Kr): a lesson about pacemaker function learned from ischemia-induced bradycardia. J Mol Cell Cardiol. 2007;42:289–94.

Maltsev VA, Lakatta EG. The funny current in the context of the coupled-clock pacemaker cell system. Heart Rhythm. 2012;9:302–7.

Maltsev VA, Vinogradova TM, Lakatta EG. The emergence of a general theory of the initiation and strength of the heartbeat. J Pharmacol Sci. 2006;100:338–69.

Maltsev VA, Yaniv Y, Maltsev AV, Stern MD, Lakatta EG. Modern perspectives on numerical modeling of cardiac pacemaker cell. J Pharmacol Sci. 2014;125:6–38.

Mangoni ME, Nargeot J. Genesis and regulation of the heart automaticity. Physiol Rev. 2008;88: 919–82.

Marcotti W, Johnson SL, Kros CJ. A transiently expressed SK current sustains and modulates action potential activity in immature mouse inner hair cells. J Physiol. 2004;560:691–708.

Marionneau C, Abriel H. Regulation of the cardiac Na channel Na1.5 by post-translational modifications. J Mol Cell Cardiol. 2015;82:36–47.

Markwalder J, Starling EH. On the constancy of the systolic output under varying conditions. J Physiol. 1914;48:348–56.

Marston SB, Redwood CS. Modulation of thin filament activation by breakdown or isoform switching of thin filament proteins: physiological and pathological implications. Circ Res. 2003;93:1170–8.

McDonald SJ, Middleton P, Dowswell T, Morris PS. Effect of timing of umbilical cord clamping of term infants on maternal and neonatal outcomes. Cochrane Database Syst Rev 2013(7): CD004074.

McLain LG. Hypertension in childhood: a review. Am Heart J. 1976;92:634–47.

McNally EM, Barefield DY, Puckelwartz MJ. The genetic landscape of cardiomyopathy and its role in heart failure. Cell Metab. 2015;21:174–82.

Mesirca P, Torrente AG, Mangoni ME. T-type channels in the sino-atrial and atrioventricular pacemaker mechanism. Pflugers Arch. 2014;466:791–9.

Mesirca P, Torrente AG, Mangoni ME. Functional role of voltage gated Ca(2+) channels in heart automaticity. Front Physiol. 2015;6:19.

Meuwly C, Golanov E, Chowdhury T, Erne P, Schaller B. Trigeminal cardiac reflex: new thinking model about the definition based on a literature review. Medicine. 2015;94:e484.

Meyrelles SS, Bernardes CF, Modolo RP, Mill JG, Vasquez EC. Bezold-Jarisch reflex in myocardial infarcted rats. J Auton Nerv Syst. 1997;63:144–52.

Mikawa T, Hurtado R. Development of the cardiac conduction system. Semin Cell Dev Biol. 2007;18:90–100.

Mitchell JR, Wang JJ. Expanding application of the Wiggers diagram to teach cardiovascular physiology. Adv Physiol Educ. 2014;38:170–5.

Molnar C, Nemes C, Szabo S, Fulesdi B. Harvey Cushing, a pioneer of neuroanesthesia. J Anesth. 2008;22:483–6.

Motloch LJ, Larbig R, Gebing T, Reda S, Schwaiger A, Leitner J, Wolny M, Eckardt L, Hoppe UC. By regulating mitochondrial Ca2+–uptake UCP2 modulates intracellular Ca2. PLoS One. 2016;11:e0148359.

Myslivecek J, Trojan S. Regulation of adrenoceptors and muscarinic receptors in the heart. Gen Physiol Biophys. 2003;22:3–14.

Nagappan R, Arora S, Winter C. Potential dangers of the Valsalva maneuver and adenosine in paroxysmal supraventricular tachycardia – beware preexcitation. Crit Care Resusc. 2002;4: 107–11.

Nakanishi T, Seguchi M, Takao A. Development of the myocardial contractile system. Experientia. 1988;44:936–44.

National High Blood Pressure Education Program Working Group on High Blood Pressure in Children and Adolescents. The fourth report on the diagnosis, evaluation, and treatment of high blood pressure in children and adolescents. Pediatrics. 2004;114:555–76.

Neves JS, Leite-Moreira AM, Neiva-Sousa M, Almeida-Coelho J, Castro-Ferreira R, Leite-Moreira AF. Acute myocardial response to stretch: what we (don't) know. Front Physiol. 2015;6:408.

Nevzorov IA, Levitsky DI. Tropomyosin: double helix from the protein world. Biochemistry (Mosc). 2011;76:1507–27.

Nishikawa KC, Monroy JA, Uyeno TE, Yeo SH, Pai DK, Lindstedt SL. Is titin a 'winding filament'? A new twist on muscle contraction. Proc Biol Sci. 2012;279:981–90.

Noori S, Wlodaver A, Gottipati V, McCoy M, Schultz D, Escobedo M. Transitional changes in cardiac and cerebral hemodynamics in term neonates at birth. J Pediatr. 2012;160:943–8.

Ohtsuki I, Morimoto S. Troponin: regulatory function and disorders. Biochem Biophys Res Commun. 2008;369:62–73.

Ono K, Iijima T. Cardiac T-type Ca(2+) channels in the heart. J Mol Cell Cardiol. 2010;48:65–70.

Papaioannou VE, Verkerk AO, Amin AS, de Bakker JM. Intracardiac origin of heart rate variability, pacemaker funny current and their possible association with critical illness. Curr Cardiol Rev. 2013;9:82–96.

Parham WA, Mehdirad AA, Biermann KM, Fredman CS. Hyperkalemia revisited. Tex Heart Inst J. 2006;33:40–7.

Park WK, Kim MH, Ahn DS, Chae JE, Jee YS, Chung N, Lynch 3rd C. Myocardial depressant effects of desflurane: mechanical and electrophysiologic actions in vitro. Anesthesiology. 2007;106:956–66.

Patterson SW, Piper H, Starling EH. The regulation of the heart beat. J Physiol. 1914;48:465–513.

Pavlovic M, Schaller A, Pfammatter JP, Carrel T, Berdat P, Gallati S. Age-dependent suppression of SERCA2a mRNA in pediatric atrial myocardium. Biochem Biophys Res Commun. 2005;326:344–8.

Periasamy M, Bhupathy P, Babu GJ. Regulation of sarcoplasmic reticulum Ca2+ ATPase pump expression and its relevance to cardiac muscle physiology and pathology. Cardiovasc Res. 2008;77:265–73.

Pilowsky PM, Goodchild AK. Baroreceptor reflex pathways and neurotransmitters: 10 years on. J Hypertens. 2002;20:1675–88.

Porth CJ, Bamrah VS, Tristani FE, Smith JJ. The Valsalva maneuver: mechanisms and clinical implications. Heart Lung. 1984;13:507–18.

Prabhakar NR, Semenza GL. Regulation of carotid body oxygen sensing by hypoxia-inducible factors. Pflugers Arch. 2016;468:71–5.

Prakash YS, Seckin I, Hunter LW, Sieck GC. Mechanisms underlying greater sensitivity of neonatal cardiac muscle to volatile anesthetics. Anesthesiology. 2002;96:893–906.

Pyle WG, Solaro RJ. At the crossroads of myocardial signaling: the role of Z-discs in intracellular signaling and cardiac function. Circ Res. 2004;94:296–305.

Qu Y, Karnabi E, Ramadan O, Yue Y, Chahine M, Boutjdir M. Perinatal and postnatal expression of Cav1.3 alpha1D Ca(2)(+) channel in the rat heart. Pediatr Res. 2011;69:479–84.

Quinn TA, Kohl P, Ravens U. Cardiac mechano-electric coupling research: fifty years of progress and scientific innovation. Prog Biophys Mol Biol. 2014;115:71–5.

Rabe H, Diaz-Rossello JL, Duley L, Dowswell T. Effect of timing of umbilical cord clamping and other strategies to influence placental transfusion at preterm birth on maternal and infant outcomes. Cochrane Database Syst Rev 2012(8):CD003248.

Rabi Y, Yee W, Chen SY, Singhal N. Oxygen saturation trends immediately after birth. J Pediatr. 2006;148:590–4.

Racca AW, Klaiman JM, Pioner JM, Cheng Y, Beck AE, Moussavi-Harami F, Bamshad MJ, Regnier M. Contractile properties of developing human fetal cardiac muscle. J Physiol. 2016;594:437–52.

Rain S, Bos Dda S, Handoko ML, Westerhof N, Stienen G, Ottenheijm C, Goebel M, Dorfmuller P, Guignabert C, Humbert M, Bogaard HJ, Remedios CD, Saripalli C, Hidalgo CG, Granzier HL, Vonk-Noordegraaf A, van der Velden J, de Man FS. Protein changes contributing to right ventricular cardiomyocyte diastolic dysfunction in pulmonary arterial hypertension. J Am Heart Assoc. 2014;3:e000716.

Redwood C, Robinson P. Alpha-tropomyosin mutations in inherited cardiomyopathies. J Muscle Res Cell Motil. 2013;34:285–94.

Ribaric S, Kordas M. Simulation of the frank-starling law of the heart. Comput Math Methods Med. 2012;2012:267834.

Robbins MS, Robertson CE, Kaplan E, Ailani J, Charleston L, Kuruvilla D, Blumenfeld A, Berliner R, Rosen NL, Duarte R, Vidwan J, Halker RB, Gill N, Ashkenazi A. The sphenopalatine ganglion: anatomy, pathophysiology, and therapeutic targeting in headache. Headache. 2016;56(2):240–58.

Robertson D, Hollister AS, Forman MB, Robertson RM. Reflexes unique to myocardial ischemia and infarction. J Am Coll Cardiol. 1985;5:99B–104.

Rozanski A, Nichols K, Yao SS, Malholtra S, Cohen R, DePuey EG. Development and application of normal limits for left ventricular ejection fraction and volume measurements from 99mTc-sestamibi myocardial perfusion gates SPECT. J Nucl Med. 2000;41:1445–50.

Salo LM, Woods RL, Anderson CR, McAllen RM. Nonuniformity in the von Bezold-Jarisch reflex. Am J Physiol Regul Integr Comp Physiol. 2007;293:R714–20.

Sasse S, Brand NJ, Kyprianou P, Dhoot GK, Wade R, Arai M, Periasamy M, Yacoub MH, Barton PJ. Troponin I gene expression during human cardiac development and in end-stage heart failure. Circ Res. 1993;72:932–8.

Schultz HD. Angiotensin and carotid body chemoreception in heart failure. Curr Opin Pharmacol. 2011;11:144–9.

Schultz HD, Li YL. Carotid body function in heart failure. Respir Physiol Neurobiol. 2007;157:171–85.

Schultz HD, Marcus NJ. Heart failure and carotid body chemoreception. Adv Exp Med Biol. 2012;758:387–95.

Schultz HD, Sun SY. Chemoreflex function in heart failure. Heart Fail Rev. 2000;5:45–56.

Schultz HD, Del Rio R, Ding Y, Marcus NJ. Role of neurotransmitter gases in the control of the carotid body in heart failure. Respir Physiol Neurobiol. 2012;184:197–203.

Schultz HD, Marcus NJ, Del Rio R. Role of the carotid body chemoreflex in the pathophysiology of heart failure: a perspective from animal studies. Adv Exp Med Biol. 2015;860:167–85.

Schwan J, Campbell SG. Prospects for in vitro myofilament maturation in stem cell-derived cardiac myocytes. Biomark Insights. 2015;10:91–103.

Seckin I, Sieck GC, Prakash YS. Volatile anaesthetic effects on Na+–Ca2+ exchange in rat cardiac myocytes. J Physiol. 2001;532:91–104.

Shah SP, Waxman S. Two cases of Bezold-Jarisch reflex induced by intra-arterial nitroglycerin in critical left main coronary artery stenosis. Tex Heart Inst J. 2013;40:484–6.

Shah AB, Hashmi SS, Sahulee R, Pannu H, Gupta-Malhotra M. Characteristics of systemic hypertension in preterm children. J Clin Hypertens (Greenwich, Conn). 2015;17:364–70.

Shareef MA, Anwer LA, Poizat C. Cardiac SERCA2A/B: therapeutic targets for heart failure. Eur J Pharmacol. 2014;724:1–8.

Sharir T, Kang X, Germano G, Bax JJ, Shaw LJ, Gransar H, Cohen I, Hayes SW, Friedman JD, Berman DS. Prognostic value of poststress left ventricular volume and ejection fraction by gated myocardial perfusion SPECT in women and men: gender-related differences in normal limits and outcomes. J Nucl Cardiol. 2006;13:495–506.

Sharpey-Schafer EP. Effects of Valsalva's manoeuvre on the normal and failing circulation. Br Med J. 1955;1:693–5.

Shi WY, Li S, Collins N, Cottee DB, Bastian BC, James AN, Mejia R. Peri-operative levosimendan in patients undergoing cardiac surgery: an overview of the evidence. Heart Lung Circ. 2015;24(7):667–72.

Shieh HH, Barreira ER, Bousso A, Ventura AC, Troster EJ. Update of the pediatric hypotension graphic adjusted for gender and height percentiles: diastolic blood pressure for girls, 1 to 17 years old. Crit Care. 2013;17 Suppl 3:23.

Smith G. Management of supraventricular tachycardia using the Valsalva manoeuvre: a historical review and summary of published evidence. Eur J Emerg Med. 2012;19:346–52.

Sobie EA, Song LS, Lederer WJ. Restitution of Ca(2+) release and vulnerability to arrhythmias. J Cardiovasc Electrophysiol. 2006;17 Suppl 1:S64–70.

Solaro RJ. Remote control of A-band cardiac thin filaments by the I-Z-I protein network of cardiac sarcomeres. Trends Cardiovasc Med. 2005;15:148–52.

Solaro RJ. Mechanisms of the Frank-Starling law of the heart: the beat goes on. Biophys J. 2007; 93:4095–6.

Solaro RJ, Rosevear P, Kobayashi T. The unique functions of cardiac troponin I in the control of cardiac muscle contraction and relaxation. Biochem Biophys Res Commun. 2008;369:82–7.

Solaro RJ, Henze M, Kobayashi T. Integration of troponin I phosphorylation with cardiac regulatory networks. Circ Res. 2013;112:355–66.

Stehle R, Solzin J, Iorga B, Poggesi C. Insights into the kinetics of Ca2 +–regulated contraction and relaxation from myofibril studies. Pflugers Arch. 2009;458:337–57.

Tanaka Y, Nakamura K, Kuroiwa N, Odachi M, Mawatari K, Onimaru M, Sanada J, Arima T. Isovolumetric relaxation flow in patients with ischemic heart disease. J Am Coll Cardiol. 1993;21:1357–64.

Teerlink JR, Metra M, Zaca V, Sabbah HN, Cotter G, Gheorghiade M, Cas LD. Agents with inotropic properties for the management of acute heart failure syndromes. Traditional agents and beyond. Heart Fail Rev. 2009;14:243–53.

Teerlink JR, Clarke CP, Saikali KG, Lee JH, Chen MM, Escandon RD, Elliott L, Bee R, Habibzadeh MR, Goldman JH, Schiller NB, Malik FI, Wolff AA. Dose-dependent augmentation of cardiac systolic function with the selective cardiac myosin activator, omecamtiv mecarbil: a first-in-man study. Lancet. 2011;378:667–75.

Thomas GD. Neural control of the circulation. Adv Physiol Educ. 2011;35:28–32.

Trippodo NC, Coleman TG, Cowley Jr AW, Guyton AC. Angiotensin II antagonists in dehydrated rabbits without baroreceptor reflexes. Am J Physiol. 1977;232:H110–3.

Tsai JC, Heitz JW. Oculocardiac reflex elicited during debridement of an empty orbit. J Clin Anesth. 2012;24:426–7.

Tskhovrebova L, Trinick J. Roles of titin in the structure and elasticity of the sarcomere. J Biomed Biotechnol. 2010;2010:612482.

van Vonderen JJ, Te Pas AB. The first breaths of life: imaging studies of the human infant during neonatal transition. Paediatr Respir Rev. 2015;16:143–6.

van Vonderen JJ, Roest AA, Siew ML, Blom NA, van Lith JM, Walther FJ, Hooper SB, te Pas AB. Noninvasive measurements of hemodynamic transition directly after birth. Pediatr Res. 2014a;75:448–52.

van Vonderen JJ, Roest AA, Siew ML, Walther FJ, Hooper SB, te Pas AB. Measuring physiological changes during the transition to life after birth. Neonatology. 2014b;105:230–42.

Vasquez EC, Meyrelles SS, Mauad H, Cabral AM. Neural reflex regulation of arterial pressure in pathophysiological conditions: interplay among the baroreflex, the cardiopulmonary reflexes and the chemoreflex. Braz J Med Biol Res. 1997;30:521–32.

Vatner SF, Zimpfer M. Bainbridge reflex in conscious, unrestrained, and tranquilized baboons. Am J Physiol. 1981;240:H164–7.

Veenhuyzen GD, Simpson CS, Abdollah H. Atrial fibrillation. CMAJ. 2004;171:755–60.

Vittorini S, Storti S, Parri MS, Cerillo AG, Clerico A. SERCA2a, phospholamban, sarcolipin, and ryanodine receptors gene expression in children with congenital heart defects. Mol Med. 2007;13:105–11.

Wan WH, Ang BT, Wang E. The Cushing Response: a case for a review of its role as a physiological reflex. J Clin Neurosci. 2008;15:223–8.

Wang Z, Yuan LJ, Cao TS, Yang Y, Duan YY, Xing CY. Simultaneous beat-by-beat investigation of the effects of the Valsalva maneuver on left and right ventricular filling and the possible mechanism. PLoS One. 2013;8:e53917.

Weisbrod D, Peretz A, Ziskind A, Menaker N, Oz S, Barad L, Eliyahu S, Itskovitz-Eldor J, Dascal N, Khananshvili D, Binah O, Attali B. SK4 Ca2+ activated K+ channel is a critical player in cardiac pacemaker derived from human embryonic stem cells. Proc Natl Acad Sci U S A. 2013;110:E1685–94.

Wetzel GT, Chen F, Klitzner TS. L- and T-type calcium channels in acutely isolated neonatal and adult cardiac myocytes. Pediatr Res. 1991;30:89–94.

Williams GS, Smith GD, Sobie EA, Jafri MS. Models of cardiac excitation-contraction coupling in ventricular myocytes. Math Biosci. 2010;226:1–15.

Wolf CM, Berul CI. Molecular mechanisms of inherited arrhythmias. Curr Genomics. 2008;9:160–8.

Xie LH, Shanmugam M, Park JY, Zhao Z, Wen H, Tian B, Periasamy M, Babu GJ. Ablation of sarcolipin results in atrial remodeling. Am J Physiol Cell Physiol. 2012;302:C1762–71.

Xin M, Olson EN, Bassel-Duby R. Mending broken hearts: cardiac development as a basis for adult heart regeneration and repair. Nat Rev Mol Cell Biol. 2013;14:529–41.

Yang L, Katchman A, Morrow JP, Doshi D, Marx SO. Cardiac L-type calcium channel (Cav1.2) associates with gamma subunits. FASEB J. 2011;25:928–36.

Yaniv Y, Spurgeon HA, Lyashkov AE, Yang D, Ziman BD, Maltsev VA, Lakatta EG. Crosstalk between mitochondrial and sarcoplasmic reticulum Ca2+ cycling modulates cardiac pacemaker cell automaticity. PLoS One. 2012;7:e37582.

Yaniv Y, Lakatta EG, Maltsev VA. From two competing oscillators to one coupled-clock pacemaker cell system. Front Physiol. 2015;6:28.

Yigit M, Kowalski W, Hutchon D, Pekkan K. Transition from fetal to neonatal circulation: modeling the effect of umbilical cord clamping. J Biomech. 2015;48(9):1662–70.

Zile MR, Baicu CF, Ikonomidis JS, Stroud RE, Nietert PJ, Bradshaw AD, Slater R, Palmer BM, Van Buren P, Meyer M, MR M, AB D, LG H, LeWinter MM. Myocardial stiffness in patients with heart failure and a preserved ejection fraction: contributions of collagen and titin. Circulation. 2015;131:1247–59.

Zimmer HG. Heinrich Ewald Hering and the carotid sinus reflex. Clin Cardiol. 2004;27:485–6.

Zuber M, Cuculi F, Oechslin E, Erne P, Jenni R. Is transesophageal echocardiography still necessary to exclude patent foramen ovale? Scand Cardiovasc J. 2008;42:222–5.

Zubrow AB, Hulman S, Kushner H, Falkner B. Determinants of blood pressure in infants admitted to neonatal intensive care units: a prospective multicenter study. Philadelphia Neonatal Blood Pressure Study Group. J Perinatol. 1995;15:470–9.

Chapter 4
Cardiovascular Pharmacology in Pediatric Patients with Congenital Heart Disease

Ali Dabbagh, Zahra Talebi, and Samira Rajaei

Vasoactive Agents

Based on a general classification, the vasoactive agents could be categorized in two main subclasses:

- Vasoactive agents which affect the arterial system or the venous bed (either vasopressors or vasodilators)
- Inotropes (positive or negative inotropes)

So, the main cardiovascular drugs discussed in this chapter belong to one of the following classes; however, this classification is not comprehensive and also, there may be some overlaps; in fact, most of the currently available pharmaceutical agents of these groups share some aspects of each category in variable amounts

A. Dabbagh, MD (✉)
Cardiac Anesthesiology Department, Anesthesiology Research Center,
Shahid Beheshti University of Medical Sciences, Tehran, Iran
e-mail: alidabbagh@yahoo.com; alidabbagh@sbmu.ac.ir

Z. Talebi, Pharm D
Anesthesiology Research Center, Shahid Beheshti University of Medical Sciences,
Tehran, Iran
e-mail: zahra.tlb@gmail.com

S. Rajaei, MD, PhD
Department of Immunology, School of Medicine, Tehran University of Medical Science,
Tehran, Islamic Republic of Iran
e-mail: samirarajaei@tums.ac.ir

© Springer International Publishing Switzerland 2017
A. Dabbagh et al. (eds.), *Congenital Heart Disease in Pediatric and Adult Patients*, DOI 10.1007/978-3-319-44691-2_4

(Holmes 2005; Bangash et al. 2012; Bracht et al. 2012; Noori and Seri 2012; Jentzer et al. 2015):

1. Pure vasopressors, i.e., *pure vasoconstrictors* (phenylephrine and vasopressin)
2. Inoconstrictors *which have both vasoconstrictor and inotropic activity* (mainly epinephrine, dopamine, and norepinephrine)
3. Inodilators *which have both vasodilator and inotropic activity* (mainly milrinone, dobutamine, and levosimendan)
4. Pure vasodilators which affect the arterial system (arterial dilators) and/or the venous system (venodilators); these agents have no inotropic activity (including mainly nitroglycerin, hydralazine, alprostadil, sodium nitroprusside, phentolamine mesylate)

When assessing different vasoactive drugs, it is often useful to consider specific receptor responses based on different organs and tissues. The following Tables 4.1 and 4.2 are a summary of some of the routinely affected organs (Kee 2003; Trappe et al. 2003; Bangash et al. 2012).

Table 4.1 Receptor types targeted by current vasoactive pharmaceuticals

Specific adrenoceptor	The main target organ(s)	Clinical response
$\alpha1$ (including α_{1A}, α_{1B}, α_{1D})	Arteries, arterioles, veins; however, α effects predominate over β in splanchnic circulation	Arterial constriction
$\alpha2$ (including α_{2A}, α_{2B}, α_{2C})	Gastrointestinal (GI) tract Cutaneous circulation	Decreased GI tone Decreased motility Decreased amount of GI secretions
$\beta1$	Heart (β 1>> β 2 in coronary circulation)	Increased heart rate Augmented myocardial contractility
$\beta2$	The vessels of the skeletal muscles	Dilation of the vessels
	Coronary arterial bed	Dilation of the vessels
	Smooth muscles in the tracheobronchial tree	Relaxation of the smooth muscles
$\beta3$	Adipose tissue	Enhancement of lipolysis in adipose tissue, thermogenesis in skeletal muscle

Modified from Fellin (2014). Published with kind permission of © Springer, 2014. All Rights Reserved

Table 4.2 Myocardial receptors characterized by their properties

Receptor type	Inotropy	Chronotropy	Dromotropy	Lusitropy	Bathmotropy
β_1	+	+	+	+	+
M_2	−	−	−	−	−

$-$ = decrease; $+$ = increase

Pure Vasopressors (Pure Vasoconstrictors)

Phenylephrine

Drug Name Phenylephrine hydrochloride

Class Alpha-adrenergic agonists

CAS Number 61-76-7

Mechanism of Action Phenylephrine is a sympathomimetic amine that acts by direct stimulation of peripheral $\alpha 1$-adrenergic receptors. It is used as a bolus or an infusion in acute management of low systemic blood pressure. The vasoconstriction effect of $\alpha 1$ adrenoceptors may result in a reflex bradycardia; although the situation is rarely seen in young children, the patient's heart rate should be carefully monitored when large doses of phenylephrine are administrated.

Phenylephrine has many indications including these:

- *The most important indication for pediatric patients* is raising SVR in CHD conditions when either ventricle is suffering from an outflow obstruction which is exacerbated with low SVR, such as tetralogy of Fallot (TOF), in which low SVR can cause cyanosis during a "tet spell," hypertonic cardiomyopathy, etc.
- It is also indicated in patients with partial obstruction in systemic to pulmonary shunt or single ventricle patients with pulmonary stenosis to improve oxygenation.
- Hypotension during anesthesia.
- Septic shock.
- Prolongation of the effects of local anesthetics.
- Prevention and treatment of nasal congestion.
- Hemorrhoids.

Dosing The common dose of phenylephrine in pediatric patients is as follows: bolus dosing, 0.5–5 µg/kg or higher, and infusion dosing (when frequent bolus doses are needed), 0.02–0.3 µg/kg/min, which should be administrated through a central venous catheter if possible.

Common Adverse Effect of Phenylephrine

- Vasoconstriction of peripheral vascular beds, including the skeletal muscle, skin, renal, and mesenteric which can be severe and compromise the blood flow in vital organs, limiting its use in extreme situations
- Nausea
- Vomiting
- Headache
- Nervousness

Cautions Extravasation into skin and subcutaneous tissues is the main caution when administrating phenylephrine; this can result in ischemia, necrosis, and even tissue loss. Also the sulfite in phenylephrine formulations can cause hypersensitivity reactions in susceptible individuals.

Vasopressin

Name of Drug Vasopressin

Class Pituitary

CAS Number 11000-17-2

Vasopressin is a vasopressor drug acting through specific vasopressin receptors. Vasopressin should be used after hemodynamic stability and is usually used in vasodilatory shock, usually when other agents are irresponsive (Holmes et al. 2003, 2004; Stahl et al. 2010; Sharawy 2014).The effects of vasopressin in refractory shocks have been studied, and many believe that low-dose vasopressin is a useful drug for septic shocks patients who have already received drugs like norepinephrine infusion (Russell 2011).

Mechanism of Action Vasopressin is the exogenous antidiuretic hormone (ADH) and as a vasopressor which produces intense vasoconstriction (through V1 receptors); also, it has antidiuretic effects (V_2 receptors). When the therapeutic doses of catecholamines are acutely or chronically elevated and, hence, adrenergic receptors mare downregulated, impaired signal transmission in adrenergic receptors occurs, especially when there is concomitant metabolic acidosis; this is why using vasopressin is advantageous in such situations. On the other hand, another potential advantage of vasopressin is that V_2 receptors help create vasodilation in order to lessen the end-organ hypoperfusion; often, epinephrine or norepinephrine administration may lead to end-organ hypoperfusion in some of the visceral organs (Holmes et al. 2003, 2004; Meyer et al. 2008).

Indications Vasopressin has many indications in pediatric population including:
- Diabetes insipidus
- Polyuria
- CPR
- Abdominal radiographic procedures
- Diagnostic procedures
- Gastrointestinal hemorrhage
- Vasodilatory shock

Its use in treating refractory vasodilatory shock in pediatric patients with cardiogenic and septic etiologies is gaining day-to-day importance (Biban and

Gaffuri 2013; Okamoto et al. 2015). Vasopressin is especially useful in cases of low systemic vascular resistance (SVR) brought on by excessive α-adrenergic blockade, such as with phentolamine or phenoxybenzamine (Motta et al. 2005; Mossad et al. 2008; Gordon 2016).

The usual dose of vasopressin administrated is 0.2–2 milliunits/kg/min infusion, which can be titrated to achieve desired effect; however, the dose should be weaned and discontinued as soon as possible. 4–8 milliunits/kg/min doses have been reported in some clinical trials to treat vasodilatory shock (Choong and Kissoon 2008; Singh et al. 2009).

Adverse effects associated with low doses of vasopressin are infrequent and mild; however, they increase in frequency and severity with higher doses.

Hypertension and bradycardia may occur due to severe vasospasm and the resulting hypertension which induces baroreceptor reflex. Arrhythmia is infrequent. Also, peripheral vasoconstriction may lead to distal limb ischemia. If extravasation occurs, skin necrosis is possible. Hyponatremia is common with vasopressin infusions when prolonged periods of drug infusion are used; therefore, serum sodium should be measured at least daily to prevent this untoward effect. Vasopressin can cause hypersensitivity reactions in susceptible individuals and should be administrated with caution in older children (Sharawy 2014).

Finally, it seems strongly logic to use *vasopressin as a rescue therapy* and the *last-resort treatment* in children with refractory shock (unresponsive to norepinephrine and epinephrine); of course, its use should be individualized and with considerations regarding the underlying clinical state (Meyer et al. 2008; Brissaud et al. 2016).

Terlipressin is another analogue of vasopressin with higher selectivity for V1 receptors; also, it has a longer half-life compared to vasopressin; terlipressin is triglycyl lysine vasopressin and is used in norepinephrine-resistant shocks with different ranges of doses varying from 7 mcg/kg twice a day to 2 mcg/kg every 4 h; however, its pharmacology is not well studied in pediatric and neonatal patients, and also, it is not available in some countries; there are still no firm recommendations for using terlipressin in severe shock in pediatric patients (O'Brien et al. 2002; Leone and Martin 2008; Meyer et al. 2011; Biban and Gaffuri 2013).

Inoconstrictors

In evaluation of catecholamines, one should always keep in mind that the density of adrenoceptors and their response to catecholamines are all markedly affected by a number of factors; among them, the two have utmost importance:

- The underlying disease
- The ongoing catecholamine treatment (Bangash et al. 2012; Bracht et al. 2012)

Epinephrine

Name of Drug Epinephrine (Adrenalin)

CAS Number 51-43-4

Drug Group α- and β-adrenergic receptor agonist

Mechanism of Effect Epinephrine affects all adrenergic receptors including α1, α2, β1, β2, and β2; also, the clinical effects of epinephrine are similar to the effects of sympathetic stimulation with all of its clinical presentations being seen except for its effects on facial arteries and the effects on sweating; epinephrine is assumed as the most potent α-adrenergic agonist (Cooper 2008; Jentzer et al. 2015).

Low-dose epinephrine infusions affect mainly the β-adrenoceptors. This is why doses of <0.1–0.2 mcg/kg/min are usually considered as "pure" inotropic dose, which could improve pump failure after cardiac surgery. However, with increasing the dose, the vasoconstrictor effects of epinephrine are presented much more (Bangash et al. 2012; Noori and Seri 2012; Jentzer et al. 2015).

Epinephrine affects the smooth muscles of bronchi and pupils and leads to bronchial dilation and iris dilation. Glycogenolysis is speeded up in liver due to epinephrine effects leading to increased blood level of glucose. Epinephrine could induce myocardial ischemia, tachyarrhythmia, pulmonary hypertension, hyperglycemia, and lactic acidosis. Epinephrine compromises hepatic and splanchnic perfusion, lactate clearance, and oxygen exchange. The decrease in hepaticosplanchnic perfusion in addition to increased hepatic metabolic workload, hypermetabolism, impairment of oxygen exchange, glycolysis, and suppression of insulin release are the main etiologic causes for lactic acidosis and hyperglycemia. Also, epinephrine acts as antagonist of histamine (Trappe et al. 2003; Bangash et al. 2012; Bracht et al. 2012).

Indications
- *Cardiopulmonary resuscitation and rhythm disturbances*: they are used to increase coronary perfusion pressure and cerebral perfusion pressure, mainly through α1-adrenergic activity, which increases the diastolic perfusion pressure. However, β-adrenergic activity increases the myocardial load and decreased subendocardial perfusion; so, these effects are not optimal effects; if the patient is in shock due to cardiac problems, epinephrine should be used cautiously due to adverse myocardial effects. Epinephrine is considered as the first-line catecholamine agent which is used in cardiopulmonary resuscitation and, also, in anaphylactic shock (Kee 2003; Bangash et al. 2012; de Caen et al. 2015; Maconochie et al. 2015).
- *Bronchospasm*: it acts as a rapid bronchodilator in acute bronchospasm and bronchial asthma; however, its unwanted effects on the cardiovascular system mandate using selective β2 agonists in such cases.
- *Anaphylaxis and anaphylactoid reactions*: during life-threatening anaphylaxis reactions and emergencies, the drug is used; subcutaneous route is usually used

in such circumstances; however, in life-threatening emergencies, cautious intravenous supplements may be considered (Simons and Sampson 2015).

- *Gastrointestinal and renal bleeding*: local intra-arterial administration into the celiac trunk, inferior mesenteric artery, or superior mesenteric artery could be used.
- *As adjunct to local anesthetics*: it could decrease local absorption of the drug.
- *Other uses*: radiation nephritis, control of local skin and/or mucosal bleeding, premature labor, treatment of severe hypoglycemia, as adjuvant to radiocontrast dyes.

Routes of Administration Epinephrine could be administered through the following routes (Cooper 2008; de Caen et al. 2015; Jentzer et al. 2015):

- Intravenous
- Intramuscular
- Subcutaneous
- Infusion through intravenous line or central line
- Intra-arterial (very rarely; e.g., in radiographic assessments)
- Through endotracheal tube in cardiopulmonary bypass
- Intraosseous
- Inhalational through pulmonary devices like metered dose inhalers or nebulizers (usually used for children above 4 years)
- Local administration in control for mucosal or skin bleeding

Epinephrine Dose in Pediatric Cardiac Surgery

Very low-dose epinephrine is defined as 0.01–0.05 mcg/kg/min. This dose of epinephrine does not raise plasma epinephrine levels significantly in such a way to induce major cardiovascular responses; if any response is seen, it will be predominantly due to β-adrenoceptor effects (Kee 2003; Maslov et al. 2015).

Low-dose epinephrine is considered as infusion between 0.05 and 0.1 mcg/kg/min (Maslov et al. 2015). Low-dose epinephrine causes $\beta 2$ adrenergic effects ($\beta 2 > \beta 1 > \alpha 1$). The result is decrease in both systemic vascular resistance (SVR) and blood pressure; however, myocardial contractility increases. As mentioned above, low-dose epinephrine infusions are usually considered as "pure" inotropic dose; this dose improves pump failure after cardiac surgery mainly through β-adrenoceptors. Of course, pharmacodynamics studies have demonstrated that heart rate should raise first before any inotropic effect of epinephrine could be exerted (Maslov et al. 2015; Lucas et al. 2016).

Moderate-dose epinephrine infusion is between 0.1 and 0.5 mcg/kg/min, though this dose is not exactly the same in all classifications (Watt et al. 2011). In this dose, $\alpha 1$ effects are much more pronounced than the lower doses.

High-dose epinephrine infusion is between 0.5 and 1 mcg/kg/min. in this higher dose, $\alpha 1 > \beta 1$, $\beta 2$ leading to increased SVR and increased cardiac index; among the clinical results is significant increase in diastolic blood pressure. Also, systolic, diastolic, and mean arterial blood pressures are elevated. This dose range may lead to increased plasma levels of glucose and lactate (Clutter et al. 1980; Cooper 2008; Jentzer et al. 2015).

Very high-dose epinephrine is when epinephrine infusion dose increases above 1.5 mcg/kg/min; as a result, SVR increases significantly, resulting in significant decrease of cardiac index. Meanwhile, pulmonary vascular resistance and right ventricular afterload are increased. These events lead to increased myocardial oxygen demand due to increased heart rate and stroke work (Maslov et al. 2015).

During cardiac arrest, the doses of epinephrine are needed that vasoconstrictive α-effects predominate, in order to increase diastolic pressure in the root of aorta leading to improved myocardial perfusion pressure. The desired dose of epinephrine in CPR will be intravenous bolus of 0.01–0.03 mg/kg every 3–5 min. It is not recommended to use doses higher than 1 mg in every 3–5 min interval. In refractory bradycardia after cardiac arrest, 0.1–0.2 mcg/kg/min as intravenous infusion could be used. Also, intraosseous dose for pediatric cardiac arrest is 0.1 mg/kg up to 1 mg which could be repeated every 3–5 min. Endotracheal tube administration of epinephrine should be with ten times higher than IV doses (0.1 mg/kg) which could be repeated up to a total dose of 10 mg; the dose could be repeated every 3–5 min during the course of CPR; however, endotracheal dose of epinephrine should be diluted in 5 mL normal saline followed by five manual ventilation maneuvers to augment its absorption (Kleinman et al. 2010; Atkins et al. 2015; de Caen et al. 2015; Maconochie et al. 2015).

Cautions Epinephrine could lead to dangerous side effects if it is not delivered cautiously; very high blood pressure, myocardial ischemia and chest pain, aortic injures and disruption, or even rupture of cerebral arteries may ensue due to inadvertent injection of the drug, leading to CNS injuries. For inpatients with underlying arrhythmia, hypertension, or hyperthyroidism, more caution is necessary. Patients undergoing general anesthesia with volatile agents are at risk of arrhythmias. In patients receiving MAO inhibitors, simultaneous administration of epinephrine needs extreme caution. Acute angle glaucoma may worsen due to epinephrine. However, in life-threatening conditions, there is no absolute contraindication.

Dopamine

Name of Drug Dopamine hydrochloride

CAS Number 62-31-7

Drug Group Selective agonist of β-1 adrenergic receptors

Mechanism of Effect Dopamine is a natural catecholamine which is produced in the following famous chain:

L-Phenylalanine is converted to L-tyrosine, and then it is converted to L-DOPA (L-3,4-dihydroxyphenylalanine). Then DOPA is changed to dopamine through the enzyme "DOPA decarboxylase."

Dopamine is one of the precursors of norepinephrine. Also, dopamine acts as a neurotransmitter in some of the sympathetic pathways. Besides, dopamine is a major neurotransmitter in some parts of the CNS like nigrostriatal pathway.

Dopamine has both positive chronotropic and inotropic effects on myocardium; so, it increases heart rate and myocardial contractility. These effects of dopamine are done through two mechanisms:

- Direct effect which is produced by agonistic effects of dopamine on beta adrenoceptors
- Indirect effect which is produced due to the effect of dopamine in releasing norepinephrine from its storage sites in sympathetic nerve endings

Clinical Effects of Dopamine

Often, dopamine is clinically considered as a vasoconstrictor and as an inotrope (i.e., inoconstrictor); however, the effects of dopamine on alpha- and beta-adrenergic receptors are weaker than epinephrine or norepinephrine. The clinical effects of dopamine are highly dose dependent, and also, there is interindividual variability in clinical response. Besides, in different clinical conditions of the same patient, there may be altered responses to dopamine. Keeping these in mind, we may classify the effects of dopamine based on the dose (Kee 2003; Trappe et al. 2003; Cooper 2008; Bangash et al. 2012; Bracht et al. 2012):

- *Low-dose dopamine* (0.5–2 µg/kg/min): it causes vasodilation which seems to be due to the selective effects of the drug on dopamine receptors which are different from its effects on α- and β-adrenoceptors (mainly on mesenteric, renal, intracerebral, and coronary vascular beds); haloperidol acts as antagonist to these receptors. Increased glomerular filtration rate, increased renal blood flow, increased renal excretion of sodium, and increased urine flow are among the main results of this dopamine dose; often, increased renal blood flow does not affect urine osmolality. However, the so-called renal-dose dopamine which is the same as low-dose dopamine is not supported by evidence for renal protection. Total peripheral vascular resistance is usually not altered so much in this dose (0.5–2 µg/kg/min) because it would be raised by alpha activity.
- *Medium-dose dopamine* (2–10 µg/kg/min): it mainly stimulates β1 adrenoceptors and increases myocardial contractility. Also, this dose augments stimulation of the sinoatrial node and increases impulse conduction in myocardial tissue. β2 adrenoceptors, which cause peripheral vasodilation, are usually not stimulated by this dose (i.e. 2–10 µg/kg/min). However, the degree of increased myocardial oxygen consumption by dopamine is less than isoproterenol. Also, dopamine increases systolic blood pressure and pulse pressure while diastolic blood pressure is not much affected. As mentioned, in low to moderate doses of dopamine, total peripheral vascular resistance is usually not altered so much (because it would be raised by alpha activity). So, as a result of relatively constant vascular resistance and increased cardiac output, perfusion in the vascular bed is increased

with 2–10 µg/kg/min dose. Often, tachyarrhythmia is not a frequent result of dopamine use.

- *High-dose dopamine* (10–20 µg/kg/min): the effects of dopamine in these doses are mainly α-adrenoceptor stimulation; the clinical result is vasoconstriction and increased blood pressure. Vasoconstrictive effect is first seen in muscular arterial tone; however, renal and mesenteric vessels are affected afterwards and with increased dose of drug. Very high dopamine doses (especially doses above 20 µg/kg/min) may lead to ischemia in the aforementioned organs, including limbs; so, doses above 20 µg/kg/min may compromise the circulation of the limbs, and we may consider the effects of this very high dose as similar to the effects of norepinephrine.

Dopaminergic activity; its effect on the immunologic and neurohormonal systems There is increasing evidence that there are very important interactions between dopaminergic system and many aspects of the neurohormonal system including a decline in secretion of prolactin, thyroid, and growth hormones and increased synthesis of the glucocorticoid hormones; these effects are especially important in the critically ill and septic patients (Van den Berghe and de Zegher 1996; Bailey and Burchett 1997).

Besides, there are great interactions between dopamine and the immunologic system, both in health and disease. In fact, dopamine could play a crucial role in modulation of the immunologic and inflammatory response. These immunomodulatory effects of dopamine are dose dependent and mediated though different dopamine receptors:

- The first family of dopaminergic-like receptors is known as D1 receptors and includes D1 and D5; and the second family of dopaminergic-like receptors is known as D2 receptors and includes D2, D3, and D4; besides, these immunomodulatory effects are mediated though α- and β-adrenergic receptors (Elenkov et al. 2000; Beck et al. 2004; Franz et al. 2015; Levite 2016).
- Dopamine affects the cytokine network, leading to decreased expression of adhesion molecules, suppression of the production trend in cytokine and chemokine network, decreased potency of neutrophil in producing chemotaxis, and impaired proliferation of T-cell population (Elenkov et al. 2000; Beck et al. 2004; Franz et al. 2015; Levite 2016).
- Dopamine receptors are expressed in T lymphocytes leading to modulation of this cell population; this effect is mediated through both the dopaminergic D1 receptors (D1/D5) and the dopaminergic D2 receptors (D2/D3/D4) (Elenkov et al. 2000; Zhao et al. 2013; Franz et al. 2015).
- The cytotoxic effects of natural killer cells are highly affected by dopamine receptors: D1 receptors (D1/D5) facilitate the activity of natural killer cells; however, D2 receptors (D2/D3/D4) suppress the activity of natural killer cells (Zhao et al. 2013; Franz et al. 2015).
- Dendritic cells (DCs) are a main part of innate immunity system; also they act as a very important linker between innate and adaptive immune system with a very

crucial role in activation of the adaptive immune system. DCs affect the whole dopaminergic system in nearly all aspects which yields to increased production and storage of dopamine; in turn, DCs stimulate the D1 and D2 receptors in an autocrine manner (Prado et al. 2013; Pacheco et al. 2014; Franz et al. 2015; Herrera et al. 2015; Levite 2016).

- Dopamine could augment differentiation of CD4 (+) T cells to T helper 1, T helper 2, and T helper 17 cell lines; these are inflammatory T cells (Prado et al. 2013; Franz et al. 2015; Herrera et al. 2015; Levite 2016).
- On the other hand, regulatory T cells may lead to release of large amounts of dopamine which can also release high amounts of dopamine; then, dopamine, in an autocrine/paracrine manner, through dopamine receptors, suppresses the effects of regulatory T cells; this effect of dopamine through regulatory T cells is in favor of inflammatory process and autoimmunity (Pacheco et al. 2014; Franz et al. 2015; Herrera et al. 2015; CID = 681 2016; Levite 2016) (Table 4.3).

Time of Effect During the first 5 min after commencing dopamine infusion, its effects are started; meanwhile, the plasma half-life of dopamine is about 2 min; so, it takes less than 10 min for systemic effects of dopamine to be disappeared. In patients using monoamine oxidase (MAO) inhibitors, the drug effect may be as long as 1 h, which mandates careful attention.

Indications

1. Shock: to increase cardiac output, blood pressure, and urinary flow; of course, volume replacement should be done first. Also, dopamine is used to increase systemic vascular resistance in these patients.
2. Acute renal failure: though doses less than 5 µg/kg/min affect the dopaminergic receptors and may increase renal and mesenteric perfusion, no improvements in glomerular filtration rate (GFR) are seen; no significant evidence is available that dopamine could improve oliguric state in the critically ill patients.
3. Hepatorenal syndrome: as part of the therapeutic protocol in such patients; however, long-term treatment is not associated with significant effects.
4. Cirrhosis: as part of the therapeutic regime is used; no proof for its long-term effects.
5. Cardiopulmonary resuscitation: as part of advanced cardiac life support (ACLS) to increase cardiac output and blood pressure.
6. Heart failure: in refractory cases with no significant improvement with cardiac glycosides and diuretics, dopamine could be used in short term to increase cardiac output and blood pressure.

Dopamine Dose and Administration Dopamine is usually administrated by intravenous infusion (bolus administration should be avoided); however, in certain situations, where intravenous infusion is not possible, it might be administrated through intraosseous infusion.

The intravenous infusion of dopamine should be done through central or at least large peripheral veins, preferably the antecubital vein; also, it is better to use an

Table 4.3 A summary of the effects of dopamine stimulation with different doses

Dose of dopamine	Type of affected receptor(s)					
	$\alpha1$ adrenoceptor	$\alpha2$ adrenoceptor	$\beta1$ adrenoceptor	$\beta2$ adrenoceptor	Dopamine 1 receptor (D1)	Dopamine 2 receptor (D2)
0.5–2 μg/kg/min	0	0	+	0	+++	+++
2–10 μg/kg/min	+	+	+++	+++	++++	++++
10–20 μg/kg/min	+++	+	+++	+	++++	++++

+ = increase, − = decrease, 0 = no change

infusion pump to control the rate of flow; the dorsal veins of hand and ankle can increase the risk of extravasations and therefore should be avoided; usually, DW5 % is used to dilute dopamine and achieve subsequent concentrations of 400, 800, 1600, and 3200 mcg/mL of dopamine. The 3200 mcg/mL concentration is used when higher concentrations are needed in patients with fluid restriction (Kee 2003; Jentzer et al. 2015; CID = 681 2016; Rizza et al. 2016).

Specific Considerations for Children Dopamine can be used in any age, the rate of administration is different in every individual, and it should be titrated to reach the desired response. The usual rate of administration in pediatric shock and CPR, and as an inotropic agent to assist weaning from cardiopulmonary bypass in children, and in the early postoperative period is starting with 2–5 mcg/kg/min and then increasing the dose 1–4 mcg/kg/min every 10–30 min to achieve the optimal response. Most patients are controlled with 5–15 mcg/kg/min. infusion rates higher than 20 mcg/kg/min which can cause excessive vasoconstriction.

Clearance of dopamine is not predictable in young children, especially neonates, and it can be up to two times higher in children younger than 2 years old. Neonates are also more sensitive to vasoconstrictor properties of dopamine. Occasionally doses as high as 50 mcg/kg/min are needed for younger children. Some clinicians avoid dopamine due to its potential to cross the blood–brain barrier and suppress pituitary hormones like thyroid-releasing hormone, in pediatric patients. These potential adverse effects are not seen with other natural or synthetic catecholamines.

Common Adverse Effects Tachycardia, angina, palpitation, vasoconstriction, hypotension, dyspnea, nausea, vomiting, and headaches.

Warnings and Contraindications

- In patients who have been previously (within 2–3 weeks of dopamine administrations) treated with MAOIs, dopamine dose should be reduced.
- Patient's plasma volume and electrolytes should be monitored to avoid overhydration while administrating IV fluids.
- Sensitive reactions are probable in patients allergic to sulfite (present in some formulations) or corn products (present in dextrose IV solutions)
- Dopamine is contraindicated in patients with pheochromocytoma or uncorrected tachyarrhythmias or VF.

General Precautions The patients' general condition, ECG, BP, and urine flow, and also preferably cardiac output and pulmonary wedge pressure should be monitored carefully before and during the treatment with dopamine to avoid the incidence or exacerbation of any of the following conditions: extravasation; hypovolemia; hypoxia, hypercapnia, and acidosis; vasoconstriction; hypotension; occlusive vascular disease; ventricular arrhythmias; ischemic heart disease; and diabetes mellitus (caution in administrating dextrose).

In order to discontinue dopamine infusion, dose of dopamine should be decreased gradually while expanding blood volume with IV fluids to prevent a recurrence of hypotension.

Norepinephrine

Name of Drug Norepinephrine bitartrate (Levophed)

Class Alpha- and beta-adrenergic agonists

CAS Number 69815-49-2

Norepinephrine is a natural occurring catecholamine, and it is mainly released by the postganglionic adrenergic nerve endings and the adrenal medulla (10–20 %). Norepinephrine, like epinephrine, works by stimulating the β1 adrenoceptors on the heart and therefore increasing the myocardial contractility.

The variation in the clinical use of epinephrine and norepinephrine is due to their difference in peripheral function. Norepinephrine is a potent α1 agonist with little to no effects on β2 receptors responsible for vasodilatation; therefore, it increases the SVR and blood pressure even with low doses. Cardiac output is usually decreased or unchanged, and heart rate may be reduced as a result of reflex increase in vagal tone. Both drugs can cause hyperglycemia in prolonged infusions, with norepinephrine causing these effects at much higher doses than epinephrine.

Indications The main indication of epinephrine is in treatment of disease states when other vasopressor agents fail and there is a need for a very potent vasoconstrictor; the main examples are refractory shock due to any cause or vasoplegia syndrome (including vasoplegia syndrome after cardiopulmonary bypass); the following is a list of indications for norepinephrine use (De Backer et al. 2010; Mossad et al. 2011; Bangash et al. 2012; Vasu et al. 2012; Mehta et al. 2013; Rizza et al. 2016; Rossano et al. 2016):

- Shock: for vasoconstriction and cardiac stimulation in the treatment of shock that persists after adequate fluid volume replacement and in cases of profound vasodilatory shock unresponsive to high doses of dopamine or dobutamine, such as sepsis in neonates.
- Anaphylactic shock: vasopressor agents, such as norepinephrine, can be used for maintaining blood pressure in patients with anaphylactic shock, but epinephrine is the drug of choice in these situations.
- Myocardial infarction: to treat the hypotension in selected cases.
- CPR: may be used for ACLS when severe hypotension (e.g., SBP <70 mmHg) and low total peripheral resistance persist with less potent drugs.
- Hypotension during anesthesia: is among a list of alternatives; however, agents like intravenous ephedrine or phenylephrine or other vasopressors are used much more commonly.
- Adjunct to local anesthetics: to decrease the rate of vascular absorption of the anesthetic, hence increasing the duration of anesthesia; however, epinephrine is used much more commonly for this purpose.
- GI hemorrhage: intraperitoneally or via a nasogastric tube as a hemostatic agent for severe upper GI bleeding.
- Pericardial tamponade to temporarily increase cardiac filling pressure and cardiac output.

Dose and Administration Administration is done by intravenous (IV) infusion using an infusion pump or other apparatus to control the rate of flow and into the antecubital vein of the arm or femoral vein. Norepinephrine should not be administered in the same IV line as alkaline solutions, which may inactivate the drug. Extravasation may result in local necrosis and must be carefully avoided. It is suggested to change the injection site periodically in prolonged therapy.

Dose range of norepinephrine infusion in pediatric cardiac patients varies from 0.02 to 0.2 mcg/kg/min. And it is better to be administered in the lowest effective dosage for the shortest possible time.

In shock usually a dose of 2 mcg/min or, alternatively, 2 mcg/m^2 per minute is administrated. In Pediatric Advanced Life Support (PALS) during CPR, 0.1–2 mcg/kg/min is infused intravenously as an adjunct to therapy until reaching the optimum blood pressure and perfusion (De Backer et al. 2010; Mossad et al. 2011; Vasu et al. 2012; Rossano et al. 2016).

Warnings and Contraindications Norepinephrine is contraindicated during anesthesia with cyclopropane or halogenated hydrocarbon general anesthetics, though they are rarely used in the current era. Also use in fingers, toes, ears, nose, or genitalia in conjunction to local anesthetics is contraindicated.

The following conditions should be thoroughly monitored in patients treated with norepinephrine: hypovolemia, as vasopressor therapy is not a substitute for replacement of blood, plasma, fluids, and/or electrolytes; hypoxia, hypercapnia, and acidosis; extravasation (injection into leg veins should be avoided, especially in geriatric patients or those with occlusive vascular diseases, arteriosclerosis, diabetes mellitus, or Buerger's disease); hypertensive or hyperthyroid patients (increased risk of adverse reactions due to hypersensitivity to this drug); peripheral or mesenteric vascular thrombosis; and sensitivity reactions (in sulfite-sensitive patients because the formulation contains sulfites).

General Precautions The following are the main precautions in using norepinephrine (De Backer et al. 2010; Mossad et al. 2011; Bangash et al. 2012; Vasu et al. 2012; Mehta et al. 2013; Rizza et al. 2016; Rossano et al. 2016):

- Prolonged administration: as it may cause decreased cardiac output, edema, hemorrhage, focal myocarditis, subpericardial hemorrhage, necrosis of the intestine, or hepatic and renal necrosis which is seen mostly in patients with severe shock and can be due to the shock itself.
- Cardiovascular and renal effects: severe vasoconstriction and limiting the blood flow in vital organs.
- Increases myocardial oxygen consumption and the work of the heart.
- Venous return to the heart may be reduced due to increased peripheral vascular resistance, which can ultimately reduce cardiac output.
- Arrhythmias: especially likely to occur in patients with acute MI, hypoxia, or hypercapnia or those receiving other drugs increasing cardiac irritability such as cyclopropane or halogenated hydrocarbon general anesthetics.
- Common adverse effects: dizziness, tremor, respiratory difficulty, headaches (Table 4.4).

Table 4.4 A summary of the main vasopressor agents

Drug	Dose	Receptors	Inotropy	HR[a]	SVR	PVR	Renal vascular resistance	Half-life	Adverse effects
Epinephrine	Cardiac arrest: Children: IV bolus: 0.01 mg/kg every 3–5 min Low cardiac output: Continuous IV infusion: 0.01–1 µg/kg/min	Lower doses: $\beta_1,\beta_2 > \alpha_1$ Higher doses: $\alpha_1 > \beta_1,\beta_2$	+ +	+ +	0, – +	0, – +	– +	<2 min	Tachyarrhythmias If extravasation occurs, skin necrosis is possible
Norepinephrine	Continuous IV infusion: 0.05–0.3 µg/kg/min (maximum dose: 2 µg/kg/min)	$\alpha_1 > \beta_1,\beta_2$	+	+	+	+	–	<2 min	Hypertension Bradycardia Myocardial ischemia If extravasation occurs, skin necrosis is possible
Dopamine	Continuous IV infusion: 2–5 µg/kg/min 5–10 µg/kg/min 10–20 µg/kg/min	DA$_1$, DA$_2$ $\beta_1,\beta_2 > \alpha_1$ $\alpha_1 > \beta_1,\beta_2$	0 + +	0 + +	0 0, – +	0 0 +	– 0 +	2 min	Hypertension, tachyarrhythmias
Dobutamine	Continuous IV infusion: 2–20 µg/kg/min	$\beta_1 > \alpha_1,\beta_2$	+	+	–	–	0	2 min	Tachyarrhythmias
Isoproterenol	Continuous IV infusion: 0.01–0.2 µg/kg/min	β_1,β_2	+	+	–	–	–	8–50 min	Tachyarrhythmias

Calcium Chloride	5–10 mg/kg IV bolus; 10 mg/kg/h infusion 20 mg/kg intracardiac (in ventricular cavity)	Contractile proteins	+	0,–	+	0,+	0	N/A	Hypertension
Milrinone	Continuous IV infusion: 0.25–0.75 μg/kg/min	Phosphodiesterase III, inhibitor/↑ cAMP	+	+	–	–	–	Infants: 3.15 0 2 h Children: 1.86 0 2 h	Hypotension, ventricular arrhythmias, headache
Nesiritide	Continuous I.V. Infusion: 0.01 μg/kg/min; if necessary, titrate by 0.005 μg/kg/min every 3 h to maximum of 0.03 μg/kg/min[b]	B-Natriuretic peptide	0	0	–	–	+	60 min	Hypotension, increased levels of serum creatinine
Levosimendan	6–12 μg/kg load; 0.05–0.1 μg/kg/min	Troponin C, increasing Ca^{2+} sensitivity; ATP-sensitive K^+ channels for vasodilation	+	0	–	–	–	1 h	Hypotension, tachyarrhythmias, nausea, headache
Digoxin	Oral: 5–15 mcg/kg/d divided every 12 h IV: 4–12 mcg/kg/day divided every 12 h	Inhibition of the Na+/K+ ATPase in myocardium	+	–	–	–	–	Infants: 18–25 h Children: 35 h	Nausea and vomiting Dizziness, headache, dysrhythmia

(continued)

Table 4.4 (continued)

Drug	Dose	Receptors	Inotropy	HR[a]	SVR	PVR	Renal vascular resistance	Half- life	Adverse effects
Phenylephrine	Bolus intravenous dose: 5–20 mcg/kg which could be repeated every 10–20 min Intravenous infusion dose: 0.1–0.5 mcg/kg/min Increase/decrease rate of infusion by minimum of 10 mcg/min at intervals no longer than Q 15 min Titration parameter: MAP; SBP adjusted for age	Selective α1 agonist	0/+	0/– May decrease heart rate if blood pressure goes very high	+++	0/+	++	5 min	Bradycardia, arrhythmia, myocardial ischemia If extravasation occurs, skin necrosis is possible
Vasopressin	0.04 units/min	Agonist of vasopressin 1 (V1) receptors	0	0	+	0		10–30 min	Hypertension Bradycardia Arrhythmia Vasoconstriction Distal limb ischemia If extravasation occurs, skin necrosis is possible

Modified from Fellin (2014). Published with kind permission of © Springer, 2014. All Rights Reserved

+ = increase, – = decrease, 0 = no change

[a]*v* vasopressin, *HR* heart rate, *SVR* systemic vascular resistance, *PVR* pulmonary vascular resistance, *DA* dopamine, *cAMP* cyclic adenosine monophosphate, *cGMP* cyclic guanosine monophosphate

[b]Recommended dose in Moss and Adams Heart Disease in Infants, Children, and Adolescent 2013: 1 μg/kg load; 0.1–0.2 μg/kg/min

Inodilators (Mainly Milrinone, Dobutamine, and Levosimendan)

The inodilators are primarily milrinone, dobutamine, and levosimendan. A summary of their characteristics could be found in Table 4.5.

Milrinone

Name of Drug Milrinone lactate

CAS Number 78415-72-2

Drug Group Cardiotonic drug; phosphodiesterase III inhibitor

Mechanism of Effect Milrinone is a positive inotropic agent and an arterial dilator with weak chronotropic effects; the drug mechanisms are totally different from catecholamine agents. Due to its effects, milrinone is commonly known as an "inodilator"; its mechanism of action is through inhibition of phosphodiesterase (PDE) III isoenzyme in cardiomyocytes and vascular smooth muscle cells; the action of PDE III is to degrade cAMP, and when it is inhibited, intracellular cAMP levels are peaked up which, in turn, leads to increased activation of protein kinase A (PKA). With increased action of PKA, many cellular structures of cardiomyocytes like calcium channels and contractile elements are activated. One of the most important roles of cAMP is to activate protein kinase A (PKA)-mediated phosphorylation of multiple target proteins (Knight and Yan 2012; Ferrer-Barba et al. 2016).

PDE III is one subfamily of the great family of PDEs; there are 11 subfamilies of PDEs; among them, 6 subfamilies function inside cardiac myocytes. One of the main roles of PDE family is to modulate the intracellular cyclic adenosine monophosphate (cAMP) and/or cyclic guanosine monophosphate (cGMP), in order to regulate the dynamic interactions between PDEs, cardiac β-adrenergic, PKA, and the process of "synthesis and hydrolysis" of cAMP and cGMP; these are elements of myocardial cells and the contractile processes; more details could be found in Chap. 2 "Cardiovascular Physiology" (Yan et al. 2007; Zaccolo and Movsesian 2007; Miller and Yan 2010; Zhao et al. 2015, 2016).

In smooth muscle cells of the arterial system, PKA leads to relaxation of the vessel walls. However, milrinone does not affect beta-adrenergic activity nor it blocks the activity of Na/K ATPase activity like cardiac glycosides. The positive inotropic effects of milrinone are presented as augmented myocardial contractility and improved Frank–Starling curve in patients with perioperative low cardiac output state. In addition to augmentation of systolic function, milrinone improves diastolic relaxation of the myocardial tissue, leading to improved diastolic function. The inodilator effects of milrinone are seen when the plasma level of the drug is in the range of 100–300 nanogram/mL (Begum et al. 2011; Knight and Yan 2012; Majure et al. 2013; Brunner et al. 2014; Bianchi et al. 2015; Ferrer-Barba et al. 2016; Gist et al. 2016).

Table 4.5 A summary and comparison between the main inodilators regarding their pharmacological properties in pediatrics

Drug	Dose	HR	MAP	PCWP	CO	SVR	Adverse effects
Milrinone	0.25–0.75 mcg/kg/min Increase/decrease by minimum of 0.125 mcg/kg/min at intervals no longer than Q 6 h *Parameters for titration of drug*: blood pressure; CO; CI	0/+	0/–	–	+	–	Arrhythmia, thrombocytopenia, myocardial ischemia, hypotension/vasodilation *No increase* in myocardial oxygen demand
Dobutamine	2.5–20 mcg/kg/min Increase/decrease by 1 mcg/kg/min at intervals no longer than Q 30 min *Parameters for titration of drug*: blood pressure; CO; CI	0/+	0	–	+	–	Arrhythmia may potentiate hypokalemia, increases myocardial oxygen demand, and so may lead to myocardial ischemia and hypotension/vasodilation
Levosimendan	Loading dose: 6–12 µg/kg over 10 min and then intravenous infusion of 0.05–0.2 µg/kg/min	0/+	0/–	–	+		Headache and/or hypotension may be induced due to vasodilatory effects of drug *No* risk of arrhythmia *No* renal or hepatic dose adjustment needed *No increase* in myocardial oxygen demand

Modified from Fellin (2014). Published with kind permission of © Springer, 2014. All Rights Reserved
+ = increase, – = decrease, 0 = no change

Indications Milrinone is primarily used for the following uses:

- Perioperative low cardiac output state (LCOS), including systolic and/or diastolic dysfunction of the myocardial tissue.
- In heart failure patients (including cardiogenic shock), milrinone is used for acute term treatment; however, its effectiveness in long-term treatment of heart failure is not confirmed yet.
- Pulmonary hypertension, especially in cases of *perioperative pulmonary hypertensive crisis* (some studies have demonstrated inhalational use as the method of choice for such patients).

Drug Dose

- *Loading dose*: 25–75 μg/kg (in patients undergoing cardiopulmonary bypass, this loading dose is often administered as a bolus dose during CPB); however, if the patient is not under cardiopulmonary bypass, this loading dose should be administered intravenously in 10–60 min, with vigilant control of blood pressure.
- *Maintenance dose*: 0.25–0.75 μg/kg/min as intravenous continuous infusion, the loading dose can be avoided to prevent the initial hypotension, and the treatment can begin with the infusion, recognizing that therapeutic plasma levels will not be achieved for several hours.

These doses lead to the desired plasma level of 100–300 nanogram/mL; however, in patients with acute kidney injury, there should be dose modification, since milrinone is metabolized mainly through kidneys (Gist et al. 2016).

Routes of Administration Milrinone is infused primarily through intravenous route, either peripheral or central lines; however, during cardiopulmonary bypass, bolus dose of drug could be administered through the ports of bypass circuit. Some studies have demonstrated these alternative routes; their efficacy is to be determined:

- Intraosseous (e.g., during cardiopulmonary resuscitation when there is no intravenous line)
- Inhalational route, especially in pulmonary hypertension crisis and cardiac transplant patient which is selectively absorbed by the pulmonary vascular system, so preventing hypotension (Brunner et al. 2014; Ventetuolo and Klinger 2014)
- Oral route which is not a routine method since it is claimed to increase morbidity (Ogawa et al. 2014)

The primary bolus dose and then the maintenance dose of milrinone could be diluted with these solutions:

- Half saline
- Normal saline
- Normal saline with 5 % dextrose

Adverse Effects and Pharmaceutical Precautions:

- One of the main contraindications of milrinone is hypersensitivity to drug or any of its formulations.

- Obstructive valve lesions, especially diseases like hypertrophic subaortic stenosis, aortic valve stenosis, or pulmonary valve stenosis; in such patients, pending on the severity of stenosis, milrinone may be prohibited or, at least, its use must be with strict caution.
- Decreased impulse delay in atrioventricular (AV) node which might lead to increased ventricular response in patients with underlying atrial flutter or atrial fibrillation; it is recommended to start cardiac glycosides before milrinone in these patients (Fleming et al. 2008); also, it has been demonstrated that in congenital heart surgery, milrinone is "an independent risk factor for clinically significant early postoperative tachyarrhythmias" (Smith et al. 2011).
- Currently, there is not enough data to support intravenous or oral administration of milrinone for periods more than 48 h; overwhelming intracellular accumulation of cAMP has been proposed as the underlying mechanism for such untoward effects; it might lead to arrhythmias.
- In patients on diuretics, adding milrinone may lead to increased renal perfusion and potential electrolyte abnormalities.
- Decreased ventricular filling pressures may result in severe hypotension which mandates hemodynamic vigilance while starting the drug.

Dobutamine

Mechanism of Action Dobutamine, which is a synthetic congener of dopamine, mainly acts as a pure positive inotropic agent through adrenergic receptors. It has no effect on DA receptors or the release of norepinephrine from nerve endings. Dobutamine mainly targets $\beta1$ receptors and its effects on $\beta2$ or $\alpha1$ receptors are less pronounced. Dobutamine produces a reduction in systemic vascular resistance with only a modest increase in heart rate and blood pressure, which is its most important advantage over dopamine and can be beneficial in patients with ventricular dysfunction.

Indications Indicated in cardiac decompensation and shock, acute heart failure, low cardiac output state after open heart surgery, neonates with asphyxia, myocarditis, MI, and after open heart surgery.

Dosage Given as continuous IV infusion in dose of 2–20 mcg/kg/min. Doses more than 20 mcg/kg per minute may produce tachycardia and ventricular ectopy and could induce or exacerbate myocardial ischemia. The concentration used is individualized depending on each patients' drug and fluid requirements but should not exceed 5000 mcg/mL (=5 mg/mL). Infusion of dobutamine should be gradually tapered after 48–72 h of administration. In patients with hypotension, dopamine or noradrenaline infusion may be used concomitantly with dobutamine.

Side Effects Ectopic heartbeats, increased heart rate, elevations in BP, hypotension, phlebitis, local inflammatory changes

Contraindications Contraindicated in obstructive lesions of the heart, cardiac arrhythmias. Hypovolemia must be corrected prior to dobutamine administration. Compared with milrinone, dobutamine shows more profound decrease in left ventricular filling pressures and vascular resistance than the phosphodiesterase inhibitors and is more likely to increase heart rate. When compared to isoproterenol, dobutamine causes less improvement in the automaticity of the sinoatrial (SA) node (Kee 2003; Holmes 2005; Noori and Seri 2012; Jentzer et al. 2015; Rossano et al. 2016).

Levosimendan

Levosimendan is a myocyte calcium sensitizer which is used mainly for treatment of acute decompensated heart failure and/or low cardiac output states in some countries. However, in a number of other countries including the USA, levosimendan is not licensed. Also, a number of trials have been done in pediatric patients demonstrating its efficacy in pediatric congenital heart disease. Its mechanism of action is through increasing myocyte calcium sensitivity by attaching to cardiac troponin C (TnC); this effect is mediated through a calcium-dependent mechanism; but its vasodilatory effects are mediated through opening ATP-sensitive potassium channels; due to these mechanisms, levosimendan does not increase myocardial oxygen demand; instead, it has cardioprotective effects through activation of ATP-sensitive K channels in the mitochondria.

Levosimendan needs no renal or hepatic dose adjustment. Its main complications include headache and/or hypotension due to vasodilatory effects of drug; however, there is no risk of arrhythmia.

The loading dose of levosimendan is 6–12 µg/kg administered intravenously over 10 min followed by continuous intravenous infusion of 0.05–0.2 µg/kg/min; time to start of effect is 5 min, with peak effects being observed in 10–30 min; the time duration of levosimendan effects is about 1–2 h; the infusion should be continued up to 24 h.

Levosimendan may decrease the mortality rate in adult patients; however, the data in pediatric patients are not enough yet (Mebazaa et al. 2007; Landoni et al. 2012; Lechner et al. 2012; Papp et al. 2012; Nieminen et al. 2013; Li and Hwang 2015; Silvetti et al. 2015; Ferrer-Barba et al. 2016; Kushwah et al. 2016; Rizza et al. 2016).

Pure Vasodilators

Nitroglycerin

Nitroglycerin (NTG) and nitroprusside are nitric oxide (NO) donors; however, NTG is predominantly a venodilator, while nitroprusside is a preferential arterial dilator. Besides, the release of NO after NTG administration is mediated through enzymatic pathways. Venodilation due to NTG leads to decrease in preload which decreases in turn the myocardial wall stress; the final result is improved oxygen balance of the myocardial tissue leading to improved myocardial function. Another beneficial effect of NTG is coronary vasodilation. Therapeutic dose of NTG is 0.5–5 µg/kg/min. However, doses from 0.5 to 2 µg/kg/min lead to venodilation, while doses from 2 to 5 µg/kg/min lead to improved cardiac index and decreased pulmonary and systemic blood pressure. Dose titration is based on clinical response (Hari and Sinha 2011).

Hydralazine

Hydralazine is an antihypertensive drug. It lowers blood pressure with a peripheral vasodilating effect, brought on by interfering with the calcium flow in vascular smooth muscle. Hydralazine effect on peripheral vascular resistance is more pronounced in arterioles as opposed to veins; it decreases diastolic blood pressure more than systolic and leads to an increase in heart rate and stroke volume and cardiac output. Hydralazine has an increasing effect on renal and cerebral blood flow.

In *pediatric patients*, hydralazine is used as an oral antihypertensive agent, when BP is not sufficiently controlled by first-line antihypertensive drugs. The common oral dose in hypertension is 0.75 mg/kg daily (or 25 mg/m^2) in 4 divided doses and can be increased gradually up to 7.5 mg/kg daily (or 200 mg daily). It can also be used parenterally in severe hypertension. In this case, 0.2–0.6 mg/kg hydralazine is administrated IV or IM and can be repeated every 4 h. Hydralazine is contraindicated in patients with mitral valvular rheumatic heart disease and CAD. It can cause pyridoxine insufficiency and peripheral neuritis and blood dyscrasias. Patients CBC and neurological symptoms should be monitored during treatment (Hari and Sinha 2011; Watt et al. 2011; Ostrye et al. 2014; Flynn et al. 2016).

Alprostadil

Alprostadil (prostaglandin E1) has various pharmacological effects including vasodilation, stimulation of smooth muscle contraction in intestine and uterus, inhibition of platelet aggregation, and so on. Its vasodilatory effect is shown with doses of 1–10 mcg/kg and can reduce blood pressure and, in reflex, increase cardiac output and heart rate.

Since smooth muscles in ductus arteriosus are especially sensitive to alprostadil, and based on animal studies, there are evidence that alprostadil can reopen closing ductus in newborns; the drug has been investigated in infants with congenital defects with restricted pulmonary or systemic blood flow who depend on a patent ductus arteriosus for sufficient oxygenation and perfusion.

In such pediatric patients, alprostadil infusion was associated with at least a 10 torr increase in blood pO_2 (mean increase about 14 torr and mean increase in oxygen saturation about 23 %) in about 50 % of the patients. Patients with low pretreatment blood pO_2 who were 4 days old or less seem to have the best response to alprostadil.

Alprostadil can improve acidosis in patients with restricted systemic blood flow. It can also increase systemic blood pressure and decrease the ratio of pulmonary artery pressure to aortic pressure.

Alprostadil is administrated as intravenous or intra-arterial infusion, and the common dose of this drug in patients with ductus arteriosus-dependent congenital heart disease is described here.

In neonates, 0.05–0.1 mcg/kg/min is the starting dose which can be increased gradually to ≤0.4 mcg/kg/min. After therapeutic response achieved, the dosage can be reduced for maintenance from 0.1 downward in a stepwise method, 0.05, 0.025, and finally to 0.01 mcg/kg/min, until lowest effective dose is achieved. The treatment should be continued until surgical repair is complete (usually ≤24–48 h). Arterial pressure should be monitored intermittently, and the infusion rate should be decreased immediately if the pressure drops significantly. Response can be monitored by measuring blood oxygenation or pH (Carroll et al. 2006; Cuthbert 2011; Strobel and Lu le 2015; Lakshminrusimha et al. 2016).

Sodium Nitroprusside

Sodium nitroprusside (SNP) like nitroglycerin is a nitric oxide (NO) donor. Inside the tissues, SNP reacts with physiologic sulfhydryl groups, and the final result is release of NO which in turn increases tissue levels of cGMP, especially in the arterial and venous system; the final result would be smooth muscle relaxation in the walls of the arterial and venous vessels. Physiologically speaking, SNP decreases afterload of left ventricle leading to improved cardiac output, though some degrees of hypotension occur; however, the improved cardiac output, especially in patients with depressed cardiac function, compensates for the hypotension, unless there is profound preexisting hypovolemia or the patient has underlying obstructive diseases like hypertrophic obstructive cardiomyopathy, aortic stenosis, or mitral stenosis (Friederich and Butterworth 1995; Moffett and Price 2008; Thomas et al. 2009).

There is a major concern for SNP toxicity in long-term or large dose infusions; reaction of SNP with oxyhemoglobin leads to formation of methemoglobin, with its final by-product, cyanide anions. Cyanide may be metabolized in the liver, or it could be accumulated in erythrocytes; however, none are greatly toxic. But if cyanide accumulates in the tissues, it could be attached to tissue cytochrome oxidase, which results in toxic impairment of oxidative phosphorylation. To prevent this side effect, we should care about cyanide accumulation, and for this purpose, infusion of large doses of the drug for long time periods should be prohibited (Moffett and Price 2008; Thomas et al. 2009; Hottinger et al. 2014).

The recommended drug dose for intravenous infusion starts at 0.3–0.5 mcg/kg/min up to a maximum of 10 mcg/kg/min; however, increasing drug dose should be cautiously performed, and effect titration should be the basic monitoring tool for increasing the drug dose to prevent hypotension and toxicity. The best predictor for SNP toxicity is its mean dose which predicts elevated cyanide levels better than any other adverse events of cyanide toxicity, especially in postoperative care of pediatric patients undergoing cardiac surgical procedures (Moffett and Price 2008; Thomas et al. 2009; Moffett et al. 2016).

The onset of action of SNP is within seconds, with its duration to be about 1–2 min and its plasma half-life about 3–4 min (Varon and Marik 2003).

In doses above 3 mcg/kg/min, doses more than 48–72 h, or in patients with renal insufficiency, the risk of drug toxicity increases significantly. There are studies that suggest that in pediatric cardiac surgery, the desired effects of SNP could be gained with 1 mcg/kg/min of the drug and doses above 2 mcg/kg/min should be preferably avoided (Friederich and Butterworth 1995; Hottinger et al. 2014; Drover et al. 2015).

Inhalational forms of SNP have been produced to prevent its toxicity especially in patients with pulmonary hypertension.

Phentolamine Mesylate (Regitine)

Phentolamine mesylate is a nonselective alpha-adrenergic blocker of relatively short duration. Its other less pronounced effects include a direct positive inotropic and chronotropic effects on cardiac muscle and vasodilator effects on vascular smooth muscle. Blocking the presynaptic α_2-adrenergic receptors can be the cause of tachycardia and arrhythmias seen with high doses of these drugs.

Phentolamine produces a decrease in systemic vascular resistance that results in an increase in cardiac output. It also reduces pulmonary vascular resistance and pulmonary arterial pressure. The common doses for this drug can be found in Table 4.6. The most important side effects of this drug are significant sinus tachycardia, arrhythmias, and excessive hypotension (Allen et al. 2013).

Antihypertensive Agents

Hypertension in pediatric patients may lead to organ damage. Currently, a wide range of antihypertensive agents are available in adult that the majority of them could be used in pediatric patients (Flynn 2011; Chu et al. 2014; Dhull et al. 2016). On the other hand, treatment of neonatal hypertension is a great challenge and needs sophisticated care (Sharma et al. 2014; Sharma et al. 2016).

The current antihypertensive pharmaceutical agents could be categorized mainly in the following subclasses:

Angiotensin-converting enzyme (*ACE*) inhibitors: among them, captopril, enalapril, lisinopril, and ramipril are the commonly used agents; however, among other members of the group, fosinopril, perindopril, quinapril, trandolapril, and benazepril could be mentioned. The main ACE inhibitors are summarized in Table 4.7 and nearly all of them are safe for treatment of pediatric hypertension (Chaturvedi et al. 2014a, b; Dhull et al. 2016).

Angiotensin II receptor antagonists (ARBs): losartan and valsartan are the prototype drugs in this group; however, other members of the group include: candesartan, eprosartan, irbesartan, olmesartan, and telmisartan. The main ARBs are presented in Table 4.8. Nearly all of ARBs are safe in pediatric patients (Chaturvedi et al. 2014a, b; Dhull et al. 2016).

Table 4.6 A summary of vasoactive drugs including vasodilator and vasoconstrictor drugs used in congenital heart diseases

Drug	Dose	Receptors	Indication	Half-life (duration)	Adverse effects/notes
Vasopressin	0.01–0.05 U/kg/h	V_1, V_2	Refractory hypotension after conventional drugs have failed, heart failure, vasodilatory shock, e.g., septic shock	10–30 min	Splanchnic ischemia due to its vasoconstrictor action
Phenylephrine	0.02–0.3 µg/kg/min	α_1	Hypotension during anesthesia	5 min	Nausea, vomiting, headache, nervousness
Nitroglycerin	0.2–10 µg/kg/min	Vascular myocyte/ guanylyl cyclase, cGMP ↑	Post cardiac surgery for valvular regurgitation; cardiac surgeries where coronaries are involved, e.g., arterial switch operation, Ross operation and repair for anomalous left coronary artery from pulmonary artery, and systemic hypertension	1–4 min	Hypotension, tachycardia, methemoglobinemia leading to cyanosis, acidosis, convulsions, and coma
Nitroprusside	0.2–5 µg/kg/min	Vascular myocyte/ guanylyl cyclase, cGMP ↑	Systemic hypertension, e.g., after repair of coarctation of aorta, malignant hypertension of renal vascular origin, acute and severe valvular regurgitation, low cardiac output state following cardiac surgery, especially after valvular surgery, acute heart failure	2 min	Excessive hypotension, cyanide toxicity
Inhaled nitric oxide	10–40 ppm	Vascular myocyte/ cGMP ↑	Pulmonary hypertension of the newborn	2–6 s	Nitric oxide should not be used for long term, as it results in methemoglobinemia

(continued)

Table 4.6 (continued)

Drug	Dose	Receptors	Indication	Half-life (duration)	Adverse effects/notes
Prostaglandin E1	0.01–0.4 µg/kg/min	Vascular myocyte/ cAMP ↑	In newborns who have congenital heart defects (e.g., pulmonary stenosis, tricuspid atresia) and who depend on patent ductus for survival	0.5–10 min	Hypotension, cardiac arrest, edema
Fenoldopam	0.025–0.3 µg/kg/ min initial dose, titrate to maximum dose 0.8 µg/kg/min	DA-1, α2	Severe hypertension	3–5 min	Hypotension, tachycardia
Nicardipine	1–3 µg/kg/min IV infusion, maximum 15 mg/h	Calcium channel antagonist	Severe hypertension	14.4 h	Headache, hypotension, nausea/vomiting, tachycardia
Phentolamine mesylate	1 mg, 0.1 mg/kg, or 3 mg/m^2	α-adrenergic blocking agent, an imidazoline	Hypertension crisis, hypertension in pheochromocytoma, extravasation of catecholamines, pulmonary artery hypertension	15–30 min	Abdominal pain, nausea, vomiting, diarrhea, exacerbation of peptic ulcer, orthostatic hypotension

Table 4.7 The main ACE inhibitors in pediatric patients

Drug	Dose	Half-life	Adverse effects
Captopril	Oral: 0.3–2.5 mg/kg/day divided every 8–12 h In infants and 0.3–6 mg/kg/day divided every 8–12 h in children and adolescents	Infants: 3.3 h Children: 1–2.3 h	Hypotension Dizziness Headache Rash Hyperkalemia Cough Angioedema
Enalapril	Oral: 0.1–0.5 mg/kg/day divided every 12 h IV (as enalaprilat): 5–10 µg/kg/dose every 8–24 h	Neonates: 10.3 h Infants and children: 2.7 (1.3–6.3) h Enalaprilat: Neonates: 11.9 (5.9–15.6) h Infants and children: 11.1 (5.1–20.8) h	
Lisinopril	Oral: initial, 0.07–0.1 mg/kg/dose once daily ≤0.5–0.6 mg/kg/day	11–13 h	
Ramipril	Oral: 2–6 mg/m2 daily ≤10 mg daily	Ramiprilat: 13–17 h	

Table 4.8 The main ARBs used in pediatric patients

Drug	Dose	Half-life	Adverse effects
Losartan	Oral: initial, 0.5 mg/kg once daily not to exceed Up to 1.4 mg/kg once daily; should not exceed 150 mg/day	1.5–2 h Active metabolite: 6–9 h	Hypotension Dizziness Headache Hyperkalemia Hypoglycemia Diarrhea
Valsartan	1–5 years: oral dose, 0.4–3.4 mg/kg once daily 6–16 years: initial oral dose, 1.3 mg/kg/dose once daily ≤2.7 mg/kg/dose once daily	4–5 h	

Calcium channel blockers (CCBs): they are categorized in two main subgroups including dihydropyridines and non-dihydropyridines; these are safe agents for treatment of pediatric hypertension (Chaturvedi et al. 2014a, b; Dhull et al. 2016). The main CCBs are summarized in Table 4.9.

Diuretics Diuretic agents are mainly classified in four subgroups which are discussed in Tables 4.10, 4.11, and 4.12 (Dhull et al. 2016; McCammond et al. 2016):

- *Loop* diuretics (bumetanide, ethacrynic acid, furosemide, torsemide)
- *Potassium-sparing* diuretics (mineralocorticoid "aldosterone" receptor antagonists) which include spironolactone, amiloride, and triamterene
- *Thiazide* diuretics (epitizide, hydrochlorothiazide and chlorothiazide, bendroflumethiazide)
- *Thiazide-like* diuretics (indapamide, chlorthalidone, metolazone)

Table 4.9 The main calcium channel blockers used in pediatric patients

Drug	Dose	Half-life	Adverse effects
Amlodipine	Children 6–17 years: 2.5–5 mg once daily or divided every 12 h	30–50 h	Edema, dizziness, flushing, palpitations, fatigue, nausea, abdominal pain, somnolence
Nifedipine	Initially, 0.25–0.5 mg/kg daily given in 1 dose or 2 divided doses up to a maximum dosage of 3 mg/kg (up to 120 mg) daily, given in 1 dose or 2 divided doses	2–7 h	
Isradipine	Initially, 0.15–0.2 mg/kg daily given in 3–4 divided doses up to a maximum dosage of 0.8 mg/kg (up to 20 mg) daily	Biphasic; initial half-life 1.5–2 h, terminal elimination half-life approximately 8 h	

Table 4.10 The main loop diuretics

Drug	Dose	Half-life	Adverse effects
Bumetanide	IV, intramuscular, or oral dose: 0.015–0.1 mg/kg/dose every 6–24 h	Neonates: 6 h Infants: 2.4 h	Hyperuricemia Hypomagnesemia Hyponatremia
Ethacrynic acid	Oral: 0.5–1 mg/kg/dose every 6–12 h IV: 1–2 mg/kg/dose every 8–12 h	2–4 h	Hypokalemia Metabolic alkalosis
Furosemide	Oral: 1–2 mg/kg/dose every 6–24 h IV, intramuscular: 0.5–2 mg/kg/dose every 6–24 h Continuous IV infusion: 0.1–0.4 mg/kg/h	0.5–2 h; 9 h in end-stage renal disease	

Modified from Fellin (2014). Published with kind permission of © Springer, 2014. All Rights Reserved
IV intravenous

Table 4.11 Spironolactone: the main mineralocorticoid (aldosterone) receptor antagonist

Drug	Dose	Half-life	Adverse effects
Spironolactone	Oral: initial 1 mg/kg/day in divided doses every 6–24 h ≤ 12.5 to 25 mg/day Maximum: 3.3–6 mg/kg/day divided every 6–24 h; should not exceed 100 mg/day	1.4 h; active metabolites: 12–20 h	Diarrhea Nausea Vomiting Dizziness Hyperkalemia Gynecomastia

Table 4.12 Thiazide and thiazide-like diuretics

Drug	Dose	Half-life	Adverse effects
Chlorothiazide	Oral: 10–40 mg/kg/day in divided doses every 12 h IV: 4–10 mg/kg/day divided every 12–24 h (maximum 20 mg/kg/day or 500 mg)	45–120 min	Hyperuricemia Hypomagnesemia Hyponatremia Hypokalemia
Hydrochlorothiazide	Oral: 1–4 mg/kg/day in divided doses every 12–24 h	6–15 h	
Metolazone	Oral: 0.2–0.4 mg/kg/day divided every 12–24 h	6–20 h	

Modified from Fellin (2014). Published with kind permission of © Springer, 2014. All Rights Reserved

Adrenergic receptor antagonists (alpha and/or beta blockers): some of these agents are discussed under the antiarrhythmic categories; however, some other are presented in Table 4.13.

Vasodilators These include arterial and/or venodilators. Nitroglycerin, nitroprusside, hydralazine, and minoxidil are among common vasodilators. Nitroglycerin and nitroprusside are discussed in the previous parts of the chapter, while hydralazine and Minoxidil are summarized in Table 4.14. Evidence shows that these agents are applicable in treatment of systemic hypertension in pediatric patients (Hari and Sinha 2011; Ostrye et al. 2014; Dhull et al. 2016; Flynn et al. 2016).

Drugs Used in Pulmonary Hypertension

For a detailed review on right ventricular failure and pulmonary hypertension treatment, the audience is suggested to refer to Chap. 32, Pulmonary Hypertension, and Chap. 33, Right Ventricular Failure. However, a brief review of the drugs used in pulmonary hypertension in congenital heart surgery is presented in the next paragraphs and in Table 4.15.

The only FDA-approved pharmaceutical specifically for treatment of pulmonary hypertension in children is inhaled nitric oxide (iNO) which is administered through the lungs. The other FDA-approved drugs for treatment of pulmonary hypertension used in adults are often based on the pathways related to the endothelial cells, including prostacyclin analogues (epoprostenol, iloprost, treprostinil), phosphodiesterase 5 inhibitors (sildenafil and tadalafil), phosphodiesterase 3 inhibitors (mainly milrinone), endothelin receptor antagonist (bosentan, ambrisentan, and macitentan), and soluble guanylate cyclase stimulator (riociguat) (Poor and Ventetuolo 2012; Ventetuolo and Klinger 2014; Abman et al. 2015; Jentzer and Mathier 2015; Kim et al. 2016).

Table 4.13 A number of adrenoceptor blocking agents

Drug	Dose	Half-life	Adverse effects
β-blockers			
Metoprolol	Initial oral dose: 0.1–0.25 mg/kg/dose twice daily, not to exceed 12.5–25 mg; up to a maximum daily dose of 1–2 mg/kg/dose twice daily, not to exceed 100 mg twice daily	3–4 h (7–9 h in poor CYP2D6 metabolizers)	Brady-arrhythmias Hypotension Headache Dizziness Fatigue
Esmolol	IV Children and adolescents 1–17 years of age: 100–500 mcg/kg per minute as constant infusion	4–7 min	The effects due to β1 selective actions
Propranolol	2–4 mg/kg daily in 2 equally divided doses up to 16 mg/kg daily	3–6 h	
Mixed alpha + beta blocker			
Carvedilol	Initial oral dose: 0.1 mg/kg/day divided twice daily Not to exceed 3.125 mg Up to a maximum daily dose of 0.8–1 mg/kg/day; divided twice daily; not to exceed 25 mg twice daily		
Labetalol	Oral Initially, 1–3 mg/kg daily given in 2 divided doses. Maximum: 10–12 mg/kg or 1.2 g daily given in 2 divided doses IV injection (severe hypertension) Children 1–17 years of age: 0.2–1 mg/kg up to maximum of 40 mg per dose by direct IV injection. Alternatively, 0.25–3 mg/kg/h by continuous IV infusion	5.5 h after IV administration and 6–8 h after oral administration	The effects due to intrinsic sympathomimetic action, α1 receptor antagonist
Peripheral alpha blockers			
Prazosin	Initially, 0.05–0.1 mg/kg daily given in 3 divided doses up to 0.5 mg/kg daily in 3 doses	2–4 h	Dizziness, lightheadedness, headache, drowsiness, lack of energy, weakness, palpitation, nausea
Terazosin	1–20 mg once daily	Approximately 12 h	

Table 4.13 (continued)

Drug	Dose	Half-life	Adverse effects
Alpha-2 adrenergic agonists			
Clonidine	Initially, 0.05–0.1 mg, may repeat up to maximum of 0.8 mg	6–20 h	Dry mouth Dizziness Drowsiness
Methyldopa	Initial oral dose: 10 mg/kg daily given in 2–4 divided doses Intravenous dose: 20–40 mg/kg per day which should be administrated every 6 h, with max dose of 65 mg/kg or 3 g per day	2–8 h after single oral dose or 4–12 h multiple oral doses	Sedation Constipation Major depression (for methyldopa)

(Driscoll et al. 2015; Xue et al. 2015; Klugman et al. 2016; McCammond et al. 2016; Rossano et al. 2016; Zou et al. 2016)

Table 4.14 Common vasodilators used in pediatric patients

Drug	Dose	Half-life	Adverse effects

Hydralazine	Oral
	  0.75–7.5 mg/kg/day; given in 4 divided doses, max 200 mg/day
	IM or IV
	  Usual dosage: 1.7–3.5 mg/kg/day or 50–100 mg/m2/day, which should be given in 4–6 divided doses (max dose on first dose 20 mg)
	Severe hypertension: IV or IM
	  Children and adolescents (1–17 years of age): 0.2–0.6 mg/kg per dose; administer every 4 h when given by intravenous bolus injection
		2–4 h	Retention of salt and water
			Reflex tachycardia
			Headache
			Palpitation

Minoxidil	0.25–1 mg/kg/day in 1 or 2 doses up to a maximum dosage of 50 mg/day	4 h	Hypertrichosis Retention of salt and water Nausea and vomiting Pericardial effusion

Modified from Fellin (2014). Published with kind permission of © Springer, 2014. All Rights Reserved

Nitric Oxide

Nitric oxide commonly known as NO is a very small lipophilic molecule, with very crucial role in intracellular signaling mechanisms in many of the cells. NO is synthetized inside the cells from transformation of L arginine; nitric oxide synthase (NOS) is the enzyme that catalyzes production of NO.

Table 4.15 Pharmacological agents used in management of pulmonary hypertension (Abman et al. 2015; Latus et al. 2015; Hansmann et al. 2016; Kim et al. 2016; Moffett et al. 2016)

Drug	Recommended dose	Adverse effects	Clinical considerations
Inhaled nitric oxide (iNO): mechanism of action is increasing cGMP, leading to smooth muscle relaxation and, subsequently, pulmonary vasodilation			
iNO	2–5 ppm to a maximum of 40 ppm	Lung injury Increased methemoglobin levels Rebound severe pulmonary hypertension due to abrupt iNO withdrawal	The only FDA-approved agent for pediatric pulmonary hypertension Should not be over administered to prevent side effects Its cost may suggest to consider the drug as the last choice
Prostacyclin/prostacyclin analogues: their mechanism of action is pulmonary and systemic vasodilation through increasing cAMP, also antiplatelet aggregation			
Epoprostenol	*Initial* infusion rate: 1–3 ng/kg/min *Maintenance* infusion rate: 50–80 ng/kg/min	Flushing, headache, nausea, diarrhea, jaw discomfort, rash, hypotension, thrombocytopenia	Potential risk of hypotension and bleeding in children receiving drugs, such as anticoagulants, platelet inhibitors, or other vasodilators
Iloprost	*Initial* dose: 2.5 μg per inhalation; 6 times/day *Maintenance* dose: 5 μg per inhalation 9 times/day	Cough, wheeze, headache, flushing, jaw pain, diarrhea, rash, and hypotension (at higher doses)	Potential risk of exacerbation of reactive airway disease
Treprostinil (IV/subcutaneous)	*Initial* infusion rate: 1.25–2 ng/kg/min *Maintenance* infusion rate: 50–80 ng/kg/min	Flushing, headache, nausea, diarrhea, musculoskeletal discomfort, rash, hypotension, thrombocytopenia, and pain at subcutaneous infusion site	Similar to epoprostenol
Treprostinil (inhaled)	*Initial* dose: 3 breaths (18 μg)/4 times/day *Maintenance* dose: 9 breaths (54 μg) 4 times/day	Cough, headache, nausea, dizziness, flushing, and throat irritation	Reactive airway symptoms and hypotension may occur at high doses
Treprostinil (oral)	*Initial* dose: 0.25 mg PO BID *Maintenance* dose: determined by tolerability	Headache, nausea, diarrhea, jaw pain, extremity pain, hypokalemia, abdominal discomfort, and flushing	If "twice daily" dosing is not tolerated, consider "three times daily" dosing

PDE 5 inhibitors: inhibit phosphodiesterase 5, leading to pulmonary vasodilation and inhibition of vascular remodeling			
Sildenafil	*Oral* dose: 0.25–0.5 mg/kg/q4-8 h *Intravenous* dose: loading dose 0.4 mg/kg over 3 h Maintenance: continuous infusion of 1.5 mg/kg/day	Headache, flushing, rhinitis, dizziness, hypotension, peripheral edema, dyspepsia, diarrhea, myalgia, and back pain	Coadministration of nitrates is contraindicated. Sensorineural hearing loss and ischemic optic neuropathy have been reported
Tadalafil	Oral dose: 1 mg/kg per day (single daily dose), preliminary studies	Similar to sildenafil No significant effect on vision	Similar to sildenafil
Antagonists of endothelin receptor: counteract with the effects of both endothelin receptors (ET$_A$ and ET$_B$), vasodilation of the pulmonary vascular system, and vascular remodeling inhibition			
Ambrisentan	Body weight<20 kg: 2.5–5 mg PO/4 times daily Body weight>20 kg: 5–10 mg PO/4 times daily	Peripheral edema, nasal congestion, headache, flushing, anemia, nausea, and decreased sperm count	Baseline liver enzymes and hemoglobin are needed Monitor based on clinical parameters
Bosentan	2 mg/kg per dose PO, two times daily If body weight is 10–20 kg: 31.25 mg PO, two times daily If body weight is 20–40 kg: 62.5 mg PO, two times daily If body weight is>40 kg: 125 mg PO two times daily	Pediatric abdominal pain, vomiting, extremity pain, fatigue, flushing, headache, edema, nasal congestion, anemia, and decreased sperm count Potential risk of dose-dependent increases in amino-transaminase levels	Liver enzymes and hemoglobin levels should be monitored; in patients with moderate or severe degrees of hepatic impairment, it should be used cautiously Also, concomitant use of CYP3A4 inducers and inhibitors should be considered as important caution
Macitentan	10 mg PO, four times daily	Nasal congestion, headache, flushing, anemia, and decreased sperm count	The incidence of serum aminotransferase elevation is low Obtain baseline liver enzymes and hemoglobin and monitor as clinically indicated Teratogenicity REMS*
sGC stimulator: its action mechanism is stimulation of soluble guanylate cyclase leading to pulmonary vasodilation associated with inhibition of vascular remodeling			
Riociguat	*Initial* dose: 0.5–1 mg PO *Maintenance* dose: 2.5 mg PO, three times daily	Headache, dizziness, dyspepsia, nausea, diarrhea, hypotension, vomiting, anemia, gastroesophageal reflux, and constipation	Coadministration of nitrates and/or PDE 5 inhibitors is contraindicated In growing rats, effects on bone formation were observed Teratogenicity is a potential risk

Visit www.adempasREMS.com

When used as an inhaled drug, NO is readily absorbed through the pulmonary system and, after local absorption, produces considerable amounts of cGMP inside the smooth muscle cells; this cellular process leads to smooth muscle relaxation especially in pulmonary blood vessels, and subsequently, pulmonary blood pressure drops; the resulting pulmonary vasodilation is a real achievement in treatment of acute right heart failure especially when weaning from cardiopulmonary bypass is difficult due to pulmonary hypertension or when the patient is in critical pulmonary hypertension crisis and/or acute right heart failure in the intensive care setting.

The molecules of NO when administered through the pulmonary route are called inhaled NO (briefly iNO). iNO is transported very fast through the alveolar–capillary membranes, and then, its molecules are rapidly metabolized by circulating erythrocytes. This rapid process of absorption and metabolism takes just a few seconds time and so makes iNO an ideal drug; inhalational route is among the best appropriate targeted therapies in pulmonary hypertension which acts exactly on the specific site of action (pulmonary vascular system), while there are least possible systemic side effects (Kim et al. 2016; Moffett et al. 2016).

Dose: iNO is administered through endotracheal tube, face mask, or nasal cannula. It is started with the lowest possible doses, from 2 to 5 ppm to a maximum of 40 ppm; higher doses are both ineffective and may cause side effects. iNO needs specific delivery instruments, its costs are really high, and very high doses may lead to lung injury and/or increased methemoglobin levels, mandating routine monitoring of methemoglobin levels. iNO should *not* be withdrawn abruptly, or there would be severe rebound pulmonary hypertension (Atz and Wessel 1997; Mossad 2001; Gao and Raj 2010; Pritts and Pearl 2010; Abman et al. 2015; Latus et al. 2015; Hansmann et al. 2016; Kim et al. 2016; Moffett et al. 2016).

Phosphodiesterase 5(PDE 5) Inhibitors These include sildenafil, tadalafil, and vardenafil; among them, sildenafil and tadalafil are the most commonly used agents for pulmonary hypertension.

Sildenafil

Sildenafil is one of the classes of drugs known as phosphodiesterase 5 (PDE 5) inhibitors. PDE 5 degrades cGMP and when it is inhibited by sildenafil, accumulation of PDE 5 in smooth muscles of the pulmonary system leads to pulmonary vasodilation and improves pulmonary hypertension, both in acute and chronic pulmonary hypertension. It is available both as oral and intravenous forms. However, its use should be associated with extreme caution especially in the critical patients to prevent any potential life-threatening hypotension. In European Union, sildenafil has approval for treatment of pediatric patients between 1 and 17 years. However, in the USA, there are still some concerns regarding safety of sildenafil in pediatric pulmonary hypertension, especially for high doses of sildenafil and also for its application in term and preterm infants, when iNO is available. That means, currently iNO is the only formally approved agent for treatment of pulmonary hypertension in infants and neonates with pulmonary hypertension in the USA, while sildenafil is used in other places for the same indication. The recommended oral dose of sildenafil is 0.25–0.5 mg/kg every 4–8 h, with a maximum dose of 2 mg/kg every 4 h; titration of the dose should be based on clinical response; intravenous dose could be found in Table 4.15. These data are in large the same for tadalafil, except for its does which could be found in Table 4.15 (Shah and Ohlsson 2011; Beghetti et al. 2014; Vorhies and Ivy 2014; Wang et al. 2014; Dodgen and Hill 2015; Perez and Laughon 2015; Lakshminrusimha et al. 2016).

Endothelin Receptor Blockers (ET Blockers)

Endothelin receptor antagonists block endothelin receptors on endothelium and vascular smooth muscle (stimulation of these receptors is associated with vasoconstriction). Bosentan, an endothelin receptor antagonist, can inhibit both ET_A and ET_B receptor activities, with a slightly higher affinity for the A subtype; therefore, it lowers pulmonary artery pressure (PAP) and pulmonary vascular resistance (PVR); so, it improves exercise tolerance in adults with pulmonary arterial hypertension. Same results can be expected to be seen in children.

In patients treated with ET-1 antagonists, monitoring of the hepatic function should be considered seriously (Liu et al. 2013). The same is correct about bosentan: elevated hepatic aminotransferase levels are the main concern with the drug occurring in approximately 11 % of adults and 3 % of children treated with bosentan. Bosentan is approved for use in children over 12 years in the USA and in children over 3 years in Canada. The common dosing for bosentan is as follows:

- 10 to 20 kg: Initial, 31.25 mg once daily for 4 weeks; increase to maintenance dose of 31.25 mg twice daily
- >20 to 40 kg: Initial, 31.25 mg twice daily for 4 weeks; increase to maintenance dose of 62.5 mg twice daily
- >40 kg: Initial, 62.5 mg twice daily for 4 weeks; increase to maintenance dose of 125 mg twice daily

Other common adverse effects of bosentan include headache, flushing, lower limb edema, hypotension, palpitations, dyspepsia, and anemia (Allen et al. 2013).

Milrinone
It is discussed in previous sections under "inodilators."

Antiarrhythmic Agents (Moffett et al. 2016)
The antiarrhythmic agents are based on the following classification which is known as Vaughan Williams Classification of Antiarrhythmic Agents. This classification depends mainly on cellular physiology of myocardial cells, discussed fully in Chap. 3. A schematic picture of the myocardial action potential is demonstrated here which helps understand the mechanism of these agents (Fig. 4.1). The Vaughan Williams Classification of Antiarrhythmic Agents is described in brief in Table 4.16. Also, detailed description of selected agents is described in Table 4.17.

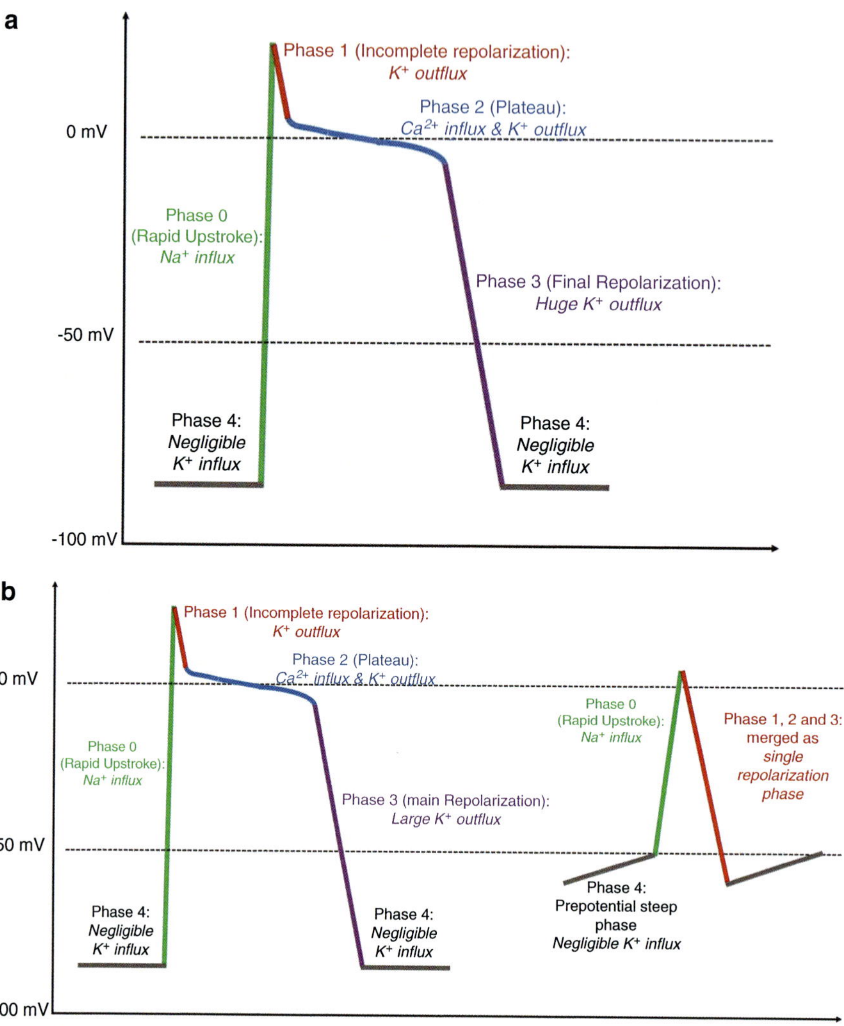

Fig. 4.1 (**a**) Progress of action potential phases in normal myocardial cells; (**b**) comparison of action potential phases between normal myocardial cells and pacemaker cells (Marcotti et al. 2004; Parham et al. 2006; Wolf and Berul 2008; Amanfu and Saucerman 2011; Marionneau and Abriel 2015)

Analgesic Agents, Sedative Drugs, and Intravenous Anesthetic Agents

Analgesia is one of the most mandatory needs during perioperative period in pediatric cardiac surgery. In fact, the children are threatened when they are separated from the parents. Even, for routine visits, anxiety and fear may disturb the child. Add to this the pain due to surgical procedure, suffering from procedures like tracheal suctioning, chest tube manipulations, and dressing change (Lucas et al. 2016).

Table 4.16 Vaughan Williams classification of antiarrhythmic agents (Vaughan Williams 1989, 1992; Zipes et al. 2006; Moffett et al. 2016)

Class of drugs	Mechanism of action	Drugs (alphabetic order)
Class Ia	*Fast Na channel blockers*: depress phase 0, prolonging repolarization	Disopyramide, procainamide, quinidine
Class Ib	*Fast Na channel blockers*: selectively depress phase 0 in abnormal/ischemic tissue, shorten repolarization	Lidocaine, mexiletine, phenytoin, tocainide
Class Ic	*Fast Na channel blockers*: markedly depress phase 0, with minimal effect on repolarization	Flecainide, moricizine, propafenone
Class II	Beta blockers: decreases slope of phase 4	Atenolol, bisoprolol, carvedilol, esmolol, metoprolol, propranolol, timolol
Class III	Potassium (K) channel blockers which prolong the cardiac action potential: mainly prolong phase 3	Amiodarone, dofetilide, ibutilide, sotalol
Class IV	Slow calcium (Ca) channel blockers: prolong phase 2	Diltiazem, verapamil
Class V	Variable mechanism	Adenosine, digoxin, magnesium sulfate

Clinical assessment of pain and sedation level is among the most basic skills needed in perioperative period. A full description of these tools and skills is described in Chap. 9 "Central Nervous System Monitoring in Pediatric Cardiac Surgery." However, to just mention the titles, the most commonly used sedation scales in these setting are:

- Ramsay Sedation Scale (Ramsay)
- Sedation Agitation Scale (SAS)
- Richmond Agitation Sedation Scale (RASS)

The very low cardiorespiratory reserve of children and infants with congenital heart diseases makes perioperative sedation and analgesia a great challenge for the caregivers that need sophisticated vigilance and exact monitoring. Overtreatment and undertreatment both have their own problems. Also, in the current era of fast-track extubation, real-time continuous monitoring is the cornerstone of postoperative care for congenital heart disease patients. These mandate appropriate choice of analgesic/sedative agents. And if the patient is going to be mechanically ventilated due to any underlying problem including hemodynamic instability, use of assist devices, pulmonary insufficiencies, or CNS insults, careful use of muscle relaxants is often among the needed ingredients of the sedation/analgesia care. Volatile anesthetics, though are not usual in the postoperative care, have a crucial role in the operating room and also could be used for some procedures (including but not limited to using sevoflurane for echocardiography in a restless baby). Tables 4.18, 4.19, 4.20, and 4.21 describe in brief the most common analgesics, sedatives, muscle relaxants, and anesthetic gases used in perioperative care of

Table 4.17 Individual antiarrhythmic agents (Moffett et al. 2016)

Medication	Dosing	Indication	Adverse events	Specific clinical considerations
Class Ia				
Procainamide	IV loading dose: 3–6 mg/kg per dose Maximum dose: 100 mg per dose (total maximum dose, 15 mg/kg) IV: continuous infusion, 20–80 mcg/kg/min	Atrial tachycardia, JET, VT	Hypotension and pro-arrhythmia	Procainamide and NAPA Concentrations are used as serum markers of therapy
Disopyramide	<1year of age 10–30 mg/kg 1–4years of age: 10–20 mg/kg 4–12 years of age: 10–15 mg/kg 12–18 years of age: 6–15 mg/kg	Ventricular arrhythmias	Anticholinergic effects	May be ineffective in patients with hypokalemia and toxic effects may be enhanced in patients with hyperkalemia
Quinidine	Oral dose: 30 mg/kg/day or 900 mg/m^2/day given in five daily doses Range: 15–60 mg/kg/day in four or five divided doses IV dose: 2–10 mg/kg per dose every 3–6 h as needed	SVT, VT, atrial tachycardia, ventricular premature complexes	Hypotension (particularly with IV formulation)	Drug level monitoring typically not performed There are two forms of drug available (sulfate and gluconate) IV route is not routinely recommended because of hypotension
Class Ib				
Lidocaine	IV bolus: 1 mg/kg per dose IV continuous infusion: 20–50 mcg/kg/min	PVCs, VT, VF	Hypotension and numbness	
Mexiletine	Adults: 400 mg loading dose (in rapid control) followed by 200 mg in 8 h	Ventricular arrhythmias	Development or exacerbation of arrhythmias and hypotension	Limit use to those with life-threatening arrhythmias, lack of evidence for improved survival for class I antiarrhythmic agents

Phenytoin	Adults: Oral 100 mg 2–4 times daily IV 100 mg by direct IV injection at 5-min intervals until a total of 1 g is given	VT, PAT	Hypotension, severe cardiotoxic reactions (e.g., decreased cardiac output, atrial or ventricular conduction depression, ventricular depression)	IV use contraindicated in patients with sinus bradycardia, SA block, second- or third-degree AV block, or Adams–Stokes syndrome
Tocainide: no longer sold in the USA				
Class Ic				
Flecainide	Oral: starting dose, 1–3 mg/kg/day or 50–100 mg/m2/day Maximum oral dose: 8 mg/kg/day or 200 mg/m2/day divided by three times/day	SVT	Potential for pro-arrhythmia in patients with congenital heart disease	Caution use in patients with congenital heart disease; milk feeds may decrease absorption; level monitoring may assist in guiding therapy
Moricizine: withdrawn from the market				
Propafenone	Oral: 200–300 mg/m^2/day (max 600 mg/m^2/day) divided three or four times/day	Paroxysmal atrial fibrillation/flutter and paroxysmal supraventricular tachyarrhythmias, VT, atrial fibrillation	Bradycardia and pro-arrhythmia	
Class II (beta blockers)				
Atenolol	Oral: 0.5–1 mg/kg/d given one or two times/day (max 2 mg/kg/d or 100 mg/d)	SVT, VT	Bradycardia, hypotension, and hypoglycemia	
Bisoprolol: no indication in arrhythmia				
Carvedilol: no indication in arrhythmia				
Esmolol	IV: bolus, 100–500 μg/kg per dose IV: continuous infusion, 300–1,000 μg/kg/min	Sinus tachycardia; atrial and ventricular tachyarrhythmias	Bradycardia, hypotension, and hypoglycemia	

(continued)

Table 4.17 (continued)

Medication	Dosing	Indication	Adverse events	Specific clinical considerations
Metoprolol	Oral: children 1–17 years, 1–2 mg/kg/day given twice daily (max 6 mg/kg/day or 200 mg/day)	SVT, VT	Bradycardia, hypotension, and hypoglycemia	
Propranolol	Oral: neonates, 0.25 mg/kg per dose every 6 h (max 5 mg/kg/day) Oral: infants and children, 0.5–1 mg/kg/day in divided doses every 6–8 h (max 60 mg/day)	SVT, VT	Bradycardia, hypotension, and hypoglycemia	

Timolol: no indication in arrhythmia

Class III

Medication	Dosing	Indication	Adverse events	Specific clinical considerations
Amiodarone	IV: bolus, 5 mg/kg per dose up to 15 mg/kg IV: continuous infusion, 10–20 mg/kg/day or 5–15 μg/kg/min Oral: 10–20 mg/kg/day or 600–800 mg/m ^{2}/day one or two times/day	Atrial tachycardia, flutter, and fibrillation; JET; VT and VF	Bradycardia, hypotension, torsade de pointes, hepatotoxicity, thyroid dysfunction, skin color alteration, corneal deposits, and pulmonary fibrosis	Patients may require 1–2 weeks of loading dose (higher doses) at the beginning of therapy due to the long half-life of amiodarone Extensive laboratory monitoring at baseline required due to high incidence of adverse events
Dofetilide	Adults: Initially, 500 mcg twice daily; modify dosage according to Clcr and QTc interval	SVT	Arrhythmias (torsade de pointes)	Arrhythmogenic, contraindicated in congenital or acquired long QT syndromes; baseline QT or QTc interval >440 ms (500 ms in patients with ventricular conduction abnormalities) Severe renal impairment (calculated Clcr <20 mL/min)

Ibutilide	*Atrial flutter and/or fibrillation* IV *Adults* weighing ≥60 kg: initially, 1 or 2 mg Adults weighing <60 kg: initially, 0.01 mg/kg (10 mcg/kg) Repeat after 10 min if needed, *atrial flutter and/or fibrillation following coronary bypass graft or valvular surgery* IV Adults weighing ≥60 kg: 1 or 2 infusions of 0.5 mg each (given 10 min apart) Adults weighing <60 kg: 1 or 2 infusions of 0.005 mg/kg (5 mcg/kg) each (given 10 min apart)	SVT, atrial flutter and/or fibrillation following coronary bypass graft or valvular surgery	Arrhythmia, CHF, renal failure	Atrial arrhythmias of not so recent onset are less likely to respond to the drug. Efficacy not determined in atrial arrhythmias of >90 days' duration (AHFS 2016)
Sotalol	Oral: children ≤2 years, 30 mg/m2 per dose every 8 h adjusted per age nomogram or 2 mg/kg/day divided every 8 h or 80–200 mg/m2/day divided every 8 h Oral: children >2 years, 80–200 mg/m2 per dose divided every 8 h	Atrial arrhythmia, VT	Bradycardia, hypotension, hypoglycemia, and torsade de pointes	Dosing for infants <2 years is controversial; ECG monitoring for QT prolongation necessary; women at greater risk for TdP than men

(continued)

Table 4.17 (continued)

Medication	Dosing	Indication	Adverse events	Specific clinical considerations
Class IV				
Diltiazem	Adults: IV Initially, 15–20 mg (or 0.25 mg/kg) by direct IV injection over 2 min 20–25 mg (or 0.35 mg/kg) can be administrated 15 min after the initial if needed Maintenance infusion: 5–15 mg/h; titrate dose to heart rate	SVT	Hypotension, renal or hepatic injury, slowing cardiac conduction, possible transient VPB on conversion of PSVT to sinus rhythm	IV diltiazem contraindicated in patients with VT Patients with atrial flutter or fibrillation with an accessory pathway If concurrent or recent (e.g., within a few hours) administration of IV β-adrenergic blockers
Verapamil	IV: children 1–15 years, 0.1–0.3 mg/kg per dose; max, 5 mg per dose Oral: 4–8 mg/kg/day in three divided doses or 1–5 years, 40–80 mg every 8 h, and >5 years, 80 mg every 6–8 h	SVT	Hypotension and bradycardia	IV use is not recommended in patients who are <1 year old because of the risk of cardiovascular collapse
Class V				
Adenosine	IV: 0.1 mg/kg per dose; subsequent doses, 0.2 mg/kg per dose, up to 0.3 mg/kg per dose	SVT	Gasping, chest pain, flushing, and wide complex tachycardia	Rapid flush required immediately after adenosine infusion Should be given at a site closest to the heart Life support equipment should be nearby when administering adenosine

Digoxin	Oral and IV: loading doses and maintenance doses have considerable variation depending on age and range from 5 to 50 mcg/kg per dose given in three divided doses. Historically, oral maintenance doses have ranged from 5 to 10 µg/kg/day divided twice daily	Atrial fibrillation and flutter, sinus tachycardia, paroxysmal supraventricular tachycardias	Bradycardia, nausea/vomiting, and visual disturbances	Adverse events from digoxin toxicity may occur in patients with kidney dysfunction, electrolyte disturbances, or drug interactions
Magnesium sulfate	IV: 25–50 mg/kg per dose infusion for torsade de pointes	VT (torsade de pointes) Prevention of JET	Hypotension Muscle weakness, sedation	May cause hypotension on infusion; rate of infusion should be dictated by patient condition

IV intravenous, *SVT* supraventricular tachycardia, *AV* atrioventricular, *JET* junctional ectopic tachycardia, *VT* ventricular tachycardia, *VF* ventricular fibrillation, *PVC* premature ventricular contraction

Table 4.18 Analgesic agents (opioids and non-opioids)

Medication	Dosing	Indication	Adverse events and specific clinical considerations
Fentanyl (opioid)	Bolus: 1–2 µg/kg Infusion: 1–10 µg/kg/h *Transdermal* fentanyl patches are available but should be avoided in children<2 years due to thin stratum corneum of the skin and increased body surface area ratio which enhance transdermal absorption	Analgesia	Chest wall rigidity with rapid bolus or high doses; rapid tolerance with infusion, respiratory depression, depressed consciousness, hallucinations, hypotension, nausea/vomiting, decreased GI motility/ileus, urinary retention Withdrawal symptoms when moderate to high doses are used for up to or more than one week Preferred for a rapid onset of analgesia in acutely distressed patients Individualize dose for each patient Virtually devoid of histamine-releasing properties More rapid onset of action and a shorter half-life than morphine Renal failure does not appear to largely affect pharmacokinetics Onset: 30 s Duration: 30–45 min
Remifentanil (opioid)	Bolus: 1–3 µg/kg/dose Infusion (preferred): 0.4–1 µg/kg/min	Analgesia	Half-life: 10–15 min, has been associated with bradycardia and hypotension particularly during rapid infusion Has no liver or renal elimination
Morphine (opioid)	Bolus: 0.05–0.1 mg/kg Infusion: 0.025–0.1 mg/kg/h Single dose: 0.1 mg/kg	Analgesia	Peak: 20 min Respiratory depression, depressed consciousness, hallucinations, hypotension, nausea/vomiting, decreased GI motility/ileus, urinary retention, histamine release, flushing, tachycardia, and pruritus may occur Withdrawal symptoms when moderate to high doses are used for up to or more than one week
Methadone (opioid)	0.1–0.2 mg/kg q 8–12 h	Analgesia, opioid tolerance	Use for opioid wean protocol

Hydromorphone	*Oral*: 0.03–0.08 mg/kg/dose q 4 h *Single IV* dose: 0.01–0.02 mg/kg q 4 h *Continuous IV* infusions: 1 mcg/kg/h Titration parameter: pain scale	Analgesia	Respiratory depression, depressed consciousness, hallucinations, hypotension, nausea/vomiting, decreased GI motility/ileus, urinary retention Individualize dose for each patient Available as PCA Effect of renal insufficiency on the elimination of hydromorphone is unknown More rapid onset of action and a shorter half-life than morphine Withdrawal symptoms when moderate to high doses are used for up to or more than one week
Acetaminophen (non-opioid: inhibits prostaglandin synthesis)	10–15 mg/kg q 6 h	Non-opioid analgesia	Do not use when there is significant hepatic disease
Ketorolac (non-opioid: nonsteroidal anti-inflammatory agent (cyclooxygenase-1 and 2 inhibitor))	0.5 mg/kg q 6 h; max 30 mg; do not administer for more than 48–72 h	Non-opioid analgesia	Injection site pain, abdominal pain, constipation, diarrhea, flatulence, indigestion, nausea/vomiting, headache Inhibition of platelet function: may cause bleeding Use with caution in patients with preexisting renal insufficiency Use lowest effective dose for the shortest period of time

Table 4.19 Sedative drugs and intravenous anesthetics (Friesen and Williams 2008; Verghese and Hannallah 2010; Galante 2011; Twite and Friesen 2014; Lucas et al. 2016; Maldifassi et al. 2016)

Medication	Mechanism of action	Dosing	Indication	Adverse events and specific clinical considerations
Propofol	Modulation of $GABA_A$ receptor complex	Bolus: 1–3 mg/kg Infusion: 100–200 µg/kg/min for procedural sedation	Procedural sedation	Do not use for prolonged ICU sedation, i.e., >4 h (risk of propofol infusion syndrome)
Midazolam	Modulation of $GABA_A$ receptor complex	Infusion: 0.025–0.1 mg/kg/h average, 0.05–0.1 mg/kg/h	Amnesia, sedation, anxiolysis	Rapid tolerance with infusion Onset: 1–5 min Duration: 20–30 min
Lorazepam	Modulation of $GABA_A$ receptor complex	Bolus: 0.025–0.1 mg/kg q 4 h Infusion:0.025 mg/kg/h	Amnesia, sedation, anxiolysis	Risk of tolerance with infusion Onset: 1–5 min Duration: 20–30 min
Dexmedetomidine	Synthetic central α2 agonist (purely α2; vs. clonidine)	0.3–0.7 µg/kg/h	Sedation; some analgesia	For short-term ICU sedation; bradycardia and heart block in infants Half-life: 6–12 min
Clonidine	α1 and α2 adrenoceptor agonist (90 % α2 with some α1 activity)	Infusion: 0.25–1 µg/kg/h	Analgesia, sedation	Does not cause significant respiratory depression May lead to hypotension
Etomidate	Modulation of $GABA_A$ receptor complex	Children >10 years of age: 0.3 mg/kg (0.2–0.6 mg/kg)	Sedation	Onset: 1 min Duration: 3–5 min
Ketamine	NMDA receptor antagonist	Bolus: 1.5–2 mg/kg May administer incremental doses of 0.5–1 mg/kg every 5–15 min as needed	Analgesia, sedation	Hallucinations, dysphoria Excessive salivation, tachycardia Onset: 3–5 min duration, 20–30 min

Table 4.20 Volatile anesthetics (Friesen and Williams 2008; Verghese and Hannallah 2010; Galante 2011; Twite and Friesen 2014; Lucas et al. 2016; Maldifassi et al. 2016)

Drug	MAC value %	Comments
Isoflurane	1.6 (newborn) 1.87 (1–6 months) 1.8 (0.5–1 year) 1.6 (1–12 years)	Irritates the respiratory tract, which may lead to laryngospasm in children
Sevoflurane	3.3 (newborn) 3.1 (1–6 months) 2.7 (0.5–1 year) 2.55 (1–12 years)	A good choice for mask induction in pediatric anesthesia Decreases the chance of postoperative nausea and vomiting Shortened recovery time and more rapid recovery of perception, which might produce a state of restlessness
Desflurane	9.2 (newborn) 9.4 (1–6 months) 9.9 (0.5–1 year) 8.0–8.7 (1–12 years)	Not suitable for mask induction in pediatric anesthesia because of its pungent smell, respiratory tract irritation, apnea, and laryngospasm
Xenon	71	When a mixture of 30 vol.% oxygen and 70 vol.% xenon is used, the analgesic effect is excellent Extremely costly Increases pulmonary artery pressure
Nitrous oxide	105, so could never be a sole anesthetic agent	Not widely used in cardiac surgery and *should not be used* on newborns and children with pulmonary infections In combination with other agents, reduces the need for volatile anesthetics *Should not be used* on newborns and children with pulmonary infections
Enflurane	1.7 (1–12 years) 1.6 (adult)	Not used in pediatric anesthesia due to possible epileptic effects and the possibility of raising hepatic enzymes
Halothane	0.87 (newborn) 1.2 (1–6 months) 0.97 (0.5–1 year) 0.89 (1–12 years)	Side effect: increased sensitivity of myocardium to circulating catecholamines Rise in hepatic enzymes May lead to increased occurrences of intraoperative arrhythmia

MAC minimum alveolar concentration

patients with congenital heart disease (Friesen and Williams 2008; Verghese and Hannallah 2010; Galante 2011; Twite and Friesen 2014; Lucas et al. 2016; Maldifassi et al. 2016).

Drugs for Pediatric Delirium

Postoperative delirium after pediatric cardiac surgery is a challenging issue; the current recommendations are based on consensus than pure evidence. So, there are at times some extrapolations from adult cardiac surgery to pediatric cardiac surgery;

Table 4.21 Neuromuscular blocking agents (depolarizing, non-depolarizing)

	Succinylcholine	Pancuronium	Vecuronium	Cisatracurium	Atracurium	Rocuronium
Initial dose	1–2 mg/kg	0.06–0.15 mg/kg	0.08–0.1 mg/kg	0.1–0.15 mg/kg	0.4–0.5 mg/kg (0.3 to 0.4 mg/kg for 1 month to 2 years of age)	0.6–1.2 mg/kg
Onset of effect	<1 min	2–5 min	1–3 min	1–3 min	1–3 min	<1 min
Duration	10 min	90–100 min	35–45 min	45–60 min	25–35 min	26–40 min
Continuous infusion dose	N/A	1–2 mcg/kg/min	0.8–1.2 mcg/kg/min	1–10 mcg/kg/min	2–12 mcg/kg/min	10–12 mcg/kg/min
Recovery	10–20 min	120–180 min	45–60 min	90 min	40–60 min	30–60 min
Renal failure	No change	Increased effect	Increased effect	No change	No change	No change
Hepatic failure	Increased effect (decrease dose)	Mild increased effect	Variable	Minimal to no change	Minimal to no change	30 % increased effect
Active metabolites	Yes	Yes	Yes	No	No	Yes
Adverse effects	Apnea bradyarrhythmia Cardiac arrest Cardiac dysrhythmia Hyperkalemia Hypersensitivity reaction Malignant hyperthermia Prolonged neuromuscular block Respiratory depression Rhabdomyolysis tachyarrhythmia	Apnea Bronchospasm Hypertension Prolonged neuromuscular block Respiratory failure tachyarrhythmia	Anaphylaxis Apnea Bronchospasm Hypotension muscle weakness Prolonged neuromuscular block Tachyarrhythmia	Bradyarrhythmia Bronchospasm Hypotension	Anaphylaxis Bradyarrhythmia Bronchospasm Edema Erythema Hives Hypersensitivity reaction Hypotension, at larger than recommended doses Laryngeal spasm Muscle weakness Paralysis Tachyarrhythmia, at higher doses	Hypotension Hypertension Tachycardia Pruritus Nausea Wheezing Allergic reactions

for example, benzodiazepines are not recommended for treatment of postoperative delirium after pediatric cardiac surgery because these drugs are potentially deliriogenic in adult patients.

The general consensus is that if non-pharmacological treatments of delirium and agitation go unsuccessful, pharmacological treatment should be started in order to prevent the child from discomforting or endangering himself/herself; in other words, a delirious child interferes with the treatment process, while a well-treated child opens "appropriate environment" for the parents to take part in the process of care, also risk of unplanned events like unwanted endotracheal extubation or failure of intravenous lines, arterial line, or central line withdrawal (Malarbi et al. 2011).

In general, appropriate pharmacological treatment of a delirious child in the postoperative period of cardiac surgery improves the overall course of treatment; so, pediatric delirium, when recognized, responds well to treatment (Schieveld et al. 2007; Madden et al. 2011; Hipp and Ely 2012).

Treatment of hyperactive delirium should be based on a number of principles:

- Some of the pharmacological agents have delirium-preventing effects; for example, premedication with clonidine (4 µg/kg), propofol, ketamine, halothane, dexmedetomidine, or opioids (e.g., fentanyl) has possible prophylactic effects in prevention of delirium or decreasing the chance and/or severity of postoperative delirium in children undergoing general anesthesia (Dahmani et al. 2010; Costi et al. 2014; Lambert et al. 2014; van Hoff et al. 2015).
- On the other hand, there might be increased occurrence of delirium after anesthesia with some gases like sevoflurane especially when the patient is not premedicated (Messieha 2013).
- Pharmacological treatment, when started, should be continued until the clinical signs persist or until any risk factor for delirium continues to exist; also, after healing, pharmacological agents should not be abruptly "turned off"; instead gradual tapering and drug weaning are the preferred routes.
- Intravenous haloperidol and oral risperidone are the main drugs used for pharmacological treatment, which is the common route for many critical patients; however, adverse events of risperidone are less than haloperidol (Warshaw and Mechlin 2009; Powney et al. 2012).
- Risperidone does not have intravenous form; but its oral form is available and is the preferred choice whenever it is possible to use oral medication and symptoms are not severe; also, in the first opportunity, haloperidol should be replaced with risperidone to decrease the chance of adverse events of haloperidol (Madden et al. 2011; McPheeters et al. 2011).
- Routine delirium scoring, at least three times a day, should be done as long as pharmacological treatment is continued (van Dijk et al. 2012).
- Adverse events of pharmacological treatment are especially seen when escalating doses are increased suddenly and abruptly; instead, gradual commencement of the drug and gradual weaning after termination of the clinical signs are the preferred methods.
- The main complications of pharmacological treatment with antipsychotics include extrapyramidal symptoms and long QTc interval.

- Extrapyramidal symptom (including dystonia, akathisia, hyperpyrexia, etc.) should be monitored and treated with anticholinergics like biperiden with a dose of 50 mcg/kg which is administered slowly through an intravenous line; also, the dose of antipsychotics should be reduced (Satterthwaite et al. 2008).
- Another main complication is lengthening of QTc interval which might lead to lethal torsade de pointes; performing ECG monitoring and recording the results for more comparisons are needs that should be fulfilled before, during, and after antipsychotic treatment (Brahmbhatt and Whitgob 2016).

A detailed list of drugs used for treatment of pediatric ICU delirium is presented in Table 4.22, and its data are based on the recent advances related to pharmacotherapy of postoperative delirium (Schieveld et al. 2007; Schieveld et al. 2009; Maglione et al. 2011; Loy et al. 2012; Asmal et al. 2013; Baron et al. 2015; Joyce et al. 2015; Masi et al. 2015; Smith et al. 2016).

Table 4.22 Drugs for pediatric ICU delirium

Drug	Onset	Dosing	Adverse effects/comments
Haloperidol (Haldol®)	3–20 min	IV: *Age*: 0–1 or body weight = 3.5–10 kg Loading: 0.05 mg in 30 min Maintenance: 0.01–0.05 mg/kg/day, divided into 2–4 times daily *Age*:1–3 or body weight = 10–15 kg Loading: 0.15–0.25 mg in 30 min Maintenance: 0.05–0.5 mg/kg/24 h divided into 2–4 times daily Age: 3–18 or body weight > 15 kg Loading: 0.3–0.5 mg in 30 min Maintenance: 0.05–0.5 mg/kg/24 h divided into 2–4 times daily *Age*: 16 years or older: 5 mg per day divided into 2–4 doses *Discontinue in patients with QTc > 500 ms*	Monitor for electrocardiographic changes QT interval prolongation and arrhythmias Extrapyramidal side effects Neuroleptic malignant syndrome (rare) Lowers seizure threshold Causes sedation
Risperidone (Risperdal®)	30–60 min	Drug form: 0.25, 0.5, 1, 2, 3, and 4 mg standard oral tablets *Patients 15–20 kg*: daily dose is 0.25 mg/day orally *Patients >20 kg*: 0.1–0.2 mg oral; maintenance, 0.2–2.0 mg/24 h	Has ORAL form only Extrapyramidal side effects Risk of seizure Sedation, drowsiness Weight gain and increased appetite Feeling hot or cold Headache, dizziness Restlessness feeling Sleep abnormalities GI problems

Table 4.22 (continued)

Drug	Onset	Dosing	Adverse effects/comments
Olanzapine[b] (off-label use)	≤60 min	2.5–5 mg PO QHS 5–10 mg IM	Monitor for electrocardiographic changes QT interval prolongation and arrhythmias Extrapyramidal side effects Lowers seizure threshold Hyperglycemia Peripheral edema Causes sedation
Quetiapine[b] (Seroquel) (off-label use)	No data	Median daily dose : 1–1.5 mg/kg/day Duration of treatment: up to 12 days	Quetiapine produces less Parkinson-like effects than ziprasidone, risperidone, and olanzapine Monitor for electrocardiographic changes QT interval prolongation and arrhythmias Extrapyramidal side effects Neuroleptic malignant syndrome (rare) Lowers seizure threshold Neutropenia Hyperglycemia Causes sedation

Modified from Fellin (2014). Published with kind permission of © Springer, 2014. All Rights Reserved
[a]There is limited trial data establishing safety, efficacy, or appropriate dosing of atypical antipsychotics
[b]Olanzapine and quetiapine are not among the commonly used drugs for postoperative delirium and should be used cautiously, if needed at all

Stress Ulcer Prevention and Treatment

In postoperative pediatric patients, the chance for postoperative stress ulcer is always a real potential threat (Griffin 1998; Langford and Mehta 2006). Pharmacological therapy is still used for many of the drugs in pediatric perioperative care as off-label use; no significant data is still available regarding the appropriate or the selected agent for pediatric critical care. Some of the selected agents are presented here in Table 4.23 (Reveiz et al. 2010; Giglia et al. 2016).

Anticoagulation and Thrombolysis Drugs

These drugs could be divided to four main subclasses (Ageno et al. 2012; Moffett et al. 2016):

- Anticoagulants (oral and parenteral forms)
- Antiplatelet agents
- Thrombolytic agents

Table 4.23 Stress ulcer prevention and treatment drugs

Agent	Dosing	Adverse effects/comments
H2 blockers		
Ranitidine	Children 1 month to 16 years of age: 2–4 mg/kg twice daily	Headache, dizziness, mental status changes, thrombocytopenia
Famotidine	Oral 0.5 mg/kg once daily at bedtime or in 2 divided doses daily (maximum 40 mg daily); up to 1 mg/kg daily has been used	Dose adjustment needed for renal dysfunction Potential increased risk of nosocomial pneumonia Efficacy not established for stress ulcer prophylaxis
Proton pump inhibitors (PPI)		
Omeprazole	5 to <10 kg, 5 mg once daily 10 to <20 kg, 10 mg once daily ≥20 kg, 20 mg once daily	Respiratory effects, fever (in children 1–2 years of age), accidental injuries (in children 2–16 years of age)
Esomeprazole	Oral Children 1–11 years of age: 10 mg once daily for up to 8 weeks Adolescents 12–17 years of age: 20 or 40 mg once daily for up to 8 weeks IV infants 1 month to <1 year of age: 0.5 mg/kg once daily	No adjustment needed for renal or liver dysfunction Potential increased risk of nosocomial pneumonia Potential increased risk of *Clostridium difficile* infection Many drug interactions IV administration *only* for patients who cannot tolerate PO/NG administration
Lansoprazole	Children 1–11 years of age: ≤30 kg, 15 mg once daily >30 kg, 30 mg once Children 12–17 years of age: 15 mg daily	

Modified from Fellin (2014). Published with kind permission of © Springer, 2014. All Rights Reserved

- Novel oral anticoagulants

Oral Anticoagulants

During the recent years, use of anticoagulants (especially oral anticoagulants) in pediatric cardiac surgery has increased, mainly in the following patient groups (Moffett et al. 2006; Jain and Vaidyanathan 2010; Donadini et al. 2012; Douketis et al. 2012; Salvin et al. 2016):

- Prophylaxis of thromboembolic events after Fontan surgery
- Mechanical prosthetic valves which are much more increasingly used in pediatric patients
- Kawasaki disease having large aneurysms
- Primary pulmonary hypertension
- Dilated cardiomyopathy patients who have severe left ventricular dysfunction

For these indications, warfarin is the most commonly used drug; however, other agents (including dabigatran, rivaroxaban, and apixaban) are not yet available for pediatric labeling, *but may be used in adult patients with congenital heart disease.* Their properties are presented in Tables 4.24, 4.25, 4.26, and 4.26.

Antiplatelet Agents

These agents are used extensively in adult patients, especially in those with acute coronary syndrome, cerebral vascular events, and thromboembolic events; however, in pediatric patients, these agents are used mainly to suppress platelet aggregation with an increasing trend especially and mainly in the following patients (Finkelstein et al. 2005; Soman et al. 2006; Mertens et al. 2008; Monagle et al. 2008; Maltz et al. 2009; Gentilomo et al. 2011; Jennings et al. 2012; Monagle et al. 2012; Mohanty and Vaidyanathan 2013; Moffett et al. 2016):

- Hypoplastic left heart syndrome
- Pulmonary artery anomalies (the latter two are the most common in pediatric cardiac surgery patients)
- Systemic to pulmonary artery shunts
- Kawasaki disease
- Primary prophylaxis for thromboembolic events in Fontan surgery in children
- Prevention of thrombosis in prosthetic heart valves
- Intracardiac devices or stents (e.g., after transcatheter closure of atrial septal defect, until endothelialization of blood exposed parts is complete)
- Dilated cardiomyopathy (these patients are predisposed to thromboembolic events due to low cardiac output, poor contractility, and concomitant atrial fibrillation)
- Childhood arterial ischemic stroke: which may be due to some etiologies like sickle cell disease, congenital heart disease, arterial dissection, prothrombotic conditions, preceding viral infections, or idiopathic
- In patients with left ventricular assist device
- For treatment of vasculitis

The antiplatelet drugs could be divided into the following categories based on their mechanism of action:

- *Salicylic acid family* including aspirin and triflusal:

  Aspirin is an irreversible cyclooxygenase inhibitor (inhibition of COX-1 and COX-2 activity).

  Triflusal (Disgren®) is a salicylate different from aspirin, which blocks cyclooxygenase, preserves vascular prostacyclin, and blocks phosphodiesterase.
- *Adenosine diphosphate (ADP) receptor inhibitors* which block P2Y12 component of ADP receptor on platelet surface (including *clopidogrel* "Plavix®," *prasugrel* "Effient®," *ticagrelor* "Brilinta®," and *ticlopidine* "Ticlid®").
- *Phosphodiesterase inhibitors* leading to increased plasma level of cellular cAMP, finally blocking platelet aggregation in response to ADP like *cilostazol* (Pletal®)

Table 4.24 Oral anticoagulant dosing, monitoring, and preoperative discontinuation

Anticoagulant	Half-life ($t_{1/2}$)/dose	Monitoring	Discontinue prior to surgery (days)/reversal agent	Mechanism of action
Warfarin (Coumadin®) http://packageinserts.bms. com/pi/pi_coumadin.pdf. *Accessed April 9, 2016*	20–60 h Individualized dosing Initial bolus dosing of 0.2 mg/kg (maximum initial dose 10 mg) with adjustments on subsequent days based on daily INR Alternative regime without bolus: age 2–12 years old, 0.09 mg/kg/day; age more than 12 years old, 0.08 mg/kg/day	PT/INR	Minimum of 5 days without reversal agents Reversal agents Vitamin K 10 mg PO/IVPB for emergent *normalization* of PT/INR; IVPB initial effect at 2 h and full correction within 24 h 5 mg PO and 1 mg IVPB produce similar effects on INR at 24 h 0.5–1 mg orally for reducing PT/INR into *therapeutic range* (for <2.5 mg use IV form administered orally) Ineffective in hepatic disease due to inability to produce factors *Oral* route not effective in biliary disease SQ not recommended due to unpredictable absorption and reversal characteristics *Prothrombin complex concentrate* (PCC, Factor IX complex, Profilnine®) 25–50 units/kg *with* vitamin K to prevent rebound increase in INR *Recombinant activated factor VII* For intracranial hemorrhage – doses vary; 20–40 µg/kg has been used; available as 1-, 2-, 5-, and 8-mg vial sizes; use lowest dose rounded to nearest vial size and repeat if needed due to risk of arterial and venous thrombotic and thromboembolic events	Inhibits vitamin K epoxide reductase; in this way, warfarin prevents vitamin K1 regeneration after γ-carboxylation *Pediatric labeling is available*

| Dabigatran (Pradaxa®) https://www.pradaxa.com/ *Accessed April 9, 2016* | 12–17 h in healthy subjects CrCl > 30 ml/min: 150 mg BID CrCl 30–50 ml/ min + dronedarone or ketoconazole: 75 mg BID CrCl 15–30 ml/min: 75 mg BID | No readily available method   Activated partial   thromboplastin   time (aPTT)   demonstrates   presence but not   degree of   anticoagulation   Prothrombin time   (PT) insensitive   Thrombin time   (TT) – normal   value rules out   presence of   dabigatran   Ecarin clotting time   (ECT) – linear dose   relationship; not   routinely available | CrCl ≥50 ml/min: 1–2 days CrCl 30-50 ml/min: 2–4 days CrCl <30 ml/min: ≥5 days Dialysis may remove up to 62 % within 2 h pINN: idarucizumab (dabigatran antidote) has been approved in 2015 by the FDA (Glund et al. 2015; Pollack et al. 2015) | Dabigatran is among direct thrombin inhibitors (DTIs) *Pediatric labeling not available yet* |
| Rivaroxaban (Xarelto®) http://www.xareltohcp. com/ *Accessed April 9, 2016* | 5–9 h in healthy subjects Atrial fibrillation VTE prophylaxis VTE treatment | No readily available method   Prolongs aPTT,   PT/INR   No direct effect   on platelet   aggregation | At least 1 day (24 h) No reversal agent available and unlikely to be dialyzable due to high protein binding | Direct factor Xa inhibitor (orally active) *Pediatric labeling not available yet* |

(continued)

Table 4.24 (continued)

Anticoagulant	Half-life ($t_{1/2}$)/dose	Monitoring	Discontinue prior to surgery (days)/reversal agent	Mechanism of action
Apixaban (Eliquis®) http://packageinserts.bms.com/pi/pi_eliquis.pdf *Accessed April 9, 2016*	~12 h following repeated dosing Atrial fibrillation	No readily available method Prolongs aPTT, PT/INR No direct effect on platelet aggregation	24–48 h prior to surgery depending on risk, location, and ability to control bleeding No reversal agent and unlikely to be dialyzable due to high protein binding Activated charcoal may be useful in overdose situations	Direct factor Xa inhibitor *Pediatric labeling not available yet*

Modified from Martin-Stone (2014). Published with kind permission of © Springer, 2014. All Rights Reserved

CrCl **clearance of creatinine,** *VTE* **venous**

Table 4.25 Parenteral anticoagulant dosing and monitoring *in adults*

Anticoagulant	Half-life ($t_{1/2}$)/dose	Monitoring	Discontinue prior to surgery (hours)/ reversal agent
Unfractionated heparin (UFH)	60–90 min VTE: 80 unit/kg bolus and then 18 units/kg/h ACS: 60 unit/kg bolus and then 12 units/kg/h Prophylaxis: 5000 units SQ BID or TID	aPTT Anti-Xa activity level (UFH levels) Activated clotting time (ACT; intraoperatively)	4–6 h Protamine 1 mg/100units of heparin (max 50 mg at a rate not to exceed 5 min) Dose adjustment based on time since heparin held: >60 min, 0.5 mg/100units; >2 h, 0.25 mg/100units
Low molecular weight heparin Dalteparin (Fragmin®) *www.pfizer.* *com/files/products/uspi_fragmin.pdf* *Accessed 18 July* Enoxaparin (Lovenox®) *http://products.sanofi.* *us/lovenox/lovenox.* *html#section-14.1* *Accessed 18 July*	4.5–7 h *VTE treatment:* *Dalteparin*: 200 units/kg SQ daily *Enoxaparin*: 1 mg/kg SQ BID or 1.5 mg/kg SQ daily *VTE prophylaxis* *Dalteparin* 5000 units SQ daily *Enoxaparin* 30 mg SQ BID or 40 mg SQ daily *ACS* *Dalteparin*120 units/kg SQ every 12 h *Enoxaparin* 1 mg/kg SQ every 12 h	Anti-Xa activity level (LMWH level) Dalteparin treatment doses should not be used in patients with CrCl ≤ 30 ml/min Enoxaparin 1 mg/kg SQ daily may be considered in patients with chronic stable kidney disease and CrCl ≤ 30 ml/min who are not dialysis dependent; anti-Xa and serum creatinine monitoring is highly recommended	24 h Protamine <8 h after last dose: 1 mg/1 mg enoxaparin or per 100 units of dalteparin 8–12 h after last dose or if repeat is necessary: 0.5 mg/1 mg enoxaparin or per 100 units of dalteparin >12 h after last dose: administration of protamine may not be necessary The anti-factor Xa activity is never completely reversed (typically 60 % is reversed)

(continued)

Table 4.25 (continued)

Anticoagulant	Half-life ($t_{1/2}$)/dose	Monitoring	Discontinue prior to surgery (hours)/ reversal agent
Direct thrombin inhibitors Argatroban® *http://us.gsk.com/products/assets/us_ argatroban.pdf Accessed 31 July 2012* Bivalirudin (Angiomax®) *www.angiomax.com/Downloads/Ang iomax_PI_2010_PN1601-12.pdf. Accessed 18 July 2012*	*Argatroban* 50 min *Treatment of HIT*: 2 mcg/kg/min initial dose; adjust for hepatic insufficiency and critically ill patients with multisystem organ failure *Bivalirudin* 25 min *CPB dosing in setting of HIT*: *On pump*: 1 mg/kg bolus, 50 mg for pump and then 2.5 mg/kg/h; goal ACT >2.5× baseline *Off pump*: 0.75 mg/kg bolus, 1.75 mg/kg/h: goal ACT >300 s	aPTT	2 h No reversal agent Case reports suggest that recombinant factor VIIa 90 µg/kg ×1 may reverse the anticoagulant effect (Schulman and Bijsterveld)
Factor Xa Inhibitor Fondaparinux (Arixtra®) *http://us.gsk. com/products/assets/us_arixtra.pdf Accessed 31 July 2012*	17–21 h VTE *Prophylaxis*: 2.5 mg SQ daily *Treatment*: <50 kg: 5 mg SQ daily 50–100Kg: 7.5 mg SQ daily >100Kg: 10 mg SQ daily	Not routinely available. International standards for anti-Xa activity for UFH/ LMWH do not apply	48 h No reversal agent Case reports suggest that recombinant factor VIIa 90 µg/kg x 1 may reverse the anticoagulant effect (Schulman and Bijsterveld)

Modified from Martin-Stone (2014)

Table 4.26 Parenteral anticoagulant dosing and monitoring in *children* (Moffett et al. 2006; Monagle et al. 2008, 2012)

Drug	Mechanism of action	Dose	Half-life	Monitor/reversal
Anticoagulants				
Unfractionated heparin (UFH)	UFH acts as an anticoagulant protein by binding to antithrombin And potentiating its anticoagulant activity over 1,000-fold, inactivating coagulant factors IIa (thrombin), Xa, XIa, and XIIa	Initial loading bolus (if indicated): 75 U/kg over 10 min Followed by age ≤1 year old: continuous rate 28 U/kg/h Age >1 year old: continuous rate 20 U/kg/h	1.5±0.5 h	Monitor: activated partial thromboplastin Time (aPTT) and the UFH anti-Xa level Reversal: Full reversal with protamine sulfate Approximately 1 mg of protamine will neutralize 100 U of UFH. Calculations based on the total amount of heparin received in the prior 2–2.5 h
Low molecular weight heparin: enoxaparin	Similar to UFH, LMWH exerts an anticoagulant effect through binding antithrombin and potentiating the antithrombin anticoagulant activity, but compared with UFH, there is a reduced inhibitory activity against factor IIa (thrombin) relative to factor Xa	Initial enoxaparin dose. Less than 3 months old: 1.7 mg/kg SC every 12 h Three months–2 years old: 1.2 mg/kg SC every 12 h More than 2 years old: 1 mg/kg subcutaneously every 12 h Obese patients approximately 0.8 mg/kg SC every 12 h to maximum dose of 170 mg	3–6 h	Monitor: routine, same as heparin reversal. LMWH can be partially reversed (≈70 %) with protamine LMWH is easier to use in pediatric patients because it does not require a dedicated line, and frequent monitoring is not needed
Fondaparinux	Synthetic analog of the antithrombin-binding penta-saccharide found in heparin and LMWH, enhances affinity for antithrombin, has no inhibitory activity against factor IIa (thrombin), and only inactivates factor Xa	0.1 mg/kg subcutaneous daily	17 h	Reversal: no reversal agents available
Argatroban *Parental DTIs*	A univalent DTI, reversibly inhibits thrombin's catalytic site	Initial infusion rate : 0.25–1 µg/kg/min	39–51 min	Monitor: aPTTs every 2–4 h to aim for an aPTT 1.5–2.5×normal
Bivalirudin *Parental DTIs*	Is bivalent DTIs and binds the active catalytic site of thrombin, as well as the thrombin/fibrinogen binding site	Bloused at 0.125 mg/kg IV and then an infusion of 0.125 mg/kg/h is initiated	25 min	Reversal: the definitive reversal therapy is renal replacement therapy

which is a selective *phosphodiesterase 3* inhibitor or *dipyridamole* "Persantine®" which is both a *phosphodiesterase 5* inhibitor and an adenosine deaminase inhibitor; dipyridamole leads to adenosine and cyclic AMP accumulation, finally inhibiting platelet aggregation (Gresele et al. 2011).

- *Glycoprotein IIB/IIIA inhibitors* which are for intravenous use only and include *abciximab* "ReoPro®," *eptifibatide* "Integrilin®," and *tirofiban*" Aggrastat®."
- *Protease-activated receptor-1 (PAR-1) antagonists*, mainly *vorapaxar* "Zontivity®," which prevent thrombin generation through blockade of thrombin-responsive receptor in platelets and vascular cells; pediatric label is not available yet (Capodanno et al. 2012; Wang 2015).
- *Thromboxane inhibitors* which include thromboxane synthase inhibitors and thromboxane receptor antagonists like *terutroban.*

A detailed pharmacological description of some selected antiplatelet agents is presented in Tables 4.27, 4.28, and 4.29 (Dixon et al. 2009; Capodanno et al. 2012; Mauri et al. 2014; Giglia et al. 2016).

Antifibrinolytic Agents

Currently there are two main available antibrinolytics agents:

- Tranexamic acid
- ε-Aminocaproic acid (EACA)

Both are recommended for perioperative use in pediatric and adult cardiac patients in order to reduce perioperative bleeding. Their mechanism of action is primarily a competitive binding to lysine-binding location of plasminogen; the final result will be competitive prevention of plasma attachment to fibrin, and so, the process of fibrin degradation (called fibrinolysis) will be prevented. A detailed discussion on these agents is presented in Chap. 39 – Postoperative Bleeding and Coagulation Management. Also, a brief review is presented in Table 4.30 (Eaton 2008; Schouten et al. 2009; Faraoni and Goobie 2014).

Antibiotic Prophylaxis in Perioperative Period

The primary goal in antibiotic prophylaxis is to prevent surgical site infection using reliable, safe, cost-effective, and appropriate spectrum antimicrobial agent(s) which could cover all common pathogens during perioperative period. There should be assurance that the plasma and tissue level of such an antibiotic has reached the necessary level before starting the operation.

Cardiothoracic surgeries are often considered as clean surgeries, and in nearly all the patients, risk of superimposed perioperative infection is low. On the other hand, organ infection or deep surgical infections, surgical site infection (SSI), in cardiac surgery patients (e.g., mediastinitis or prosthetic valve endocarditic),

Table 4.27 Oral and intravenous antiplatelet agents

Antiplatelet agent	Mechanism of action	Dose	Duration of effect	Half-life	Discontinue prior to surgery/monitor/reversal
Oral antiplatelet agents					
Aspirin	Cyclooxygenase inhibitor (irreversible inhibition of COX-1 and COX-2 activity) Inhibiting formation of thromboxane (TXA2) Inhibiting platelet activation and aggregation)	1–5 mg/kg/day (maximum: 91 mg)	7 days (since the affected platelets should be replaced)	5–20 min	3–5 days is needed before surgery to discontinue the drug, of course depending on residual aspirin effect desired No routine monitor No reversal agent available For reversal, platelets (4–20 U/kg) may be given to counteract the platelet aggregation inhibition from ASA
Clopidogrel (Plavix®) http://www.plavix.com/Index.aspx *Accessed April 9, 2016*	Irreversibly blocks P2Y12 component of ADP receptor on platelet surface; also, platelet aggregation is prevented	≤2 years old: initial dose is 0.2 mg/kg/dose, once daily ≥2 years old: initial dose is 1 mg/kg/day; titrate to response 1–6 mg/kg/day for periods between 1 and 6 months	7 days (since the affected platelets should be replaced)	The t½ of the parent drug is around 6 h; however, t½ of the active thiol metabolite is about 30 min	5–7 days No routine monitor No reversal agent available, platelets 4–20 U/kg
Prasugrel (Effient®) http://www.effient.com/Pages/index.aspx *Accessed April 9, 2016*	Irreversibly blocks P2Y12 component of ADP receptor on platelet surface		7 days (since the affected platelets should be replaced)		7 days
Ticagrelor (Brilinta®) http://www.brilinta.com/ *Accessed April 9, 2016*	Reversibly blocks P2Y12 component of ADP receptor on platelet surface		48 h ($t_{1/2}$ 6–13 h including active metabolite)		3–5 days

(continued)

Table 4.27 (continued)

Antiplatelet agent	Mechanism of action	Dose	Duration of effect	Half-life	Discontinue prior to surgery/monitor/reversal
Intravenous antiplatelet agents					
Abciximab (Reopro®) http://www.reopro.com/Pages/index.aspx *Accessed August 8, 2012*	Irreversible glycoprotein IIb/IIIa inhibitor		24 h		24 h
Eptifibatide (Integrilin®) http://www.integrilin.com/integrilin/index.html *Accessed August 8, 2012*	Reversible glycoprotein IIb/IIIa inhibitor	180 mcg/kg bolus followed by infusion of 2 mcg/kg/min If clearance of creatinine is <50 ml/min, 180 mcg/kg bolus followed by infusion of 1 mcg/kg/min	4 h		4 h
Tirofiban (Aggrastat®) http://www.aggrastat.com/ *Accessed August 8, 2012*	Reversible glycoprotein IIb/IIIa inhibitor	0.4 μg/kg/min × 30 min and then 0.1 μg/kg/min If clearance of creatinine is <30 ml/min, reduce dose by 50 %	4 h		4 h
Dipyridamole; both IV and oral (Persantine®)	Inhibition of the activity of adenosine deaminase Another mechanism is to inhibit phosphodiesterase activity so the plasma level of cellular cAMP increases leading to blockade of platelet aggregation in response to ADP	1–5 mg/kg/day	40 min	10–12 h	No routine monitoring No reversal agent available, platelets 10–20 U/kg

Table 4.28 Thrombolytic agents

Thrombolytic agent	Mechanism of action	Dose	Half-life	Discontinue prior to surgery/monitor/ reversal
Thrombolytic therapy				
Alteplase (TPA) Reteplase Tenecteplase Urokinase Streptokinase	These are recombinant DNA-based products; biosynthetic forms of the enzyme *human tissue-type plasminogen activator* (tPA)	*Urokinase* loading: 4,400u/kg Maintenance: 4,400 u/kg/h for 6–12 h *Streptokinase* loading: 2,000 u/kg Maintenance: 2,000 u/kg/h for 6–12 h *tPA* 0.1–0.6 mg/ kg/h for 6 h	5–10 min	Monitor: fibrinogen, TCT, PT, aPTT No reversal agent available

Table 4.29 Blood-related products (Groom et al. 1996; Curley et al. 2014; Durandy 2015; Jobes et al. 2015; Lei and Xiong 2015; Payani et al. 2015; Remy et al. 2015)

Agent	Indication	Dose
Red packed cells	Perioperative bleeding	Estimated blood volume × (ideal hematocrit − actual hematocrit)/ hematocrit 1 unit packed red blood cells
Platelets	*Qualitative or quantitative* platelet deficiency *Acute bleeding* and platelets below 50,000 mm^3 *Invasive procedures* and platelets under 50,000 mm^3 *Central nervous system* procedures and platelets under 100,000 mm^3	1–2 unit/10 kg or 10–15 cm^3/kg
Fresh frozen plasma	Coagulation factors deficiency (liver disease, vitamin K deficiency, malabsorption syndrome, atresia of the extra hepatic biliary tract) Disseminated intravascular coagulation Emergency reversal of warfarin Dilutional coagulopathy in massive transfusion Replacement of specific coagulation factors (factors II, V, X, XI, XIII) Hereditary angioedema Microvascular bleeding with PT and extended TPT	Unit/10 kg or 10–15 cc/kg

(continued)

Table 4.29 (continued)

Agent	Indication	Dose
Cryoprecipitate: Contains factor VIII (80 units), von Willebrand factor, factor XIII, fibrinogen (150–250 mg), and fibronectin	*Concentration* of fibrinogen less than 150 mg/dl and microvascular bleeding *Massive* transfusion with fibrinogen concentration under 150 mg/dl and active bleeding *Deficiency* of fibrinogen, dysfibrinogenemia, and afibrinogenemia	1 unit/5–10 kg
Desmopressin	*Congenital disorders*: von Willebrand disease: type I, contraindicated in type 2B; ineffective in type III Mild hemophilia: Effective for minor procedures or dental extractions *Platelet function congenital disorders*: Bernard–Soulier syndrome *Vascular disorders*: Ehlers–Danlos and Marfan syndrome Acquired disorders: Acquired von Willebrand syndrome:	Dose 0.3 mcg/kg through intravenous line
Fibrinogen concentrate	Hemorrhagic diathesis in congenital disorders such as hypofibrinogenemia, dysfibrinogenemia, and afibrinogenemia; acquired hypofibrinogenemias such as synthesis disorders, increased intravascular consumption, and hyperfibrinolysis	30–50 mg/kg
Prothrombin complex	Reverse warfarin and for the treatment of bleeding in hemophilic patients with inhibitors and deficiency of specific coagulation factors; perioperative bleeding refractive to the use of fresh frozen plasma, platelets, and cryoprecipitate	20–30 UI/kg calculated with factor II
Activated recombinant factor 7	Perioperative intractable bleeding when other measures have failed to control hemostasis	Dose: 40–80 µg/kg (off-label dose in cardiac patients)
Concentrates of coagulation factors (like PCC, FEIBA, etc.)	Selective replacement of coagulation factors in uncontrollable postoperative bleeding leading to more direct and rapid correction of factor deficiencies	*PCC* (human prothrombin complex): which has factor IX with varying doses of other coagulation factors II, VII, and X *FEIBA*: factor eight inhibitor bypass activity

Table 4.30 Dosing antifibrinolytic agents

Agent	Indication	Dose regimen
Epsilon-aminocaproic acid (Amicar®)	Perioperative bleeding in major pediatric cardiac surgery	100 mg/kg of body weight or 3 g/m2 of body surface area during the first hour, followed by 33.3 mg/h or 1/g/m2/h Total dose should not exceed 18 g/m2/day No dose ranging study available
Tranexamic acid (Cyklokapron®)	Perioperative bleeding in major pediatric cardiac surgery	20–30 mg/kg loading dose IV and then 10–15 mg/kg/h infusion

Modified from Martin-Stone (2014). Published with kind permission of © Springer, 2014. All Rights Reserved

though not so much frequent, constitute a major condition which may at times lead to catastrophic outcomes with very high morbidity and mortality rate. However, if we include superficial SSI, greater percentages of patients are involved with postoperative SSI.

In pediatric cardiac surgical patients, there are a number of risk factors for SSI. Though risk factors for superficial SSI are not exactly the same as risk factors for deep SSI (e.g., mediastinitis), a brief list of all these risk factors is presented here (Mehta et al. 2000; Allpress et al. 2004; Nateghian et al. 2004; Lepelletier et al. 2005; Iarussi et al. 2008; Costello et al. 2010; Bucher et al. 2011; Vijarnsorn et al. 2012):

- Younger patients (lower age)
- Longer surgical procedures (i.e., duration of surgery)
- More units of postoperative blood transfusions
- Infancy (age <1 month)
- Underlying failure to thrive
- Higher classes of ASA (American Society of Anesthesiologist) score
- Prolonged preoperative stay
- Prolonged ICU stay (>3 days)
- Prolonged intubation
- Prolonged inotropic support in ICU
- Prolonged mechanical ventilation (>2 days)
- Prolonged hospital length of stay (>14 days)
- Prolonged postoperative hospital stay
- Reopen procedures
- Extubation failure (especially when repeated failure occurs)
- Increased leukocyte band cell counts during preoperative period and on first postoperative day
- Elevated serum lactate levels in the first postoperative day

In Tables 4.31 and 4.32, a brief description of the commonly used antibiotic prophylaxis regimens is presented.

Table 4.31 Antibiotic prophylaxis for pediatric cardiac surgeries

Procedure	Common pathogens	Recommended antibiotic prophylaxis	Postoperative duration of antibiotic treatment
Congenital cardiac procedures (including but not limited to patent ductus arteriosus, atrial/ventricular septal defects, Glenn shunt, valve repair/replacement, prosthetic graft insertion, aortic reconstruction)	*S. epidermidis*, *S. aureus* *Coagulase-negative Staphylococcus* *Escherichia coli* *Pseudomonas aeruginosa* *Haemophilus influenzae non-type b*	*Cefazolin* or *vancomycin* for known MRSA or high risk for MRSA or major reaction to beta-lactams	Discontinue within 48–72 h of surgical end time
Ventricular assist devices (VADs)	*S. epidermidis* *S. aureus* *Streptococcus* *Corynebacteria* Enteric Gram-negative bacilli *Candida*	Vancomycin 15 mg/kg IV within 60 min prior to surgical incision and q12h × 48 h Piperacillin–tazobactam 3.375 g IV within 60 min prior to surgical incision and q6h × 48 h Fluconazole 400 mg IV within 60 min prior to surgical incision and q24h × 48 h Mupirocin (Bactroban®) 2 % nasal ointment applied to nares the night before and morning of surgery (if nasal culture is positive for *S. aureus*)	Gram-negative coverage tailored to patient flora and/or institutional susceptibility × 48 h Mupirocin (Bactroban®) 2 % nasal ointment to nares BID for 5 days (if nasal culture is positive for *S. aureus*)

Modified from Fellin (2014)

S. epidermidis, *S. aureus*, *Streptococcus*, *Corynebacteria*, enteric Gram-negative bacilli

Table 4.32 Commonly used antibiotics for prophylaxis in cardiac surgical patients

Antibiotic agent	Intraoperative redosing with normal renal function	Timing of the first dose	Time for effect	Redosing time (minutes)
Cefazolin	25 mg/kg q 6–8 h (max 1000 mg; if greater than 80 kg, use 2000 mg)	Begin 60 min or less before incision	30	Every 6–8 h
Cefotaxime	20–30 mg/kg	Begin 60 min or less before incision	30	Every 6 h
Cefuroxime	50 mg/kg	within 1 h prior to incision	15–60	Every 4 h
Clindamycin	5–10 mg/kg up to 900 mg	Begin 60 min or less before incision	30	Every 6–8 h
Vancomycin	10 mg/kg (up to 1000 mg if > 50 kg)	Begin 60–120 min before incision	60	Every 6 h

Modified from Fellin (2014)

References

Abman SH, Hansmann G, Archer SL, Ivy DD, Adatia I, Chung WK, Hanna BD, Rosenzweig EB, Raj JU, Cornfield D, Stenmark KR, Steinhorn R, Thebaud B, Fineman JR, Kuehne T, Feinstein JA, Friedberg MK, Earing M, Barst RJ, Keller RL, Kinsella JP, Mullen M, Deterding R, Kulik T, Mallory G, Humpl T, Wessel DL. Pediatric pulmonary hypertension: guidelines from the American heart association and American thoracic society. Circulation. 2015;132:2037–99.

Ageno W, Gallus AS, Wittkowsky A, Crowther M, Hylek EM, Palareti G. Oral anticoagulant therapy: antithrombotic therapy and prevention of thrombosis, 9th ed: American college of chest physicians evidence-based clinical practice guidelines. Chest. 2012;141:e44S–88.

Allen HD, Driscoll DJ, Shaddy RE, Feltes TF. Moss & Adams' heart disease. In: Infants, children, and adolescents: including the fetus and young adult. Philadelphia: Lippincott Williams & Wilkins; 2013.

Allpress AL, Rosenthal GL, Goodrich KM, Lupinetti FM, Zerr DM. Risk factors for surgical site infections after pediatric cardiovascular surgery. Pediatr Infect Dis J. 2004;23:231–4.

Amanfu RK, Saucerman JJ. Cardiac models in drug discovery and development: a review. Crit Rev Biomed Eng. 2011;39:379–95.

Asmal L, Flegar SJ, Wang J, Rummel-Kluge C, Komossa K, Leucht S. Quetiapine versus other atypical antipsychotics for schizophrenia. Cochrane Database Syst Rev. 2013;11:CD006625.

Atkins DL, Berger S, Duff JP, Gonzales JC, Hunt EA, Joyner BL, Meaney PA, Niles DE, Samson RA, Schexnayder SM. Part 11: Pediatric Basic Life Support and Cardiopulmonary Resuscitation Quality: 2015 American Heart Association Guidelines Update for Cardiopulmonary Resuscitation and Emergency Cardiovascular Care. Circulation. 2015;132:S519–25.

Atz AM, Wessel DL. Inhaled nitric oxide in the neonate with cardiac disease. Semin Perinatol. 1997;21:441–55.

Bailey AR, Burchett KR. Effect of low-dose dopamine on serum concentrations of prolactin in critically ill patients. Br J Anaesth. 1997;78:97–9.

Bangash MN, Kong ML, Pearse RM. Use of inotropes and vasopressor agents in critically ill patients. Br J Pharmacol. 2012;165:2015–33.

Baron R, Binder A, Biniek R, Braune S, Buerkle H, Dall P, Demirakca S, Eckardt R, Eggers V, Eichler I, Fietze I, Freys S, Frund A, Garten L, Gohrbandt B, Harth I, Hartl W, Heppner HJ,

Horter J, Huth R, Janssens U, Jungk C, Kaeuper KM, Kessler P, Kleinschmidt S, Kochanek M, Kumpf M, Meiser A, Mueller A, Orth M, Putensen C, Roth B, Schaefer M, Schaefers R, Schellongowski P, Schindler M, Schmitt R, Scholz J, Schroeder S, Schwarzmann G, Spies C, Stingele R, Tonner P, Trieschmann U, Tryba M, Wappler F, Waydhas C, Weiss B, Weisshaar G. Evidence and consensus based guideline for the management of delirium, analgesia, and sedation in intensive care medicine. Revision 2015 (DAS-Guideline 2015) - short version. Ger Med Sci. 2015;13:Doc19. doi: 10.3205/000223. eCollection 2015.

Beck G, Brinkkoetter P, Hanusch C, Schulte J, van Ackern K, van der Woude FJ, Yard BA. Clinical review: immunomodulatory effects of dopamine in general inflammation. Crit Care. 2004;8: 485–91.

Beghetti M, Wacker Bou Puigdefabregas J, Merali S. Sildenafil for the treatment of pulmonary hypertension in children. Expert Rev Cardiovasc Ther. 2014;12:1157–84.

Begum N, Shen W, Manganiello V. Role of PDE3A in regulation of cell cycle progression in mouse vascular smooth muscle cells and oocytes: implications in cardiovascular diseases and infertility. Curr Opin Pharmacol. 2011;11:725–9.

Bianchi MO, Cheung PY, Phillipos E, Aranha-Netto A, Joynt C. The effect of milrinone on splanchnic and cerebral perfusion in infants with congenital heart disease prior to surgery: an observational study. Shock (Augusta, Ga). 2015;44:115–20.

Biban P, Gaffuri M. Vasopressin and terlipressin in neonates and children with refractory septic shock. Curr Drug Metab. 2013;14:186–92.

Bracht H, Calzia E, Georgieff M, Singer J, Radermacher P, Russell JA. Inotropes and vasopressors: more than haemodynamics! Br J Pharmacol. 2012;165:2009–11.

Brahmbhatt K, Whitgob E. Diagnosis and management of delirium in critically Ill infants: case report and review. Pediatrics. 2016;137:1–5.

Brissaud O, Botte A, Cambonie G, Dauger S, de Saint Blanquat L, Durand P, Gournay V, Guillet E, Laux D, Leclerc F, Mauriat P, Boulain T, Kuteifan K. Experts' recommendations for the management of cardiogenic shock in children. Ann Intens Care. 2016;6:14.

Brunner N, de Jesus Perez VA, Richter A, Haddad F, Denault A, Rojas V, Yuan K, Orcholski M, Liao X. Perioperative pharmacological management of pulmonary hypertensive crisis during congenital heart surgery. Pulm Circ. 2014;4:10–24.

Bucher BT, Warner BW, Dillon PA. Antibiotic prophylaxis and the prevention of surgical site infection. Curr Opin Pediatr. 2011;23:334–8.

Capodanno D, Bhatt DL, Goto S, O'Donoghue ML, Moliterno DJ, Tamburino C, Angiolillo DJ. Safety and efficacy of protease-activated receptor-1 antagonists in patients with coronary artery disease: a meta-analysis of randomized clinical trials. J Thromb Haemost: JTH. 2012;10:2006–15.

Carroll SJ, Ferris A, Chen J, Liberman L. Efficacy of prostaglandin E1 in relieving obstruction in coarctation of a persistent fifth aortic arch without opening the ductus arteriosus. Pediatr Cardiol. 2006;27:766–8.

Chaturvedi S, Lipszyc DH, Licht C, Craig JC, Parekh R. Pharmacological interventions for hypertension in children. Cochrane Database Syst Rev. 2014a;2:Cd008117.

Chaturvedi S, Lipszyc DH, Licht C, Craig JC, Parekh R. Pharmacological interventions for hypertension in children. Evid Based Child Health: Cochrane Review J. 2014b;9:498–580.

Choong K, Kissoon N. Vasopressin in pediatric shock and cardiac arrest. Pediatr Crit Care Med. 2008;9:372–9.

Chu PY, Campbell MJ, Miller SG, Hill KD. Anti-hypertensive drugs in children and adolescents. World J Cardiol. 2014;6:234–44.

CID=681 NCfBIPCD. 2016. Dopamine.

Clutter WE, Bier DM, Shah SD, Cryer PE. Epinephrine plasma metabolic clearance rates and physiologic thresholds for metabolic and hemodynamic actions in man. J Clin Invest. 1980;66:94–101.

Cooper BE. Review and update on inotropes and vasopressors. AACN Adv Crit Care. 2008;19:5–13; quiz 14–5.

Costello JM, Graham DA, Morrow DF, Morrow J, Potter-Bynoe G, Sandora TJ, Pigula FA, Laussen PC. Risk factors for surgical site infection after cardiac surgery in children. Ann Thorac Surg. 2010;89:1833–41; discussion 1841–32.

Costi D, Cyna AM, Ahmed S, Stephens K, Strickland P, Ellwood J, Larsson JN, Chooi C, Burgoyne LL, Middleton P. Effects of sevoflurane versus other general anaesthesia on emergence agitation in children. Cochrane Database Syst Rev. 2014;9:Cd007084.

Curley GF, Shehata N, Mazer CD, Hare GM, Friedrich JO. Transfusion triggers for guiding RBC transfusion for cardiovascular surgery: a systematic review and meta-analysis*. Crit Care Med. 2014;42:2611–24.

Cuthbert AW. Lubiprostone targets prostanoid EP(4) receptors in ovine airways. Br J Pharmacol. 2011;162:508–20.

Dahmani S, Stany I, Brasher C, Lejeune C, Bruneau B, Wood C, Nivoche Y, Constant I, Murat I. Pharmacological prevention of sevoflurane- and desflurane-related emergence agitation in children: a meta-analysis of published studies. Br J Anaesth. 2010;104:216–23.

De Backer D, Biston P, Devriendt J, Madl C, Chochrad D, Aldecoa C, Brasseur A, Defrance P, Gottignies P, Vincent JL. Comparison of dopamine and norepinephrine in the treatment of shock. N Engl J Med. 2010;362:779–89.

de Caen AR, Berg MD, Chameides L, Gooden CK, Hickey RW, Scott HF, Sutton RM, Tijssen JA, Topjian A, van der Jagt EW, Schexnayder SM, Samson RA. Part 12: Pediatric Advanced Life Support: 2015 American Heart Association Guidelines Update for Cardiopulmonary Resuscitation and Emergency Cardiovascular Care. Circulation. 2015;132:S526–42.

Dhull RS, Baracco R, Jain A, Mattoo TK. Pharmacologic treatment of pediatric hypertension. Curr Hypertens Rep. 2016;18:32.

Dixon BS, Beck GJ, Vazquez MA, Greenberg A, Delmez JA, Allon M, Dember LM, Himmelfarb J, Gassman JJ, Greene T, Radeva MK, Davidson IJ, Ikizler TA, Braden GL, Fenves AZ, Kaufman JS, Cotton Jr JR, Martin KJ, McNeil JW, Rahman A, Lawson JH, Whiting JF, Hu B, Meyers CM, Kusek JW, Feldman HI. Effect of dipyridamole plus aspirin on hemodialysis graft patency. N Engl J Med. 2009;360:2191–201.

Dodgen AL, Hill KD. Safety and tolerability considerations in the use of sildenafil for children with pulmonary arterial hypertension. Drug Healthc Patient Saf. 2015;7:175–83.

Donadini MP, Ageno W, Douketis JD. Management of bleeding in patients receiving conventional or new anticoagulants: a practical and case-based approach. Drugs. 2012;72:1965–75.

Douketis JD, Spyropoulos AC, Spencer FA, Mayr M, Jaffer AK, Eckman MH, Dunn AS, Kunz R. Perioperative management of antithrombotic therapy: Antithrombotic Therapy and Prevention of Thrombosis, 9th ed: American College of Chest Physicians Evidence-Based Clinical Practice Guidelines. Chest. 2012;141:e326S–50.

Driscoll A, Currey J, Tonkin A, Krum H. Nurse-led titration of angiotensin converting enzyme inhibitors, beta-adrenergic blocking agents, and angiotensin receptor blockers for people with heart failure with reduced ejection fraction. Cochrane Database Syst Rev. 2015;12:Cd009889.

Drover DR, Hammer GB, Barrett JS, Cohane CA, Reece T, Zajicek A, Schulman SR. Evaluation of sodium nitroprusside for controlled hypotension in children during surgery. Front Pharmacol. 2015;6:136.

Durandy Y. Use of blood products in pediatric cardiac surgery. Artif Organs. 2015;39:21–7.

Eaton MP. Antifibrinolytic therapy in surgery for congenital heart disease. Anesth Analg. 2008;106:1087–100.

Elenkov IJ, Wilder RL, Chrousos GP, Vizi ES. The sympathetic nerve--an integrative interface between two supersystems: the brain and the immune system. Pharmacol Rev. 2000;52:595–638.

Faraoni D, Goobie SM. The efficacy of antifibrinolytic drugs in children undergoing noncardiac surgery: a systematic review of the literature. Anesth Analg. 2014;118:628–36.

Fellin R. "Cardiovascular pharmacology". In: Dabbagh A, Esmailian F, Aranki SF, editors. Postoperative critical care for cardiac surgical patients. Heidelberg: Springer; 2014. p. 41–72.

Ferrer-Barba A, Gonzalez-Rivera I, Bautista-Hernandez V. Inodilators in the management of low cardiac output syndrome after pediatric cardiac surgery. Curr Vasc Pharmacol. 2016;14: 48–57.

Finkelstein Y, Nurmohamed L, Avner M, Benson LN, Koren G. Clopidogrel use in children. J Pediatr. 2005;147:657–61.

Fleming GA, Murray KT, Yu C, Byrne JG, Greelish JP, Petracek MR, Hoff SJ, Ball SK, Brown NJ, Pretorius M. Milrinone use is associated with postoperative atrial fibrillation after cardiac surgery. Circulation. 2008;118:1619–25.

Flynn JT. Management of hypertension in the young: role of antihypertensive medications. J Cardiovasc Pharmacol. 2011;58:111–20.

Flynn JT, Bradford MC, Harvey EM. Intravenous hydralazine in hospitalized children and adolescents with hypertension. J Pediatr. 2016;168:88–92.

Franz D, Contreras F, Gonzalez H, Prado C, Elgueta D, Figueroa C, Pacheco R. Dopamine receptors D3 and D5 regulate CD4(+)T-cell activation and differentiation by modulating ERK activation and cAMP production. J Neuroimmunol. 2015;284:18–29.

Friederich JA, Butterworth JF. Sodium nitroprusside: twenty years and counting. Anesth Analg. 1995;81:152–62.

Friesen RH, Williams GD. Anesthetic management of children with pulmonary arterial hypertension. Paediatr Anaesth. 2008;18:208–16.

Galante D. Intraoperative management of pulmonary arterial hypertension in infants and children-corrected and republished article. Curr Opin Anaesthesiol. 2011;24:468–71.

Gao Y, Raj JU. Regulation of the pulmonary circulation in the fetus and newborn. Physiol Rev. 2010;90:1291–335.

Gentilomo C, Huang YS, Raffini L. Significant increase in clopidogrel use across U.S. children's hospitals. Pediatr Cardiol. 2011;32:167–75.

Giglia TM, Witmer C, Procaccini DE, Byrnes JW. Pediatric cardiac intensive care society 2014 consensus statement: pharmacotherapies in cardiac critical care anticoagulation and thrombolysis. Pediatr Crit Care Med. 2016;17:S77–88.

Gist KM, Goldstein SL, Joy MS, Vinks AA. Milrinone dosing issues in critically Ill children with kidney injury: a review. J Cardiovasc Pharmacol. 2016;67:175–81.

Glund S, Moschetti V, Norris S, Stangier J, Schmohl M, van Ryn J, Lang B, Ramael S, Reilly P. A randomised study in healthy volunteers to investigate the safety, tolerability and pharmacokinetics of idarucizumab, a specific antidote to dabigatran. Thromb Haemost. 2015;113:943–51.

Gordon NKGR. The organelle of differentiation in embryos: the cell state splitter. Theor Biol Med Model. 2016;13:35.

Gresele P, Momi S, Falcinelli E. Anti-platelet therapy: phosphodiesterase inhibitors. Br J Clin Pharmacol. 2011;72:634–46.

Griffin MR. Epidemiology of nonsteroidal anti-inflammatory drug-associated gastrointestinal injury. Am J Med. 1998;104:23S–9; discussion 41S–2S.

Groom RC, Akl BF, Albus R, Lefrak EA. Pediatric cardiopulmonary bypass: a review of current practice. Int Anesthesiol Clin. 1996;34:141–63.

Hansmann G, Apitz C, Abdul-Khaliq H, Alastalo TP, Beerbaum P, Bonnet D, Dubowy KO, Gorenflo M, Hager A, Hilgendorff A, Kaestner M, Koestenberger M, Koskenvuo JW, Kozlik-Feldmann R, Kuehne T, Lammers AE, Latus H, Michel-Behnke I, Miera O, Moledina S, Muthurangu V, Pattathu J, Schranz D, Warnecke G, Zartner P. Executive summary. Expert consensus statement on the diagnosis and treatment of paediatric pulmonary hypertension. The European Paediatric Pulmonary Vascular Disease Network, endorsed by ISHLT and DGPK. Heart. 2016;102 Suppl 2:ii86–100.

Hari P, Sinha A. Hypertensive emergencies in children. Indian J Pediatr. 2011;78:569–75.

Herrera AJ, Espinosa-Oliva AM, Carrillo-Jimenez A, Oliva-Martin MJ, Garcia-Revilla J, Garcia-Quintanilla A, de Pablos RM, Venero JL. Relevance of chronic stress and the two faces of microglia in Parkinson's disease. Front Cell Neurosci. 2015;9:312.

Hipp DM, Ely EW. Pharmacological and nonpharmacological management of delirium in critically ill patients. Neurotherapeutics: J Am Soc Exper NeuroTherapeut. 2012;9:158–75.

Holmes CL. Vasoactive drugs in the intensive care unit. Curr Opin Crit Care. 2005;11:413–7.

Holmes CL, Landry DW, Granton JT. Science review: vasopressin and the cardiovascular system part 1 – receptor physiology. Crit Care. 2003;7:427–34.

Holmes CL, Landry DW, Granton JT. Science review: vasopressin and the cardiovascular system part 2 - clinical physiology. Crit Care. 2004;8:15–23.

Hottinger DG, Beebe DS, Kozhimannil T, Prielipp RC, Belani KG. Sodium nitroprusside in 2014: a clinical concepts review. J Anaesthesiol Clin Pharmacol. 2014;30:462–71.

Iarussi T, Marolla A, Pardolesi A, Patea RL, Camplese P, Sacco R. Sternectomy and sternum reconstruction for infection after cardiac surgery. Ann Thorac Surg. 2008;86:1680–1.

Jain S, Vaidyanathan B. Oral anticoagulants in pediatric cardiac practice: a systematic review of the literature. Ann Pediatr Cardiol. 2010;3:31–4.

Jennings LK, Michelson AD, Jacoski MV, Tyagi A, Grgurevich S, Li JS, Picolo I. Pharmacodynamic effects of clopidogrel in pediatric cardiac patients: a comparative study of platelet aggregation response. Platelets. 2012;23:430–8.

Jentzer JC, Coons JC, Link CB, Schmidhofer M. Pharmacotherapy update on the use of vasopressors and inotropes in the intensive care unit. J Cardiovasc Pharmacol Ther. 2015;20: 249–60.

Jentzer JC, Mathier MA. Pulmonary hypertension in the intensive care unit. J Intensive Care Med. 2015;31:369–85.

Jobes DR, Sesok-Pizzini D, Friedman D. Reduced transfusion requirement with use of fresh whole blood in pediatric cardiac surgical procedures. Ann Thorac Surg. 2015;99:1706–11.

Joyce C, Witcher R, Herrup E, Kaur S, Mendez-Rico E, Silver G, Greenwald BM, Traube C. Evaluation of the safety of quetiapine in treating delirium in critically Ill children: a retrospective review. J Child Adolesc Psychopharmacol. 2015;25:666–70.

Kee VR. Hemodynamic pharmacology of intravenous vasopressors. Crit Care Nurse. 2003;23: 79–82.

Kim JS, McSweeney J, Lee J, Ivy D. Pediatric cardiac intensive care society 2014 consensus statement: pharmacotherapies in cardiac critical care pulmonary hypertension. Pediatr Crit Care Med. 2016;17:S89–100.

Kleinman ME, Chameides L, Schexnayder SM, Samson RA, Hazinski MF, Atkins DL, Berg MD, de Caen AR, Fink EL, Freid EB, Hickey RW, Marino BS, Nadkarni VM, Proctor LT, Qureshi FA, Sartorelli K, Topjian A, van der Jagt EW, Zaritsky AL. Part 14: pediatric advanced life support: 2010 American Heart Association Guidelines for Cardiopulmonary Resuscitation and Emergency Cardiovascular Care. Circulation. 2010;122:S876–908.

Klugman D, Goswami ES, Berger JT. Pediatric cardiac intensive care society 2014 consensus statement: pharmacotherapies in cardiac critical care antihypertensives. Pediatr Crit Care Med. 2016;17:S101–8.

Knight WE, Yan C. Cardiac cyclic nucleotide phosphodiesterases: function, regulation, and therapeutic prospects. Hormone Metabol Res. 2012;44:766–75.

Kushwah S, Kumar A, Sahana KS. Levosimendan. A promising future drug for refractory cardiac failure in children? Indian Heart J. 2016;68 Suppl 1:S57–60.

Lakshminrusimha S, Mathew B, Leach CL. Pharmacologic strategies in neonatal pulmonary hypertension other than nitric oxide. Semin Perinatol. 2016;40:160–73.

Lambert P, Cyna AM, Knight N, Middleton P. Clonidine premedication for postoperative analgesia in children. Cochrane Database Syst Rev. 2014;1:Cd009633.

Landoni G, Biondi-Zoccai G, Greco M, Greco T, Bignami E, Morelli A, Guarracino F, Zangrillo A. Effects of levosimendan on mortality and hospitalization. A meta-analysis of randomized controlled studies. Crit Care Med. 2012;40:634–46.

Langford RM, Mehta V. Selective cyclooxygenase inhibition: its role in pain and anaesthesia. Biomed Pharmacother. 2006;60:323–8.

Latus H, Delhaas T, Schranz D, Apitz C. Treatment of pulmonary arterial hypertension in children. Nat Rev Cardiol. 2015;12:244–54.

Lechner E, Hofer A, Leitner-Peneder G, Freynschlag R, Mair R, Weinzettel R, Rehak P, Gombotz H. Levosimendan versus milrinone in neonates and infants after corrective open-heart surgery: a pilot study. Pediatr Crit Care Med. 2012;13:542–8.

Lei C, Xiong LZ. Perioperative Red Blood Cell Transfusion: What We Do Not know. Chin Med J (Engl). 2015;128:2383–6.

Leone M, Martin C. Role of terlipressin in the treatment of infants and neonates with catecholamine-resistant septic shock. Best Pract Res Clin Anaesthesiol. 2008;22:323–33.

Lepelletier D, Perron S, Bizouarn P, Caillon J, Drugeon H, Michaud JL, Duveau D. Surgical-site infection after cardiac surgery: incidence, microbiology, and risk factors. Infect Control Hosp Epidemiol. 2005;26:466–72.

Levite M. Dopamine and T cells: dopamine receptors and potent effects on T cells, dopamine production in T cells, and abnormalities in the dopaminergic system in T cells in autoimmune, neurological and psychiatric diseases. Acta Physiol (Oxf). 2016;216:42–89.

Li MX, Hwang PM. Structure and function of cardiac troponin C (TNNC1): implications for heart failure, cardiomyopathies, and troponin modulating drugs. Gene. 2015;571:153–66.

Liu C, Chen J, Gao Y, Deng B, Liu K. Endothelin receptor antagonists for pulmonary arterial hypertension. Cochrane Database Syst Rev. 2013;2:Cd004434.

Loy JH, Merry SN, Hetrick SE, Stasiak K. Atypical antipsychotics for disruptive behaviour disorders in children and youths. Cochrane Database Syst Rev. 2012;9:Cd008559.

Lucas SS, Nasr VG, Ng AJ, Joe C, Bond M, DiNardo JA. Pediatric cardiac intensive care society 2014 consensus statement: pharmacotherapies in cardiac critical care: sedation, analgesia and muscle relaxant. Pediatr Crit Care Med. 2016;17:S3–15.

Maconochie IK, de Caen AR, Aickin R, Atkins DL, Biarent D, Guerguerian AM, Kleinman ME, Kloeck DA, Meaney PA, Nadkarni VM, Ng KC, Nuthall G, Reis AG, Shimizu N, Tibballs J, Pintos RV. Part 6: pediatric basic life support and pediatric advanced life support: 2015 international consensus on cardiopulmonary resuscitation and emergency cardiovascular care science with treatment recommendations. Resuscitation. 2015;95:e147–68.

Madden K, Turkel S, Jacobson J, Epstein D, Moromisato DY. Recurrent delirium after surgery for congenital heart disease in an infant. Pediatr Crit Care Med. 2011;12:e413–5.

Maglione M, Maher AR, Hu J, Wang Z, Shanman R, Shekelle PG, Roth B, Hilton L, Suttorp MJ, Ewing BA, Motala A, Perry T. AHRQ comparative effectiveness reviews. In: Off-label use of atypical antipsychotics: an update. Rockville: Agency for Healthcare Research and Quality (US); 2011.

Majure DT, Greco T, Greco M, Ponschab M, Biondi-Zoccai G, Zangrillo A, Landoni G. Meta-analysis of randomized trials of effect of milrinone on mortality in cardiac surgery: an update. J Cardiothorac Vasc Anesth. 2013;27:220–9.

Malarbi S, Stargatt R, Howard K, Davidson A. Characterizing the behavior of children emerging with delirium from general anesthesia. Paediatr Anaesth. 2011;21:942–50.

Maldifassi MC, Baur R, Sigel E. Functional sites involved in modulation of the GABA receptor channel by the intravenous anesthetics propofol, etomidate and pentobarbital. Neuropharmacology. 2016;105:207–14.

Maltz LA, Gauvreau K, Connor JA, Jenkins KJ. Clopidogrel in a pediatric population: prescribing practice and outcomes from a single center. Pediatr Cardiol. 2009;30:99–105.

Marcotti W, Johnson SL, Kros CJ. A transiently expressed SK current sustains and modulates action potential activity in immature mouse inner hair cells. J Physiol. 2004;560:691–708.

Marionneau C, Abriel H. Regulation of the cardiac Na channel Na1.5 by post-translational modifications. J Mol Cell Cardiol. 2015;82:36–47.

Martin-Stone S. Postoperative bleeding disorders after cardiac surgery. In: Dabbagh A, Esmailian F, Aranki SF, editors. Postoperative critical care for cardiac surgical patients. Berlin: Springer; 2014. p. 161–96. Published with kind permission of © Springer, 2014. All Rights Reserved.

Masi G, Milone A, Veltri S, Iuliano R, Pfanner C, Pisano S. Use of quetiapine in children and adolescents. Paediatr Drugs. 2015;17:125–40.

Maslov MY, Wei AE, Pezone MJ, Edelman ER, Lovich MA. Vascular Dilation, Tachycardia, and Increased Inotropy Occur Sequentially with Increasing Epinephrine Dose Rate, Plasma and Myocardial Concentrations, and cAMP. Heart Lung Circ. 2015;24:912–8.

Mauri L, Kereiakes DJ, Yeh RW, Driscoll-Shempp P, Cutlip DE, Steg PG, Normand SL, Braunwald E, Wiviott SD, Cohen DJ, Holmes Jr DR, Krucoff MW, Hermiller J, Dauerman HL, Simon DI, Kandzari DE, Garratt KN, Lee DP, Pow TK, Ver Lee P, Rinaldi MJ, Massaro JM. Twelve or 30 months of dual antiplatelet therapy after drug-eluting stents. N Engl J Med. 2014;371:2155–66.

McCammond AN, Axelrod DM, Bailly DK, Ramsey EZ, Costello JM. Pediatric cardiac intensive care society 2014 consensus statement: pharmacotherapies in cardiac critical care fluid management. Pediatr Crit Care Med. 2016;17:S35–48.

McPheeters ML, Warren Z, Sathe N, Bruzek JL, Krishnaswami S, Jerome RN, Veenstra-Vanderweele J. A systematic review of medical treatments for children with autism spectrum disorders. Pediatrics. 2011;127:e1312–21.

Mebazaa A, Nieminen MS, Packer M, Cohen-Solal A, Kleber FX, Pocock SJ, Thakkar R, Padley RJ, Poder P, Kivikko M. Levosimendan vs dobutamine for patients with acute decompensated heart failure: the SURVIVE Randomized Trial. JAMA. 2007;297:1883–91.

Mehta PA, Cunningham CK, Colella CB, Alferis G, Weiner LB. Risk factors for sternal wound and other infections in pediatric cardiac surgery patients. Pediatr Infect Dis J. 2000;19:1000–4.

Mehta S, Granton J, Gordon AC, Cook DJ, Lapinsky S, Newton G, Bandayrel K, Little A, Siau C, Ayers D, Singer J, Lee TC, Walley KR, Storms M, Cooper DJ, Holmes CL, Hebert P, Presneill J, Russell JA. Cardiac ischemia in patients with septic shock randomized to vasopressin or norepinephrine. Crit Care. 2013;17:R117.

Mertens L, Eyskens B, Boshoff D, Gewillig M. Safety and efficacy of clopidogrel in children with heart disease. J Pediatr. 2008;153:61–4.

Messieha Z. Prevention of sevoflurane delirium and agitation with propofol. Anesth Prog. 2013;60:67–71.

Meyer S, Gortner L, McGuire W, Baghai A, Gottschling S. Vasopressin in catecholamine-refractory shock in children. Anaesthesia. 2008;63:228–34.

Meyer S, McGuire W, Gottschling S, Mohammed Shamdeen G, Gortner L. The role of vasopressin and terlipressin in catecholamine-resistant shock and cardio-circulatory arrest in children: review of the literature. Wie Med Wochenschr. 2011;161:192–203.

Miller CL, Yan C. Targeting cyclic nucleotide phosphodiesterase in the heart: therapeutic implications. J Cardiovasc Transl Res. 2010;3:507–15.

Moffett BS, Parham AL, Caudilla CD, Mott AR, Gurwitch KD. Oral anticoagulation in a pediatric hospital: impact of a quality improvement initiative on warfarin management strategies. Qual Saf Health Care. 2006;15:240–3.

Moffett BS, Price JF. Evaluation of sodium nitroprusside toxicity in pediatric cardiac surgical patients. Ann Pharmacother. 2008;42:1600–4.

Moffett BS, Salvin JW, Kim JJ. Pediatric cardiac intensive care society 2014 consensus statement: pharmacotherapies in cardiac critical care antiarrhythmics. Pediatr Crit Care Med. 2016;17:S49–58.

Mohanty S, Vaidyanathan B. Anti-platelet agents in pediatric cardiac practice. Ann Pediatr Cardiol. 2013;6:59–64.

Monagle P, Chalmers E, Chan A, DeVeber G, Kirkham F, Massicotte P, Michelson AD. Antithrombotic therapy in neonates and children: American College of Chest Physicians Evidence-Based Clinical Practice Guidelines (8th Edition). Chest. 2008;133:887s–968.

Monagle P, Chan AK, Goldenberg NA, Ichord RN, Journeycake JM, Nowak-Gottl U, Vesely SK. Antithrombotic therapy in neonates and children: Antithrombotic Therapy and Prevention of Thrombosis, 9th ed: American College of Chest Physicians Evidence-Based Clinical Practice Guidelines. Chest. 2012;141:e737S–801.

Mossad E, Motta P, Sehmbey K, Toscana D. The hemodynamic effects of phenoxybenzamine in neonates, infants, and children. J Clin Anesth. 2008;20:94–8.

Mossad EB. Pro: intraoperative use of nitric oxide for treatment of pulmonary hypertension in patients with congenital heart disease is effective. J Cardiothorac Vasc Anesth. 2001;15:259–62.

Mossad EB, Motta P, Rossano J, Hale B, Morales DL. Perioperative management of pediatric patients on mechanical cardiac support. Paediatr Anaesth. 2011;21:585–93.

Motta P, Mossad E, Toscana D, Zestos M, Mee R. Comparison of phenoxybenzamine to sodium nitroprusside in infants undergoing surgery. J Cardiothorac Vasc Anesth. 2005;19:54–9.

Nateghian A, Taylor G, Robinson JL. Risk factors for surgical site infections following open-heart surgery in a Canadian pediatric population. Am J Infect Control. 2004;32:397–401.

Nieminen MS, Fruhwald S, Heunks LM, Suominen PK, Gordon AC, Kivikko M, Pollesello P. Levosimendan: current data, clinical use and future development. Heart Lung Vessel. 2013;5:227–45.

Noori S, Seri I. Neonatal blood pressure support: the use of inotropes, lusitropes, and other vasopressor agents. Clin Perinatol. 2012;39:221–38.

O'Brien A, Clapp L, Singer M. Terlipressin for norepinephrine-resistant septic shock. Lancet. 2002;359:1209–10.

Ogawa R, Stachnik JM, Echizen H. Clinical pharmacokinetics of drugs in patients with heart failure: an update (part 2, drugs administered orally). Clin Pharmacokinet. 2014;53:1083–114.

Okamoto Y, Nohmi T, Higa Y, Seki K, Yamashita A. Vasopressin does not raise cardiac enzymes following cardiac surgery: a randomized double-blind clinical trial. J Cardiothorac Vasc Anesth. 2015;29:46–51.

Ostrye J, Hailpern SM, Jones J, Egan B, Chessman K, Shatat IF. The efficacy and safety of intravenous hydralazine for the treatment of hypertension in the hospitalized child. Pediatr Nephrol (Berlin, Germany). 2014;29:1403–9.

Pacheco R, Contreras F, Zouali M. The dopaminergic system in autoimmune diseases. Front Immunol. 2014;5:117.

Papp Z, Edes I, Fruhwald S, De Hert SG, Salmenpera M, Leppikangas H, Mebazaa A, Landoni G, Grossini E, Caimmi P, Morelli A, Guarracino F, Schwinger RH, Meyer S, Algotsson L, Wikstrom BG, Jorgensen K, Filippatos G, Parissis JT, Gonzalez MJ, Parkhomenko A, Yilmaz MB, Kivikko M, Pollesello P, Follath F. Levosimendan: molecular mechanisms and clinical implications: consensus of experts on the mechanisms of action of levosimendan. Int J Cardiol. 2012;159:82–7.

Parham WA, Mehdirad AA, Biermann KM, Fredman CS. Hyperkalemia revisited. Tex Heart Inst J. 2006;33:40–7.

Payani N, Foroughi M, Dabbagh A. The effect of intravenous administration of active recombinant factor VII on postoperative bleeding in cardiac valve reoperations: a randomized clinical trial. Anesth Pain Med. 2015;5:e22846.

Perez KM, Laughon M. Sildenafil in term and premature infants: a systematic review. Clin Ther. 2015;37:2598–607. e2591.

Pollack Jr CV, Reilly PA, Eikelboom J, Glund S, Verhamme P, Bernstein RA, Dubiel R, Huisman MV, Hylek EM, Kamphuisen PW, Kreuzer J, Levy JH, Sellke FW, Stangier J, Steiner T, Wang B, Kam CW, Weitz JI. Idarucizumab for Dabigatran Reversal. N Engl J Med. 2015;373:511–20.

Poor HD, Ventetuolo CE. Pulmonary hypertension in the intensive care unit. Prog Cardiovasc Dis. 2012;55:187–98.

Powney MJ, Adams CE, Jones H. Haloperidol for psychosis-induced aggression or agitation (rapid tranquillisation). Cochrane Database Syst Rev. 2012;11:Cd009377.

Prado C, Bernales S, Pacheco R. Modulation of T-cell mediated immunity by dopamine receptor d5. Endocr Metab Immune Disord Drug Targets. 2013;13:184–94.

Pritts CD, Pearl RG. Anesthesia for patients with pulmonary hypertension. Curr Opin Anaesthesiol. 2010;23:411–6.

Remy KE, Natanson C, Klein HG. The influence of the storage lesion(s) on pediatric red cell transfusion. Curr Opin Pediatr. 2015;27:277–85.

Reveiz L, Guerrero-Lozano R, Camacho A, Yara L, Mosquera PA. Stress ulcer, gastritis, and gastrointestinal bleeding prophylaxis in critically ill pediatric patients: a systematic review. Pediatr Crit Care Med. 2010;11:124–32.

Rizza A, Bignami E, Belletti A, Polito A, Ricci Z, Isgro G, Locatelli A, Cogo P. Vasoactive drugs and hemodynamic monitoring in pediatric cardiac intensive care: an Italian survey. World J Pediatr Congenit Heart Surg. 2016;7:25–31.

Rossano JW, Cabrera AG, Jefferies JL, Naim MP, Humlicek T. Pediatric cardiac intensive care society 2014 consensus statement: pharmacotherapies in cardiac critical care chronic heart failure. Pediatr Crit Care Med. 2016;17:S20–34.

Russell JA. Bench-to-bedside review: vasopressin in the management of septic shock. Crit Care. 2011;15:226.

Salvin JW, Bronicki R, Costello JM, Moffett B, Procaccini D. Pediatric cardiac intensive care society 10th international conference 2014 consensus statement: pharmacotherapies in cardiac critical care. Pediatr Crit Care Med. 2016;17:S1–2.

Satterthwaite TD, Wolf DH, Rosenheck RA, Gur RE, Caroff SN. A meta-analysis of the risk of acute extrapyramidal symptoms with intramuscular antipsychotics for the treatment of agitation. J Clin Psychiatry. 2008;69:1869–79.

Schieveld JN, Leroy PL, van Os J, Nicolai J, Vos GD, Leentjens AF. Pediatric delirium in critical illness: phenomenology, clinical correlates and treatment response in 40 cases in the pediatric intensive care unit. Intensive Care Med. 2007;33:1033–40.

Schieveld JN, van der Valk JA, Smeets I, Berghmans E, Wassenberg R, Leroy PL, Vos GD, van Os J. Diagnostic considerations regarding pediatric delirium: a review and a proposal for an algorithm for pediatric intensive care units. Intensive Care Med. 2009;35:1843–9.

Schouten ES, van de Pol AC, Schouten AN, Turner NM, Jansen NJ, Bollen CW. The effect of aprotinin, tranexamic acid, and aminocaproic acid on blood loss and use of blood products in major pediatric surgery: a meta-analysis. Pediatr Crit Care Med. 2009;10:182–90.

Shah PS, Ohlsson A. Sildenafil for pulmonary hypertension in neonates. Cochrane Database Syst Rev. 2011;8:Cd005494.

Sharawy N. Vasoplegia in septic shock: do we really fight the right enemy? J Crit Care. 2014;29:83–7.

Sharma D, Farahbakhsh N, Shastri S, Sharma P. Neonatal hypertension. J Matern Fetal Neonatal Med. 2016;1–34. http://www.ncbi.nlm.nih.gov/pubmed/27072362. doi: 10.1080/14767058.2016.1177816.

Sharma D, Pandita A, Shastri S. Neonatal hypertension: an underdiagnosed condition, a review article. Curr Hypertens Rev. 2014;10:205–12.

Silvetti S, Silvani P, Azzolini ML, Dossi R, Landoni G, Zangrillo A. A systematic review on levosimendan in paediatric patients. Curr Vasc Pharmacol. 2015;13:128–33.

Simons FE, Sampson HA. Anaphylaxis: unique aspects of clinical diagnosis and management in infants (birth to age 2 years). J Allergy Clin Immunol. 2015;135:1125–31.

Singh VK, Sharma R, Agrawal A, Varma A. Vasopressin in the pediatric cardiac intensive care unit: myth or reality. Ann Pediatr Cardiol. 2009;2:65–73.

Smith AH, Owen J, Borgman KY, Fish FA, Kannankeril PJ. Relation of milrinone after surgery for congenital heart disease to significant postoperative tachyarrhythmias. Am J Cardiol. 2011;108:1620–4.

Smith HA, Gangopadhyay M, Goben CM, Jacobowski NL, Chestnut MH, Savage S, Rutherford MT, Denton D, Thompson JL, Chandrasekhar R, Acton M, Newman J, Noori HP, Terrell MK, Williams SR, Griffith K, Cooper TJ, Ely EW, Fuchs DC, Pandharipande PP. The preschool confusion assessment method for the ICU: valid and reliable delirium monitoring for critically Ill infants and children. Crit Care Med. 2016;44:592–600.

Soman T, Rafay MF, Hune S, Allen A, MacGregor D, deVeber G. The risks and safety of clopidogrel in pediatric arterial ischemic stroke. Stroke. 2006;37:1120–2.

Stahl W, Bracht H, Radermacher P, Thomas J. Year in review 2009: critical care–shock. Crit Care. 2010;14:239.

Strobel AM, le Lu N. The critically Ill infant with congenital heart disease. Emerg Med Clin North Am. 2015;33:501–18.

Thomas C, Svehla L, Moffett BS. Sodium-nitroprusside-induced cyanide toxicity in pediatric patients. Expert Opin Drug Saf. 2009;8:599–602.

Trappe HJ, Brandts B, Weismueller P. Arrhythmias in the intensive care patient. Curr Opin Crit Care. 2003;9:345–55.

Twite MD, Friesen RH. The anesthetic management of children with pulmonary hypertension in the cardiac catheterization laboratory. Anesthesiol Clin. 2014;32:157–73.

Van den Berghe G, de Zegher F. Anterior pituitary function during critical illness and dopamine treatment. Crit Care Med. 1996;24:1580–90.

van Dijk M, Knoester H, van Beusekom BS, Ista E. Screening pediatric delirium with an adapted version of the Sophia Observation withdrawal Symptoms scale (SOS). Intensive Care Med. 2012;38:531–2.

van Hoff SL, O'Neill ES, Cohen LC, Collins BA. Does a prophylactic dose of propofol reduce emergence agitation in children receiving anesthesia? A systematic review and meta-analysis. Paediatr Anaesth. 2015;25:668–76.

Varon J, Marik PE. Clinical review: the management of hypertensive crises. Crit Care. 2003;7:374–84.

Vasu TS, Cavallazzi R, Hirani A, Kaplan G, Leiby B, Marik PE. Norepinephrine or dopamine for septic shock: systematic review of randomized clinical trials. J Intensive Care Med. 2012;27:172–8.

Vaughan Williams EM. Relevance of cellular to clinical electrophysiology in interpreting antiarrhythmic drug action. Am J Cardiol. 1989;64:5j–9.

Vaughan Williams EM. The relevance of cellular to clinical electrophysiology in classifying antiarrhythmic actions. J Cardiovasc Pharmacol. 1992;20 Suppl 2:S1–7.

Ventetuolo CE, Klinger JR. Management of acute right ventricular failure in the intensive care unit. Ann Am Thorac Soc. 2014;11:811–22.

Verghese ST, Hannallah RS. Acute pain management in children. J Pain Res. 2010;3:105–23.

Vijarnsorn C, Winijkul G, Laohaprasitiporn D, Chungsomprasong P, Chanthong P, Durongpisitkul K, Soonswang J, Nana A, Subtaweesin T, Sriyoschati S, Pooliam J. Postoperative fever and major infections after pediatric cardiac surgery. J Med Assoc Thai. 2012;95:761–70.

Vorhies EE, Ivy DD. Drug treatment of pulmonary hypertension in children. Paediatr Drugs. 2014;16:43–65.

Wang A. Review of vorapaxar for the prevention of atherothrombotic events. Expert Opin Pharmacother. 2015;16:2509–22.

Wang RC, Jiang FM, Zheng QL, Li CT, Peng XY, He CY, Luo J, Liang ZA. Efficacy and safety of sildenafil treatment in pulmonary arterial hypertension: a systematic review. Respir Med. 2014;108:531–7.

Warshaw G, Mechlin M. Prevention and management of postoperative delirium. Int Anesthesiol Clin. 2009;47:137–49.

Watt K, Li JS, Benjamin Jr DK, Cohen-Wolkowiez M. Pediatric cardiovascular drug dosing in critically ill children and extracorporeal membrane oxygenation. J Cardiovasc Pharmacol. 2011;58:126–32.

Wolf CM, Berul CI. Molecular mechanisms of inherited arrhythmias. Curr Genomics. 2008;9:160–8.

Xue H, Lu Z, Tang WL, Pang LW, Wang GM, Wong GW, Wright JM. First-line drugs inhibiting the renin angiotensin system versus other first-line antihypertensive drug classes for hypertension. Cochrane Database Syst Rev. 2015;1:Cd008170.

Yan C, Miller CL, Abe J. Regulation of phosphodiesterase 3 and inducible cAMP early repressor in the heart. Circ Res. 2007;100:489–501.

Zaccolo M, Movsesian MA. cAMP and cGMP signaling cross-talk: role of phosphodiesterases and implications for cardiac pathophysiology. Circ Res. 2007;100:1569–78.

Zhao CY, Greenstein JL, Winslow RL. Interaction between phosphodiesterases in the regulation of the cardiac beta-adrenergic pathway. J Mol Cell Cardiol. 2015;88:29–38.

Zhao CY, Greenstein JL, Winslow RL. Roles of phosphodiesterases in the regulation of the cardiac cyclic nucleotide cross-talk signaling network. J Mol Cell Cardiol. 2016;91:215–27.

Zhao W, Huang Y, Liu Z, Cao BB, Peng YP, Qiu YH. Dopamine receptors modulate cytotoxicity of natural killer cells via cAMP-PKA-CREB signaling pathway. PLoS One. 2013;8:e65860.

Zipes DP, Camm AJ, Borggrefe M, Buxton AE, Chaitman B, Fromer M, Gregoratos G, Klein G, Moss AJ, Myerburg RJ, Priori SG, Quinones MA, Roden DM, Silka MJ, Tracy C, Smith Jr SC, Jacobs AK, Adams CD, Antman EM, Anderson JL, Hunt SA, Halperin JL, Nishimura R, Ornato JP, Page RL, Riegel B, Priori SG, Blanc JJ, Budaj A, Camm AJ, Dean V, Deckers JW, Despres C, Dickstein K, Lekakis J, McGregor K, Metra M, Morais J, Osterspey A, Tamargo JL, Zamorano JL. ACC/AHA/ESC 2006 guidelines for management of patients with ventricular arrhythmias and the prevention of sudden cardiac death: a report of the American College of Cardiology/American Heart Association Task Force and the European Society of Cardiology Committee for Practice Guidelines (Writing Committee to Develop Guidelines for Management of Patients With Ventricular Arrhythmias and the Prevention of Sudden Cardiac Death). J Am Coll Cardiol. 2006;48:e247–346.
Zou Z, Yuan HB, Yang B, Xu F, Chen XY, Liu GJ, Shi XY. Perioperative angiotensin-converting enzyme inhibitors or angiotensin II type 1 receptor blockers for preventing mortality and morbidity in adults. Cochrane Database Syst Rev. 2016;1:Cd009210.

Part II
Diagnostics and Monitoring

Chapter 5
Perioperative Care of the Congenital Cardiac Patient in the Cardiac Catheterization Laboratory

Lorraine Lubin and Robert Wong

Introduction

New innovative techniques in cardiac catheterization (cath) procedures and advances in technology in the field have created an environment in which the primary objective has advanced from diagnostics to a minimally invasive therapeutic intervention. These advances and new devices have provided nonsurgical alternatives for the treatment of congenital heart disease which in many instances have replaced open cardiac surgery and decreased the morbidity and mortality for multiple goals of therapy. While the ultimate outcome for the patient is a more minimally invasive therapy, the catheterization lab has taken on more of an operating room setting requiring more intensive monitoring and higher-acuity anesthetic management. With the survival of congenital heart patients increasing and creating a situation in which there are more adults with congenital heart disease than pediatric patients, the patient population of the pediatric cath lab reflects the demographics of the specialty. The pediatric cath lab is now more correctly referred to as the congenital cardiac cath lab with the capability of caring for all patients, irrelevant of age by a single group of providers.

In the past years, anesthesia providers were not significantly involved in the care of patients in the congenital cath lab, and cardiologists were responsible for prescribing the sedation medications used during the procedure. However, as the acuity of the interventions has increased and hybrid operating rooms have emerged, the cath lab has morphed into a near-operating room setting in which anesthesia machines, medication carts, and airway equipment have come to

L. Lubin, MD (✉) • R. Wong, MD
Cedars Sinai Medical Center, Department of Anesthesiology,
8700 Beverly Blvd, Suite 8211, Los Angeles, CA 90048, USA
e-mail: Lorraine.Lubin@cshs.org; Robert.Wong@cshs.org

© Springer International Publishing Switzerland 2017
A. Dabbagh et al. (eds.), *Congenital Heart Disease in Pediatric and Adult Patients*, DOI 10.1007/978-3-319-44691-2_5

essentially every room. With respect to the perioperative risks in the cardiac cath lab, the data from the Pediatric Perioperative Cardiac Arrest Registry has shown that approximately one-third of cardiac arrests occur in children with congenital heart disease (CHD), of which 17 % occur during cardiac cath procedures. With this in mind, the anesthesiologist must not only be familiar with the patient's congenital physiology, but it is also critical for the appropriate monitoring equipment, blood availability, surgical backup, and postoperative disposition be arranged.

The Cath Lab Environment

The environment of the cath lab differs from the operating room environment in important ways with respect to the anesthesia and surgical setting. The procedures include both adults and children with varying levels of acuity which range from outpatient procedures to the hybrid cases and care of patients on significant forms of medical and device support. The staff in the cath lab is generally not trained in open surgical procedures and is very focused with respect to their scope of practice. More and more anesthesia providers are becoming the mainstay of the cath lab as the procedures become more invasive such as valve implantation, surgical pacemaker implantation, complex percutaneous coronary interventions (PCI), ventricular assist device placement, aortic interventions, and hybrid procedures. Hybrid procedures involve varying levels of open surgical intervention and catheter-based intervention and also rely on multiple imaging techniques such as echocardiography and fluoroscopy. One of the many challenges of the cath lab apart from the evolving new technology and roles of various specialties is the work space. Due to the fluoroscopy equipment, the space for anesthesia providers is limited, and special equipment and support personnel are not readily available. This makes emergent resuscitation more difficult. In modern-day facilities, the cath lab is designed to be adjacent to or relatively near the cardiac operating rooms. The advent of hybrid suites which are larger than the average cath lab suite is also being developed. Hybrid suites encompass equipment needed for both catheter-based interventions and open cardiac surgical procedures. Hybrid suites contain supporting equipment for perfusionist such as the cardiopulmonary bypass (CPB) machine and extracorporeal membrane oxygenation (ECMO). Since a hybrid room is designed for open cardiac procedures, the room must meet the standards of an operating room-anesthetizing location with appropriate air exchange, gases, electrical outlets, gas scavenging, suction and room for the CPB machine, and anesthesia machine and medication/supply cart as well as important equipment such as echocardiography machines.

MRI scanners are also becoming a more important imaging modality and are replacing cardiac cath in some diagnostic situations. If MRI is part of the cath plan, the patients are frequently moved under the same anesthetic and monitoring equipment, and timing is crucial. The patient must be kept in a MRI-compatible gurney, and monitoring equipment as well as infusion pumps must also be MRI compatible.

Radiation safety is another important consideration in the cath lab environment. Cardiac catheterization which uses cine fluoroscopy can deliver relatively high doses of radiation. There is no known safe exposure for either patients or providers which are accepted to decrease cancer risk. It is recommended to wear dosimeter badges and follow the radiation safety principles advised to reduce the occupational exposure: (1) Wear proper radiation lead clothing shields and protective lead eyewear. (2) Minimize exposure time. (3) Maintain the maximal distance acceptable to the source of the radiation, and use lead screens whenever possible. With respect to the risk to the patient, there is an increased risk with increasing dose, and the average dose used during both diagnostic and therapeutic cases remains relatively high with the youngest patients frequently receiving the highest exposures. In 2006, a study was released which looked at the chromosomal damage in patients with CHD; there was a distinct correlation that cardiac cath was associated with long-term chromosomal damage.

The Goals of Congenital Cardiac Catheterization

Diagnostic catheterization for patients with CHD is important to further delineate the patient's anatomy, physiology or hemodynamics, biventricular function, and responsiveness to medications as well as respiratory interventions. The information obtained from catheterization data is vital in many cases for appropriate surgical decision-making in a relatively fragile patient population. The circumstances in which the cath data is obtained are extremely important due to its effects on the calculated hemodynamic data. For example, hemodynamic data is acquired on room air settings, and dissolved oxygen is minimized or accounted for in the calculated data. The effects of positive-pressure ventilation, sedation, or other inotropic or vasoactive medications must also be factored in when accessing the final data and imaging. The communication between the anesthesiologist and interventional cardiologist is vital in the management of these patients.

Diagnostic cath is only one of multiple imaging modalities used to correctly access the congenital heart patient's anatomy and physiology and in many cases is not necessary for many patients requiring surgery. Advances in other imaging techniques most notably echocardiography, and MRI compared to the invasive nature of cardiac cath and its associated complications such as vascular compromise, require that significant consideration must be given to the indications for diagnostic catheterization.

In 2011, the American Heart Association put forth their recommended indications for diagnostic congenital cardiac catheterization which comprise the following indications:

1. To perform the measurement of central and peripheral intravascular pressures and derive hemodynamic information including pulmonary vascular resistance (PVR), systemic vascular resistance (SVR), shunt fractions, oxygen consumption, and cardiac output.
2. To define cardiac and vascular anatomy. Cardiac catheterization in conjunction with echocardiography and MRI may be needed in patients with complex anatomy and in previously operated patients in whom the anatomy is not known from operative reports.
3. To evaluate myocardial function and assess the effects of respiratory interventions and medications on the cardiovascular system. These types of diagnostic catheterizations are frequently performed on patients who have single-ventricle anatomy when deciding upon the timing of the procedure or its appropriateness. It is also common for patients with pulmonary hypertension or as part of a transplantation evaluation to undergo this type of diagnostic cath.
4. Coronary artery angiography, endocardial biopsies, and evaluation of myocardial function are parts of the routine surveillance of patients following cardiac transplantation. Endocardial biopsy is also indicated in the face of acute cardiac decompensation from possible viral myocarditis or other forms of myocarditis or cardiomyopathy.
5. To obtain a diagnostic evaluation as part of an interventional procedure.

Procedural Vascular Access and the Approach

The routine approach for vascular access and diagnostic cath in patients with biventricular hearts is to cannulate the femoral vein and artery using the Seldinger technique. For patients with univentricular hearts, access is frequently obtained by the internal jugular or subclavian vein in order to evaluate the pulmonary arteries subsequent to cavopulmonary connections or Glenn procedures. After placement of appropriate-sized sheaths, the catheters are advanced through the vascular and heart chambers where pressures and oxygen saturation measurements are made in the appropriate sequence. The oxygen saturation measurements of the cardiac chambers and vasculature will facilitate the detection of shunts and allow the calculation of shunt fractions, oxygen consumption, cardiac output, and pulmonary blood flow. The oxygen saturation data is obtained on room air to avoid error in the calculations, and the angiograms are generally performed after the physiologic measurements have been made.

In patients with CHD, vascular access can be extremely challenging. Vascular thrombosis and injury are common sources of morbidity in this population which includes neonates and the adult congenital patients. With the advancement of interventional procedures including occluder devices and transcatheter valves, much larger vascular sheaths are required to deploy these devices and increase the risk of vascular injury.

Anesthetic Considerations in Diagnostic and Interventional Cardiac Cath Procedures

Procedures both diagnostic and interventional in the cath lab differ from open surgical cases in a number of important ways. Cath procedures in general are not associated with major fluid shifts, significant systemic inflammatory responses, or severe postoperative pain. The most stimulating portion of the procedure with respect to pain occurs during the attaining of vascular access, and in many cases the procedure can be performed as a same-day procedure. However, unlike patients who generally have outpatient surgery, the patients presenting to the congenital cath lab frequently have severe underlying cardiac disease and other significant comorbidities. The underlying illness as well as the proposed procedure with significant frequency can result in severe, life-threatening events which require the expertise of a congenital cardiac anesthesiologist working with the interventional cardiologist to ensure perioperative hemodynamic stability.

In the past years, a topic of controversy has been which provider is responsible for the administration of sedation and monitoring for patients undergoing congenital cardiac catheterization. Prior to anesthesia providers being responsible for the management of patients in the cath lab, the respective cardiologist was in charge of ordering nurse-administered sedation with variable levels of success and morbidity. While this practice may be adequate for an adult patient whom may be cooperative during a limited diagnostic catheterization, congenital heart patients require a different approach. The challenge of vascular access, younger patients who are unable to cooperate, patients with severe life-threatening comorbidities, and the risk of severe hemodynamic instabilities, has created a medical scenario in which anesthesiologists are considered essential members of the congenital cath lab team. In recent years the American Society of Anesthesiologists published guidelines which state that any provider of sedation must be able to rescue the patient if the level of sedation be deeper than intended. It is also required that any provider of sedative medications has knowledge of the pharmacology of the medications used and any potential interactions with the underlying disease and multi-organ system dysfunction as well as the ability to manage the airway on a wide variety of patients which may have coexisting syndromes that affect the airway anatomy. With this in mind, anesthesia providers considered the standard of care for congenital heart patients undergoing cardiac catheterization. These patients irrespective of the anesthesia technique chosen require the same perioperative assessment and intra-procedure monitoring which are comparable to that of an operative case.

In the United Kingdom, all children undergoing cardiac catheterization receive a general anesthetic for the procedure. In the United States, the technique employed is based on the needs of the procedure and the underlying illness of the patient. There are instances where conscious sedation may be appropriate for a diagnostic procedure where the patient can cooperate, and the data required may be more optimal in the case of a spontaneous breathing patient. However, endotracheal intubation is recommended for most interventional cath procedures especially when the patient may be at risk for ventilatory failure due to illness, underlying disease state, and prematurity, risk of hemoptysis; risk of significant hemodynamic disturbances exist; the need for suspension of respirations such as in 3D reconstruction imaging; the need for TEE; and the risk of patient movement or coughing during a critical point in the procedure.

Premedication for diagnostic or interventional catheterization procedure is recommended for patients who require medication for procedural anxiety. Midazolam 0.5–0.75 mg/kg orally is considered safe and effective and generally has a rapid onset. For adult congenital patients who require pre-procedural premedication, midazolam given by slow IV titration is recommended. These patients may be very medically fragile with multi-organ system dysfunction and require vigilance with respect to sedation medication and their hemodynamic response.

Preoperative Assessment

The preoperative assessment for the patient undergoing cardiac cath should be as comprehensive as that for any operative procedure with focus on the cardiovascular system. Any signs and symptoms of worsening heart failure or cyanosis should be elicited such as shortness of breath, diaphoresis, tachypnea, fatigue, poor feeding or feeding intolerance, and decrease in baseline saturations. It is even more crucial in the patient with CHD to review any perioperative respiratory illnesses as this can lead to severe perioperative respiratory compromise and increase in PVR above baseline. If a history of perioperative respiratory infection is elicited, the case should be rescheduled for an appropriate future date. The airway assessment is extremely important as the risk of concomitant syndromes in patients with CHD remains significant. Airway equipment should be appropriately sized and available in the cath lab prior to induction. If the patient is undergoing a mask induction and IV access is to be obtained after general anesthesia is induced, it is advised that ultrasound and other equipment useful in obtaining IV access are readily available. Difficult IV access is a recognized problem in this patient population, and a review of previous operative reports or cath reports is recommended to help delineate what access sites are potentially available.

Intraoperative Management

The type of anesthetic and the induction technique employed are dependent on the nature of the procedure planned and baseline functional state of the patient. Inhalational induction with sevoflurane is generally well tolerated when titrated to effect and IV access is obtained in an expeditious fashion. There are patients who are considered extremely medically fragile, and preinduction IV access is considered the safest plan. This can frequently be achieved with mild oral sedation with midazolam and ketamine or other non-IV regimens and topical EMLA cream. If a hybrid procedure is planned or there is a need for perioperative invasive monitoring, an arterial line and CVP can be placed with avoidance of the site required for the procedure. Positioning also needs to be considered for the CHD patient undergoing cath in that the arms are usually placed above the head to optimize the cardiac biplane imaging and 3D reconstructions. Vigilance is needed to avoid brachial plexus injury in this scenario, and the arms must be checked frequently and intermittently relaxed and repositioned.

The hemodynamic changes which accompany the induction and maintenance of anesthesia need to be appreciated when interpreting the data acquired from a diagnostic cath and in ensuring hemodynamic stability for an interventional cath. While the anatomy of a given patient will not be altered by anesthetic manipulations and medication, the physiology of a patient is affected in a dose-dependent and generally predictable manner. The measurements obtained must be interpreted in the context in which they were obtained with appreciation given to the hemodynamic effects of the respective anesthetics used as well as any vasoactive medications and the manner of ventilation employed. Careful selection of the agents used and appropriate titration will help minimize untoward hemodynamic affects. The most common hemodynamic effects of anesthetic medications during a congenital heart cath are depression of the systemic blood pressure, changes in arterial saturation and carbon dioxide concentration, decreases in SVR, and changes in PVR, cardiac output, oxygen consumption, and shunt flow. Maintaining systemic blood pressure under anesthesia can be a challenge as most anesthetic agents cause a direct reduction in SVR, and a reduction in cardiac output can also result from the negative inotropic and chronotropic effects of these agents and from decrease preload secondary to vasodilation and positive-pressure ventilation. The hemodynamic effects of anesthetics tend to be more significant in sicker patients with less ability to compensate. Careful dosing of all agents is recommended as well as judicious fluid management. If vasopressors are required, the use should be communicated with the cardiologist as they will influence the obtained data. In addition, cardiac output will decrease under general anesthesia secondary to a reduction in whole-body oxygen consumption.

Another important consideration is the manner in which a patient is ventilated. A recent study reported a transition from positive-pressure ventilation to negative-pressure ventilation or spontaneous breathing, increasing the cardiac output by 11 % in otherwise healthy children, 28 % in postoperative cardiac patients, and 54 % in patients with Fontan physiology. High oxygen concentrations in patients with large left-to-right shunts can significantly lower the PVR, therefore increasing the left-to-right shunt with a significant increase in the Qp:Qs ratio. Additionally, changes in arterial carbon dioxide concentrations or pH will significantly affect pulmonary blood flow. Also, small changes in pulmonary vein oxygen saturations will create large changes in the calculation of the shunt fraction. The advantages and disadvantages of positive- versus negative-pressure ventilation are numerous and relatively predictable. With respect to acquiring the most accurate cath data and optimizing cardiac output, a patient would be spontaneously breathing, on room air with an unobstructed airway and an intact respiratory drive. However, this is rarely possible in an operative or procedural situation, and the best decision is generally one in which the patient has an unobstructed airway or protected airway with controlled ventilation which prevents hypercapnia and atelectasis. Consistency in the approach to the ventilation is important in the management of these patients, with respect to the interpretation of the data among the treatment team.

Anesthetic Agents Used in Congenital Cardiac Catheterization

Many different regimens of anesthetic agents have been used in congenital cardiac cath cases as a single agent or as a combination. At this time there is no ideal agent that has been identified that can be used in all cases. The following is a discussion of a variety of agents and their known hemodynamic effects and advantages and disadvantages.

Volatile Anesthetic Agents

The volatile anesthetic agents have been used safely in congenital heart patients of all ages for many years despite the concerns of depressed contractility and decreased SVR. These agents are known to decrease blood pressure in a dose-dependent fashion and attenuate hypoxic pulmonary vasoconstriction, thereby worsening V/Q mismatch. The most commonly used agents in the United States are isoflurane which is thought to have the least myocardial depression and sevoflurane which also has a relatively safe hemodynamic profile. The advantage of sevoflurane is the ability to use it during a mask induction in conjunction with nitrous oxide and later as a maintenance agent. The actual MAC of the volatile agent may be just enough to ablate awareness and can be used in combination with narcotic medication, benzodiazepine and muscle relaxant. Nitrous oxide is frequently used during the initial mask induction and then discontinued due to the potential for significant increases in PVR in adult patients with pulmonary hypertension. There has not been evidence to show deleterious effects of nitrous oxide on the pulmonary hemodynamics in infants with or without pulmonary hypertension. Nitrous oxide is also used with caution in this patient population due to the risk of paradoxical emboli and the risk of worsening a venous air embolism which can occur as a result of air introduced with central venous cannulation.

Propofol

Propofol has been used safely with efficacy in the congenital cardiac population during cath lab procedures and induction. Propofol has less emergence delirium and offers more rapid recovery. The antiemetic properties also help decrease the incidence of postoperative nausea and vomiting. There are dose-dependent decreases in SVR, blood pressure, heart rate, and contractility which make it a less favorable agent in patients with fragile hemodynamics. It has no effect on PVR or pulmonary artery pressure (PAP). Caution must be exercised when considering the use in patients with aortic stenosis, systemic-to-pulmonary artery shunts, pulmonary hypertension, diminished ventricular function, and single-ventricle physiology. Propofol is an IV general anesthetic and causes respiratory depression and loss of airway reflexes which can lead to airway obstruction and hypercarbia in unintubated patients and result in hemodynamic compromise.

Opiate Medications

Opiate medications do not have amnestic properties and cannot be used as a single anesthetic agent alone but are efficacious analgesics which are part of a balanced anesthetic. Opiates such as fentanyl have minimal hemodynamic effects and have been used safely for patients with CHD. They are recognized to be efficacious in attenuating the pulmonary vasoconstrictive response to noxious stimuli. Opiates are known to have associated bradycardia and significant respiratory depression which cause hypoventilation and hypercarbia. Opiates such as morphine which causes significant histamine release can adversely affect the PVR. Remifentanil which is used as an infusion and titrated to effect has been used with hemodynamic stability but at higher doses has been noted to cause problems with electrophysiological cases due to slowing of the sinus node function and atrioventricular node function. Fentanyl is the most commonly used opiate in pediatric congenital cardiac surgery and is frequently used as an infusion and later after extubation is switched to a longer-acting opiate medication such as morphine or Dilaudid. Opiates are associated with postoperative nausea and vomiting and require antiemetic medications to be used in conjunction in many patients.

Benzodiazepines

Benzodiazepines are anxiolytic medications which have been used with good efficacy in patients with CHD and in the setting of the cath lab are frequently used as a premedication. In general, the class has minimal hemodynamic and respiratory depression when appropriately titrated. In pediatric patients oral midazolam is frequently used as a premedication, while in older patients it is given in the IV form. Midazolam is also used as an intraoperative sedative in cooperative patients and to prevent intraoperative awareness in the setting of cardiac surgery due to its amnestic properties. When used with volatile agents such as sevoflurane, midazolam can attenuate emergence delirium, dysphoria, and hallucination caused by ketamine. When used in combination with opiate medications, there can be significant respiratory depression, and appropriate titration and monitoring are warranted.

Ketamine

Ketamine is used for both procedural sedation and being an important induction agent and premedication. Ketamine is unique in that it has profound analgesic properties as well as being a powerful sedative hypnotic that actually allows preservation of airway reflexes and ventilatory drive. The most important characteristic regarding ketamine is the preservation of stable hemodynamics. Isolated myocardium shows a negative inotropic effect; however, the sympathomimetic effects of ketamine offset the potential negative inotropic effect which is not generally appreciated clinically. Ketamine does increase oxygen consumption which can create a potential error in the hemodynamic calculations unless the oxygen consumption is directly measured. Ketamine is also unique in that PVR and PAP remain essentially unchanged in patients with pulmonary hypertension. The disadvantages of ketamine include increased salivation, nausea, dysphoria, prolonged wake-up, and myoclonus. The stable hemodynamics on induction make it a preferred agent with the side effects frequently offset with antiemetic medications such as ondansetron and anti-sialagogue effects of glycopyrrolate which also prevents bradycardia associated with direct laryngoscopy. The potential dysphoria or hallucinations can be offset with midazolam or propofol which is frequently used in conjunction with ketamine.

Dexmedetomidine

Dexmedetomidine is a potent, new medication which can be given by bolus and more frequently as an infusion. It is a sedative, centrally acting alpha-2 agonist which causes sedation, anxiolysis, and mild analgesia with some moderate hemodynamic effects. Significant respiratory depression is generally avoided; however, there is considerable sinus node and atrioventricular node depression with resultant bradycardia in a dose-dependent manner. Dexmedetomidine is generally not recommended for electrophysiological cases, and its bradycardic side effects are frequently utilized in instances of dysrhythmia such as junctional ectopic tachycardia and other forms of tachycardia. It is generally not recommended in patients at risk for heart block or bradycardia as well as patients who are rate dependent such as neonates and patients with single-ventricle physiology, impaired ventricular function, and significant regurgitant lesions.

Complications in the Congenital Cath Lab

The incidence of significant complications in the congenital cath lab is reported to be between 7 and 24 % with complications being more frequent in the interventional procedures relative to the diagnostic cases. Mortality in the congenital cath lab remains reported at less than 1 %. The most commonly reported complications are vascular injuries and dysrhythmias. Less commonly reported but significant complications include bleeding, stroke, vascular rupture, cardiac tamponade, valvular damage, vascular thrombosis, air embolus, retained foreign body/catheter, device embolus, contrast reaction or anaphylaxis, and brachial plexus injury. The most significant risk factors for major morbidity or complication in the cath lab include age less than one year, smaller patient size, and complexity of intervention. Arrhythmias are common and generally transient. Risk factors for arrhythmias include hypercarbia, electrolyte disturbances, catheter manipulation, cardiac ischemia, drugs, coronary air embolus, and myocardial and conduction tissue damage. Pacing capability should be available as well as defibrillators and antiarrhythmic medications. Patients with severe pulmonary hypertension are also at significant risk for mortality in the cath lab. The risk of periprocedural cardiac arrest is well documented in patients with CHD. The Pediatric Perioperative Cardiac Arrest Registry shows that approximately one-third of cardiac arrests occur in children with CHD of which 17 % occur during cardiac cath procedures. The risk factors for procedural cardiac arrest in the cath lab include age less than one year, single-ventricle physiology, and preoperative cath procedures. The risk of cardiac decompensation in the congenital cath lab requires that surgical backup be immediately available for potential rescue and rapid deployment of mechanical circulatory support.

Hybrid Procedures

Hybrid procedures incorporate both surgical and transcatheter techniques as part of a single operative procedure to treat CHD. Most frequently, hybrid procedures are employed to treat hypoplastic left heart syndrome (HLHS) in which a PDA stent is deployed and bilateral PA bands are placed with an open sternotomy. The use of CPB is deferred as well as aortic cross clamping which avoids the myocardial injury and inflammatory response associated with open heart procedures as well as possible neurologic injury. Hybrid procedures are also used to close VSDs, implant pulmonary valves, and branch PA stents as well as a number of other minimally invasive procedures. The anesthetic management of a hybrid procedure is dictated by the nature of the procedure. The hybrid suite is an operating room with full cath lab capabilities as well as cardiac operating room capabilities. The ability to attempt a catheter-based intervention with conversion to open surgery is another advantage of the hybrid suite.

Conclusion

The congenital cardiac cath lab has moved to a new era of therapeutic intervention with patients being intervened on at younger ages and with more invasive procedures with potential for significant hemodynamic instability. The anesthetic challenges of the congenital cath lab include the frequently remote location of the suite, sicker and younger patients, higher potential for respiratory and cardiac instability, as well as environmental issues such as significant radiation exposure. The importance of communication with the interventional cardiologist is a vital factor regarding patient status during a procedure, and the availability of surgical backup and mechanical circulatory support is essential considering the risk of cardiac instability. Multidisciplinary team collaboration as well as vigilance and preparation create the safest atmosphere to provide the patient with CHD a good procedural outcome.

Bibliography

Abbas SM, Rashid A, Latif H. Sedation for children undergoing cardiac catheterization: a review of the literature. J Pak Med Assoc. 2012;62:159–63.

Andreassi MG. Radiation risk from pediatric cardiac catheterization: friendly fire on children with congenital heart disease. Circulation. 2009;120:1847–9.

Bergersen L, Marshall A, Gauvreau K, et al. Adverse event rates in congenital cardiac catheterization a multi-center experience. Catheter Cardiovasc Interv. 2010;75:389–99.

Mehta R, Lee KJ, Chaturvedi R, et al. Complications of pediatric cardiac catheterization: a review in the current era. Catheter Cardiovasc Interv. 2008;72:278–85.

Odegard DK, BergerDSEN K, Thiagarajan R, et al. The frequency of cardiac arrests in patients with congenital heart disease undergoing cardiac catheterization. Anesth Analg. 2014;118:175–82.

Ramamoorthy C, Haberkern C, Bhananker SM, et al. Anesthesia-related cardiac arrest in children with heart disease: data from the pediatric perioperative cardiac arrest (POCA) registry. Anesth Analg. 2010;110:1376–82.

Tobias J, Gupta P, Naguib A, et al. Dexmedetomidine: applications for the pediatric patient with congenital heart disease. Pediatr Cardiol. 2011;32:1075–87.

White M. Approach to managing children with heart disease for non-cardiac surgery. Pediatr Anesth. 2011;21:522–9.

Wong J, Steil G, Curtis M, et al. Cardiovascular effects of Dexmedetomidine sedation in children. Anesth Analg. 2012;22:1042–52.

Chapter 6
Perioperative Imaging

Ruchira Garg and Lorraine Lubin

Echocardiography, or cardiac ultrasound, is a modality that readily lends itself to periprocedural imaging: the portability, lack of radiation, noninvasive, or minimally invasive nature of this modality is ideal for the pediatric population. Traditionally, one considers transesophageal echocardiography (TEE) as the mainstay of intraoperative imaging; however, intracardiac, epicardial, and even transthoracic imaging have important roles in the operating room and/or catheterization laboratory. Even the smallest babies benefit from TEE in the operating room with miniaturization of echo technology, but epicardial echocardiography provides information in those even too small for the microprobes.

The initial postnatal transthoracic echocardiogram provides a comprehensive assessment of cardiac anatomy and physiology to guide intervention and surgical decision-making, with rare exception: critical lesions may require immediate postnatal surgical intervention based on limited or no postnatal imaging. A patient with transposition and known restrictive atrial septum may have scheduled delivery in the catheterization laboratory to provide the opportunity for balloon atrial septostomy under transthoracic echocardiography guidance (Fig. 6.1a–c); a fetus with complete heart block may be best delivered in the operating room for emergent pacemaker placement, or surgical intervention may be required within hours of birth to relieve obstructed total anomalous pulmonary venous return. Imaging should to be directed and brief.

R. Garg, MD (✉)
Congenital Non-Invasive Cardiology in the Congenital Heart Program, Cedars-Sinai Heart Institute, 127 S. San Vicente Boulevard, Suite A3600, Los Angeles, CA 90048, USA
e-mail: Ruchira.Garg@cshs.org

L. Lubin, MD
Congenital Cardiac Anesthesiology, Operative Transesophageal Echocardiography, Cedars Sinai Medical Center, Department of Anesthesiology,
8700 Beverly Blvd, Suite 8211, Los Angeles, CA 90048, USA
e-mail: Lorraine.Lubin@cshs.org

© Springer International Publishing Switzerland 2017
A. Dabbagh et al. (eds.), *Congenital Heart Disease in Pediatric and Adult Patients*, DOI 10.1007/978-3-319-44691-2_6

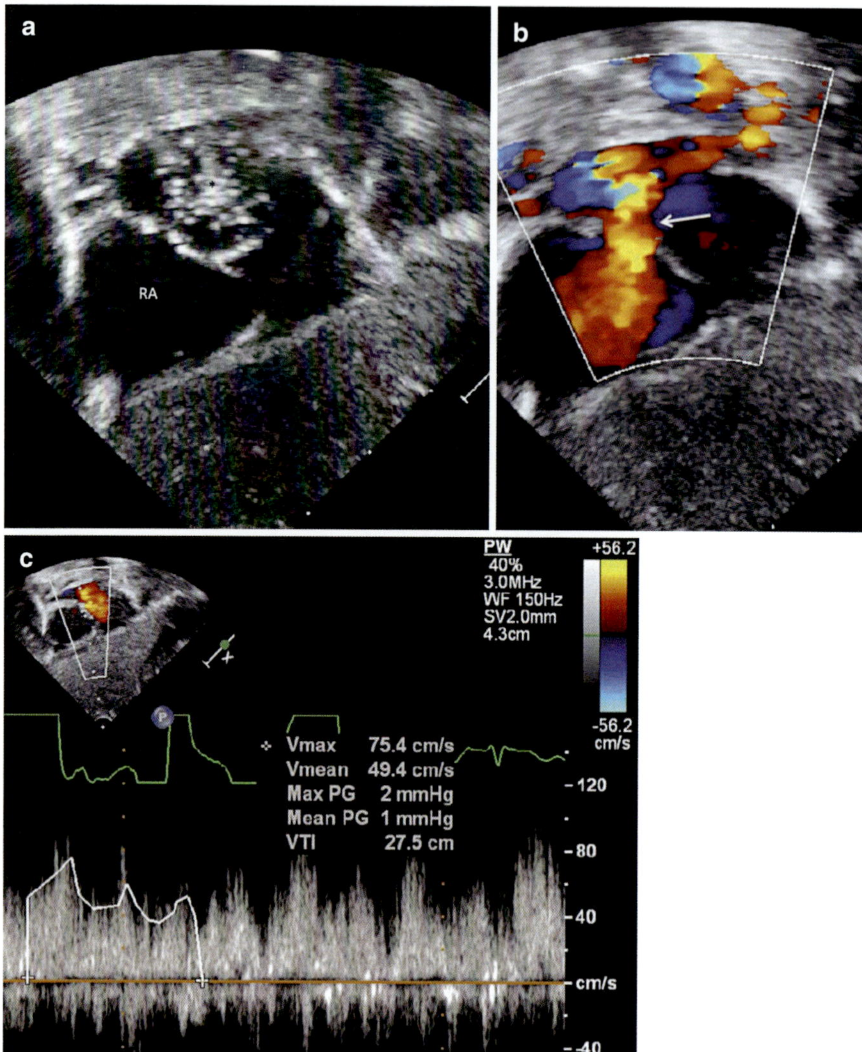

Fig. 6.1 Transthoracic subxiphoid (subcostal) long-axis 2D image (**a**) of the atrial septum and a balloon atrial septostomy catheter (*) inflated in the left atrium. Immediately after septostomy pullback, the color Doppler image (**b**) shows laminar left-to-right shunting (*arrow*) and a negligible residual mean interatrial gradient of 1 mmHg (**c**). (*RA* right atrium)

Excluding these rare lesions transthoracic imaging remains the mainstay of ambulatory, preoperative assessment of congenital heart disease in all ages. The goal of the preoperative or preprocedural echocardiogram is complete delineation of the primary anatomic defect and physiology, identification of any coexisting lesions, and baseline cardiac function. For the past two decades transthoracic echocardiographic assessment has been deemed sufficient for a complete repair of even major congenital heart defects (Tworetzky et al. 1999). As such, this preoperative echocardiogram must achieve complete delineation of cardiac anatomy prior to entering the operating room. Conscious sedation can be necessary in young, noncooperative children; sedation risk assessment, including the American Society of Anesthesiology (ASA) score, can identify those at higher risk for sedation-related complications (Hoffman et al. 2002) to modify the sedation plan or appropriately refer for deep sedation if required for a complete echocardiogram. Cardiac MRI and MRA can be used selectively in patients in whom congenital lesions cannot be fully delineated by echocardiography. This includes patients with venous, arch, and other vascular anomalies but also quantifies valvular regurgitation and biventricular systolic function.

Transesophageal echocardiography (TEE) is rarely used as a diagnostic modality in pediatric-aged patients: thoracic imaging windows are frequently sufficient, and deep sedation, usually with anesthesia, is required to safely perform TEE in children. The vast majority of lesions can be adequately managed with less-invasive imaging, and TEE is often reserved for preoperative/preintervention imaging to further refine the diagnosis prior to the procedure. TEE can be superior to TTE for imaging valvular disease, atrial and ventricular septal defects, intracardiac vegetations or thrombus, and postsurgical anatomy when scar tissue can further compromise acoustic windows, typically in the older patient who can tolerate moderate sedation for a diagnostic study.

Once the decision is finalized to pursue surgery and/or transcatheter intervention, imaging plays a direct role in the procedural suite. As the modalities utilized vary somewhat between the procedural sites, they will be discussed under the respective locations.

Catheterization Laboratory

Numerous periprocedural imaging modalities are available to the interventionalist: intracardiac, transesophageal, and transthoracic echocardiography all have standard 2D and 3D options which complement fluoroscopy and 3D rotational angiography. The interventionalist acquires fluoroscopic and rotational angiography images and typically manipulates the intracardiac imaging probe. In many congenital programs, procedural echocardiographic imaging in the catheterization suite is performed and interpreted by a congenital imaging specialist. This is often a pediatric/congenital echocardiographer with specialized noninvasive imaging training, but can also be a cardiac anesthesiologist or any physician comfortable with the equipment and complexity of congenital heart disease. As such, the room configuration must account for the physical and viewing needs of all the participating providers. Echocardiographic images should display alongside fluoroscopic images, allowing the interventionalist to simultaneously gauge the status of his instruments and devices in the heart. Similarly, the imager must be able to view fluoroscopy to keep abreast of the ongoing procedure as he/she acquires images. A TEE probe can easily obscure a device at the most crucial point of the procedure; this is easily avoided if the imager has real-time access to fluoroscopic images.

The imager and interventionalist likely began a dialogue at the time of patient selection, well before meeting in the catheterization laboratory. A shared understanding of the characteristics of the lesion, expectations for the procedure, and open and timely communication throughout the case provide the best chance for a successful complex congenital intervention (Kutty et al. 2013).

Intracardiac Echocardiography

The emergence of intracardiac echocardiography (ICE) in 2006 was perfectly suited to the growing volume of device implantations. This technology places a miniaturized single-plane ultrasound element at the tip of a moderately flexible and drivable 8- or 10-French multiuse catheter (Fig. 6.2). The sheath is placed in the groin, either alongside the procedural sheath or in the contralateral groin. In a cooperative patient, the interventionalist can perform the entire procedure with local anesthetic injection and anxiolysis, rather than general anesthetic which is usually required for TEE. The catheter is guided, typically by the interventionalist, into the right atrium under fluoroscopy with the ability to rotate the catheter along its axis, flex and anteflex the tip, as well as tilt the catheter right and left. The small size of the catheter tip does not permit a biplane crystal to be utilized, so the operator uses a combination of the above maneuvers to orient the crystals into the ideal imaging plane to visualize the relevant structures. There is no thermistor on the probe as the continuous flow of blood prevents any risk of thermal injury from probe heating, permitting continuous imaging throughout the procedure.

Atrial septal defect (ASD) closure is a primary indication for ICE (Assaidi et al. 2014). ICE is used to define the pulmonary venous return, the tricuspid and mitral

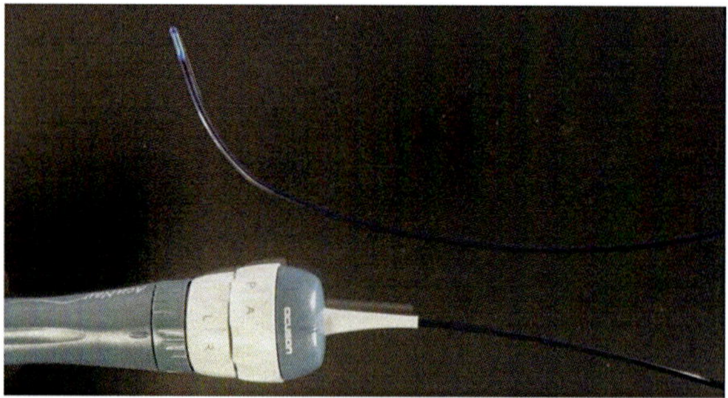

Fig. 6.2 An 8-F AcuNav catheter (Siemens Inc., Erlangen, Germany) is shown with the tip in a flexed position. The catheter can be tilted in either the anteroposterior (AP) or left-right (LR) planes and rotated along the long axis by the operator. The catheter is predominantly used for intracardiac echocardiography but has also been used for transesophageal imaging

valve regurgitation, and the ASD features: the number of defects, size of each, location, and integrity of the rims are all defined with the probe positioned in the right atrium. Balloon sizing, when performed, uses a compliant balloon inflated across the defect until there is no residual atrial shunting. The narrowest diameter, or "waist," is measured by both fluoroscopy and ICE to select an appropriately-sized device. During device deployment, ICE is used to document disk capture of all defect rims, residual shunting, and stability of the device prior to and after device release. This entire procedure is typically performed with administration of local anesthetic and anxiolysis to the older patient, but under general anesthesia in the smaller child. Most operators will use ICE in children older than 2 years of age, or greater than 15 kg; in younger children, both sheath size and space in the heart for manipulation of the probe alongside intervention catheters can be challenging.

Another use for ICE in the catheterization laboratory includes assessment of the pulmonary valve in patients undergoing transcatheter valve replacement (Whiteside et al. 2015; Awad et al. 2014). The operator can steer the catheter into the right ventricle to provide images of the diseased pulmonary valve and the newly replaced valve. Angiographic assessment of pulmonary valve regurgitation can be confounded by exaggerated catheter-related regurgitation when an injection is performed in the main pulmonary artery. In contrast, ICE can be performed after removal of any devices and catheters that may disrupt the normal excursion and competence of the pulmonary valve. The post-procedural gradient and mechanism of residual stenosis can also be delineated by ICE (Whiteside et al. 2015). Similar preliminary interest and experience are present for transcatheter aortic valve (Bartel et al. 2015) placement in adults instead of TEE, which typically requires endotracheal intubation and deep sedation or anesthesia.

The ICE probe has also been used off-label as a transesophageal imaging solution when infant biplane probes cannot be passed due to their comparatively larger sizes (Fig. 6.3). Using a 10-F AcuNav catheter, 22 studies were performed in infants ranging from 2.1 to 5.6 kg with no hemodynamic compromise, airway resistance, or postoperative esophageal complication including insignificant heating of the tip (Bruce et al. 2002). It has also been used as an alternative to conventional TEE or ICE in adult patients with PFO (Mitchell-Heggs et al. 2010) to avoid the need for endotracheal intubation and deep sedation. The limitations of an ICE probe placed in the esophagus include lack of biplane imaging and difficulty in obtaining transgastric imaging due to limitations in probe flexion. With the advent of the micromini probe (Fig. 6.3b), a miniaturized biplane transesophageal probe, there is now rarely a need to use the ICE probe for this purpose.

Transthoracic Echocardiography

Transthoracic echocardiography has little utility in the operating room unless being used for epicardial imaging. There is similarly limited utility in the catheterization suite; nonetheless, we always keep a machine and probe available. An urgent pericardial effusion evaluation is best performed with TTE, rather than struggling with the ICE catheter or emergently placing a TEE probe. Also, in our experience, the catheterization lab can be an excellent opportunity to perform a complete transthoracic study on a toddler to avoid duplicate sedation, both to confirm the referral diagnosis and exclude any additional lesions.

In our experience, there are two ideal uses for transthoracic-guided catheterization intervention: balloon atrial septostomy and closure of the hemodynamically significant ductus arteriosus in neonates. Both of these procedures are performed in very small patients, where passage of a TEE probe may not be possible and certainly comes with increased risk. TTE is thus ideally suited to both interventions and can be performed either bedside or in the catheterization suite.

In patients with transposition of the great arteries or other cardiac defects that require unrestrictive atrial mixing, transthoracic subcostal/subxiphoid imaging delineates the plane of the interatrial septum (Fig. 6.1). The interventionalist passes a balloon atrial septostomy catheter from the femoral or umbilical vein into the heart. Under continuous TTE guidance, the balloon catheter is visualized crossing the restrictive atrial septum (Fig. 6.1a). After balloon inflation and confirmation of positioning in the left atrium, a vigorous "pull-back" septostomy is performed to tear the thin septum primum and allow unrestrictive mixing of blood in these cyanotic patients (Fig. 6.1b, c). Occasionally, transthoracic echocardiography will also be used to guide static balloon dilatation and stent placement in thicker atrial septums where a conventional septostomy cannot be performed.

We have recently published our experience with transcatheter closure of patent ductus arteriosus (PDA) in neonates, including premature infants, ranging from 700 gm to 4000 gm. While this technique has been used for decades in older children and adults, neonates have been historically excluded due to concerns about damage to groin access vessels, and device obstruction to pulmonary or aortic blood flow. Surgical ligation has been the mainstay of treatment for the persistent and hemodynamically important ductus arteriosus in the premature infant but comes with important morbidity and mortality (Roze et al. 2015; Hamrick and Hansmann 2010). We have found that TTE combined with judicious use of fluoroscopy allows us, in real time, to visualize device placement and impact of the device on descending aortic and left pulmonary artery flow (Zahn et al. 2015). We have had a procedural success of 88 % with no complications and no mortality and excellent midterm follow-up (pending publication).

Transesophageal Echocardiography

Despite the advent of new technology, TEE retains a firm footing in the catheterization laboratory. TEE provides excellent delineation of the entirety of the intracardiac anatomy, without compromising the sterile field. The operator remains at the head of the bed, often performing a complete anatomic study at the onset of the case, and can then provide real-time feedback throughout the intervention including information about cardiac function and pericardial effusion. Guidelines for TEE performance, indications, contraindications, etc. were recently published as a joint statement from the American Society of Echocardiography and the Society of Cardiovascular Anesthesiologists (Hahn et al. 2014). The pediatric patient with congenital heart disease presents unique indications for TEE, safety issues, and technical considerations necessitating additional operator training for TEE compared with adult TEE (Ayres et al. 2005). Commercially available TEE probes (Fig. 6.3) range from micro-TEE probes which are approved for use in babies >2.5 kg, mini-TEE probes approved for weights >5.0 kg, and adult probes, including 3D-TEE probes, for patients >18–25 kg. Adverse events related to TEE are more prevalent in smaller children (Stevenson 1999); fortunately, the safety profile and image quality of the micro-TEE probe (Zyblewski et al. 2010; Pavithran et al. 2014) have allowed this probe to be used successfully in neonates and small infants.

Atrial septal defect closure in the smaller patient, or for complex atrial anatomy, is an ideal application for TEE. Figures 6.4a–d are from a 9.5-kg infant, too small for the ICE probe, with complex atrial anatomy and failure to thrive. The secundum atrial septal defect was complicated by the additional presence of a large tunnel-type patent foramen ovale created by leftward insertion of the septum primum. Upon initial attempts to close the defect with a 12-mm Amplatzer septal occluder,

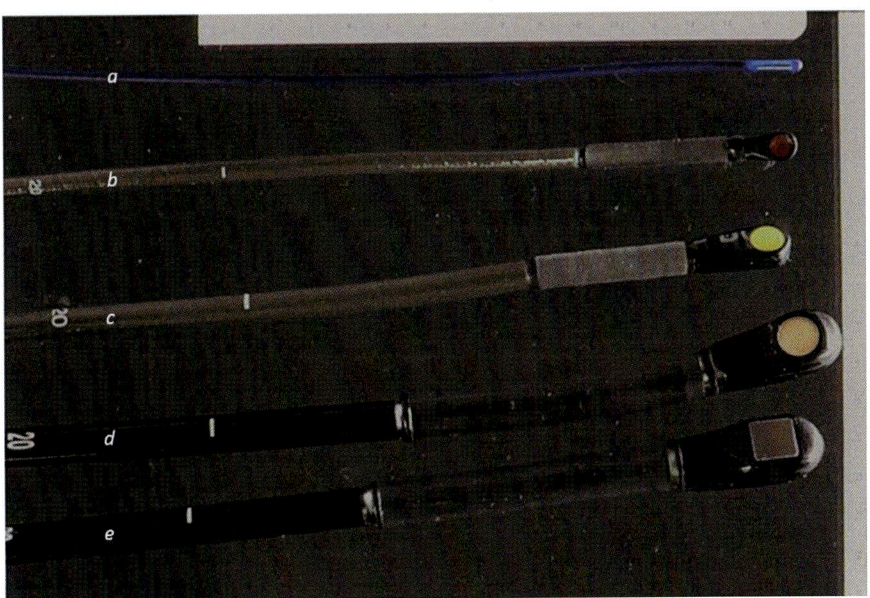

Fig. 6.3 This image demonstrates a sample of the various probe sizes that can be used for transesophageal echocardiography (TEE). Probe *a* is the 8-F AcuNav catheter (Siemens Inc., Erlangen, Germany) also depicted in Fig. 6.2. The remaining probes *b* through *e* are Philips medical probes designed for transesophageal use: probe *b* is a micro-TEE S8-3 t TEE probe, approved for use in babies >2.5 kg; probe *c* is a mini-TEE S7-3 t sector array probe for infants >5.0 kg, *d* is an adult omniplane probe, and *e* is the 3D X7-2 t adult xMATRIX array TEE probe

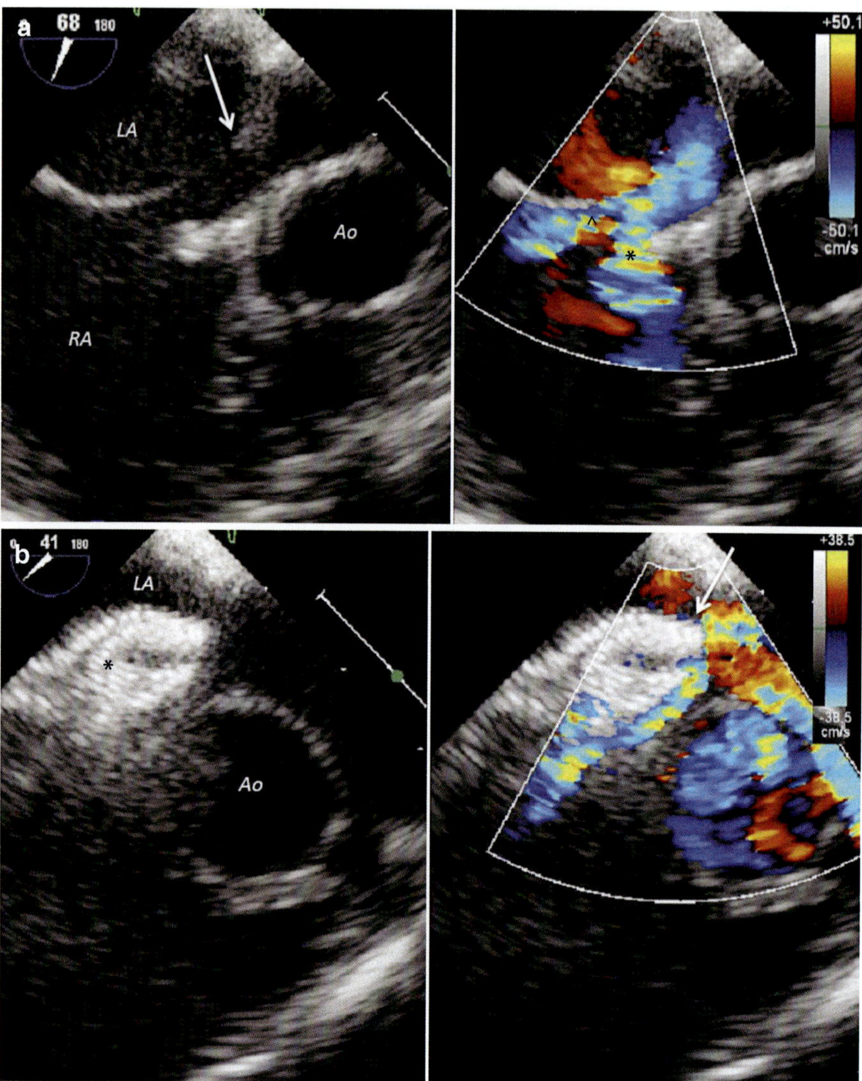

Fig. 6.4 TEE images in a 9.5-kg infant with complex atrial anatomy and failure to thrive. (**a**) The secundum atrial septal defect (*) was complicated by the additional presence of a large tunnel-type patent foramen ovale (^) created by leftward insertion of the septum primum (*arrow*). (**b**) Upon initial attempts to close the defect with a 12-mm Amplatzer septal occluder (*), the anterior superior aspect of the device prolapsed into the left atrium, behind the aortic root (*arrow*). (**c**) Upon recognizing this unique anatomy by TEE, the previous device was removed and a 30-mm Amplatzer Cribriform Device was selected. Note that the thin septum primum (*thin arrow*) and thick septum secundum (*thick arrow*) are successfully captured by the left atrial disk (*) as the right atrial disk (^) is partially deployed. (**d**) After device release the left and right atrial disks are now in appropriate position, straddling the aortic root (*Ao*), and there is no residual shunting

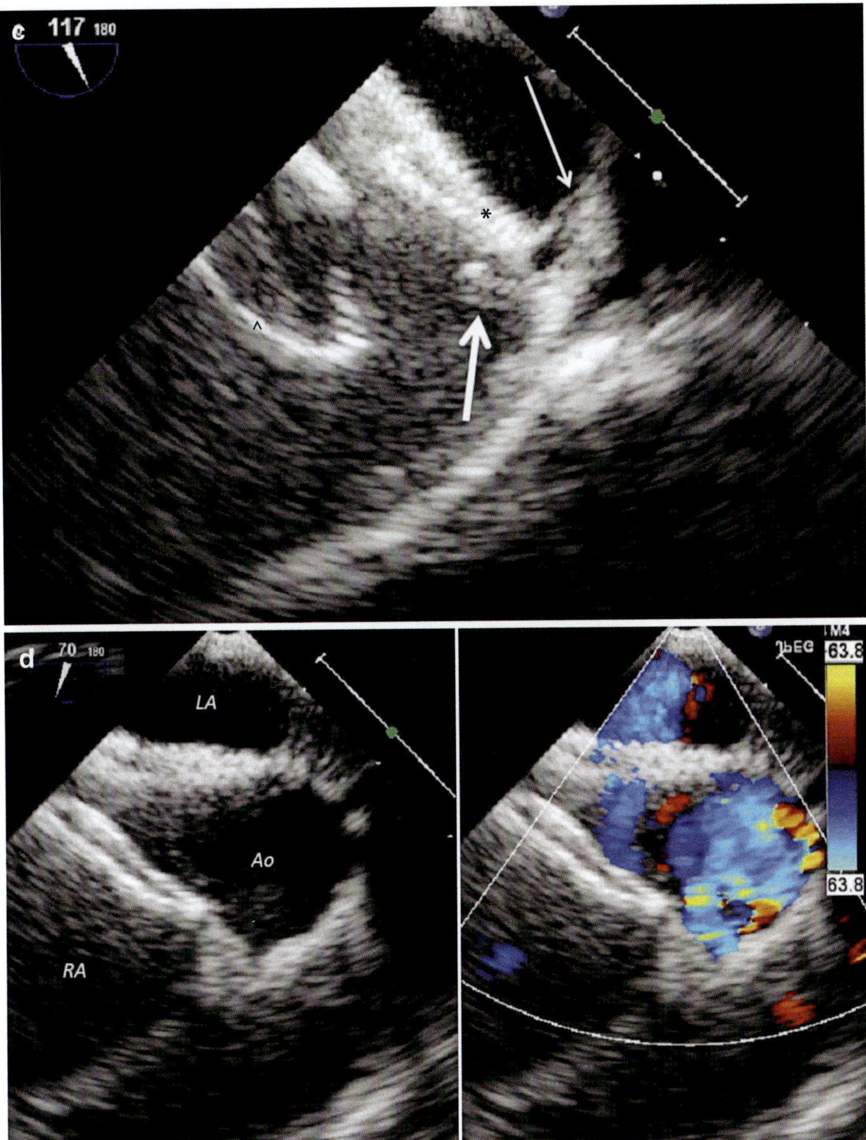

Fig. 6.4 (continued)

the anterior superior aspect of the device prolapsed into the left atrium, behind the aortic root. Upon recognizing this unique anatomy by TEE, the previous device was removed, and a more appropriate device (30-mm Amplatzer cribriform device) was selected and successfully deployed to close the defect with good position behind the aortic root and no residual shunting.

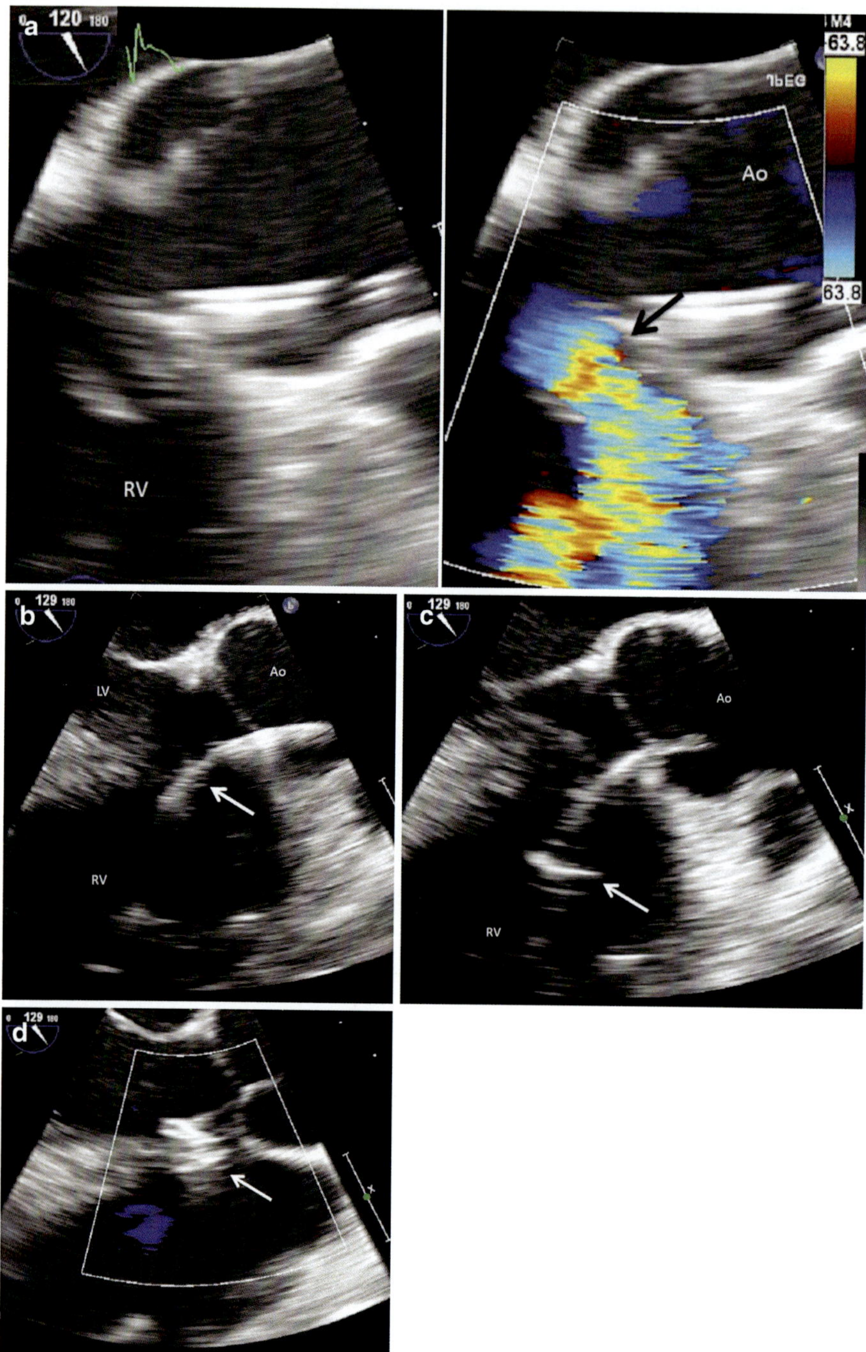

Fig. 6.5 (**a**) Color compare image with the *dark arrow* demonstrating the left-to-right ventricular septal defect immediately below the aortic valve and root (*Ao*). The *white arrows* (**b, c**) show wire position and device position, respectively, as the device is being deployed. The final image (**d**) shows the device (*white arrow*) released from the delivery cable with no significant residual shunting on color Doppler interrogation. (*RV* right ventricle, *LV* left ventricle)

TEE is routinely used for transcatheter ventricular septal defect closure. Biplane and/or 3D imaging provided by the echocardiographer gives the interventionalist freedom from manipulation of the ICE catheter. The interventionalist can thereby focus on passing catheter equipment and watching fluoroscopic images, while the TEE is adjacently displayed (Fig. 6.5a–d) to obtain challenging wire and device position. Once the device is visualized in appropriate position, without compromising aortic valve or tricuspid valve function, the device is released and TEE is used to assess for final device position, residual shunting, and valvular regurgitation.

There are many additional utilities for TEE in the catheterization laboratory, with 3D TEE playing a prominent role, in particular, for adult structural interventions (Faletra et al. 2014). 2D and 3D TEE have been found to be useful in percutaneous aortic valve replacement (Smith et al. 2013; Hahn et al. 2015), left atrial appendage occlusion procedures, and transseptal puncture to obtain catheter access to the left atrium or create a new atrial septal defect (Bayrak et al. 2012), guidance for intracardiac balloon angioplasty, or stent placement. The complete list of indications is too exhaustive to cover in this chapter; suffice it to say that TEE and/or ICE is utilized whenever imaging can aid in diagnosis or intervention in the catheterization laboratory.

Operating Room

TEE is the primary modality for perioperative imaging. A complete preoperative transesophageal is performed prior to cardioplegia and ideally prior to incision to avoid electrocautery device artifact. This requires close communication and collaboration with the operative team and expeditious imaging to avoid any surgical delays. After conveying the results of this study to both anesthesia and the surgeon, the imager (when different from the anesthesiologist) leaves, expecting to return after the surgery is completed, and there is resumption of cardiac activity.

Postoperatively, before separation from cardiopulmonary bypass, frequently the TEE is used to assess for residual air bubbles within the left side of the heart. Once the patient is weaned off bypass, the postoperative assessment provides information about the intervention(s) performed, any residual lesions with an assessment of their hemodynamic importance, and evaluation of cardiac function. Based on the findings, a decision is made whether to continue with closure versus to return to bypass to address any important residual lesions. An important advantage of intraoperative post-procedural imaging includes this ability to re-intervene immediately based on TEE results before chest closure. This certainly reduces morbidity with shorter lengths of stay and also reduces cost (Mayer 1998; Nathan et al. 2014).

Valvuloplasty, with repair of a dysplastic and regurgitant valve, is one of many examples where a surgeon relies on the hemodynamic assessment of postoperative TEE to determine whether he/she has sufficiently reduced valvular regurgitation without creation of unacceptable valvular stenosis—a fine balance that is incredibly difficult to predict in the empty and arrested heart. 3D TEE is a useful adjunct to 2D imaging, especially for valvular disease, though unfortunately not commercially available for pediatric probes.

Transesophageal Echocardiography Safety and Complications

TEE in the congenital heart patient population has been used extensively with the complication rate related to TEE reported to be approximately 1–3 %. The incidence of serious complications is extremely rare. Compromise of vascular structures causing hemodynamic instability and the airway is the most commonly encountered complication especially in small infants. Probe manipulation which causes aortic compression or distortion may also influence accurate arterial line measurements and blood pressure interpretation.

In patients with an anomalous subclavian artery origination with a retroesophageal course, the arterial line pressure tracing may be lost or dampened with placement or manipulation of the TEE probe. This occurs because the probe compresses the vessel as it passes behind the esophagus. The diagnosis of these aberrant vessels may actually be made when the echo probe is placed in the operating room. It is recommended to place the arterial line in an extremity not supplied by the aberrant vessel to avoid loss of the pressure tracing. In operative cases in which these aberrant vascular connections are planned to be repaired, TEE is of little benefit and may actually cause respiratory compromise due to airway compression. In patients who are undergoing repair of anomalous pulmonary venous connections, there may be compression of the posteriorly located venous confluence by the echo probe, and hemodynamic instability may occur. Epicardial imaging is generally recommended for these patients.

Inadvertent extubation of the endotracheal tube is another problem with manipulation of the echo probe intraoperatively. Capnography can help alert the anesthesiologist to this problem. If desaturation occurs or there is difficulty with ventilation, the position of the echo probe should be adjusted and in some instances may need to be removed. At the time of probe removal, the endotracheal tube should be secured to avoid extubation. A low threshold should exist to adjust, remove the echo probe, or suspend imaging if hemodynamic or respiratory compromise is noted with probe manipulation.

Postoperative swallowing difficulties, mild mucosal injury, and soft palate bruising have been noted by upper endoscopy in some patients. Unrecognized esophageal perforation has been reported due to intraoperative TEE as well as inadvertent surgical stomach laceration due to an anterior-positioned probe during transgastric imaging during surgical incision. These cases emphasize the need for extreme care with placement and manipulation of the echo probe especially in fragile newborns and infants.

Contraindications to Transesophageal Echocardiography

In preparation for the use of intraoperative TEE, a complete review of relevant clinical history should be made including previously reported imaging studies. TEE is a semi-invasive procedure with the abovementioned associated risks. However, it provides frequently crucial perioperative information regarding the nature of the surgical repair. This being said, the benefits of the procedure must always be weighed against the possible risks or complications. The most general contraindications to TEE involve esophageal pathology, inadequate airway control, or severe respiratory decompensation. Other significant considerations include coagulopathy, cervical spine injury or severe cervical spine deformity, and oropharyngeal pathology. There are many congenital heart patients who have previously had esophageal surgery and later undergone uncomplicated TEE exams. However, the timing regarding safe instrumentation has not been firmly established, and preoperative esophagoscopy may be prudent to confirm proper healing and integrity of the esophagus. Alternative imaging methods exist; therefore, TEE can be declined if there is concern for potential injury.

Relative and Absolute Contraindications to TEE

Relative Contraindications to TEE

1. Prior esophageal surgery
2. Esophageal varices or diverticulum
3. Oropharyngeal pathology
4. Severe coagulopathy
5. Cervical spine injury, instability, or anomaly
6. Vascular ring or aberrant aortic arch vessels
7. Potential airway compromise

Absolute Contraindications to TEE

1. Poor airway control or injury
2. Severe respiratory distress, depression, or potential compromise
3. Uncooperative or unconsented patient
4. Active gastrointestinal bleeding
5. Perforated hollow viscus
6. Esophageal stricture or obstruction
7. Unrepaired or recently repaired tracheoesophageal fistula

Epicardial Echocardiography

When faced with the rare patient who has contraindication to TEE placement, or cannot have successful passage of a TEE probe due to small size, airway compromise, or hemodynamic instability, some centers, including ours, have used epicardial echocardiography. This involves placement of a high-frequency transthoracic probe (with the smallest footprint) in a sterile sleeve, directly on the anterior surface

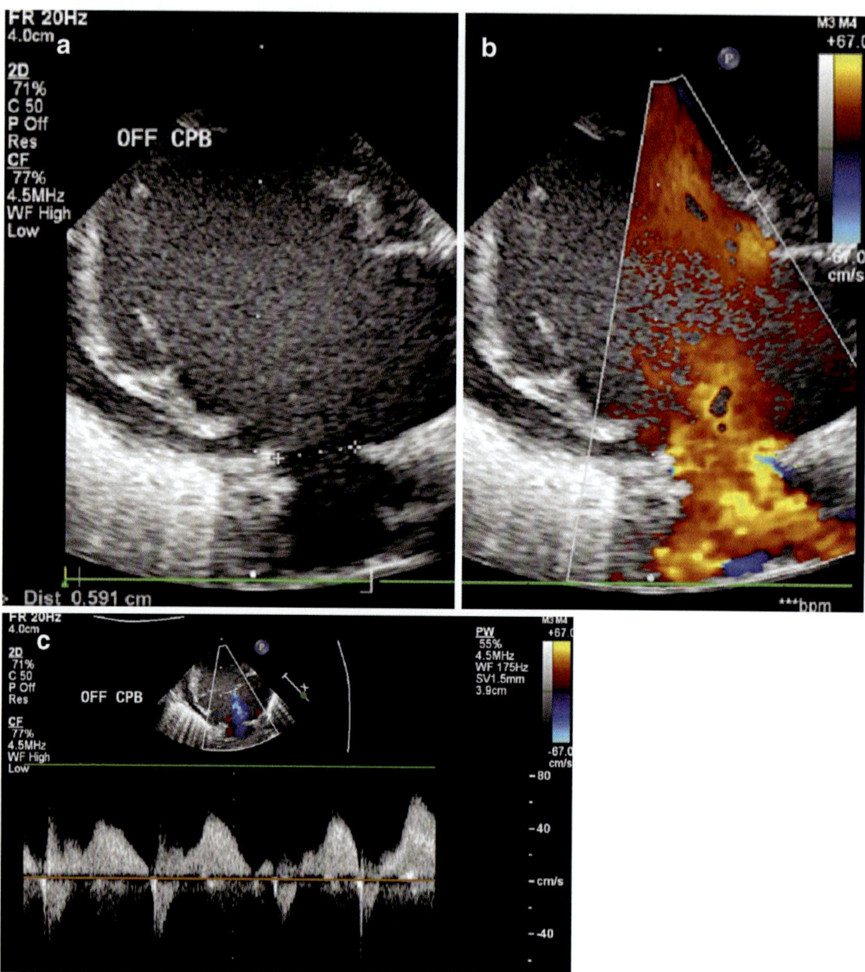

Fig. 6.6 (**a**) Epicardial color compare image obtained with a high-frequency transthoracic probe within a sterile sleeve positioned at the cardiac apex by the surgeon. The patient has heterotaxy syndrome with surgical repair of obstructed infradiaphragmatic total anomalous pulmonary venous connection. (**b**) Color Doppler demonstrates laminar flow into the near common atrium. (**c**) Pulse Doppler interrogation of the right lower pulmonary vein by epicardial echocardiography demonstrates a phasic, normal flow profile, drastically improved from the continuous low-flow Doppler profile seen preoperatively by TTE

of the heart. The surgeon manipulates the probe under the guidance of the echocardiographer, who is operating the echocardiography machine. These images are typically obtained postoperatively, after separation from bypass, such as the images seen in Fig. 6.6a–c after infradiaphragmatic total anomalous pulmonary venous connection repair. As there is direct contact with the heart, these studies are brief and focused to evaluate specific lesions and function, to minimize hemodynamic instability from cardiac compression.

Conclusion

Real-time, high-fidelity imaging assists the surgeon to reconstruct complex congenital hearts and the interventionalist to deploy ever-evolving cardiac devices safely and effectively. As with any medical technology, there are unique strengths, risks, and limitations inherent to each of our imaging modalities. As an imager, one should have a comprehensive understanding of each modality of the congenital cardiac lesions and the nature of the interventions to be performed. It is this knowledge that gives the surgeon confidence that his/her repair is good, and whether further surgical intervention is required. The partnership between imaging and intervention is crucial to obtain optimal surgical and catheter-based interventions.

References

Assaidi A, Sumian M, Mauri L, Mancini J, Ovaert C, Salaun E, Habib G, Fraisse A. Transcatheter closure of complex atrial septal defects is efficient under intracardiac echocardiographic guidance. Arch Cardiovasc Dis. 2014;107:646–53.

Awad SM, Masood SA, Gonzalez I, Cao Q-L, Abdulla R-I, Heitschmidt MG, Hijazi ZM. The use of intracardiac echocardiography during percutaneous pulmonary valve replacement. Pediatr Cardiol. 2014;36:76–83.

Ayres NA, Miller-Hance W, Fyfe DA, et al. Indications and guidelines for performance of transesophageal echocardiography in the patient with pediatric acquired or congenital heart disease. J Am Soc Echocardiogr. 2005;18:91–8.

Bartel T, Edris A, Velik-Salchner C, Müller S. Intracardiac echocardiography for guidance of transcatheter aortic valve implantation under monitored sedation: a solution to a dilemma? Eur Heart J Cardiovasc Imaging. 2015;8:280–8.

Bayrak F, Chierchia G-B, Namdar M, et al. Added value of transoesophageal echocardiography during transseptal puncture performed by inexperienced operators. Europace. 2012;14:661–5.

Bruce CJ, O'Leary P, Hagler DJ, Seward JB, Cabalka AK. Miniaturized transesophageal echocardiography in newborn infants. J Am Soc Echocardiogr. 2002;15:791–7.

Faletra FF, Pedrazzini G, Pasotti E, Muzzarelli S, Dequarti MC, Murzilli R, Schlossbauer SA, Slater IP, Moccetti T. 3D TEE during catheter-based interventions. JACC Cardiovasc Imaging. 2014;7:292–308.

Hahn RT, Abraham T, Adams MS, et al. Guidelines for performing a comprehensive transesophageal echocardiographic examination. Anesthesia Analgesia. 2014;118:21–68.

Hahn RT, Gillam LD, Little SH. Echocardiographic imaging of procedural complications during self-expandable transcatheter aortic valve replacement. JACC Cardiovasc Imaging. 2015;8:319–36.

Hamrick SEG, Hansmann G. Patent ductus arteriosus of the preterm infant. Pediatrics. 2010;125:1020–30.

Hoffman GM, Nowakowski R, Troshynski TJ, Berens RJ, Weisman SJ. Risk reduction in pediatric procedural sedation by application of an American Academy of Pediatrics/American Society of Anesthesiologists process model. Pediatrics. 2002;109:236–43.

Kutty S, Delaney JW, Latson LA, Danford DA. Can we talk? reflections on effective communication between imager and interventionalist in congenital heart disease. J Am Soc Echocardiogr. 2013;26:813–27.

Mayer JEJ. Utility of intraoperative transesophageal echocardiography in the assessment of residual cardiac defects. Pediatr Cardiol. 1998;19:346–51.

Mitchell-Heggs L, Lim P, Bensaid A, et al. Usefulness of trans-oesophageal echocardiography using intracardiac echography probe in guiding patent foramen ovale percutaneous closure. Eur J Echocardiogr. 2010;11:394–400.

Nathan M, Gauvreau K, Liu H, Pigula FA, Mayer JE, Colan SD, Del Nido PJ. Outcomes differ in patients who undergo immediate intraoperative revision versus patients with delayed postoperative revision of residual lesions in congenital heart operations. J Thorac Cardiovasc Surg. 2014;148:2540–6.e1–5.

Pavithran S, Natarajan K, Vishwambaran B, Arke AD, Sivakumar K. Preliminary evaluation of a microtransesophageal probe in neonates and young infants undergoing surgery for congenital heart disease. Ann Pediatr Cardiol. 2014;7:173–9.

Roze J-C, Cambonie G, Marchand-Martin L, Gournay V, Durrmeyer X, Durox M, Storme L, Porcher R, Ancel P-Y. Association between early screening for patent ductus arteriosus and in-hospital mortality among extremely preterm infants. JAMA. 2015;313:2441–8.

Smith LA, Dworakowski R, Bhan A, Delithanasis I, Hancock J, MacCarthy PA, Wendler O, Thomas MR, Monaghan MJ. Real-time three-dimensional transesophageal echocardiography adds value to transcatheter aortic valve implantation. J Am Soc Echocardiogr. 2013;26:359–69.

Stevenson JG. Incidence of complications in pediatric transesophageal echocardiography: experience in 1650 cases. J Am Soc Echocardiogr. 1999;12:527–32.

Tworetzky W, McElhinney DB, Brook MM, Reddy VM, Hanley FL, Silverman NH. Echocardiographic diagnosis alone for the complete repair of major congenital heart defects. J Am Coll Cardiol. 1999;33:228–33.

Whiteside W, Pasquali SK, Yu S, Bocks ML, Zampi JD, Armstrong AK. The utility of intracardiac echocardiography following melody™ transcatheter pulmonary valve implantation. Pediatr Cardiol. 2015;36:1754–60.

Zahn EM, Nevin P, Simmons C, Garg R. A novel technique for transcatheter patent ductus arteriosus closure in extremely preterm infants using commercially available technology. Catheter Cardiovasc Interv. 2015;85:240–8.

Zyblewski SC, Shirali GS, Forbus GA, Hsia T-Y, Bradley SM, Atz AM, Cohen MS, Graham EM. Initial experience with a miniaturized multiplane transesophageal probe in small infants undergoing cardiac operations. Ann Thorac Surg. 2010;89:1990–4.

Chapter 7
Pediatric Cardiovascular Monitoring

Dheeraj Kumar Goswami and David Freed Vener

Continuous monitoring during anesthesia gives the practitioner information on physiologic perturbations that may require an intervention. The monitors do not make these interventions, and interpretation and action of the practitioner are still required to affect outcome. The focus of this chapter is to discuss both the noninvasive and invasive cardiac monitors that are used in cardiac surgery, risks in their placement, and the information that can be obtained from them.

A 16-year-old boy requires emergent ventricular assist device (VAD) placement for dilated cardiomyopathy. The patient has two peripheral intravenous lines and no invasive monitoring upon arrival to the operating room. The patient is transferred from the stretcher to the bed. The basic noninvasive monitors are removed and replaced by those on the operating room table. The blood pressure is 93/45 with a HR of 106; the pulse oximetry is showing low signal quality, and no value is on the monitor.

Noninvasive Monitoring

The initial monitors are often placed on the patient in the preinduction period. These monitors are a standard of care for all anesthetics but are particularly important in adult and pediatric cardiac patients due to their increased risk of cardiac arrest

D.K. Goswami, MD (✉)
Anesthesiology and Pediatric Critical Care, Johns Hopkins Hospital, Baltimore, MD, USA
e-mail:dgoswam2@jhmi.edu

D.F. Vener, MD
Pediatrics and Anesthesiology Departments, Baylor College of Medicine and Texas
Children's Hospital, Houston, TX, USA
e-mail:dfvener@texaschildrens.org

© Springer International Publishing Switzerland 2017
A. Dabbagh et al. (eds.), *Congenital Heart Disease in Pediatric and Adult Patients*, DOI 10.1007/978-3-319-44691-2_7

(Morray et al. 2000; Nashef et al. 2002). These standard monitors include a pulse oximeter, a 5-lead continuous electrocardiogram (ECG) leads, a noninvasive blood pressure, an end-tidal CO_2, and a temperature (ASA standards of care: Monitoring).

Pulse Oximetry

Pulse oximetry was invented in the early 1970s, but it was not until the early 1980s that there was widespread adoption in the operating room (Severinghaus and Honda 1987). Pulse oximetry takes advantage of the fact that both oxy- and deoxyhemoglobin are chromophores. Chromophores are molecules that absorb and reflect certain wavelengths of light. The pulse oximetry probes transmit both red and infrared light to the pulsatile component of blood supply. The wavelengths that pass through are measured, and the oxygenation saturation is calculated continuously by measuring and comparing pulsatility changes.

The use of the pulse oximeter can be complicated in some cardiac or perfusion abnormalities as it is dependent on pulsatility and can be altered by profound hypoxia. Therefore, the pulse oximeter can be inaccurate due to poor flow to extremities in shock states or peripheral vasoconstriction due to the use of potent vasoconstrictors and hypothermia. This can also be a concern in patients who have a VAD or are placed on extracorporeal membrane oxygenation (ECMO) due to the lack of pulsatility with these devices (Trivedi et al. 1997a, b). The placement of the probe in a central location (e.g., the nose, ear, forehead) may improve accuracy in these low-flow states. There is no way of improving the accuracy during profound hypoxia though the most common concern is an underestimation of oxygen saturation (Severinghaus et al. 1989). Care must be taken when placing pulse oximeter probes on distal extremities in patients with low-flow states to avoid ischemic injury to the underlying skin and tissues.

5-Lead Electrocardiogram

There are three types of ECG most commonly used in anesthesia: 3-, 5-, and 12-lead. The purpose of the ECG is to help the anesthesia provider define the rhythm and to monitor heart strain or ischemia. The 5-lead ECG is most commonly used in the cardiac operating room as it provides information regarding the anterior, lateral, and inferior portions of the heart and can generally be placed without affecting the surgical field. The 12-lead ECG is rarely used in the operating room environment but is more commonly utilized in the ICU and gives more detailed information.

Ventricular tachycardia and ventricular fibrillation are easier to diagnose and can often be seen in any lead. The visualization of a P wave can be difficult. This difficulty can be exacerbated in children in whom the normal heart rate is often greater than 100 bpm. The "easiest" lead to visualize a P wave is lead II in all three varieties of ECG. Care and consideration should be taken in congenital heart patients with abnormal heart positioning such as dextrocardia. A full discussion on this topic could be found in Chap. 8. In rare circumstances it might be useful to utilize either an esophageal or epicardial electrode to help diagnose atrial dysrhythmias.

Blood Pressure

Noninvasive automated blood pressure monitoring has been used in the operating room for over 40 years. The most common monitoring system uses the oscillometric method via a size- and age-appropriate cuff (Frohlich 1988). The oscillometric method initially has the cuff achieve a pressure above the systolic pressure of the patient. The pressure gradually decreases and the artery will expand and contract secondary to pulsatile blood flow. The peak amplitude of the expansion and contraction is approximately the mean arterial pressure (MAP) (Graettinger et al. 1988). Individual companies have proprietary algorithms to compute systolic, mean, and diastolic pressures.

Noninvasive blood pressure monitoring is reasonably accurate and usually within 5 % of intra-arterial monitoring in a hemodynamically stable patient. Despite the accuracy, the algorithms that compute the pressures are fallible with extremes in pulse pressure, heart rate, and arterial stiffness (O'Brien et al. 2001; van Montfrans 2001). The blood pressure cuffs must also be placed at the correct locations and be sized appropriately. The cuff should cover approximately 80 % of the circumference of the upper arm and two-thirds the distance from the elbow to the shoulder. The placement of the cuff in the lower extremity is commonly done but may lead to inaccuracy in the reading.

Near-Infrared Spectroscopy Monitors

Near-infrared spectroscopy (NIRS) monitors are routinely used at many cardiac surgery centers, both in pediatric and adult patients. They can be both a neurologic and a cardiac monitor as the NIRS can be considered a surrogate for the mixed venous saturation of the brain. A full discussion on this topic can be found in Chap. 9 Neurologic Monitoring.

The pulse oximeter probe is adjusted and placed on the ear and the signal strength improves and the reading is 99 % on facemask oxygen supplementation. Induction is completed with etomidate, fentanyl, and rocuronium, and vital signs remain stable with intubation and the transition to positive pressure ventilation. Arterial line placement is successful with ultrasound guidance in the right radial artery. The arterial line waveform is dampened and there is poor blood return. The arterial line was placed on the first attempt.

Invasive Monitoring

The weak peripheral pulse oximetry signal and the poor blood return on the peripheral radial arterial line are likely due to poor peripheral blood flow. A femoral arterial line is placed with an improved waveform and much improved blood return. The waveform still has a very rounded upstroke concerning for poor cardiac output. The BP reading on the radial line is 66/54 while on the femoral line is 95/43.

Arterial Line

Arterial line access is routinely obtained in cardiac surgery for beat-to-beat pressure monitoring, for monitoring of pressure on cardiopulmonary bypass (CPB), and for obtaining blood for laboratory analysis from the patient. Percutaneous access by ultrasound or palpation is often the first choice technique particularly in neonates, but a surgical cutdown may be preferred or required at times. The most common location for arterial access is the radial artery, but the ulnar, axillary, brachial, and femoral arteries and the umbilical artery (in newborns) may also be considered.

The most concerning complication from arterial access is distal ischemia. Most anesthesiologists prefer cannulating vessels with significant collateral circulation. The brachial artery is often thought of as having less collateral flow and is only used as an option of last resort in children but is more commonly utilized in adults. The radial artery has ulnar circulation to the hand, and the Allen's test is often used to reconfirm though studies have questioned its need and efficacy in routine use (Slogoff et al. 1983; Bertrand et al. 2014). Pseudoaneurysms are another rare complication of arterial cannulation occurring at a rate of 0.09–0.3 % depending on the location of cannulation (femoral being the highest risk). Local and systemic infection is also uncommon, less than 1 % regardless of location in a review from Scheer et al. (2002).

The umbilical artery is the optimal site for neonates in the perinatal period. It is relatively easy to place catheters in the umbilical artery under direct visualization, and they have low complication rates. Peripherally placed arterial catheters in children and, specifically, neonates are associated with increased risks, and temporary ischemia was reported to be over 4 % in one study by Hack et al. (1990). It is important to closely monitor the extremity in which the catheter is placed during and after surgery. Catheter choice can be difficult especially in neonates. 24 g catheters are frequently used in patients under 5 kg, but they are unreliable and easily kinked and may not last for the entire perioperative period. 22 g catheters are commonly used in patients up to 20–30 Kg patients and 20 g catheters are used for larger patients. Some practitioners advise on rewiring to specific arterial line catheters, 2.5 Fr for neonates and infants and 3 Fr for larger patients. These catheters have the advantage of being more easily sutured in place.

There are special considerations that should be taken into account with arterial line placement and interpretation. The femoral artery may be preferred in cases of poor distal perfusion. Radial arterial cannulation may be difficult in neonates, and its accuracy can come under question because of changes in vascular tone and intravascular volume when coming off bypass. Dampening and resonance can effect arterial line transmission. Dampening usually occurs when the energy given by the pulse is lost in the transduction system. This can occur when the line is kinked, if it has an air bubble or clot inside it, or if there are any loose connections. Resonance occurs when the oscillatory frequency of the system is the same as that of the arterial waveform. This can be improved by using a stiffer connector or a shorter and wider transduction system. Dampening and resonance are less likely to occur in femoral arterial lines than in radial arterial lines.

An accurate waveform can give a significant amount of information to cardiac rhythm and function of the heart. The area under the systolic portion of the curve is proportional to the stroke volume (Bourgeois et al. 1976). Some studies have stated that cardiac output (CO) can be estimated using the waveform and a rounded upstroke could be a sign of worsening function (Tartiere et al. 2007). The location of the catheter will also impact the waveform due to increasing wave reflection in distal smaller arteries (O'Rourke 1990). The peak of the systolic wave will be higher and there will also be a lower diastolic pressure.

Overall, arterial cannulation can be done safely and can be an excellent source of hemodynamic and laboratory monitoring. Patient age and perfusion status should be considered when discussing location for placement, and distal perfusion should be closely monitored if there are any concerns.

Central Venous Lines

The patient is 16 years old, 164 cm tall and also weighs 74 kg. The decision is made to attempt a central venous line in the right internal jugular vein. The line is placed via ultrasound with the Seldinger technique while the patient is in Trendelenburg position. There was ectopy with placement of the wire that improves after pulling the wire back two centimeters. A 7 Fr 15 cm triple lumen line is then placed over the wire with good blood return in all lumens.

Central venous lines are routinely placed in most patients undergoing cardiac surgery. The most common reasons are central venous pressure (CVP) monitoring, medication administration, and difficult peripheral access. The placement of these lines is generally safe especially in well-trained hands. These lines often have multiple lumens to be able to monitor CVP and administer medications or draw blood at the same time (Fig. 7.1).

There are three primary veins for line placement, internal jugular (IJV), subclavian (SCV), and femoral (FV). All three locations have benefits and risks. The FV is thought of as the easiest to cannulate and the least likely to cause major injury with initial line placement. However, femoral line placement has a much higher infection risk in adult patients, though the data are not as clear in pediatrics (O'Grady et al. 2011). The IJV has a slightly higher complication rate than FV cannulation with carotid cannulation/injury and pneumothorax being the most concerning. The SCV has the highest complication rate due to arterial injury and pneumothorax, but also has the lowest infection rate of the three (Kornbau et al. 2015), and is thought to be the most comfortable for the patient postoperatively. Additionally, the SCV

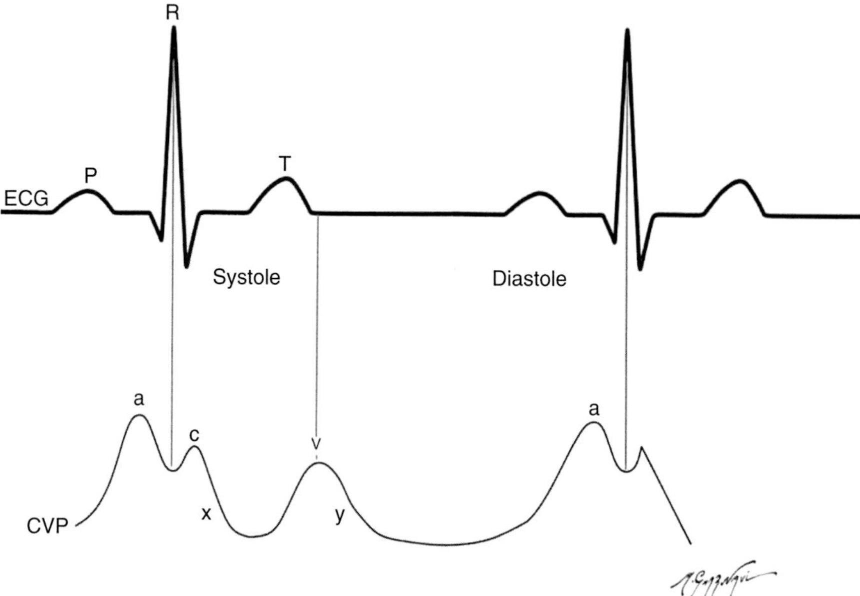

Fig. 7.1 CVP waves and the relation with ECG (Modified from Dabbagh (2014). Published with kind permission of © Springer, 2014. All Rights Reserved)

Table 7.1 Two alternative formulas for calculating length of catheter placement via right internal jugular vein approach (Andropoulos et al. 2001; Yoon et al. 2006)

1. Andropoulos et al. 2001	2. Yoon et al. 2006
(Ht/10-1) cm if HT < 100 cm (Ht/10-2) cm if HT > 100 cm	(0.07 × Ht) + 1.7

catheter may become occluded during the operative procedure when sternal retraction is utilized and the catheter is "pinched" between the clavicle and first rib.

Routine use of ultrasound has become common and is the standard of care for placement in the IJV according to the ASA guidelines and a recent study by Reusz and Csomos (2015). Multiple studies have shown a decrease in the complication rate when ultrasound is used though it does take some training to become facile (Hind et al. 2003). Line length can also be difficult to estimate for pediatric patients. Two studies have come up with specific formulas based on the height in cm for right internal jugular vein catheter placement (Andropoulos et al. 2001; Yoon et al. 2006) (Table 7.1).

For example, an 80 cm patient should have a 7 cm line placed per formula 1 in the right internal jugular vein and a 7 cm line placed per formula 2. Our patient who is 164 cm should have a 14 cm line placed per formula 1 while a 13 cm line placed per formula 2. While not perfect, these estimates can give a practitioner a general sense of the optimal length of the line. Line placement should be confirmed at the earliest possible time by chest x-ray. Optimal position is generally felt to be with the tip of the catheter located at the SVC – right atrial junction.

Table 7.2 Common CVP changes in tracing in different cardiac condition

Cardiac condition	Change in CVP tracing
Atrial fibrillation	Loss of A wave
A-V dyssynchrony/A-V block	Cannon A waves
Tricuspid regurgitation	Large V wave
Cardiac tamponade	Loss of Y descent

Long-term complications from CVL placement may include infection, clot formation, and vessel stenosis or obstruction – particularly in patients with poor cardiac output and blood flow and the infusion of more sclerotic agents such as calcium chloride. Placement should be completed under sterile conditions and following appropriate CVL bundle guidelines, including chlorhexidine skin preparation, full gown and gloves for the provider, and whole body draping for the patient.

CVP is the primary hemodynamic measure that is obtained by placement of a central venous line. The pressure reading gives information regarding the venous system as a whole. The waveform is created by the transmission of energy during events through the cardiac cycle. There are many variables that affect the waveform leading to a number of different manifestations. A few abnormalities are common, and their effects on the waveform should be known. Dampening and resonance are rarely a problem with CVP monitoring since it is a low-pressure system. However, the line is also more likely to be located against a vessel wall for that same reason. In this case, the CVP monitoring will not be accurate, and the line position may need to be adjusted (Table 7.2).

Pulmonary Artery Catheter

The cardiac surgeon states that he would like a pulmonary artery catheter (PAC) instead of the central venous line. He would like to know the pulmonary artery pressure and monitor it during the placement of the VAD and in the immediate postoperative period. A wire is placed in sterile fashion through the most distal lumen of the CVL. The CVL is then removed and the PAC is placed via a sheath introducer and the catheter is attempted to be floated in the pulmonary artery. The patient develops ectopy and subsequently ventricular tachycardia that does not improve with removal of the catheter from the ventricle. The patient is immediately cardioverted and no further attempts are made to float the Swan–Ganz at this time.

Pulmonary artery catheters (PAC) have been used in cardiac surgery for measuring cardiac output (CO), mixed venous saturation, direct pulmonary artery pressures, and pulmonary capillary wedge pressure. They were routinely used until a number of studies including a Cochrane review and the ESCAPE trial questioned their effectiveness in the ICU and in the operating room (Pulmonary Artery Catheter Consensus conference: consensus statement 1997; Binanay et al. 2005; Rajaram et al. 2013). These studies, among many others, have resulted in a marked reduction in the number of PACs placed, though many institutions still place them routinely

(Marik 2013b). The placement of a PAC in children is very uncommon and is often complicated by sheath size and intracardiac shunting that make the readings unreliable or inaccurate. Though now almost 20 years old, the Pulmonary Artery Consensus Conference recommended the use of PA catheters in children suffering from shock refractory to fluids and vasopressors, pulmonary hypertension, and acute lung injury when attempting to decipher cardiogenic from non-cardiogenic causes. A recent review supported this statement and discussed the lack of evidence for their use (Perkin and Anas 2011). There is much more variability in adult patients, but a major meta-analysis looked at 13 randomized studies in ICU, surgical, and cardiac settings showed no significant improvement in any major outcome associated with PAC usage (Shah et al. 2005). In a recent study, the benefits of PACs were discussed in very specific cases including acute heart failure requiring inotropes (Sotomi et al. 2014). Many experts also believe that there are patient-specific situations where placement of a PAC may help management where no guidelines are in place (Kahwash et al. 2011).

When placed, a PAC can give information that cannot be accurately obtained from any other monitor system. CO monitoring can be completed via two means, thermodilution and oxygen consumption. Thermodilution is usually favored in adult patients due to its ease and immediate value obtained without practitioner calculation. In this method, a known volume at a known temperature is injected into the patient via the catheter itself. The thermistor then reads the temperature downstream, and the CO is calculated, dependent on the temperature change and using the patient's body surface area (Ganz and Swan 1972). The thermistor placed on the catheter requires a larger sheath and, therefore, is often difficult to place in children and infants. Thermodilution is also not accurate when there is intracardiac shunting as seen in many congenital heart patients (Freed and Keane 1978). The Fick method of oxygen saturation sampling is instead routinely used. The Fick method requires the sampling of oxygen saturation at the pulmonary artery (venous oxygenation) and pulmonary vein (arterial oxygenation) with an estimated oxygen consumption based on the size of the patient to calculate CO (Rutledge et al. 2010). The peripheral artery oxygenation is often used as a surrogate for the pulmonary vein, but this assumes no significant intracardiac shunting:

$$\text{Cardiac Output} = \frac{\text{Oxygen consumption}}{\text{arteriovenous oxygen difference}}$$

or

$$\text{CO} = \frac{\text{VO}_2}{\text{Ca} - \text{Cv}}$$

PACs can directly obtain the pressure of the pulmonary artery in adults and children. This is often beneficial in patients with pulmonary hypertension though the risk in obtaining them especially in children is high (Carmosino et al. 2007). However, there currently are no other means to obtain accurate pressure measurements across the capillary bed, making placement a necessity. The PA catheter also has a balloon at the end and can be wedged in a peripheral pulmonary artery allowing for an indirect measurement of left atrial (LA) pressure. This can help decipher cardiac vs. noncardiac lung injury.

The placement of a PA catheter is generally safe but includes all the risk of IJV placement and, additionally, the increased risk of placing a large catheter from the right atrium across the tricuspid valve into the right ventricle and then into the pulmonary artery. Care should be taken not to cannulate or dilate the carotid artery as severe injury could occur due to the large sheath and catheter size. The placement of the catheter can cause conduction problems, arrhythmias, and injury to the valves, and there are case reports of it knotting requiring surgical removal (Graybar et al. 1983; Perkin and Anas 2011). The most concerning complication is pulmonary artery hemorrhage that may occur when obtaining a wedge pressure. The hemorrhage is often difficult to stop and is a mortality risk (Hannan et al. 1984). A PA catheter may be placed directly by the surgeon in the operating room if that information is considered important for intra- and postoperative management. Depending upon the catheter type chosen, it is possible to also make use of a continuous mixed venous oximetry catheter to be utilized to help guide postoperative inotropic, transfusion, and volume therapy.

PACs can give information that is difficult if not impossible to achieve through any other monitoring system. They are not without their risks, however, and these risks frequently outweigh any benefit in routine cardiac cases. There are certain patients and medical situations where a PAC is not only warranted but potentially required and great care should be used in its placement and interpretation.

The PAC is floated right before bypass initiation with assistance by the surgeon guiding it manually to minimize the risk of arrhythmias during placement. The wedge pressure is 22, with PA pressures of 54/32 mean of 41 with a mean systemic pressure of 62. The wedge pressure is 8 with a mean PA pressure of 30 compared to the systolic mean of 58 after VAD initiation (Fig. 7.2).

Minimally Invasive Cardiac Output Monitors

Minimally invasive cardiac output monitors are defined as any device placed that can measure cardiac output without the placement of a PAC. The benefits of CO monitoring without the risks of PAC placement are very appealing. There are multiple devices that have been developed with a great deal of variability in their science and accuracy. Many of these devices require some invasive catheters including arterial, CVL, or both. We will discuss only a few on the many types of minimally invasive monitors in this chapter.

  D.K. Goswami and D.F. Vener

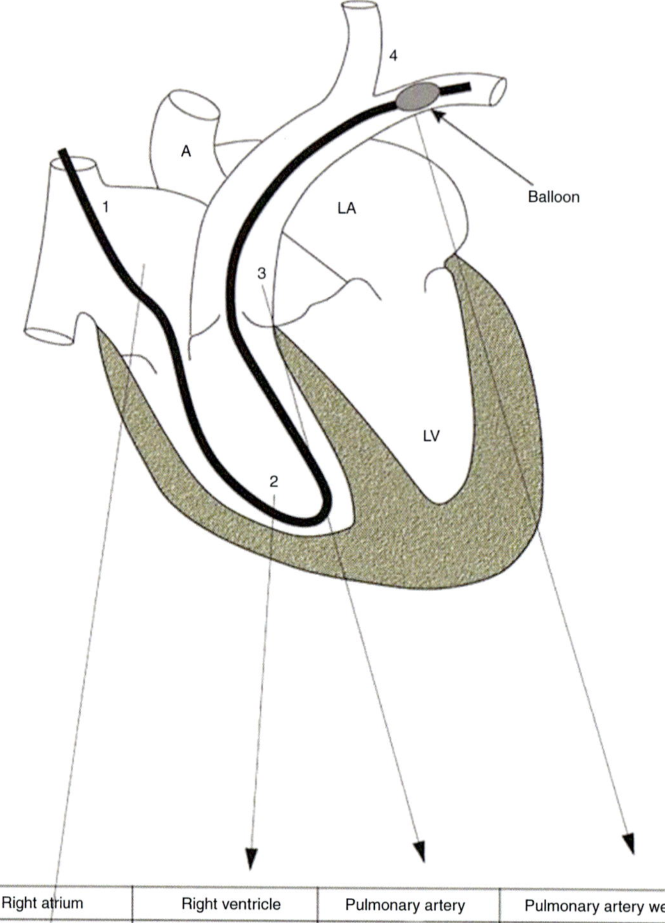

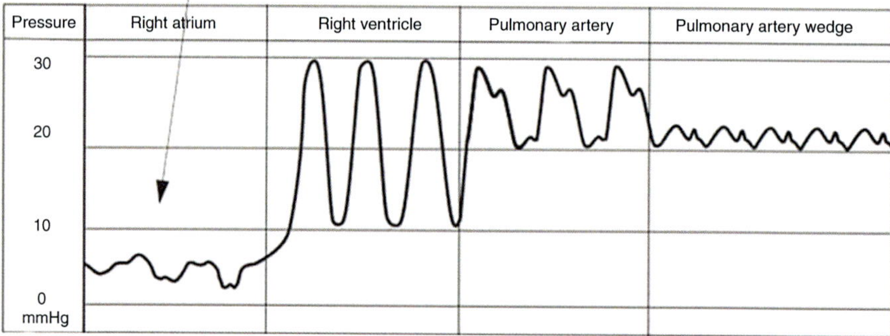

Fig. 7.2 A schematic presentation of the PAC course and its related pressure waveforms in cardiac chambers, pulmonary artery, and main left pulmonary artery (Modified from Dabbagh (2014). Published with kind permission of © Springer, 2014. All Rights Reserved)

Pulse Contour Analysis

The most commonly used monitors evaluate pulse contour analysis and the systolic upstroke of an arterial line to obtain stroke volume. These monitors must be calibrated, and the two most common use lithium or ice cold water to obtain a thermodilution baseline from CVL or peripheral IV[1] to arterial line. An algorithm is used, while the arterial waveform is continuously monitored, and the CO is displayed. These monitors are inaccurate when there is any dampening or resonance of the arterial signal and are also inaccurate with an aortic balloon pump, arrhythmias, or aortic insufficiency (Monnet et al. 2004; Hofer et al. 2007; Richard et al. 2011; Monnet and Teboul 2015). There is also limited number of studies in the cardiac operating room, and only two studies involve pediatric cardiac patients (Mahajan et al. 2003; Sander et al. 2005, 2006; Fakler et al. 2007; Phan et al. 2011; Broch et al. 2015). The majority of these studies showed relative inaccuracies of the monitors compared to the gold standard methods (Fick or thermodilution). The risk factor of these catheters is minimal and is the same as the risk of the invasive lines needed for them.

Ultrasound

The ultrasound technique of noninvasive cardiac monitoring is a by-product of the development of routine transesophageal echocardiography (TEE) used in cardiac and other major surgical cases. TEE is able to estimate CO by obtaining the instantaneous blood flow through a specific cross-sectional diameter of the descending aorta multiplied by the heart rate. The probes used in the minimally invasive technique are much smaller and portable compared to the TEE probes. Each has a different method in obtaining the flow and diameter, and general validation to the gold standard has been poor in most studies (Valtier et al. 1998; Chand et al. 2006; Chatti et al. 2009; Phan et al. 2011).

There is some benefit however in following trends despite the lack of absolute accuracy when compared to thermodilution. The major concerns are the toleration and difficulty with precise placement with the intraesophageal type. The extrathoracic version uses nomograms, which may further decrease accuracy. Both types use the assumption that blood flow is the same in the carotids and the descending aorta, which is not necessarily the case in sick patients (Marik 2013a). The studies in children are extremely poor with no studies including patients with shunts or significant congenital heart disease (Wongsirimetheekul et al. 2014; Beltramo et al. 2016). The risk factors for placement of these devices are minimal for the intraesophageal (similar to OG tube placement) and virtually nonexistent for the extrathoracic version.

---

[1] The LIDCO monitor uses lithium dilution and can be done via a peripheral line.

Bioimpedance/Bioreactance

Bioimpedance cardiac monitors are the least invasive of the devices discussed in this chapter. Electrodes are placed on a patient that both give and receive electrical signal. The primary component of variable impedance (what is altering the signal) is blood flow in the aorta. An algorithm is used to compute cardiac output from this change in impedance. These monitoring devices would seem to have the poorest correlation with the gold standard of thermodilution (Marik et al. 1997; Critchley et al. 2000; Spiess et al. 2001; Sageman et al. 2002; Gujjar et al. 2008). Pediatric studies have used these devices clinically, showing CO changes with interventions and correlation with TEE, but there was poor correlation with thermodilution (Schubert et al. 2008; Cote et al. 2015). The placement of these devices involves simple electrodes and is without any significant risk.

Minimally invasive cardiac output monitors are being used in many patients with variable diseases and ages. Their accuracy and validity are questioned when compared to the gold standard, but new algorithms have improved some of these concerns. They have yet to be considered part of the routine management for pediatric or adult cardiac patients.

At this time, a monitor that is without flaws and that will diagnose the hemodynamic variable that it is monitoring has not been developed. It is imperative that the practitioner understand how a specific monitor works and its limitations and the risks with its placement before deciding on its use. The interpretation of the monitor and the practitioners' response will always be the most important component in patient management (Tables 7.3 and 7.4).

Table 7.3 Normal range of blood pressure in *BOYS* with especial focus on *"The fourth report on the diagnosis, evaluation, and treatment of high blood pressure in children and adolescents"* of the *"National High Blood Pressure Education Program Working Group on High Blood Pressure in Children and Adolescents"* (McLain 1976; Blumenthal et al. 1977; Horan and Sinaiko 1987; Feld and Springate 1988; Brzezinski 1990; Zubrow et al. 1995; Bartosh and Aronson 1999; 2004; Dionne et al. 2012; Bonafide et al. 2013; Heys et al. 2013; Shieh et al. 2013; Bassareo and Mercuro 2014; Ingelfinger 2014; Shah et al. 2015)

	DBP mmHg		SBP mmHg		MAP mmHg	
Age (year)	50 % DBP	95 % DBP	50 % SBP	95 % SBP	50 % MAP	95 % MAP
1	34–39	54–58	80–89	98–106	49–55	69–75
2	39–44	59–63	84–92	101–110	54–60	73–79
3	44–48	63–67	86–95	104–112	58–64	77–82
4	47–52	66–71	88–97	106–115	61–67	79–86
5	50–55	69–74	90–98	108–116	63–69	82–88
6	53–57	72–76	91–100	109–117	66–71	84–90
7	55–59	74–78	92–101	110–119	67–73	86–92
8	56–61	75–80	94–102	111–120	69–75	87–93
9	57–62	76–81	95–104	113–121	70–76	88–94
10	58–63	77–82	97–106	115–123	71–77	90–96
11	59–63	78–82	99–107	117–125	72–78	91–97

Table 7.3 (continued)

| Age (year) | DBP mmHg | | SBP mmHg | | MAP mmHg | |
	50% DBP	95% DBP	50% SBP	95% SBP	50% MAP	95% MAP
12	59–64	78–83	101–110	119–127	73–79	92–98
13	60–64	79–83	104–112	121–130	75–80	93–99
14	60–65	80–84	106–115	124–132	76–82	95–100
15	61–66	81–85	109–117	126–135	77–83	96–102
16	63–67	82–87	111–120	129–137	79–85	98–104
17	65–70	84–89	114–122	131–140	81–87	100–106

Table 7.4 Normal range of blood pressure in *GIRLS* with especial focus on *"The fourth report on the diagnosis, evaluation, and treatment of high blood pressure in children and adolescents"* of the *"National High Blood Pressure Education Program Working Group on High Blood Pressure in Children and Adolescents"* (McLain 1976; Blumenthal et al. 1977; Horan and Sinaiko 1987; Feld and Springate 1988; Brzezinski 1990; Zubrow et al. 1995; Bartosh and Aronson 1999; National High Blood Pressure Education Program Working Group on High Blood Pressure in Children and Adolescents 2004; Dionne et al. 2012; Heys et al. 2013; Bassareo and Mercuro 2014; Ingelfinger 2014; Shah et al. 2015)

| Age (year) | DBP mmHg | | SBP mmHg | | MAP mmHg | |
	50% DBP	95% DBP	50% SBP	95% SBP	50% MAP	95% MAP
1	38–42	56–60	83–90	100–107	53–58	71–76
2	43–47	61–65	85–91	102–109	57–62	75–80
3	47–51	65–69	86–93	104–110	60–66	78–83
4	50–54	68–72	88–94	105–112	63–67	80–85
5	52–56	70–74	89–96	106–114	64–69	82–87
6	54–58	72–76	91–98	108–115	66–71	84–89
7	55–59	73–77	92–101	110–119	67–73	85–91
8	57–60	75–78	94–102	111–120	69–74	87–92
9	58–61	76–79	95–104	113–121	70–75	88–93
10	59–62	77–80	97–106	115–123	72–77	90–94
11	60–63	78–81	99–107	117–125	73–78	91–96
12	61–64	79–82	102–109	119–126	75–79	92–97
13	62–65	80–83	104–110	121–128	76–80	94–98
14	63–66	81–84	106–112	123–129	77–81	95–99
15	64–67	82–85	107–113	124–131	78–82	96–100
16	64–68	82–86	108–114	125–132	79–83	96–101
17	64–68	82–86	108–115	125–132	81–84	96–101

References

Andropoulos DB, Bent ST, Skjonsby B, Stayer SA. The optimal length of insertion of central venous catheters for pediatric patients. Anesth Analg. 2001;93:883–6.

Bartosh SM, Aronson AJ. Childhood hypertension. An update on etiology, diagnosis, and treatment. Pediatr Clin North Am. 1999;46:235–52.

Bassareo PP, Mercuro G. Pediatric hypertension: an update on a burning problem. World J Cardiol. 2014;6:253–9.

Beltramo F, Menteer J, Razavi A, Khemani RG, Szmuszkovicz J, Newth CJ, Ross PA. Validation of an ultrasound cardiac output monitor as a bedside tool for pediatric patients. Pediatr Cardiol. 2016;37:177–83.

Bertrand OF, Carey PC, Gilchrist IC. Allen or no Allen: that is the question! J Am Coll Cardiol. 2014;63:1842–4.

Binanay C, Califf RM, Hasselblad V, O'Connor CM, Shah MR, Sopko G, Stevenson LW, Francis GS, Leier CV, Miller LW. Evaluation study of congestive heart failure and pulmonary artery catheterization effectiveness: the ESCAPE trial. JAMA. 2005;294:1625–33.

Blumenthal S, Epps RP, Heavenrich R, Lauer RM, Lieberman E, Mirkin B, Mitchell SC, Boyar Naito V, O'Hare D, McFate Smith W, Tarazi RC, Upson D. Report of the task force on blood pressure control in children. Pediatrics. 1977;59(I-ii):797–820.

Bonafide CP, Brady PW, Keren R, Conway PH, Marsolo K, Daymont C. Development of heart and respiratory rate percentile curves for hospitalized children. Pediatrics. 2013;131:e1150–7.

Bourgeois MJ, Gilbert BK, Von Bernuth G, Wood EH. Continuous determination of beat to beat stroke volume from aortic pressure pulses in the dog. Circ Res. 1976;39:15–24.

Broch O, Carbonell J, Ferrando C, Metzner M, Carstens A, Albrecht M, Gruenewald M, Hocker J, Soro M, Steinfath M, Renner J, Bein B. Accuracy of an autocalibrated pulse contour analysis in cardiac surgery patients: a bi-center clinical trial. BMC Anesthesiol. 2015;15:171.

Brzezinski WA. Blood pressure. In: Walker HK, Hall WD, Hurst JW, editors. Clinical methods: the history, physical, and laboratory examinations. Boston: Butterworths; 1990. Butterworth Publishers, a division of Reed Publishing.

Carmosino MJ, Friesen RH, Doran A, Ivy DD. Perioperative complications in children with pulmonary hypertension undergoing noncardiac surgery or cardiac catheterization. Anesth Analg. 2007;104:521–7.

Chand R, Mehta Y, Trehan N. Cardiac output estimation with a new Doppler device after off-pump coronary artery bypass surgery. J Cardiothorac Vasc Anesth. 2006;20:315–9.

Chatti R, de Rudniki S, Marque S, Dumenil AS, Descorps-Declere A, Cariou A, Duranteau J, Aout M, Vicaut E, Cholley BP. Comparison of two versions of the Vigileo-FloTrac system (1.03 and 1.07) for stroke volume estimation: a multicentre, blinded comparison with oesophageal Doppler measurements. Br J Anaesth. 2009;102:463–9.

Cote CJ, Sui J, Anderson TA, Bhattacharya ST, Shank ES, Tuason PM, August DA, Zibaitis A, Firth PG, Fuzaylov G, Leeman MR, Mai CL, Roberts Jr JD. Continuous noninvasive cardiac output in children: is this the next generation of operating room monitors? Initial experience in 402 pediatric patients. Paediatr Anaesth. 2015;25:150–9.

Critchley LA, Calcroft RM, Tan PY, Kew J, Critchley JA. The effect of lung injury and excessive lung fluid, on impedance cardiac output measurements, in the critically ill. Intensive Care Med. 2000;26:679–85.

Dabbagh A. Cardiovascular monitoring. In: Dabbagh A, Esmailian F, Aranki SF, editors. Postoperative critical care for cardiac surgical patients. Berlin: Springer; 2014. p. 77–127.

Dionne JM, Abitbol CL, Flynn JT. Hypertension in infancy: diagnosis, management and outcome. Pediatr Nephrol (Berlin, Germany). 2012;27:17–32.

Fakler U, Pauli C, Balling G, Lorenz HP, Eicken A, Hennig M, Hess J. Cardiac index monitoring by pulse contour analysis and thermodilution after pediatric cardiac surgery. J Thorac Cardiovasc Surg. 2007;133:224–8.

Feld LG, Springate JE. Hypertension in children. Curr Probl Pediatr. 1988;18:317–73.

Freed MD, Keane JF. Cardiac output measured by thermodilution in infants and children. J Pediatr. 1978;92:39–42.

Frohlich ED. Recommendations for blood pressure determination by sphygmomanometry. Ann Intern Med. 1988;109:612.

Ganz W, Swan HJ. Measurement of blood flow by thermodilution. Am J Cardiol. 1972;29:241–6.

Graettinger WF, Lipson JL, Cheung DG, Weber MA. Validation of portable noninvasive blood pressure monitoring devices: comparisons with intra-arterial and sphygmomanometer measurements. Am Heart J. 1988;116:1155–60.

Graybar GB, Adler E, Smith W, Puyau FA. Knotting of a Swan-Ganz catheter. Chest. 1983;84:240.

Gujjar AR, Muralidhar K, Banakal S, Gupta R, Sathyaprabha TN, Jairaj PS. Non-invasive cardiac output by transthoracic electrical bioimpedance in post-cardiac surgery patients: comparison with thermodilution method. J Clin Monit Comput. 2008;22:175–80.

Hack WW, Vos A, Okken A. Incidence of forearm and hand ischaemia related to radial artery cannulation in newborn infants. Intensive Care Med. 1990;16:50–3.

Hannan AT, Brown M, Bigman O. Pulmonary artery catheter-induced hemorrhage. Chest. 1984;85:128–31.

Heys M, Lin SL, Lam TH, Leung GM, Schooling CM. Lifetime growth and blood pressure in adolescence: Hong Kong's "Children of 1997" birth cohort. Pediatrics. 2013;131:e62–72.

Hind D, Calvert N, McWilliams R, Davidson A, Paisley S, Beverley C, Thomas S. Ultrasonic locating devices for central venous cannulation: meta-analysis. BMJ (Clinical research ed). 2003;327:361.

Hofer CK, Ganter MT, Zollinger A. What technique should I use to measure cardiac output? Curr Opin Crit Care. 2007;13:308–17.

Horan MJ, Sinaiko AR. Synopsis of the report of the second task force on blood pressure control in children. Hypertension. 1987;10:115–21.

http://www.asahq.org/quality-and-practice-management/standards-and-guidelines.

Ingelfinger JR. Clinical practice. The child or adolescent with elevated blood pressure. N Engl J Med. 2014;370:2316–25.

Kahwash R, Leier CV, Miller L. Role of the pulmonary artery catheter in diagnosis and management of heart failure. Cardiol Clin. 2011;29:281–8.

Kornbau C, Lee KC, Hughes GD, Firstenberg MS. Central line complications. Int J Crit Illn Inj Sci. 2015;5:170–8.

Mahajan A, Shabanie A, Turner J, Sopher MJ, Marijic J. Pulse contour analysis for cardiac output monitoring in cardiac surgery for congenital heart disease. Anesth Analg. 2003;97:1283–8.

Marik PE. Noninvasive cardiac output monitors: a state-of-the-art review. J Cardiothorac Vasc Anesth. 2013a;27:121–34.

Marik PE. Obituary: pulmonary artery catheter 1970 to 2013. Ann Intensive Care. 2013b;3:38.

Marik PE, Pendelton JE, Smith R. A comparison of hemodynamic parameters derived from transthoracic electrical bioimpedance with those parameters obtained by thermodilution and ventricular angiography. Crit Care Med. 1997;25:1545–50.

McLain LG. Hypertension in childhood: a review. Am Heart J. 1976;92:634–47.

Monnet X, Teboul JL. Minimally invasive monitoring. Crit Care Clin. 2015;31:25–42.

Monnet X, Richard C, Teboul JL. The pulmonary artery catheter in critically ill patients. Does it change outcome? Minerva Anestesiol. 2004;70:219–24.

Morray JP, Geiduschek JM, Ramamoorthy C, Haberkern CM, Hackel A, Caplan RA, Domino KB, Posner K, Cheney FW. Anesthesia-related cardiac arrest in children: initial findings of the Pediatric Perioperative Cardiac Arrest (POCA) Registry. Anesthesiology. 2000;93:6–14.

Nashef SA, Roques F, Hammill BG, Peterson ED, Michel P, Grover FL, Wyse RK, Ferguson TB. Validation of European System for Cardiac Operative Risk Evaluation (EuroSCORE) in North American cardiac surgery. Eur J Cardiothorac Surg. 2002;22:101–5.

National High Blood Pressure Education Program Working Group on High Blood Pressure in Children and Adolescents. The fourth report on the diagnosis, evaluation, and treatment of high blood pressure in children and adolescents. Pediatrics. 2004;114:555–76.

O'Brien E, van Montfrans G, Palatini P, Tochikubo O, Staessen J, Shirasaki O, Lipicky R, Myers M. Task Force I: methodological aspects of blood pressure measurement. Blood Press Monit. 2001;6:313–5.

O'Grady NP, Alexander M, Burns LA, Dellinger EP, Garland J, Heard SO, Lipsett PA, Masur H, Mermel LA, Pearson ML, Raad II, Randolph AG, Rupp ME, Saint S. Summary of recommendations: guidelines for the prevention of intravascular catheter-related infections. Clin Infect Dis Off Publ Infect Dis Soc Am. 2011;52:1087–99.

O'Rourke M. Arterial stiffness, systolic blood pressure, and logical treatment of arterial hypertension. Hypertension. 1990;15:339–47.

Perkin RM, Anas N. Pulmonary artery catheters. Pediatr Crit Care Med. 2011;12:S12–20.

Phan TD, Kluger R, Wan C, Wong D, Padayachee A. A comparison of three minimally invasive cardiac output devices with thermodilution in elective cardiac surgery. Anaesth Intensive Care. 2011;39:1014–21.

Pulmonary Artery Catheter Consensus conference: consensus statement. Crit Care Med. 1997;25:910–25.

Rajaram SS, Desai NK, Kalra A, Gajera M, Cavanaugh SK, Brampton W, Young D, Harvey S, Rowan K. Pulmonary artery catheters for adult patients in intensive care. Cochrane Database Syst Rev. 2013;(2):CD003408.

Reusz G, Csomos A. The role of ultrasound guidance for vascular access. Curr Opin Anaesthesiol. 2015;28:710–6.

Richard C, Monnet X, Teboul JL. Pulmonary artery catheter monitoring in 2011. Curr Opin Crit Care. 2011;17:296–302.

Rutledge J, Bush A, Shekerdemian L, Schulze-Neick I, Penny D, Cai S, Li J. Validity of the LaFarge equation for estimation of oxygen consumption in ventilated children with congenital heart disease younger than 3 years – a revisit. Am Heart J. 2010;160:109–14.

Sageman WS, Riffenburgh RH, Spiess BD. Equivalence of bioimpedance and thermodilution in measuring cardiac index after cardiac surgery. J Cardiothorac Vasc Anesth. 2002;16:8–14.

Sander M, von Heymann C, Foer A, von Dossow V, Grosse J, Dushe S, Konertz WF, Spies CD. Pulse contour analysis after normothermic cardiopulmonary bypass in cardiac surgery patients. Crit Care. 2005;9:R729–34.

Sander M, Spies CD, Grubitzsch H, Foer A, Muller M, von Heymann C. Comparison of uncalibrated arterial waveform analysis in cardiac surgery patients with thermodilution cardiac output measurements. Crit Care. 2006;10:R164.

Scheer B, Perel A, Pfeiffer UJ. Clinical review: complications and risk factors of peripheral arterial catheters used for haemodynamic monitoring in anaesthesia and intensive care medicine. Crit Care. 2002;6:199–204.

Schubert S, Schmitz T, Weiss M, Nagdyman N, Huebler M, Alexi-Meskishvili V, Berger F, Stiller B. Continuous, non-invasive techniques to determine cardiac output in children after cardiac surgery: evaluation of transesophageal Doppler and electric velocimetry. J Clin Monit Comput. 2008;22:299–307.

Severinghaus JW, Honda Y. History of blood gas analysis. VII. Pulse oximetry. J Clin Monit. 1987;3:135–8.

Severinghaus JW, Naifeh KH, Koh SO. Errors in 14 pulse oximeters during profound hypoxia. J Clin Monit. 1989;5:72–81.

Shah MR, Hasselblad V, Stevenson LW, Binanay C, O'Connor CM, Sopko G, Califf RM. Impact of the pulmonary artery catheter in critically ill patients: meta-analysis of randomized clinical trials. JAMA. 2005;294:1664–70.

Shah AB, Hashmi SS, Sahulee R, Pannu H, Gupta-Malhotra M. Characteristics of systemic hypertension in preterm children. J Clin Hypertens (Greenwich). 2015;17:364–70.

Shieh HHBE, Bousso A, Ventura AC, Troster EJ. Update of the pediatric hypotension graphic adjusted for gender and height percentiles: diastolic blood pressure for girls, 1 to 17 years old. Crit Care. 2013;17 Suppl 3:23.

Slogoff S, Keats AS, Arlund C. On the safety of radial artery cannulation. Anesthesiology. 1983;59:42–7.

Sotomi Y, Sato N, Kajimoto K, Sakata Y, Mizuno M, Minami Y, Fujii K, Takano T. Impact of pulmonary artery catheter on outcome in patients with acute heart failure syndromes with hypotension or receiving inotropes: from the ATTEND Registry. Int J Cardiol. 2014;172:165–72.

Spiess BD, Patel MA, Soltow LO, Wright IH. Comparison of bioimpedance versus thermodilution cardiac output during cardiac surgery: evaluation of a second-generation bioimpedance device. J Cardiothorac Vasc Anesth. 2001;15:567–73.

Tartiere JM, Logeart D, Beauvais F, Chavelas C, Kesri L, Tabet JY, Cohen-Solal A. Non-invasive radial pulse wave assessment for the evaluation of left ventricular systolic performance in heart failure. Eur J Heart Fail. 2007;9:477–83.

Trivedi NS, Ghouri AF, Lai E, Shah NK, Barker SJ. Pulse oximeter performance during desaturation and resaturation: a comparison of seven models. J Clin Anesth. 1997a;9:184–8.

Trivedi NS, Ghouri AF, Shah NK, Lai E, Barker SJ. Effects of motion, ambient light, and hypoperfusion on pulse oximeter function. J Clin Anesth. 1997b;9:179–83.

Valtier B, Cholley BP, Belot JP, de la Coussaye JE, Mateo J, Payen DM. Noninvasive monitoring of cardiac output in critically ill patients using transesophageal Doppler. Am J Respir Crit Care Med. 1998;158:77–83.

van Montfrans GA. Oscillometric blood pressure measurement: progress and problems. Blood Press Monit. 2001;6:287–90.

Wongsirimetheekul T, Khositseth A, Lertbunrian R. Non-invasive cardiac output assessment in critically ill paediatric patients. Acta Cardiol. 2014;69:167–73.

Yoon SZ, Shin TJ, Kim HS, Lee J, Kim CS, Kim SD, Park CD. Depth of a central venous catheter tip: length of insertion guideline for pediatric patients. Acta Anaesthesiol Scand. 2006;50:355–7.

Zubrow AB, Hulman S, Kushner H, Falkner B. Determinants of blood pressure in infants admitted to neonatal intensive care units: a prospective multicenter study. Philadelphia Neonatal Blood Pressure Study Group. J Perinatol. 1995;15:470–9.

Chapter 8
Electrocardiography: Basic Knowledge with Focus on Fetal and Pediatric ECG

Majid Haghjoo and Mohammadrafie Khorgami

Although the basic principles of electrocardiogram (ECG) interpretation in children are identical to those in adults, pediatric ECGs are more challenging to read as compared to adult ECGs. These difficulties are mainly related to progressive changes in normal cardiac anatomy and physiology between birth and adolescence. Furthermore, structural and hemodynamic changes in congenital heart disease (CHD) may affect nearly all aspect of the surface ECG.

There are many reasons for ECG recording in children, including chest pain, syncope, and suspected arrhythmia. Recording of an artifact-free ECG is the first step in correct interpretation of the pediatric ECGs. This may be real challenge in agitated infants or active children. To obtain an artifact-free ECG recording, distracters such as cartoons, movies, and stickers would be highly helpful. Some children in outpatient setting have sinus tachycardia due to anxiety that should be taken into consideration. Because of right ventricular (RV) dominance in infancy, some pediatric cardiologists prefer to obtain 15-lead ECG, including leads V3R, V4R, and V7. The normal neonatal ECG has more high-frequency details because of higher voltage and shorter QRS duration; therefore, the American Heart Association recommended 150 Hz for minimum bandwidth cutoff and 500 Hz for minimum sampling rate (Bailey et al. 1990).

The second step in correct pediatric ECG interpretation is to consider the clinical condition at the time of recording. Many of the noncardiac diseases in children may have important effects on the normal ECG; therefore, abnormal ECGs do not always equal to the heart disease.

The normal ECG values in pediatrics are age and heart rate dependent. The most changes occur in the first year of life. In the fetal life, circulatory system is primarily dependent on the RV. As a result, at birth the RV is larger and thicker than the left

M. Haghjoo, MD, FESC, FACC (✉) • M. Khorgami, MD
Department of Cardiac Electrophysiology, Rajaie Cardiovascular Medical and Research Center, Iran University of Medical Sciences, Tehran, Iran
e-mail: majid.haghjoo@gmail.com; rafikhorgami@gmail.com

ventricle (LV). This produces ECG pattern reminiscent of RV hypertrophy (RVH) in adult. During infancy, progressive decrease in pulmonary vascular resistance and closure of PDA shifts physiological stress to the left side, and the LV force becomes predominant by 6 months (O'Connor et al. 2008).

The systematic approach for pediatric ECG interpretation includes evaluation for heart rate, rhythm, QRS axis, conduction intervals, and chamber hypertrophy and enlargement.

Heart Rate

The heart rate variation during childhood is significant. The age, body mass index, metabolic states, and other variables influence the heart rate. The standard ECG is usually recorded at paper speed of 25 mm/s; therefore, small box equals to 0.04 s (40 ms), and large box equals to 0.2 s (200 ms). Atrial and ventricular rates should be calculated separately if they are different. There are several methods for calculating heart rate (Fig. 8.1):

1. Dividing the number of large boxes between two consecutive R waves by 300
2. Dividing the number of small boxes between two consecutive R waves by 1500
3. Dividing R-R interval (in ms) by 60,000
4. For irregular rhythms: multiplying number of QRS complexes recorded during the 10-s rhythm strip by 6

Neonatal heart rate varies between 150 and 230 beats/min especially during crying. The heart rate reaches a peak between 1 and 2 months of life and then decreases gradually until 6 months. Between 6 months and first year of life, it tends to reach a plateau, and after that it decreases gradually to reach the adult heart rate (Schwartz et al. 2002).

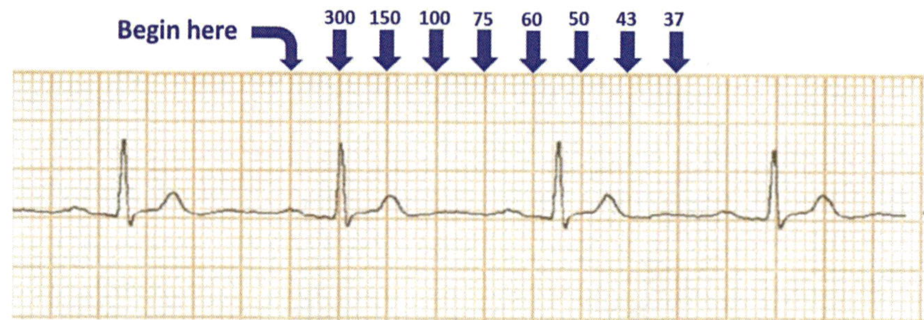

Fig. 8.1 Rapid heart rate calculation by dividing the number of large boxes between two consecutive R waves by 300

Rhythm

For determination of heart rhythm, it is important to determine the exact origin of cardiac impulses. During normal sinus rhythm (NSR), the sinus node is responsible for electrical impulse generation. This impulse depolarized atrial myocytes from superior-right to inferior-left direction. Consequently, the P-wave axis would be between zero and +90°, and the P-wave morphology would be positive in leads I, II, and aVF and biphasic in lead V1. If the P-wave origin is from other atrial locations, the P-wave morphology would be different, for example, left atrial rhythm shows a negative P-wave in leads I and aVL and low RA rhythm exhibits a negative P-wave in leads II, III, and aVF. Therefore, NSR is characterized by a normal P-wave (positive I, II, and aVF) before each QRS complex with a constant PR interval and a heart rate within the normal range for age.

QRS Axis

Frontal QRS axis vector is the means of the ventricular wave fronts direction in frontal plan. There are several methods to estimate the QRS axis:

1. *Quadrant method*: polarity of QRS complexes in leads I and aVF is determined. Based on polarity of these two leads, four quadrants and corresponding QRS axis are defined. If the leads I and aVF are both positive, axis is definitely normal. Otherwise, there is some kind of axis deviation. Negative QRS in both leads indicates an "extreme axis deviation." Positive QRS in lead I and negative in lead aVF point to a possible left axis deviation (LAD), and reverse configuration shows right axis deviation (RAD) (Fig. 8.2).
2. *Isoelectric lead*: Isoelectric lead is characterized by either a biphasic QRS with equal R- and S-wave amplitude or a flatline QRS. If the QRS is isoelectric in any given lead, the axis is perpendicular to this lead.
3. *Positive lead*: Other method is to find the lead with tallest R wave. The axis is roughly in the same direction as this lead.

Normal neonatal QRS axis is between + 55 and +200 because of RV dominancy and decreases to +160 by 1 month. However, in preterm infant, normal frontal axis is between + 65 and +174 (Schwartz et al. 2002). Parallel to cardiac changes during the first 1–3 years of life, ECG pattern changes from RV dominance to LV dominance. As a result, QRS axis will shift from right to more leftward axis (−30 to +100) (O'Connor et al. 2008).

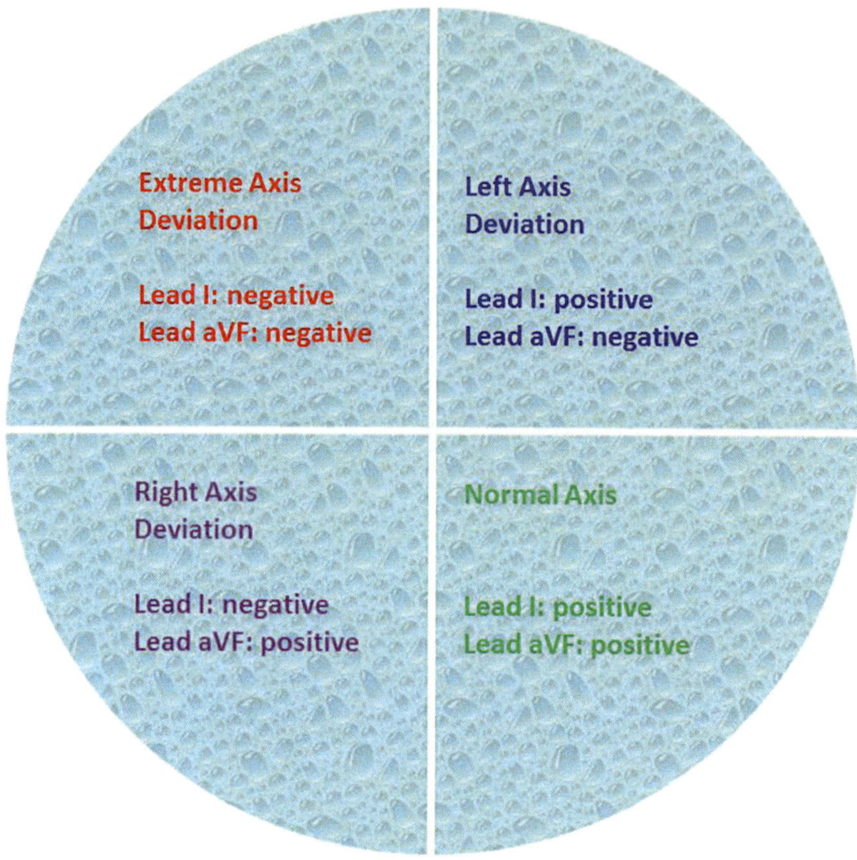

Fig. 8.2 QRS axis determination by quadrant method

Conduction Intervals

PR Interval

The PR interval represents electrical impulse conduction from sinus node through atria, atrioventricular (AV) node, His bundle, bundle branches, and Purkinje system to ventricular myocyte (Fig. 8.3). PR interval measured from onset of P-wave to the onset of QRS complex, usually in lead II. Normal AV conduction defined as normal PR interval and normal association of each P-wave to the following QRS complex.

Normal PR interval duration is shorter in children and changes with age and heart rate. This finding may be due to the smaller cardiac mass in children. The neonatal PR interval may vary between 70 ms and 140 ms with mean of 100 ms (Schwartz et al. 2002). Therefore, AV conduction abnormality in young children may present with normal-appearing PR interval.

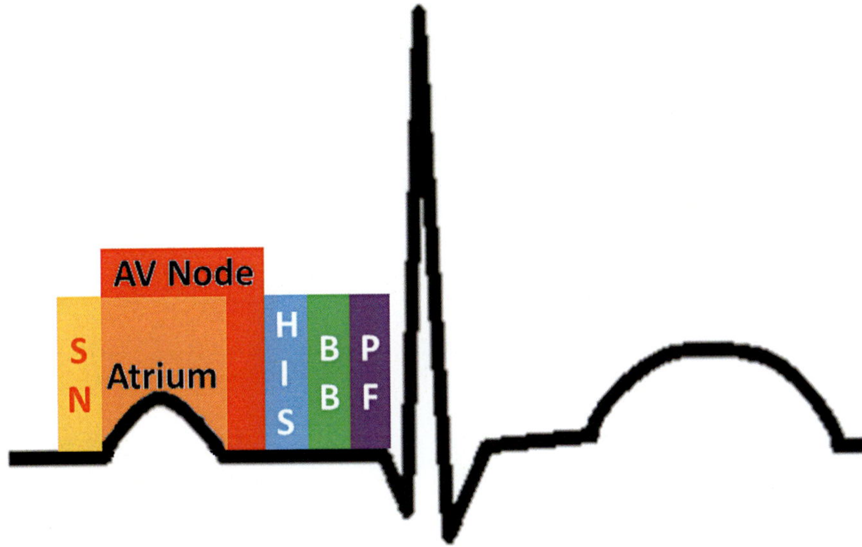

Fig. 8.3 PR interval components

Short PR interval indicates that impulse generates from locations other than normal pacemaker (sinus node), the presence of accessory AV connections, or facilitated AV node conduction. PR prolongation represents impaired AV conduction. Injury to normal conduction pathway in atrium, AV node, His bundle, and bundle branches could increase PR duration.

For PR analysis, association of each QRS to previous P-wave is necessary. P-QRS evaluation in consecutive beats could help us to detect dissociation of the P-wave and QRS complex in disorders such as junctional rhythm and AV blocks.

QT Interval

QT interval reflects both ventricular depolarization and repolarization. It is measured from the onset of Q-wave to the end of T wave usually in leads II, V5, or V6 (Schwartz et al. 2002). QT is age and heart rate dependent. The increase of heart rate results in shorter QT interval. In the cases that T and U waves have overlap and discrimination of two waves is difficult or P-wave superimposes on T wave (usually in infant with higher heart rate), a line is drawn from the peak of the T-wave tangential to its downslope until it intersects the isoelectric line, and this point is considered as the end of T wave (Fig. 8.4).

For elimination of R-R interval variation on QT interval, QT should be corrected (QTc). Bazett's formula is a practical method for QTc calculation: $QTc = QT$ interval (ms)/$\sqrt{R\text{-}R}$ interval (sec) (Bazett 1920).

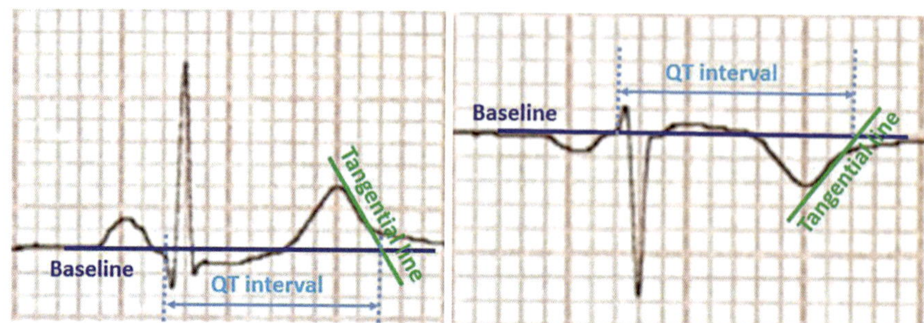

Fig. 8.4 QT measurement using tangential method. In this method, the end of the T wave is determined by the intersection of a tangent line extrapolated from the T wave at the point of maximum downslope to the isoelectric baseline

Multiple studies were done to determinate cutoff point for QT prolongation. In first few days of neonatal period, upper limit (2 standard deviation above mean or 97.5 percentile) for QTc is 440 ms. After this period, there is an increase in QT interval duration. In the first 6 months of life, QTc interval can be as long as 490 ms; however, after 6 months the cutoff point for normal QTc is 440 ms (O'Connor et al. 2008). Anyway, if the QTc is greater than 50 % consecutive R-R interval, it is considered as abnormal.

The QT interval calculation is important because the presence of long QT predisposes the patients into malignant arrhythmia, i.e., torsades de pointes. The QT prolongation may have congenital and acquired types. Before evaluation for congenital disorders, acquired causes such as drugs and electrolyte abnormalities should be ruled out. In the presence of bundle branch block, JT segment is calculated, but there is a question about the accuracy of this measurement.

Morphology

P Wave

The P wave displays atrial depolarization. The first 0.04–0.06 s of the P-wave is related to RA depolarization and remainder related to the LA. RA enlargement is defined as tall and peaked P-wave in lead II. In infant and children, P-wave amplitude greater than 2.5–3.0 mV is considered abnormal. LA enlargement is characterized by a broad (≥0.12 s) and notched P-wave in lead II or wide (>0.04 s) and deep (>0.1 mV) terminal component (negative phase) in lead V1. In biatrial enlargement, both criteria for atrial enlargement are present.

QRS Complex

The measurement of R-wave amplitude and QRS duration especially in precordial leads reflects ventricular depolarization status. Because of lower ventricular mass, the QRS duration is usually shorter in children than in adult: under 4 years of age, it is less than 0.09 s, less than 0.10 s up to 16 years of age, and less than 0.11 s by late adolescence (Deal et al. 2004).

Thin chest and proximity of the heart to ribs in neonate cause tall R or S wave in precordial leads in comparison to limb leads. Low QRS voltage may indicate myocarditis, pericardial effusion, and hypothyroidism.

Fetal circulation is mainly dependent on RV function; therefore, in neonatal period RV muscle mass increased in comparison to LV. This change on surface ECG reflects as high amplitude R wave in right precordial lead with R/S > 1 and deep S wave in left precordial leads with R/S < 1. Gradually after 1 month, the RV loses its dominancy and the LV is the dominant ventricle by the end of the first year of life. As a result, the R-wave amplitude will decrease in right precordial leads and increase in left precordial leads with advancing age (S-wave changes are reverse). Therefore, age-related R- and S-wave amplitude changes in precordial leads should be considered while assessing the ECG for ventricular hypertrophy.

T Wave

The T-wave morphology and axis are changing during childhood. T wave represents ventricular repolarization. As opposed to ventricular depolarization, repolarization begins from the epicardium to the endocardium (QRS-T axis concordance). More than 90° difference between two axes may indicate myocardial injury. The T-wave amplitude value may vary from 0.5 mV in limb leads to 10 mV in precordial leads (Coviello 2016).

In the first week of life, T wave is upright in leads V1 and V3R. Then, it becomes inverted until 8 years and even may be continued to adolescence. In the first 3–5 years of life, 50 % of children have inverted T wave in lead V2, but this value decreases to 5–10 % in 8–12 years (Dickinson 2005). Persistent positive T wave after the first week may represent RVH. T wave is usually positive in left precordial leads in childhood except for the first few days of life that T wave may be flat or inverted. Although ST-T segment changes are nonspecific, but evaluation for diseases such as myocarditis, cardiomyopathy, pericarditis, and electrolyte disorders should be done.

In children especially during tachycardia, P wave may be superimposed on T wave. Comparison of serial T-wave morphology in long strip of the ECG may be helpful. Notched T wave in leads V2 and V3 can be a normal variant in the children. It may be misdiagnosed with 2:1 atrioventricular block, but with careful examination, this pattern is not observed in other leads. Hyperkalemia causes tall and peaked T wave (tented T wave) in surface ECG.

ST Segment

It is measured from the end of the QRS complex to the onset of the T wave. J point is the beginning of ST segment. It represents termination of depolarization with onset of ventricular repolarization. It is elevated when it is at least 1 mm above the isoelectric line and depressed when it is 0.5 mm below the isoelectric line (Deal et al. 2004). ST-segment elevation as J-point elevation is very common in adolescents. It is related to early depolarization and may be considered in differential diagnosis of other diseases especially pericarditis. In early repolarization, ST segment returns to the baseline with exercise. Early repolarization usually better observed in mid-precordial leads. Special forms of the early repolarization may be a risk factor for sudden death. ST-segment elevation in children is usually related to the pericarditis; however, less common causes such as myocardial ischemia should be considered.

Chamber Hypertrophy

Right Ventricular Hypertrophy

RVH in children mostly results from congenital heart diseases with pressure and volume overload mechanisms. Other causes include cardiomyopathy, hereditary myocardial disease, pulmonary vascular disease, and respiratory disease.

The ECG criteria for RVH (Table 8.1) include R wave >98th percentile in V1, S wave >98th percentile in V6, R/S ratio >98th percentile in V1, RAD according to age, upright T wave in V1 between the first week and 8 years, specific morphologies of QRS (R, QR, RsR) in right precordial leads, and neonatal R-wave progression in precordial leads in older children (Fig. 8.5) (Davignon et al. 1979). As a criterion for RVH, RAD should be considered with other criteria. In combination with right atrial enlargement and deep S wave in V6, cor pulmonale should be suspected.

Diagnosis of RVH in neonate may be difficult, but signs of RVH include QR complex in V1, upright T wave in V1 after the first week of life, increased R-wave amplitude in V1, and decreased S-wave amplitude in V6.

Table 8.1 Right ventricular hypertrophy voltage criteria

R wave >98th percentile in lead V1
S wave >98th percentile in lead V6
R/S ratio >98th percentile in lead V1
Right axis deviation (>98th percentile of QRS in frontal plane)
Upright T wave in V1 (1 week old to 8 years old)
qR pattern in V1
rsR' pattern in lead V1, where R' >15mm (<1 year old) or R' >10 mm (>1 year old)
Neonatal R-wave progression in precordial leads in older children

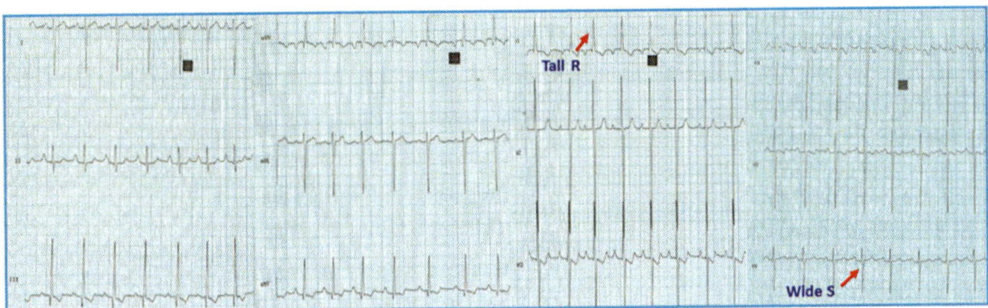

Fig. 8.5 Right ventricular hypertrophy. Typical ECG features are tall R wave in V1, deep S wave in V6, and right axis deviation

Table 8.2 Left ventricular hypertrophy voltage criteria

R wave > 98th percentile in lead V6
S wave > 98th percentile in lead V1
R/S ratio > 98th percentile in lead V6
Q wave > 98th percentile in lead V6 or lead III
Inverted T wave in left precordial leads
Increased T-QRS angle (> 100°)
Increased inferior forces
Decreased RV dominancy (neonate)
Normal adult ECG pattern (neonate)

Left Ventricular Hypertrophy

Left ventricular hypertrophy (LVH) interpretation at surface ECG is based on voltage and repolarization criteria. ECG criteria of the LVH (Table 8.2) include R wave > 98th percentile in V6, S wave > 98th percentile in V1, R/S ratio > 98th percentile in V6, Q wave > 98th percentile in V6 or lead III, inverted T wave in left precordial leads, increased T-QRS angle (>100°), and increased inferior forces (low specificity) (Fig. 8.6).

In normal conditions T-wave and QRS complex axes have similar directions, but two axes would shift to opposite directions in LVH. It is important to note that LAD in children is not a criterion for LVH. Although ST-segment and T-wave changes are nonspecific markers for myocardial disease, they should be considered as the signs of LVH after excluding ischemic and myocardial diseases.

In neonate the decreased RV dominancy may be the only sign of LVH; therefore, normal adult ECG pattern in neonate is indicative of the LVH. Of course in preterm infant, the LV force is more prominent.

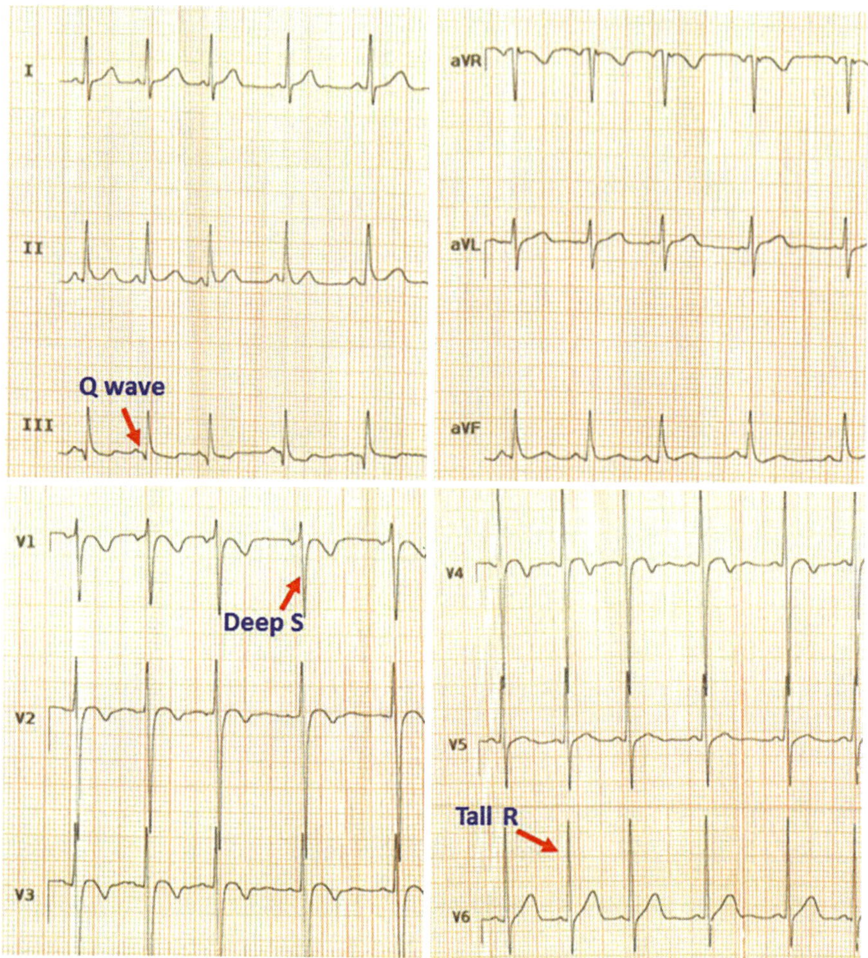

Fig. 8.6 Left ventricular hypertrophy. Typical ECG features consist of tall R wave in V6, deep S wave in V1, Q wave in lead III, and increased inferior forces

Biventricular Hypertrophy

Biventricular hypertrophy (BiVH) should be considered when criteria for both RVH and LVH are present (Table 8.3). In BiVH, increased R-wave and S-wave voltages are observed in leads V1 and V6. High amplitude R and S wave in mid-precordial leads may be seen in children with thin chest wall. If combination of R- and S-wave amplitudes in leads V3 and V4 is more than 60 mm, BiVH should be considered (Katz and Wachtel 1937).

Table 8.3 Biventricular hypertrophy voltage criteria

Increased R-wave and S-wave voltages in lead V1 and lead V6
High amplitude R and S wave in mid-precordial leads
Combination of R- and S-wave amplitudes in leads V3 or V4 > 60 mm

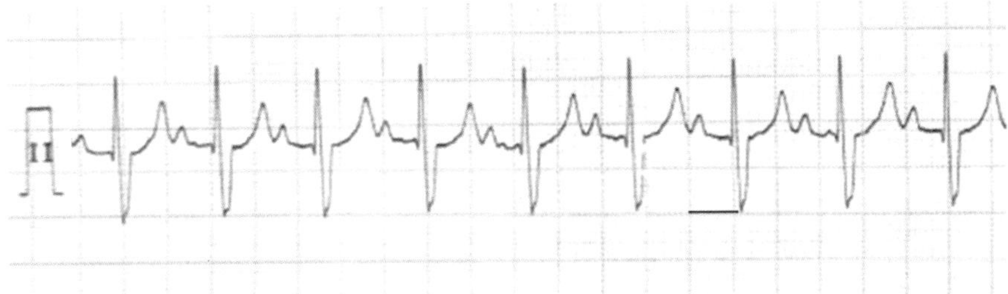

Fig. 8.7 First-degree atrioventricular block is characterized by PR interval prolongation (more than 200 ms)

Conduction Abnormalities

Atrioventricular Block

AV block can occur in children as well as in adult. Underlying causes may be congenital or acquired. Based on the severity of conduction system disease, AV block is divided into first, second, and third degree.

First-degree AV block, defined as PR interval prolongation, is a benign condition in children. As it was mentioned before, PR interval is shorter in children than adult; therefore, a normal-appearing PR interval may be indicative of conduction system disease. This form of AV block is usually asymptomatic and no treatment is necessary (Fig. 8.7).

Second-degree AV block is characterized by intermittent failure of atrial impulse conduction to the ventricles (Fig. 8.8). There are two types of second-degree AV block: Mobitz type I (Wenckebach) and Mobitz type II. Mobitz type I AV block is defined as progressive prolongation of AV conduction leading up to a nonconducted P wave. This kind of AV block is usually located in the AV node and needs no treatment. Mobitz type II AV block is present when there is sudden loss of AV conduction without prior PR elongation. This type of AV block is usually located more distally in the His bundle, bundle branches, and Purkinje system. The treatment is pacemaker implantation.

Third-degree or complete AV block is presented by lack of association between atrial and ventricular depolarization (Fig. 8.9). In this situation, atrial activity will be faster than ventricular response with no clear association. The treatment is pacemaker implantation.

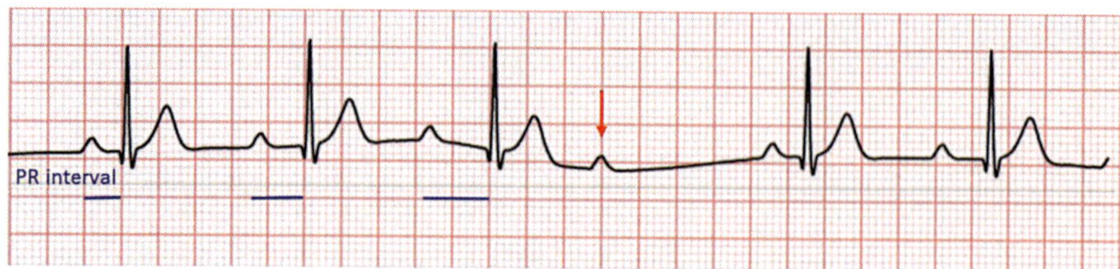

Fig. 8.8 Mobitz type I AV block is characterized by progressive prolongation of atrioventricular conduction leading up to a nonconducted P wave (*red arrow*)

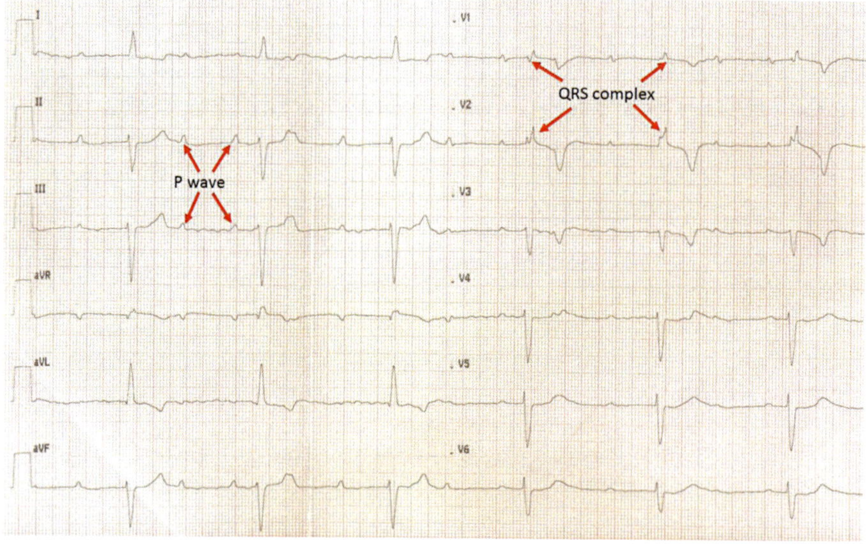

Fig. 8.9 Complete atrioventricular block presented by lack of association between atrial (*P waves*) and ventricular depolarization (*QRS complexes*)

Intraventricular Conduction Defect

His bundle divided into left and right bundle branches. Left bundle is sheetlike structure that is divided to left anterior fascicle and left posterior fascicle. Right bundle branch is cord-like structure that runs along moderator band to anterior portion of RV. Impulse conduction in left bundle and its branches is faster compared with right-sided counterpart. Consequently depolarization of both ventricles is nearly simultaneous and QRS complex is narrow. Injury to bundle branches may cause ventricular conduction delay and wide QRS.

Table 8.4 Right bundle branch block criteria

Wide QRS according to age
rsR' in V1
Wide S wave in lead I, inferior leads, and left precordial leads

Right Bundle Branch Block

In right bundle branch block (RBBB), RV depolarizes through myocardium; therefore, ventricle depolarization is sequential from LV to RV through interventricular septum. Normal LV conduction gives rise to normal initial component of QRS, but the second component is slurred and wide due to delayed RV activation.

ECG characteristics of RBBB include wide QRS according to age, rsR' in V1, wide S wave in lead I, inferior leads, and left precordial leads (Table 8.4).

Surgical closure of congenital heart disease especially VSD closure in tetralogy of Fallot is the most common cause of RBBB (Fig. 8.10). Compared with RBBB in adult population, usually there is no inverted T-wave and ST-segment depression. Isolated rsR' pattern with normal QRS complex duration in right precordial leads is termed incomplete RBBB. This pattern does not necessarily implicate disease and may be seen in normal children, but evaluation for atrial septal defect (ASD) should be considered.

Left Bundle Branch Block

In left bundle branch block (LBBB), interventricular depolarization is from right to left in reverse manner, and initial force (Q wave) in left precordial leads is not observed. Because of LV anatomical position, slow conduction direction is left and posteroinferior.

ECG characteristics of LBBB (Table 8.5) include wide QRS according to age, absent Q wave in leads V5 and V6, notched slurred R in leads I, aVL, V5, and V6, broad S wave in leads V1 and V2, and ST depression with inverted T wave in left precordial leads (Fig. 8.11). LBBB is less common than RBBB. The most common cause is aortic valve and left ventricular outflow tract (LVOT) surgical repair. Other causes include hypertrophic cardiomyopathy, dilated cardiomyopathy (DCM), and myocarditis.

Left Fascicular Block

Left anterior hemiblock (LAHB) is rare in children. In this type of block, QRS is normal. Last portion of LV depolarization is directed toward anterosuperior region and, therefore, causes LAD and rS pattern in inferior leads. Some causes of LAHB include ventricular septal defect (VSD) closure, LVOT surgical repair, tricuspid atresia, endocardial cushion defects, and cardiomyopathy. LAHB diagnosis in infants needs serial ECG evaluation.

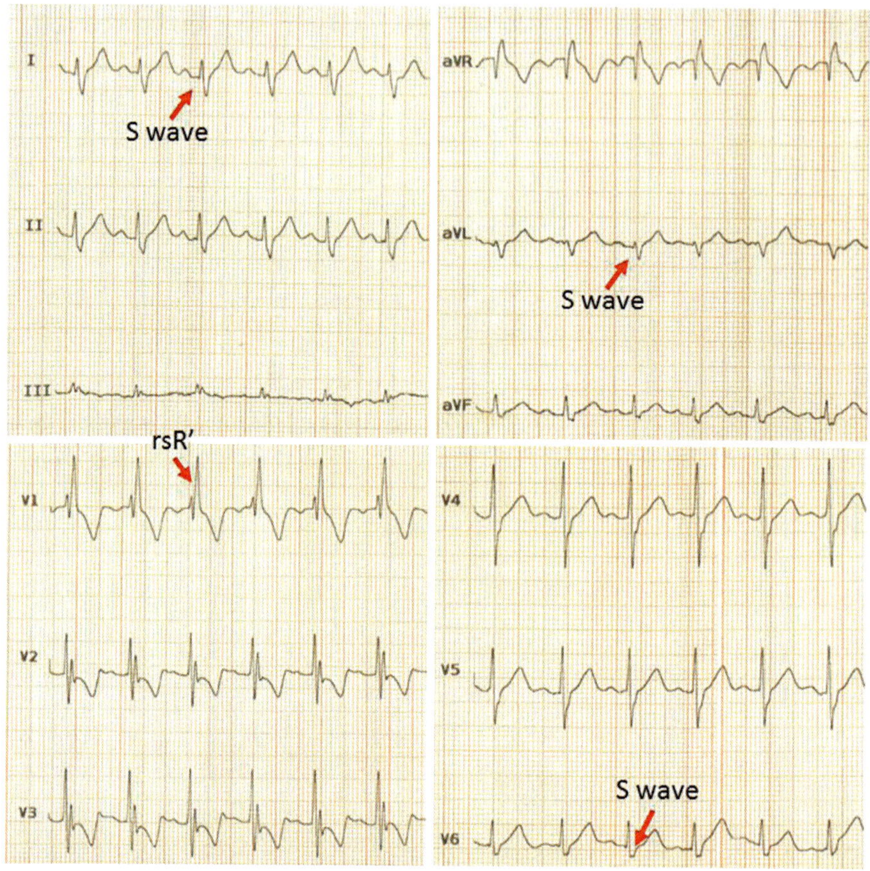

Fig. 8.10 Right bundle branch block. Note that there is rsR' in lead V1 and deep S waves in leads I, aVL, and V6

Table 8.5 Left bundle branch criteria

Wide QRS according to age
Absent Q wave in leads V5 and V6
Notched slurred R in leads I, aVL, V5, and V6
Broad S wave in leads V1 and V2
ST depression with inverted T wave in left precordial leads

In left posterior hemiblock (LPHB), LV depolarize from anterosuperior to posteroinferior direction. The ECG characteristics of LPHB include normal QRS duration, RAD (RVH should be ruled out), and QS pattern in inferior leads.

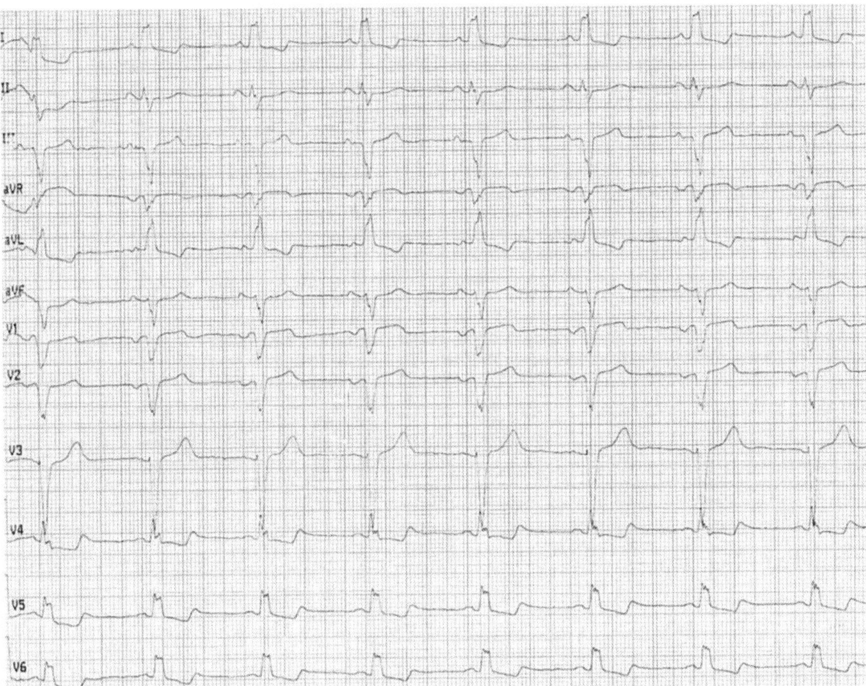

Fig. 8.11 Left bundle branch block. Typical features are the absence of Q wave in leads V5 and V6, notched slurred R in leads I, aVL, V5, and V6, broad S wave in leads V1 and V2, ST depression with inverted T wave in left precordial leads

Multifascicular Block

Bifascicular block refers to the presence of conduction abnormality in two of the three main fascicles of the His-Purkinje system. Bifascicular block is defined as the complete LBBB or the combination of RBBB with either LAFB or LPFB. Most cases were seen after tetralogy of Fallot repair.

Trifascicular block is an electrical disorder in all three fascicles of the conduction system. This abnormality is diagnosed by the presence of alternating bundle branch block (alternating RBBB and LBBB or RBBB with alternating LAHB or LPHB). Bifascicular block with first-degree atrioventricular (AV) block is not necessarily indicative of trifascicular block because PR prolongation is related to the AV nodal disease in majority of the cases.

Cardiac Tachyarrhythmias

Supraventricular Tachycardias

Supraventricular tachycardias (SVT) are a common problem in children who are presenting in emergency department. In addition to cardiac arrhythmia, a fast heart rate can be a physiological response to pain, dehydration, and fever. SVT is the most common tachycardia in pediatric patients. It occurs with a frequency of 1 in 250 to 1 in 1000. Clinical presentation varies from poor feeding or lethargy in infants to palpitation, dyspnea, dizziness, and chest pain in older children.

Several mechanisms are responsible for SVT in children. Different types of pediatric SVTs are listed in Table 8.6. The most common type of the pediatric SVT is orthodromic atrioventricular reciprocating tachycardia (AVRT) using an accessory pathway. The characteristic ECG findings for orthodromic AVRT (Fig. 8.12) are the presence of P wave in the ST segment during tachycardia (QRS-P interval > 0.07 s), ST-segment depression in inferior and left precordial leads, ST-segment elevation in lead aVR, and Wolff-Parkinson-White pattern (short PR, wide QRS complex, and delta wave) in NSR (Fig. 8.13). The heart rate is typically more than 220 beats/min (bpm) in infants and more than 180 bpm in children.

Ventricular Tachycardias

Although pediatric tachycardias are more likely to be from a supraventricular origin, tachycardias from a ventricular origin do occur. Ventricular tachycardia (VT) usually presents with wide QRS tachycardia in ECG (Fig. 8.14). It is important to note that QRS complex duration is shorter in children than adult; therefore, a tachycardia with slightly prolonged QRS may represent a VT or SVT with aberrancy. VT can go unrecognized for a while before presenting with syncope, heart failure, or cardiac arrest.

Table 8.6 Supraventricular tachycardias in children	
	Sinus tachycardia (ST)
	Orthodromic atrioventricular reciprocating tachycardia (O-AVRT)
	Permanent form of junctional reciprocating tachycardia (PJRT)
	Antidromic reciprocating tachycardia (A-AVRT)
	Atrioventricular nodal reentrant tachycardia (AVNRT)
	Junctional ectopic tachycardia (JET)
	Focal atrial tachycardia (FAT)
	Multifocal atrial tachycardia (MAT)
	Atrial flutter (AFL)
	Atrial fibrillation (AF)

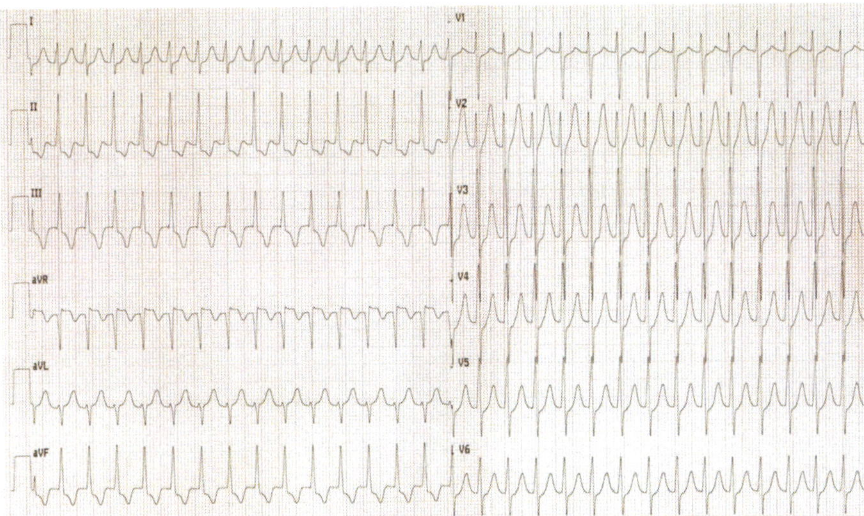

Fig. 8.12 Orthodromic atrioventricular reciprocating tachycardia. Note that there marked ST-segment depression in inferior and left precordial leads and ST-segment elevation in lead aVR

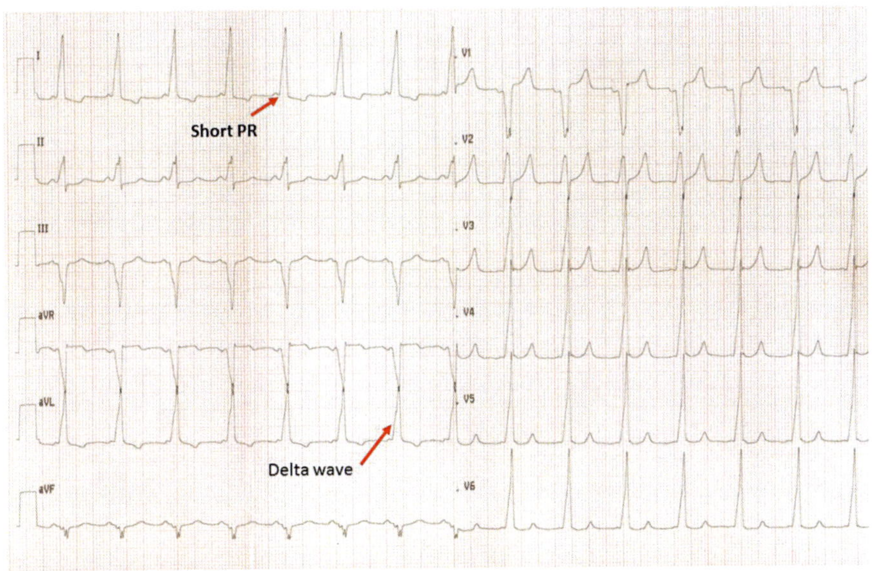

Fig. 8.13 Wolff-Parkinson-White syndrome. Characteristic features are short PR interval, delta wave (initial slurring of QRS complex), and QRS widening

In surface ECG, VT is characterized by a series of three or more repetitive ventricular extrasystole with heart rate of > 120 bpm. It is highly important to remember the age-related QRS complex duration changes in children. In infants, the QRS complex duration in VT is more than 0.08 s, and in children older than 3 years is

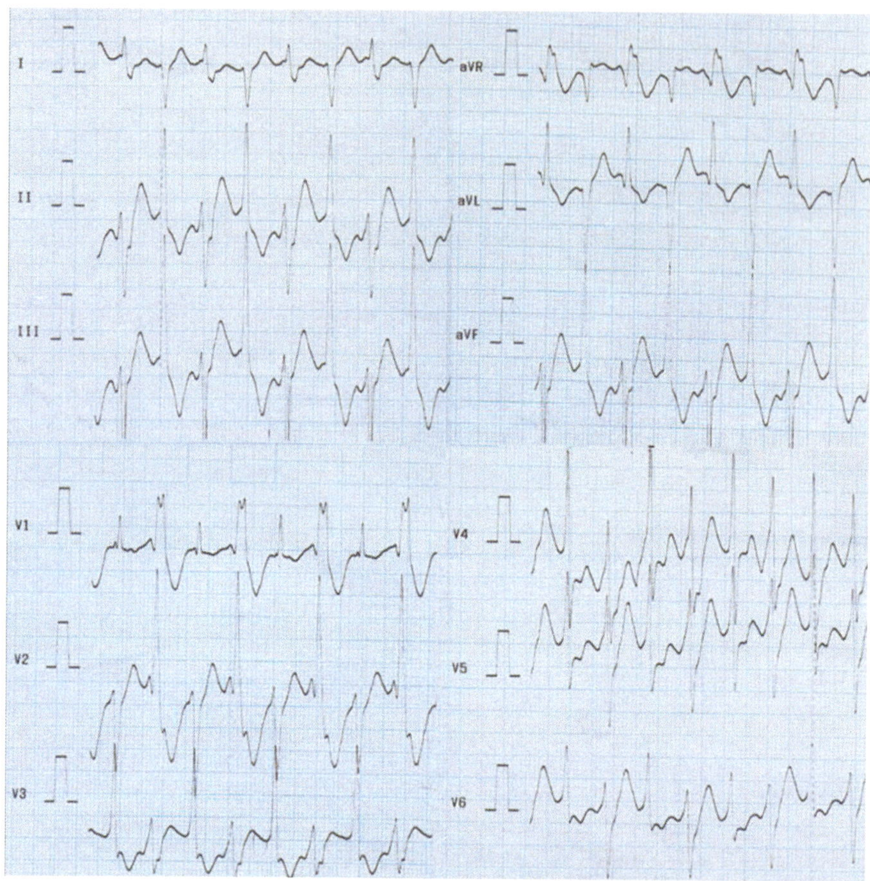

Fig. 8.14 Ventricular tachycardia. This ECG shows bidirectional ventricular tachycardia with characteristic alternating QRS axis and right bundle branch block type morphology

more than 0.09 s. Therefore, it is highly likely to misdiagnose the VT as SVT. To ensure proper diagnosis of VT, other useful criteria such as AV dissociation, capture, and fusion beats should be considered in these situations.

Congenital Heart Disease

Atrial Septal Defect

Atrial septal defect (ASD) is a congenital heart disease with left to right shunt. The ECG pattern mainly results from volume overload that related to ASD size: in small ASD, ECG is usually normal; however, in the larger ASD, there is rsR' pattern in

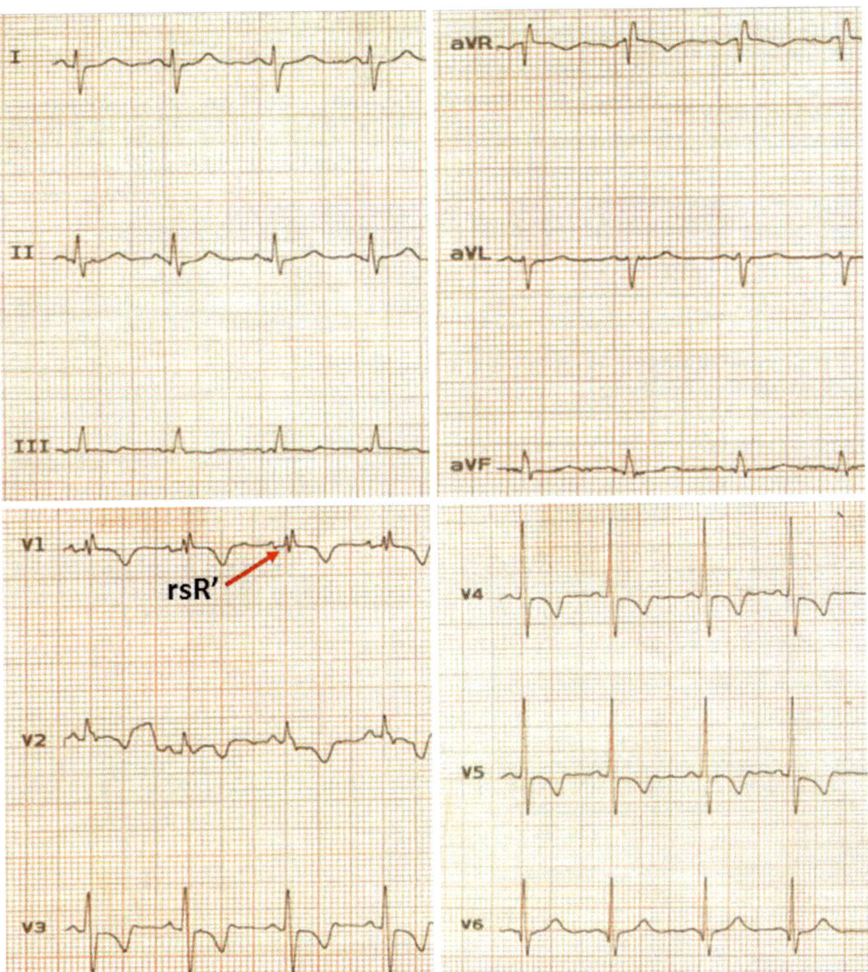

Fig. 8.15 Atrial septal defect. The rsR' pattern in lead V1 and right axis deviation are typical characteristics

right precordial leads including V4R and V1 due to volume overload and RV conduction delay (Fig. 8.15). This ECG finding may be helpful in asymptomatic children as a clue for further evaluation for ASD but also may be observed in normal children. The P-wave axis is usually between 90 and 120° (Zufelt et al. 1998). Frontal right axis deviation is observed in medium and large ASD (Fig. 8.15). The other types of ASDs have appropriate ECG finding. In sinus venosus ASD, the P-wave axis may be less than 30° or in ASD primum the frontal left axis deviation is seen (Davia et al. 1973).

Ventricular Septal Defect

ECG finding in VSD determines the size and degree of interventricular shunts. Because of limited left to right shunt in small VSD, ECG is normal or minimal change is seen. In moderate and large size VSD, left to right shunt degree is significant. Volume overload causes dilation and hypertrophy of LA and LV. Frontal axis deviates to the left and counterclockwise rotation occurred. LA enlargement causes broad notched P wave in lead II (Fig. 8.16). A characteristic finding of large VSD is sign of RVH on ECG. Latter finding becomes more prominent with increase in pulmonary vascular resistance.

In neonate and infants with large VSD, excessive amount of blood flow to pulmonary circulation prevents natural decrease in pulmonary vascular resistance to occur in first months of life. As a result RV dominancy and RVH continue beyond neonatal period. Patients with pulmonary vascular obstructive disease initially demonstrate biventricular hypertrophy (Fig. 8.16) and gradually progress to RVH only.

Atrioventricular Septal Defect

Failure of the endocardial cushion development to complete atrial and ventricular septation results in atrioventricular septal defect (AVSD). Complete form of AVSD is characterized by ASD premium and inlet VSD. The AV node displaces from its normal position in Koch triangle in posteroinferior direction. The bundle has a longer course and descends along the crest of ventricular septum. The superior axis deviation is one of the main ECG features of the AVSD (Fig. 8.17), and the axis is between −40 and −150 (Gamboa et al. 1966). The intra-atrial conduction delay results in PR prolongation. The RVH pattern in ECG is a constant finding (Fig. 8.17). LVH may also be observed.

In partial AVSD, left axis deviation is observed and frontal axis usually is between -30 and -150°. The PR prolongation may be seen in about 50 % due to increased intra-atrial conduction time (Park 2014). Other ECG findings include RVH pattern, rsR in right precordial leads, RBBB, and tall or broad and notched P-wave due to RA or LA enlargement.

Patent Ductus Arteriosus

The patent ductus arteriosus (PDA) has slightly different appearances in preterm and full-term neonates. In preterm infant, lung disease causes persistence of RV dominancy and the ECG may be confusing. Similar to other congenital heart disease with left to right shunt, left to right shunt and severity of LV volume overload determine ECG pattern. In moderate-sized and large PDA, ECG pattern of LVH is

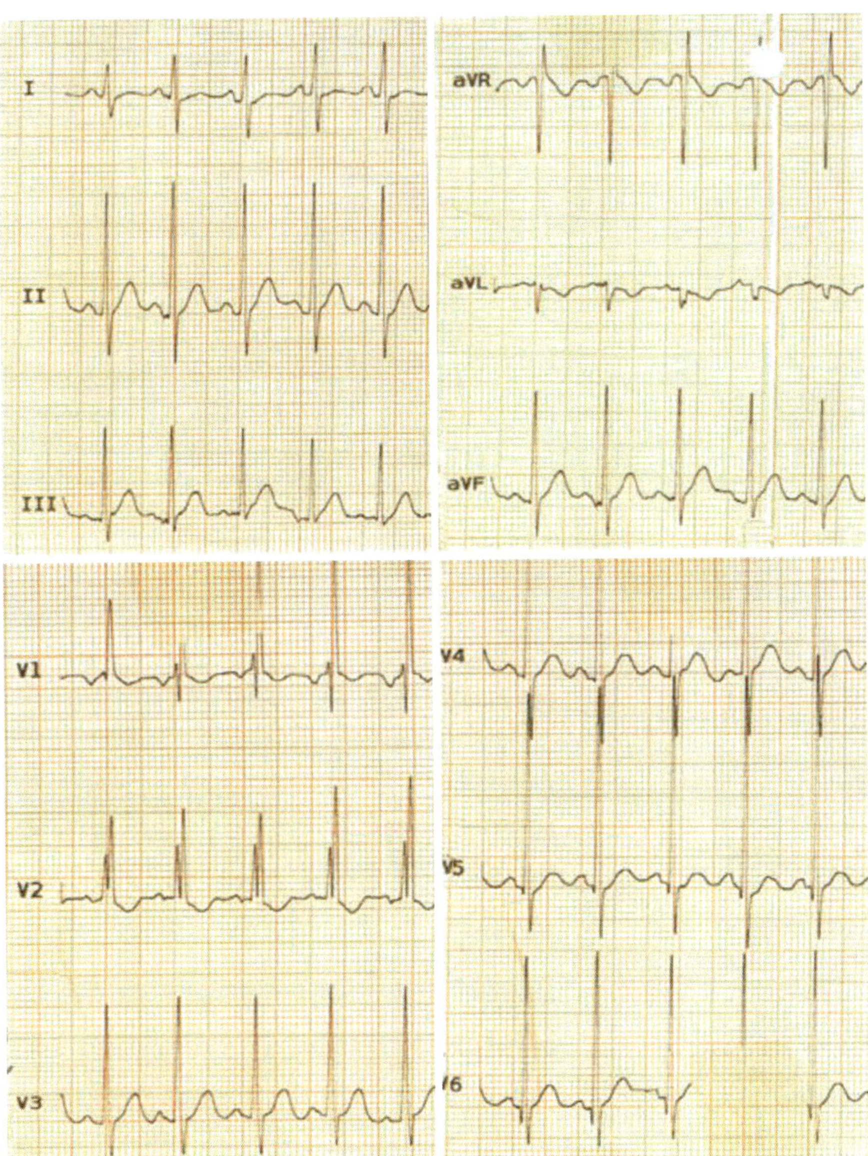

Fig. 8.16 Ventricular septal defect with pulmonary vascular disease. This ECG shows biventricular hypertrophy and left atrial abnormality

manifested by tall R wave and deep Q wave in inferior leads and leads V5–V6 (Fig. 8.18). There is also LA abnormality with broad biphasic P wave. Without intervention and resulting increase in pulmonary pressure, ECG patterns of RVH and RA enlargement will be appeared.

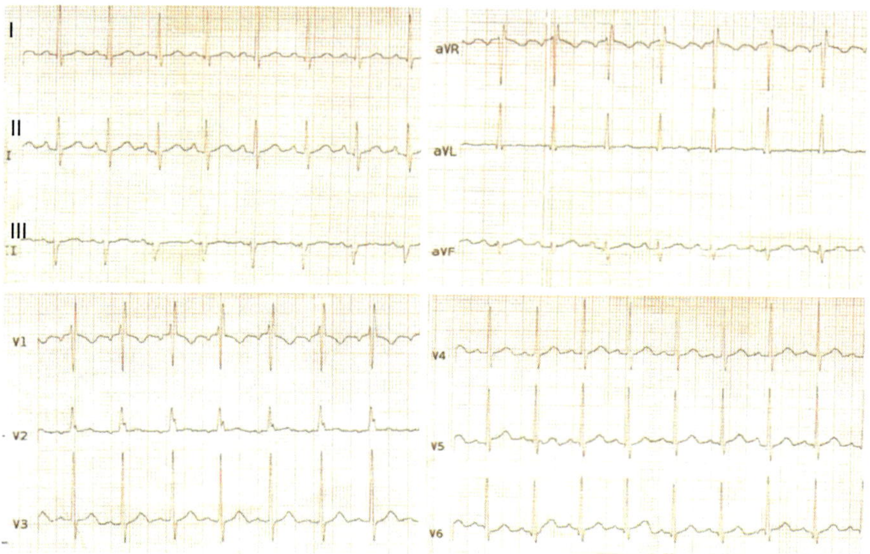

Fig. 8.17 Complete atrioventricular septal defect. Note that there is left axis deviation, incomplete right bundle branch block, and biventricular hypertrophy

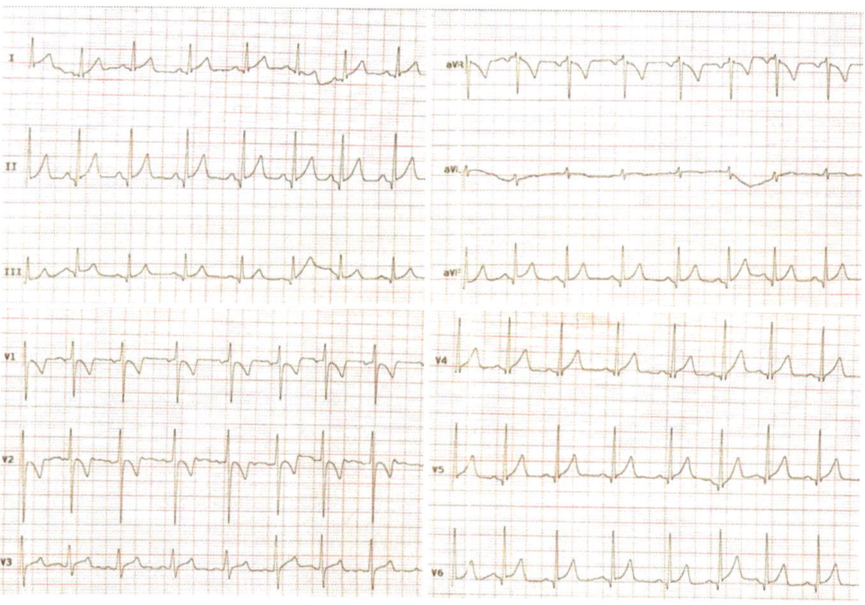

Fig. 8.18 Patent ductus arteriosus. There is typical left ventricular hypertrophy pattern with tall R wave and deep Q wave in inferior leads and leads V5–V6 and left atrial abnormality

Truncus Arteriosus

In truncus arteriosus, a single great artery with single semilunar valve arises from the heart, and this artery is the origin of aorta, pulmonary, and coronary arteries. The ventricular septal defect is a constant finding. The baseline normal sinus rhythm was usual because the AV node is located in normal position. Similar to other congenital heart disease with left to right shunt, there is ECG pattern of LVH and LA enlargement. Gradually, the BVH pattern may be seen.

Partially and Totally Anomalous Pulmonary Venous Returns

Total anomalous pulmonary venous connection or TAPVC manifested with anomalous drainage of pulmonary vein to right atrium or any pathway that terminated to RA. As a result a huge blood volume loads to the right side of the heart that increases pulmonary blood flow. Severe RA and RV enlargement and RVH are present. The ECG finding includes frontal prominent R wave in right precordial leads, upright T wave in leads V4R and V1, and tall P wave in lead II.

In TAPVC with obstruction, ECG shows RVH and right axis deviation because of pulmonary hypertension. The ECG finding of partially anomalous pulmonary venous return (anomalous connection of one to three pulmonary veins) with ASD resembles isolated ASD. In PAPVC with intact ventricular septum, ECG is normal.

Tricuspid Atresia

Tricuspid atresia is classified based on the position of great arteries and present of VSD. The AV node is located in the muscular floor of the right atrium and bundle of His descends along the posterior rim of the VSD near to the acute cardiac margin. As opposed to other cyanotic congenital heart disease, frontal axis deviates to left superior because of decreased RV dominancy. The ECG sign of RA enlargement appeared few months after birth.

In patients with large VSD and increased pulmonary blood flow, tall R wave and deep Q wave in left precordial lead were seen (Gamboa et al. 1966). Chronic RA stretching predisposes heart to atrial arrhythmia such as atrial tachycardia and flutter.

Pulmonary Valve Stenosis and Pulmonary Valve Atresia

Based on severity of RV outlet obstruction, the spectrum of disorders from mild valvular stenosis to severe pulmonary atresia with RV hypoplasia is observed. In mild pulmonary valve stenosis, ECG may be normal, but in moderate and severe stenosis, right axis deviation and RVH are usually seen (Fig. 8.19). One practical

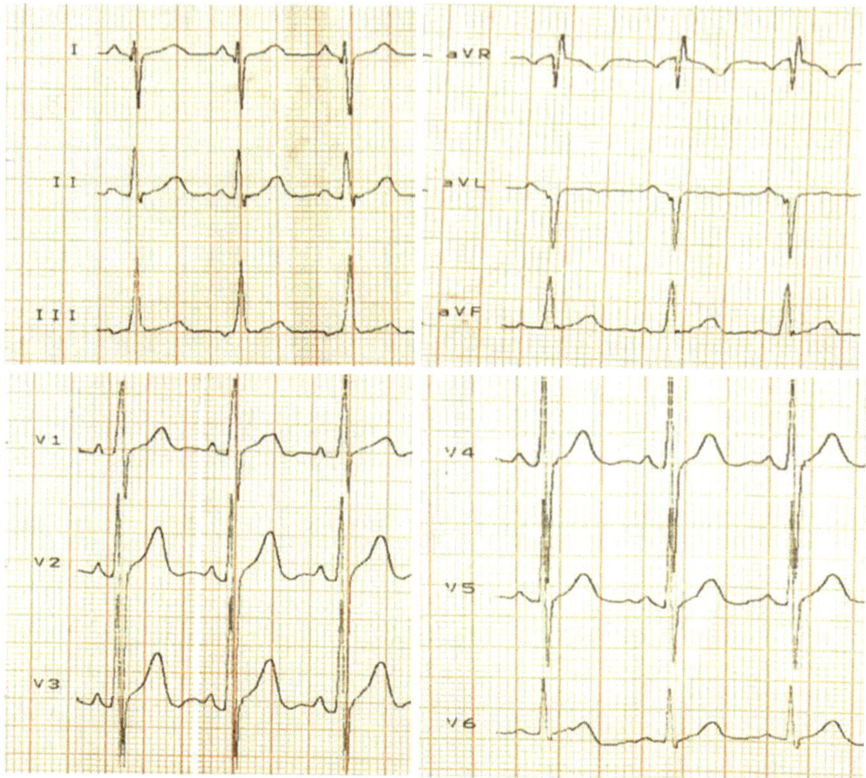

Fig. 8.19 Pulmonary valve stenosis. ECG shows right atrial abnormality (lead V1), right axis deviation, and right ventricular hypertrophy pattern

formula for calculation of RV systolic pressure in the presence of pure R wave in V1 is (Dick et al. 1975) RV systolic pressure (mmHg) = R wave height (mm) × 5.

In severe form, the frontal axis is more than 110°. Other ECG findings include RBBB, QR wave in right precordial leads. If there is the left axis deviation and LVH in critical PS, more evaluation for diagnosis of Noonan syndrome is recommended.

Pulmonary atresia with intact ventricular septum results in underdevelopment and hypoplasia of RV. As opposed to other cyanotic heart disease, the right and anterior forces are decreased. Neonate with LVH findings on ECG and significant cyanosis raises the suspicion of diagnosis of pulmonary atresia and intact ventricular septum. The ASD or PFO is always present and ECG shows RA enlargement. Due to coronary arteries involvement and ventriculocoronary connections, ischemic patterns of ST-T changes may be seen in these patients.

In the presence of the VSD, RV pressure overloads occurred and ECG shows right axis deviation and RVH. In rare cases that multiple and large collaterals result in increased pulmonary blood flow, LVH and LA enlargement are seen in ECG.

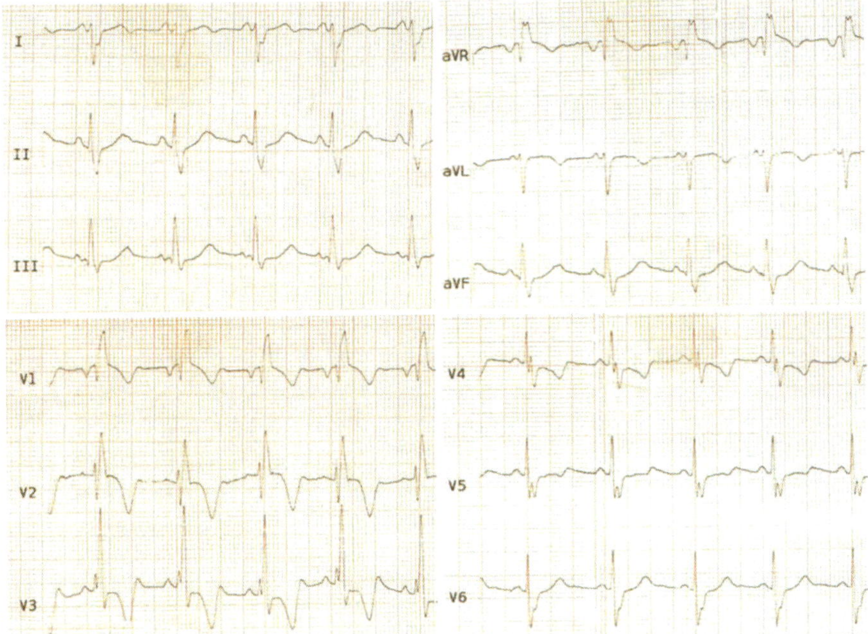

Fig. 8.20 Tetralogy of Fallot after surgical repair. Typical sign is right bundle branch block

Tetralogy of Fallot

Deviation of infundibular septum in fetal period begins the complex pathology of TOF. This anomaly includes pulmonary stenosis and VSD that results in right axis deviation and RVH in ECG. The SA node and AV node are intact, but cases of complete AV block were seen.

After conventional surgical repair, one of the well-known ECG patterns is RBBB (Fig. 8.20). Association of RBBB with left anterior fascicular block may also occur. The effects of the pulmonary valve insufficiency (PI) in long time period on RV remodeling and LV function necessitate regular evaluation of PI severity after surgery. The length of QRS complex is one of the markers that predict severity of pulmonary insufficiency, needs for pulmonary valve replacement, and adverse outcome. The QRS duration equal to or more than 180 ms predisposes these patients to ventricular tachyarrhythmia. In multicenter studies on 800 patients with TOF, the QRS duration equal to or more than 180 ms or more than 5 ms annual increase was a predictor for sudden cardiac death (Gatzoulis et al. 1995). The progressive ventricular fibrosis and dilation are the natural course of TOF, and unoperated older age patient exhibits ventricular ectopy. The SVT including atrial arrhythmias, atrial flutter, and fibrillation has also been reported after total correction in long-term follow-up.

Ebstein Anomaly

The Ebstein's anomaly is characterized by some degree of tricuspid valve displacement toward RV cavity. The addition of atrialized RV to RA chamber changes the electroanatomical map of the right atrium. The intra-atrial conduction delay results in PR prolongation in approximately 40 % of patients. The RA enlargement and tricuspid valve regurgitation result in tall-peaked P wave in ECG especially lead II and increase in duration of P wave. Other ECG findings include RBBB and Q wave in right precordial leads. The disruption of the atrioventricular fibrosis tissue that separates atrium from ventricles electrically predisposes this anomaly to muscle bridge connections termed accessory pathway. These pathways bypass normal conduction system and result in preexcitation and WPW syndrome.

Cappato and coworkers studied 21 patients with Ebstein's anomaly and AV reciprocating tachycardia. All accessory pathways were right sided typically in the posteroseptal, posterior, and posterolateral positions (Cappato et al. 1996). Multiple accessory pathways have been reported in 6–36 % patients with WPW syndrome. Reich et al. investigated 59 patients with Ebstein's anomaly and AP-mediated arrhythmias (Reich- et al. 1998). They found multiple accessory pathways in 33 % pathways and 96 % pathways were right sided.

In Ebstein's anomaly, other tachyarrhythmias are also common. These arrhythmias include atrial tachycardia, atrial flutter, atrial fibrillation, and ventricular tachycardia. The SVT in the presence of rapid conducting accessory pathways could deteriorate unstable hemodynamic state of patients with severe Ebstein's anomaly. Radiofrequency ablation for elimination of all accessory pathways is recommended before corrective surgery of tricuspid valve; however, recurrence rate is high.

Aortic Valve Stenosis

Such as other left-sided obstructive disease, aortic valve stenosis presents with pressure overload and LVH. Both voltage and repolarization criteria in ECG are useful for identifying the LVH. With progression to severe stenosis, signs of subendocardial ischemia and strain pattern as inverted T-wave and ST-segment depressions in left precordial leads appear. Even in severe aortic valve stenosis, the resting ECG may be normal, and appropriate tests include exercise test and 24-h ECG Holter monitoring. During exercise test, significant ST-segment changes are observed in severe form of the disease.

Wagner et al. reported that patients with severe AS (peak-to-peak pressure gradient more than 80 mmHg) did not present with ECG finding on ECG, and T-wave morphology in lead V6 was only discriminatory ECG finding in 2–21-year-old patients (Wagner et al. 1977). Wolf et al. reported that the prevalence of ventricular ectopy and ventricular arrhythmias is higher in 24-h Holter monitoring of patients with aortic valve stenosis (Wolfe et al. 1993).

Coarctation of Aorta

The COA usually present in adolescence with systemic hypertension. The ECG finding of LVH is usual and LA abnormality is also observed in chronic untreated COA (Fig. 8.6). In neonate and infancy, the COA is asymptomatic and ECG is usually normal. It is important to note that the presence of LVH in this period necessitate ruling out of other left-sided obstructive disease including aortic valve stenosis.

Transposition of the Great Arteries

In TGA, aorta origin arises from morphological RV and pulmonary artery origin arises from morphological LV. Therefore, there is the parallel circulation, and the desaturated venous blood returns to systemic circulation, and saturated pulmonary venous blood returns to pulmonary artery. In the neonatal period, the RV pressure is normally high and after this period with reducing pulmonary vascular resistance gradually decreased to normal value. In TGA, the RV should pump blood against systemic circulation, and the ECG finding of RVH is present after the first week along with right axis deviation (Fig. 8.21). In the presence of the VSD, biventricular hypertrophy is observed.

The typical ECG finding of TGA may be not found in the presence of other anomalies such as pulmonary stenosis or atrioventricular septal defect.

Congenitally Corrected Transposition of the Great Arteries

In congenitally corrected transposition of the great arteries (CCTGA), the right-sided and anterosuperior ventricle has LV morphology, and left-sided and postero-inferior ventricle has RV morphology, but the atria and great arteries connect normally with inverted ventricles. This atrioventricular and ventriculoarterial discordance results in normal circulation physiology, but there are conduction system disorder and associated structural disease because of improper roles of LV and RV.

In CCTGA, the SA node inserts in the SVC-RA junction in normal position, and the atrial conduction directs from right and anterior to left and posterior; therefore the P-wave axis and morphology are normal. The main factor that determinates the AV node location is the presence or absence of atrioventricular concordance. In CCTGA the AV node is located in RA wall and anterosuperior quadrant of mitral valve. The bundle runs between mitral valve and valve of posterior great artery and descends anterior to outflow tract of posterior great artery. In the presence of the VSD, the location of nonbranching bundle in relation to VSD is anterosuperior. The left bundle descends in right side of the interventricular septum and right bundle penetrates septum and shifts to left (Ho and Anderson 1985).

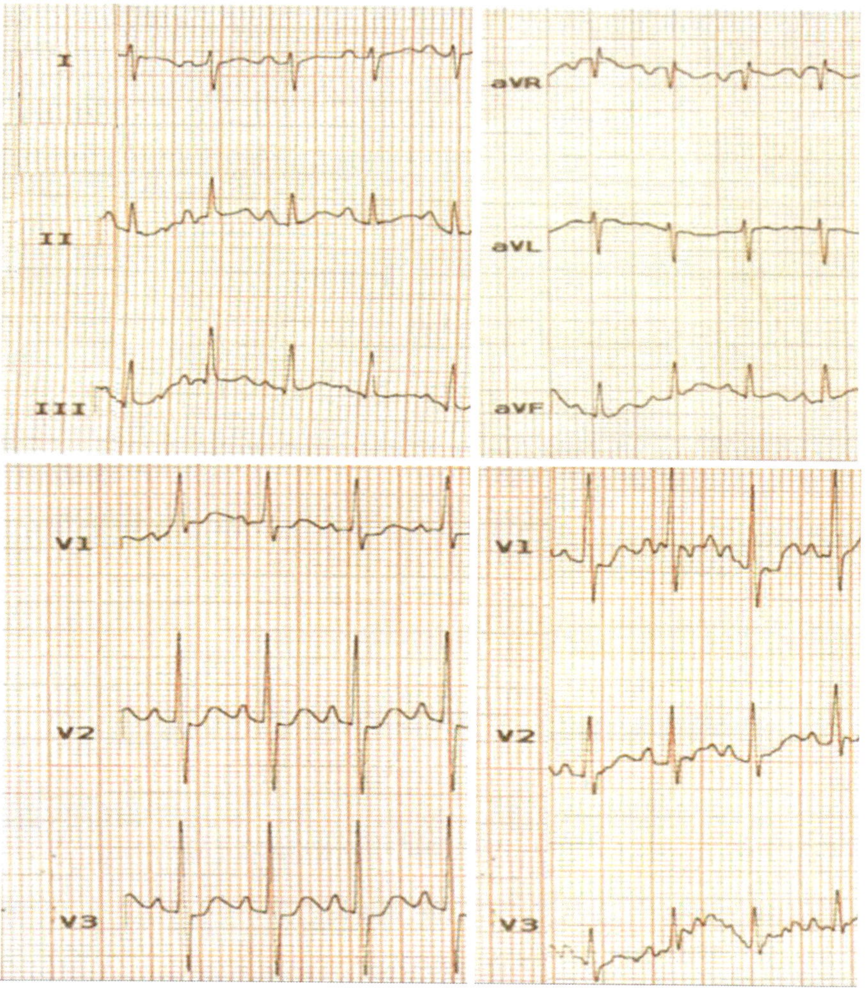

Fig. 8.21 Transposition of great arteries. This ECG shows right axis deviation and right ventricular hypertrophy pattern

In normal structural heart, the initiation of ventricular depolarization is from left to right of the interventricular septum. Because the mean frontal conduction axis is away from left and inferior precordial leads, the initial QRS force is negative, and Q wave in leads V5 and V6 is observed. In CCTGA, the initial depolarization direction reversed because of inverted left and right bundle branches. The ECG finding includes the absence of Q wave in leads V5 and V6 and the presence of QS complex in leads V4R and V1, large Q wave in leads III and aVF, left axis deviation, and first-degree AV block present in 50 % of patients.

The CCTGA can also present with complete AV block. Complete AV block occurs in 4 % newborns with CCTGA that may be progressive and lifetime incidence is 20–30 % (Huhta et al. 1983). CCTGA is also on the top list of postsurgical complete AV block. The presence of accessory pathway and WPW syndrome is more common in CCTGA.

Cardiomyopathy

Hypertrophic Cardiomyopathy

Hypertrophic cardiomyopathy (HCM) is characterized by LVH without any obvious cause. The ECG patterns of HCM are nonspecific. The voltage criteria of LVH including tall R wave in left precordial leads and deep S wave in right precordial leads are usually observed. The ST-T changes and LA enlargement are other ECG findings. These criteria did not correlate well with severity of LVH and LV outflow tract obstruction.

With progression of disease, the ischemic ECG pattern as deep Q wave in inferior and left lateral precordial leads appears. Interestingly, the ECG pattern of RVH may be seen in an infant with HCM. In the presence of giant negative T waves in left precordial leads, apical HCM should be considered.

Chronic pressure overload on ischemic LV myocardium predisposes patient to ventricular tachyarrhythmia and ectopy. Preexcitation is reported in some form of HCM with genetic basis. In addition, other supraventricular tachyarrhythmias, including atrial tachycardia, atrial flutter, and atrial fibrillation, have been reported.

Dilated Cardiomyopathy

The DCM is the primary myocardial involvement with dilatation of LA and LV. In DCM, ECG shows LVH and LA enlargement. The nonspecific ST-T changes were seen. Several types of supraventricular and ventricular arrhythmias are seen in DCM, and ventricular arrhythmia is one of the main causes of death.

Arrhythmogenic Right Ventricular Cardiomyopathy/Dysplasia

Arrhythmogenic right ventricular cardiomyopathy/dysplasia (ARVC/D) is the genetic disorder with fibrofatty replacement of the myocardial tissue that involves mainly the right ventricle. The disease is usually inherited as autosomal dominant.

ECG usually shows depolarization and repolarization abnormalities. These patients may be present with ventricular arrhythmia, syncope, and sudden cardiac death. Epsilon wave (any deflection between end of QRS complex and onset of T

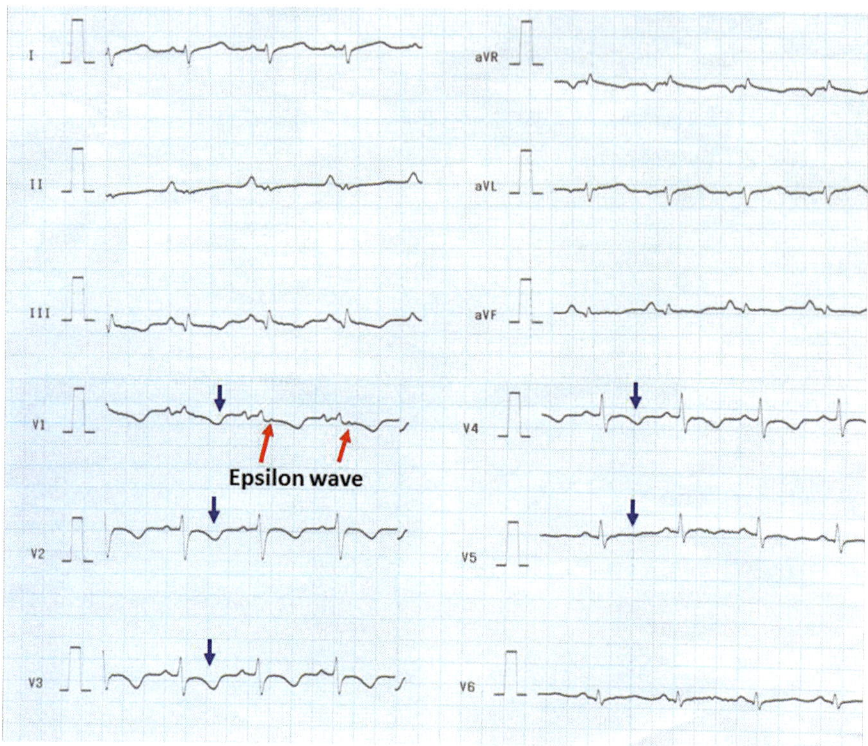

Fig. 8.22 Arrhythmogenic right ventricular cardiomyopathy/dysplasia. Pathognomonic signs are epsilon waves (*red arrows*) and T-wave inversion in leads V1–V3 and beyond

wave in leads V1–V3) is the characteristic ECG finding on ECG (Fig. 8.22) (Marcus et al. 2010). Epsilon wave is more common in children than adult. Isolated wide QRS complexes in right precordial leads and T-wave inversion in leads V1–V3 and beyond are other characteristic findings; however, negative T wave in leads V1 and V2 may be normal variant in children.

Due to progressive nature of myocardium disease, ventricular arrhythmias are more common in ARVD/C and may be life threatening. VT usually has left bundle branch block pattern but other forms such as polymorphic VT and VF were also observed.

Restrictive Cardiomyopathy

The RCM is a myocardial disease that is characterized with restricted ventricular filling. Severe biatrial enlargement with small-sized ventricles is typical echocardiographic findings. The constant ECG findings are LA enlargement, RA enlargement, or both. Other ECG finding includes LVH, RVH, ST-T changes, and ST-segment depression.

Due to the nature of the RCM, arrhythmias are common. Atrial flutter is the most common type of arrhythmia in these patients. Other types of atrial arrhythmias are also observed. AV block was also reported especially in familial RCM (Fitzpatrick et al. 1990; Walsh et al. 2012).

Dystrophies

Duchenne Muscular Dystrophy

In Duchenne muscular dystrophy (DMD), progressive myocardial fibrosis results in severe heart failure. ECG finding includes short PR interval, deep Q waves in lateral and left precordial leads, and RVH pattern (Perloff et al. 1967). A prolonged QT interval was reported in some patients. Supraventricular and ventricular arrhythmia are common in end stage of disease. Becker muscular dystrophy is other dystrophinopathy that has slower progressive pattern, and ECG finding is similar to DMD.

Myotonic Muscular Dystrophy

Myotonic muscular dystrophy (MMD) is the most common type of muscular dystrophy with autosomal dominant inheritance (Pelargonio et al. 2002). In contrast to other muscular dystrophies, MMD is manifested by progressive conduction system abnormalities. Therefore, different types of conduction abnormalities, including first-degree AV block, second- and third-degree AV blocks, and wide QRS, may be observed.

These patients have slower rate in comparison to other normal children. The QT interval is prolonged and predisposes patients to torsades de pointes. Ventricular arrhythmia, atrial flutter, and atrial fibrillation may occur in this disorder (Facenda-Lorenzoa et al. 2013).

Inflammatory Conditions

Kawasaki Disease

Kawasaki disease is an autoimmune heart disease that is characterized by coronary vasculitis and may result in aneurysmal formation, thrombosis, and myocardial infarction.

In acute phase, ECG finding of myocarditis is usually observed. Low-voltage QRS complexes, ST-T changes, and sinus tachycardia may occur. Aneurysmal formation in coronary artery may lead to thrombosis and myocardial infarction. The posterior wall myocardial infarction occurred following RCA involvement that characterized by deep Q-waves and ST-segment elevation in inferior leads (Surnitorno et al. 2008).

Pericarditis

Pericarditis is an inflammatory disease of the pericardium. Pericarditis is the most common cause of ST elevation in children. ECG is a useful tool for evaluation of pericarditis. In pericarditis, ECG changes are usually classified to four stages:

1. *Stage 1*: ST-segment elevation appears in almost all leads, especially lateral and inferior leads with PR interval depression.
2. *Stage 2*: ST- and PR-segment returns to normal baseline.
3. *Stage 3*: Diffuse T-wave inversion.
4. *Stage 4*: ECG returns to normal usually 2–4 weeks after onset of disease.

Massive pericardial effusion with low-voltage QRS and QRS alternans are other ECG findings in pericarditis. QRS alternans is defined as periodic change in QRS amplitude.

Myocarditis

The myocarditis is an inflammatory myocardial process that terminated in myocardial necrosis. The primary change in ECG is sinus tachycardia. The low-voltage QRS complex and ST-T changes are seen due to diffuse damage to myocardium. The PR prolongation and increased QT interval may be seen. Q waves indicate acute myocardial necrosis. The myocardium inflammation predisposes these patients to several ventricular and supraventricular arrhythmias.

Acute Rheumatic Fever

Acute rheumatic fever (ARF) is a cardiac inflammatory process following pharyngeal streptococcus infection. PR interval prolongation is one of the well-known diagnostic criteria for ARF.

In chronic rheumatic heart disease with mild valvulitis, the ECG usually will be normal. The ECG finding in chronic mitral regurgitation shows LA enlargement and LVH. LA enlargement will be significant in mitral stenosis and also RVH gradually appeared. Atrial enlargement is a substrate for supraventricular arrhythmia. Aortic valve is the second common valve that involved in ARF. Aortic regurgitation manifested with LVH on ECG.

Cardiac Tumors

Rhabdomyoma

Rhabdomyoma is the most common type of cardiac tumor in children. The ECG pattern depends on the size of tumor and proximity to conduction system. In large rhabdomyomas, ECG shows ventricular hypertrophy and ST-T changes. Conduction system compression by tumor may produce AV block and bundle branch block.

Effects of tumor on hemodynamic condition and conduction system involvement predisposed these patients to supraventricular or ventricular tachyarrhythmias. Preexcitation has also been reported. Rhabdomyomas may regress with time; therefore, preexcitation and other arrhythmia may resolve spontaneously.

In some patients, ventricular arrhythmia may be sustained and resistance to drug therapy and radiofrequency catheter ablation. In this condition, tumor resection is the only definite way for treatment (Miyake et al. 2011).

Fibroma

Fibroma is the single intramural tumor most commonly found in the LV. The ECG pattern is similar to rhabdomyomas. Arrhythmia is usually presented as ventricular tachycardia that may be fatal in some cases (Miyake et al. 2011).

Myxoma

Myxoma is the single left atrium tumor that may be obstructing LV inflow. ECG showed LA enlargement and in large tumors RVH gradually appeared because of pulmonary hypertension. Tumor embolization to pulmonary artery also results in RVH pattern on ECG (Zitnik and Giuliani 1970).

References

Bailey JJ, Berson AS, Garson A. Recommendations for standardization and specifications in automated electrocardiography: bandwidth and digital signal processing. Circulation. 1990;81: 730–9.

Bazett HC. An analysis of the time-relations of electrocardiograms. Heart. 1920;7:353–70.

Cappato R, Schluter M, Weiss C, et al. Radiofrequency current catheter ablation of accessory atrioventricular pathways in Ebstein's anomaly. Circulation. 1996;94:376–83.

Coviello SJ. ECG interpretation made incredibly easy. 6th ed. Philadelphia: Wolters Kluwer; 2016, NLM ID: 101658311.

Davia JE, Cheitlin MD, Bedynek JL. Sinus venosus atrial septal defect: analysis of fifty cases. Am Heart J. 1973;85:177–85.

Davignon A, Rautaharju P, Boisselle E. Normal ECG standards for infants and children. Pediatr Cardiol. 1979;1:123–31.

Deal BJ, Johnsrude CL, Buck SH. Pediatric ECG Interpretation: a illustrative guide. Wiley-Blackwell | ISBN: 1405117303 | 2004-07-30.

Dick M, Fyler DC, Nadas AS. Tricuspid atresia: the clinical course in 101 patients. Am J Cardiol. 1975;36:327–37.

Dickinson DF. The normal ECG in childhood and adolescence. Heart. 2005;91:1626–30.

Facenda-Lorenzoa M, Hernández-Afonsoa J, Rodríguez-Estebana M. Cardiac manifestations in myotonic dystrophy type 1 patients followed using a standard protocol in a specialized unit. Rev Esp Cardiol. 2013;66:193–7.

Fitzpatrick AP, Shapiro LM, Rickards AF, et al. Familial restrictive cardiomyopathy with atrioventricular block and skeletal myopathy. Br Heart J. 1990;63:114–8.

Gamboa R, Gersony WM, Nadas AS. The electrocardiogram in tricuspid atresia and pulmonary atresia with intact ventricular septum. Circulation. 1966;34:24–37.

Gatzoulis M, Till J, Somerville J. Mechanoelectrical interaction in tetralogy of Fallot QRS prolongation relates to right ventricular size and predicts malignant ventricular arrhythmias and sudden death. Circulation. 1995;92:231–7.

Ho SY, Anderson RH. Conduction tissue in congenital heart surgery. World J Surg. 1985;9:550.

Huhta C, Maloney D, Ritter DC. Complete atrioventricular block in patients with atrioventricular discordance. Circulation. 1983;67:1374–7.

Katz LN, Wachtel H. The diphasic QRS type of electrocardiogram in congenital heart disease. Am Herat J. 1937;13:202–6.

Marcus F, McKenna W, Sherrill D. Diagnosis of arrhythmogenic right ventricular cardiomyopathy/dysplasia proposed modification of the task force criteria. Circulation. 2010;121:1533–41.

Miyake C, Del Nido P, Alexander M. Cardiac tumors and associated arrhythmias in pediatric patients, with observations on surgical therapy for ventricular tachycardia. J Am Coll Cardiol. 2011;58(18):1903–9.

O'Connor M, McDaniel N, Brady WJ. The pediatric electrocardiogram. Part I: age-related interpretation. Am J Emerg Med. 2008;26:221–8.

Park MK. Park's pediatric cardiology for practitioners. 6th ed. 2014, ISBN: 978-0-323-16951-6.

Pelargonio G, Russo D, Sanna T. Myotonic dystrophy and the heart. Heart. 2002;88(6):665–70.

Perloff K, Roberts WC, deLeon AC. The distinctive electrocardiogram of Duchenne's progressive muscular dystrophy. An electrocardiographic pathologic correlative study. Am J Med. 1967;42:179–88.

Reich- JD, Auld D, Hulse E. The Pediatric Radiofrequency Ablation Registry's experience with Ebstein's anomaly. Pediatric Electrophysiology Society. J Cardiovasc Electrophysiol. 1998;9:1370–7.

Schwartz PJ, Garson Jr A, Paul T. Guidelines for the interpretation of the neonatal electrocardiogram. A Task Force of the European Society of Cardiology. Eur Heart J. 2002;23:1329–44.

Surnitorno N, Karasawa K, Taniguchi K, et al. Association of sinus node dysfunction, atrioventricular node conduction abnormality and ventricular arrhythmia in patients with Kawasaki disease and coronary involvement. Circ J. 2008;72:274–80.

Wagner HR, Weidman WH, Ellison RC. Indirect assessment of severity in aortic stenosis. Circulation. 1977;56:120–3.

Walsh M, Grenier M, Jefferies J. Conduction abnormalities in pediatric patients with restrictive cardiomyopathy. Circ Heart Fail. 2012;5:267–73.

Wolfe RR, Driscoll DJ, Gersony WM. Report from the Second Joint Study on the Natural History of Congenital Heart Defects (NHS-2): arrhythmias in patients valvar aortic stenosis, pulmonary stenosis, and ventricular septal defects: results of twenty-four ECG monitoring. Circulation. 1993;87:189–1101.

Zitnik RS, Giuliani ER. Clinical recognition of atrial myxoma. Am Heart J. 1970;80:689–700.

Zufelt K, Rosenberg HC, Li MD. The electrocardiogram and the secundum atrial septal defect: a reexamination in the era of echocardiography. Can J Cardiol. 1998;14(2):227–32.

Chapter 9
Central Nervous System Monitoring in Pediatric Cardiac Surgery

Ali Dabbagh and Michael A.E. Ramsay

Introduction: The Role of CNS Monitoring in Pediatric Cardiac Surgery

During the last decades, significant improvements have been gained in general surgical outcome of congenital heart surgeries, especially in the neonates and younger children. However, these improvements have led us to focus more on clinical outcome of these patients, especially regarding neurodevelopmental indices. In fact, with improved surgical techniques, postoperative CNS outcome is one of the most important long-term concerns and one of the most important outcome surrogates for CHD surgeries. Postoperative neurologic complications could be potentially more frequent and much more serious as much as the age of surgery declines, usually neonates being the most vulnerable patient group (Ghanayem et al. 2010; Snookes et al. 2010).

On the other hand, among perioperative CNS injuries, nowadays, we focus on impairments more than just seizures and focal lesions, while these are still considered significant. Reports have demonstrated the incidence of major CNS lesions after CHD surgeries not more than 10 %, while the incidence of cognitive impairments is up to 50 %, based on the center and the duration of follow-up years (Markowitz et al. 2007; Ghanayem et al. 2010).

A. Dabbagh, MD, FCA (✉)
Cardiac Anesthesiology Department, Anesthesiology Research Center,
Shahid Beheshti University of Medical Sciences, Tehran, Iran
e-mail: alidabbagh@yahoo.com, alidabbagh@sbmu.ac.ir

M.A.E. Ramsay, MD, FRCA
Texas A&M Health Science Center, Baylor University Medical Center and
President of Baylor Research Institute, Dallas, TX, USA
e-mail: michaera@BaylorHealth.edu

© Springer International Publishing Switzerland 2017
A. Dabbagh et al. (eds.), *Congenital Heart Disease in Pediatric
and Adult Patients*, DOI 10.1007/978-3-319-44691-2_9

"

Postoperative cognitive impairments (POCI) in pediatric CHD surgeries could be categorized into these subgroups:

- Cognitive dysfunction (including language impairments)
- Impairments in organization of motor functions (including fine and gross motor impairments, visual-spatial dysfunctions, etc.)
- Emotional health dysfunction and functional limitations including attention deficit disorder, behavioral impairments, internalizing problems, externalizing problems, functional limitations in socialization, impairments in daily living skills, defects in communication, and impairments in adaptive behavior (Bellinger et al. 1997; Limperopoulos et al. 2001; Markowitz et al. 2007; Majnemer et al. 2008)

Clinical Assessment of Pain and Sedation in Postoperative Period in Children

Pediatric patient arousal state and responsiveness are always a clinical challenge. Many pediatric sedation assessment scales have been clinically used for many years; however, the core outcome measured by each of them is not the same.

When dealing with CNS, both the *level of consciousness* and the *pain state* are important.

Assessment of Pain

The reader is referred to the chapter dealing with *postoperative pain in pediatric cardiac anesthesia* in this book; however, a brief summary of the most commonly used scales is presented here. More than 20 observational *pain scales* have been assessed and reviewed in two systematic reviews (von Baeyer and Spagrud 2007; McGrath et al. 2008). Based on these studies and other similar ones, the following five scales are much more suitable for pediatric patients undergoing cardiac surgery:

The Children's Hospital of Eastern Ontario Pain Scale (CHEOPS)
The Face, Legs, Activity, Cry, Consolability Scale (also modified FLACC)
The COMFORT Scale
The Toddler Preschool Postoperative Pain Scale (TPPPS)
The Parents' Postoperative Pain Measure (PPPM)

The Children's Hospital of Eastern Ontario Pain Scale: CHEOPS

First introduced in 1985 by McGrath et al., CHEOPS is an observational pain assessment tool in 1–7-year-old children. This scale has well-established reliability and validity. CHEOPS has six items scored 0–3 and the final score ranges from 4 to 13, with final score of 4–6 denoting "no pain." The items assessed in CHEOPS are:

- Cry (1–3)
- Facial expression (1–3)
- Verbalization (0–2)
- Activity of torso (1–2)
- Touch (1–2)
- Response of legs (1–2)

The scale is more appropriate for *postoperative pain* assessment and *procedural pain* assessment (McGrath PJ et al. 1985; Merkel et al. 1997; von Baeyer and Spagrud 2007; McGrath et al. 2008).

Face, Legs, Activity, Cry, Consolability Scale (FLACC)

It was first described by Merkel et al. in 1997. FLACC is the acronym for ingredients of pain assessment checklist. In fact, the items used in FLACC are much similar to CHEOPS but are designed in 0–10 metrics to make it easier to use. FLACC includes five items, each scoring 0–2 with a total score range of 0–10 with 0 representing no pain; it is applicable for children in 4–18 years old. Also, FLACC could be used in children with cognitive impairment. The items assessed in FLACC are:

- Face (0–2)
- Legs (0–2)
- Activity (0–2)
- Cry (0–2)
- Consolability (0–2)

FLACC has relatively fair reliability but moderate validity and is appropriate for assessment of *postoperative pain in hospital* and *procedural pain*; however, Crellin et al. questioned using FLACC in all circumstances and populations to which is currently applied (Merkel et al. 1997; Malviya et al. 2006; von Baeyer and Spagrud 2007; McGrath et al. 2008; Verghese and Hannallah 2010; Voepel-Lewis et al. 2010; Crellin et al. 2015).

COMFORT Scale

First described by Ambuel et al. in 1992, currently COMFORT is the only scale available for *children on ventilator* or in *critical care setting*. It is composed of eight items; each item could be ranked 0–5, and the final score will be from a minimum of 8 up to a maximum of 40. Among the items, 2 of 8 are directly hemodynamic variables; the items assessed in COMFORT are:

- Alertness (1–5)
- Calmness/agitation (1–5)
- Respiratory response (1–5)
- Physical movement (1–5)
- Blood pressure (1–5)

- Heart rate (1–5)
- Muscle tone (1–5)
- Facial tension (1–5)

COMFORT is one of the best available scales for assessment of sedation in *mechanically ventilated* patients, especially in patients undergoing cardiac surgery. It has good reliability and internal consistency (Ambuel et al. 1992; Johansson and Kokinsky 2009; Lamas and Lopez-Herce 2010; Voepel-Lewis et al. 2010).

Toddler Preschool Postoperative Pain Scale (TPPPS)

TPPPS was first described by Tarbell et al. in 1992; the scale is most applicable for children aged 1–5 years. TPPPS is consisted of 3 main pain categories:

- Vocal expression of pain (composed of 3 pain behaviors)
- Facial expression of pain (composed of 3 pain behaviors)
- Bodily expression of pain (composed of 1 pain behavior)

Minimum score in TPPPS would be 0 (no pain) and maximum score 7 (most severe pain). It is best used for *postoperative pain* with satisfactory reliability and good validity (Tarbell et al. 1992; von Baeyer and Spagrud 2007; McGrath et al. 2008).

Parents' Postoperative Pain Measure (PPPM)

PPPM was introduced in 1996 by Chambers et al. and is used for 2–12-year-old children. It includes 15 items each scored 0 or 1 (a dichotomal approach using *YES* or *NO* basis for parents); hence, the scores will range from a minimum of 0 to a maximum of 15. PPPM has good reliability and high validity. Its unique feature is that PPPM measures *postoperative pain at home* using parents' assessments with high reliability and good validity (Chambers et al. 1996; von Baeyer and Spagrud 2007; McGrath et al. 2008).

Assessment of Sedation

The scales used for assessment of sedation in the clinical setting of pediatric ICU are numerous; however, these scales are the main scales used for this purpose:

Ramsay Sedation Scale (Ramsay)
Sedation Agitation Scale (SAS)
Richmond Agitation Sedation Scale (RASS)

The scales are clinical assessment scales; it means that patient arousal state and responsiveness are the basis for their assessment.

Ramsay Sedation Scale (Ramsay)

Ramsay Sedation Scale was first introduced in 1974 and has been widely used thereafter. In this scale, six scores are arranged from 1 to 6 (Table 9.1). The "cooperative, orientated, and tranquil" patient is scored 2 (Ramsay et al. 1974).

Richmond Agitation Sedation Scale (RASS)

RASS needs minimal training, and less than 1 min is needed for assessment of the patient using this scale. However, RASS should be determined in the very first assessment of patient arousal state to see if the patient is "alert and calm" equaling "zero." Then, throughout ICU care, the patient should be reassessed using Confusion Assessment Method in the ICU (CAM-ICU) and be rechecked (Table 9.2). In brief, RASS has ten grades ranging from +4 to −5:

- +4 to +1: combative to restless stages
- 0 (zero score): "alert and calm" patient
- −1 to −5: drowsy to unarousable patient

Table 9.1 A summary of Ramsay Sedation Scale

Score	Clinical description
1	Patient anxious and agitated or restless or both
2	Patient cooperative, orientated, and tranquil
3	Patient asleep, *responds* to commands
4	Patient asleep, with *brisk* response to light glabellar tap or loud auditory stimulus
5	Patient asleep, with *sluggish* response to light glabellar tap or loud auditory stimulus
6	*Unresponsive* to any stimulus

Modified from Ramsay et al. (1974)

Table 9.2 A summary of the Richmond Agitation Sedation Scale (RASS)

Score	Clinical term	Stimulus
+4	Combative	VOICE (verbal stimulation)
+3	Very agitated	
+2	Agitated	
+1	Restless	
0	Alert and calm	
−1	Drowsy	
−2	Light sedation	
−3	Moderate sedation	
−4	Deep sedation	TOUCH (physical stimulation)
−5	Unarousable	

Modified from Dabbagh (2014) (Published with kind permission of © Springer, 2014. All Rights Reserved)

The interested reader could find the full scale in Sessler et al. and Ely et al. (Sessler et al. 2002; Ely et al. 2003).

Sedation Agitation Scale (SAS)

SAS is shorter than RASS; it starts from 1 and leads to 7. SAS has seven scores (without negative scores), while score 4 stands exactly at the middle and is for the "calm and cooperative patient" (Table 9.3) (Riker et al. 1999; Simmons et al. 1999).

Near Infrared Spectroscopy (NIRS)

Though introduced in laboratory studies for nearly 40 years, this is just about a decade that NIRS has been used in the clinical setting for CNS monitoring.

Nearly 40 years has passed from the time that Professor "Frans Jöbsis" introduced the technology of *near infrared spectroscopy* (NIRS) for clinical application as a monitor in 1977 (Wolf et al. 2007).

The monitor is at times known as cerebral oximetry because the frontal area of the cortex is the most common site for its application; however, other parts of the body, for example, the flanks, have been used frequently during the previous years as an index of somatic perfusion and oxygenation status; hence, NIRS is often the general accepted term.

NIRS is used in many clinical states and procedures including cardiac surgery; in cardiac surgery, NIRS is an important component of *perioperative multimodal CNS monitoring*.

Both animal models and human studies have demonstrated its usefulness; though some controversies may exist, including some types of cyanotic patients, these studies at times question the effect of NIRS application on patient outcome (especially the systematic review recently published by Zheng et al. (2013)). Also, other studies have some other considerations especially for pediatric congenital heart surgery patients (Gottlieb and Mossad 2014).

Table 9.3 A summary of the Sedation Agitation Scale (SAS)

Score	Clinical term
7	Dangerous agitation
6	Very agitated
5	Agitated
4	Calm and cooperative
3	Sedated
2	Very sedated
1	Unarousable

Modified from Dabbagh (2014) (Published with kind permission of © Springer, 2014. All Rights Reserved)

NIRS has these advantages:

- Monitoring is noninvasive, providing real-time, continuous data.
- Monitors not only the CNS status but also some aspects of hemodynamics since it monitors both oxygenation and perfusion status (i.e., mandates appropriate hemodynamic of CNS).
- During all the perioperative period, NIRS has its merits.
- During cardiopulmonary bypass or during cardiac arrest, NIRS still works, not needing a pulsatile flow like pulse oximetry.

Technology of NIRS: near infrared (NIR) light in the range of 700–1000 nm is radiated through self-adhesive optodes; then, penetration, passage, and reflection of NIR light are through the skull or other underlying tissues; specific calculations are used for estimation of NIRS. However, the NIR light, when penetrated through, for example, the skull bone, is partly absorbed by biologic chromophores like oxyhemoglobin (OHb), deoxyhemoglobin (HHb), and cytochrome oxidase, while the rest of the light is returned back and is used for data measurement and calculations of the software to demonstrate the final refracted number of the oximetry; the calculations are based on the "modified Beer-Lambert law."

Light reflection is the basic mechanism of NIRS, while light transmission through, for example, the fingertip is used in pulse oximetry; this technology difference is the reason why we can attach the optodes of NIRS to the skull (for cerebral oximetry) or flank (for somatic and visceral oximetry), finally demonstrating the figures of rSO_2 on the monitor screen. The NIRS optodes have a number of "light emitting diodes" (LEDs) (Fig. 9.1).

> The differential absorption of near infrared light in the range of 700–1000 nm through the skin, bone, or other underlying tissues is used for NIRS.

NIRS compares each patient with himself/herself; it means that for each patient, a baseline is measured at the first time; then, on a real-time basis, any subsequent change is compared with the baseline: more than 20% change is considered as a significant change needing some intervention to restore NIRS numbers to normal. Also, the absolute number for NIRS is defined from 40 to 90 (Fig. 9.2).

What Really NIRS Measures NIRS measures O_2 content of the target tissue; the final figures are the result of balance between tissue oxygen supply and consumption (Fig. 9.1); in other words, the trend of NIRS shows the trend of changes in tissue oxygen content. But what factors affect tissue oxygen content?

In the brain tissue, the following factors are among the main ones affecting cerebral oxygen content:

- *Cerebral tissue oxygen delivery* to the organ through the blood which is determined by arterial oxygen saturation, hemoglobin, and arterial oxygen content.
- *Cerebral hemodynamics.* A number of factors alter cerebral hemodynamics:

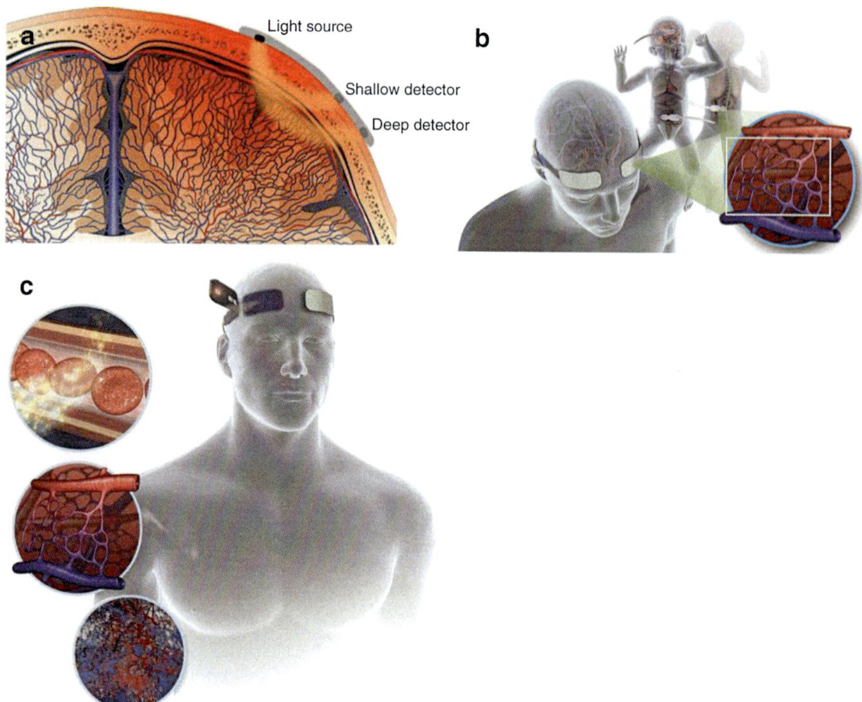

Fig. 9.1 (**a**) Schematic drawing of light transmission through skull with two depth of light penetration with resultant regional values; (**b**): the final figures of NIRS are the result of balance between tissue oxygen supply and consumption; (**c**) mechanism of NIRS in microvasculature (Published with kind permission of © Medtronic, 2016. All Rights Reserved)

Fig. 9.2 Intraoperative bilateral NIRS for cerebral oxygenation monitoring (Published with kind permission of © Medtronic, 2016. All Rights Reserved)

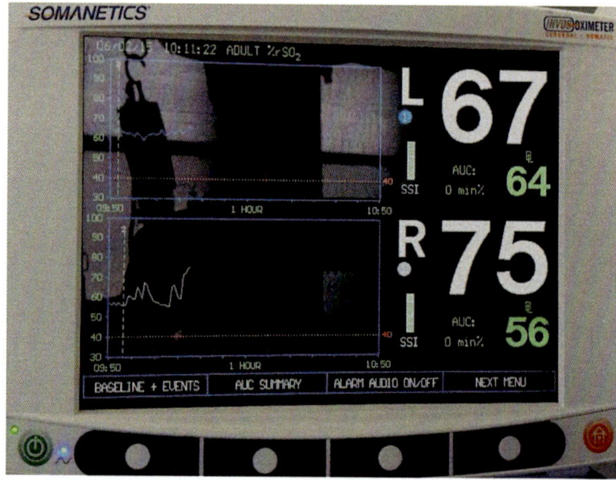

1. *Systolic, diastolic, and mean arterial pressure*; hypotension decreases tissue oxygen delivery; carotid stump pressure is the most important pressure.
2. *Patency of cerebral arteries* due to any underlying obstruction (permanent or transient), for example, extraordinary rotation of the head could affect tissue oxygen delivery, and mechanical impedance against blood flow decreases tissue oxygen delivery.
3. *Vasoactive drugs* strongly affect cerebral blood and oxygen delivery.
4. *Cerebral venous drainage* (including any hindrance in cerebral veins) decreases tissue oxygen delivery.

- *Cerebral tissue oxygen expenditure* which is determined by cerebral tissue metabolism:

  1. *Seizure* activity or *fever* increases tissue oxygen consumption.
  2. *Level of anesthesia* (including sedation or consciousness state) affects the level of cerebral activity; the deeper the patient, the less oxygen demand; insufficient anesthesia level increases tissue oxygen consumption.
  3. *Tissue temperature* affects tissue metabolism and hypothermia decreases tissue oxygen demand.

Practical notes for using cerebral NIRS: there are a number of notes that one should consider during clinical practice for using cerebral NIRS:

- Correct attachment of the probes: the underneath of the probes should be fine with no hair beneath; also, when using two probes, they should be symmetrical.
- For neonates and small children, either neonatal probes should be used or one probe should be attached to the frontal area; however, when one probe is used, the differentiation property between right and left perfusion through carotids is not well gained; this is why using separate probes for each side of the frontal area is recommended.
- Baseline figures should be taken for each patient and they are very important; each patient is compared with its baseline.
- NIRS has been traditionally known as a CNS monitor; however, it has recently been used in pediatric patients and neonates as a *somatic monitor*; so it could monitor other tissues to check if their oxygenation is appropriate in some parts of the body like splanchnic perfusion, renal perfusion, and spinal cord perfusion (Fig. 9.3). The difference between somatic and cerebral NIRS should not be more than 15–20; increased difference suggests a drop in cerebral tissue oxygen content, and its etiology should be sought. Usually, somatic NIRS reading is higher than cerebral NIRS, but if somatic NIRS drops, there is something wrong in somatic perfusion mandating a revision of whole body perfusion state. This is why both cerebral and somatic NIRS could be used as appropriate surrogates for treatment of perfusion impairments, for both regional and global impairments (Nelson et al. 2008; Murkin and Arango 2009; Tweddell et al. 2010; Gil-Anton et al. 2015).

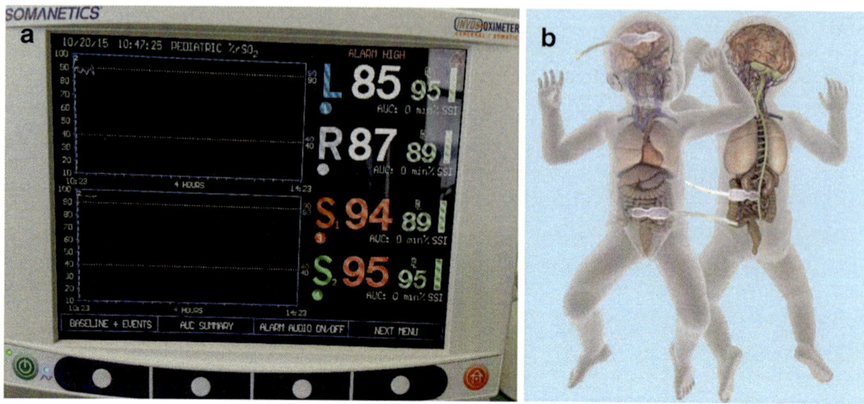

Fig. 9.3 (**a**) Intraoperative NIRS demonstrating both cerebral and somatic NIRS; the lower half of the monitor panel shows the results of somatic optodes (S_1 and S_2); (**b**) schematic drawing of cerebral and somatic NIRS (Published with kind permission of © Medtronic, 2016. All Rights Reserved)

- When considering the *postoperative period*, acceptable NIRS results (cerebral and especially somatic) could be good predictors for successful weaning and extubation (Gil-Anton et al. 2015).
- In patients with extracorporeal support devices (including ECMO, RV, or LV assist devices), NIRS could be of very good benefit (Papademetriou et al. 2012).
- Some species of *hemoglobin* (like sickle cell) or very high concentration of hemoglobin (e.g., patients with severe polycythemia) might have interference with real results of cerebral NIRS; other factors like skin pigmentation, ambient light, or injected dyes might produce interference (Gottlieb and Mossad 2014).
- Underlying cardiopulmonary impairments, anemia, or vascular diseases might be confounders of NIRS readings.

In clinical practice, any decline in regional cerebral NIRS reading often needs an algorithmic approach involving the following steps (Denault et al. 2007; Murkin and Arango 2009):

1. Turn position of the head to a neutral position to relieve any underlying mechanical obstruction due to excessive lateral rotation.
2. Ask surgeon to control the position of arterial and/or venous cannula to relieve obstructions in blood flow.
3. Correct hypotension (especially mean arterial pressure).
4. Diagnose and treat any underlying systemic desaturation (blood gas and/or pulse oximetry).
5. Correct excessive hyperventilation; $PaCO_2$ especially below 35 mmHg should be corrected.
6. Diagnose and treat anemia especially when hematocrit is below 30 %.
7. Check cerebral oxygen consumption state, treat any underlying seizure or convulsive activity, detect any episodes of hyperthermia or fever and treat them, check the level of anesthesia or sedation, and add the depth of anesthesia or sedate the patient more as needed.

8. Diagnose and treat any underlying pump failure, including possible failing heart or inadequate flow of pump or inadequate perfusion by assist devices; modalities like echocardiography, jugular venous blood oxygen saturation ($SjVO_2$), or metabolic assessments like lactate level could be useful guides.
9. Diagnose and treat any possible etiologies causing cerebral edema and/or increased intracranial pressure; diagnose with imaging modalities or intracranial pressure monitors and treat increased ICP with positioning and medical treatments.

Electroencephalography (EEG) Including Traditional EEG, qEEG, and CCEEG

History of EEG

EEG is an invention by the German psychiatrist Hans Berger who described the electrical recordings of the brain in 1926 for the first time; his records are still valid. Nowadays, after decades and also with improvements in this technology, EEG is still a very useful diagnostic and monitoring tool, though it is considered a *good* CNS monitoring but not a *perfect* one.

Here we discuss EEG in two main topics:

1. The basic standards of EEG including basic technical requirements and how EEG works
2. Using EEG in perioperative period as continuous CNS monitor

In both of the above segments, we will always consider two age ranges:

1. Adult and older pediatric patients
2. Neonates and small pediatric group

The current discussion on EEG has contributions from two main sources:

- The guidelines published by American Clinical Neurophysiology Society (1994, 2006a, b; Herman et al. 2015a, b); list of the guidelines and statements of the American Clinical Neurophysiology Society is available at its website: https://www.acns.org/practice/guidelines.
- The guidelines and statements released by American Society of Neurophysiological Monitoring (Isley et al. 2009); their position statements are available at http://www.asnm.org/.

What Are the Applications of EEG in the Perioperative Period?

There are a number of main reasons for using EEG in the *perioperative period*, including (Isley et al. 2009; Edmonds et al. 2011):

Detection and diagnosis of any *underlying CNS pathology* or any *baseline disorder*; for this purpose, it is important to have a baseline EEG for further assessments and documentations; this is especially a major consideration in patients with underlying disease or potential risk factors for ischemia.

Detection and documentation of any *new abnormality* in CNS function in the perioperative period; these new findings should be diagnosed and if needed, be treated soon.

As a *continuous monitoring device* and a real-time neurologic assessment tool and a *diagnostic tool* for detection of seizure or other CNS events like coma, brain death, drug toxicities, or possibility of residual anesthetic effects.

Titrating the dosage of *anesthetics* and *sedatives* during perioperative period.

During early *rewarming from cardiopulmonary bypass*, often an imbalance between brain oxygen demands and oxygen delivery occurs which could be a potential etiology for brain ischemia.

A *therapy tailoring guide* which is used for monitoring the dosage of anticonvulsants and their efficacy in controlling clinical and subclinical seizure activity; so EEG works as a guide for titration of drug dosage (like anticonvulsant dose) in order to guarantee drug efficacy.

In barbiturate-induced or hypothermia-induced coma, when we need objective confirmation of *cortical silence* which needs monitoring the efficacy of cerebral protection strategies during the perioperative period.

Tailoring appropriate critical perioperative care in patients at risk of even borderline ischemic events; for example, prevention of adverse effects of *hyperventilation* on cerebral perfusion, prevention of deleterious effects of acute *hemodilution* (both intraoperative, during cardiopulmonary bypass, or postoperative), and prevention of adverse effects during *rewarming* from cardiopulmonary bypass or hyperthermia in postoperative period.

How EEG Works (Including 10/20 System and the Waves)

The standard electrode system is the 10/20 electrode system of the International Federation of Clinical Neurophysiology and American Clinical Neurophysiology Society (Klem et al. 1999; 2006e; Isley et al. 2009).

The main source for EEG waves is the postsynaptic activity of cortical neurons; these neurons, called "pyramid" cortical cells or "Betz" cells, are located in the outermost layer of the brain cortex just underneath and perpendicular to the skull. Having very long axons extending toward the inner parts of the brain, EEG is the summative activity of millions of these pyramids; i.e., only the *postsynaptic* electrical currents of pyramids (both excitatory and inhibitory functions) accumulate and create EEG waves; however, the axonal activity does not contribute in production of EEG waves. Often, the following characteristics are considered as the main features of EEG waves:

1. *Frequency*: the number of time that each wave occurs in each second, presented as Hz; each EEG wave is usually consisted of at least two basic waves which are

overlapped together and compose the final waves; the composing waves could be analyzed by Fourier analysis; Table 9.4 is a summary of basic EEG waves; we could use this mnemonic for EEG waves GBATDS.

2. *Time*: is demonstrated on horizontal axis of EEG records.
3. *Amplitude*: EEG waves have an amplitude between 10 and 100 100 µV, which is about 100 times less than the amplitude of electrocardiography waves; with increasing age, the amplitude of EEG waves decreases.

Table 9.4 Normal EEG rhythms; i.e., EEG waves (mnemonics: GBATDS)

Wave category	Symbol	Frequency	Amplitude and/or voltage	Related activity	Clinical equivalent
Gamma rhythm	γ	25.1–55 Hz	High voltage and amplitude	Corticothalamic perception; both during wakefulness and sleep	Engaged in: Sensory processing activities Perception process
Beta rhythm	β	12.6–25 Hz	In adults 10–20 µV	Cortico-cortical network	Fully awake patient with: Open eyes Mental activity
Alpha rhythm	α	8–12.5 Hz	Relatively high voltage and amplitude: 30–50 µV In adults: 10–20 µV	Mainly composed of electrical activity emerged from parietal and occipital lobes of the corticothalamic network	Awake, but relaxed individual with closed eyes Equals drowsy state
Theta rhythm	θ	4–8 Hz	50–100 µV In adults: 10–20 µV	Often seen in temporal lobes in the awake state but sleepy and relaxed And corticothalamic activity and limbic activity	Equals stage 2 of sleep (i.e., light sleep) or drowsy state Also, frequently seen in young children
Delta rhythm	δ	1–4 Hz	High amplitude 100–200 µV	Corticothalamic dissociation	Equals deep dreamless sleep (stage 3 of non-REM sleep); so helps defining the depth of sleep Another name is slow wave sleep Also, seen during coma or other brain disorders Finally, seen in infancy
Slow rhythm		<1Hz			

4. *Symmetry*: one should always seek for symmetry in EEG waves between the two hemispheres even in an anesthetized patient.
5. *Voltage*: the EEG electrodes record the difference in their voltage between two electrodes across the time scale; in other words, deflections above or below the horizontal scale are the result of voltage difference between the two electrodes: negative "voltage difference" between the first and the second electrodes would be demonstrated as *above the scale deflection* (i.e., up deflection), while positive difference between the first and the second electrodes would appear as *below the scale deflection* (i.e., down deflection) on EEG.

EEG function is composed of thousands of EEG *epochs*; each epoch is an interval of "few seconds," which records electrical activity in this time domain and is usually 2–4 s; then, the electrical activity of each epoch is analyzed by the device microprocessor and demonstrated as EEG waves on a time-based scale.

Electrode Arrangement on the Scalp The standard order of EEG electrode arrangement on the scalp is named *montage of electrodes*. Basically, four main anatomic landmarks are used for electrode attachment over the scalp:

- Anterior location: nasion
- Posterior location: occipital or inion
- Two preauricular locations

The above locations combined with alphanumeric coding are used to name the standard electrode positions, which help us locate the lesions and, also, to compare similar anatomical points on the two hemispheres (Fig. 9.4):

- F: frontal electrodes.
- O: occipital electrodes.
- P: parietal electrodes.
- T: temporal electrodes.
- C: central electrodes.
- A: auricular electrodes.
- M: mastoid electrodes.
- Even numbers as subscripts demonstrate right hemisphere.
- Odd numbers as subscripts demonstrate left hemisphere.
- z as subscript demonstrates midline electrodes (z: zero).

Guideline 5 of the American Clinical Neurophysiology Society describes the standard electrode position nomenclature (2006e).

The Standard Electrode System The standard 10/20 electrode system could be used to have the standard 16 channel systems in recording conventional EEG; for intraoperative or postoperative CNS recording, we usually use 2–8 channels, and even many times during the perioperative period, only three electrodes are used which are attached to the frontal area: two of them are used to record the neuronal electrical activity as "differential amplifier with voltage difference," while the third electrode is the "mandatory reference signal" electrode, although some authors believe

Fig. 9.4 The EEG
electrode arrangement on
the scalp

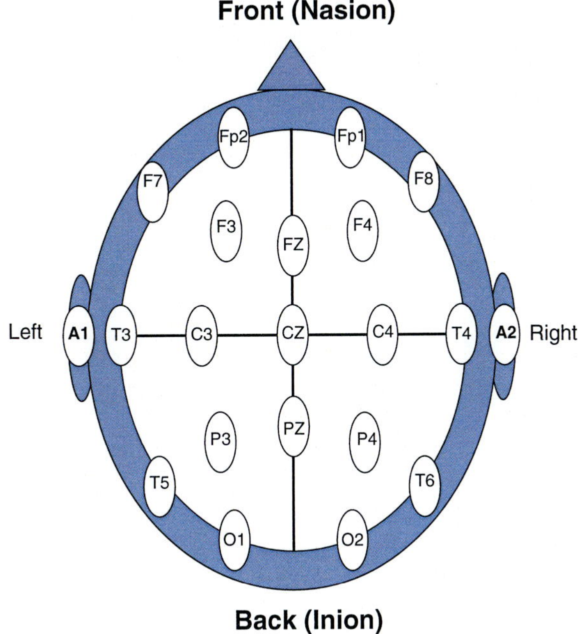

that at least eight channels should be used. How we use the electrodes for electrode montage is described fully in Guideline 6 of the American Clinical Neurophysiology Society: A proposal for standard montages to be used in clinical EEG (2006f).

Grounding Electrode According to the American Clinical Neurophysiology Society guideline (2008 version), except for a number of situations, we should always use a grounding electrode; these exceptions include those patients in which other electrical equipment are attached to the patient (like operating room or intensive care units); in these latter patients, we should avoid double grounding.

Different types of electrodes are available. However, it is more important to follow instructions for use more than just the electrode type; i.e., a constant type of electrode should be used for electrode *montage*; for artifact prevention, the electrodes should be well attached, appropriate electrode quality should be guaranteed, and, finally, enough gel should be pasted to prevent any extra resistance and guarantee low amount of impedance. The three electrode types are cup electrodes, silver-silver chloride electrodes, and needle electrodes:

- "Cup" electrodes which are usually made from "tin, silver, or gold."
- "Silver-silver chloride" electrodes are the third type of EEG electrodes.
- Gold disks or silver-silver chloride disks adhered to collodion are the best options, while other good-quality electrodes are acceptable.
- Needle electrodes are not recommended unless in very special condition with related precautions.

- All these three types of electrodes should be free of inherent noise; keep electrodes clean to decrease noise.
- Besides good quality of electrodes, guaranteed adhesion with enough gel, and keeping electrodes clean, the EEG cables and wires should be avoided from the vicinity of other cables to prevent noise and improve signal quality; shielding the EEG leads also could improve the quality.
- Special care should be given to prevent transmission of contagious diseases like HIV, Creutzfeldt-Jakob disease, viral hepatitis, or other similar agents.

Interpretation of EEG

For EEG interpretation, a number of variables should be considered, though this is far beyond the scope of this book; however, a summary of those indices which suggest abnormality is mentioned here:

- *Asymmetry*: there should be symmetry between right and left hemispheres; asymmetry is suggestive of pathology; asymmetry could be sign of ischemia or arterial occlusion.
- *Spikes*: the spike waves are suggestive of seizure activity which may or may not be accompanied with clinical convulsion.
- *Decreased frequency, decreased voltage, and decreased amplitude*: during early stages of ischemia, frequency of waves decreases, while the voltage is preserved; in early ischemia, decreased frequency of waves is seen, while the voltage of EEG waves is preserved; however, with more severe ischemic time, both wave frequency and voltage are depressed; if there is an EEG *amplitude* drop more than 30 % or there is more than *30 s* time interval of EEG changes, it should be considered with great caution as important indicators of ischemia.
- *Normal EEG waves seen in abnormal states*: this could also be a sign of pathology (e.g., if appearance of delta waves in unusual state could be an indicator of a brain lesion).

The abnormal EEG changes are often specifically seen as significant decrease in "beta and the alpha" waves. Also, the following abnormal characteristics are seen in these patients:

- Newly occurred abnormalities are often seen in the left hemisphere in the postoperative period.
- More invasive, more complex, or longer procedure creates much severe postoperative changes.
- Postoperative CNS ischemia (CBF<22 mL/100 g/min) changes EEG waves from normal to ischemic pattern; this ischemic pattern occurs whenever cerebral blood flow drops below this critical threshold.
- One should always consider the effects of altered hemodynamic status, temperature, and anesthetic drugs on EEG findings especially when interpreting abnormal waves.
- Injuries due to cardiac surgery are similar in EEG to "organic brain syndrome" findings.

How to Report EEG

Based on Guideline 7 of American Clinical Neurophysiology Society, each report is recommended to be prepared under four main subclasses; a full description could be found in the guideline text (2006g); however, briefly speaking, the following items are the main components of an EEG record:

1. *Basic patient information*: including age, sex, name, and EEG identification number.
2. *Introduction of report*: how the patient was prepared, including any received drugs for sedation, sleep deprivation, fasting state, how many electrodes from the standard 21 electrodes of the 10/20 system were used, and how long was the total recording time.
3. *Description of the report*: should include all findings, both normal and abnormal, away from interpretation; this interpretation should include all the findings in such a way that whenever another clinician reads the record, they could reach a decision even without looking at the EEG recordings.
4. *Interpretation of the report*: interpretation should be prepared having these two parts: *impression* and *clinical correlation*.

    Impression is the subjective finding of the interpreter about *normality or abnormality of EEG*; it should not be too long, and if it has any abnormality, it should contain the main 2–3 findings.

    Clinical correlation is the other part that should be mentioned in *interpretation of EEG*, and it should correlate the EEG findings with clinical picture. If the EEG findings are mild, the phrase *minor irregularities in cerebral function* is suggested in the report; however, if it is more than mild, the term *cerebral dysfunction* is appropriate for the interpretation of the report. These terms are appropriate for using in the record: *findings of EEG are consistent with the diagnosis, or supportive of the diagnosis, or compatible with clinical findings*. If EEG findings are not compatible with clinical findings, it should be stated cautiously, in order not to directly question the clinical diagnosis. Also, if any medication has been used before EEG, it should be mentioned in the interpretation. Some samples of EEG could be added to the record, especially when using electronic recording.

Limitations of EEG

There are a number of limitations for EEG, and this is why we believe EEG is a *good* CNS monitoring but not a *perfect* one (Constant and Sabourdin 2012):

- EEG works through electrodes which are usually attached to the scalp. These electrodes report the electrical activity of the cortex, i.e., the neurons located just beneath the cortical layer; however, this electrical activity does not include the full activity of the subcortical parts of the brain including the nuclei; hence, it could not alarm ischemia in subcortical regions.

- Using conventional EEG in the perioperative period, especially inside the OR, is a difficult task due to its technical complexities; it is sometimes really cumbersome and inconvenient, though newer modalities of EEG are much more used especially in the postoperative period.
- EEG is a biorhythm; so it will be affected like other biorhythms like age, environment, and circadian variations.
- Ischemia in the perioperative period does not always present itself in the same manner; in other words, if the inhibitory neurons of the CNS suffer an ischemic insult, the result in EEG would be as EEG overactivity.
- EEG could detect abnormalities including ischemia; however, it could not detect location of ischemia (ischemic site), definite mechanism of ischemia (the exact etiology), or the anatomic zone of ischemia (the scope of injury).

EEG Considerations in Pediatric and Neonatal Group

The basic principles are the same; especially, EEG in older children and adolescents has many similarities to adult EEG; however, neonates, infants, and younger pediatric patients need special consideration regarding the age-specific interpretations (De Weerd et al. 1999; Husain 2005).

Amplitude Integrated EEG: aEEG

This version of EEG is used much more recently in critical care of CNS; aEEG is a bedside tool for neurophysiologic assessment and uses fewer channels than a standard EEG; so aEEG is much easier, both regarding its use and interpretation, and could help earlier diagnosis much more than conventional EEG; however, standard EEG is more sensitive for the diagnosis of seizure. However, it is not mandatory that aEEG be interpreted by a neurologist. Of course, standard EEG remains the decisive method of diagnosis for neurophysiologic assessments. In neonatal ICU, unless we use aEEG in NICU, a considerable part of patients with neonatal seizure would be undetected (Boylan et al. 2015; Kang and Kadam 2015).

EEG Spectrogram This method has been introduced as a new processing method to describe the effects of different anesthetics as EEG waves; however, a three-dimensional model is used which describes power, amplitude, and frequency of EEG waves; power is calculated as 10 log10 (amplitude) and changes the resulting three-dimensional graph as a 2D colored graph; the three-dimensional graph is named as compressed spectral array (CSA). In these records, each of the spectra is calculated on based on 3 s interval, while each two adjacent spectra have overlaps of 0.5 s (Purdon et al. 2013; Ching and Brown 2014; Purdon et al. 2015).

For more detailed information, the interested author could refer to "minimum technical standards for EEG recording in suspected cerebral death" which is discussed in detail in Guideline 3 (2006c). Also, "Standards of Practice in Clinical Electroencephalography" are discussed in detail in Guideline 4 (2006d). Besides, Guideline 7 is the guideline discussing fully the method of writing EEG reports (2006g).

Transcranial Doppler: TCD

TCD was first described in 1982 by Rune Aaslid. It is a noninvasive neuromonitoring device which measures the velocity of blood flow through cerebral arteries. When invented, TCD was designed to be a simple device with simple technology, which could be frequently used for neuromonitoring; however, not many people can be considered as enough skilled in using the device. TCD has the following characteristics:

- Noninvasive neuromonitoring
- High temporal resolution
- Continuous, frequent, repeatable, and reproducible measurements of CBF velocity
- Rapid and accurate assessments with high probability
- Real-time monitoring (which could be used easily at bedside or in the operating theater)
- Never reported to have any complication
- Relatively low price
- May be used as a monitoring for up to several hours (including the postoperative period)

How TCD Works Low-frequency (1–2 MHz) ultrasonic Doppler signal is used in TCD through a pulse-waved Doppler; the Doppler beam calculates the blood flow velocity based on "Doppler shift." Doppler waves are projected from the piezoelectric crystal in TCD probe toward the tissue; then, these waves are reflected back to the crystal; finally, the movement of RBCs inside arterial lumen causes the Doppler shift. The angle of insonation is a very important factor.

TCD calculates blood flow velocity in different CNS arterial system, including anterior, middle, and posterior cerebral arteries (i.e., ACA, MCA, and PCA) and, also, internal carotid arteries (ICA) (Alexandrov et al. 2012).

Blood flow velocity especially in the middle cerebral artery (V_{MCA}) is the main index measured by TCD when used for monitoring in perioperative period of cardiac surgery.

The following variables are measured by TCD for each of the insonated arteries (Nelson et al. 2008; Wang et al. 2010):

(i) *Peak systolic velocity* (PSV).
(ii) *End diastolic velocity* (EDV), which is often 25–50 % of PSV.
(iii) *Mean velocity* (MV) is calculated using this formula:

$$MV = \left[PSV + \left(2 \times EDV \right) \right] / 2$$

(iv) *Pulsatility index* (*PI*) also known as Gosling's pulsatility index is the resistance in each cycle of blood flow through cerebral arteries; for calculation of PI, this formula is used:

$$PI = \left(PSV - EDV \right) / MV$$

PI values could be assessed with TCD (Fig. 9.9). Normal value for PI is from 0.5 to 1.19. If PI is below 0.5, it demonstrates proximal arterial occlusion or stenosis; the occlusion or stenosis in proximal arteries causes arteriolar vasodilation and decreases the above ratio which calculates PI. On the other hand, if any occlusion, stenosis, or vasoconstriction occurs in distal arterial segments, PI increases above 1.19. Another clinical state decreasing PI to less than 0.5 is "arteriovenous malformation (AVM)"; in AVM, the distal connection to venous system decreases distal resistance, and PI goes well below 0.5. On the other hand, increased intracranial pressure (increased ICP) increases PI; so ICP and PI have same directions for change; each 1 mmHg increase in ICP causes 2.4 % increase in PI (Nicoletto and Burkman 2009a, b).

(v) *Resistance index* (*RI*) also known as Pourcelot resistance index is used for calculation of arterial resistance to blood flow and is calculated by this formula:

$$RI = \left(PSV - EDV \right) / PSV$$

Normally, an RI > 0.8 is an index of increased resistance, and the diagnosis list for increased RI is similar to PI (White and Venkatesh 2006; Naqvi et al. 2013).

When we think about the final CNS outcome, one should always consider the relationship between oxygen supply-demand with special attention to critical situations like the period of cardiopulmonary bypass (CPB). Though the innate cerebral autoregulation mechanisms protect the brain during blood pressure "ups" and "lows," these *safety mechanisms* could be impaired in special situations: *they may be impaired to varying degrees during and, somewhat, after CPB*. Among all neuromonitoring modalities, TCD measures cerebral blood flow (CBF) during and after CPB. CBF is a function of cerebral perfusion pressure (CPP) and cerebral vascular resistance (CVR). Meanwhile, CPP is the algebraic result of the mean arterial pressure (MAP) minus intracranial pressure (ICP); i.e., CPP = MAP–ICP. So we will have

$$CBF = \left(MAP - ICP \right) / CVR$$

Among all cerebral arteries, often, the best waveform pattern is gained through middle cerebral artery (MCA), because of better bony window through temporal bone especially in adults and the children with closed fontanels. Measurement of the "angle-corrected flow velocity" is usually not as much exact for ACA and PCA as the MCA measurements; this is an important reason that why in the majority of patients, we use MCA for perioperative TCD monitoring (Hayashida et al. 2004).

Based on clinical and experimental studies on cerebral arterial system, the following factors are considered as the confounders of the blood velocity calculated by TCD; they might affect blood velocity calculated by TCD and should be considered during TCD (Brass et al. 1988; Vriens et al. 1989; 1993; Trindle et al. 1993; Poulin et al. 1996; Torbey et al. 2001; Kassab et al. 2007; Rasulo et al. 2008; Purkayastha and Sorond 2012; Naqvi et al. 2013):

- *Age*: in human brain circulation, the lowest CBF is after birth which is about 25 cm/s; however, CBF increases to its peak at 4–6 years after birth, peaking up to 100 cm/s; between 20 and 70 years, CBF decreases with a steady state slope, decreasing 0.3–0.5 % per year, and finally reaches to 40 cm/s at the seventh decade of life.
- *Hematocrit*: has an inverse relationship with CBF, drops in hematocrit increase CBF up to 20 %.
- *Gender*: CBF is a bit higher (10–15 %) in premenopausal women, possibly to compensate for lower hematocrit levels.
- *$PaCO_2$* (arterial pressure of CO_2): when $PaCO_2$ decreases, some degrees of cerebral vasoconstriction happen and cause increased CVR leading to decreased CBF; also, CBF increases in response to hypercapnia.
- *MAP*: the underlying hemodynamic (especially MAP) status affects CBF; the relationship between MAP and CBF is linear.
- *ICP (intracranial pressure)*: affects CBF directly.
- *Blood viscosity*: when blood viscosity increases, velocity of CBF decreases and vice versa.
- *Depth of anesthesia* and level of consciousness, including administration of analgesic agents or anesthetic drugs, could affect CBF and TCD results.
- *Diurnal time pattern* affects TCD through diurnal changes in blood pressure and CNS perfusion: the lowest CBF are seen about 11 AM.
- *Patient posture* affects the CBF: it is different in the seating position compared to supine position.

Before fontanel closure, other arteries except for MCA could be used since their windows are pretty well. Add to this point that in neonates and small children, the difficulties in using TCD are less also due to the smaller skull bone layer and the smaller distance from probe contact surface to the point of velocity calculation.

Indications for Using TCD   There are a wide range of indications for using TCD; a detailed list of TCD standards and guidelines is available describing the physical and clinical standards and the requirements for using the device; however, for *perioperative neuromonitoring* of pediatric cardiac surgery patients, TCD is mainly used for the following reasons (Iida et al. 1997; Hoffman 2006; Alexandrov et al. 2007, 2012; Edmonds et al. 2011; Ghazy et al. 2016):

- *Perioperative monitoring*: increasing attention has been drawn to TCD as one of the choices of neuromonitoring modalities in patients undergoing DHCA and antegrade cerebral perfusion, especially in pediatric cardiac surgery and especially for checking the CNS autoregulatory response due to effects of stimuli like hypercapnia or blood pressure fluctuations.
- *Assessment of cerebral blood flow for prevention of hypo- or hyperperfusion*: detection of adequate cerebral blood flow during selective cerebral perfusion and antegrade cerebral perfusion especially associated with DHCA and low-flow perfusion bypass for special procedures like aortic reconstruction and, also, measurement of cerebral flow rates during other modes of CPB. Besides, for adequacy of blood flow to CNS, TCD could be used for checking the correct position of *arterial or venous cannula* during CPB. Another application is assessment of hyperemia: a low CBF velocity ratio of MCA/ICA with a high mean flow velocity of the MCA could be predictive for critical hyperemia especially in patients with critical state.
- Evaluation of cerebrovascular *autoregulation.*
- *Detection of embolism*: detection of microemboli load during CPB which are usually directed from aorta to the brain circulation through MCA; during the post-DHCA period, there is increased likelihood for embolic load to CNS, and TCD could help for its detection.
- Detection of possible *thrombosis.*
- *Detection of arterial stenosis*: stenotic regions inside the intracranial arterial system could be detected by TCD.
- Monitoring intracranial pressure (*ICP*) by a noninvasive method.
- Measurement of effective downstream pressure.
- Diagnosis of *brain death.*
- *Assessment of vasospasm*: evaluation of patency in CNS arterial system and to detect any underlying CNS arterial vasospasm.
- Assessing the *efficacy of antithrombotic therapies* in reducing the platelet embolic load sent to CNS.

Windows for TCD Signal Acquisition

TCD windows are divided into two main time intervals: before closure of fontanels and after closure of fontanels.

Before fontanels are closed, the following windows are recommended; of course the probe used in such state is a fine bar-shaped probe, pretty much smaller than the conventional probes of TCD (Correa et al. 2004; Enriquez et al. 2006; Brennan and Taylor 2010; Steggerda et al. 2012):

1. *MCA* are assessed very well through the temporal bone.
2. *ACA and the circle of Willis* could be examined through anterior fontanel.

3. *Posterior cerebral circulation* could be evaluated through foramen magnum or mastoid fontanel (i.e., posterolateral fontanel) which is located anatomically posterior to mastoid process; mastoid fontanel is a good window especially in preterm and term neonates.

After closure of fontanels, the following windows are used mainly for TCD, though before closure of fontanels, the windows are much more "open" for TCD. However, these are the standard windows:

1. *Transtemporal window* is mainly located at the suprazygomatic portion of the temporal bone and is used mainly for insonation of MCA, while ACA and PCA could possibly be assessed through this window with using special maneuvers (Figs. 9.5 and 9.6); this window is used for TCD more than any other window. This window

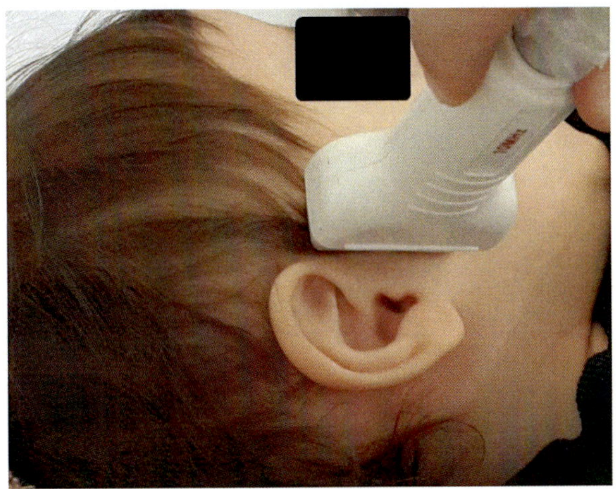

Fig. 9.5 Transtemporal window (Courtesy of Dr Tanghatari Neurology lab)

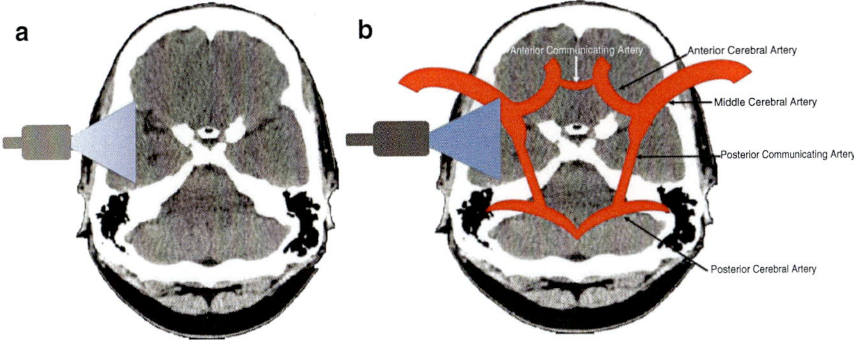

Fig. 9.6 (**a**) Schematic representation of trans-temporal window for Middle Cerebral Artery (MCA) with TCD; (**b**) a general presentation of other main cerebral arteries is demonstrated

needs supine position. The examiner should draw an arbitrary line from the tragus of the ear to the lateral canthus of the eye; there is an area extending from this line up to about 2 cm; the probe head should be inserted here gently, perpendicular to the bony plate of the temporal bone with enough probe gel; MCA blood flow has a good correlation with the total cerebral blood flow; this is among the reasons why using this window has gained great popularity. The sample volume of TCD probe should be adjusted based on the diameter of the head. In pediatric patient population, the desired depth is estimated based on the head circumference, described by Alexandrov et al. in Tables 9.2 and 9.5 (Alexandrov et al. 2007).

2. *Transorbital window* is used for insonation through the orbit, usually for the assessment of the ophthalmic arteries and, in some patients, to examine some cavernous parts of ICA (known as the carotid siphon). It is recommended to decrease 10–15 % of the probe power when using this window. The probe should be placed on the eyelid with the insonation angle a bit medial and upward (Fig. 9.7).

3. *Retromandibular window* is used to examine of cervical parts of carotid artery (Fig. 9.8).

4. *Suboccipital window* is used to assess posterior arterial system; it mainly consists of the basilar and vertebral arteries and is used for ACA and PCA. The transducer should be placed below and medial to the mastoid process, while it is recommended to turn patient to his/her side (Fig. 9.9).

Table 9.5 Desired depth of TCD insonation based on head circumference in children

Diameter of head (cm)	Proximal MCA (mm)	Distal MCA (mm)
12	30–54	30–36
13	30–58	30–36
14	34–62	34–40

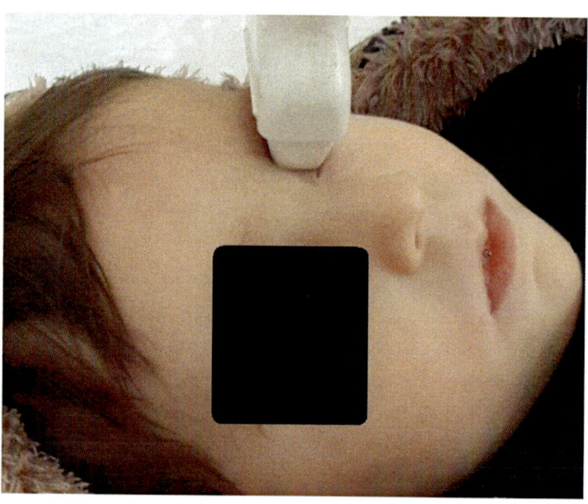

Fig. 9.7 Transorbital window (Courtesy of Dr Tanghatari Neurology lab)

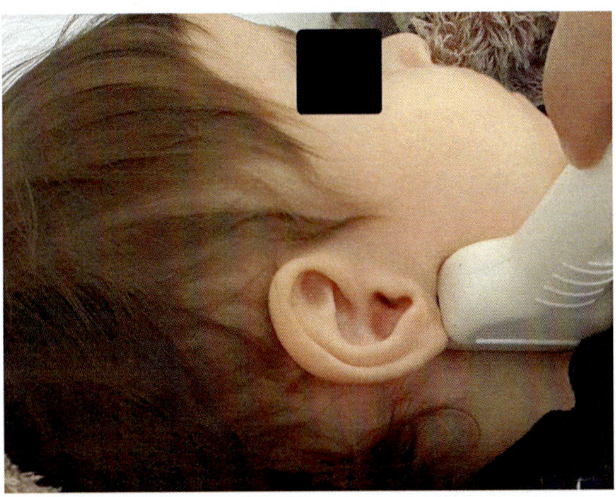

Fig. 9.8 Retromandibular window (Courtesy of Dr Tanghatari Neurology lab)

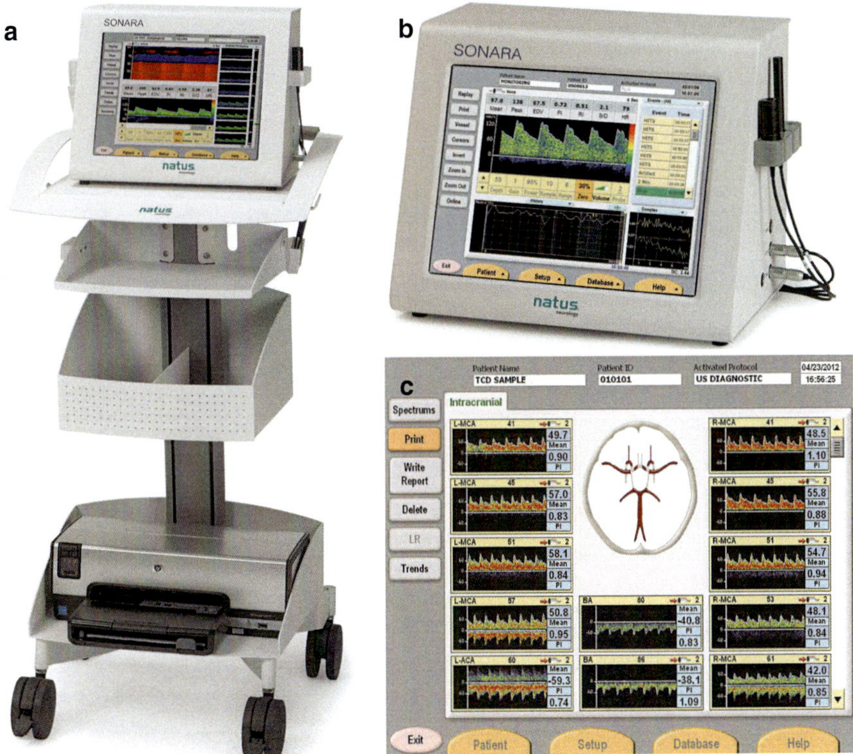

Fig. 9.9 The SONARA Transcranial Doppler (TCD) systems; (**a**) complete system; (**b**) the monitor; (**c**) the monitor panel of SONARA demonstrating Doppler waves on different arteries; (**d**) SONARA/TEK Digital TCD Module; (**e**) SONARA Doppler probes (Published with kind permission of © Natus Neurology Incorporated, 2016. All Rights Reserved)

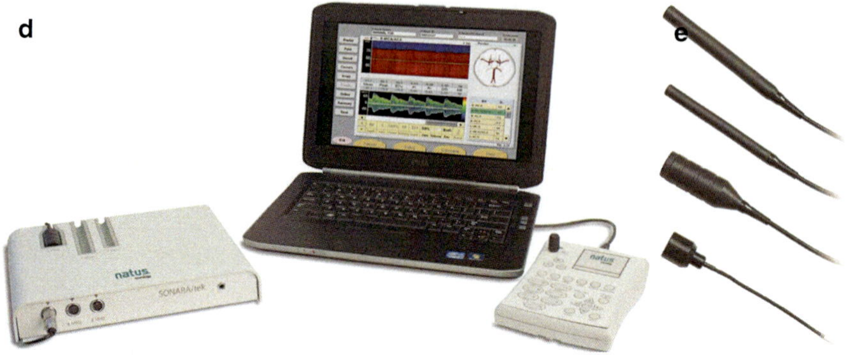

Fig. 9.9 (continued)

What Are the Main Limitations of TCD?

There are a number of difficulties which impede application of TCD especially for longer intervals:

- Difficulties in making reproducible measurements.
- Like some other devices, depends highly on the operator.
- The correct angle of insonation; if insonation is not done with a correct angle, the calculations would not be exact.
- Difficulties in finding an appropriate window which is seen more often in adults and older children.
- Lack of regional blood flow assessments; instead, TCD calculates CBF velocity in main CNS arteries.

Jugular Venous Oxygen Saturation (SjVO$_2$)

Assessment of the jugular oxygen saturation goes back to more than 70 years ago when the very first steps by Myerson et al. and Gibbs et al. have led gradually toward the current SjVO$_2$ monitoring. In 1942, Gibbs et al. described arterial and cerebral venous blood oxygen differences and a number of other biochemical differences; they studied 50 healthy young men (Gibbs EL 1942). Then, in 1945, Gibbs et al. demonstrated that there is no difference in oxygen saturation between simultaneous right and left jugular bulbs (Gibbs EL 1945). Then, in 1963, Datsur et al. had a much more important finding: they described SjVO$_2$ as an "indirect surrogate indicator for global oxygenation of the cortex"; also, they had another main finding; they found SjVO$_2$ as an indicator for the balance between "cerebral blood flow (CBF)" and "cerebral metabolic rate for oxygen (CMRO$_2$)" (Schell and Cole 2000; Chieregato et al. 2003).

What Does SjVO₂ Monitoring Show Us?

If we want to give a brief description, we can say: "$SjVO_2$ monitors the biochemistry profile of the venous blood draining each hemisphere." Of course, there is always some mixing between right and left internal jugular veins, in such a way that venous drainage from each hemisphere is about 70% from the ipsilateral jugular vein and 30% from the contralateral vein; however, in most patients, the right internal jugular vein is the dominant drainage vein, and this is why we usually monitor $SjVO_2$ through the right internal jugular vein. Although the right side is the dominant side, the mixing pattern between right and left hemispheres is not always the same.

Though Gibbs and colleagues measured jugular venous samples instantaneously, currently available $SjVO_2$ monitors measure the following variables based on a continuous assay method:

- Oxygen saturation in cerebral mixed venous blood, i.e., blood draining total cerebral tissue
- pH and PCO_2 in cerebral mixed venous blood
- Glucose and lactate levels in cerebral mixed venous blood

Based on the above variables and simultaneous arterial levels, the monitor calculates the following:

- Cerebral *arterial-venous O₂ difference* or "A-V O_2 gradient ($\Delta A\text{-}VO_2$)" which is the difference between brain arterial and venous oxygen, and it is a surrogate for CNS oxygen uptake; one should keep in mind that $SjVO_2$ is usually lower than simultaneous mixed venous blood taken from a pulmonary artery catheter (i.e., systemic SvO_2) since O_2 consumption in the brain tissue is higher than other tissues; so mixed venous O_2 content of jugular vein is lower than systemic mixed venous O_2 content.
- Cerebral "arterial-venous difference" for *lactate, pH,* and *PCO₂* which demonstrates the metabolic state of brain tissue.
- Cerebral "arterial-venous difference" for *glucose*; increased gradient shows increased cerebral activity.

In other words, if cerebral tissue O_2 delivery cannot meet tissue O_2 demands, the cerebral tissue would not be well oxygenated, and the result will be increased A-V gradient for oxygen. The increased $\Delta A\text{-}VO_2$ shows that inadequate brain tissue oxygenation leads to increased oxygen extraction from the arterial blood ending to "widened difference" between arterial and mixed venous oxygen saturation (Yoshitani et al. 2005).

Usually, increased A-V gradient for lactate, pH, and PCO_2 will be associated with increased "$\Delta A\text{-}VO_2$" which is an evidence for tendency to anaerobic metabolism and tissue oxygen deficiency. These parameters should be vigorously monitored in patients undergoing cardiopulmonary bypass; in cardiac surgery patients, there are episodes that need sophisticated care, like the rewarming period, patients undergoing antegrade cerebral perfusion, or patients with low-flow pump states like "deep hypothermic circulatory arrest" (Shaaban Ali et al. 2001).

SjVO₂ Catheters and the Technique Used for Their Insertion

Currently available $SjVO_2$ catheters use the reflectance oximetry technology which is the technique used in pulmonary artery catheters; these catheters are usually one of the two models: two optical fibers or three optical fibers. In the two-fiber model, light reflection to blood is through one fiber and the reflection of light is sent back to *photosensor* of the monitor by the second fiber; patient hemoglobin should be given to machine to calculate $SjVO_2$ a percentage of oxygenated Hb/total Hb. However, spectral absorption is used to calculate Hb concentration in three wavelength catheters; so in three wavelength monitors, real-time results of $SjVO_2$ are demonstrated.

In the older models of $SjVO_2$, the *conventional technique*, serial measurements of $SjVO_2$ are done which is associated with the limitation of "point checking of $SjVO_2$" mandating frequent sampling and serial measurement. Catheters with fiber-optic tips have removed the need for repeated sampling and give real-time data. Also, lateral neck rotation to either side will make erroneous or, at least, biased results because rotation of the head could affect the venous return and distort measurements (Howard et al. 1999; Schell and Cole 2000; Shaaban Ali et al. 2001).

Anatomic Approach

- Usually, the approach is the same as used for insertion of central venous catheter (CVC) through the *right internal jugular*.
- *Seldinger* technique is used needing a guidewire.
- Although the jugular bulb is located just below the skull base, the preferred site for $SjVO_2$ cannulation is the same as CVC insertion: *the anterior triangle*.
- The vein should be punctured in a *cephalad direction*; also, the guidewire should be introduced cephalad; using Doppler sonography could be a feasible guide for locating the needle and the wire; however, in the past decades, X-ray has been used for documentation.
- If the patient is awake, a sense of pressure is felt in the skull base due to the guidewire.
- The catheter is then inserted over the guidewire; Doppler sonography or an external sizer helps us determine the right location of catheter tip.
- Lateral or anteroposterior neck X-ray is the gold standard for verifying the location of the catheter tip; in X-ray results, we should look for the catheter tip to be around the mastoid process; a horizontal plane passes from the mastoid process, the first cervical spine, and the inferior margin of the orbital rim.
- Also, we could draw an imaginary line connecting right and left mastoid processes, and the catheter tip should be located just cephalad to this assumptive line.
- This technique has been used for *both pediatric and adult patients*.
- The catheter tip should be as much as possible inside or, at least, near the *bulb of jugular vein*; the optimum position is the roof of the jugular bulb which gives us the best $SjVO_2$ results.

- Another simple and acceptable method (though not as much exact as X-ray) is to use the surface landmark for jugular vein bulb which is 1 cm anterior and 1 cm below the mastoid process.
- Jugular bulb is located distal to the jugular foramen (jugular foramen is an anatomic window in the skull bone for emission of the jugular vein); this anatomic point is just located cephalad to the "common facial vein outlet."
- Before starting to measure $SjVO_2$, catheter calibration (both in vivo and in vitro) is necessary; this should be done based on manufacturer information.
- The catheter tip should not be displaced or entrapped into jugular vein wall; otherwise, if the catheter tip is displaced or has moved more than 2 cm from the bulb of jugular vein either cephalic or caudal, the results of $SjVO_2$ fall in the biased range of measurement and are not exact due to venous blood sample "contamination."
- Sampling speed should not exceed 2 mL/min; otherwise, there will be the risk of venous blood contamination because of blood mixing with extracranial venous blood and the result would be erroneous overestimation of $SjVO_2$.

Contraindications for $SjVO_2$ Catheter Insertion The following causes are considered as absolute contraindications for $SjVO_2$ catheter insertion:

- Cervical spine injuries
- Bleeding diathesis
- Local trauma of the neck
- Local infection of the neck

However, the following items are considered as relative contraindications:

- Impaired drainage of the cerebral veins
- Tracheostomy

Complications of $SjVO_2$ Catheter There are two main categories of complications related to $SjVO_2$ catheters:

- Complications of $SjVO_2$ *catheter insertion procedure* (like tissue or arterial injuries): these are similar to central venous catheter insertion complications.
- Complications of $SjVO_2$ catheter related to the *residing catheter* (to be included: increased risk of thrombosis or infection).

Data Interpretation by $SjVO_2$ Monitor The final $SjVO_2$ number depends on the following ratio:

$$CMRO_2 / CBF$$

$SjVO_2$ between 55 and 80 % is considered normal; $SjVO_2 < 50$ % is in "desaturation domain," and $SjVO_2 > 80$ % is in "luxuriant saturation" domain (Schell and Cole 2000).

However, there is another approach for interpretation of $SjVO_2$ data and that is calculation of the *arterial-jugular vein oxygen gradient* ($AjvDO_2$); this index is calculated using the following series of equations:

$$DO_2 = CBF \times CaO_2$$

$$CMRO_2 = CBF \times (CaO_2 - CjvO_2)$$

$$AjvDO_2 = CaO_2 \quad CjvO_2$$

In the above equations:

DO$_2$: Cerebral O$_2$ delivery
CBF: Cerebral blood flow
CMRO$_2$: Cerebral metabolic rate for oxygen (cerebral O$_2$ consumption)
CaO$_2$: Arterial O$_2$ content
CjvO$_2$: Jugular vein O$_2$ content
AjvDO$_2$: Arterial-jugular vein oxygen gradient

When solving the above three equations, we will have the following equation for AjvDO$_2$ which says:

$$AjvDO_2 = CaO_2 - CjvO_2$$

And finally, we reach to this formula:

$$AjvDO_2 = CMRO_2 / CBF$$

Normally, AjvDO$_2$ is between 4 and 8 mLO$_2$/100 mL of blood. However, interpretation of abnormal AjvDO$_2$ has one of the two categories:

- AjvDO$_2$ < 4 mLO$_2$/100 shows luxurious perfusion state with resulting abundance of O$_2$ in venous blood (luxurious O$_2$ delivery).
- AjvDO$_2$ > 8 mLO$_2$/100 shows inadequate oxygen delivery to brain tissue, resulting in as much as possible oxygen extraction from blood with resulting widening of arterial and venous oxygen gradient (desaturation state).

Based on the two above approaches (the absolute value of SjVO$_2$ or AjvDO$_2$), a list of differential diagnosis could be seen in Table 9.3.

Limitations of Data Interpretation for SjVO$_2$ and Methods to Correct It

SjVO$_2$ is better defined as "indirect surrogate index of global cerebral perfusion"; so SjVO$_2$ could detect global cerebral ischemia but cannot detect exactly the location of the ischemic region in cerebral hemispheres; this definition implies that:

- SjVO$_2$ has high specificity.
- SjVO$_2$ has low sensitivity (in other words, SjVO$_2$ could).
- It is affected by simultaneous hemoglobin concentration; saturation of the systemic arterial blood; core body temperature, fever, and/or hypothermia; level of CO$_2$ in the arterial blood; and level of anesthesia and/or sedation.

The following items could be very useful guides for caring the patient based on $SjVO_2$ results (Howard et al. 1999; Schell and Cole 2000; Shaaban Ali et al. 2001):

1. Determine $SjVO_2$ state (desaturated state or luxuriant state).
2. If it is desaturated (i.e., $SjVO_2 < 50\%$), check a venous blood sample (VBG) analysis using a CVC catheter.
3. If VBG O_2 saturation is $>50\%$, once again *calibrate* $SjVO_2$ monitor.
4. Correct the main determinants of *oxygen delivery*.

   - Increase *hemoglobin* above 9 mg/mL.
   - Correct *PaCO_2* above 30 Torr (to reach 35–40).
   - Increase *arterial oxygen saturation* $(SaO_2) > 90\%$.

5. Manipulate *intracranial hemodynamic status* to decrease intracranial pressure (ICP) < 20 and cerebral perfusion pressure (CPP) > 60 to have a CPP at least 60–70 mmHg; of course, mean arterial pressure (MAP) should be controlled to be above the minimum perfusing level.
6. Monitor and manipulate the underlying *metabolic state* of the brain (including temperature to prevent hypothermia, level of anesthesia to prevent wakefulness and inadequate anesthesia, EEG to prevent and treat any possibility of convulsion or electrical overactivity).
7. Rule out arterial vasospasm by TCD (Table 9.6).

Table 9.6 Differential diagnosis of cerebral perfusion state based on the absolute value of $SjVO_2$ and $AjvDO_2$ (Schell and Cole 2000)

Desaturated state ($SjVO_2 < 50\%$ or $AjvDO_2 > 8$)	Luxuriant state ($SjVO_2 > 80\%$ or $AjvDO_2 < 4$)
Decreases CBF Head injury Systemic hypotension Increased ICP (e.g., brain edema or impaired cerebral venous return) Arterial vasospasm Hyperventilation/hypocapnia Thromboembolism Arterial hypoxia (e.g., due to impaired ventilation due to lung pathology or ventilator problems, impaired hemoglobin oxygenation, or impaired transfer and delivery of oxygen to tissues including brain)	*Increased CBF* Hyperemia Arteriovenous shunts
Increased CMRO_2 Convulsion or seizure Fever/hyperthermia Inadequate anesthesia/sedation level	*Decreased CMRO_2* Anesthetic drugs which depress the level of brain function Hypothermia Brain death

Depth of Anesthesia and Sedation

Anesthesia level and sedation level are monitored using bispectral analysis index (BIS). During the perioperative period, the level of sedation/analgesia should be monitored in order to deliver adequate anesthesia/analgesia without over-administration. BIS has widespread use not only inside the operating room but also in the postoperative period inside the intensive care unit and for procedural sedation, especially in children in whom clinical assessment of consciousness is not always an easy task. On the other hand, BIS could help us create appropriate documentations for patients undergoing anesthesia/sedation for legal protection of the caregiver (Courtman et al. 2003; Johansen 2006; Lamas et al. 2009). BIS gives us a number which is categorized according to the following scale:

BIS level	Clinical state
>80	Awake
60–80	Sedation
40–60	Surgical anesthesia
<40	Deeply anesthetized

Evoked Potentials: Somatosensory Evoked Potential (SSEP), Motor Evoked Potential (MEP), Auditory Evoked Potential (AEP), and Visual Evoked Potential (VEP)

Evoked potentials provide real-time and objective data about the integrity of the nervous system which are both objective and reproducible data. For this purpose, functional integrity of the central and peripheral nervous system throughout the neural circuits and neural pathways is monitored by different modalities of evoked potentials, including SSEP, MEP, VEP, AEP, and BAEP, discussed here. Three main modalities of evoked potentials are:

Somatosensory evoked potential (SSEP): functional integrity of ascending pathways are monitored by SSEP, starting from peripheral receptors (median or ulnar nerve for upper extremity and posterior tibial nerve or peroneal nerve for lower extremity) going up to multiple spinal segments. Afterward, the neural pathway extends to the contralateral thalamus, finally ending in the cortical neurons. Visual evoked potential (VEP) is a subtype of SSEP monitoring visual stimuli as the sensory input.

Motor evoked potential (MEP) is the special modality of evoked potential for monitoring motor pathway. MEP monitors the neural process responding to the electrical motor stimuli starting from cortical neurons down to the related nuclei and corticospinal tracts and, finally, reaching peripheral motor units.

Visual evoked potential (VEP) monitors integrity and function of visual neural pathway; starting from retina, going through optic nerve, optic chiasma, optic radiation, and, finally, to the occipital cortex.

Auditory evoked potential (*AEP*) objectively monitors the neural pathway involved in hearing; this pathway starts from cochlea, going to ear, and reaches the auditory nerve (eighth cranial nerve). The final destination of this pathway is the brainstem, the related brain ganglia, and finally related cortical areas. In AEP, the first milliseconds monitor the "brainstem" function which is part of the auditory pathway; this part of AEP is called brainstem auditory evoked response (BAEP).

SSEP, MEP, VEP, AEP, and BAEP are frequently used in clinical practice including in the perioperative period of pediatric cardiac surgery patients, with the following items as the main indications for their use:

- CNS monitoring during therapeutic hypothermia; meanwhile EEG becomes but evoked potentials function well to monitor CNS integrity.
- CNS monitoring in patients with unstable hemodynamics, deep sedation, and altered consciousness states (Keenan et al. 1987; Burrows et al. 1990; Rosenblatt 1999; Freye 2005; Kunihara et al. 2007; Sloan and Jameson 2007).

The main differences between EEG and evoked potentials could be summarized as:

- Lower voltage amplitude in evoked potentials compared to EEG.
- EEG is demonstration of spontaneous electrical activity of cerebral cortical neurons, while evoked potentials are the neurologic response to a variety of stimuli by the monitor (sensory or motor).
- EEG monitors cerebral cortex exclusively, while evoked potentials could monitor cerebral cortex, deeper nuclei, parts of brainstem, spinal cord, and peripheral nerves.
- Functional integrity of the nervous system is checked by evoked potentials even during deep anesthesia or therapeutic hypothermia; in these latter clinical conditions, EEG may be flat while evoked potentials still work.

References

Alexandrov AV, Sloan MA, Wong LK, Douville C, Razumovsky AY, Koroshetz WJ, Kaps M, Tegeler CH. Practice standards for transcranial Doppler ultrasound: part I--test performance. J Neuroimaging Off J Am Soc Neuroimaging. 2007;17:11–8.

Alexandrov AV, Sloan MA, Tegeler CH, Newell DN, Lumsden A, Garami Z, Levy CR, Wong LK, Douville C, Kaps M, Tsivgoulis G. Practice standards for transcranial Doppler (TCD) ultrasound. Part II. Clinical indications and expected outcomes. J Neuroimaging Off J Am Soc Neuroimaging. 2012;22:215–24.

Ambuel B, Hamlett KW, Marx CM, Blumer JL. Assessing distress in pediatric intensive care environments: the COMFORT scale. J Pediatr Psychol. 1992;17:95–109.

Bellinger DC, Rappaport LA, Wypij D, Wernovsky G, Newburger JW. Patterns of developmental dysfunction after surgery during infancy to correct transposition of the great arteries. J Dev Behav Pediatr JDBP. 1997;18:75–83.

Boylan GB, Kharoshankaya L, Wusthoff CJ. Seizures and hypothermia: importance of electroencephalographic monitoring and considerations for treatment. Semin Fetal Neonatal Med. 2015;20:103–8.

Brass LM, Pavlakis SG, DeVivo D, Piomelli S, Mohr JP. Transcranial Doppler measurements of the middle cerebral artery. Effect of hematocrit. Stroke. 1988;19:1466–9.

Brennan CM, Taylor GA. Sonographic imaging of the posterior fossa utilizing the foramen magnum. Pediatr Radiol. 2010;40:1411–6.

Burrows FA, Hillier SC, McLeod ME, Iron KS, Taylor MJ. Anterior fontanel pressure and visual evoked potentials in neonates and infants undergoing profound hypothermic circulatory arrest. Anesthesiology. 1990;73:632–6.

Chambers CT, Reid GJ, McGrath PJ, Finley GA. Development and preliminary validation of a postoperative pain measure for parents. Pain. 1996;68:307–13.

Chieregato A, Calzolari F, Trasforini G, Targa L, Latronico N. Normal jugular bulb oxygen saturation. J Neurol Neurosurg Psychiatry. 2003;74:784–6.

Ching S, Brown EN. Modeling the dynamical effects of anesthesia on brain circuits. Curr Opin Neurobiol. 2014;25:116–22.

Constant I, Sabourdin N. The EEG signal: a window on the cortical brain activity. Paediatr Anaesth. 2012;22:539–52.

Correa F, Enriquez G, Rossello J, Lucaya J, Piqueras J, Aso C, Vazquez E, Ortega A, Gallart A. Posterior fontanelle sonography: an acoustic window into the neonatal brain. AJNR Am J Neuroradiol. 2004;25:1274–82.

Courtman SP, Wardurgh A, Petros AJ. Comparison of the bispectral index monitor with the Comfort score in assessing level of sedation of critically ill children. Intensive Care Med. 2003;29:2239–46.

Crellin DJ, Harrison D, Santamaria N, Babl FE. Systematic review of the Face, Legs, Activity, Cry and Consolability scale for assessing pain in infants and children: is it reliable, valid, and feasible for use? Pain. 2015;156:2132–51.

Dabbagh A. Postoperative Central Nervous System Monitoring". In: Dabbagh A, Esmailian F, Aranky SF, editors. Postoperative critical care for cardiac surgical patients'. Berlin: Springer; 2014. p. 129–59.

De Weerd AW, Despland PA, Plouin P. Neonatal EEG. The international federation of clinical neurophysiology. Electroencephalogr Clin Neurophysiol Suppl. 1999;52:149–57.

Denault A, Deschamps A, Murkin JM. A proposed algorithm for the intraoperative use of cerebral near-infrared spectroscopy. Semin Cardiothorac Vasc Anesth. 2007;11:274–81.

Edmonds Jr HL, Isley MR, Sloan TB, Alexandrov AV, Razumovsky AY. American society of neurophysiologic monitoring and american society of neuroimaging joint guidelines for transcranial doppler ultrasonic monitoring. J Neuroimaging Off J Am Soc Neuroimaging. 2011;21:177–83.

EL Gibbs LW, Gibbs FA. Bilateral internal jugular blood. Comparison of AV differences, oxygen-dextrose ratios and respiratory quotients. Am J Psychiatry. 1945;102:184–90.

EL Gibbs LW, Nims LF, et al. Arterial and cerebral venous blood. Arterial-venous differences in man. J Biol Chem. 1942;144:325–42.

Ely EW, Truman B, Shintani A, Thomason JW, Wheeler AP, Gordon S, Francis J, Speroff T, Gautam S, Margolin R, Sessler CN, Dittus RS, Bernard GR. Monitoring sedation status over time in ICU patients: reliability and validity of the Richmond Agitation-Sedation Scale (RASS). JAMA. 2003;289:2983–91.

Enriquez G, Correa F, Aso C, Carreno JC, Gonzalez R, Padilla NF, Vazquez E. Mastoid fontanelle approach for sonographic imaging of the neonatal brain. Pediatr Radiol. 2006;36:532–40.

Freye E. Cerebral monitoring in the operating room and the intensive care unit - an introductory for the clinician and a guide for the novice wanting to open a window to the brain. Part II: Sensory-evoked potentials (SSEP, AEP, VEP). J Clin Monit Comput. 2005;19:77–168.

Ghanayem NS, Hoffman GM, Mussatto KA, Frommelt MA, Cava JR, Mitchell ME, Tweddell JS. Perioperative monitoring in high-risk infants after stage 1 palliation of univentricular congenital heart disease. J Thorac Cardiovasc Surg. 2010;140:857–63.

Ghazy T, Darwisch A, Schmidt T, Fajfrova Z, Zickmuller C, Masshour A, Matschke K, Kappert U. Transcranial Doppler sonography for optimization of cerebral perfusion in aortic arch operation. Ann Thorac Surg. 2016;101:e15–6.

Gil-Anton J, Redondo S, Garcia Urabayen D, Nieto Faza M, Sanz I, Pilar J. Combined cerebral and renal near-infrared spectroscopy after congenital heart surgery. Pediatr Cardiol. 2015;36(6):1173–8.

Gottlieb EA, Mossad EB. Limitations of cerebral oxygenation monitoring by near-infrared spectroscopy in children with cyanotic congenital heart disease and profound polycythemia. J Cardiothorac Vasc Anesth. 2014;28:347–9.

Guideline 1: minimum technical requirements for performing clinical electroencephalography. J Clin Neurophysiology Off Publ Am Electroencephalographic Soc. 2006a; 23:86–91.

Guideline 2: minimum technical standards for pediatric electroencephalography. J Clinical Neurophysiology Off Publ Am Electroencephalographic Soc. 2006b; 23:92–6.

Guideline 3: minimum technical standards for EEG recording in suspected cerebral death. J Clin Neurophysiology Off Publ Am Electroencephalographic Soc. 2006c; 23:97–4.

Guideline 4: standards of practice in clinical electroencephalography. J Clin Neurophysiol Official Publ Am Electroencephalographic Soc. 2006d; 23:105–6.

Guideline 5: guidelines for standard electrode position nomenclature. J Clin Neurophysiol Off Publ Am Electroencephalographic Soc. 2006e. 23:107–10.

Guideline 6: a proposal for standard montages to be used in clinical EEG. J Clin Neurophysiol Off Publ Am Electroencephalographic Soc. 2006f; 23:111–7.

Guideline 7: guidelines for writing EEG reports. J Clin Neurophysiol Off Publ Am Electroencephalographic Soc. 2006g; 23:118–21.

Guideline one: minimum technical requirements for performing clinical electroencephalography. American Electroencephalographic Society. J Clinical Neurophysiol Off Publ Am Electroencephalographic Soc. 1994;11:2–5.

Hayashida M, Kin N, Tomioka T, Orii R, Sekiyama H, Usui H, Chinzei M, Hanaoka K. Cerebral ischaemia during cardiac surgery in children detected by combined monitoring of BIS and near-infrared spectroscopy. Br J Anaesth. 2004;92:662–9.

Herman ST, Abend NS, Bleck TP, Chapman KE, Drislane FW, Emerson RG, Gerard EE, Hahn CD, Husain AM, Kaplan PW, LaRoche SM, Nuwer MR, Quigg M, Riviello JJ, Schmitt SE, Simmons LA, Tsuchida TN, Hirsch LJ. Consensus statement on continuous EEG in critically ill adults and children, part I: indications. J Clin Neurophysiology Off Publ Am Electroencephalographic Soc. 2015a;32:87–95.

Herman ST, Abend NS, Bleck TP, Chapman KE, Drislane FW, Emerson RG, Gerard EE, Hahn CD, Husain AM, Kaplan PW, LaRoche SM, Nuwer MR, Quigg M, Riviello JJ, Schmitt SE, Simmons LA, Tsuchida TN, Hirsch LJ. Consensus statement on continuous EEG in critically ill adults and children, part II: personnel, technical specifications, and clinical practice. J Clin Neurophysiol Off Publ Am Electroencephalographic Soc. 2015b;32:96–108.

Hoffman GM. Neurologic monitoring on cardiopulmonary bypass: what are we obligated to do? Ann Thorac Surg. 2006;81:S2373–80.

Howard L, Gopinath SP, Uzura M, Valadka A, Robertson CS. Evaluation of a new fiberoptic catheter for monitoring jugular venous oxygen saturation. Neurosurgery. 1999;44:1280–5.

Husain AM. Review of neonatal EEG. Am J Electroneurodiagnostic Technol. 2005;45:12–35.

Iida K, Satoh H, Arita K, Nakahara T, Kurisu K, Ohtani M. Delayed hyperemia causing intracranial hypertension after cardiopulmonary resuscitation. Crit Care Med. 1997;25:971–6.

Invasive hemodynamic monitoring in obstetrics and gynecology. ACOG Technical Bulletin Number 175 – December 1992. Int J Gynaecol Obstet. 1993;42:199–205.

Isley MR, Edmonds Jr HL, Stecker M. Guidelines for intraoperative neuromonitoring using raw (analog or digital waveforms) and quantitative electroencephalography: a position statement by the American Society of Neurophysiological Monitoring. J Clin Monit Comput. 2009;23:369–90.

Johansen JW. Update on bispectral index monitoring. Best Pract Res Clin Anaesthesiol. 2006;20:81–99.

Johansson M, Kokinsky E. The COMFORT behavioural scale and the modified FLACC scale in paediatric intensive care. Nurs Crit Care. 2009;14:122–30.

Kang SK, Kadam SD. Neonatal seizures: impact on neurodevelopmental outcomes. Front pediatr. 2015;3:101.

Kassab MY, Majid A, Farooq MU, Azhary H, Hershey LA, Bednarczyk EM, Graybeal DF, Johnson MD. Transcranial Doppler: an introduction for primary care physicians. J Am Board Fam Med JABFM. 2007;20:65–71.

Keenan NK, Taylor MJ, Coles JG, Prieur BJ, Burrows FA. The use of VEPs for CNS monitoring during continuous cardiopulmonary bypass and circulatory arrest. Electroencephalogr Clin Neurophysiol. 1987;68:241–6.

Klem GH, Luders HO, Jasper HH, Elger C. The ten-twenty electrode system of the International Federation. Int Federation Clin Neurophysiol Electroencephalogr Clin Neurophysiol Suppl. 1999;52:3–6.

Kunihara T, Tscholl D, Langer F, Heinz G, Sata F, Schafers HJ. Cognitive brain function after hypothermic circulatory arrest assessed by cognitive P300 evoked potentials. Eur J Cardiothorac Surg. 2007;32:507–13.

Lamas A, Lopez-Herce J. Monitoring sedation in the critically ill child. Anaesthesia. 2010;65:516–24.

Lamas A, Lopez-Herce J, Sancho L, Mencia S, Carrillo A, Santiago MJ, Martinez V. Assessment of the level of sedation in children after cardiac surgery. Ann Thorac Surg. 2009;88:144–50.

Limperopoulos C, Majnemer A, Shevell MI, Rosenblatt B, Rohlicek C, Tchervenkov C, Darwish HZ. Functional limitations in young children with congenital heart defects after cardiac surgery. Pediatrics. 2001;108:1325–31.

Majnemer A, Limperopoulos C, Shevell M, Rohlicek C, Rosenblatt B, Tchervenkov C. Developmental and functional outcomes at school entry in children with congenital heart defects. J Pediatr. 2008;153:55–60.

Malviya S, Voepel-Lewis T, Burke C, Merkel S, Tait AR. The revised FLACC observational pain tool: improved reliability and validity for pain assessment in children with cognitive impairment. Paediatr Anaesth. 2006;16:258–65.

Markowitz SD, Ichord RN, Wernovsky G, Gaynor JW, Nicolson SC. Surrogate markers for neurological outcome in children after deep hypothermic circulatory arrest. Semin Cardiothorac Vasc Anesth. 2007;11:59–65.

McGrath PJ JG, Goodman JT, Schillinger J, Dunn J, Chapman JA. CHEOPS: a behavioral scale for rating postoperative pain in children. In: Fields HL, Dubner R, Cervero F, editors. Advances in pain research and therapy. New York: Raven; 1985. p. 395–402.

McGrath PJ, Walco GA, Turk DC, Dworkin RH, Brown MT, Davidson K, Eccleston C, Finley GA, Goldschneider K, Haverkos L, Hertz SH, Ljungman G, Palermo T, Rappaport BA, Rhodes T, Schechter N, Scott J, Sethna N, Svensson OK, Stinson J, von Baeyer CL, Walker L, Weisman S, White RE, Zajicek A, Zeltzer L. Core outcome domains and measures for pediatric acute and chronic/recurrent pain clinical trials: PedIMMPACT recommendations. J Pain Off J Am Pain Soc. 2008;9:771–83.

Merkel SI, Voepel-Lewis T, Shayevitz JR, Malviya S. The FLACC: a behavioral scale for scoring postoperative pain in young children. Pediatr Nurs. 1997;23:293–7.

Murkin JM, Arango M. Near-infrared spectroscopy as an index of brain and tissue oxygenation. Br J Anaesth. 2009;103 Suppl 1:i3–13.

Naqvi J, Yap KH, Ahmad G, Ghosh J. Transcranial Doppler ultrasound: a review of the physical principles and major applications in critical care. Int J Vasc med. 2013;2013:629378.

Nelson DP, Andropoulos DB, Fraser CD Jr. Perioperative neuroprotective strategies. Semin Thorac Cardiovasc Surg Pediatr Card Surg Annu. 2008;11(1):49–56.

Nicoletto HA, Burkman MH. Transcranial Doppler series part III: interpretation. Am J Electroneurodiagnostic Technol. 2009a;49:244–59.

Nicoletto HA, Burkman MH. Transcranial Doppler series part IV: case studies. Am J Electroneurodiagnostic Technol. 2009b;49:342–60.

Papademetriou MD, Tachtsidis I, Elliot MJ, Hoskote A, Elwell CE. Multichannel near infrared spectroscopy indicates regional variations in cerebral autoregulation in infants supported on extracorporeal membrane oxygenation. J Biomed Opt. 2012;17:067008.

Poulin MJ, Liang PJ, Robbins PA. Dynamics of the cerebral blood flow response to step changes in end-tidal PCO_2 and PO_2 in humans. J Appl Physiol (Bethesda, Md : 1985). 1996;81:1084–95.

Purdon PL, Pierce ET, Mukamel EA, Prerau MJ, Walsh JL, Wong KF, Salazar-Gomez AF, Harrell PG, Sampson AL, Cimenser A, Ching S, Kopell NJ, Tavares-Stoeckel C, Habeeb K, Merhar R, Brown EN. 2013. Electroencephalogram signatures of loss and recovery of consciousness from propofol. Proc Natl Acad Sci U S A 110:E1142–51.

Purdon PL, Sampson A, Pavone KJ, Brown EN. Clinical electroencephalography for anesthesiologists: Part I: background and basic signatures. Anesthesiology. 2015;123:937–60.

Purkayastha S, Sorond F. Transcranial Doppler ultrasound: technique and application. Semin Neurol. 2012;32:411–20.

Ramsay MA, Savege TM, Simpson BR, Goodwin R. Controlled sedation with alphaxalone-alphadolone. Br Med J. 1974;2:656–9.

Rasulo FA, De Peri E, Lavinio A. Transcranial Doppler ultrasonography in intensive care. Eur J Anaesthesiol Suppl. 2008;42:167–73.

Riker RR, Picard JT, Fraser GL. Prospective evaluation of the Sedation-Agitation Scale for adult critically ill patients. Crit Care Med. 1999;27:1325–9.

Rosenblatt B. Monitoring the central nervous system in children with congenital heart defects: clinical neurophysiological techniques. Semin Pediatr Neurol. 1999;6:27–31.

Schell RM, Cole DJ. Cerebral monitoring: jugular venous oximetry. Anesth Analg. 2000;90:559–66.

Sessler CN, Gosnell MS, Grap MJ, Brophy GM, O'Neal PV, Keane KA, Tesoro EP, Elswick RK. The Richmond Agitation-Sedation Scale: validity and reliability in adult intensive care unit patients. Am J Respir Crit Care Med. 2002;166:1338–44.

Shaaban Ali M, Harmer M, Latto I. Jugular bulb oximetry during cardiac surgery. Anaesthesia. 2001;56:24–37.

Simmons LE, Riker RR, Prato BS, Fraser GL. Assessing sedation during intensive care unit mechanical ventilation with the Bispectral Index and the Sedation-Agitation Scale. Crit Care Med. 1999;27:1499–504.

Sloan TB, Jameson LC. Electrophysiologic monitoring during surgery to repair the thoraco-abdominal aorta. J Clin Neurophysiol Off Publ Am Electroencephalographic Soc. 2007;24:316–27.

Snookes SH, Gunn JK, Eldridge BJ, Donath SM, Hunt RW, Galea MP, Shekerdemian L. A systematic review of motor and cognitive outcomes after early surgery for congenital heart disease. Pediatrics. 2010;125:e818–27.

Steggerda SJ, de Bruine FT, Smits-Wintjens VE, Walther FJ, van Wezel-Meijler G. Ultrasound detection of posterior fossa abnormalities in full-term neonates. Early Hum Dev. 2012;88:233–9.

Tarbell SE, Cohen IT, Marsh JL. The Toddler-Preschooler Postoperative Pain Scale: an observational scale for measuring postoperative pain in children aged 1–5. Preliminary report. Pain. 1992;50:273–80.

Torbey MT, Hauser TK, Bhardwaj A, Williams MA, Ulatowski JA, Mirski MA, Razumovsky AY. Effect of age on cerebral blood flow velocity and incidence of vasospasm after aneurysmal subarachnoid hemorrhage. Stroke. 2001;32:2005–11.

Trindle MR, Dodson BA, Rampil IJ. Effects of fentanyl versus sufentanil in equianesthetic doses on middle cerebral artery blood flow velocity. Anesthesiology. 1993;78:454–60.

Tweddell JS, Ghanayem NS, Hoffman GM. Pro: NIRS is "standard of care" for postoperative management. Semin Thorac Cardiovasc Surg Pediatr Card Surg Annu. 2010;13:44–50.

Verghese ST, Hannallah RS. Acute pain management in children. J Pain Res. 2010;3:105–23.

Voepel-Lewis T, Zanotti J, Dammeyer JA, Merkel S. Reliability and validity of the face, legs, activity, cry, consolability behavioral tool in assessing acute pain in critically ill patients. Am J Crit Care Off Publ Am Assoc Crit-Care Nurses. 2010;19:55–61; quiz 62.

von Baeyer CL, Spagrud LJ. Systematic review of observational (behavioral) measures of pain for children and adolescents aged 3 to 18 years. Pain. 2007;127:140–50.

Vriens EM, Kraaier V, Musbach M, Wieneke GH, van Huffelen AC. Transcranial pulsed Doppler measurements of blood velocity in the middle cerebral artery: reference values at rest and during hyperventilation in healthy volunteers in relation to age and sex. Ultrasound Med Biol. 1989;15:1–8.

Wang W, Bai SY, Zhang HB, Bai J, Zhang SJ, Zhu DM. Pulsatile flow improves cerebral blood flow in pediatric cardiopulmonary bypass. Artif Organs. 2010;34:874–8.

White H, Venkatesh B. Applications of transcranial Doppler in the ICU: a review. Intensive Care Med. 2006;32:981–94.

Wolf M, Ferrari M, Quaresima V. Progress of near-infrared spectroscopy and topography for brain and muscle clinical applications. J Biomed Opt. 2007;12:062104.

Yoshitani K, Kawaguchi M, Iwata M, Sasaoka N, Inoue S, Kurumatani N, Furuya H. Comparison of changes in jugular venous bulb oxygen saturation and cerebral oxygen saturation during variations of haemoglobin concentration under propofol and sevoflurane anaesthesia. Br J Anaesth. 2005;94:341–6.

Zheng F, Sheinberg R, Yee MS, Ono M, Zheng Y, Hogue CW. Cerebral near-infrared spectroscopy monitoring and neurologic outcomes in adult cardiac surgery patients: a systematic review. Anesth Analg. 2013;116:663–76.

Chapter 10
Respiratory Monitoring

Stacey Marr

Introduction

There is no doubt that respiratory function is one of the main functions of human being. However, when a patient, especially a child, undergoes some complex surgeries like surgery for congenital heart diseases, respiratory monitoring is much more stressed. However, this is not such a simple task. In this chapter we will discuss the main modalities for respiratory monitoring (Brochard et al. 2012).

Clinical Assessment

Clinical assessment is of great importance when assessing the child after cardiac surgery (Gazit et al. 2010). As with all monitoring, assessment parameters need to be taken in the context of the child, i.e., what is "normal" for one child will not necessarily be "normal" for another (Sivarajan and Bohn 2011). Recent work by Bonafide et al. has highlighted that the normal range for vital signs among hospitalized children can differ significantly from traditional reference ranges (Bonafide et al. 2013). A clinical assessment of a child will require using the four key skills of inspection, auscultation, palpation, and percussion.

S. Marr, MSc, RN, NP
Novick Cardiac Alliance, Memphis, TN, USA
e-mail: stacey.marr@cardiac-alliance.org

© Springer International Publishing Switzerland 2017

A. Dabbagh et al. (eds.), *Congenital Heart Disease in Pediatric and Adult Patients*, DOI 10.1007/978-3-319-44691-2_10

Inspection

This skill is useful to assess respiratory rate and pattern as well as the work of breathing, color, and emotional state of the child. This portion of the assessment requires the assessor to look at the *rate, pattern,* and *work of breathing* (WOB).

Rate Normal respiratory rates for infants and children are listed below; however, as previously discussed hospitalized children frequently do not fall within these parameters (Bonafide et al. 2013). Furthermore, children in congestive heart failure will typically have a significant faster respiratory rate than their unaffected peers. When assessing rate in children after cardiac surgery, it will be more important to review the trend of the rate rather than a single event, i.e., is the child becoming more tachypneic? A very slow respiratory rate in infants and children is a sign of imminent respiratory arrest or overdosing with narcotic agents (Davis et al. 2009) (Table 10.1).

Pattern Infants and children are nasal breathers and the ratio of inspiration to expiration is 1:2 or 1:3 in normal breathing (Brant et al. 2010; Auten et al. 2016). Regularity of breathing is particularly important to assess as apnea (cessation of breathing for 20 s or more) is a sign of significant respiratory distress in infants and neonates though neonates will often have short periods of apnea, referred to as periodic breathing, and this is normal as long as it is not associated with change in color or desaturation. On inspiration thoracic expansion and abdominal bulging ought to be seen in infants and young children, and loss of this synchrony of movement is referred to as "seesaw" breathing and is an abnormal pattern in this age group. Depth of breathing is also an important measure of effectiveness of respiration as shallow breathing leads to relatively poor gas exchange (Pasterkamp et al. 1997; Curley et al. 2005; Davis et al. 2009; Brochard et al. 2012; Oliveira and Marques 2014; Auten et al. 2016).

Work of Breathing (WOB)

The respiratory rate and pattern will give some idea of the work associated with breathing; however, describing the work of breathing in terms of the use of accessory muscles and presence of recession is a clearer indication of respiratory function.

Table 10.1 Normal age-matched respiratory rates (Davis et al. 2009; Fleming et al. 2011; Elder et al. 2013; Ross and Rosen 2014; McCollum et al. 2015; Auten et al. 2016)

Age	Normal rate
Infant	30–60
Toddler	24–40
Preschool age	20–32
School age	17–28
Adolescent	14–20

Nasal Flaring

A widening of the nostrils while breathing, this is more commonly seen in infants and young children and is a very subtle sign of respiratory distress and easily missed by practitioners (Fig. 10.1).

Recession

Infants and children have a very pliable rib cage, and when respiratory rate effort is increased, some indrawing or retraction can be seen along the costal margins where the diaphragm attaches (subcostal recession) or between the ribs (intercostal recession). In very small infants, the whole sternum may be drawn in (sternal recession), and recession above the sternum, between the clavicles, is described as a tracheal tug. As a child grows, the rib cage becomes more rigid and recession will rarely be seen, though recession in an older child (5+ years) is a sign of significant respiratory distress (Fig. 10.1).

Accessory Muscle Use

In respiratory distress a child may use accessory muscles to aid breathing; these muscles are used to increase the size of the thoracic cavity on inspiration, and the use of these muscles is a preterminal sign in infants and children as they will tire easily and have little respiratory reserve. Head bobbing in infants is only seen as the infant uses the sternocleidomastoid muscle to aid breathing (Fig. 10.1).

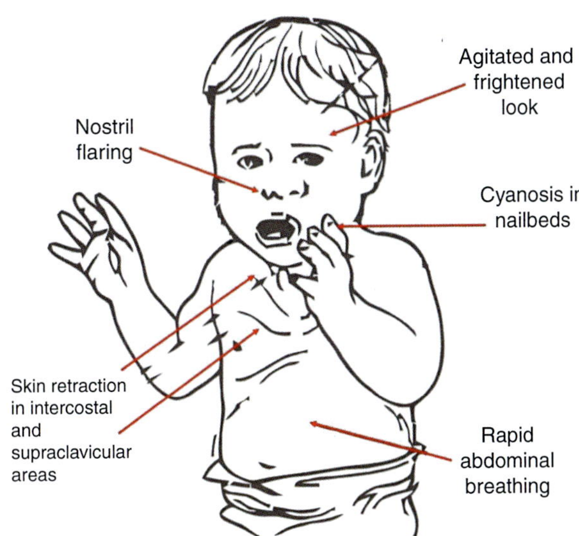

Fig. 10.1 A child with respiratory distress

Skin Color

The assessment of skin color in children with congenital heart disease is often a complex process, as children with reduced pulmonary blood flow will appear cyanosed without respiratory distress and children in congestive cardiac failure will appear pale. In normal children the presence of cyanosis is considered to be a severe sign of respiratory distress; however, for children with congenital heart disease, this may be normal. The assessment of color should be combined with activity in an awake child. A child or infant who has cyanosis from a respiratory cause, i.e., an acute reduction in available oxygen, will have an altered state of consciousness, whereas a child who has cyanosis from their cardiac lesion will most likely be sitting and playing without signs of respiratory distress. In the older child, the presence of clubbing of the fingers or toes will indicate a longer-term cyanosis.

Auscultation

Auscultation also involves listening without the stethoscope in order to hear respiratory noises and then using the stethoscope to hear breath sounds. Auscultation is a skill that develops over time and care ought to be taken to ensure the sound heard is coming from the child and not the equipment; also, an orderly performed pattern should be adopted for auscultation, both anterior side and posterior side (Fig. 10.2).

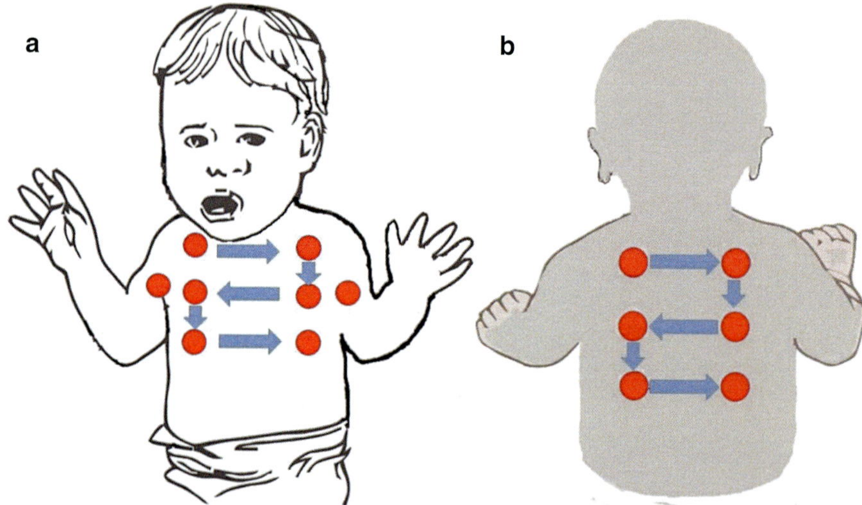

Fig. 10.2 Orderly performed auscultation; (**a**) anterior chest, from top to down and also including both armpits; (**b**) posterior chest, from top to down

Respiratory Sounds

Breath sounds are caused by vibrations against the airway walls by the turbulence of air as it passes through the airways. The sounds are produced in the large airways and transmitted via the lung tissue and rib cage to the surface and can be heard with a stethoscope.

The sounds heard on auscultation should be compared one side to the other and reported in terms of:

1. *Sound*: describe the noise heard, i.e., crackle, wheeze, or stridor.
2. *Intensity*: this refers to the pitch of the sound as high (soft) or low (loud).
3. *Timing*: does the sound occur on inspiration or expiration or is it biphasic?
4. *Quality*: is it continuous or intermittent?

Normal Breath Sounds

Bronchial sounds should be heard in the large airways – they are loud high-pitched sounds heard on inspiration and expiration. The presence of these sounds over the lung fields is an abnormal finding suggestive of consolidation or collapse of a lobe.

Vesicular sounds are heard in the smaller airways and periphery of the lung field. They should be quiet and low-pitched sounds; an increase in intensity of these sounds can also suggest pulmonary consolidation

Bronchovesicular sounds consist of a full inspiratory sound and a softer shortened expiratory sound, and they are best heard in the hilar region; an increase in intensity of these sounds can indicate consolidation.

Adventitious or Abnormal Sounds

Stridor A loud monophonic wheezing sound usually heard in the extrathoracic airways; it is associated with laryngeal or tracheal obstruction, and post extubation stridor is common in children with Down syndrome. The sound is initially heard on inspiration and as it worsens the sound will become biphasic and then silent.

Wheeze A high-pitched musical sound, most commonly heard on expiration and is often associated with a prolonged expiratory phase. This sound is produced by high-velocity flow of air through a restricted airway lumen and indicates intrathoracic airway obstruction. This sound is initially heard on expiration, but as the condition worsens, it will become biphasic and eventually silent. Children with pulmonary edema or congestive heart failure may present with an inspiratory wheeze referred to as a "cardiac wheeze."

Crackles Inspiratory high-pitched sounds like paper or hair being rubbed together, they are discontinuous sounds that originate within the airways. They are heard when an obstructed airway suddenly opens, and the pressures on either side of the obstruction suddenly equilibrate resulting in transient, distinct vibrations in the airway wall. The dynamic airway obstruction can be caused by either accumulation of secretions within the airway lumen or by airway collapse caused by the pressure from inflammation or edema in surrounding pulmonary tissue.

Grunting This sound is heard when a child is maintaining auto peep against a closed glottis.

Palpation

This skill has limited usefulness in infants though can be used to discover skeletal deformities or crepitus (crackles). Palpation of the thorax ought to give information on the position of the trachea, symmetry of chest movement, voice/breath sounds, and presence of subcutaneous emphysema.

Percussion

This skill is essential to perform an accurate respiratory assessment on infants and children. Percussion is performed by placing the middle finger of the nondominant hand flat on the patient's body and then tapping the distal joint with the middle finger of the other hand; this can be a difficult skill to master and will take time and practice. Percussion is used to determine the presence of air (high resonance on percussion), fluid, or mass (dull resonance on percussion) within the thorax (Pasterkamp et al. 1997; Oliveira and Marques 2014). In infants this skill may be the only way to determine the presence of a pneumothorax or effusion as breath sounds can be misleading in this age group as sounds are transmitted across the relatively thin-walled chest cavity.

The ability to perform and report an accurate clinical assessment of the respiratory system in children following cardiac surgery is imperative to aid management decisions. Most children with cardiac disease have few primary pulmonary problems, and thus a respiratory assessment cannot be taken in isolation from a good cardiovascular assessment nor in the absence of knowledge about cardiopulmonary interactions (Shekerdemian and Bohn 1999).

Cardiopulmonary Interactions

Cardiopulmonary interaction is a term that describes the inseparable connection between the heart and the lungs as they work to meet the tissues' oxygen demand. Any alteration or dysfunction in one system will have consequences for the other

	Action	Effects Pulmonary	Effects Cardiac
Normal Breathing	Diaphragm drops and intrathoracic pressure becomes negative	Air is sucked into the lungs to equalise pressure	Blood flows into the Right Atrium from SVC and IVC as pressure gradient decreases Transmural pressure in Thoracic Aorta increases and Left Ventricular afterload increases
	Diapragm rebounds and intrathoracic pressure become positive	Air is expelled from the lungs to equalise pressure	
Mechanical Ventilation	Ventilator delivers a postitive pressure breath	Air is delivered to the lungs under pressure	Blood flow from SVC and IVC are impeded and preload is reduced and Transmural pressure in the thoracic aorta is decreased leading to a reduction in Left Ventricular afterload
	Ventilator stops delivering positive pressure but maintains Positive End Expiratory Pressure (PEEP)	Air flows out of the lungs and alveoli are maintained open with PEEP	

Fig. 10.3 Table of cardiopulmonary interactions during normal ventilation and mechanical ventilation

system and often in intensive care interventions, which are aimed to improve the function of one system, will have a deleterious effect on another. The peripheral venous system is extrathoracic and therefore at atmospheric pressure (Shekerdemian and Bohn 1999; Bronicki and Anas 2009).

The pulmonary circulation and heart are intrathoracic and are influenced by changes to intrathoracic pressure. During normal respiration, the muscles of respiration generate a negative intrathoracic pressure; the negative pressure generated by deep inspiration maximizes the pressure gradient between the peripheral venous system and the right atrium and facilitates right atrial filling and thus preload. On the other hand, the thoracic aorta is located within the thoracic cavity and is subject to changes in pleural pressures. The difference between the pressure within the aorta and the pleural pressure is referred to as the transmural pressure. In normal respiration the pleural pressure falls during inspiration and thus increases the transmural pressure and consequently left ventricular afterload. The application of positive-pressure ventilation alters this delicate balance and can have serious consequences for children after cardiac surgery (Pinsky 1997; Thomson 1997; Tregay et al. 2016) (Fig. 10.3).

Respiratory Monitoring Adjuncts

There are many new techniques for respiratory monitoring which have become available in recent years, and the appropriate use of available monitoring procedures can improve patient safety and outcomes in intensive care (Brochard et al. 2012). In the pediatric context, some of the newer modalities are of limited usefulness or are impractical for use with our population; therefore, this chapter will limit this discussion to pulse oximetry and capnometry/capnography (Rimensberger 2009a, b; Rettig et al. 2015; Chen et al. 2016).

Pulse Oximetry

This is widely used in pediatric intensive care and by anesthetists during surgical procedures. It is a measure of the percentage of hemoglobin saturated with oxygen which is estimated by the rate of absorption of two different wavelengths of light (Sivarajan and Bohn 2011). The use of this measurement tool is widespread, and one of the advantages to its use is that most practitioners are familiar with the equipment used and the significance of the results. It is also very useful as an early warning signal and will reduce the frequency of arterial blood gas sampling (Brochard et al. 2012). The disadvantages of this measurement are that it cannot distinguish between normal hemoglobin, carboxyhemoglobin, and methemoglobin; it loses sensitivity at lower saturation levels, and movement and artifact will affect the results seen. The other point to note is that this device will measure the percentage of hemoglobin saturated with oxygen but will not distinguish a low oxygen-carrying capacity in the presence of acute anemia – for example, a child may be received from the operating room with a measured saturation of 100 % and an Hb of 14 g/dl, and if that child is bleeding and the Hb falls to 7 g/dl, the pulse oximeter will likely still measure the saturation as 100 % even though the oxygen-carrying capacity of the blood has reduced by half. It is essential that the probe fits the child as poorly fitting probes will provide inaccurate data; observing a good correlation with the heart rate measured on ECG and the pulse rate measured by the pulse oximeter will aid in determining whether the probe is reading accurately or not. As with any single parameter, it cannot be taken in isolation, and recording the saturations hourly, observing for a trend, will be more useful in aiding clinical decision-making.

Capnography and Capnometry

The measurement of end-tidal CO_2 has been available for more than 30 years and used in adult intensive care units for many of those years. Capnography works by capturing exhaled air and redirecting it into the capnography device. The air then passes between a light and a detector that measures how much light is shining on it. As the concentration of CO_2 increases, more light is absorbed by the CO_2 and less light is transmitted onto the detector plate. An initial reluctance to use this measure in children was related to the large device size and consequent increase in dead space and the lack of cuffed tubes used in this age group. However, as devices have become smaller and more accurate, this reluctance has faded, and the use of end-tidal CO_2 ($ETCO_2$) on ventilated patients in the ICU has become the "gold standard" of care. The information which can be derived from $ETCO_2$ are changes in alveolar ventilation, confirmation of endotracheal tube placement, the degree of right-to-left intracardiac shunt, change in pulmonary blood flow, and effectiveness of cardiopulmonary resuscitation. This adjunct can be used solely to measure the graphical representation of expired CO_2 (capnography), to provide a number for end-expiratory CO_2 (capnometry), or more usefully in cardiac patients to observe for differences in $PaCO_2$

and ETCO2. In cases of systemic-to-pulmonary artery shunt monitoring, the difference between $ETCO_2$ and $PaCO_2$ will provide essential information regarding shunt patency – if the shunt were to become blocked, then the $PaCO_2$ would rise with a consequent fall in the $ETCO_2$ indicating reduced pulmonary blood flow (Sivarajan et al. 2008; Clarizia et al. 2011; Sivarajan et al. 2011; Sivarajan and Bohn 2011).

References

Auten R, Schwarze J, Ren C, Davis S, Noah TL. Pediatric pulmonology year in review 2015: part 1. Pediatric pulmonol. 2016;51(7):733–9.

Bonafide CP, Brady PW, Keren R, Conway PH, Marsolo K, Daymont C. Development of heart and respiratory rate percentile curves for hospitalized children. Pediatrics. 2013;131:e1150–7.

Brant JM, Beck S, Miaskowski C. Building dynamic models and theories to advance the science of symptom management research. J Adv Nurs. 2010;66:228–40.

Brochard L, Martin GS, Blanch L, Pelosi P, Belda FJ, Jubran A, Gattinoni L, Mancebo J, Ranieri VM, Richard JC, Gommers D, Vieillard-Baron A, Pesenti A, Jaber S, Stenqvist O, Vincent JL. Clinical review: respiratory monitoring in the ICU-a consensus of 16. Crit Care. 2012;16:219.

Bronicki RA, Anas NG. Cardiopulmonary interaction. Pediatr Crit Care Med. 2009;10:313–22.

Chen F, Bajwa NM, Rimensberger PC, Posfay-Barbe KM, Pfister RE. Thirteen-year mortality and morbidity in preterm infants in Switzerland. Arch Dis Child Fetal Neonatal Ed. 2016;101:F377–83.

Clarizia NA, Manlhiot C, Schwartz SM, Sivarajan VB, Maratta R, Holtby HM, Gruenwald CE, Caldarone CA, Van Arsdell GS, McCrindle BW. Improved outcomes associated with intraoperative steroid use in high-risk pediatric cardiac surgery. Ann Thorac Surg. 2011;91:1222–7.

Curley MA, Hibberd PL, Fineman LD, Wypij D, Shih MC, Thompson JE, Grant MJ, Barr FE, Cvijanovich NZ, Sorce L, Luckett PM, Matthay MA, Arnold JH. Effect of prone positioning on clinical outcomes in children with acute lung injury: a randomized controlled trial. JAMA. 2005;294:229–37.

Davis SQ, Permutt Z, Permutt S, Naureckas ET, Bilderback AL, Rand CS, Stein BD, Krishnan JA. Perception of airflow obstruction in patients hospitalized for acute asthma. Ann Allergy Asthma Immunol Off Publ Am Coll Allergy Asthma Immunol. 2009;102:455–61.

Elder DE, Campbell AJ, Galletly D. Current definitions for neonatal apnoea: are they evidence based? J Paediatr Child Health. 2013;49:E388–96.

Fleming S, Thompson M, Stevens R, Heneghan C, Pluddemann A, Maconochie I, Tarassenko L, Mant D. Normal ranges of heart rate and respiratory rate in children from birth to 18 years of age: a systematic review of observational studies. Lancet. 2011;377:1011–8.

Gazit AZ, Huddleston CB, Checchia PA, Fehr J, Pezzella AT. Care of the pediatric cardiac surgery patient – part 2. Curr Probl Surg. 2010;47:261–376.

McCollum ED, King C, Hollowell R, Zhou J, Colbourn T, Nambiar B, Mukanga D, Burgess DC. Predictors of treatment failure for non-severe childhood pneumonia in developing countries – systematic literature review and expert survey – the first step towards a community focused mHealth risk-assessment tool? BMC Pediatr. 2015;15:74.

Oliveira A, Marques A. Respiratory sounds in healthy people: a systematic review. Respir Med. 2014;108:550–70.

Pasterkamp H, Patel S, Wodicka GR. Asymmetry of respiratory sounds and thoracic transmission. Med Biol Eng Comput. 1997;35:103–6.

Pinsky MR. The hemodynamic consequences of mechanical ventilation: an evolving story. Intensive Care Med. 1997;23:493–503.

Rettig JS, Smallwood CD, Walsh BK, Rimensberger PC, Bachman TE, Bollen CW, Duval EL, Gebistorf F, Markhorst DG, Tinnevelt M, Todd M, Zurakowski D, Arnold JH. High-frequency oscillatory ventilation in pediatric acute lung injury: a multicenter international experience. Crit Care Med. 2015;43:2660–7.

Rimensberger PC. Mechanical ventilation in paediatric intensive care. Ann Fr Anesth Reanim. 2009a;28:682–4.

Rimensberger PC. To intubate or not to intubate at birth, this is still the question! Will experimental studies give us the answer?: commentary on the article by Polglase et al. on page 67. Pediatr Res. 2009b;65:19–20.

Ross KR, Rosen CL. Sleep and respiratory physiology in children. Clin Chest Med. 2014;35: 457–67.

Shekerdemian L, Bohn D. Cardiovascular effects of mechanical ventilation. Arch Dis Child. 1999; 80:475–80.

Sivarajan VB, Best D, Brizard CP, Shekerdemian LS, d'Udekem Y, Butt W. Duration of resuscitation prior to rescue extracorporeal membrane oxygenation impacts outcome in children with heart disease. Intensive Care Med. 2011;37:853–60.

Sivarajan VB, Bohn D. Monitoring of standard hemodynamic parameters: heart rate, systemic blood pressure, atrial pressure, pulse oximetry, and end-tidal CO2. Pediatr Crit Care Med. 2011;12:S2–11.

Sivarajan VB, Chrisant MR, Ittenbach RF, Clark 3rd BJ, Hanna BD, Paridon SM, Spray TL, Wernovsky G, Gaynor JW. Prevalence and risk factors for tricuspid valve regurgitation after pediatric heart transplantation. J Heart Lung Transplant Off Publ Int Soc Heart Transplant. 2008;27:494–500.

Thomson A. The role of negative pressure ventilation. Arch Dis Child. 1997;77:454–8.

Tregay J, Brown KL, Crowe S, Bull C, Knowles RL, Smith L, Wray J. Signs of deterioration in infants discharged home following congenital heart surgery in the first year of life: a qualitative study. Arch Dis Child. 2016.

Chapter 11
Coagulation Monitoring

Antonio Pérez-Ferrer and Pablo Motta

Introduction

Hemorrhage is a common problem during and after pediatric cardiac surgery that challenges surgeons and anesthesiologist. Young age, low weight, polycythemia, deep hypothermia, and complex cardiac surgery are risk factors for severe bleeding (Miller et al. 1997a; Williams et al. 1999; Szekely et al. 2009). In addition we need to take into account the growing use of drugs that affect platelet aggregation and coagulation which if not managed correctly could increase the bleeding risk. Bleeding and transfusion of blood components is associated with a dose dependent increase in postoperative morbi-mortality (Willems et al. 2010; Wolf et al. 2014; Agarwal et al. 2015a).

The surgeon and the anesthesiologist during the preoperative evaluation should be able to estimate the patient's bleeding risk either for congenital or acquired disease so the specialist can evaluate them. In addition they should be able to diagnose and treat bleeding during and after surgery. The approach to perioperative hemorrhage should be of a multidisciplinary team including surgery, anesthesia, and nursing since it is a dynamic process triggered by surgery, but if not address early, it will turn into coagulopathy due to factor depletion.

In any hemorrhage, it is extremely important to diagnose the triggering factors as well as to monitor coagulation adequately to differentiate between surgical and medical causes of bleeding allowing a goal-directed therapy. Perioperative bleeding is not straightforward phenomenon like hemophilia (one missing factor which is

A. Pérez-Ferrer, MD, PhD. (✉)
Department of Pediatric Anesthesiology, La Paz University Hospital, Madrid, Spain
e-mail: antonioperezferrer@gmail.com

P. Motta, MD
Department of Pediatric Cardiac Anesthesia, Texas Children's Hospital,
Baylor College of Medicine, Houston, TX, USA
e-mail: pxmotta@texaschildrens.org

© Springer International Publishing Switzerland 2017
A. Dabbagh et al. (eds.), *Congenital Heart Disease in Pediatric
and Adult Patients*, DOI 10.1007/978-3-319-44691-2_11

easy to replace) and is usually a dynamic multifactorial event caused by previous exposure to anticoagulant and/or antiplatelets, dilution and/or loss coagulating factors, cellular elements during surgery, and in some situations developing hyperfibrinolysis.

Due to this fact, it is crucial to monitor the cause of coagulopathy and guide its therapy promptly (Nakayama et al. 2015).

Pediatric Hemostasis

The hemostasis is a multifaceted physiological process in which there is a complex balance between opposite mechanism of coagulation and anticoagulation, which protect the vascular system from uncontrolled bleeding, or excessive coagulation. There are three phases in the coagulation process, which under normal conditions interact together to produce clot in the injury area preserving the flow to the rest of the body. The first phase is the primary hemostasis where the platelets produce thrombi when faced to the damaged endothelium. Next, the secondary hemostasis or coagulation is when fibrinogen is transformed to fibrin in which the clot reinforces the initial thrombi. Lastly the tertiary phase of hemostasis or fibrinolysis in which the clot is degraded when no longer needed. During the last few years, important advances have been made in the knowledge of the physiology of coagulation shifting from the classic cascade model of coagulation based on laboratory testing (prothrombin time and activated partial thromboplastin time) to a different cellular model of coagulation (Hoffman and Monroe 2001). In this model tissue factor, FVIIA has a key role with other cellular elements which carry tissue factor and platelets whose surface generates large quantities of thrombin which converts fibrinogen in fibrin. The most significant maturation changes of coagulation occur during the first 6 months of life, but it continues to develop through infancy (Andrew et al. 1992; Miller et al. 1997b). The maternal coagulation factors (cF) do not cross the placenta so the amount of neonatal factors is due to synthesis which starts in the fifth week of life and peaks on the eleventh week of life.

All the components of the hemostatic system are present at birth, but neonatal hematologic system has peculiarities that need to be highlighted (Table 11.1).

Comparison Between Neonatal and Adult Hemostasis

There are qualitative and quantitative differences between neonates and adults (see Table 11.2).

Due to these developmental differences, activated partial thromboplastin time (aPTT) is prolonged during the first 3 months of life without increasing the risk of bleeding. Despite this fact, newborns have a good balance between procoagulant

Table 11.1 Neonatal hematologic system

Compensates the reduction of oxygen-carrying capacity by the anemia by increasing cardiac output (limited response)
Adaptation to the low intrauterine oxygen tension by increasing hematocrit through Hb F (70 % in the neonate). Transfusion increases the risk of retrolental fibroplasia and necrotizing enterocolitis
More catabolism linked to decreased erythropoietin production: infant physiologic anemia (8–12 weeks of life)
Immunosuppression state: maternal antibodies could create a graft-versus-host disease (GVHD) and increase risk for infection (CMV)
Risk of anemia due to multiple blood drawn. Limit the volume and number of draws
Higher susceptibility to citrate intoxication
Efforts need to be made to decrease the number of transfusions and exposure to donors (use of pediatric units)
There is a reduction in the coagulation factors—vitamin K-dependent factors, contact factors, and natural coagulation inhibitors
Hypofibrinolysis and primary hemostasis are enhanced besides a deficient platelet function
Hemostatic balance is adequate besides prolonged cephaline time during the first 3–6 months of life

Table 11.2 Comparison between neonatal and adult hemostasis

Component	Neonatal function	Effect on the hemostasis
Coagulation factors	↓ F II, VII, IX, XI, XII ± Fibrinogen, F V ↑ F VIII	↓Thrombin generation
Primary hemostasis	↑vWF ↓ Platelet function	↑ Primary hemostasis
Fibrinolysis	↓ Plasminogen, t-PA, y α_2 antiplasmin ↑PAI	Hypofibrinolysis
Natural coagulation inhibitors	↓AT, proteins C y S	↓ Inhibition capacity of activated coagulation proteins

F factor, *vWF* von Willebrand factor, *t-PA* tissue plasminogen activator, *PAI* plasminogen activator inhibitor, *AT* antithrombin

factors and natural anticoagulants with adequate hemostasis that allows undergoing surgery without an increased risk of bleeding. Other coagulation test like bleeding time is decreased, while the thromboelastogram shows a hypercoagulable trace with shortening of the reaction time (Miller et al. 1997b).

Congenital Heart Disease and Coagulation

Congenital heart disease is associated with coagulation anomalies. Platelets turnover anomalies with increased peripheral destruction and a higher rate of young "sticky" platelets associated with significantly reduced levels of large multimer von Willebrand factor that improve postcorrective surgery.

Cyanotic heart disease has been particularly associated with defects in coagulation. The increase red cell production secondary to chronic hypoxemia decreases platelet synthesis in an inverse related ratio. In addition, platelet life span is shorter with a decreased adhesion and aggregation properties. Recently, Gertler et al. (2014) in a study of platelet function in cyanotic pediatric patients by multiple electrode aggregometry showed that there was no clinically significant effect of cyanosis on baseline and perioperative platelet function, chest tube drain, and the number of exposures to blood products. The authors concluded that children under 1 year of age do not require a different approach with regard to platelet transfusions, independent of cyanosis.

Low cardiac output and liver congestion can decrease the production of coagulation factors especially the vitamin K-dependent ones (II, VII, IX y X). This deficit is also associated with reduced fibrinogen levels, antithrombin III (ATIII), factors V and VII, and proteins C and S that has been seen in patients with hypoplastic left heart syndrome usually before first-stage palliation but occasionally post Fontan completion. Controversy exists regarding the hypocoagulable state in pediatric patients with congenital heart disease. Is it real of just a technical artifact from traditional coagulation test and/or thromboelastogram (Spiezia et al. 2013). The fact is that the quantity of plasma, coagulation factors, and anticoagulant proteins in these patients is decreased in relationship with polycythemia. The reduction of pro- and anticoagulant factors associated with the peculiar physiology has a higher incidence of both thromboembolic events and bleeding complications. Due to this fact, this patient population requires a heightened vigilance and proactive therapy (Eaton and Iannoli 2011).

Clinical Evaluation and Preoperative Laboratory Testing

The most common laboratory testing used to evaluate coagulation in our patients is the PT, INR, aPTT, fibrinogen, and platelet count. During the perioperative period, the use of these testing has been questioned since they are not predictive of perioperative hemorrhage (Dzik 2004; Chee et al. 2008; Samkova et al. 2012). The abnormal results rate of "traditional" testing is 0.4–46 % which changes patient management in only 0–7 % and detects complications in only 0–8 % of the patients. There is no evidence in adult and pediatric medical literature that these preoperative testing improves patients outcome. In addition in major pediatric surgery, 64 % of PT and 94 % of aPTT of intraoperative measurements were outside the reference range, while impaired CT was observed in 13 and 6.3 % of ExTEM and InTEM ROTEM clotting times. The correlation between PT and aPTT to ExTEM and InTEM was poor. The recommended thresholds for PT and aPTT might overestimate the need for coagulation therapy (Haas et al. 2012). A good structured questionnaire about bleeding history has a better predictive value for perioperative hemorrhage than any other coagulation testing (Chee et al. 2008).

Coagulopathy and Cardiac Bypass

Cardiac surgery is one of the surgical procedures that affect more the hemostatic milieu. Patients with cardiomyopathy are hypercoagulable and require anticoagulant and/or antiplatelet therapy, which need to be held in the preoperative period. Following cardiopulmonary bypass (CPB), the balance is shifted to coagulopathy. Recent advances in CPB circuits reduce the inflammatory activation, but they still remain profoundly nonphysiologic. High-dose heparin avoids thrombosis of the CPB circuit, but low level of intravascular and intracircuit coagulation continues through bypass. The exposure of blood to the negatively charged surfaces of the CPB circuit triggers fibrinogen binding to the circuit, platelet, and coagulation activation (via factor XII). Once the platelets have been activated, they are not functional for the postoperative hemostasis. The extrinsic pathway is activated through the release of tissue factor during surgery in the surgical field. Both coagulation pathways activate thrombin with thrombotic and antithrombotic effects (Eaton and Iannoli 2011). The mechanical effect caused by the pump turbulence and active oxidation damages platelets and consumes coagulating factors. In addition the hemodilution effect by the CPB priming on the coagulating factors and platelets produces a hypocoagulable state upon CPB wean and through the postoperative period. In 5–7 % of the CPB runs the endothelium reacts to the surgical trauma releasing TPA (tissue plasminogen activator), which in hypocoagulable state causes a state of primary fibrinolysis. The activation of the coagulation by the CPC circuit, microembolic production, and tissue debris makes the patient prone to hypercoagulable state after heparin reversal with protamine and blood product use. CPB is a profoundly pro-inflammatory state with activation of multiple inflammatory humoral (e.g., interleukins, complement, etc.) and cellular mediators (e.g., monocytes and neutrophils). The inflammatory system and coagulation interact at many different levels by reducing inflammation, which reduces the activation of coagulation and vice versa (Cappabianca et al. 2011).

Monitoring of Coagulation

Laboratory-Based Coagulation Test

As previously stated, during the perioperative period, the use of traditional laboratory testing has been questioned since they are not predictive of perioperative hemorrhage. Furthermore, traditional testing in the perioperative period has been questioned due to the slow turnover (45–60 min) which by the time the results are back the patient situation may be completely different due to empiric administration of blood products and medication. It should not come to a surprise since traditional coagulation testing was not designed for quick coagulation diagnosis in the surgical period. The purpose of traditional testing is to predict isolated coagulation defects

Fig. 11.1 The coagulation factors plasma level necessary to keep a normal hemostasis in vivo. *PT* prothrombin time, *aPTT* activated partial thromboplastin time, *NA* not affected, *vWF* von Willebrand factor (Modified from Tanaka et al. 2009)

Factor	PT	aPTT	*In vivo*
Fibrinogen (mg/ dL)	100	60	50–100
Prothrombin (%)	50	15	20–30
Factor V (%)	50	40	20
Factor VII (%)	50	NA	10
Factor X (%)	60	25 %	20
Factor VIII (%)	NA	35 %	40
Factor IX (%)	NA	20 %	30
Factor XI (%)	NA	30 %	50
Factor XII (%)	NA	20 %	0
Factor XIII (%)	NA	NA	5
vWF (%)	NA	NA	30

such as hemophilia (aPTT) and/or treatment with oral anticoagulants vitamin K antagonist (PT/INR). Prothrombin time and aPTT are based on nonphysiological situation, testing ex vivo fibrin formation after artificial stimulation. Citrated blood is centrifuged; plasma is recalcified and activated in a crystal tube in which several optic measurements detect the beginning of the coagulation process or fibrin formation. The velocity of thrombus formation, strength, and tendency to dissolution cannot be extrapolated from traditional testing. The effect of platelet, VWF, FXIII inhibitors, and cellular components does not affect traditional testing. Recent hemostasis model highlights the importance of platelet activation and amplification in its surface in live models of coagulation (Hoffman and Monroe 2001). Due to this fact, the role of traditional testing is limited in the live coagulation process.

Figure 11.1 shows the coagulation factors plasma level necessary to keep normal hemostasis in vivo. The relationship between coagulation time and coagulating factors is not lineal; it is exponential (Dzik 2004). Due to this fact, abnormal coagulation testing is not necessarily associated with critical plasma level of coagulation factors. Plasma levels of 20–30 % of coagulating factors are necessary to achieve a normal hemostasis, but it will require plasma levels of 40–50 % for traditional coagulation testing to be normal. Blood loss equivalent to 50 % of the blood volume replaced by crystalloids (dilution) is associated with abnormal coagulation testing but is not always associated higher propensity to bleeding. This is due to the fact that PT and aPTT are more affected by moderated decrease (to 75 %) of several factors than the decrease of an isolated factor below 50 % of its level.

In the perioperative period, rarely there is an isolated decrease of a single factor; instead, usually there is generalized decrease of all factors including fibrinogen. Fibrinogen level is severalfold above the critical value of 100 mg/dl; below that is associated with bleeding tendency. This critical value is reached when there is a blood loss of 1.4 of the blood volume. When blood loss is about 2 blood volumes, critical levels of platelets and other coagulating factors is reached, and the tendency to further bleeding is enhanced (Hiippala et al. 1995). The recommended fibrinogen levels by most guidelines are higher (150–200 mg/dl) than the critical value described by the Hiippala et al. study in 1995 and are achieved sooner with lesser amount of hemodilution (Kozek-Langenecker et al. 2013; Spahn et al. 2013). It is difficult to picture that a complex process like the coagulation which requires

Table 11.3 Limitations of conventional laboratory coagulation analyses

Performed at a standardized temperature (37 °C) impeding the detection of coagulopathies induced by hypothermia
The global test (aPTT, INR/Quick) reflects only the initial formation of thrombin in plasma and is unaffected by any of the corpuscular elements of the blood
Conventional coagulation test does not provide any information about clot stability over time or regarding fibrinolysis
The platelet count is purely quantitative and cannot detect preexisting, drug-induced, or perioperatively acquired platelet dysfunction
Performing conventional laboratory analyses and reporting coagulation test results take 40–90 min after blood drawing

changes in the physical properties of the blood from liquid to solid (coagulation) and from solid to liquid (fibrinolysis) can be characterized with only two coagulation tests, platelet count and fibrinogen level and D-dimer. These traditional tests do not evaluate the whole hemostatic process but only just some punctual aspects of it.

In the clinical setting either in the operating room or the intensive care unit when we are faced to a hemorrhagic patient, two questions need to be answered. First, what is the cause of the hemorrhage? Second, how can we fix it? Oftentimes this question is addressed based only on traditional coagulation testing, and the treatment is mostly empiric with overuse of blood product, which is not free of risks (Karam et al. 2015). Many times the lonely clinician is unable to answer these two questions with the right tools to achieve a goal-directed therapy with medication and/or blood products

Table 11.3 summarizes the limitations of conventional coagulation laboratory testing (Weber et al. 2013).

Point-of-Care Monitoring

Thromboelastography (TEG®) and Thromboelastometry (ROTEM®)

The TEG/ROTEM attempt to address the initial two questions (What is the cause of the hemorrhage? How can we fix it?) by detecting the changes in the physical properties of the blood that reflect the hemostasis as a whole by the interaction of the whole blood components (Fig. 11.2).

The coagulation process can be divided into four phases that correspond with the current coagulation process:

1. Primary hemostasis is the interaction between the vascular components, platelets and vWF.
2. Second is the thrombin production triggered by the activation of factor X through the tissue factor (TF)-activated factor VII (FVIIa) complex.
3. Third is the thrombus formation by the polymerization of fibrin and finally the clot stabilization by the factor XIII.
4. Clot lysis.

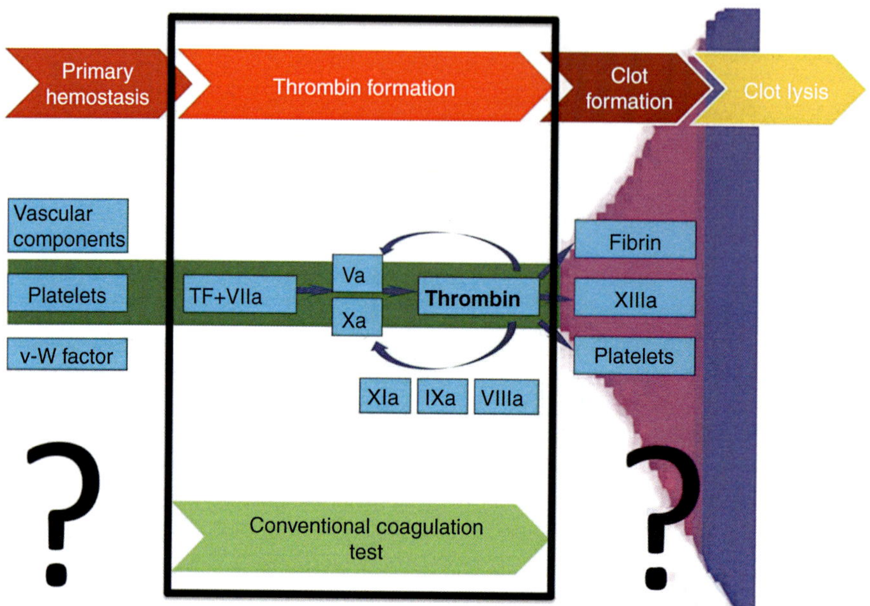

Fig. 11.2 Diagram of the coagulation process showing the areas that are unseen by conventional testing (*question mark*)

Traditional coagulation testing (PT and aPTT) just reflects the beginning of thrombin generation (Fig. 11.2). Conventional coagulation testing cannot assess primary hemostasis, clot formation, and clot lysis.

History and Nomenclature

The thromboelastography (TEG®) was described first by Hellmut Hartert in 1948 in Heidelberg, before the introduction of aPTT in clinical practice. It was fairly popular in the 1980s as a useful technique to assess the hemostatic process particularly in the beginning of liver transplant programs. In Fig. 11.3 the different stages of coagulation can be compared between traditional testing (green arrow inside the black square) and TEG®/ROTEM® which in addition assess the thrombin formation; it also shows the developing of the clot and its strength linked to platelet function, fibrin, and factor XIII. Finally, TEG®/ROTEM® shows the lysis of the clot (long arrow).

Even though TEG® was noted to be useful since the beginning, it was troublesome for clinical use due to the management complexity and extreme sensitivity to vibration. In 1993 Haemoscope Corporation IL, USA, patented the term TEG and currently Haemoscope is a division of Haemonetics Corporation (Fig. 11.4).

Latterly Pentapharm GMBH, Munich, patented a new device based on similar principles and used the term ROTEM (rotational thromboelastometry) (Fig. 11.5). Both tests are similar; some have the TEG ending (thromboelastography, thromboelastogram) and others the TEM ending (thromboelastometry, themogram).

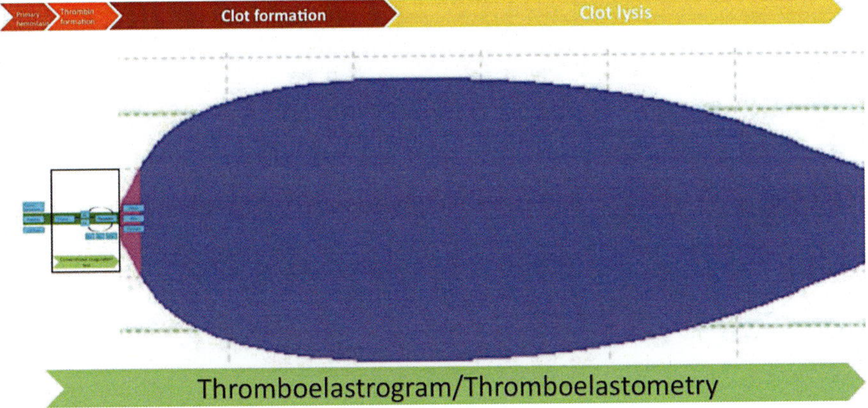

Fig. 11.3 Coagulation process (*above*). Conventional testing only reports the beginning of thrombin generation (*Black Square*). TEG®/ROTEM® report in addition to thrombin generation, clot formation, and lysis

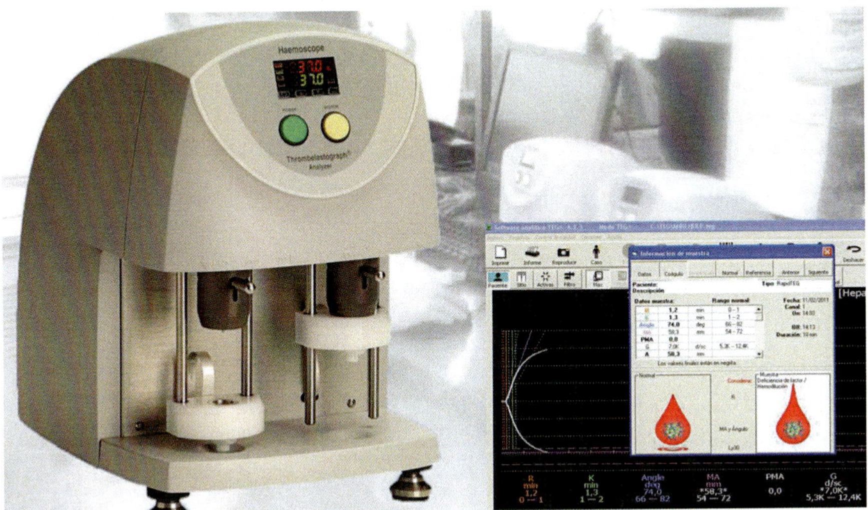

Fig. 11.4 Photograph of the TEG® 5000 hemostasis analyzer and related software screenshot (Used by permission of Haemonetics Corporation)

Currently, the technology has improved. Management is easier and less sensitivity to vibration, so it can be used in the surgical suite.

Operation Principles

Both devices had a similar operation principles based on measuring the changes of the viscoelastic properties of the clot associated with the polymerization of fibrin. The blood sample is placed in the tray with other reagents. In the TEG® the hanging pin is

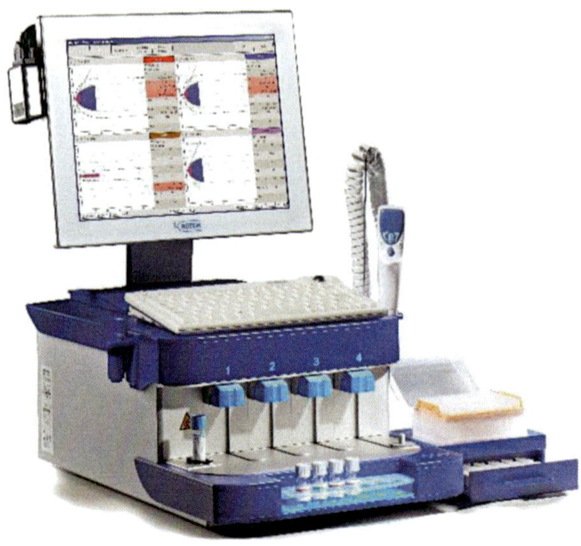

Fig. 11.5 Photograph of the ROTEM® delta hemostasis analyzer (Used by permission of Tem international GmbH)

still, detecting the movement of the tray that rotates from right to left 4.75 ° on the longitudinal axis. In the ROTEM® the tray is immobile and the hanging pin spins. Once the coagulation process starts with the production of fibrin, there is a restriction of the pin on the tray that is integrated electronically and represented in a graph, which has higher amplitude when there is higher resistance to movement (Fig. 11.6).

Graph Analysis and Parameters

We are going to describe the different parameters to interpret the ROTEM® (Fig. 11.7) and TEG® (Fig. 11.8).

The time it takes since the measurement starts to the beginning of clot formation is called *R* (*reaction time*) *in TEG®* and *CT* (*clotting time*) *in ROTEM®*. It is the line since the start of the graph until it reaches 2 mm in amplitude. It is measured in seconds, and it shows the speed in fibrin formation. It is affected by plasma coagulation factors and circulating anticoagulants.

The time it takes between the amplitude of the graph to increase from 2 to 20 mm wide is called *K* (*clot kinetics*), *α angle in TEG®, and CFT* (*clot formation time*) *in ROTEM®*. It is also measured in seconds, and it relates the information about the kinetics of the clot formation. It is a nonspecific parameter since it is influenced by coagulating factors, anticoagulants, fibrin polymerization, and clot stability (platelets, fibrin, and FXIII).

Maximal graph amplitude (MA in TEG®) or maximum clot firmness (MCF in ROTEM®). It is measured in mm and is one of the most important parameters since it reports the maximal clot firmness through the increase in fibrin polymerization, platelets, and FXIII. The use of FIBTEM or functional fibrinogen can differentiate between the platelets or fibrinogen contribution to the clot firmness.

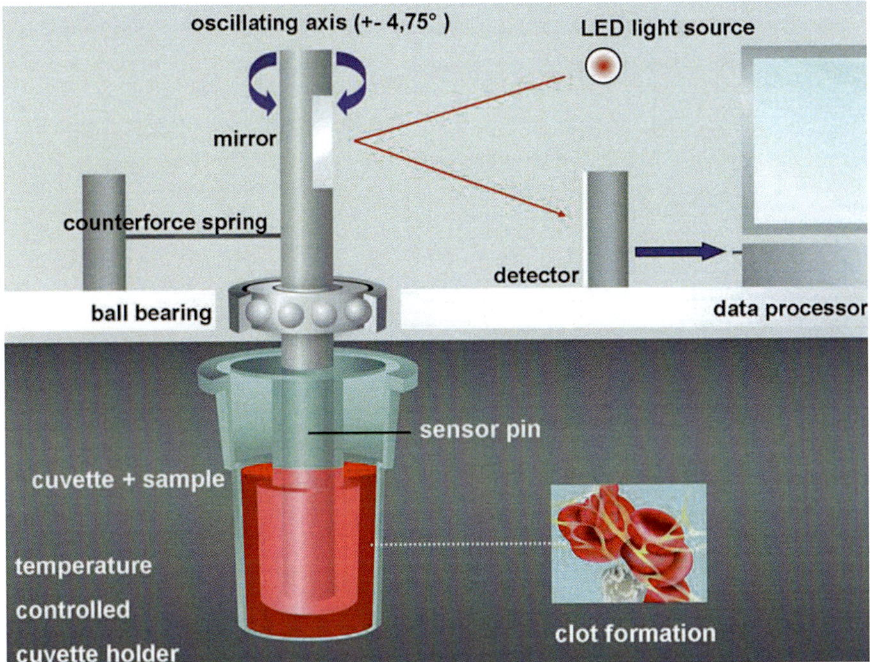

Fig. 11.6 Illustration of the ROTEM® detection principle (Used by permission of TEM international GmbH). A whole blood sample is placed into a cuvette and a cylindrical pin is immersed. Between pin and cuvette remains a gap of 1 mm, bridged by the blood. The pin is rotated by a spring to the right and the left. As long as the blood is liquid, the movement is unrestricted. When blood starts clotting, the clot increasingly restricts the rotation of the pin with rising clot firmness. This kinetic is detected mechanically and calculated by an integrated computer to the typical curves and numerical parameters. In TEG® the principle is similar, but the tray spins while the pin is fixed (adapted from image authorized by ROTEM®).

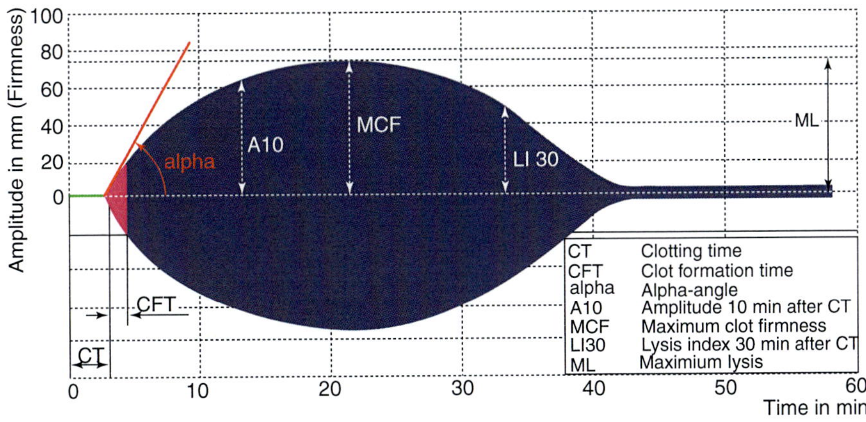

Fig. 11.7 ROTEM® graph and parameters (TEMogram) (Used by permission of Tem International GmbH)

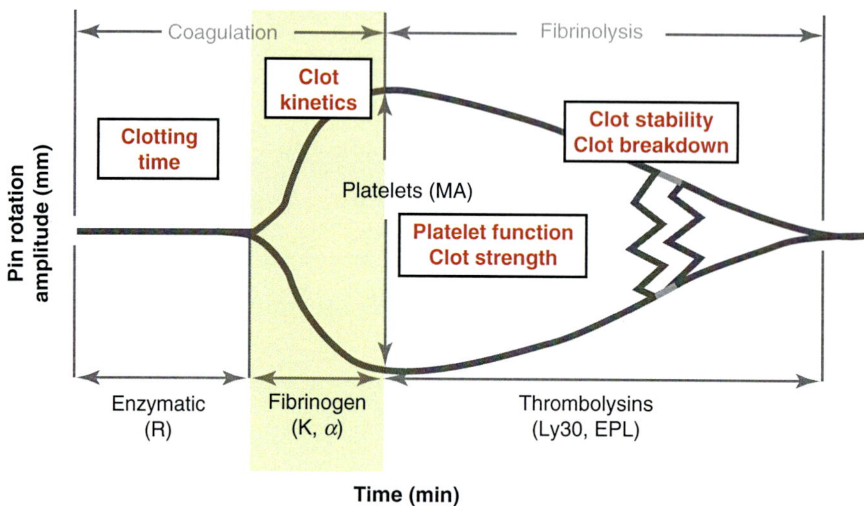

Fig. 11.8 TEG® hemostasis analyzer graph and parameters (Image used by permission of Haemonetics Corporation)

ML (*maximum lysis in ROTEM®*) is the reduction on clot firmness after MCF in relationship with time. It is presented in a percentage of the MCF. If the clot is stable, the ML is < 15 %. Fibrinolysis is considered when the ML > 15 %. In the *TEG®* the parameters *LY30 and LY60* measure the percentage of lysis at 30 and 60 min. LY30 is considered abnormal when > 7.5 %.

In TEG®, there is a hemostatic index (*CI, coagulation index*) that integrates R, K, α, and MA. Normal range for CI is −3 to +3, values < −3 represent hypocoagulable, and > 3 is hypercoagulable states.

Table 11.4 shows normal values for TEG® and Table 11.5 for ROTEM®.

Types of Testing

ROTEM® The testing is performed in citrated blood that implies the citrate reversal by the addition calcium chloride to the blood sample. The ROTEM pipetting is automatic, which facilitates the process. The new ROTEM needs a sample of whole citrated blood decreasing the pipetting and sample manipulation. The samples need to be run ideally within 2 h of the sample extraction to a maximum time of 4 h.

EXTEM is an in vitro semiquantitative testing on citrated blood recalcified through the activation of the extrinsic pathway by the thromboplastin (tissue factor). It measures from the start of the coagulation pathway to the clot formation and subsequent fibrinolysis (factors involved VII, X, V, II, I and platelets and fibrinolysis).

Table 11.4 TEG® hemostasis analyzer table of normal values used by permission of Haemonetics Corporation

	R (min)	α (degree)	K (min)	MA (mm)	LY30 (%)	CI (coagulation index)
Kaolín	4–8	47–74	0–4	54–72	>7.5 % fibrinolysis	< −3 hypocoagulability > +3 hypercoagulability
R-TEG	0–1	66–82	1–2	54–72	>7.5 % fibrinolysis	
FF	n.d.	n.d.	n.d.	9–29	n.d.	n.d.

R-TEG rapid TEG, *FF* functional fibrinogen, *min* minutes, *mm* millimeters, *n.d* no data

Table 11.5 ROTEM® table of normal values used by permission of Tem International GmbH

	CT (sg)	α-angle (°)	CFT (sg)	A10(mm)	*MCF(mm)*	LI30(%)	ML(%)
INTEM	100–240	70–83	30–110	44–66	50–72	94–100	0–15
EXTEM	38–79	63–83	34–160	43–65	50–72	94–100	0–15
FIBTEM	n.d.	n.d.	n.d.	7–23	9–25	n.d.	n.d.
HEPTEM	100–240	70–83	30–110	44–66	50–72	94–100	0–15
APTEM	38–79	63–83	34–160	43–65	50–72	94–100	0–15

sg seconds, *mm* millimeters, *n.d* no data

INTEM is an in vitro semiquantitative testing on citrated blood recalcified through the activation of the intrinsic pathway by the ellagic acid. It measures since the start of the coagulation pathway to the clot formation and subsequent fibrinolysis (factors involved XII, XI, IX, VII, X, V, II, I and platelets and fibrinolysis).

FIBTEM monitors specifically fibrinogen function. The activation of coagulation is similar to EXTEM but the reactants contain cytochalasin D that inactivates the platelets. The clot formed depends only in polymerization and fibrin formation. If we compare it with EXTEM, we can estimate the contribution of the platelets to the maximal clot firmness.

APTEM The coagulation is activated like in the EXTEM, but the reactants contain aprotinin which causes an in vitro inactivation of the fibrinolysis. Comparing EXTEM with APTEM results, it can be inferred if there is fibrinolysis if the APTEM results improve the EXTEM ones.

HEPTEM It is similar coagulation activation like INTEM but the reactant has heparinase. Comparing the INTEM with HEPTEM, we can detect if the coagulation anomalies are related to heparin and can be corrected with protamine.

NATEM It is global in vitro semiquantitative testing on citrated blood recalcified without a coagulation activator. The coagulation gets activated through the contact between the pin and the tray. Similar testing can be done in the TEG®.

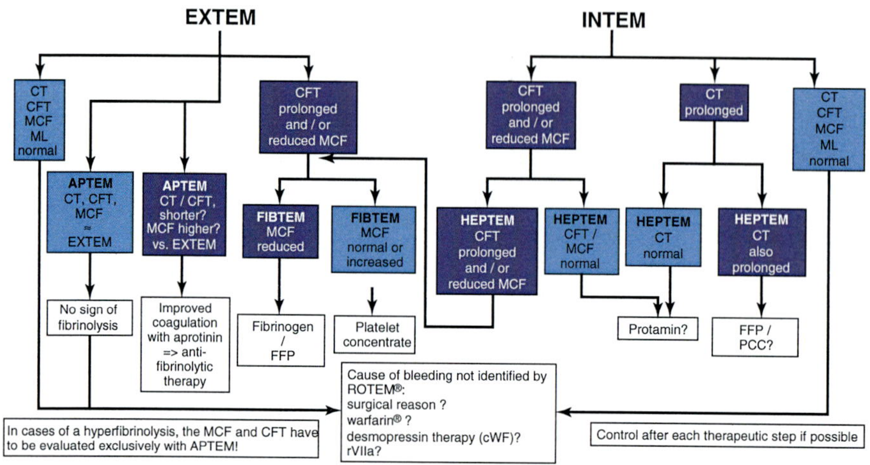

Fig. 11.9 Differential diagnosis and therapeutic ROTEM® algorithm used in the clinic cologne-merheim (Vorweg et al. 2001), and reproduced in ROTEM promotional material (Calatzis et al. 2013) (Reproduced with permission of TEM International GmbH)

Testing without coagulation activators are of little clinical use since there is a long latency before the results and has no advantages with traditional coagulation testing.

The ROTEM® has four channels, and it can run four simultaneous tests that need to be chosen depending on the clinical setting and the expected coagulation problem. Usually we run EXTEM, INTEM, and FIBTEM saving the last channel for the HEPTEM in patients who have been heparinized, or there is a suspected alteration of the intrinsic pathway (e.g., heparinized patient or unclamping of liver transplant). APTEM is used in patients that we suspect fibrinolysis. Figure 11.9 shows a diagnostic and treatment algorithm based on ROTEM®.

TEG® The TEG® can run on citrated blood in case the sample cannot be processed immediately, or it can be run immediately after blood is drawn (within 4 min from extraction). If citrated blood is used, it needs to be reversed with 20 μl calcium chloride 0,2 M to the tray. In TEG® 5000 pipetting is manual, and the testing is as follows:

Kaolin It is a global test activated by kaolin. It measures the coagulation activation, clot consolidation, and later fibrinolysis (Fig. 11.10).

- *Heparinase*: it measures the heparin effect comparing with normal kaolin testing. The test is similar to kaolin test but using a blue tray with heparinase.

- *Functional fibrinogen assay*: adds to the blood sample tissue factor and platelet inhibitor to separate the fibrinogen and platelet function. It estimates the fibrinogen function.

- *Rapid TEG*: speeds the coagulation process by triggering the intrinsic and extrinsic coagulation pathways by adding to the sample tissue factor, kaolin, and phospholipids. The result turnover is quicker and also monitors heparin anticoagulation by a specific TEG ACT. It is used for rapid coagulation evaluation in the multiple trauma setting.
- *Platelet mapping*: allows antiplatelet agents monitoring. It activates platelets by adding ADP, arachidonic acid, or both. It is especially useful to detect the risk of bleeding in the anti-aggregated surgical patient.

The equivalence between TEG® and ROTEM® is shown in Fig. 11.11. Even though there is similarity between TEG® and ROTEM® measurements, they are not completely interchangeable (Venema et al. 2010; Solomon et al. 2012).

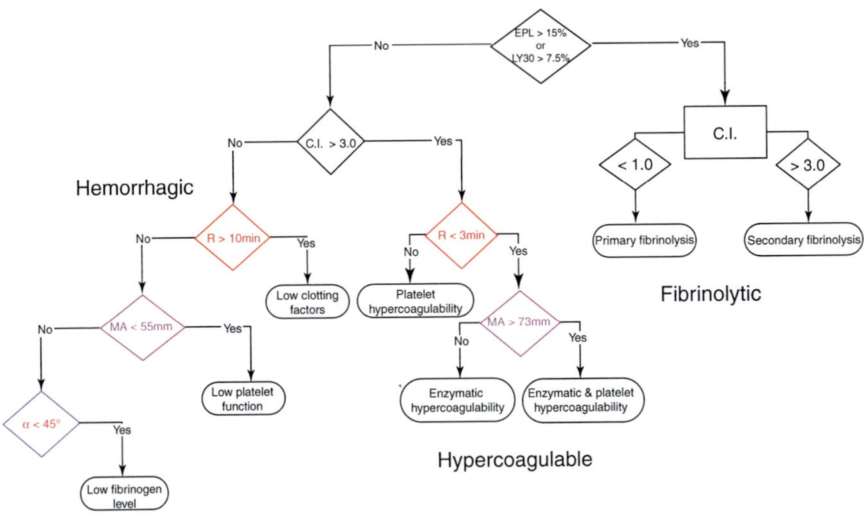

Fig. 11.10 TEG® interpretation algorithm (Used by permission of Haemonetics Corporation)

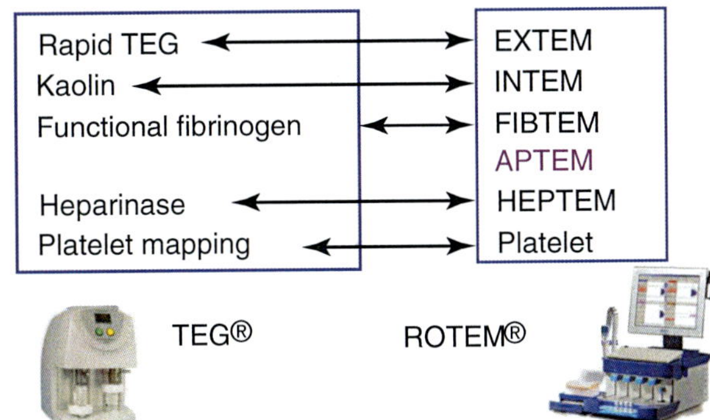

Fig. 11.11 Approximate equivalence between TEG® and ROTEM® testing

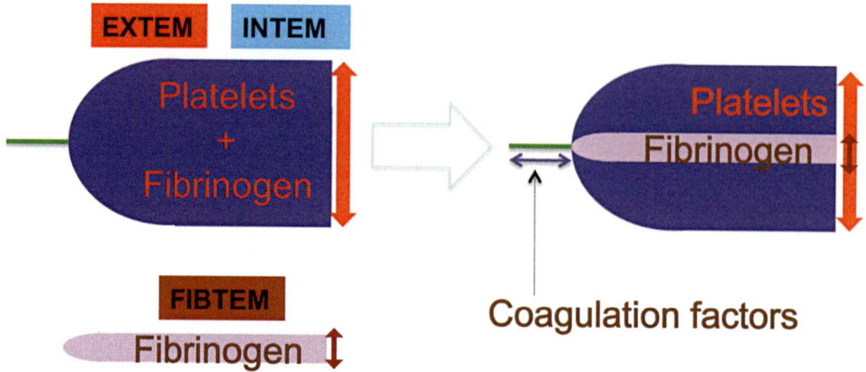

Fig. 11.12 ROTEM® graph interpretation

Result Interpretation

It may be intimidating for the neophyte with this technology, but the interpretation of the results is easy and intuitive. An experimented physician only seeing the graph without the values can have an estimation of the patient hemostasis. Figure 11.12 shows a graph display of TEG® and ROTEM® that helps to easily understand coagulation evaluation.

In summary to facilitate understanding, TEG® and ROTEM® testing assess individually coagulation factors (individual green line), platelet function, and fibrinogen. The last two are measured together in global testing in both systems, but fibrinogen can be assessed individually along with fibrinolysis (FIBTEM or functional fibrinogen). Global tests such as EXTEM or INTEM (navy blue graph) and the isolated fibrinogen function test (pink graph) are found on the left side of Fig. 11.12. There is no isolated platelet function testing, but if you subtract to the global testing graph the fibrinogen testing, you can estimate the platelet function (right side graph). Fibrinolysis can be observed by the graph tapering in form of teardrop.

Of course, in clinical practice the initial impression of reviewing the graph display should be verified with the numeric data.

Lately TEG® and ROTEM® testing have improved their technology to become more user-friendly and less sensible to vibration. ROTEM® has added to the ROTEM® *delta* system a platelet module (the ROTEM® *platelet*) working by impedance aggregometry and measuring platelet function in whole blood. Both TEG® and ROTEM® are about to launch new fully automated systems: *TEG®6 s* (resonance method) and *ROTEM® sigma* systems that have avoided the need for manual, controlled pipetting or prior manipulation of reagents. The only requirement is to transfer a small amount of blood to the loaded cartridge and wait for the trace (Fig. 11.13).

Indications and Limitations of Thromboelastography and Thromboelastometry

Since the beginning thromboelastography has been used in the operating room and ICU especially in cardiac surgery and liver transplantation. Currently, its use has been expanded to any bleeding situation where coagulopathy is involved and prompt

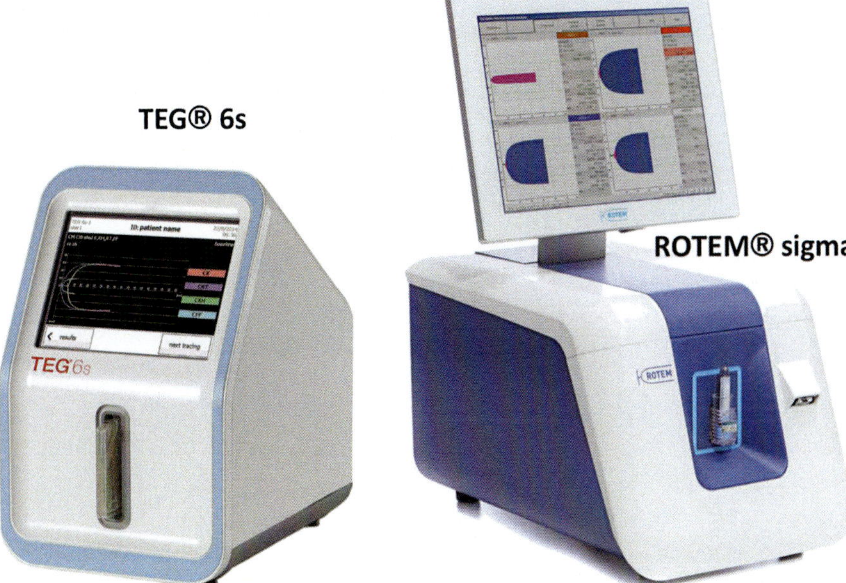

Fig. 11.13 Photographs of the latest devices developed by TEG® and ROTEM® (Published with permission of Haemonetics Corporation and Tem International GmbH)

Table 11.6 Common indications of viscoelastic testing

Major surgery
Cardiac surgery
Liver transplant
Scoliosis
Vascular surgery
Major bleeding
Multiple trauma
Obstetric hemorrhage
Severe burn
Heparinized patients: ECMO and VAD (ventricular assist device)
Acute normovolemic hemodilution
Medical disorders: hemopoyetic, liver, and renal disease

diagnosis and guided treatment is beneficial (Table 11.6). The clinical evidence for its use is still limited (Haas et al. 2014).

Even though these tests are performed in whole blood and currently is the best test available, it must be kept in mind that it is still an "in vitro" test that does not account for fluid dynamics in the vessels and endothelial interaction. For example, these are not useful for von Willebrand disease. In addition the coagulation activators added induce coagulation without participation of primary hemostasis. The primary hemostasis and platelet function cannot be evaluated by viscoelastic testing, and it is released in the ROTEM® fact sheet. The effect of aspirin and ADP antagonist (clopidogrel or ticlopidine) can only be

Table 11.7 Indications and limitations of viscoelastic testing

Indications of thromboelastography and thromboelastometry use
Bedside testing with short turnover
Global test of coagulation in whole blood
Easy model of interpretation of coagulation
Guided treatment (blood products and medications)
Cardiac surgery and liver transplant
Massive hemorrhage: multiple trauma and obstetric hemorrhage
Procoagulant state diagnosis and anti-procoagulant treatment diagnosis
Thromboelastography limitations
Static in vitro testing
Does not asses primary hemostasis (von Willebrand disease)
Difficulties in standardize the sample processing
Different equipment with different activators
Limited sensitivity to anti-aggregant treatment
Requires individual training to run testing
Needs quality control by personnel outside the laboratory

evaluated by specific testing. When there is a severe alteration of platelet function through glycoprotein IIb/IIIa inhibition either pharmacological or congenital (Glanzmann thrombasthenia), it could affect the maximal amplitude of the trace and the clot firmness. Another limitation is the low sensitivity to oral anticoagulant (e.g., Coumadin) or low molecular weight heparin administration. For these drugs there is specific testing including INR and anti-Xa activity, respectively. The indications and limitations of viscoelastic testing are summarized in Table 11.7.

Platelet Function Testing

Numerical and functional platelet disorders are common among pediatric cardiac surgery patients. Platelet function test can be useful to screen high-risk patients.

PFA-100® The PFA-100 (Siemens Healthcare, Malvern, PA, USA) is a system for analyzing platelet function in which citrated whole blood is aspirated at high shear rates through disposable cartridges containing an aperture within a membrane coated with either collagen and epinephrine (CEPI) or collagen and ADP (CADP). These agonists induce platelet adhesion, activation, and aggregation leading to rapid occlusion of the aperture and cessation of blood flow termed the closure time (CT). The PFA-100 can be useful in screening patients with von Willebrand disease or a platelet GpIb defect (Bernard-Soulier syndrome) and is often used to establish the presence or absence of aspirin resistance. The PFA-100 has a high negative predictive value (98 %) to identify patients not needing platelet transfusions post cardiac bypass (Slaughter et al. 2001). If the PFA-100 gives a normal result (78–199 s for the CEPI cartridge, 55–137 s for the CADP cartridge), then (with some exceptions: storage pool deficiency, primary secretion defects, mild type 1 vWD) primary hemostasis is intact and so may obviate further screening of platelet function defects. However, its use in a bleeding and coagulopathic patient is not well characterized as many of these tests may not work with dilutional coagulopathy (Theusinger et al. 2015).

VerifyNow System (Accumetrics, Inc., San Diego, CA) and ***whole blood impedance aggregometry*** (Multiplate, DynaByte, Munich, Germany) are used increasingly to monitor therapeutic responses to aspirin, P_2Y_{12} antagonists (ticlopidine, clopidogrel, prasugrel, ticagrelor, etc.), and GP IIB/IIIa inhibitors (abciximab or eptifibatide).

The VerifyNow® System is a whole blood, point-of-care test, which measures platelet-induced aggregation as an increase in light transmittance. It detects platelet activity by measuring in vitro platelet aggregation in a blood sample exposed to specific agonists. This includes inhibition of platelet activity in response to antiplatelet therapies. There are three types of VerifyNow tests: Aspirin, PRUTest (P2Y12), and IIb/IIIa. Each test device contains a lyophilized preparation of human fibrinogen-coated beads and a platelet agonist. The platelet agonist varies by test type. Each test is based upon the ability of GP IIb/IIIa receptors on activated platelets to bind to fibrinogen-coated beads. When the activated platelets are exposed to the fibrinogen-coated beads, aggregation occurs in proportion to the number of available platelet receptors. The instrument is designed to measure this aggregation as an increase in light transmittance allowing detection and quantification of the effect of antiplatelet medication.

The Multiplate analyzer® is a POC impedance aggregometer to detect and quantify the effect of antiplatelet medication. The device consists of five channels for contemporary tests, an integrated computer, and guided automatic pipetting. The principle of measurement of the Multiplate device is electrical impedance. An electrical current passes through individual sets of electrodes. When the electrodes come into contact with a whole blood sample, platelets bind to and cover the electrodes in a small monolayer. As the platelets become activated after exposure to a specific platelet agonist, the platelets strongly adhere to the electrodes and begin to aggregate. An increase in the number of platelets adhering to the electrodes increases the resistance (impedance) between the pair of electrodes. The Multiplate records platelet aggregation at approximately 0.5 s interval, and its software plots these changes as a curve. Three parameters are calculated: aggregation, area under the curve (AUC), and velocity. The most important parameter is the area under the aggregation curve (AUC). AUC is recorded as units or U. It is affected by the total height of the aggregation curve as well as by its slope and is best suited to express the overall platelet activity. The aggregation (in AU) is the maximum height of the curve during the measurement period and the velocity (in AU/min) is the maximum slope of the curve (Table 11.8).

Table 11.8 Test available for Multiplate analyzer

Test	Activation	Sensitivity	Not sensitive for
ASPI test	Arachidonic acid: is converted to TXA2 by platelet-own cyclooxygenase	Aspirin, Gp IIb/IIIa antagonists	Clopidogrel, vWF
ADP test	ADP: binds onto platelet ADP receptors	Clopidogrel, Gp IIb/IIIa antagonists	Aspirin, vWF
ADP test HS	ADP + prostaglandin E1 (prostaglandin is a natural inhibitor and enhances the sensitivity of the assay for clopidogrel)	Clopidogrel, Gp IIb/IIIa antagonists	Aspirin, vWF
TRAP test	TRAP-6 (thrombin receptor activating peptide): TRAP-6 is a potent agonist which mimics the platelet-activating action of thrombin	Gp IIb/IIIa antagonists	vWF, aspirin, clopidogrel (weak effect on TRAP test)
COL test	Collagen: collagen activates platelet and triggers a release of arachidonic acid from the platelet membrane, which is converted to TXA2 by the cyclooxygenase	Aspirin, Gp IIb/IIIa antagonists	Clopidogrel, vWF
RISTO test	Ristocetin: vWF dependent platelet activation via the GpIb receptor	Bernard-Soulier syndrome, severe vWD, aspirin	Mild vWD

TXA2 thromboxane A2, *Gp* glycoprotein, *vWF* von Willebrand factor, *ADP* adenosine diphosphate

TEG® Platelet Mapping The whole blood Thrombelastograph (TEG®) Platelet Mapping assay (Haemoscope Corporation, Niles, Illinois, US) measures clot strength and maximal amplitude (MA), reflects maximal platelet function, and detects the reduction in platelet function, presented as percentage inhibition, by both aspirin (Tantry et al. 2005) and clopidogrel. The TEG® Platelet Mapping assay relies on evaluation of clot strength to enable a quantitative analysis of platelet function. Platelet mapping is a modification of TEG allowing a specific examination of platelet function relating to two different agonists, arachidonic acid (AA) and adenosine-5-diphosphate (ADP). Thrombin activation (initiated in the TEG assay by contact with kaolin) of platelets is so powerful that it masks any effect of secondary platelet activators. Therefore, this reaction is carried out in the setting of heparinized blood to block thrombin activation. Factor XIII is added to generate a baseline fibrin meshwork (generates fibrin) and represents minimal platelet activation. The contribution of the ADP or thromboxaneA2 (TxA2) receptors to the clot formation is provided by the addition of ADP or AA. The curves generated are compared to standard TEG trace. Platelet Mapping™ has shown a statistically significant correlation to optical platelet aggregation as the gold standard assay (Craft et al. 2004).

Platelet mapping is useful for the evaluation of adequate platelet inhibition by aspirin or clopidogrel (Craft et al. 2004), and it is useful in percutaneous coronary angioplasty (PTCA). During these procedures due to the endothelial damage and clot rupture in the coronary artery, the coagulation cascade is activated and platelets have a key role in the ischemic complications after PTCA. Platelet inhibition by GPIIb/IIIa receptor inhibitors is a potent therapy to reduce the risk of myocardial infarction and death. There are several types of drugs that can be monitored by this test to secure adequate anti-aggregation avoiding excessive inhibition that could derive in bleeding. In fact, TEG® Platelet Mapping was able to predict excessive postoperative chest tube bleeding and the need for platelet transfusion (Chowdhury et al. 2014).

The ROTEM® *platelet* ROTEM® *delta* system incorporates a platelet module that works by impedance aggregometry, measuring platelet function in whole blood. With the influence of von Willebrand factor (vWF) at the place of the injury, the platelet stick to the exposed collagen (= adhesion), leading to activation of further platelets. Fibrinogen plays a key role at the aggregation of platelets. The detection method works placing a whole blood sample into a cuvette with two electrodes. After the addition of the reagent, the platelets are activated, aggregating to the electrodes within the next minutes. The measured impedance between the electrodes increases and is graphically displayed as a curve. The result is represented via three parameters:

- *A6* (Ohm): *A6* shows the measured impedance at the measurement time of 6 min as amount of platelet aggregation.
- *Maximum slope* (Ohm/min): *MS* is the maximum slope of the aggregation graph and a measurement rate of aggregation.
- *Area under the curve* (Ohm*min): *AUC* contains the area under the aggregation curve from the start of measurement to 6 min and provides information on the overall platelet aggregation.

With the ROTEM® *platelet*, differential diagnosis, and the tests ADPTEM, TRAPTEM, and ARATEM, the reason for a decreased platelet aggregation can be determined. A disturbed platelet aggregation is indicated by a decreased amplitude (curve). As causes, the intake of drugs that are influencing the platelet function or platelet dysfunctions due to, e.g., extracorporeal assist devices, surgery, or others has to be considered. Drugs, which can influence the platelet aggregation, are cyclo-oxygenase inhibitors (e.g., patient treatment with acetylsalicylic acid), GP IIb/IIIa receptor blockers (e.g., patient treatment with GP IIb/IIIa antagonists), or ADP receptor blocker (e.g., patient treatment with thienopyridines or direct ADP receptor antagonists). The results are available fast, and therefore a difference between surgical bleeding and platelet dysfunction can be made, and the monitoring of a platelet therapy is possible.

Monitoring Integration in Clinical Care

In cardiac surgery post-CPB, there is a limited predictive capability with the available testing, but there is high negative predictive value. In other words, if the TEG® is normal, it rules out coagulopathy, and surgical causes of bleeding should be explored (Cammerer et al. 2003). The use of TEG® helps to achieve prompt diagnosis and treatment of the postoperative hemorrhage in cardiac surgery (Despotis et al. 2009). Once the patient is on CPB, there is decrease in the maximal amplitude in all tests without platelet inhibitor (e.g., ROTEM® EXTEM and TEG® kaolín with heparinase) due to the effect of hemodilution by the prime of the CPB circuit that reduces the platelet and fibrinogen function. This effect is also seen in test with platelet inhibitor FIBTEM (ROTEM®) and functional fibrinogen (TEG®) that shows fibrinogen dilution. Platelet dysfunction worsens with CBP duration. During full heparinization on CPB, the trace of the tests that are susceptible to anticoagulation with heparin such as INTEM (ROTEM®) and kaolín (TEG®) will be a flat line. To obtain a meaningful test on CPB, heparinase is needed to neutralize the heparin effect such as HEPTEM (ROTEM®) and heparinase (TEG®). These testing will also detect the presence of fibrinolysis and its response to treatment. Thromboelastography and thromboelastometry are the gold standard for the fibrinolysis diagnosis since it is more specific in the surgical patient than the fibrin degradation products and/or D-dimer (increased in the setting of trauma, tumor, or orthopedic surgery). Fibrinolysis diagnosis is made by the lysis times reviewed previously on this chapter. It can easily been noticed by thinning at the end of the graph. Figure 11.4 shows a pediatric patient undergoing a heart transplant who developed fibrinolysis.

Post protamine administration, the comparison between test with and without heparinase could tell us the need of additional protamine if the traces are different (Mittermayr et al. 2009). At this time the need for platelets, fibrinogen, and other blood products needs to be assessed. It must be kept in mind that activated clotting time (ACT) not only depends on heparin administration, but it is also affected by hemodilution, low platelet count, hipofibrinogenemia, and/or protamine overdose. Repeated doses of protamine prolong the ACT and cause additional platelet dysfunction. Usually protamine is administered far too much to treat bleeding in patients who really do not need it. The erroneous approach is to treat ACT values, not unreversed heparin (Levy and Tanaka 2009).

Recent guidelines from the European Society of Anaesthesiology in management of severe perioperative bleeding (Kozek-Langenecker et al. (2013) recommend that fibrinogen concentrate infusion guided by point-of-care viscoelastic coagulation monitoring should be used to reduce perioperative blood loss in complex cardiovascular surgery (1B level of evidence), suggesting the use of fibrinogen concentrate or cryoprecipitate to increase plasma fibrinogen concentrations above trigger values of 1.5–2.0 g/L or FIBTEM MCF>7 in bleeding children (2C).

During the prolonged exposure to artificial surfaces like mechanical valves, artificial hearts, and/or assist devices, there is a hypercoagulable state beyond the CPB period. This continuous exposure enhanced by turbulent flows activates platelets causing white thrombi. In addition if the intrinsic and/or extrinsic coagulation pathways are activated, red thrombi can be produced as well. Big thrombi can obstruct the flow to vital organs and if fragmented can embolize distally. To avoid this hypercoagulable state, this patient population requires anticoagulant and anti-aggregant treatment that can be monitored by thromboelastogram and platelet function monitors. Heparin anticoagulation increases the R-value and platelet function inhibition is adjusted with specific testing.

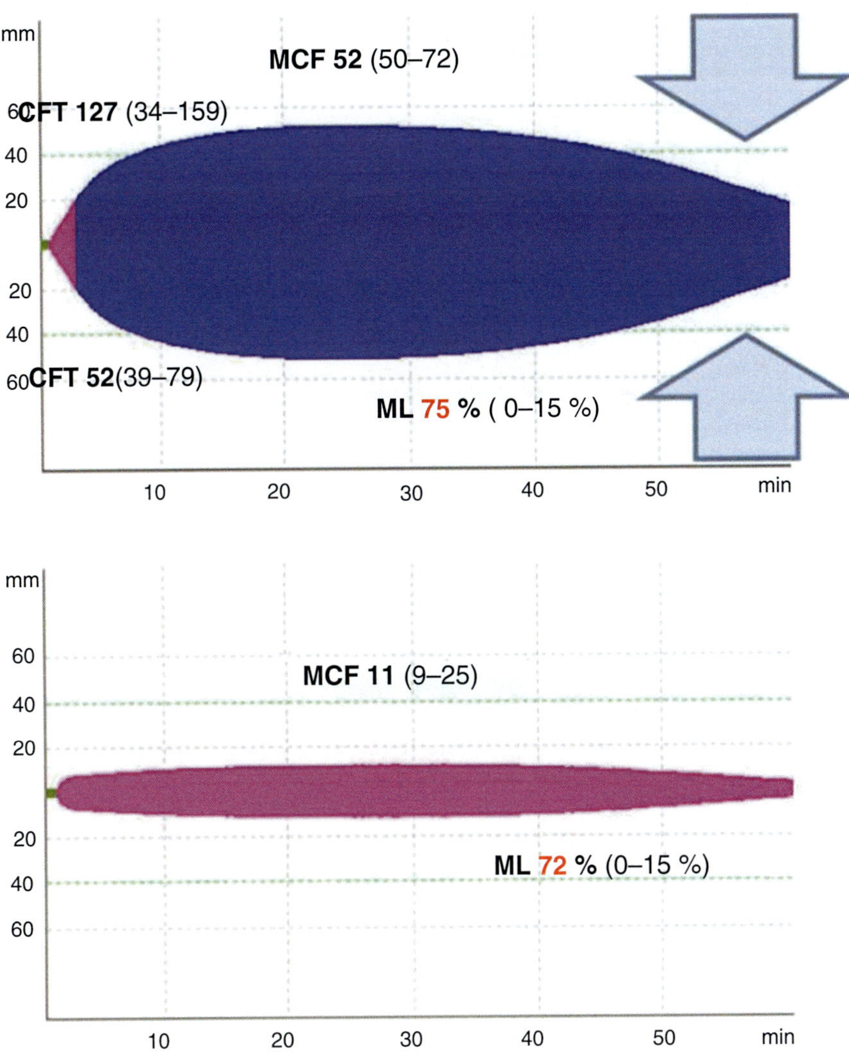

Fig. 11.14 EXTEM graph (*above*) and FIBTEM graph (*below*) showing thinning at the end of the graph (*arrows*) suggestive of hyperfibrinolysis

ROTEM® and TEG® have developed algorithm to be used in cardiac surgery and are summarized in Table 11.9:

Clinical guidelines by the Society of Thoracic Surgeons and the Society of Cardiovascular Anesthesiologist published in 2007 addressing the need of bedside coagulation monitoring should guide blood product administration. Through the guideline there is discussion about the validity of methods and algorithm to guide blood and blood product use. Interestingly enough in Chap. 7, reviewing the use of ROTEM® and/or TEG® for bedside monitoring of hemostasis and decrease blood product in cardiac surgery use, the level of evidence was A (based on prospective

Table 11.9 Protocol of test to be measured in cardiac surgery

Sample times	ROTEM®[b]	TEG®
Anesthesia (before CPB)	INTEM EXTEM FIBTEM	Kaolin ± Rapid TEG Functional fibrinogen
Late phase of *CPB* (rewarming)	HEPTEM EXTEM FIBTEM	Heparinase ± rapid TEG Functional fibrinogen
10 min after *Protamine*	HEPTEM + INTEM[a] FIBTEM	Kaolin + heparinase[a] Functional fibrinogen
ICU	EXTEM	± Rapid TEG

[a]CT_{INTEM}/CT_{HEPTEM} or kaolin/heparinase = 1.0 for optimizing heparin neutralization
If there is suspicion of hyperfibrinolysis: + APTEM
After each treatment: repeat test with abnormal results
Platelet function test (Platelet Mapping or ROTEM Platelet) should be considered in patients who recently used aspirin and P_2Y_{12} antagonists
[b]*Note*: This recommendation is based on liquid ROTEM® reagents. The heparin sensitive single use reagents fib-tem S, ex-tem S, and ap-tem S are not used for testing during CPB

randomized studies). In June 2008 NHS Quality Improvement Scotland published recommendation regarding the effectiveness of ROTEM® and TEG®. This report was built with health technology assessment tool, which reviews the evidence base in four aspects:

1. Clinical effectiveness: the report concluded that viscoelastic testing reduces the number of blood transfusion, complications, and infections from isolated clinical management.
2. Costs and benefits: improves quality of life and is cost-effective. ROTEM® and TEG® even though more expensive than traditional testing but save blood, blood product administration, hospital stay, and short- and long-term complications.
3. Organizing aspects: differences exist in the way different hospitals use ROTEM® and TEG®.
4. Patient benefits: avoiding transfusion is welcomed by patients.

Based on this evidence, the NHS Quality Improvement Scotland recommended the use of ROTEM® and TEG® instead of traditional coagulation testing to identify bleeding during or after cardiac surgery or liver transplant (Craig et al. 2008).

The publications show that there is a reduction of blood product use in cardiac surgery which is guided by thromboelastogram or thromboelastometry algorithm versus the use of clinical judgment and traditional testing (Nuttall et al. 2001; Agarwal et al. 2015b). In addition there is a reduction in the surgical re-exploration in cardiac surgery once thromboelastography has been introduced in clinical practice (Spiess et al. 1995).

Individualized goal-directed hemostatic therapy seems to be safer and most effective approach to stop bleeding in cardiac surgery. The POC algorithm guided by thromboelastometry and whole blood impedance aggregometry based on first-line therapy with fibrinogen and prothrombin complex has reduced the use of blood transfusion, reduced the incidence of thrombotic/thromboembolic and transfusion-related adverse events, decreased cost, and improved patient outcomes (Görlinger et al. 2013b). A recent National Institute for Health and Care Excellence (NICE), UK, diagnostic guideline recommends viscoelastic devices (ROTEM and TEG) to help monitor blood clotting during and after cardiac surgery, because the use of viscoelastometric POC testing devices was shown to be "associated with lower mortality, a reduced probability of experiencing complications, and less transfusion and hospitalization" (NICE 2014). Furthermore, when coagulopathy is suspected, the American Society of Anesthesiologists (ASA) advocates the use of POC testing devices to identify and treat the cause of bleeding (ASA 2015).

Görlinger et al. 2013a, in a large retrospective study that reviewed 14,162 ROTEM assays obtained from adults undergoing noncardiac surgery observed that early values of clot firmness, measured as soon as 5 min after clotting time, were strongly correlated (r>0.9) with the maximum clot firmness (MCF). In another study performed on 437 ROTEM® obtained from adults undergoing cardiac surgery with cardiopulmonary bypass, Dirkmann et al. (2013) confirmed the strong correlations between A5, A10, A15, and MCF, both before and after protamine administration. Perez-Ferrer et al. (2015) in a large multicenter retrospective study that analyzed data from 4762 ROTEM® obtained in children who underwent cardiac or noncardiac surgeries demonstrated a strong correlation between early values of clot amplitudes (e.g., A5, A10, A15) and maximum clot firmness (MCF). These results confirmed that the use of early thromboelastometry parameters (as soon as 5 min after clotting time) allows for an early goal-directed hemostatic therapy in bleeding children, as demonstrated by Nakayama et al. (2015) in 100 pediatric cardiac patients, using early thromboelastometric variables (EXTEM-A10 and INTEM-A10) in the ROTEM algorithm and comparing with conventional care, reduced bleeding, red cell transfusion, and critical care duration.

The number of patients treated with antiplatelet drugs due to cardiovascular disease is continuously increasing, even in pediatric patients. New ADP receptor antagonists are being developed with different pharmacokinetic and pharmacodynamic profile which its antiplatelet effect needs to be assessed. POC testing may be desired to guide a bridging protocol when one or two of the antiplatelet drugs are to be discontinued. Moreover, patients not responding to antiplatelet drugs can be identified. However, some institutions treat these patients without using these devices and the standard of care has to be determined yet (Theusinger et al. 2015). POC testing allows monitoring the hemostasis which is one of the most worrisome aspects of any surgery. These are global coagulation testing run at the bedside (e.g., operation room and ICU) that allows managing ongoing coagulopathy.

The use of POC devices integrated in evidence-based algorithms is one of the important mechanisms to limit blood product exposure, avoiding transfusion-related adverse events. POC-based algorithms allow goal-directed transfusions of blood products and better-targeted factor concentrate substitutions.

References

Agarwal HS, Barrett SS, Barry K, et al. Association of blood products administration during cardiopulmonary bypass and excessive post-operative bleeding in pediatric cardiac surgery. Pediatr Cardiol. 2015a;36:459–67.

Agarwal S, Johnson RI, Shaw M. Preoperative point-of-care platelet function testing in cardiac surgery. J Cardiothorac Vasc Anesth. 2015b;29:333–41.

American Society of Anesthesiologists Task Force on Perioperative Blood Management. Practice guidelines for perioperative blood management: an updated report by the American Society of Anesthesiologists Task Force on Perioperative Blood Management*. Anesthesiology. 2015;122:241–75.

Andrew M, Vegh P, Johnston M, Bowker J, Ofosu F, Mitchell L. Maturation of the hemostatic system during childhood. Blood. 1992;80(8):1998–2005.

Calatzis A, Spannagl M, Vorweg M. ROTEM® analysis targeted treatment of acute haemostatic disorders. ROTEM Promotional Analysis Booklet; 2013.

Cammerer U, Dietrich W, Rampf T, et al. The predictive value of modified computerized thromboelastography and platelet function analysis for postoperative blood loss in routine cardiac surgery. Anesth Analg. 2003;96(1):51–7.

Cappabianca G, Rotunno C, de Luca Tupputi Schinosa L, et al. Protective effects of steroids in cardiac surgery: a meta-analysis of randomized double-blind trials. J Cardiothorac Vasc Anesth. 2011;25(1):156–65.

Chee YL, Crawford JC, Watson HG, Greaves M. Guidelines on the assessment of bleeding risk prior to surgery or invasive procedures. British Committee for Standards in Haematology. Br J Haematol. 2008;140(5):496–504.

Chowdhury M, Shore-Lesserson L, Mais AM, et al. Thromboelastograph with Platelet Mapping (TM) predicts postoperative chest tube drainage in patients undergoing coronary artery bypass grafting. J Cardiothorac Vasc Anesth. 2014;28(2):217–23.

Craft RM, Chavez JJ, Bresee SJ, et al. A novel modification of the Thromboelastograph assay, isolating platelet function, correlates with optical platelet aggregation. J Lab Clin Med. 2004;143:3001–9.

Craig J, Aguiar-Ibanez R, Bhattacharya S, et al. HTA Programme: health technology assessment report 11 – the clinical and cost effectiveness of thromboelastography/thromboelastometry. NHS Quality Improvement Scotland. 2008. www.nhshealthquality.org. Accessed Aug 2015.

Despotis G, Avidan M, Eby C. Prediction and management of bleeding in cardiac surgery. J Thromb Haemost. 2009;7 Suppl 1:111–7.

Dirkmann D, Gorlinger K, Dusse F, et al. Early thromboelastometric variables reliably predict maximum clot firmness in patients undergoing cardiac surgery: a step towards earlier decision making. Acta Anaesthesiol Scand. 2013;57:594–603.

Dzik WH. Predicting hemorrhage using preoperative coagulation screening assays. Curr Hematol Rep. 2004;3(5):324–30.

Eaton MP, Iannoli EM. Coagulation considerations for infants and children undergoing cardiopulmonary bypass. Paediatr Anaesth. 2011;21(1):31–42.

Gertler R, Hapfelmeier A, Tassani-Prell P, et al. The effect of cyanosis on perioperative platelet function as measured by multiple electrode aggregometry and postoperative blood loss in neonates and infants undergoing cardiac surgery. Eur J Cardiothorac Surg. 2014. pii: ezu412.

Görlinger K, Dirkmann D, Solomon C, et al. Fast interpretation of thromboelastometry in non-cardiac surgery: reliability in patients with hypo-, normo-, and hypercoagulability. Br J Anaesth. 2013a;110:222–30.

Görlinger K, Shore-Lesserson L, Dirkmann D, et al. Management of hemorrhage in cardiothoracic surgery. J Cardiothorac Vasc Anesth. 2013b;27(4 Suppl):S20–34.

Haas T, Spielmann N, Mauch J, et al. Comparison of thromboelastometry (ROTEM®) with standard plasmatic coagulation testing in paediatric surgery. Br J Anaesth. 2012;108(1):36–41.

Haas T, Görlinger K, Grassetto A, et al. Thromboelastometry for guiding bleeding management of the critically ill patient: a systematic review of the literature. Minerva Anestesiol. 2014;80(12):1320–35.

Hiippala ST, Myllylä GJ, Vahtera EM. Hemostatic factors and replacement of major blood loss with plasma-poor red cell concentrates. Anesth Analg. 1995;81(2):360–5.

Hoffman M, Monroe 3rd DM. A cell-based model of hemostasis. Thromb Haemost. 2001;85:958–65.

Karam O, Demaret P, Shefler A, et al. Indications and effects of plasma transfusions in critically ill children. Am J Respir Crit Care Med. 2015;191(12):1395–402.

Kozek-Langenecker SA, Afshari A, et al. Management of severe perioperative bleeding: guidelines from the European Society of Anaesthesiology. Eur J Anaesthesiol. 2013;30(6):270–382.

Levy JH, Tanaka KA. Anticoagulation and reversal paradigms: is too much of a good thing bad? Anesth Analg. 2009;108(3):692–4.

Miller BE, Mochizuki T, Levy JH, et al. Predicting and treating coagulopathies after cardiopulmonary bypass in children. Anesth Analg. 1997a;85:1196–202.

Miller BE, Bailey JM, Mancuso TJ, Weinstein MS, Holbrook GW, Silvey EM, Tosone SR, Levy JH. Functional maturity of the coagulation system in children: an evaluation using thrombelastography. Anesth Analg. 1997b;84(4):745–8.

Mittermayr M, Velik-Salchner C, Stalzer B, et al. Detection of protamine and heparin after termination of cardiopulmonary bypass by thrombelastometry (ROTEM): results of a pilot study. Anesth Analg. 2009;108(3):743–50.

Nakayama Y, Nakajima Y, Tanaka KA, et al. Thromboelastometry-guided intraoperative haemostatic management reduces bleeding and red cell transfusion after paediatric cardiac surgery. Br J Anesth. 2015;114:91–102.

National Institute for Health and Care Excellence. Detecting, managing and monitoring haemostasis: viscoelastometric point-of-care testing (ROTEM, TEG and Sonoclot systems). 2014. https://www.nice.org.uk/guidance/dg13. Accessed Aug 2015.

Nuttall GA, Oliver WC, Santrach PJ, et al. Efficacy of a simple intraoperative transfusion algorithm for nonerythrocyte component utilization after cardiopulmonary bypass. Anesthesiology. 2001;94:773–81.

Perez-Ferrer A, Vicente-Sanchez J, Carceles-Baron MD, et al. Early thromboelastometry variables predict maximum clot firmness in children undergoing cardiac and non-cardiac surgery. Br J Anaesth. 2015;115(6):896–902.

Samkova A, Blatny J, Fiamoli V, Dulicek P, Parizkova E. Significance and causes of abnormal preoperative coagulation test results in children. Haemophilia. 2012;18(3):e297–301.

Slaughter TF, Sreeram G, Sharma AD, et al. Reversible shear-mediated platelet dysfunction during cardiac surgery as assessed by the PFA-100 platelet function analyzer. Blood Coagul Fibrinolysis. 2001;12(2):85–93.

Solomon C, Sørensen B, Hochleitner G, et al. Comparison of whole blood fibrin-based clot tests in thrombelastography and thromboelastometry. Anesth Analg. 2012;114(4):721–30.

Spahn DR, Bouillon B, Cerny V, et al. Management of bleeding and coagulopathy following major trauma: an updated European guideline. Crit Care. 2013;19(2):R76.

Spiess BD, Gillies BS, Chandler W, et al. Changes in transfusion therapy and reexploration rate after institution of a blood management program in cardiac surgical patients. J Cardiothorac Vasc Anesth. 1995;9(2):168–73.

Spiezia L, Campello E, Simioni P. "Hypocoagulable" thromboelastography profiles in patients with cyanotic congenital heart disease: facts or technical artifacts? Int J Cardiol. 2013;168(3):2914.

Szekely A, Cserep Z, Sapi E, et al. Risks and predictors of blood transfusion in pediatric patients undergoing open heart operations. Ann Thorac Surg. 2009;87:187–97.

Tanaka KA, Key NS, Levy JH. Blood coagulation: hemostasis and thrombin regulation. Anesth Analg. 2009;108(5):1433–46.

Tantry US, Bliden KP, Gurbel PA. Overestimation of platelet aspirin resistance detection by thrombelastograph platelet mapping and validation by conventional aggregometry using arachidonic acid stimulation. J Am Coll Cardiol. 2005;46:1705–9.

Theusinger OM, Stein P, Levy JH. Point of care and factor concentrate-based coagulation algorithms. Transfus Med Hemother. 2015;42(2):115–21.

Venema LF, Post WJ, Hendriks HG, et al. An assessment of clinical interchangeability of TEG and RoTEM thromboelastographic variables in cardiac surgical patients. Anesth Analg. 2010;111(2):339–44.

Vorweg M, Hartmann B, Knüttgen D, et al. Management of fulminant fibrinolysis during abdominal aortic surgery. J Cardiothorac Vasc Anesth. 2001;15(6):764–7.

Weber CF, Klages M, Zacharowski K. Perioperative coagulation management during cardiac surgery. Curr Opin Anaesthesiol. 2013;26(1):60–4.

Willems A, Harrington K, Lacroix J, et al. Comparison of two red-cell transfusion strategies after pediatric cardiac surgery: a subgroup analysis. Crit Care Med. 2010;38:649–56.

Williams GD, Bratton SL, Ramamoorthy C. Factors associated with blood loss and blood product transfusions: a multivariate analysis in children after open-heart surgery. Anesth Analg. 1999;89:57–64.

Wolf MJ, Maher KO, Kanter KR, et al. Early postoperative bleeding is independently associated with increased surgical mortality in infants after cardiopulmonary bypass. J Thorac Cardiovasc Surg. 2014;148:631–6.

Part III
Preoperative Considerations

Chapter 12
Preoperative Evaluation

Ramin Baghaei Tehrani

Introduction

Evaluation of the patient with congenital cardiac lesion consists of complete understanding of the anatomic detail of the lesion as well as its pathophysiological impact. To achieve this goal, the clinician should first gather information from medical history, physical examination, and paraclinical studies. Then, he or she can interpret patient's information in the context of making an accurate diagnosis. This chapter describes sequential steps of a rational preoperative evaluation in patients with congenital cardiac disease.

Medical History

The first step for approach to the patient suspected of having a congenital heart disease is a thorough medical history. Data collection should be returned back to the fetal life. Some information related to the mother's pregnancy could be very important. For example, infants born of mothers with diabetes mellitus may have different kinds of congenital heart defects (Rowland et al. 1973). According to one study, the incidence of congenital heart disease in this group is 4 %, which is five times the incidence in the general population (Mace et al. 1979). The defects are of a wide variety, but the most common lesion is the transposition of the great arteries (Driscoll et al. 1960). History of maternal systemic lupus erythematosus is also important because of its association with congenital cardiac disorders in the fetus.

R. Baghaei Tehrani, MD (✉)
Cardiac Surgery Department, Modarres Hospital, School of Medicine,
Shahid Beheshti University of Medical Sciences, Tehran, Iran
e-mail: baghaei.ramin@gmail.com

© Springer International Publishing Switzerland 2017
A. Dabbagh et al. (eds.), *Congenital Heart Disease in Pediatric and Adult Patients*, DOI 10.1007/978-3-319-44691-2_12

Other maternal historical notes which are of diagnostic importance are rubella syndrome babies, premature infants, and children who were born and lived at high altitude. In all three situations, patent ductus arteriosus is possible (Moss 1992).

A history of maternal exposure to alcohol or drugs may provide a clue to diagnose the cardiac defect. A variety of drugs may cause different types of malformations in the offspring.

The physician should also ask about perinatal history that includes premature rupture of membrane, gestational age and Apgar score, asphyxia and cyanosis at birth, and any defects (even not heart-related) diagnosed at birth.

Another aspect of history taking is the family history. The presence of a congenital heart disease in a first-degree relative may be very important. According to Nora, the recurrence rate in a first-degree relative is 1–4% (Nora and Nora 1976). The atrial septal defect, tetralogy of Fallot, ventricular septal defect, and patent ductus arteriosus are the most recurring lesions.

Now the physician should focus on the patient's condition. The growth and development of the child should be considered very carefully. Height and weight gain can be affected by poor cardiac function, pulmonary edema, or a left-to-right shunt.

Inappropriate sweating has been frequently seen in infants with large left-to-right shunt. It is generally accepted that inappropriate sweating in an infant, particularly while feeding, is a reliable sign of overt or impending heart failure.

Syncope of cardiac origin is relatively rare in infants and children. When it occurs, it is almost always due to an arrhythmia (Nora 1968; Nora and Nora 1976; Moss 1992).

Endurance and exercise tolerance may be affected by underlying cardiac diseases, especially those involving obstructive lesions such as aortic and pulmonic stenosis.

Chest pain may be a symptom of congenital heart disease in children, although it is not common. The pain character can be atypical. It is usually induced by effort, but it can occur at rest. Aortic stenosis, pulmonic stenosis, mitral valve prolapse, and primary pulmonary hypertension are some congenital cardiac causes of chest discomfort (Selbst et al. 1990).

In the past, history of squatting was very common in patients with tetralogy of Fallot. Nowadays, this sign has been found infrequently.

Also, the physician should ask about palpitation. This can suggest sinus tachycardia, supraventricular or ventricular arrhythmia, and other irregular rhythms.

Physical Examination

Each examiner should follow five steps in order to perform a complete cardiac physical examination: vital signs, inspection, palpation, percussion, and auscultation.

The first step is vital sign assessment. Heart rate and respiratory rate changes can be the first clues of myocardial failure, pulmonary congestion, or arrhythmia, well before changes in blood pressure occur. On the initial visit, blood pressures should be measured in both upper extremities and one lower extremity. Blood pressure measurement in young infants is achieved by following a special maneuver (Cobben et al. 2014; Strobel and Lu le 2015; Thomas and Battle 2015).

Each patient should be inspected for general appearance, nutritional status, skin color, and any kind of discomfort. All of the abovementioned items may be very important in diagnosis of underlying disease.

Cyanosis could be an important sign of cardiac lesion. It is categorized as peripheral and central cyanosis. Central cyanosis, which is due to the lesions of the lungs or the heart, involves the skin and the mucosa, in contrast to peripheral cyanosis. The differentiating point between pulmonary cyanosis and cardiac cyanosis is that the first diminishes with oxygen and crying. Cyanosis is clinically detectable when arterial saturation is less than 80 % to 85 % unless the patient is anemic. Cyanosis is a helpful clue because it places the defect within the cyanotic group of heart diseases (Moss 1992). The age at which cyanosis is first observed has important diagnostic implications. For example, most neonates with transposition of great arteries have obvious cyanosis in the first days of life, but in tetralogy of Fallot, cyanosis may be delayed for weeks or months (Levin et al. 1977).

Palpation is one of the most important parts of physical examination. Peripheral pulses, the chest, the abdomen, and the back should be palpated in each cardiac examination.

Visible or palpable pulsations sometimes provide a helpful clue to diagnosis, for example, pulsations in the suprasternal notch can occur with aortic stenosis or insufficiency. On the other hand, a diminished pulsation in the lower extremity is the hallmark of coarctation.

Percussion is primarily used to evaluate the total span of the liver. Chest percussion can detect pulmonary consolidation or effusion.

Auscultation is the final and probably most important step in physical examination. The examiner should recognize heart sounds and describe murmurs in terms of location, timing, severity, and radiation. The analysis of auscultation findings may lead to diagnosis of heart lesion.

The signs of congestive heart failure should be sought. These include pallor, sweating, cool extremities, tachypnea, tachycardia, jugular venous distention, hepatomegaly, edema, and ascites.

The association between cardiac defects and some genetic syndromes should be considered. The knowledge that some specific heart lesions predominate in some syndromes helps to provide the diagnosis (Grifka 1999).

Timing of Signs and Symptoms Age at which a murmur first appears can be helpful in diagnosis. The murmur of a ventricular septal defect is not audible at birth. It may be delayed for several hours to a few weeks.

Cardiac failure due to a congenital heart defect occurs mainly during infancy. At a given age, certain defects predominate. Thus, the age when heart failure begins is a helpful clue to diagnosis (Moss 1992).

Para Clinical Diagnostic Tests

Chest Radiography

Chest X-ray is a useful diagnostic tool in the evaluation of patients with congenital heart disease. Abdominal situs, position of the aortic arch, size and shape of the cardiac silhouette, and pulmonary vascularity are all important clues in the evaluation of a patient suspected of having a congenital cardiac anomaly.

The position of the cardiac apex, stomach bubble, and liver determines the splanchnic situs of the patient. Isolated dextrocardia is often associated with congenital heart disease, while situs inversus totalis has a low incidence of cardiac anomalies (Jacobs 2015).

Cardiac shape has some clues to the underlying pathophysiological defects. Cardiomegaly is seen with volume loading lesions or valvular insufficiency. Some specific features implicate specific disorders, for example, a boot-shaped heart is typically seen in patients with tetralogy of Fallot, or a narrow mediastinum is characteristic of transposition of great arteries (TGA) because of anteroposterior orientation of the aorta and pulmonary artery.

Consideration of the pulmonary vascularity is also very important while evaluating the chest radiography. Left-to-right shunts result in cardiomegaly and increased pulmonary vascularity. On the other hand, cyanotic lesions with a component of pulmonary stenosis show decreased pulmonary vascular markings. Features of pulmonary edema are seen in left-sided heart failure or obstruction in the pulmonary venous pathway (i.e., obstructive total anomalous pulmonary venous connection).

Electrocardiography

Electrocardiography (ECG) is one of the important steps in preoperative evaluation. The clinician should follow a systematic approach for evaluation of ECG. It means that the items listed below should be evaluated sequentially: heart rate, heart rhythm, axis, and intervals (PR, QRS, etc.). Then, size and shape and any changes of specific waves (P, R, Q, T) should be considered.

The enlargement or hypertrophy of cardiac chambers, dysrhythmia, and ischemic changes which are shown in the patient's ECG could provide helpful clues for the diagnosis or the degree of progression of the cardiac lesion (Baik et al. 2015; Gorges et al. 2015).

Echocardiography

Today, the accuracy of echocardiography as the sole method of preoperative anatomic evaluation is validated. It is obvious that full anatomic details should be delineated before surgery for appropriate planning. A complete echocardiographic report consists of atrial situs, looping of ventricles, atrioventricular and ventriculoarterial concordance or discordance, the position and intactness of the atrial and ventricular septa, inflow and outflow tracts of ventricles, function of ventricles, shape and function of atrioventricular and ventriculoarterial valves, the anatomy of venae cavae, pulmonary veins, and aorta. The changes due to previous operations should also be evaluated (Marek et al. 1995).

Transesophageal echocardiography is a valuable means for evaluating patients, not only in the operating room but also in the intensive care units. It is useful for obtaining further details of complex congenital heart lesions and assessing postoperative results (Bengur et al. 1998; Stevenson 2003; Kamra et al. 2011).

Computerized Tomography

Multislice computerized tomography has provided images with very high resolution. This test could be performed extremely fast. Computed tomography can be used for anatomic evaluation and three-dimensional reconstruction of cardiac and extra-cardiac structures.

The short acquisition time and the obviation of the need for sedation are advantages compared with MRI; however, there are concerns with radiation exposure and the use of nephrotoxic contrast agents (Einstein 2009).

Cardiac Magnetic Resonance Imaging (cMRI)

Cardiac MRI can be utilized as an imaging modality when specific anatomic and functional study is needed. It provides detailed information about cardiac structure, especially in patients with complex congenital lesions. It can be used to evaluate intracardiac shunts and quantify ventricular volumes. The need for sedation in young children and inability to use in the presence of metal implants are the limitations of cardiac MRI (Constantine et al. 2004).

Cardiac Catheterization and Angiography

The role of cardiac catheterization and angiography as a diagnostic tool has changed during the past decades. Today, the indications of catheterization are limited. The three major indications for performing a cardiac catheterization are the following:

- A complete anatomic diagnosis or necessary hemodynamic information cannot be obtained by noninvasive methods.
- Clinical signs and symptoms are not consistent with a patient's diagnosis.
- A patient's clinical course is not progressing as expected.

Anticipatory preparation for all catheterizations must include a complete history, review of all previous cardiac catheterizations and surgeries, physical examination, and review of all pertinent noninvasive studies.

Cardiac catheterization mainly consists of the measurements of different physiologic variables. These include the measurement of pressures, saturations and intracardiac shunts, cardiac output, and vascular resistance.

Sometimes cardiac catheterization should be performed as a kind of preoperative intervention. Balloon atrial septostomy may be needed in neonates with transposition of the great arteries to improve intracardiac mixing and thus tissue oxygenation. Patients with pulmonary atresia, ventricular septal defect, and multiple aortopulmonary collaterals may also undergo preoperative cardiac catheterization to determine the anatomy of their collateral flow and whether they can be occluded prior to surgery (El-Said et al. 2000; Rutledge et al. 2002; Carlson et al. 2005; Grifka et al. 2008; Butera et al. 2015; Rihal et al. 2015a, b).

Conclusion

The art of making accurate diagnosis and appropriate surgical planning demands a meticulous preoperative evaluation. This process consists of definitive components; each of them has its specific importance. Scientific analysis of information gathered from medical history, physical examination, and diagnostic tests could guide the surgeon to choose the best management plan.

References

Baik N, Urlesberger B, Schwaberger B, Freidl T, Schmolzer GM, Pichler G. Cardiocirculatory monitoring during immediate fetal-to-neonatal transition: a systematic qualitative review of the literature. Neonatology. 2015;107:100–7.

Bengur AR, Li JS, Herlong JR, Jaggers J, Sanders SP, Ungerleider RM. Intraoperative transesophageal echocardiography in congenital heart disease. Semin Thorac Cardiovasc Surg. 1998;10:255–64.

Butera G, Morgan GJ, Ovaert C, Anjos R, Spadoni I. Recommendations from the Association of European Paediatric Cardiology for training in diagnostic and interventional cardiac catheterisation. Cardiol Young. 2015;25:438–46.

Carlson KM, Justino H, O'Brien RE, Dimas VV, Leonard Jr GT, Pignatelli RH, Mullins CE, Smith EO, Grifka RG. Transcatheter atrial septal defect closure: modified balloon sizing technique to avoid overstretching the defect and oversizing the Amplatzer septal occluder. Catheter Cardiovasc Interv Off J Soc Cardiac Angiography Interv. 2005;66:390–6.

Cobben JM, Oostra RJ, van Dijk FS. Pectus excavatum and carinatum. Eur J Med Genet. 2014;57:414–7.

Constantine G, Shan K, Flamm SD, Sivananthan MU. Role of MRI in clinical cardiology. Lancet. 2004;363:2162–71.

Driscoll SG, Benirschke K, Curtis GW. Neonatal deaths among infants of diabetic mothers. Postmortem findings in ninety-five infants. Am J Dis Children. 1960;100:818–35.

Einstein AJ. Radiation protection of patients undergoing cardiac computed tomographic angiography. JAMA. 2009;301:545–7.

El-Said HG, Ing FF, Grifka RG, Nihill MR, Morris C, Getty-Houswright D, Mullins CE. 18-year experience with transseptal procedures through baffles, conduits, and other intra-atrial patches. Catheter Cardiovasc Interv Off J Soc Cardiac Angiography Interv. 2000;50:434–9; discussion 440.

Gorges M, Whyte SD, Sanatani S, Dawes J, Montgomery CJ, Ansermino JM. Changes in QTc associated with a rapid bolus dose of dexmedetomidine in patients receiving TIVA: a retrospective study. Paediatr Anaesth. 2015;25:1287–93.

Grifka RG. Cyanotic congenital heart disease with increased pulmonary blood flow. Pediatr Clin North Am. 1999;46:405–25.

Grifka RG, Fenrich AL, Tapio JB. Transcatheter closure of patent ductus arteriosus and aorto-pulmonary vessels using non-ferromagnetic Inconel MReye embolization coils. Catheter Cardiovasc Interv Off J Soc Cardiac Angiography Interv. 2008;72:691–5.

Jacobs JP. The science of assessing the outcomes and improving the quality of the congenital and paediatric cardiac care. Curr Opin Cardiol. 2015;30:100–11.

Kamra K, Russell I, Miller-Hance WC. Role of transesophageal echocardiography in the management of pediatric patients with congenital heart disease. Paediatr Anaesth. 2011;21:479–93.

Levin DL, Paul MH, Muster AJ, Newfeld EA, Waldman JD. d-Transposition of the great vessels in the neonate. A clinical diagnosis. Arch Intern Med. 1977;137:1421–5.

Mace S, Hirschfield SS, Riggs T, Fanaroff AA, Merkatz IR. Echocardiographic abnormalities in infants of diabetic mothers. J Pediatr. 1979;95:1013–9.

Marek J, Skovranek J, Hucin B, Chaloupecky V, Tax P, Reich O, Samanek M. Seven-year experience of noninvasive preoperative diagnostics in children with congenital heart defects: comprehensive analysis of 2,788 consecutive patients. Cardiology. 1995;86:488–95.

Moss AJ. Clues in diagnosing congenital heart disease. West J Med. 1992;156:392–8.

Nora JJ. Multifactorial inheritance hypothesis for the etiology of congenital heart diseases. The genetic-environmental interaction. Circulation. 1968;38:604–17.

Nora JJ, Nora AH. Genetic and environmental factors in the etiology of congenital heart diseases. South Med J. 1976;69:919–26.

Rihal CS, Naidu SS, Givertz MM, Szeto WY, Burke JA, Kapur NK, Kern M, Garratt KN, Goldstein JA, Dimas V, Tu T. 2015 SCAI/ACC/HFSA/STS Clinical Expert Consensus Statement on the Use of Percutaneous Mechanical Circulatory Support Devices in Cardiovascular Care: Endorsed by the American Heart Association, the Cardiological Society of India, and Sociedad Latino Americana de Cardiologia Intervencion; Affirmation of Value by the Canadian Association of Interventional Cardiology-Association Canadienne de Cardiologie d'intervention. J Am Coll Cardiol. 2015a;65:e7–26.

Rihal CS, Naidu SS, Givertz MM, Szeto WY, Burke JA, Kapur NK, Kern M, Garratt KN, Goldstein JA, Dimas V, Tu T. 2015 SCAI/ACC/HFSA/STS Clinical Expert Consensus Statement on the Use of Percutaneous Mechanical Circulatory Support Devices in Cardiovascular Care: Endorsed by the American Heart Association, the Cardiological Society of India, and Sociedad Latino Americana de Cardiologia Intervencionista; Affirmation of Value by the Canadian Association of Interventional Cardiology-Association Canadienne de Cardiologie d'intervention. J Am Coll Cardiol. 2015b;65:2140–1.

Rowland TW, Hubbell Jr JP, Nadas AS. Congenital heart disease in infants of diabetic mothers. J Pediatr. 1973;83:815–20.

Rutledge JM, Mullins CE, Nihill MR, Grifka RG, Vincent JA. Initial experience with intratherapeutics Intrastent Doublestrut LD stents in patients with congenital heart defects. Catheter Cardiovasc Interv Off J Soc Cardiac Angiography Interv. 2002;56:541–8.

Selbst SM, Ruddy R, Clark BJ. Chest pain in children. Follow-up of patients previously reported. Clin Pediatr. 1990;29:374–7.

Stevenson JG. Utilization of intraoperative transesophageal echocardiography during repair of congenital cardiac defects: a survey of North American centers. Clin Cardiol. 2003;26:132–4.

Strobel AM, Lu le N. The critically ill infant with congenital heart disease. Emerg Med Clin North Am. 2015;33:501–18.

Thomas MJ, Battle RW. Something old, something new: using family history and genetic testing to diagnose and manage athletes with inherited cardiovascular disease. Clin Sports Med. 2015;34:517–37.

Chapter 13
Anesthetic Management of Adults with Congenital Heart Disease

Lorraine Lubin and Robert Wong

Congenital heart defects constitute the most common type of birth defects and occur in approximately 8 in 1000 live births. With the exclusion of bicuspid aortic valve disease, the majority of untreated patients born with congenital heart disease (CHD) expire in childhood with approximately 15–25 % surviving into adulthood. Significant advances in prenatal diagnosis, interventional cardiology techniques, congenital heart surgery, anesthesiology, and critical care have allowed approximately 90 % of these patients to survive into adulthood. The profile of patients with congenital heart disease has evolved, and now there are estimates to suggest that in the United States, there are more adults than children living with congenital heart disease. Most of these patients will require additional interventional cardiology or cardiac surgical procedures either palliative or curative during adulthood. Although major studies evaluating this population have not been done, adults with CHD are a medically fragile group, which have an increased risk for perioperative morbidity and mortality. Formal guidelines which direct the management of these patients have not been developed; however, the American College of Cardiology recommends that adult patients with moderate to severe CHD be referred to a center specializing in the care of these patients and receive expert consultation with the appropriate care providers such as adult congenital heart cardiologists, surgeons, and anesthesiologists prior to undergoing procedures.

L. Lubin, M.D. (✉)
Cedars Sinai Medical Center, Department of Anesthesiology,
8700 Beverly Blvd, Suite 8211, Los Angeles, CA 90048, USA
e-mail: Lorraine.Lubin@cshs.org

R. Wong, M.D.
Cedars Sinai Medical Center, Department of Anesthesiology,
8700 Beverly Blvd, Rm 4209, West Hollywood, Los Angeles,
CA 90048, USA
e-mail: Robert.Wong@cshs.org

© Springer International Publishing Switzerland 2017
A. Dabbagh et al. (eds.), *Congenital Heart Disease in Pediatric
and Adult Patients*, DOI 10.1007/978-3-319-44691-2_13

When caring for adult patients with CHD undergoing procedures requiring anesthesia, it is imperative that the providers appreciate the anatomy and physiology which may be relatively unique to each patient. A team approach is required, and the providers should communicate regarding the risks of the procedure, the procedural techniques anticipated, and the ability or lack thereof to compensate for any hemodynamic or physiologic perturbations such as hypovolemia/hypervolemia, anemia, and hypotension.

Epidemiology of Adult Congenital Heart Disease

Approximately 25 % of adult patients with structural heart disease have not undergone repair of their lesion because they were not considered to have hemodynamic compromise worthy of intervention. Other patients may be diagnosed in adulthood when seeking medical attention for another condition such as pregnancy. Another subset of adult patients with unrepaired CHD have incurred severe physiologic perturbations as sequelae of their CHD and are no longer candidates for repair of their structural heart lesions. Of the patients with mild unrepaired CHD, the most common lesions include mild aortic valve stenosis secondary to a bicuspid aortic valve, atrial septal defects, small restrictive ventricular septal defects, mild pulmonary valve stenosis, mitral valve prolapse, and isolated congenitally corrected transposition of the great arteries. The majority of patients evaluated in the outpatient setting have previously undergone surgical or interventional catheter-based procedures. Adults who have undergone repair of what are considered uncomplicated lesions such as atrial septal defects (ASDs) or patent ductus arteriosus (PDA) may be indiscernible from unaffected patients. These same lesions if left unrepaired may result in pulmonary vascular disease/pulmonary hypertension or Eisenmenger syndrome. Patients with pulmonary vascular disease/pulmonary hypertension or Eisenmenger syndrome especially with cyanosis constitute an extremely high-risk population.

Cyanotic heart disease includes structural heart defects that result in a decrease in pulmonary blood flow or result in mixing of oxygenated and deoxygenated blood. These conditions lead to reduced blood oxygen content and cyanosis. The majority of patients with adult cyanotic congenital heart disease will have had previous surgical interventions as children. The most frequently encountered cyanotic defects managed in the adult congenital heart patient population include tetralogy of Fallot, D-transposition, single-ventricle anatomy, truncus arteriosus, total anomalous pulmonary venous return, and double outlet right ventricle (Table 13.1).

Major Categories of Congenital Cardiac Structural Defects

Adult congenital heart disease (ACHD) is composed of a variety of structural anomalies with hemodynamic consequences, which result from both the native anatomy and compensatory physiology. Due to the multitude of structural malformations, including complex forms with combined lesions, a classification system based on

Table 13.1 Most commonly encountered adult congenital heart lesions

Tetralogy of Fallot, truncus arteriosus, and double outlet right ventricle with conotruncal anomalies postrepair
Secundum atrial septal defect
Ventricular septal defect
Complex single ventricles post-Fontan procedure
Coarctation of the aorta postrepair
Congenital aortic valve stenosis
Atrioventricular canal defects postrepair
Congenitally corrected transposition of the great arteries
Sinus venosus atrial septal defects with partial anomalous pulmonary venous return
Transposition of the great arteries after atrial or arterial switch

physiologic effects is the most useful. *The four categories, which are most commonly used, include shunt lesions, mixing lesions, obstructive lesions, and regurgitant lesions.* Over time, a compensatory physiology will evolve and produce aberrant loading conditions and potential impairment in ventricular function. In some patients, the compensatory changes are imperceptible and may cause little impairment in functions, while other lesions or their combined anatomy may cause significant cardiovascular compromise.

Shunt Lesions

Shunt lesions result in an aberrant communication between cardiac structures. The direction and volume of blood flow depends on the diameter and length of the communication and its relative position in the heart. The shunt lesion can occur at the level of the atria, ventricles, and great vessels or even be extra-cardiac. The flow of blood across the shunt or a vascular structure is determined by a number of factors, including the pressure drop across the structure, length, radius, resistance, and fluid viscosity. Poiseuille's law describes this relationship in the following equation:

$$\Delta P \qquad Q \quad P_1 \qquad P_2 \qquad L$$

POISEUILLE'S LAW

$$Q = \frac{\Delta P \cdot r^4 \cdot \pi}{\eta L \cdot 8}$$

where Q=blood flow, ΔP=pressure change in the fluid as it flows across the shunt, r=radius of the structure, L=length of the structure, and n =the viscosity of blood. From this equation, it is seen that blood flow increases dramatically with increases in radius, increases to a lesser degree with increase in the pressure gradient across the structure, and decreases with an increase in length of the structure and blood viscosity. With a decrease in radius, a consequential decrease in blood flow to the fourth power is observed. Ohm's law describes the change in pressure, blood flow, and vascular resistance by the following equation:

$$Q = P/R$$

In this equation, P=the pressure generated within the cardiac chamber, Q=flow, and R=vascular resistance.

The direction and magnitude of shunt defects at the ventricular level and at the level of the great vessels, for example, a PDA, are determined by the radius of the defect and the difference in pulmonary and systemic vasculature resistance. For shunts at the level of the atrium, the ventricular diastolic pressure must also be taken into account. For small shunts, which persist into adulthood, the indication for repair is based on the potential risk of strokes from paradoxical emboli and the occurrence of bacterial endocarditis. Moderate to large shunt defects can lead to ventricular failure due to volume overload. Shunt lesions that result in chronic increases in pulmonary blood flow may result in Eisenmenger syndrome. Eisenmenger syndrome is an irreversible increase in pulmonary vascular resistance (PVR) that ultimately leads to pulmonary hypertension, right-sided heart failure, and right-to-left shunting. An anesthetic consideration regarding right-to-left shunting is that inhalation inductions may be delayed. However, these delays may be more marked with larger shunts and insoluble anesthetic gases.

Mixing Lesions

Mixing lesions occur when blood from the pulmonary and systemic circulations combine to create a mixture of oxygenated and deoxygenated blood. As with shunt lesions, mixing defects may occur at the level of the atria, ventricles, or great vessels. The ratio of pulmonary and systemic flow is again based on vascular resistance. Increased pulmonary blood flow results with elevated systemic vascular resistance (SVR). This flow pattern results in ventricular volume overload and pulmonary hypertension. Vascular medial hypertrophy of the pulmonary vessels occurs and results in increased PVR and pulmonary hypertension. In severe cases of pulmonary overcirculation, systemic malperfusion occurs with resulting metabolic acidosis, shock, and cardiovascular collapse. Conversely, elevated PVR results in increased systemic flow, decreased pulmonary flow, hypoxemia, and cyanosis. Depending on the underlying anatomy, most patients with mixing defects receive palliation or complete repair in the neonatal period. Patients with ductal-dependent lesions frequently require a mixed circulation before repair. D-Transposition of the great vessels is a defect in which a mixing lesion is required for survival and an atrial septal defect may need to be created by the Rashkind procedure (balloon atrial septostomy) to allow mixing at the atrial level and prevent a circulation in parallel. Depending on the degree of systemic hypoxemia secondary to mixing of saturated and desaturated blood, deficits in oxygen delivery may exist with resulting compensatory mechanisms, including erythrocytosis and polycythemia with resulting hyperviscosity. Patients with mixing lesions are also at risk for bacterial endocarditis and paradoxical emboli and stroke. Other considerations for patients with mixing lesions include the degree of biventricular dysfunction and loading conditions as well as the function of other organ systems.

Obstructive Lesions

Obstructive or stenotic lesions impose a ventricular pressure load proximal to the defect that results in increased intracavitary pressure and concentric ventricular hypertrophy. Initially, the wall stress is preserved; however, over time the vascular supply becomes inadequate to support the hypertrophied ventricle. The ventricle becomes relatively ischemic and dilated with increased wall tension and decreased contractility. Chronic obstructive lesions also lead to decreased ventricular compliance and diastolic dysfunction, even in cases with preserved systolic function. Patients with obstructive lesions are extremely preload dependent for adequate diastolic filling and cardiac output. Lesions, which are severely obstructive, can present with inadequate cardiac output and perfusion of the pulmonary, coronary, cerebral, and peripheral tissue beds. Significant decreases in exercise tolerance and cardiovascular reserve may be seen in patients with obstructive lesions.

Regurgitant Lesions

In general, regurgitant lesions do not usually exist as primary defects. They more commonly develop as sequelae or as a result of intervention secondary to CHD. However, worsening valvular incompetence or regurgitation results in decreases in ventricular ejection volume and function. The compensatory mechanisms to increase stroke volume cause ventricular dilation with increased wall tension and a propensity for ventricular failure. A significant number of interventional cardiac catheter-based procedures and even cardiac surgical interventions are preformed to correct lesions such as pulmonary regurgitation after tetralogy of Fallot repair in the adult congenital heart population.

Acyanotic Congenital Heart Disease

Dextrocardia

Dextrocardia is usually described as the heart having a mirror-image location in the right hemithorax. Dextrocardia with situs inversus is a mirror-image location of the intrathoracic structures as well as the intra-abdominal structures. This cardiac anomaly causes the heart to lie in the right hemithorax with the liver and gallbladder under the left portion of the diaphragm. The stomach is located under the right portion of the diaphragm and the appendix is located in the left lower quadrant. Dextrocardia with situs inversus may be functionally normal. Isolated dextrocardia with normally related abdominal viscera frequently indicates the presence of CHD. In some patients, the stomach bubble may be indistinguishable from large bowel gas because the stomach is not in its usual position, either left or right, and the liver appears to be uniformly distributed across the right and left diaphragm. This suggests visceral heterotaxy or situs ambiguous, associated with either polysplenia or asplenia and a high incidence of congenital heart malformations. In these patients, the apex may point to the left, right, or anteriorly and is referred to as mesocardia or atrial isomerism.

Dextrocardia with situs inversus usually exists in otherwise structurally and functionally normal hearts. These patients will generally have their congenital malpositioning noted when they present for noncardiac-related medical attention. The risk of noncardiac surgery in patients with dextrocardia with situs inversus and otherwise structurally normal hearts is the same as for patients with situs solitus (normally positioned abdominal viscera) and normally positioned hearts. The importance of diagnosing this anomaly lies in the correct interpretation of symptoms related to the underlying anatomic location of the organ in question. For example, patients with dextrocardia with situs inversus will experience the pain of acute appendicitis in the left lower quadrant rather than the right lower quadrant. The diagnostic importance of recognizing this anomaly has obvious surgical implications.

Congenitally Corrected Transposition of the Great Vessels

In uncorrected D-transposition of the great vessels (D-TGV), the aorta arises from the anatomic right ventricle; in corrected L-transposition of the great vessels (L-TGV), the venae cavae drain into the right atrium, which empties into an anatomic left ventricle through a mitral valve. The anatomic left ventricle ejects into the pulmonary artery (PA). In this form of transposition, the atrioarterial connections are concordant, and therefore systemic venous return enters the lung for oxygenation, and pulmonary venous return enters the left atrium and passes into an anatomic right ventricle through a tricuspid valve. Saturated blood then enters the aorta from the anatomic right ventricle. Without another major structural anomaly such as a ventricular septal defect (VSD) with or without pulmonic stenosis, patients with L-TGA may be entirely asymptomatic. There may be people with L-TGA who remain undiagnosed. However, there are a number of known associations with L-TGA, including complete heart block, VSD, pulmonic stenosis, left-sided atrioventricular (AV) valve regurgitation, Ebstein's anomaly of the tricuspid valve, and other complex lesions. Complete heart block may result from the abnormal alignment of the ventricles and interventricular septum. This malalignment of the connection between the bundle of His and the AV node may worsen as the heart grows with a loss of continuity between the two structures and resulting third-degree or complete heart block. Eventually, these patients may require a permanent pacemaker. With L-TGA, the morphologic right ventricle (systemic ventricle) is at risk of depressed function. There is also a risk of bacterial endocarditis secondary to left AV valve regurgitation. The long-term function of the anatomic right ventricle as the systemic ventricle remains controversial. By 45 years of age, 67 % of adults with L-TGA with associated anomalies such as ASD or VSD have developed congestive heart failure (CHF). Even without associated anomalies, approximately 25 % of patients with L-TGA will have developed CHF by 45 years of age. To decrease complications from L-TGA, the "double switch" procedure can be performed in which the venous return is transposed using an atrial switch procedure and either the ventricular or arterial connections are transposed via a Rastelli procedure or an arterial switch procedure. In caring for the patient with L-TGA undergoing noncardiac surgery, one must consider the possibilities for disturbances in AV conduction, the ventricular function, and the risk of endocarditis. A preoperative ECG should be obtained, with intraoperative and postoperative ECG monitoring performed. For patients with 2:1 heart block (second-degree block), it may be prudent to place a temporary transvenous or transesophageal pacemaker. If the ventricular function is impaired, arterial line and/or transesophageal echocardiographic monitoring may be warranted.

Congenitally Bicuspid Aortic Valve

A congenitally bicuspid aortic valve may result from abnormal differentiation of the primitive truncal valve, leaving two of the aortic valve cusps fused together, producing a bicuspid instead of tricuspid valve. The bicuspid aortic valve orifice is eccentric and opens in an abnormal fashion. The abnormal orifice produces varying degrees of obstruction, which results in stenosis and increased flow velocity with a systolic ejection murmur. The risk to the patient with a bicuspid aortic valve undergoing noncardiac surgery is determined by the degree of stenosis of the valve and the ventricular function. Bacterial endocarditis is also a risk factor and prophylactic antibiotics should be considered. For patients with severe bicuspid aortic stenosis, balloon valvuloplasty may substantially reduce the gradient across the valve and offer significant symptomatic relief. Balloon valvuloplasty is only an option if the valve is thin and mobile. Adult patients with severe fibrocalcific bicuspid aortic stenosis account for 50 % of the surgically significant cases of aortic stenosis. These patients are similar to patients with acquired aortic stenosis with calcific disease of a trileaflet valve and incur similar surgical risks and anesthetic management. Calcific bicuspid aortic stenosis is even less amenable to balloon valvuloplasty than a calcified, stenotic trileaflet valve. However, in the age of transcatheter aortic valve replacement (TAVR), these patients may be candidates for a minimally invasive replacement which leaves them open in the future for a valve in a valve replacement with the deferral of open cardiac surgical intervention. As with all adults with congenital heart disease, it is important to consider the possibility of acquired coronary artery disease (CAD), and it is advisable to screen these patients for CAD. It needs to be determined whether angina is secondary to CAD or solely to the aortic stenosis with the increased oxygen demands of the hypertrophied left ventricle. For patients with bicuspid aortic stenosis, appropriate preoperative evaluation and optimization will help decrease the perioperative risk factors. Intraoperative management should be guided by the patient's functional status and the complexity of the surgical procedure. Conventional monitoring and the use of arterial line, pulmonary artery catheter (PAC), and transesophageal echocardiography may be useful in guiding perioperative therapy. Patients must be monitored for signs of ischemia and ventricular dysfunction. Also, acute decreases in SVR will not be compensated by an increase in stroke volume secondary to the fixed left ventricular outflow tract (LVOT) obstruction.

Volume losses and hypotension must be promptly treated. Volume replacement should be pursued cautiously to avoid pulmonary edema which may result depending on the functional status of the left ventricle or systemic ventricle. Pharmacologic support of SVR and ventricular dysfunction may be necessary with inotropes. The requirement of inotropic support is best guided by the previously mentioned monitoring modalities.

Patients with bicuspid aortic stenosis are also at risk for aortic regurgitation secondary to the thickened, calcified leaflets that may become incompetent secondary to their immobile nature. The bicuspid aortic valve may also become incompetent secondary to poststenotic aortic root dilatation. Aortic regurgitation imposes a volume load on the already pressure-overloaded systemic ventricle, which may further impair ventricular function and increase the risk of bacterial endocarditis. In patients with impaired ventricular function, the mode of aortic valve replacement needs to be considered with either surgical replacement or TAVR.

Coarctation of the Aorta

Coarctation of the aorta occurs in 8–10 % of all congenital heart defects. It is more common in males than females, with a ratio of 2:1. Patients with Turner's syndrome have a 30 % incidence of coarctation. Coarctation is an obstructive lesion that may present early and acutely in the neonatal period as critical coarctation (approximately 9 % of coarctation cases) or may be detected later in life as an incidental finding, manifesting as right upper extremity hypertension with diminished lower extremity pulses. The majority of coarctations are located close to the insertion of the ductus arteriosus into the aorta. These juxtaductal coarctations are thought in some way to be produced by contraction of the arterial wall musculature that occurs with constriction of the ductus early in the neonatal period. This may account for the acute presentation of systemic hypoperfusion in affected neonates. Other forms of coarctation are not as easily explained. Coarctation may have only mild gradients at rest, but the gradient will significantly increase with any hyperdynamic state. Unrelieved coarctation leads to upper extremity hypertension, and the consequence of sustained hypertension secondary to coarctation is that the arteries of the head and neck as well as the coronary arteries are exposed to an increased risk of developing atherosclerotic changes. The ventricular myocardium also hypertrophies, increasing the demands on the coronary arteries. The diminished pulsatility of the blood flow distal to the coarctation promotes renal secretion of renin and angiotensin, which may further promote hypertension. The most common sequelae are systolic hypertension, recurrent or residual coarctation, aortic aneurysm, aortic dissection, intracranial aneurysm, and intracranial hemorrhage secondary to intracranial aneurysm formation and sudden death. Due to the significant long-term sequelae and potential disastrous comorbidities, it is of the upmost importance to repair coarctation in a timely fashion. The longer the delay in treatment, the greater the risk of persistent hypertension after the repair. Additionally, the actual life expectancy is significantly reduced, the longer the lesion is left untreated. The overall survival after repair is 91 % at 10 years, 84 % at 20 years, and 76 % at 30 years. For patients who have undergone surgical repair, 30 % will have hypertension with a higher incidence than those repaired within the first years of life. If a coarctation is treated within the first few years of life and no significant gradient persists, the patients are expected to be able to lead essentially normal lives.

The surgical approaches to coarctation repair include resection of the stenotic area with direct end-to-end anastomosis, subclavian flap aortoplasty, or aortoplasty with a homograft or synthetic graft material. All of these techniques require the use of aortic cross clamping around the area of coarctation, with the surgical risks of paraplegia or paresis secondary to spinal cord ischemia. Residual obstruction or re-coarctation occurs in 6–33 % of all patients. The manner in which residual obstruction or re-coarctation is treated is dictated by the severity and anatomic location of the stenosis. Minimally invasive, catheter-based techniques have become the standard of care and are frequently required more than once in a given patient. Stented graft placement and balloon angioplasty of the aorta are the most common therapy required after the initial surgical repair.

Patients with a history of coarctation both unrepaired and repaired also require the following issues to be considered perioperatively:

- The potential presence and functional status of a concomitant bicuspid aortic valve (as many as 85 % of patients with coarctation will have a bicuspid aortic valve)
- The presence of hypertension
- Systemic ventricular function
- The potential for premature or concomitant CAD
- The need for lifelong bacterial endocarditis prophylaxis

In addition to a complete history and physical examination, an ECG, echocardiogram, and ventricular stress test will provide a preoperative assessment of myocardial function, ventricular hypertrophy, and potential for ischemia. The patient with coarctation at the highest risk undergoing a procedure is the older patient with coexisting stenotic or an incompetent bicuspid aortic valve, depressed systemic ventricular function, and acquired CAD. If the patient is to undergo a surgical procedure and it is not urgent, intervention including coarctation repair, aortic valve replacement, coronary artery bypass or angioplasty/stenting, and medical management of the hypertension and depressed ventricular function may be undertaken to decrease the operative risk and provide optimal patient management. In patients with sequelae secondary to coarctation including systemic hypertension and depressed ventricular function, an arterial line and PAC placement are recommended to guide perioperative management. Depending on the degree of ventricular function impairment, intraoperative transesophageal echocardiography (TEE) may be helpful.

Pulmonic Stenosis

Pulmonic stenosis (PS) is an obstructive lesion of the right ventricular outflow tract that produces a pressure overload situation and compensatory changes associated with such lesions. Pulmonic stenosis may be subvalvular, valvular, or supravalvular. PS may also occur near the bifurcation and involve the branch pulmonary arteries. PS may be an isolated lesion or occur as an associated lesion with other complex malformations (tetralogy of Fallot) or as part of a syndrome such as Williams syndrome or Rubella syndrome and others. Mild PS generally causes no major hemodynamic perturbations. However, if the stenosis is severe, right ventricular hypertrophy and dysfunction may ensue. Most importantly for the patient undergoing a procedure is the limitations of compensatory responses of the systemic circulation to critical hemodynamic changes such as hypovolemia. In the case of mild PS, the risk of endocarditis exists with little hemodynamic compromise. However, for patients with severe PS and with impaired right ventricular function, their hemodynamics may be significantly improved with balloon valvuloplasty if the lesion is amenable to intervention. For emergent procedures in patients with severe pulmonic stenosis, perioperative arterial line monitoring and central venous pressure monitoring may be beneficial. Intraoperative transesophageal echocardiography (TEE) should be used for patients with PS and right ventricular or biventricular dysfunction in which loading conditions and ventricular function monitoring are required but in whom a PAC is not an option.

Primary Pulmonary Hypertension and Pulmonary Vascular Disease

Primary pulmonary vascular disease or primary pulmonary hypertension (PPH) is characterized by a decrease in the cross-sectional area of the pulmonary vascular bed caused by pathologic changes in the vascular tissue. PPH is characterized by progressive, irreversible vascular changes similar to those seen in Eisenmenger syndrome but without intracardiac anomalies. PPH is extremely rare in pediatric patients and is primarily a condition of adulthood and is more prevalent in women. It has a poor prognosis and may progress to a cyanotic condition with biventricular heart failure. Pulmonary vascular disease results from any process that produces prolonged elevation of PA pressure, such as large left-to-right shunts, obstructive airway disease, and chronic lung disease with hypoxia, and causes progressive medial hypertrophy of the pulmonary vasculature with an ultimate decrease in the cross-sectional area. The cause of PPH is not fully understood, but endothelial dysfunction of the pulmonary vascular bed may be an important factor. If severe pulmonary hypertension develops suddenly in the face of an unprepared or non-hypertrophied right ventricle (RV), right-sided heart failure will result. In patients with chronic pulmonary hypertension, gradual hypertrophy and dilatation of the RV develop and the RV pressure may ultimately exceed the systemic pressure.

A decrease in cardiac output may result from at least two mechanisms: (1) A volume and pressure overload of the RV impairs cardiac function, primarily by impaired coronary perfusion of the hypertrophied and dilated RV and decreased left ventricular (LV) function resulting from the dramatic leftward shift of the interventricular septum caused by increasing RV volume. The latter also alters LV structures and decreases LV compliance, resulting in an increase in both LV end-diastolic pressure and left atrial (LA) pressure. (2) The second mechanism may result if a sudden increase in PVR occurs with decreased pulmonary venous return to the LA and hypotension and circulatory shock results as a consequence. Pulmonary edema can occur with or without elevation of the LA pressure. Direct disruption of the walls of the small arterioles proximal to the hypoxic/constricted arterioles may be responsible similar to the mechanism which is proposed for high-altitude pulmonary edema.

Irrelevant of the cause, the clinical manifestations of pulmonary hypertension are similar when significant hypertension exists. The patient's history will often reveal dyspnea, fatigue, and syncope on exertion. A history of CHD or CHF in infancy is present in most cases of Eisenmenger syndrome. Some patients may have a history of angina and headache. Hemoptysis is a late and occasionally fatal manifestation. Cyanosis with or without clubbing may be present. The neck veins may be distended with signs of right-sided heart failure such as hepatomegaly and ankle edema. The ECG will likely show right-axis deviation secondary to RVH, and right atrial enlargement may manifest as arrhythmias occurring in the later stage.

PPH and other types of pulmonary vascular disease are difficult to treat and nearly impossible to reverse unless the etiology is eliminated. Measures to remove or treat the underlying cause include timely surgical correction of the congenital heart defects such as ventricular septal defects (VSDs) or patent ductus arteriosus (PDA) before obstructive anatomic changes occur in the pulmonary vessels. The anesthetic management of pulmonary hypertension is guided by the underlying cause. Strategies for the intraoperative management including cases requiring cardiopulmonary bypass (CPB) and non-bypass cases need individualized assessment. The incidence of symptomatic pulmonary hypertension after repair of an intracardiac lesion does not often justify the placement of pulmonary artery catheters (PACs); however, centers that are familiar with their use have low associated morbidity. The most common strategies to manage pulmonary hypertension include avoiding maneuvers which elicit vasoconstrictive responses, maintaining oxygenation to lower pulmonary vascular resistance (PVR), maintaining alkaline pH, minimizing tidal volumes or using spontaneous modes of ventilation, and the use of pulmonary vasodilators such as nitric oxide, inhaled prostacyclin (PGI_2), and, in the ICU, oral sildenafil. Nitric oxide is a direct pulmonary vasodilator with no significant systemic effect as it is rapidly metabolized by red blood cells. Nitric oxide is administered by inhalation with a special delivery system which can be added to a ventilator or anesthesia machine.

Noncardiac surgery or procedures for patients with PPH, PH, or PVD can be formidable. Fixed or elevated PVR may limit perioperative hemodynamic compensation. The potential for hypotension, RV or biventricular dysfunction, and hemodynamic instability is significant. An abrupt fall in systemic vascular resistance (SVR) may precipitate intense cyanosis. An intraoperative arterial line and PAC monitoring are recommended. In patients in whom placing a PAC is not feasible or in whom the risk of arrhythmia, RA/RV perforation, or PA rupture is believed to be unacceptably high, a TEE may be important in accessing loading conditions, in evaluating biventricular function and the magnitude of right-to-left shunting and air embolism, and in estimating PA pressures from the tricuspid regurgitant jet. TEE must be performed and interpreted by a qualified practitioner in all settings. The perioperative assessment of volume status and necessity for circulatory with inotropes is critically important in the patient with PH. The use of regional anesthesia for patients with pulmonary hypertension is recommended if appropriate for a given procedure as long as the patient does not have associated sedation which incurs significant hypoventilation. In the case of a general anesthetic, appropriate hemodynamic monitoring, airway and ventilatory management along with an appropriate depth of anesthesia will decrease the risk of perioperative instability.

Left-to-Right Shunt Lesions

Patent Ductus Arteriosus

A patent ductus arteriosus (PDA) is a persistent communication between the left PA and the descending aorta, which is approximately 5–10 mm distal to the origin of the left subclavian artery. It is a normal fetal structure and generally undergoes functional closure in the early neonatal period and becomes the ligamentum arteriosum. If the PDA does not close, persistent shunting occurs between the aorta and the PA. A PDA occurs in 5–10 % of all congenital heart lesions, excluding premature infants. It is more common in females than males, with a male-to-female ratio of 1:3. A PDA is an extremely common problem among premature infants as a component of persistent fetal circulation and may require interventional catheter-based closure or surgical ligation if it results in respiratory failure or CHF. Patients are generally asymptomatic if the ductus is small. However, a large shunt may predispose patients to lower respiratory tract infections, atelectasis, pulmonary hypertension, bacterial endocarditis, and CHF. Adult patients with PDAs may have developed pulmonary hypertension and pulmonary vascular disease with right-to-left shunting and cyanosis. Paradoxical emboli and stroke are also significant risks for patients with PDA. Therefore, the existence of a PDA is an indication for closure either by transcatheter approach or surgical ligation. The presence of severe pulmonary vascular disease and PH may be a contraindication for closure.

Atrial Septal Defects

Atrial septal defects (ASDs) or ostium secundum ASD occurs as an isolated anomaly in 5–10 % of all CHD. It is more common in females than males with a male-to-female ratio of 1:2. Thirty to fifty percent of pediatric patients with CHD have an ASD as an associated defect. Three types of ASDs exist, including secundum, primum, and venosus defects. A patent foramen ovale (PFO) in ordinary circumstances does not cause intracardiac shunting although in certain conditions such as high right-sided heart pressures it may. Ostium secundum defects are the most common type of ASD, accounting for 50–70 % of all ASDs. This defect allows for left-to-right shunting of blood from the LA to the RA. Primum defects occur in approximately 30 % of all ASDs, including those existing as complete endocardial cushion defects. Isolated primum defects occur in approximately 15 % of ASDs. Sinus venosus defects occur in about 10 % of all ASDs and are most commonly located at the entry of the superior vena cava (SVC) into the RA. The right pulmonary veins may anomalously drain into the RA and rarely at the entry site of the inferior vena cava (IVC). Spontaneous closure occurs before 18 months of age in more than 80 % of patients with defects less than 8 mm. An ASD with a diameter greater than 8 mm rarely closes spontaneously. If a defect is left untreated, CHF and pulmonary hypertension may develop in adults in their 20s and 30s. Patients are at risk for atrial arrhythmias such as atrial fibrillation or flutter, paradoxical emboli and stroke, and rarely bacterial endocarditis.

Device or surgical closure is indicated for patients with left-to-right shunts with a (Q_p/Q_s) of more than 1.5:1. Some physicians consider a smaller shunt to be an indication for intervention because of a risk for paradoxical emboli and stroke. Severe pulmonary vascular disease or high PVR is considered a contraindication for closure. An isolated secundum ASD occurring in an otherwise healthy young adult without pulmonary vascular disease/pulmonary hypertension incurs little additional risk during noncardiac surgery. However, there are two conditions in which difficulties could arise: paradoxical embolization of air or other materials which could stream across the ASD into the system and potentially cerebral circulation. Also, in response to hemorrhage or hypovolemia, there is a compensatory increase in SVR with the decrease in venous return; this situation could worsen a left-to-right shunt.

With time, the large left-to-right shunt decreases pulmonary compliance and increases the work of breathing. The right side of the heart becomes enlarged with both diastolic and systolic dysfunction developing. The LV becomes less distensible and this may worsen the left-to-right shunt. In the fourth decade of life, there is an increase in the incidence in atrial arrhythmias especially atrial fibrillation, atrial flutter, and supraventricular tachycardia. A baseline ECG should be obtained in patients with a history of ASD. The majority of adults older than 35 years of age will frequently be symptomatic from a secundum ASD with at least moderate PH or PVD and RV dysfunction as a result of the chronic left-to-right shunt. For adult patients undergoing cardiac surgery for repair of an ASD, an arterial line, central venous line, and TEE monitoring are recommended. For patients undergoing device closure of their ASD, sedation with intracardiac echo may be recommended or general anesthesia with TEE monitoring may also be undertaken. An arterial line and central line are generally not necessary for device closure. For patients undergoing noncardiac surgery, the monitoring required is generally dictated by the severity of their pulmonary hypertension. For patients with severe PH undergoing a major surgical operation, an arterial line, central venous pressure monitoring, and TEE are recommended. TEE in this situation would be valuable in accessing loading conditions, biventricular function, and the presence and magnitude of shunting. PACs are generally not recommended due to the propensity to cross the atrial septal defect into the left heart. Also, patients with ASDs frequently have valvular regurgitant lesions of the tricuspid, pulmonary, and mitral valve and require bacterial endocarditis prophylaxis.

Ventricular Septal Defects

Ventricular septal defects (VSDs) are the most common form of congenital heart disease and account for 15–20 % of congenital heart defects, not including those VSDs which coexist with cyanotic heart lesions. Perimembranous defects are the most common defects accounting for 70 % of VSDs. With a small restrictive defects, patients may remain relatively asymptomatic until early adulthood. With moderate to large unrestrictive defects, patients will have delayed growth and development and decreased exercise tolerance, recurrent pulmonary infections, and CHF. Spontaneous closure occurs in 30–40 % of patients with membranous VSDs during the first 6 months of life. CHF develops in infants with large unrestrictive VSDs at approximately the first 6–8 weeks of life. Pulmonary vascular occlusive disease may begin to develop as early as 6–12 months of life in patients with unrestrictive defects, but the resulting right-to-left shunt or Eisenmenger syndrome usually does not develop until the teenage years. As mentioned earlier, VSD is the most common form of CHD in childhood. However, certain unrepaired forms of CHD are rarely found in adulthood and VSDs are among them. There are occasional instances when patients with small to moderate-sized, restrictive VSDs present in adulthood.

The repair of VSDs in the adult population may be undertaken in an open surgical fashion or more commonly with a device closure. The degree of pulmonary hypertension or pulmonary vascular occlusive disease will dictate whether the closure can be preformed. For noncardiac surgery the risk is low and related to the magnitude of the left-to-right shunt and to the compensatory response of the LV to the volume overload. Patients with unrestrictive VSDs, who have survived to adulthood, usually do so because an increase in PVR reduces the left-to-right shunt and the volume overload to the LV but achieves a reversed shunt. Very few patients with unrepaired, unrestrictive VSDs survive to adulthood due to the rapid development of PVD, Eisenmenger syndrome, and biventricular failure. Patients with repaired or unrepaired VSDs should be managed and monitored as mentioned previously in the discussion of pulmonary vascular disease. Bacterial endocarditis prophylaxis should be given to both patients with repaired and unrepaired VSDs. Patients with VSDs may have valvular heart disease as a consequence of compensatory intracardiac changes or surgical interventions. Arrhythmias and varying degrees of heart block may be present, including right bundle branch block (RBBB), which occurs in less than 10 % of patients and may be a cause of sudden death. Complete heart block occurs in less than 5 % of patients. Residual shunts occur in 20 % of repaired patients with VSDs and if hemodynamically significant may result in pulmonary hypertension.

Cyanotic Congenital Heart Disease

Patients with cyanotic CHD are hypoxemic with arterial desaturation which results from shunting of systemic venous blood into the arterial circulation. The severity of hypoxemia and desaturation is determined by the magnitude of the shunting. Most patients with cyanotic CHD do not survive to adulthood without surgical intervention or palliation. In adults with cyanotic CHD, the most common causes are tetralogy of Fallot and Eisenmenger syndrome.

Tetralogy of Fallot

Tetralogy of Fallot (TOF) occurs in 10 % of all CHD. It is the most common cyanotic heart defect seen in children after infancy and is the most common form of adult cyanotic CHD. TOF is characterized by a large subarterial VSD, an aorta that overrides the left and right ventricles, right ventricular outflow tract (RVOT) obstruction, and right ventricular hypertrophy (RVH). The RVOT obstruction may be subvalvular, valvular, and supravalvular or in the branch pulmonary arteries.

There are also several associated anomalies with TOF, including pulmonary atresia, a right-sided aorta, and ASD, which occurs in 10% of patients and is referred to as pentalogy of Fallot. Coronary anomalies occur in 10% of patients. Patients with TOF are cyanotic secondary to right-to-left shunting. Secondary to the large VSD, the right and left ventricles have equalized pressures. Right-to-left shunting of the venous blood occurs because of increased resistance to pulmonary blood flow secondary to the RVOT obstruction. The severity of the RVOT obstruction determines the magnitude of shunting and therefore cyanosis. The resistance to flow across the RVOT is relatively fixed, and thus changes in SVR affect the magnitude of right-to-left shunting. A decrease in SVR worsens the right-to-left shunt, whereas an increase in SVR decreases the right-to-left shunting. In managing a patient with TOF, it is imperative that the SVR be maintained so the hypoxemia is not worsened.

Patients with TOF generally have cyanosis starting within the first year of life. These children exhibit what is referred to "tet spells" or hypercyanotic spells. These sudden hypoxic episodes are characterized by tachypnea and severe cyanosis with occasional loss of consciousness, seizures, cerebrovascular accidents, and even death. Tet spells do not occur in adolescents or adults. Adults with TOF have dyspnea and very limited exercise tolerance. They also have multisystemic complications of chronic cyanosis, including erythrocytosis, hyperviscosity, renal dysfunction, uric acid metabolism disturbances/gout, hemostatic derangements, cerebral abscesses, strokes, and endocarditis. Most patients with TOF who have not undergone surgical repair or palliation die in childhood. The survival rate is 66% at 1 year of age, 40% at 3 years of age, 11% at 20 years of age, 6% at 30 years of age, and 3% at 40 years of age.

In the past, infants with TOF underwent one of the three palliative procedures to increase pulmonary blood flow with a direct arterial-to-venous shunt (systemic to PA). This serves to increase pulmonary blood flow, decrease cyanosis, and improve exercise tolerance. These shunt procedures included the Waterston procedure (ascending aorta to PA anastomosis), the Potts procedure (descending aorta to left PA anastomosis), and the Blalock–Taussig shunt (subclavian artery to PA anastomosis). These procedures were often associated with long-term consequences such as pulmonary hypertension, PA distortion, and LV volume overload. At present, complete surgical repair with closure of the VSD and relief of the RVOT obstruction is usually performed. Palliative shunting, balloon valvuloplasty, and RVOT stenting are generally only performed on children with unfavorable PA anatomy or those too small or ill to undergo complete repair.

Adult and pediatric patients who have undergone repair of TOF are at risk for other long-term sequelae. Pulmonary regurgitation and/or stenosis may develop as a consequence of surgical repair of the valve or the RVOT with result RVH and RV dysfunction. Repair or replacement of the pulmonary valve may be required either by a surgical approach or more commonly by a transcatheter or hybrid approach. Aneurysm formation at the site of the RVOT repair is not uncommon in repaired TOF patients and has a risk of rupturing. Patients also frequently experience residual or recurrent obstruction of the RVOT and require re-intervention either by surgical or interventional cardiology technique. Ten to twenty percent of patients with repaired TOF have residual VSDs and may be at risk for developing pulmonary hypertension and require repeat surgery. Aortic regurgitation is also a common postrepair finding secondary to the location of the subarterial VSD. Right bundle branch block and other conduction disturbances are common after TOF repair. Complete heart block is a rare complication that requires a permanent pacemaker. All patients with TOF, both repaired and unrepaired, are at risk for endocarditis and should receive SBE prophylaxis before dental or surgical procedures.

Ebstein's Anomaly

Ebstein's anomaly of the tricuspid valve occurs in less than 1 % of all congenital heart defects. Ebstein's anomaly is a congenital defect of the tricuspid valve in which the septal leaflet and occasionally the posterior leaflet are displaced into the right ventricle and the anterior leaflet is usually redundant, malformed, and abnormally adherent to the right ventricular free wall. As a result, a portion of the right ventricle is "atrialized" in that it is incorporated into the RA and a functional hypoplasia of the RV results. Redundant tricuspid valve tissues can occasionally obstruct the RVOT, and tricuspid regurgitation (TR) or tricuspid stenosis is frequently present. The RA is dilated and hypertrophied and patients are prone to arrhythmias. Eighty percent of patients with Ebstein's anomaly have an ASD or patent foramen ovale (PFO) by which right-to-left shunting may occur.

In the case of Ebstein's anomaly, the severity of the hemodynamic compromise is dependent on the functional status of the tricuspid valve leaflets. Patients with mild apical displacement of the tricuspid leaflets have virtually normal valvular function, whereas those with severe tricuspid leaflet displacement or abnormal anterior leaflet attachment, with valvular dysfunction, have elevated RA pressure and right-to-left interatrial shunting. Likewise, the clinical presentation of Ebstein's anomaly varies from severe cyanosis and heart failure in a fetus or neonate to the absence of symptoms in an adult in whom it is discovered as an incidental finding.

Intrauterine mortality is high for the fetus with Ebstein's anomaly. Neonates with severe disease have cyanosis with heart failure and a murmur noted in the first few days of life. As PVR decreases, there may be a transient improvement, but the condition worsens after the ductus arteriosus closes, thereby decreasing pulmonary blood flow. Older children with Ebstein's anomaly often come to medical attention when a murmur is found on physical exam. Adolescents and adults frequently present with supraventricular tachycardia (SVT) and other arrhythmias. For patients with paroxysmal atrial tachycardia, cyanosis, and cardiomegaly, these are the factors which are most closely associated with poor outcome. In patients with Ebstein's anomaly with ASD or PFO, there is a risk of paradoxical embolism, brain abscess, and sudden death. On physical exam patients may have severe cyanosis, hepatomegaly due to passive congestion and elevated RA pressures. Frequently, these patients have large P waves on ECG as well as right bundle branch block (RBBB) and first-degree heart block. Approximately 20 % of patients with Ebstein's anomaly have Wolff–Parkinson–White (WPW) syndrome, which is a ventricular preexcitation arrhythmia through an accessory pathway between the atrium and the ventricle. A delta wave may be present on ECG.

For adult patients with Ebstein's anomaly who are symptomatic despite medical management, it is recommended to undergo repair or replacement of the tricuspid valve and closure of the ASD. Surgery may also be recommended for patients with less severe symptoms but whom also have cardiomegaly. For patients undergoing both cardiac surgical intervention and noncardiac surgery, it is recommended that all patients have complete perioperative evaluation and optimization including appropriate imaging such as echocardiogram and/or MRI as well as ECG. Perioperative arterial line and central venous pressure monitoring are recommended as well as intraoperative TEE. TEE monitoring is recommended to evaluate anatomy, shunting, loading conditions, biventricular function, the presence of RVOT obstruction, the presence of associated anomalies, loading conditions, and the integrity of the repair in the case of cardiac surgery. PAC monitoring is not recommended as it is likely to cross the ASD into the left heart.

Transposition of the Great Arteries

D-Transposition of the great arteries (D-TGA) occurs in about 5 % of all CHD with a male predominance of three males to one female. D-TGA exists when there is an anatomic discordance between the ventricles and the great arteries, in that the morphologic RV gives rise to the aorta and the morphologic LV gives rise to the PA. The physiologic consequence, surgical plan, and long-term sequelae are contingent on the age at presentation and the associated anomalies. If the systemic and pulmonary venous returns are normal, the alternatives for surgical correction have traditionally been "switching" the circulation at the great arterial level (arterial switch or Jatene procedure) or at the atrial level (Senning or Mustard procedure). For patients with D-TGA, VSD, and subpulmonic stenosis, the Rastelli procedure realigns the ventricular septum so that the appropriate venous return is associated with the correct great vessel and the subpulmonic stenosis is resected. Patients with associated defects such as aberrant venous return and RVOT or LVOT obstruction (occurs in 30 % of patients) require a customized plan for correction or palliation. Additionally, 30 % of patients with D-TGA have coronary anomalies including the origins of the coronary arteries and the sinuses of Valsalva, which are displaced to the posterior portion of the transposed aorta. This represents a risk for coronary compromise and ischemia as a short- and long-term consequence of arterial switch procedures. VSDs of hemodynamic significance are also associated with 25 % of D-TGA patients.

Prior to the introduction of the atrial baffle procedures (Senning and Mustard operations), the 1-year mortality for patients with D-TGA was approximately 90 %. The Senning and Mustard interatrial baffle procedures were developed in the late 1950s and early 1960s and significantly improved survival for patients with

D-TGA. Many of these patients now comprise a significant portion of the adult congenital population. The procedures attempt to correct the circulation which runs parallel by redirecting venous return at the atrial level. Systemic venous blood enters the RA and is directed across the atrial septum through the baffle and across the mitral valve to the LV and into the PA. Similarly, pulmonary venous return is directed across the atrial septum through the tricuspid valve and into the RV and ejected into the aorta. The difference between the two procedures involves aspects related to the atrial septum construction and placement of the suture lines, which have had long-term sequelae.

Atrial switch procedures have a number of long-term consequences including arrhythmias, sudden death, RV (systemic ventricle) dysfunction, baffle leaks, and obstruction which impairs venous return from the respective circulation. SVT, atrial fibrillation, atrial flutter, and sinus node dysfunction are the most common arrhythmias. Pulmonary hypertension, ventricular dysfunction, and junctional rhythm are risk factors for SVT. Approximately, one third of patients with atrial switch procedures will ultimately require a permanent pacemaker secondary to sinus node dysfunction. Ten percent of patients will experience baffle obstruction of either the systemic or pulmonary venous return. The function of the RV as the systemic ventricle deteriorates with time, and sudden death is experienced in 5 % of patients and is attributable to persistent heart failure. Other causes of sudden death in these patients are attributable to arrhythmias and pulmonary hypertension.

For patients with D-TGA, VSD, and subpulmonic stenosis, the Rastelli procedure is frequently performed. In this procedure, the VSD is closed in a manner that redirects venous return to the appropriate great vessel, and an RV to PA conduit is placed to relieve the subpulmonic stenosis. Long-term follow-up in these patients reveals 74 % survival for patients operated on in the 1980s. The majority of patients require further intervention both surgical and catheter based. There is also a 5 % risk for sudden death in these patients due to ventricular dysfunction and arrhythmias.

The arterial switch operation or Jatene procedure involves transplanting the coronary arteries to the PA and connecting the proximal great vessels to the distal ends of the other vessel in an attempt to restore anatomically correct circulation. This procedure is considered superior to the atrial switch procedures in that it is physiologically correct and results in fewer long-term complications such as arrhythmias, RV failure, baffle obstruction, and TR. For patients with uncomplicated D-TGA, normal sinus rhythm is usually present, and providing good coronary blood flow, LV function is preserved. However, PA stenosis at the site of reconstruction occurs in 5–10 % of cases. Complete heart block is a risk in 5–10 % of patients, and aortic regurgitation (AR) is a late complication and occurs in 20 % of patients especially in patients who underwent PA banding in the neonatal period. An important cause of AR may be unequal size of the pulmonary valve cusps that leads to eccentric valvular coaptation. The most important life-threatening complication associated with arterial switch is the possibility of coronary obstruction which leads to myocardial ischemia, infarction, and death. Long-term outcomes continue to be accessed with many patients who have previously undergone the arterial switch procedure entering their third decade of life. The overall conclusion is that the arterial switch is the procedure of choice with preservation of physiologic circulation but that coronary obstruction, pulmonary stenosis, and aortic insufficiency remain significant problems.

Eisenmenger Syndrome

Eisenmenger syndrome develops over time as a consequence of significant, uncorrected left-to-right shunting in association with a VSD, ASD, or PDA. As discussed previously in this chapter, morphologic transformations occur in the small PAs and arterioles, leading to pulmonary hypertension and the resultant reversal of the intracardiac shunt creating cyanosis. In the small PAs and arterioles, medial hypertrophy, intimal cellular proliferation, and fibrosis lead to narrowing or closure of the vessel lumen. With sustained pulmonary hypertension, insidious atherosclerosis and calcification often develop in large PAs. The initial morphologic alterations, medial hypertrophy of the pulmonary arterioles, intimal proliferation and fibrosis, and occlusion of capillaries are potentially reversible. However, as the disease progresses, the morphologic changes including plexiform lesions and necrotizing arteritis are irreversible and result in obliteration of the pulmonary vascular bed, which leads to increased PVR. As the PVR approaches or exceeds systemic resistance, the shunt is reversed. The morphologic changes in the pulmonary vasculature that occur with Eisenmenger syndrome usually begin in childhood, but symptoms don't usually start to appear until adolescences or early adulthood when the right-to-left shunt is sustained and cyanosis appears.

Most patients have decreased exercise tolerance and dyspnea and these symptoms may be compensated for a time period. Atrial arrhythmias frequently develop such as atrial fibrillation and atrial flutter. Erythrocytosis develops due to arterial desaturation, and symptoms of hyperviscosity such as visual disturbances, fatigue, headache, dizziness, and paresthesias frequently develop. Hemoptysis secondary to rupture or infarction of dilated PAs can occur and be life-threatening. Patients who have developed cyanosis also have abnormal hemostasis and are at risk for cerebrovascular accidents which can occur due to paradoxical emboli, venous thrombosis, or intracranial hemorrhage. Patients with Eisenmenger are also at risk for brain abscess and syncope. Syncope may occur secondary to inadequate cardiac output or arrhythmias. Symptoms of heart failure are not common until the disease is in advanced stages and implies a very poor prognosis. Patients with Eisenmenger are at risk for sudden death.

Medical management of Eisenmenger syndrome is similar to that of pulmonary hypertension and includes inhaled oxygen, nitric oxide, treprostinil, and IV vasodilators such as epoprostenol. Other dilators such as sildenafil may be taken orally and used in conjunction with calcium channel blockers, endothelin receptor antagonists, anticoagulants, diuretics, and antiarrhythmics. For some patients, the ultimate therapy may be heart–lung transplantation providing other organ systems have preserved function. The effectiveness of these therapies is limited by the severity of the disease. Patients with Eisenmenger syndrome should avoid high-altitude and excessive exertion, dehydration, and the use of systemic vasodilators.

Pregnancy is associated with high maternal and fetal morbidity and mortality. The fixed PVR precludes any compensation for acute fluctuations in SVR, cardiac output, and blood volume during labor, delivery, and the peripartum period. Any acute decrease in SVR precipitates increased right-to-left shunting and results in severe cyanosis. Valsalva maneuvers during labor may acutely increase SVR, depress systemic and cerebral perfusion, and trigger fatal syncope.

Patients undergoing both cardiac and noncardiac surgery should be cared for in centers experienced in the management of such patients and require a multidisciplinary approach. The anesthesia care required is meticulous management of fluid status and both systemic and pulmonary vascular resistance. Maintenance of SVR and contractility, minimizing blood loss and intravascular volume depletion, as well as preventing paradoxical embolization are imperative. Most patients are admitted for overnight IV placement and mild hydration. Prophylactic phlebotomy is generally not done in most centers as the volume shifts may be poorly tolerated. The intraoperative management is frequently dictated by the nature of the procedure; however, most general anesthetic including cardiac procedures will necessitate arterial line and central venous pressure monitoring and TEE monitoring. PACs are not indicated due to the likelihood of crossing the shunt lesion such as an ASD or the potential for PA rupture.

Single-Ventricle Physiology and Complex Cyanotic Congenital Heart Disease

Advances in palliative and corrective heart surgery, catheter-based interventions, anesthesia, and imaging have significantly increased the number of patients with complex, cyanotic heart disease who have reach adulthood. Patients who have undergone single-ventricle palliation with a Fontan procedure illustrate the cumulative risks of dysrhythmias, decreased ventricular function, and chronic hypoxemia as well as other multi-organ system sequelae.

Many complex congenital heart lesions result in anatomic malformations that are not amenable to surgical intervention and result in a functioning biventricular circulation. These lesions include severe Ebstein's anomaly, tricuspid atresia, hypoplastic left heart syndrome (HLHS), unbalanced atrioventricular canal (AV canal), and various defects associated with heterotaxy syndrome. These forms of CHD require staged procedures that attempt to use an existing ventricle as the systemic ventricle and create a mechanism for pulmonary blood flow that may not necessarily require a pumping chamber and will likely be passive flow. The surgical plan for these patients is somewhat individualized and dependent on the native anatomy with the ultimate conformation relatively similar among patients with single-ventricle physiology. The Fontan circuit functions to direct systemic venous return via a conduit into the PA system. The circuit does not require a right-sided heart chamber, and pulmonary venous blood returns into a common atrium and flows into the systemic ventricle.

The first palliative operation for patients with single-ventricle physiology usually requires a shunt from an arterial source that provides pulmonary blood flow or a ductal stent to maintain an open PDA as the source for pulmonary blood flow in the first-stage hybrid palliation procedure. Adequate mixing at the atrial level is required with an unrestrictive ASD along with unobstructed systemic ventricular outflow. In the past, the Blalock–Taussig (BT) shunt (right subclavian to PA anastomosis) or a central shunt (aorta to PA shunt) was performed. Presently, the modified BT shunt is frequently used with a Gore-Tex conduit from the right subclavian artery to the PA to provide pulmonary blood flow. Historically, the classic BT shunt permanently compromised arterial blood flow to the right arm. The modified BT shunt is generally ligated at the time of the subsequent procedure and does not permanently compromise flow. This is relevant in that patients who have undergone a classic BT shunt will not have an accurate blood pressure measured in the right upper extremity. The BT shunt in the case of HLHS provides the pulmonary blood flow while the creation of a neo-aorta (Norwood procedure) from the proximal PA creates the manner in which systemic blood flow leaves the heart. The subsequent procedures in the palliative process attempt to route systemic blood flow to the PA vascular bed. The second-stage procedure (bidirectional Glenn shunt) involves creating a superior vena cava to PA anastomosis. The final stage, or Fontan procedure, results in the creation of an inferior vena cava to PA connection and may be undertaken in a number of ways. Fenestration of the Fontan conduit creates a functional ASD that serves as a pressure outlet in the setting of pulmonary hypertension and maintains LA filling and systemic perfusion.

Modifications and revisions of the single-ventricle palliative path have been made since their initial performance in the 1970s and decreased the incidence of adverse sequelae such as arrhythmias, pulmonary hypertension, ventricular dysfunction, and heart failure. For patients who underwent the Fontan procedure in the 1970s, the 15-year survival rate was 50–80 %. The majority of Fontan patients have NYHA class I or II symptoms and exhibit decreased exercise tolerance. Approximately 40 % of these patients require reoperation for conduit obstruction, permanent pacemaker, or AV valve repair for valvular regurgitation. Atrial arrhythmias are very common among Fontan patients, and loss of the atrial contribution to cardiac output can result in significant impairment, and patients will frequently require permanent pacing.

Another significant adverse sequelae of Fontan physiology is protein-losing enteropathy (PLE). PLE develops in 5–10 % of patients and is manifested by gastrointestinal protein malabsorption, ascites, peripheral edema, pleural effusions, and low serum protein levels. Elevated systemic venous pressure, abnormal mucosal blood flow patterns, and glycosylation of enteric proteins have been implicated as the cause of this condition. Patients with fenestrated versus non-fenestrated Fontan conduits have a decreased incidence of protein-losing enteropathy. The therapies include fenestration of the Fontan conduit, anticoagulation, dietary modifications, corticosteroids, and ultimately heart transplantation.

Following Fontan procedures, the formation of arteriovenous malformations (AVMs) has been observed, especially pulmonary AVMs in the lungs. Pulmonary AVMs produce a significant volume load on the ventricle and impair function. Shunting may also occur through the AVMs and induce parenchymal changes, hypoxia, and poor lung compliance.

The perioperative management of these patients requires attention to maintaining SVR, not increasing PVR and attention to loading conditions and fluid status. High positive pressures with ventilation or other maneuvers which decrease venous return are not recommended. The type of invasive monitoring is dictated by the procedure. For patients undergoing cardiac surgery or procedures, arterial line and central pressure monitoring is recommended. TEE is required to access ventricular function, AV valve regurgitation, potential paradoxical emboli, loading conditions, and the integrity of the repair. For patients undergoing noncardiac surgery, similar monitoring may be advised depending on the procedure. Attention needs to be paid to bleeding or other volume losses with appropriate fluid management or blood replacement. Patients are at high risk for antibodies and type-specific blood may take extra time to prepare.

Perioperative Concerns and Anesthetic Management

The perioperative strategy and management require a complete assessment and consider factors relevant to both the patient's underlying physiology as well as factors related to the proposed procedure. The patient's baseline cardiovascular reserve and underlying multi-organ system impairment must be evaluated in conjunction with the concerns specific to the CHD and potential acquired comorbidities related to aging. The techniques required for the procedure need to be considered and balanced in light of what the patient's cardiovascular reserve will tolerate. For example, a patient with a failing Fontan physiology is unlikely to tolerate high-pressure abdominal insufflation associated with numerous laparoscopic procedures currently being performed. It is recommended that adult patients with CHD be cared for in a center with a dedicated team familiar with their unique physiology and that a multidisciplinary approach be used when faced with complicated medical decisions regarding these patients.

Syndromes and Associated Anomalies

Many forms of CHD occur in association with other congenital syndromes and congenital anomalies which are noncardiac. Endocardial cushion defects such as AV canal, ASDs, and VSDs are common among patients with Down's syndrome. These patients have characteristic anomalies which impact management such as developmental delay, hypotonia, large tongue, short necks, potential for atlanto-occipital dislocation, and other features related to the syndrome. DiGeorge syndrome is another association in which conotruncal anomalies occur with abnormal calcium homeostasis, immunodeficiency, and multiple midline craniofacial anomalies. VACTERL association includes vertebral defects, anal atresia, cardiac defects, tracheoesophageal fistula, renal anomalies, and limb abnormalities. Patients with VACTERL association typically have at least three of these defects and require attention to potential other systemic involvement. However, in the adult congenital population, it is likely that other noncardiac defects would have been previously diagnosed.

Perioperative Monitoring

Perioperative monitoring must be carefully considered and appropriate for the level of baseline impairment and anticipated demands of the procedure. Arterial line, central venous pressure monitoring, and TEE monitoring may be required to ensure the most accurate assessment of loading conditions, biventricular function, direction and magnitude of shunting, and potential for paradoxical embolism. The standard monitoring equipment such as ECG, pulse oximetry, and temperature and noninvasive blood pressure monitors may also require a little extra consideration. For example, the question may arise as to where to place the ECG pads for a patient with dextrocardia or heterotaxy syndrome. The answer is that a 5-lead and 3-lead ECG placement is done in the standard fashion for all patients (baseline ECGs are also performed in the standard position). For patients who have undergone a coarctation repair incorporating the left subclavian artery, the right upper extremity will most accurately reflect the systemic blood pressure. There may also be a residual gradient between the upper and lower extremity blood pressures in these patients. For patients who have previously undergone a classic BT shunt, the ipsilateral extremity may not accurately reflect the systemic blood pressure as well as oxygen saturation, and an alternative site should be selected. For patients undergoing cardiac surgery, cerebral oximetry is also recommended and considered standard of care.

Airway and Ventilatory Management

Patients with CHD may have associated anomalies including those involving the airway. In the adult population, these anomalies may already be well documented and/or known to the patient or their families. In addition, patients who have undergone previous surgery may have experienced prolonged periods of intubation and mechanical ventilatory support, and the potential for subglottic stenosis and a history of tracheostomy are possibilities. The transition from spontaneous ventilation to positive pressure ventilation can significantly impair preload, secondary to decrease systemic venous return. This is especially important in the scenario of hypovolemia.

Patients with single-ventricle physiology are extremely sensitive to positive pressure ventilation because their pulmonary blood flow is preload dependent. Episodes of desaturation may be an indication that pulmonary blood flow is being compromised. If standard interventions are attempted such as increasing tidal volume or adding positive end-expiratory pressure (PEEP), the result may be further decrease in the saturation, secondary to further decrease in pulmonary blood flow. In the case of single-ventricle physiology, maintaining adequate intravascular volume status, limiting the peak inspiratory pressure, and avoidance of PEEP will facilitate pulmonary blood flow and preserve oxygenation.

Intravenous Access Considerations

Intravenous access can often present a significant problem in patients with CHD, especially those who have undergone multiple procedures or who have significant peripheral collateralization secondary to cyanotic heart disease or venous obstruction. A careful examination of the patient may reveal previously cannulated or cutdown sites as well as a review of previous operative reports and cath reports. Ultrasound of the potential sites as well as angiography in the cath lab will help in identifying sites available for vascular cannulation. Patients with right-to-left shunts are at risk for paradoxical embolization of air or particles, even when infused into peripheral lines and vigilance and the use of infusion filters is recommended to decrease the possibility of emboli.

Perioperative Fluid Management and NPO Intervals

Standard NPO intervals in healthy adult patients with normal cardiovascular reserve generally have little impact. However, for patients with cardiac anatomy dependent on adequate filling pressures, even minor decreases in preload can have adverse effects. Patients with single-ventricle physiology, cyanotic patients with erythrocytosis, patients with Eisenmenger physiology, and patients with volume-dependent obstructive lesions are extremely sensitive to acute decreases in preload. Decreased preload and the vasodilating effects of anesthetic agents can lead to acute circulatory collapse even in patients who seem well compensated prior to induction. Ensuring adequate preload prior to induction and judicious titration of anesthetic agents can facilitate preservation of cardiac output in the previously described patients. Management of perioperative volume losses should be guided by the monitoring of vital signs, arterial line pressure, central venous pressure, hematocrit, urine output, acid–base status, and electrolytes.

Third-space losses, especially in the case of patients with protein-losing enteropathy, must be considered. PLE results in hypoalbuminemia, ascites, and pericardial and pleural effusion and is associated with high systemic venous pressures and ventricular dysfunction of the single ventricle. These patients are frequently total volume fluid overloaded with third-space sequestered volume and intravascular space depleted with poor cardiovascular reserve. This clinical situation implies extremely poor cardiac reserve, and the ability to tolerate or compensate for intravascular depletion, vasodilating anesthetics, and positive pressure ventilation is exceptionally limited. Medication doses should be reduced to account for the effect of hypoalbuminemia, and all medications should be titrated to effect with hemodynamic monitoring. Appropriate first-case scheduling, minimizing NPO intervals, or preoperative hospital admission with IV hydration should be considered in this group of patients, to avoid the risks of intravascular volume depletion.

Hematocrit and Perioperative Transfusion Management

Patients with chronic cyanosis will compensate for their hypoxemia with a baseline erythrocytosis in an attempt to increase oxygen delivery. If a chronically cyanotic patient is found to have a normal range hematocrit, a coexisting anemia, usually iron deficiency, should be considered. Erythrocytosis predisposes patients to complications of hyperviscosity. A hematocrit of greater than 40 % is generally considered to provide an adequate red cell mass for oxygen delivery. However, the patient's own baseline hematocrit will frequently serve as a guide, providing they are not anemic.

Extra consideration must be given to the situation in which a transfusion is required in that many patients with CHD require special preparation of blood products. Patients with DiGeorge syndrome or who are immunosuppressed require cytomegalovirus (CMV)-negative blood that has been irradiated and leukocyte filtered. This is done to decrease the potential transmission of CMV and prevent graft-versus-host disease, along with other leukocyte-mediated transfusion reactions. If a question arises regarding the type of blood products required for a specific condition, a hematologist or blood bank pathologist should be consulted. Additionally, the majority of adult congenital heart patients have undergone previous heart surgery with the concomitant exposure to blood products and previous transfusion. It is extremely common for these patients to have developed antibodies that may complicate the cross-match process, and extra time must be allowed in order to prepare type-specific blood products. Attention must also be paid to patients that may in the future require heart transplantation. Limiting transfusions and therefore antibody formation is vital for these patients. Adult congenital heart patients should also receive leukocyte-depleted blood to also help decrease antibody formation.

Antibiotic Prophylaxis

The requirement for SBE prophylaxis is dictated by the underlying cardiac disease and anatomy as well as the type of procedure being performed. The American Heart Association offers a comprehensive list with specific recommendations for patients with CHD on their website www.americanheart.org. Most patients with CHD have significant graft material and prosthetic valves as well as intracardiac shunts and regurgitant or stenotic valves. They are at high risk for endocarditis and it is a frequent complication for many patients with CHD.

Pacemakers and Arrhythmias

Arrhythmias are among the most prevalent and complex sequelae for patients with adult CHD. The arrhythmias and common rhythm disturbances associated with each defect has been previously discussed and can be found with the respective lesion discussion. Many patients with adult CHD require antiarrhythmic therapy that should be reviewed before surgery. The side effects and interactions of these medications should be known. A baseline ECG is recommended before all procedures, and if arrhythmias do arise in the perioperative period, a rapid diagnosis should be made and therapy should be instituted. The underlying etiology should be considered in each case with respect to the circumstances and underlying anatomy and physiology. For example, D-TGA with atrial switch anatomy is known to be associated with atrial arrhythmias. Electrolyte disturbances especially secondary to diuretic therapy, hypercarbia, acidosis, severe hypoxia, and antiarrhythmic agents can also produce arrhythmias. Medications that blunt vagal tone should be used with extreme caution.

Many patients with adult CHD have permanent pacemakers and implantable cardiac defibrillators (ICD). The settings and the underlying rhythm should be known. A magnet for conversion to the asynchronous mode should be available, and the therapy mode of the ICD may need to be deactivated to avoid triggering inappropriately in the operative setting.

Postoperative Considerations

In the immediate postoperative period, extreme vigilance and similar levels of monitoring which were employed during the operative period should be continued. The level of postoperative monitoring should be appropriate for the patient's baseline physiology and the nature of the surgical procedure and its anticipated postoperative sequelae. Many patients with adult CHD will continue to need arterial line and CVP monitoring in the postoperative period and may require management in the intensive care unit that an otherwise normal cardiovascular status patient undergoing the same procedure would not require.

Pain management and postoperative nausea and vomiting are important considerations. Appropriate analgesia including narcotic medications, regional anesthesia which does not impair SVR, acetaminophen derivatives, and nonsteroidal anti-inflammatory medications are all used with success in patients with CHD. Analgesia facilitates improved respiratory mechanics and decreases oxygen consumption.

However, respiratory depression, hypercarbia, and airway obstruction must be avoided secondary to their significant effects on increasing PVR. The management of postoperative nausea and vomiting is crucial for oral hydration and the ability to resume medication regimens especially antiarrhythmic and anticoagulation medications.

Conclusion

Adult patients with CHD represent an ever-increasing group of patients with complex cardiac anatomy and physiology as well as acquired comorbidities. These patients represent a challenge to the medical community and require a multidisciplinary team approach with comprehensive perioperative planning. At this time, there are no evidence-based guidelines for the perioperative management of adult patients with CHD. Large-scale clinical trials are required to demonstrate the optimal management strategies, and it is recommended that these patients be cared for in cardiac centers with congenital heart specialists who are familiar with their physiology. An appreciation of the previously discussed principles will assist the provider in evaluating a multitude of structural lesions based on their underlying physiologic effects. Ultimately, an understanding of the patient's unique physiology and multi-organ system sequelae will enhance the likelihood of perioperative cardiovascular stability.

Case Study: Anesthetic Management of a Hybrid Approach to Transcatheter Pulmonary Valve Replacement in a Previously Repaired Patient with Tetralogy of Fallot

A 15-year-old male with a history of TOF s/p transannular patch repair as an infant presents with severe pulmonary valve regurgitation (PR) and right heart dilatation. Although asymptomatic from a cardiac standpoint, he did have severe right ventricular dilation on MRI (RVEDV = 180 ml/m^2). After careful discussion about treatment options, the patient decided on a transcatheter Melody valve. A diagnostic angiogram showed an extremely enlarged and tortuous pulmonary artery not amenable to a Melody valve. 3D reconstruction of the patient's PA was used to further evaluate the anatomy for other possible interventions. After careful planning and several virtual implants, a hybrid procedure was decided upon in which a Melody valve could be placed within a pulmonary artery stent. In preparation for the hybrid procedure, the patient was premedicated with midazolam and induced with etomidate and cisatracurium for general endotracheal anesthesia. A radial arterial line and right internal jugular central line were placed. Both OR staffing and a perfusionist were on standby to go on cardiopulmonary bypass and convert to an open procedure

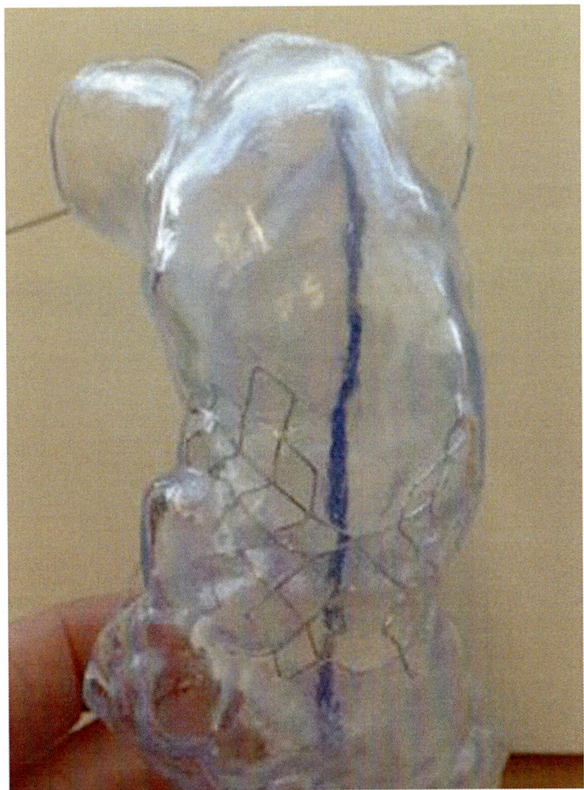

Fig. 13.1 3D reconstruction of pulmonary artery

if necessary. Access for stent delivery was achieved through a subxiphoid incision by a cardiothoracic surgeon. Under fluoroscopy and transesophageal echocardiogram (TEE), a covered stent and landing stent were placed with vascular plugs along the tortuous pulmonary artery taking care not to compromise the branch pulmonary arteries and ensuring good flow through the RVOT. After confirmation of proper seating of the stents, the Melody valve was delivered through the subxiphoid incision and deployed within the landing zone stent in the pulmonary artery. Postdeployment intracardiac echo (ICE), TEE, and angiogram showed no PR and no compromise to the branch pulmonary arteries. The patient was transferred to the PICU where he was extubated after several hours and discharged home the next day (Figs. 13.1, 13.2, 13.3, and 13.4).

Case Discussion

Surgical repair of TOF has been occurring for about 50 years with excellent outcomes. However, with longer survival, we are seeing more long-term complications of these repairs, specifically pulmonary valve regurgitation. Untreated PR in these patients can result in right-sided remodeling, which if left untreated can lead to right heart failure. Previously, that intervention was not recommended until the patient became symptomatic from the pulmonary regurgitation. However, several

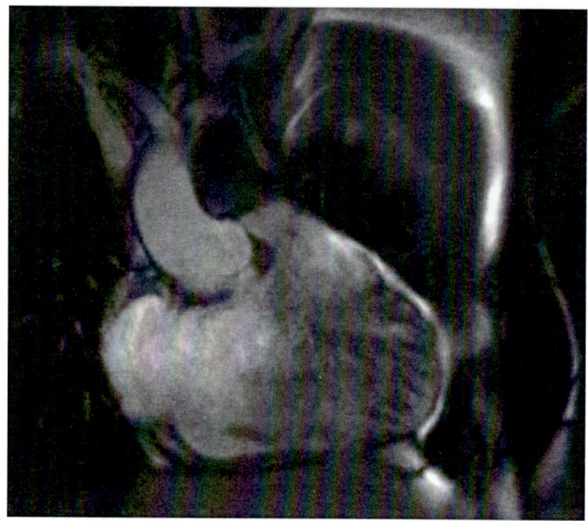

Fig. 13.2 Cardiac MRI showing dilated right ventricle

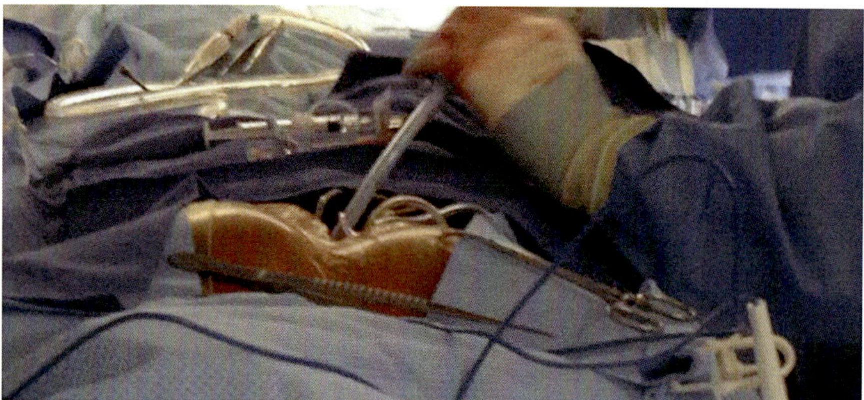

Fig. 13.3 Subxiphoid access for stent delivery

studies have shown that early repair of pulmonary valve regurgitation can prevent long-term right heart remodeling.

Currently, cardiac MRI is the gold standard for measuring right ventricular volume and pulmonary regurgitation. The precise timing of when to intervene is unclear, but studies seem to show remolding of the RV when RVEDV >150 ml/m^2. Despite the overall good outcomes with surgical repair for these patients with pulmonary regurgitation, it is not without its risk factors. Most patients will have significant scar tissue formation with adherent right ventricle to the chest wall, making entering the chest extremely high risk. There are some limitations secondary to unfavorable PA anatomy which may require a hybrid approach with access through a subxiphoid incision to allow for multiple large stent placement and/or

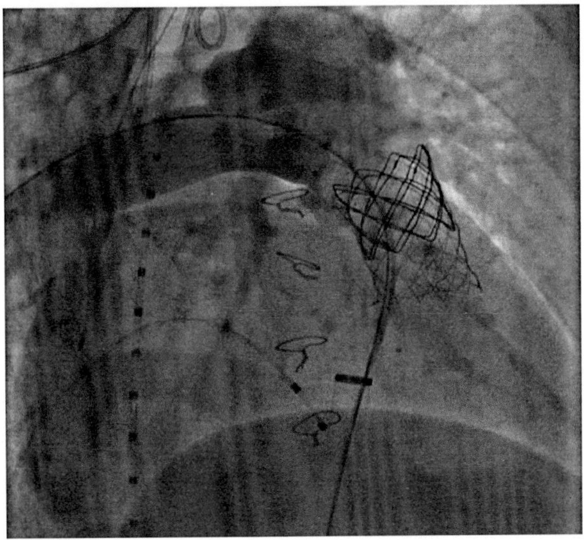

Fig. 13.4 Angiogram showing post-Melody valve deployment with no pulmonary regurgitation

better trajectory of valve deployment. General anesthesia and arterial line are mandatory, while central access should be considered depending on the patient's venous access and baseline cardiac function. TEE is used to monitor function, access the pre- and postimplant anatomy, access loading conditions, guide the procedure, and monitor for pericardial effusion. The usual goals for PR physiology should be applied for these cases. Perfusionists and surgical staff should be readily available to go on bypass and convert to an open procedure should complications arise. Complications include bleeding, pulmonary artery rupture, cracked stents, compression of coronary vessels, arrhythmias, pulmonary regurgitation, and stent migration and embolism. Early extubation in the cath lab has been described; however, it may be prudent to leave the patient intubated if there are concerns for bleeding or if there are large fluid shifts related to volume resuscitation. The Melody valve and other transcatheter valves have made repair of pulmonary regurgitation in previously repaired TOF patients much less invasive and ultimately safer. It is important to be aware of the complications that can occur with the hybrid procedure.

Bibliography

Baum VC, Perloff JK. Anesthetic implications of adults with congenital heart disease. Anesth Analg. 1993;76:1342.

Brickner ME, Hillis LD, Lange RA. Congenital heart disease in adults. Part one & two. N Engl J Med. 2000;342:334–42.

Cannesson M, Earing M, Collange V. Anesthesia for noncardiac surgery in adults with congenital heart disease. Anesthesiology. 2009;111(2):432–40.

Hosking MP, Beynen FM. The modified Fontan procedure: physiology and anesthetic implications. J Cardiothorac Vasc Anesth. 1992;6:465–75.

Hucin B, Voriskova M, Hruda J, et al. Late complications and quality of life after atrial correction of transposition of the great arteries in 12 to 18 year follow up. J Cardiovasc Surg. 2000;41: 233–9.
Khairy P, Poirier N, Mercier LA. Univentricular heart. Circulation. 2007;115:800–12.
Landzberg MJ, Murphy Jr DJ, Davidson Jr WR, Jarcho JA, Krumholz HM, Mayer Jr JE, Mee RB, Sahn DJ, Van Hare GF, Webb GD. Task force 4: organization of delivery systems for adults with congenital heart disease. J Am Coll Cardiol. 2001;37:1187–93.
Marelli AJ, Mackie AS, et al. Congenital heart disease in the general population: changing prevalence and age distribution. Circulation. 2007;115:163–72.
Perloff JK, Child JS. Congenital heart disease in adults. 3rd ed. Philadelphia: WB Saunders; 2008.
Perloff JK, Warner CA. Challenges posed by adults with repaired congenital heart disease. Circulation. 2001;103:2637–43.

Chapter 14
Medical Facility Infrastructure Considerations

Antonio Hernandez Conte

During the mid-1800s in the United States, it was recognized that medical and surgical care for the pediatric patient required facilities that were altogether different than those utilized to care for the adult patient. The forward-thinking pediatricians, surgeons, and anesthesiologists of the 1800s would be satisfied to know that their vision of a medical facility dedicated to pediatric is just as applicable in the twenty-first century as it was in the 1800s. The process for identifying pediatric patients, evaluating their health status, and ultimately treating their conditions has grown into a most complex endeavor and requires a vast array of infrastructural considerations. This chapter will outline the various processes, guidelines, and facility infrastructure requirements that are necessary to optimally care for the pediatric patient with congenital heart disease.

Identification of Pediatric Patients and Referral Management

In the United States, more than one-third of patients are referred to a specialist each year, and specialist visits constitute more than one-half of outpatient visits. Despite the frequency of referrals and the importance of the specialty referral process, the process itself has been a long-standing source of frustration among both primary care physicians (PCPs) and specialists. These statistics hold true for both the adult and pediatric populations. Numerous strategies have been developed and tested in an effort to improve the specialty referral process; these may include the utilization of "gatekeepers of care" or specialty referral guidelines (Mehrotra et al. 2011).

A. Hernandez Conte, MD, MBA
Division of Cardiac Anesthesiology, Kaiser Permanente Los Angeles Medical Center,
Cedars-Sinai Medical Center, Los Angeles, CA, USA
e-mail: sedated@bellsouth.net; antonio.conte@kp.org

© Springer International Publishing Switzerland 2017
A. Dabbagh et al. (eds.), *Congenital Heart Disease in Pediatric and Adult Patients*, DOI 10.1007/978-3-319-44691-2_14

PCPs vary in their threshold for referring a patient, which results in both the underuse and the overuse of specialists. Many referrals do not include a transfer of information, either to or from the specialist, and when they do, the transfer materials often contain insufficient data for medical decision-making. Making matters more complicated, care across the primary care-specialty interface is poorly integrated. Additionally, PCPs often do not know whether a patient actually went to the specialist or what the specialist recommended. PCPs and specialists also frequently disagree on the specialist's role during the referral episode (e.g., single consultation or continuing co-management). Therefore, typically a referral for specialty assessment may lead to a dilemma for parents or caregivers of the pediatric patient. To further complicate the scenario, a significant portion of healthcare delivery systems in the United States are not horizontally or vertically integrated. Therefore, referral processes are even more complex, and information transfer is poor in these instances which can lead to delays in assessment and ultimately life-changing care.

Academic medical centers, traditionally tertiary and quaternary care centers housed within a centralized medical facility and associated with a medical school, have been viewed as slightly more integrated models of care. However, many of these centers receive transfers and referrals from outside community hospitals so many of the same problems exist. One particular academic institution developed and implemented a networking strategy specifically for pediatric surgery (Coran et al. 1999). The major changes were the addition of a satellite facility, as well as the incorporation of four additional external practices to the existing university practice. To assess the impact on financial status of the new networking paradigm upon clinical activity, education, and academic productivity, the following parameters were analyzed: gross and net revenue, surgical cases, clinic visits, ranking of the pediatric surgery residency, publications, grant support, and development and endowment funds. Overall, clinical revenue increased over the period of 5 years, surgical cases and clinic visits increased, and additional facility were hired to more than double the number of physicians. Additionally, faculty and resident satisfaction increased due to the improved clinical working model.

For pediatric patients, care and referrals in the United States are further exacerbated by the lack of insurance for pediatric patients. Therefore, state and local social work agency administrations must coordinate funding mechanisms and these must be put into place prior to any care delivery can occur. As a leader in pediatric specialty care since the 1800s, the Johns Hopkins Medical Center set about trying to determine the referral patterns and obstacles inherent in pediatric primary care referral to specialists (Forrest et al. 1999). Their study demonstrated that most pediatricians typically referred patients for assistance in diagnosing a particular sign or symptom and were less likely to do so unless the parents specifically requested a secondary referral or opinion during a telephone call. Referrals to outside specialists dramatically increased if it would likely lead to a surgical or procedural intervention.

Linking pediatric patients to specific care has been a major area of focus for the last two decades. While multiple strategies are being tested by pediatricians and others working in child health, to date there has been no study with a primary focus on how pediatric practices link young children and their families to services and support systems. Placing the three major components of care all in the same vertically and

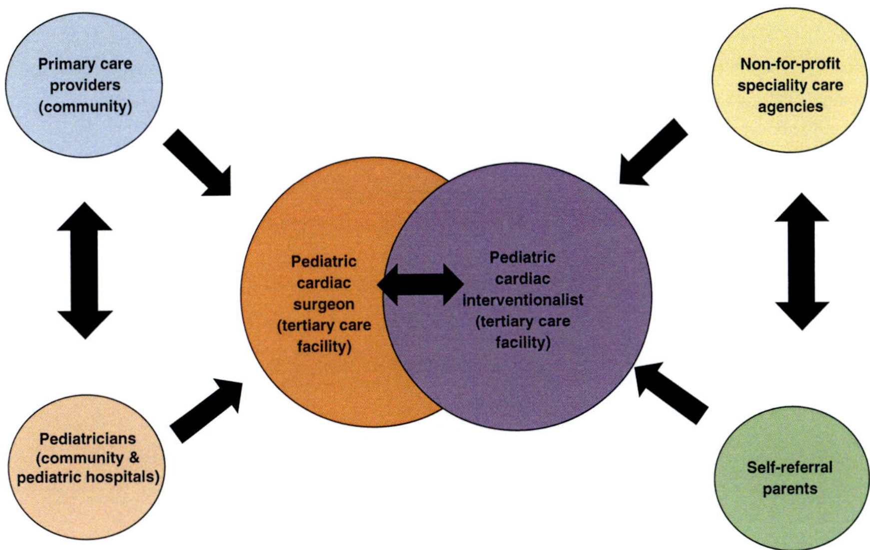

Fig. 14.1   Venn diagram demonstrating the multi-faceted flow patterns for referral and evaluation of pediatric and congenital heart patients

horizontally integrated structure holds the greatest promise in ameliorating pediatric linkage deficits particularly for the pediatric congenital population. Coordination would maximize utilization of co-location, co-management, and networking/information sharing—these would help use existing resources more effectively and improve the quality of care by reducing barriers to care; promoting early referral, linkage, and follow-up; promoting cross-discipline problem-solving and family-centered care; and reducing duplication and fragmentation of services. Service provider networking and information sharing can help uncover gaps in services and can also set the stage for collaborative efforts to address gaps (e.g., coalitions to change policies and programs). Initiating and maintaining regular, multi-sector, or multiagency service provider networking sessions generally exceed the capacity of individual pediatric practices, requiring commitment and funding from others in the community or beyond (Fig. 14.1).

The referral of pediatric patients to highly specialized centers providing cardiac and congenital evaluation and treatment poses even larger barriers to patients and pediatricians as few centers are capable of providing the high level of care necessary, and a referral may involve coordination over large geographic distances and the ability to bypass multiple obstacles.

Evaluation Coordination

Centers providing evaluation and treatment of pediatric cardiac and congenital issues must at a minimum possess a wide array of resources involving technological investments and a broad group of highly specialized personnel. Some of the referral tools are based upon marketing in a geographic catchment area. Pediatricians and parents may learn about particular services through media outlets such as television, radio, and print advertisements. While media outlets are helpful, they do not allow for differentiation of the end-product (high-quality care) and the equitable dissemination of resources being made available to all needy parties.

In the U.S. marketplace, almost every major city has a children's hospital that typically mounts media campaigns to promote the availability of particular medical service resources. Additionally, pediatricians may oftentimes meet pediatric specialists at continuing medical education events in their local community; these are designed to expose primary care providers to new service lines and highly trained pediatric specialists in their community. Otherwise, pediatricians and patients living in less urban or more rural areas face increased barriers to entry for proper care.

Focus-specific care groups, such as the Pediatric Congenital Heart Association (PCHA), provide large platforms to distribute information to both healthcare providers and patients directly. Groups such as PCHA possess the ability to reach large populations of patients through coordinated communication systems. Unfortunately, in the United States, rapid coordination and referral to an appropriate congenital pediatric specialist remain a byzantine process that delays evaluation and care.

Optimal and highly organized care would allow initial evaluation with multiple specialists all in one centralized setting. The advantage of this "setup" is that the evaluation team members can confer with one another and provide a higher level of assessment during one single encounter with the patient and family members (Fig. 14.2). After the initial assessment has been completed, additional diagnostic testing can be coordinated during a follow-up visit. Again, it is advantageous to schedule the follow-up testing on a single day or sequential days to minimize the disruption to the patient and family while also yielding a short period of evaluation and assessment so that interventions can be planned if necessary.

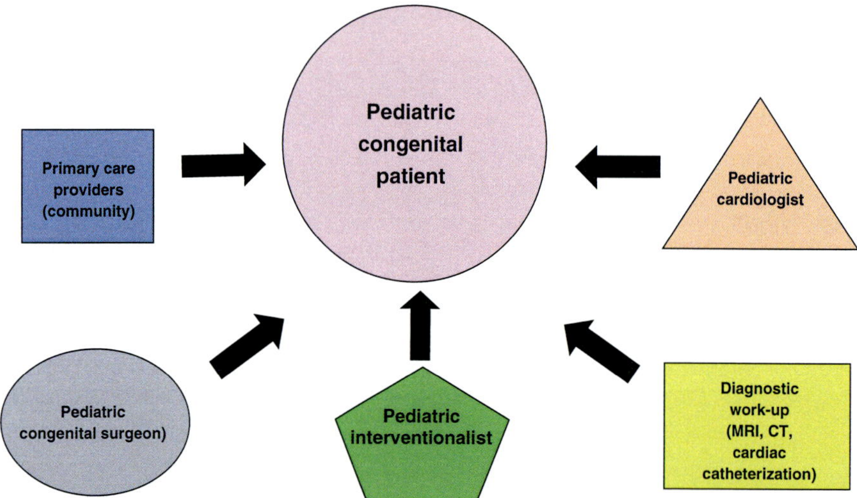

Fig. 14.2 Venn diagram displaying primary and secondary referral sources contributing to full evaluation of pediatric and congenital patients

Surgical and Cardiologic Interventional Issues

Teams The formation of teams within an institution in order to provide services and treatment interventions to the pediatric patient undergoing congenital surgery is a large undertaking. The medical facility must meet an array of minimum threshold standards pertaining to nursing requirements, physician training requirements, technologic equipment inspection, and local/state inspection for provision of specific services.

Nursing personnel must meet advanced educational and levels of experience commensurate with care of complex pediatric patients. Many nursing personnel must have had previous experience in an intensive care unit or surgical setting with particular exposure to neonates, infants, and children. Physician personnel from the fields of anesthesiology, critical care, cardiology, surgery, radiology, and imaging must all possess the requisite training for their respective fields and be board certified in order to manage a wide range of pediatric anomalies. Additionally, some states in the United States require a minimum number of cases be performed annually at centers so that a baseline level of proficiency within the institution is maintained. Additionally, training programs must be accredited by the national oversight and reviewing organizations (i.e., American Council for Graduate Medical Education) for each specialty. It is beyond the scope of this chapter to recommend or outline specific requirements as those may vary by state, country, and/or locale in the United States, Europe, and Asia.

Pediatric Surgeon Versus Adult Surgeon Traditionally, the definition of pediatric patients has been those whom are under the age of 18 years. Therefore, medical and surgical care was confined to pediatric medical centers. However, currently there has been an increase in the number of pediatric patients living into adulthood, and those patients may require additional interventional or surgical congenital procedures past the age of 18. In the United States, there is some controversy as to whether the patient should continue to be treated at a children's hospital versus an adult hospital that may or may not provide pediatric services. As recently as 2009, a group of researchers set about to explore the risk factors and outcomes regarding adult patients undergoing congenital surgery in an adult hospital versus a children's hospital (Kogon et al. 2009). The researchers determined that congenital heart surgery can be performed in adults with reasonable morbidity and mortality. Caring for an anticipated aging adult congenital population with increasingly numerous coexisting medical problems and risk factors is best facilitated in an adult hospital setting. Also, when surgery becomes necessary, these adult patients are best served by a congenital heart surgeon.

Another study evaluated the same issue and determined that pediatric patients within specific diagnostic groups are more likely to undergo operation by pediatric heart surgeons (PHS), whereas adult patients with congenital heart disease patients within the same diagnostic groups are more likely to undergo operation by non-PHSs. In-hospital death rates are lower for adult congenital heart patients operated on by PHSs; therefore, adult patients with congenital heart disease should be only

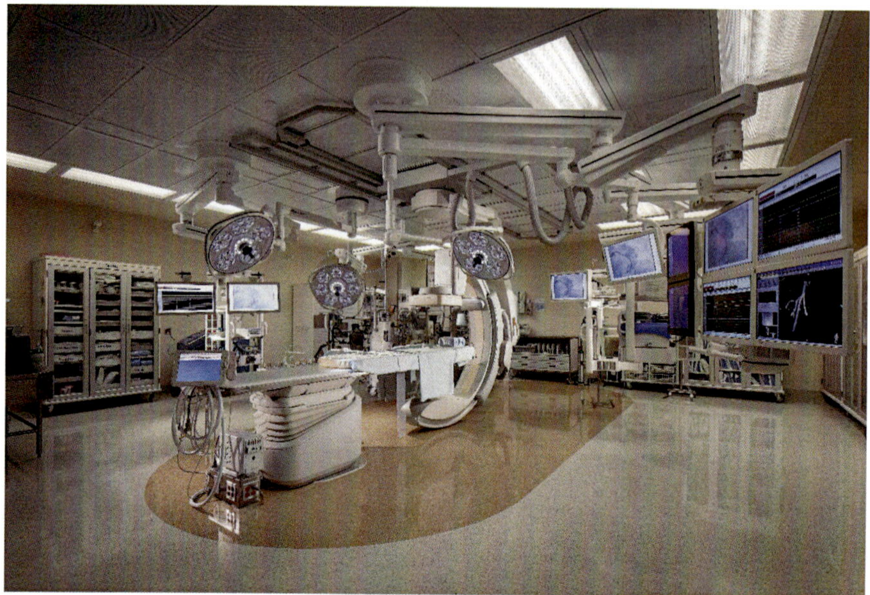

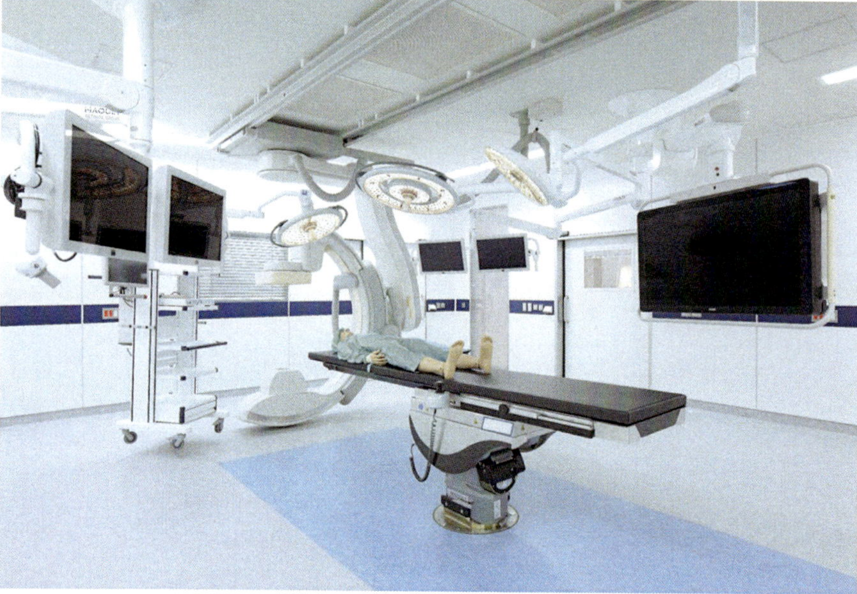

Fig. 14.3 Two types of "hybrid" suite with imaging compatible table, mobile fluoroscopic C-arm, large monitors, and anesthesia machine (Note: Cardiopulmonary bypass unit is not pictured, but should be readily available)

analyzed whether or not the primary surgeon was pediatric trained versus non-pediatric trained, and it did not analyze location in an adult hospital versus a children's hospital.

Quality Assurance Regardless of location, quality assurance and performance improvement measures should be defined so that continual monitoring of care delivered can be assessed. Additionally, participation in a large database submission site (i.e., Society of Thoracic Surgeons—STS) is encouraged so that further knowledge can be obtained from multiple institutional experience. The STS database offers specific site for congenital heart surgery (http://www.sts.org/national-database/database-managers/congenital-heart-surgery-databas).

"Hybrid" Suites Medical facilities in the United States offering interventions and surgery for congenital heart surgery have now migrated to a "hybridized" environment that blends components from traditional operating rooms with those of cardiac interventional suites (see Fig. 14.3). The "hybrid" environments include an array of personnel from both sectors and heavily rely upon the ability to provide fluoroscopic imaging throughout the procedure along with technical specialists to offer potential use of cardiopulmonary bypass and/or assist devices.

The "hybrid" suites may contain a patient table that is compatible with imaging requirements while also containing a mobile fluoroscopic device (i.e., C-arms). Advanced hybrid suites may also contain magnetic resonance imaging and/or computed tomography capability. Additionally, the hybrid rooms have anesthesia machines and large monitors to allow monitoring from all personnel during the procedure.

References

Coran AG, Blackman PM, Sikina C, Harmon CM, Lelli Jr JL, Geiger JD, Hirschl RB, Teitelbaum DH, Polley Jr TZ, Golladay ES, Austin E, Adelman SH. Specialty networking in pediatric surgery a paradigm for the future of academic surgery. Ann Surg. 1999;230:331–9.

Forrest CB, Glade GB, Baker AE, Bocian AB, Myungsa Kang M, Starfield B. The pediatric primary-specialty care interface, how pediatricians refer children and adolescents to specialty care. Arch Pediatr Adolesc Med. 1999;153:705–14.

Kogon BE, Plattner C, Leong T, Kirshbom PM, Kanter KR, McConnell M, Book W. Adult congenital heart surgery: adult or pediatric facility? Adult or pediatric surgeon? Ann Thorac Surg. 2009;87:833–40.

Mehrotra A, Forrest CB, Lin CY. Dropping the baton: specialty referrals in the United States. Millbank Q. 2011;89:39–69.

Part IV
Intraoperative Care Including Management of Specific Pathologies

Chapter 15
Limiting the Lifetime Surgical Impact of Congenital Heart Disease and Guiding Care for the Congenital Heart Patient

Marion E. McRae and Ruchira Garg

Limiting the Lifetime Surgical Impact of Congenital Heart Disease and Guiding Care for the Congenital Heart Patient

Mortality has declined dramatically in the recent era with improvements in surgical and catheter-based intervention for congenital heart disease (CHD) as evidenced by the fact that two-thirds of individuals with congenital heart disease are now adults (Marelli et al. 2014). However, survival is rarely free of morbidity, related to underlying disease, genetic abnormalities, and the often numerous interventions required over a lifetime. These morbidities have significant long-term physiologic and psychological impact on patients and should be a focus of contemporary clinical management. The "cumulative trauma" of multiple reoperations, cardiopulmonary bypass, aortic cross-clamping, large incisions, vascular trauma, blood and antigen exposure, and radiation associated with diagnostic imaging and intervention are but a few of the hazards that can be minimized and often avoided with a comprehensive strategy designed to reduce these events.

M.E. McRae, RN, MScN, ACNP-BC (✉)
Guerin Family Congenital Heart Program, Cedars-Sinai Medical Center,
127 S. San Vicente Blvd., AHSP A3404, Los Angeles, CA 90048, USA
e-mail: Marion.mcrae@cshs.org

R. Garg, MD, FACC, FASE
Congenital Non-invasive Cardiology, Guerin Family Congenital Heart Program, Cedars-Sinai
Medical Center, 127 S. San Vicente Blvd., AHSP A3600, Los Angeles, CA 90048, USA
e-mail: Ruchira.garg@cshs.org

© Springer International Publishing Switzerland 2017
A. Dabbagh et al. (eds.), *Congenital Heart Disease in Pediatric
and Adult Patients*, DOI 10.1007/978-3-319-44691-2_15

Transcatheter Palliation

Conventional surgical techniques have been time-tested with excellent results; however, repeat sternotomies come with important morbidity and mortality. Transplant mortality increases with repeat sternotomies. Lewis et al. (2015) identified that three or more sternotomies are a predictor of mortality (HR 8.5, $p=0.02$). When intervention is required, especially in the small infant, strong consideration should be given to transcatheter techniques for palliation. Right ventricular outflow tract obstruction requiring supplemental blood flow can readily be treated in appropriate candidates with right ventricular outflow tract stenting (Dohlen et al. 2009; McMullan et al. 2014) or stenting of the ductus arteriosus (Alwi et al. 2004; Amoozgar et al. 2012) rather than surgical shunts to reduce the number of chest incisions and potential complications (McMullan et al. 2014). Extrapolating this philosophy to all ages, there are numerous opportunities to replace conventional surgical strategies with catheter-based or hybrid strategies.

Transcatheter Occlusion of Patent Ductus Arteriosus in Premature Infants

Patent ductus arteriosus (PDA) is very common in premature children (Leirgul et al. 2014). Excessive pulmonary blood flow from left to right ductal shunting overloads the underdeveloped premature neonatal lungs and can delay the normal drop in pulmonary vascular resistance. Positive pressure ventilation can be prolonged, further traumatizing the lungs. Historically, first-line treatment has been cyclooxygenase (COX) inhibitors such as indomethacin or ibuprofen. If COX inhibitors are ineffective and the ductus is hemodynamically significant, ductal ligation is traditionally pursued. This requires a left thoracotomy and can cause significant morbidity in very premature babies including phrenic nerve injury (Yon et al. 1977; Koehne et al. 2001), vocal cord paralysis (Zbar et al. 1996; Roksund et al. 2010), pneumothorax (Koehne et al. 2001), bleeding (Koehne et al. 2001), rib deformities (Seghaye et al. 1997), scoliosis (Seghaye et al. 1997), and wound infection. Catheter-based ligation has been an option only in term and older infants based on device availability. In fact, is the procedure of choice in older patients with little use of surgical ligation in the current era (El-Said et al. 2013; Baruteau et al. 2014). Concerns about risk of such procedures in very low birth weight and premature infants exist. We have refined an approach whereby transcatheter closure using a transvenous technique can be safely performed at the bedside in the neonatal intensive care unit using a micro-fluoroscopy unit and transthoracic echocardiography (Zahn et al. 2015). A Rainbow Flex Procedural Bed (NeoForce, Ivyland, PA) permits C-arm fluoroscopy while maintaining thermoregulation, which is an important consideration in maintaining stability in a premature neonate. Closure of the PDA has been achieved in 27 of 30 cases, the majority of which have been performed with the Amplatzer

Vascular Plug II device (St. Jude Medical, St. Paul, MN). We have treated infants as small as 780 g with this therapy with a high degree of success (see Fig. 15.1).

Transcatheter Valves

Many patients who have undergone repair of tetralogy of Fallot or pulmonary atresia will require pulmonary valve replacement at least once during their lifetime, for residual regurgitation and/or stenosis. Surgical pulmonary valve replacement is

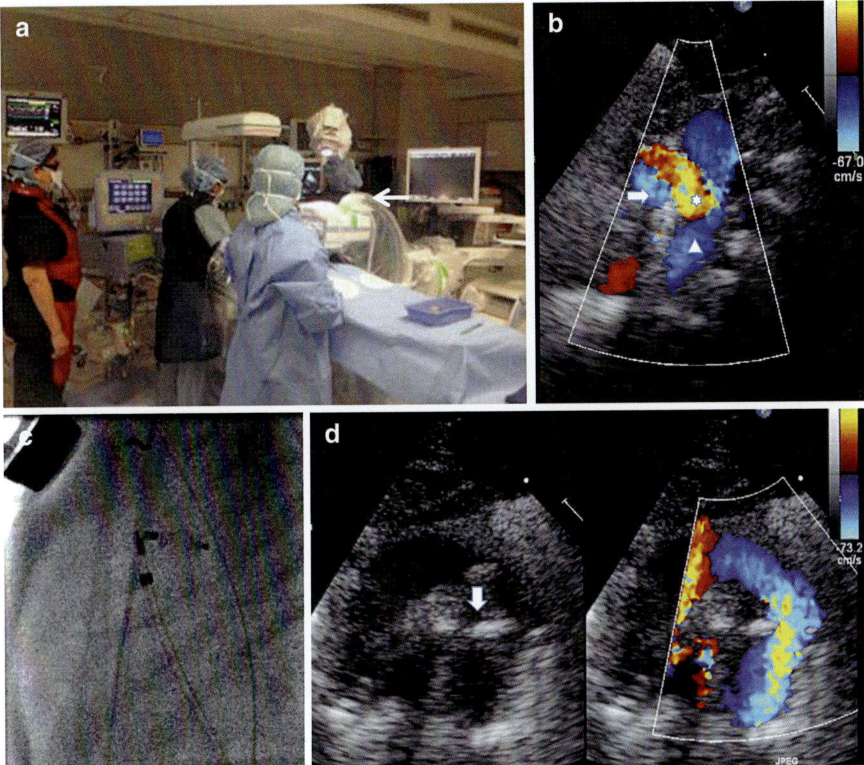

Fig. 15.1 (**a**) Transcatheter PDA closure in the NICU using rainbow flex procedural bed and micro-fluoroscopy unit (at *white arrow*) (authors). (**b**) Large PDA (*) with hemodynamically important left-to-right shunt in a 59-day-old 1200-g, former 27-week premature infant. The PDA (at *star*, descending aorta (at *triangle*)) and left pulmonary artery (*white arrow*) are demonstrated (authors). (**c**) Angiographic image of the ductal device still attached to the delivery cable. Note the transthoracic echocardiogram (used to obtain images continuously throughout the procedure) probe at the upper left corner of the photo (authors). (**d**) The PDA device (at *white arrow*) in place with no residual ductal shunting an color image (authors). (**e**) There is no gradient in the descending aorta after device placement (authors). (**f**) The left pulmonary artery (at *white arrow*) is unobstructed by the device (authors). (**g**) Spectral Doppler interrogation with the device in situ (authors)

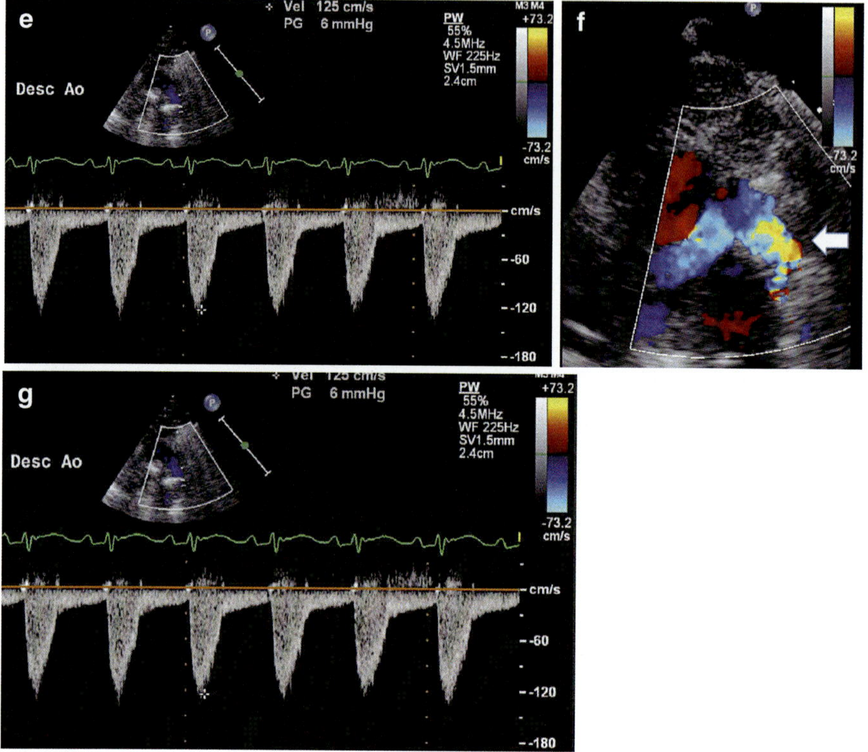

Fig. 15.1 (continued)

associated with significant pain and common complications such as pleural effusion, pericardial effusion, and arrhythmias and has a mortality of 0.5 % (Fuller et al. 2015). It is no surprise that transcatheter pulmonary valve replacement for those with appropriately configured right ventricular outflow tracts has become first-line therapy. The Melody valve (Medtronic, Minneapolis, MN) (Cheatham et al. 2015) is a bovine jugular valve that was the first transcatheter pulmonary valve placed in man (Bonhoeffer et al. 2000). It is ideally suited to the patient with a right ventricular to pulmonary artery conduit as it has a maximum inflated diameter of 24 mm. Unfortunately, the majority of patients requiring pulmonary valve replacement have a reconstructed "native" pulmonary valve that is regurgitant from initial surgical valvotomy and have diameters much larger than the capacity of the Melody valve. The Edwards SAPIEN valve (Edwards Lifesciences, Irvine, CA), a bovine pericardial stent-mounted transcatheter valve, has been successfully used for this indication in selected patients with appropriately sized right ventricular outflow tracts for this indication (Wilson et al. 2015; Phillips et al. 2016) as it is manufactured in sizes up to 29 mm. The internal diameter of the larger SAPIEN valve also increases the likelihood that multiple repeat transcatheter valve-in-valve procedures can be performed when these valves require future replacement. Sizing of the outflow tract to select appropriate patients and appropriate valves requires careful assessment. Some centers are using 3D modeling of the right ventricular outflow tract using

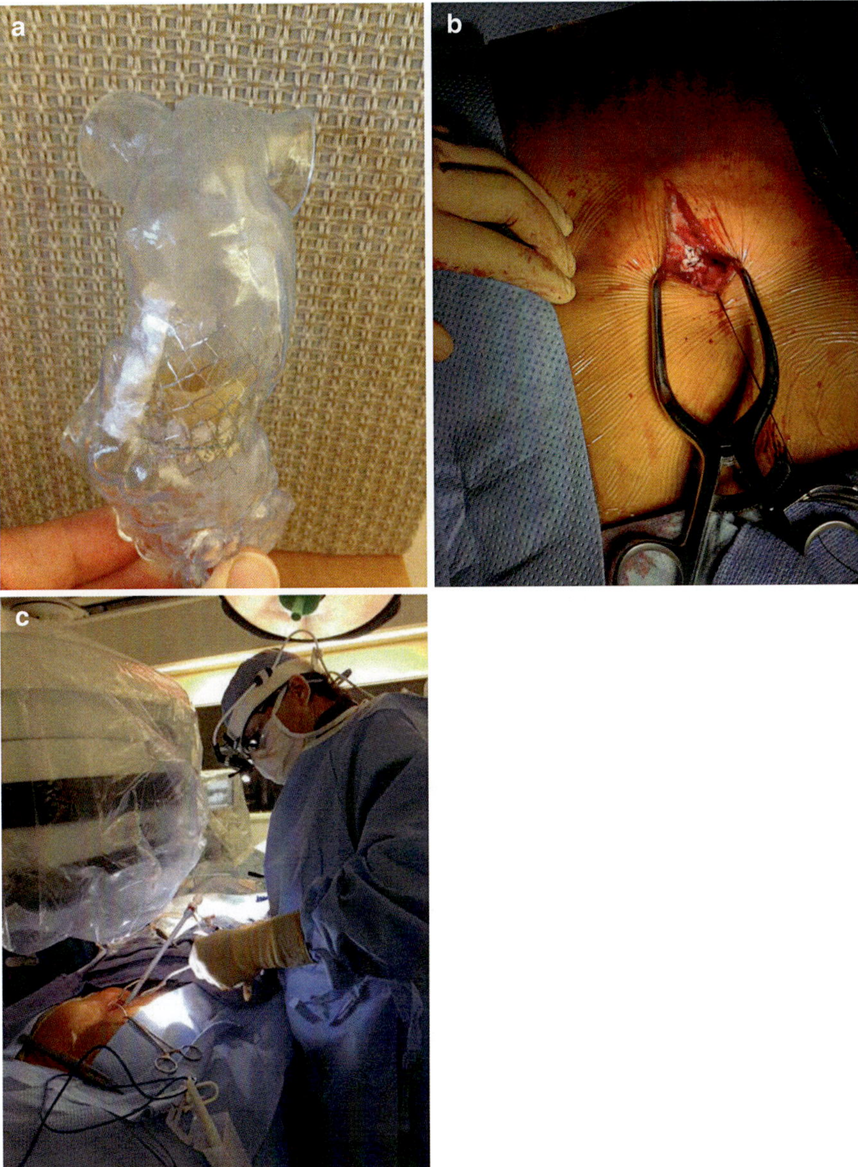

Fig. 15.2 (**a**) 3D model of a right ventricular outflow tract with an Edwards SAPIEN valve in situ with geometric remodeling of the annular area with plugged stent around the valve (authors). (**b**) Hybrid pulmonary valve incision for periventricular placement of the valve (authors). (**c**) Hybrid pulmonary valve incision with valve delivery catheter in situ (authors)

magnetic resonance imaging (MRI) (Phillips et al. 2016) to augment balloon sizing (see Fig. 15.2). Compliance of the native RVOT must also be tested with a balloon before valve placement. High compliance can be a contraindication to use of this technique, with risk of distal valve embolization (Phillips et al. 2016). Native RVOT

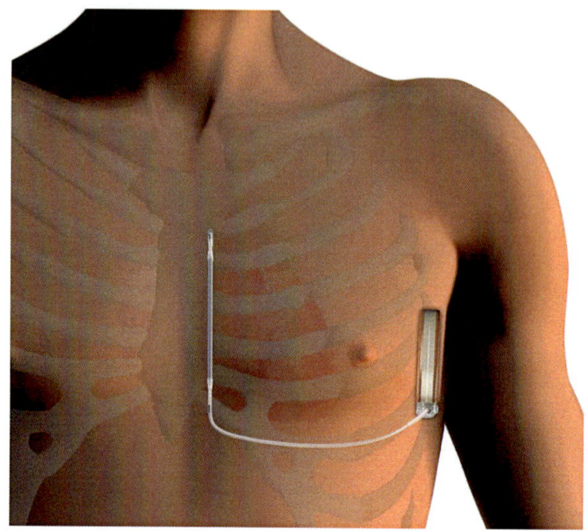

Fig. 15.3 Emblem S-ICD subcutaneous defibrillator (Image provided courtesy of Boston Scientific. © Boston Scientific Corporation. © 2016 Boston Scientific Corporation or its affiliates. All rights reserved)

pulmonary valve implantation can also be performed by hybrid technique (using a 2-inch incision at the bottom of the old sternotomy) (see Fig. 15.2) to enter the right ventricle via a periventricular approach with the delivery catheter or by surgically plicating the pulmonary artery to a size amenable to use of this valve (Travelli et al. 2014). The latter technique requires a sternotomy but not the use of cardiopulmonary bypass. For individuals with a large, irregularly shaped RVOT, internal geometric remodeling using covered stents plugged with Amplatzer vascular plug II device(s) (St. Jude Medical, St. Paul, MN) to reduce annular size can be performed (Phillips et al. 2016). Hospital discharge generally occurs at 24 h for transcatheter approaches (O'Byrne et al. 2015) and at 48 h for hybrid approaches (Phillips et al. 2016) in comparison to an average 4- to 5-day hospital stay for surgical pulmonary valve replacement (Vergales et al. 2013; McKenzie et al. 2014; O'Byrne et al. 2015).

Electrophysiologic Devices

A number of minimally invasive and alternative electrophysiologic devices have become available that may benefit selected CHD patients. Subcutaneous leadless implantable cardioverter-defibrillators (ICD) (Emblem S-ICD, Boston Scientific, Marlborough, MA; see Fig. 15.3) can be useful for adult patients with poor venous access to the heart. The extracardiac Fontan patient who requires only defibrillation and not pacing capacity is a perfect candidate for this device (Bordachar et al. 2016). Recent studies (Lambiase et al. 2014; Burke et al. 2015) have demonstrated the safety and efficacy of the subcutaneous ICD. The device requires no fluoroscopy for insertion (Bardy et al. 2010). At present, the size of the device limits the

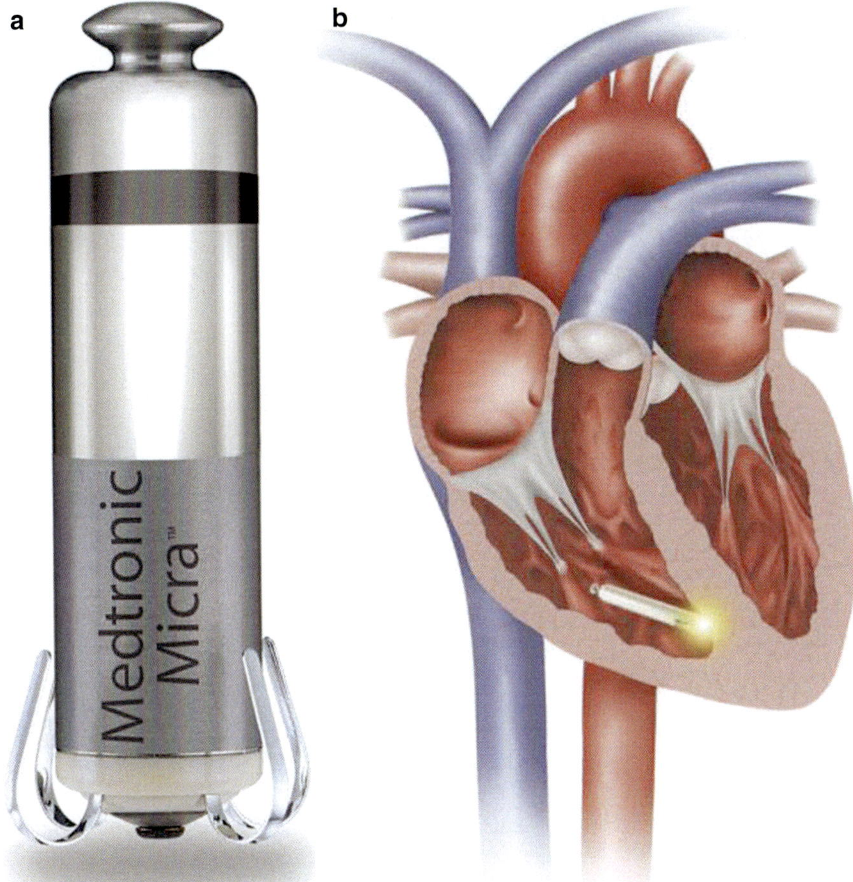

Fig. 15.4 Leadless pacemakers. (a) Medtronic Micra (Medtronic, Minneapolis, MN) (Reproduced with permission of Medtronic, Inc) (b) St. Jude Nanostim in situ in the right ventricle. St. Jude Nanostim and St. Jude Medical are trademarks of St. Jude Medical, Inc., or its related companies (Reproduced with permission of St. Jude Medical, © 2016. All rights reserved)

implantation to older children and adults. In addition, there are additional screening requirements that must be met (Bordachar et al. 2016).

Leadless pacemakers (Medtronic Micra, Medtronic, Minneapolis, MN; St. Jude Nanostim, St. Jude Medical, St. Paul, MN; see Fig. 15.3) have demonstrated early success in adult patients who require only ventricular pacing (Reddy et al. 2014, 2015; Ritter et al. 2015; Reynolds et al. 2016). The devices are lodged in the right ventricle. These devices have great potential for patients with pacemaker-related tricuspid regurgitation and pacemaker lead-related venous obstruction or those patients at higher risk for pocket complications (Reddy et al. 2014) (Fig. 15.4).

Pacemaker devices that are MRI conditional are now commercially available (Wilkoff et al. 2011; Gimbel et al. 2013). Many CHD patients require regular tomographic imaging, and MRI, in particular, provides unique information about cardiac function, flow, and anatomy that is not available by any other modality. Although patients with conventional pacemakers have been safely placed in a scanner (Pulver et al. 2009), these devices are still considered "unsafe" in a 1.5 or 3 Tesla magnet, and pacemaker-dependent patients can never undergo MRI with conventional pacemakers. Retained temporary pacemaker wires, cut at the skin, are safe for MRI scanning, but permanent epicardial pacemaker leads can heat up in the presence of energy from the magnet (Luechinger et al. 2005). Some of the current limitations of MRI examination in patients with MRI-conditional pacemakers include the necessity to reprogram into sensing mode only or an asynchronous pacing mode that some patients cannot tolerate. Due to lack of sensing, loss of AV synchrony can adversely affect cardiac output measurements made during MR examinations (Pulver et al. 2009). Patients should be screened for abandoned leads or capped leads (even MRI-conditional leads) prior to scanning due to the potential for these leads to heat up (Mattei et al. 2015).

Blood Conservation/Bloodless Cardiac Surgery

Blood transfusion during surgery can be associated with many types of adverse events including transfusion-associated lung injury, allergic reactions, antibody formation (Eder and Chambers 2007), and infection (Allain et al. 2009). Studies have demonstrated that more liberal transfusion strategies are associated with longer lengths of hospital stay (de Gast-Bakker et al. 2013; Iyengar et al. 2013), pulmonary complications (Iyengar et al. 2013; Redlin et al. 2013), infection (Szekely et al. 2009), and renal failure (Iyengar et al. 2013). Sensitization, often a result of blood transfusion, is of concern for CHD patients who may be candidates for transplantation in the future. Jehovah's Witness patients may decline transfusion for themselves or their children based on religious beliefs. Therefore, an approach that avoids or minimizes blood transfusion is part of a comprehensive strategy to reduce cumulative risk.

Adherence to the Society of Thoracic Surgeons and International Society for Minimally Invasive Cardiothoracic Surgery guidelines for blood conservation (Society of Thoracic Surgeons Blood Conservation Guideline Task Force et al. 2011; Menkis et al. 2012) helps to achieve bloodless surgery. For Jehovah's Witness patients, this includes the use of erythropoietin (Alghamdi et al. 2006) (300–500 units per kilogram of body weight) injected subcutaneously twice weekly for 2–4 weeks. Supplementation with therapeutic doses of folate, iron, and a daily multivitamin is also used. One should aim to get the preoperative hemoglobin to at least 16–17 g/dL on acyanotic patients. The cardiopulmonary bypass circuit size is minimized to limit prime volumes (Kim et al. 2016). Retrograde autologous priming of the cardiopulmonary bypass circuit (Hou et al. 2009), venous antegrade prime, the use of acute normovolemic hemodilution, dilutional or balanced ultrafiltration during cardiopulmonary bypass, and modified ultrafiltration (Olshove et al. 2010) are also recommended for blood conservation (Society of Thoracic Surgeons Blood Conservation Guideline Task Force et al. 2011; Menkis et al. 2012). Cell saver autologous transfusion is also useful in reducing blood exposure (Wang et al. 2009) and can be used in Jehovah's Witness patients if it is kept directly connected in circuit with the patient's circulation. Thromboelastogram-directed transfusion is used in non-Jehovah's Witness patients to allow earlier detection and treatment of bleeding. It may allow more targeted transfusion to treat bleeding (Niebler et al. 2012) and is associated with reduced transfusion prevalence (Romlin et al. 2011; Kane et al. 2016).

Intraoperative and postoperative point-of-care testing should be used as much as possible to limit blood sampling to a drop or two. All labs that cannot be performed with point-of-care testing should be drawn in pediatric tubes, even for adult patients. The need for lab tests should be reassessed daily to avoid excessive blood draws.

Pain Management

Poor pain management can cause a great deal of psychological and physiologic stress postoperatively. Therefore, strategies to prevent pain and minimize inflammation can be beneficial to early mobility and psychological recovery. Around-the-clock dosing of intravenous acetaminophen 15 mg/kg every 6 h for 72 h and intravenous ketorolac for 48 h (0.5 mg/kg every 6 h except in patients with low platelets or neonates) can be beneficial in reducing the need for narcotics in surgical CHD patients without significantly increased risk of bleeding or creatinine rise (Lieh-Lai et al. 1999; Gupta et al. 2004; Dawkins et al. 2009; Inoue et al. 2009). It also has the potential to reduce delirium associated with narcotics although this has not yet been demonstrated in a study. Local anesthetic regional nerve blockade can also reduce the need for narcotics immediately after surgery although there are no studies demonstrating this at present.

The use of intravenous dexmedetomidine has been demonstrated in a meta-analysis (Pan et al. 2016) to shorten mechanical ventilation times, lower narcotic needs, reduce stress responses as evidenced by lower blood glucose and serum cortisol levels, reduce delirium, and reduce agitation. The reduced stress response has also been shown to decrease the incidence of supraventricular and ventricular tachycardias (Chrysostomou et al. 2011) as well as junctional ectopic tachycardia (Rajput et al. 2014) which can be difficult to treat. It has been demonstrated to be safe and effective even for prolonged use in CHD patients (Bejian et al. 2009). However, there are significantly increased risks of bradycardia and hypotension (Pan et al. 2016); therefore, careful dosing and monitoring are needed in patients at risk for these side effects. A detailed discussion on pain management can be found in Chap. 42, Postoperative Pain Management.

Radiation Issues

The number of imaging studies needed by CHD patients over a lifetime can amount to very significant doses of radiation. Downing et al. (2015) reported 21 % of single-ventricle palliation patients received annualized effective doses of greater than 20 millisieverts per year and well exceed the 6.20 millisievert annual background radiation exposure for the average individual (American Nuclear Society 2016). The annual allowable exposure for those working with radioactive material is a maximum of 50 millisieverts per year (American Nuclear Society 2016). The top contributor to radiation exposure is cardiac catheterization (Ait-Ali et al. 2007; Hoffmann et al. 2007; Downing et al. 2015). Gastric emptying studies (Downing et al. 2015) and computed tomography scans (Ait-Ali et al. 2007; Hoffmann et al. 2007) are also significant contributors. Studies of cancer risk among patients with congenital heart defects indicate a higher incidence of cancer over that of the general population (Olsen et al. 2014; Videbaek et al. 2016) with adjusted hazard rates of 1.19 (95 % CI 0.69–2.04) (Videbaek et al. 2016). Increasing radiation exposure at a younger age in CHD patients, a vulnerable time when exposure correlates with elevated malignancy risk has been documented over the last several decades (Beausejour Ladouceur et al. 2016). Ait-Ali et al. (2007) estimated the lifetime attributable risk of fatal and nonfatal cancer was 1.9–2 times higher when a 1-year-old child experienced the same radiation dose as a 15-year-old child.

Radiation exposure can also shorten leukocyte telomeres in CHD patients, and this is associated with biologic aging (Vecoli et al. 2016). Telomere length is also a predictor of the development of coronary artery disease after radiation therapy (M'Kacher et al. 2015). Therefore, radiation exposure in CHD patients may predispose them to coronary artery disease as they age.

Strategies to document total radiation exposure over a lifetime and limit radiation exposure are needed. The increased use of magnetic resonance imaging (MRI) can reduce the cumulative doses of radiation. Increased implementation of MRI-safe pacemakers should increase the use of MRI in patients who would otherwise require computed tomography angiography or catheterization. Cancer screening will become increasingly important in the primary care of these patients. Due to the potential risk of atherosclerosis from radiation, primary prevention of and screening for coronary artery disease will become important for ACHD specialists.

Neurodevelopmental Issues

Neurodevelopmental issues after cardiac surgery in infancy are a well-described problem (Brosig et al. 2013; Gaynor et al. 2014, 2015; Ricci et al. 2015; Sarrechia et al. 2016). These problems can be compounded when there are coexisting genetic conditions that affect neurodevelopment. A systematic review (Hirsch et al. 2012) could not find much supporting evidence for any of the current neuromonitoring and neuroprotective techniques. However, a more recent report by Hoffman et al. (2016)

showed that higher arterial saturation and narrower arterial-cerebral and arterial-somatic near-infrared spectroscopy saturation differences were associated with better or improving motor performance. Preoperative brain imaging has enlightened us to the fact that there can be abnormal brain findings in neonates born with CHD, even in the absence of intervention (Miller and McQuillen 2007; Paquette et al. 2013). Continuing work in this area to identify those individuals at greatest risk and to maximize neurodevelopmental outcomes continues. In the interim, careful assessment of these patients and early referral to occupational therapy, physiotherapy, and speech therapy will be important in trying to optimize the functioning of these individuals.

Psychological Stressors

Cumulative stressors over a lifetime can lead to maladaptive and impaired coping including post-traumatic stress disorder (PTSD) (Alonzo 2000). Surgery along with other invasive or unpleasant treatments used for CHD can precipitate maladaptive and impaired coping. Studies have demonstrated a 12 % (Connolly et al. 2004) to 29 % (Toren and Horesh 2007) incidence of PTSD in children and adolescents who have undergone CHD surgery depending on the duration of time from surgery and the instrument used to measure PTSD. In ACHD patients, Deng et al. (2016) reported an 11 % incidence of PTSD using CHD-specific PTSD measures which is significantly higher than the 3.5 % incidence in the general population. Of the traumatic events, 34 % were related to cardiac surgery, and 41 % were related other cardiovascular events including arrhythmias, heart failure, stroke, and cardiac arrest. The two factors most strongly associated with PTSD were depressive symptoms and year of most recent cardiac surgery. Earlier surgical date correlated with greater incidence of PTSD (Deng et al. 2016). In addition, 14.9 % of mothers and 9.5 % of fathers of children undergoing CHD surgery experienced PTSD 6 months postoperatively (Helfricht et al. 2008), which has the potential to impair family functioning.

Child Life Counseling/Psychological Assessment

Recognizing the high anxiety and PTSD associated with CHD surgery and intervention, the importance of adequate preparation for surgery and procedures in order to avoid traumatic experiences is important. Most pediatric centers use child life counselors to prepare children and other family members for the experience. Role-playing with props, family members, and walking through the procedure help a child and family anticipate the procedure and better cope with their emotions. If a child life counselor is not available or if the patient is an adult, patients should be referred to a psychiatrist or psychologist for pre-procedural assessment and treatment for post-traumatic events and to prepare for an upcoming procedure or surgery.

Conclusion

Thoughtful consideration of the factors discussed in this chapter should help to reduce the impact of the treatment of CHD over the course of a lifetime. This may permit improvement of both the physiological and psychological outcomes in CHD patients.

References

Ait-Ali L, Foffa I, Andreassi MG. Diagnostic and therapeutic radiation exposure in children: new evidence and perspectives from a biomarker approach. Pediatr Radiol. 2007;37:109–11.

Alghamdi AA, Albanna MJ, Guru V, Brister SJ. Does the use of erythropoietin reduce the risk of exposure to allogeneic blood transfusion in cardiac surgery? A systematic review and meta-analysis. J Card Surg. 2006;21:320–6.

Allain JP, Stramer SL, Carneiro-Proietti AB, Martins ML, Lopes da Silva SN, Ribeiro M, Proietti FA, Reesink HW. Transfusion-transmitted infectious diseases. Biologicals. 2009;37:71–7.

Alonzo AA. The experience of chronic illness and post-traumatic stress disorder: the consequences of cumulative adversity. Soc Sci Med. 2000;50:1475–84.

Alwi M, Choo KK, Latiff HA, Kandavello G, Samion H, Mulyadi MD. Initial results and medium-term follow-up of stent implantation of patent ductus arteriosus in duct-dependent pulmonary circulation. J Am Coll Cardiol. 2004;44:438–45.

American Nuclear Society. Radiation dose calculator. La Grange Park: American Nuclear Society; 2016. http://www.ans.org/pilresources/dosechart/msv.php.

Amoozgar H, Cheriki S, Borzoee M, Ajami G, Soltani M, Ahmadipour M, Peiravian F, Amirghofran A. Short-term result of ductus arteriosus stent implantation compared with surgically created shunts. Pediatr Cardiol. 2012;33:1288–94.

Bardy GH, Smith WM, Hood MA, Crozier IG, Melton IC, Jordaens L, Theuns D, Park RE, Wright DJ, Connelly DT, Fynn SP, Murgatroyd FD, Sperzel J, Neuzner J, Spitzer SG, Ardashev AV, Oduro A, Boersma L, Maass AH, Van Gelder IC, Wilde AA, van Dessel PF, Knops RE, Barr CS, Lupo P, Cappato R, Grace AA. An entirely subcutaneous implantable cardioverter-defibrillator. N Engl J Med. 2010;363:36–44.

Baruteau AE, Hascoet S, Baruteau J, Boudjemline Y, Lambert V, Angel CY, Belli E, Petit J, Pass R. Transcatheter closure of patent ductus arteriosus: past, present and future. Arch Cardiovasc Dis. 2014;107:122–32.

Beausejour Ladouceur V, Lawler PR, Gurvitz M, Pilote L, Eisenberg MJ, Ionescu-Ittu R, Guo L, Marelli AJ. Exposure to low-dose ionizing radiation from cardiac procedures in patients with congenital heart disease: 15-year data from a population-based longitudinal cohort. Circulation. 2016;133:12–20.

Bejian S, Valasek C, Nigro JJ, Cleveland DC, Willis BC. Prolonged use of dexmedetomidine in the paediatric cardiothoracic intensive care unit. Cardiol Young. 2009;19:98–104.

Bonhoeffer P, Boudjemline Y, Saliba Z, Merckx J, Aggoun Y, Bonnet D, Acar P, Le Bidois J, Sidi D, Kachaner J. Percutaneous replacement of pulmonary valve in a right-ventricle to pulmonary-artery prosthetic conduit with valve dysfunction. Lancet. 2000;356:1403–5.

Bordachar P, Marquie C, Pospiech T, Pasquie JL, Jalal Z, Haissaguerre M, Thambo JB. Subcutaneous implantable cardioverter defibrillators in children, young adults and patients with congenital heart disease. Int J Cardiol. 2016;203:251–8.

Brosig C, Mussatto K, Hoffman G, Hoffmann RG, Dasgupta M, Tweddell J, Ghanayem N. Neurodevelopmental outcomes for children with hypoplastic left heart syndrome at the age of 5 years. Pediatr Cardiol. 2013;34:1597–604.

Burke MC, Gold MR, Knight BP, Barr CS, Theuns DA, Boersma LV, Knops RE, Weiss R, Leon AR, Herre JM, Husby M, Stein KM, Lambiase PD. Safety and efficacy of the totally subcutaneous implantable defibrillator: 2-year results from a pooled analysis of the IDE study and EFFORTLESS registry. J Am Coll Cardiol. 2015;65:1605–15.

Cheatham JP, Hellenbrand WE, Zahn EM, Jones TK, Berman DP, Vincent JA, McElhinney DB. Clinical and hemodynamic outcomes up to 7 years after transcatheter pulmonary valve replacement in the US melody valve investigational device exemption trial. Circulation. 2015;131:1960–70.

Chrysostomou C, Sanchez-de-Toledo J, Wearden P, Jooste EH, Lichtenstein SE, Callahan PM, Suresh T, O'Malley E, Shiderly D, Haney J, Yoshida M, Orr R, Munoz R, Morell VO. Perioperative use of dexmedetomidine is associated with decreased incidence of ventricular and supraventricular tachyarrhythmias after congenital cardiac operations. Ann Thorac Surg. 2011;92:964–72; discussion 972.

Connolly D, McClowry S, Hayman L, Mahony L, Artman M. Posttraumatic stress disorder in children after cardiac surgery. J Pediatr. 2004;144:480–4.

Dawkins TN, Barclay CA, Gardiner RL, Krawczeski CD. Safety of intravenous use of ketorolac in infants following cardiothoracic surgery. Cardiol Young. 2009;19:105–8.

de Gast-Bakker DH, de Wilde RB, Hazekamp MG, Sojak V, Zwaginga JJ, Wolterbeek R, de Jonge E, Gesink-van der Veer BJ. Safety and effects of two red blood cell transfusion strategies in pediatric cardiac surgery patients: a randomized controlled trial. Intensive Care Med. 2013;39:2011–9.

Deng LX, Khan AM, Drajpuch D, Fuller S, Ludmir J, Qadeer A, Tobin L, Kovacs A, Kim YY. Prevalence and correlates of post-traumatic stress disorder in adults with congenital heart disease. Am J Cardiol. 2016;117(5):853–7.

Dohlen G, Chaturvedi RR, Benson LN, Ozawa A, Van Arsdell GS, Fruitman DS, Lee KJ. Stenting of the right ventricular outflow tract in the symptomatic infant with tetralogy of Fallot. Heart. 2009;95:142–7.

Downing TE, McDonnell A, Zhu X, Dori Y, Gillespie MJ, Rome JJ, Glatz AC. Cumulative medical radiation exposure throughout staged palliation of single ventricle congenital heart disease. Pediatr Cardiol. 2015;36:190–5.

Eder AF, Chambers LA. Noninfectious complications of blood transfusion. Arch Pathol Lab Med. 2007;131:708–18.

El-Said HG, Bratincsak A, Foerster SR, Murphy JJ, Vincent J, Holzer R, Porras D, Moore J, Bergersen L. Safety of percutaneous patent ductus arteriosus closure: an unselected multicenter population experience. J Am Heart Assoc. 2013;2:e000424.

Fuller SM, He X, Jacobs JP, Pasquali SK, Gaynor JW, Mascio CE, Hill KD, Jacobs ML, Kim YY. Estimating mortality risk for adult congenital heart surgery: an analysis of the Society of Thoracic Surgeons Congenital Heart Surgery Database. Ann Thorac Surg. 2015;100:1728–35; discussion 1735–1726.

Gaynor JW, Ittenbach RF, Gerdes M, Bernbaum J, Clancy RR, McDonald-McGinn DM, Zackai EH, Wernovsky G, Nicolson SC, Spray TL. Neurodevelopmental outcomes in preschool survivors of the Fontan procedure. J Thorac Cardiovasc Surg. 2014;147:1276–82; discussion 1282–1283 e1275.

Gaynor JW, Stopp C, Wypij D, Andropoulos DB, Atallah J, Atz AM, Beca J, Donofrio MT, Duncan K, Ghanayem NS, Goldberg CS, Hovels-Gurich H, Ichida F, Jacobs JP, Justo R, Latal B, Li JS, Mahle WT, McQuillen PS, Menon SC, Pemberton VL, Pike NA, Pizarro C, Shekerdemian LS, Synnes A, Williams I, Bellinger DC, Newburger JW, International Cardiac Collaborative on Neurodevelopment I. Neurodevelopmental outcomes after cardiac surgery in infancy. Pediatrics. 2015;135:816–25.

Gimbel JR, Bello D, Schmitt M, Merkely B, Schwitter J, Hayes DL, Sommer T, Schloss EJ, Chang Y, Willey S, Kanal E, Advisa MRISSI. Randomized trial of pacemaker and lead system for safe scanning at 1.5 Tesla. Heart Rhythm. 2013;10:685–91.

Gupta A, Daggett C, Drant S, Rivero N, Lewis A. Prospective randomized trial of ketorolac after congenital heart surgery. J Cardiothorac Vasc Anesth. 2004;18:454–7.

Helfricht S, Latal B, Fischer JE, Tomaske M, Landolt MA. Surgery-related posttraumatic stress disorder in parents of children undergoing cardiopulmonary bypass surgery: a prospective cohort study. Pediatr Crit Care Med. 2008;9:217–23.

Hirsch JC, Jacobs ML, Andropoulos D, Austin EH, Jacobs JP, Licht DJ, Pigula F, Tweddell JS, Gaynor JW. Protecting the infant brain during cardiac surgery: a systematic review. Ann Thorac Surg. 2012;94:1365–73; discussion 1373.

Hoffman GM, Brosig CL, Bear LM, Tweddell JS, Mussatto KA. Effect of intercurrent operation and cerebral oxygenation on developmental trajectory in congenital heart disease. Ann Thorac Surg. 2016;101:708–16.

Hoffmann A, Engelfriet P, Mulder B. Radiation exposure during follow-up of adults with congenital heart disease. Int J Cardiol. 2007;118:151–3.

Hou X, Yang F, Liu R, Yang J, Zhao Y, Wan C, Ni H, Gong Q, Dong P. Retrograde autologous priming of the cardiopulmonary bypass circuit reduces blood transfusion in small adults: a prospective, randomized trial. Eur J Anaesthesiol. 2009;26:1061–6.

Inoue M, Caldarone CA, Frndova H, Cox PN, Ito S, Taddio A, Guerguerian AM. Safety and efficacy of ketorolac in children after cardiac surgery. Intensive Care Med. 2009;35:1584–92.

Iyengar A, Scipione CN, Sheth P, Ohye RG, Riegger L, Bove EL, Devaney EJ, Hirsch-Romano JC. Association of complications with blood transfusions in pediatric cardiac surgery patients. Ann Thorac Surg. 2013;96:910–6.

Kane LC, Woodward CS, Husain SA, Frei-Jones MJ. Thromboelastography-does it impact blood component transfusion in pediatric heart surgery? J Surg Res. 2016;200:21–7.

Kim SY, Cho S, Choi E, Kim WH. Effects of mini-volume priming during cardiopulmonary bypass on clinical outcomes in low-bodyweight neonates: less transfusion and postoperative extracorporeal membrane oxygenation support. Artif Organs. 2016;40:73–9.

Koehne PS, Bein G, Alexi-Meskhishvili V, Weng Y, Buhrer C, Obladen M. Patent ductus arteriosus in very low birthweight infants: complications of pharmacological and surgical treatment. J Perinat Med. 2001;29:327–34.

Lambiase PD, Barr C, Theuns DA, Knops R, Neuzil P, Johansen JB, Hood M, Pedersen S, Kaab S, Murgatroyd F, Reeve HL, Carter N, Boersma L, Effortless Investigators. Worldwide experience with a totally subcutaneous implantable defibrillator: early results from the EFFORTLESS S-ICD Registry. Eur Heart J. 2014;35:1657–65.

Leirgul E, Fomina T, Brodwall K, Greve G, Holmstrom H, Vollset SE, Tell GS, Oyen N. Birth prevalence of congenital heart defects in Norway 1994–2009 – a nationwide study. Am Heart J. 2014;168:956–64.

Lewis M, Ginns J, Schulze C, Lippel M, Chai P, Bacha E, Mancini D, Rosenbaum M, Farr M. Outcomes of adult patients with congenital heart disease after heart transplantation: impact of disease type, previous thoracic surgeries, and bystander organ dysfunction. J Card Fail. 2015;22:578–82.

Lieh-Lai MW, Kauffman RE, Uy HG, Danjin M, Simpson PM. A randomized comparison of ketorolac tromethamine and morphine for postoperative analgesia in critically ill children. Crit Care Med. 1999;27:2786–91.

Luechinger R, Zeijlemaker VA, Pedersen EM, Mortensen P, Falk E, Duru F, Candinas R, Boesiger P. In vivo heating of pacemaker leads during magnetic resonance imaging. Eur Heart J. 2005;26:376–83; discussion 325–377.

M'Kacher R, Girinsky T, Colicchio B, Ricoul M, Dieterlen A, Jeandidier E, Heidingsfelder L, Cuceu C, Shim G, Frenzel M, Lenain A, Morat L, Bourhis J, Hempel WM, Koscielny S, Paul JF, Carde P, Sabatier L. Telomere shortening: a new prognostic factor for cardiovascular disease post-radiation exposure. Radiat Prot Dosimetry. 2015;164:134–7.

Marelli AJ, Ionescu-Ittu R, Mackie AS, Guo L, Dendukuri N, Kaouache M. Lifetime prevalence of congenital heart disease in the general population from 2000 to 2010. Circulation. 2014;130:749–56.

Mattei E, Gentili G, Censi F, Triventi M, Calcagnini G. Impact of capped and uncapped abandoned leads on the heating of an MR-conditional pacemaker implant. Magn Reson Med. 2015;73:390–400.

McKenzie ED, Khan MS, Dietzman TW, Guzman-Pruneda FA, Samayoa AX, Liou A, Heinle JS, Fraser Jr CD. Surgical pulmonary valve replacement: a benchmark for outcomes comparisons. J Thorac Cardiovasc Surg. 2014;148:1450–3.

McMullan DM, Permut LC, Jones TK, Johnston TA, Rubio AE. Modified Blalock-Taussig shunt versus ductal stenting for palliation of cardiac lesions with inadequate pulmonary blood flow. J Thorac Cardiovasc Surg. 2014;147:397–401.

Menkis AH, Martin J, Cheng DC, Fitzgerald DC, Freedman JJ, Gao C, Koster A, Mackenzie GS, Murphy GJ, Spiess B, Ad N. Drug, devices, technologies, and techniques for blood management in minimally invasive and conventional cardiothoracic surgery: a consensus statement from the International Society for Minimally Invasive Cardiothoracic Surgery (ISMICS) 2011. Innovations (Phila). 2012;7:229–41.

Miller SP, McQuillen PS. Neurology of congenital heart disease: insight from brain imaging. Arch Dis Child Fetal Neonatal Ed. 2007;92:F435–7.

Niebler RA, Gill JC, Brabant CP, Mitchell ME, Nugent M, Simpson P, Tweddell JS, Ghanayem NS. Thromboelastography in the assessment of bleeding following surgery for congenital heart disease. World J Pediatr Congenit Heart Surg. 2012;3:433–8.

O'Byrne ML, Glatz AC, Mercer-Rosa L, Gillespie MJ, Dori Y, Goldmuntz E, Kawut S, Rome JJ. Trends in pulmonary valve replacement in children and adults with tetralogy of Fallot. Am J Cardiol. 2015;115:118–24.

Olsen M, Garne E, Svaerke C, Sondergaard L, Nissen H, Andersen HO, Hjortdal VE, Johnsen SP, Videbaek J. Cancer risk among patients with congenital heart defects: a nationwide follow-up study. Cardiol Young. 2014;24:40–6.

Olshove Jr VF, Preston T, Gomez D, Phillips A, Galantowicz M. Perfusion techniques toward bloodless pediatric open heart surgery. J Extra Corpor Technol. 2010;42:122–7.

Pan W, Wang Y, Lin L, Zhou G, Hua X, Mo L. Outcomes of dexmedetomidine treatment in pediatric patients undergoing congenital heart disease surgery: a meta-analysis. Paediatr Anaesth. 2016;26:239–48.

Paquette LB, Wisnowski JL, Ceschin R, Pruetz JD, Detterich JA, Del Castillo S, Nagasunder AC, Kim R, Painter MJ, Gilles FH, Nelson MD, Williams RG, Bluml S, Panigrahy A. Abnormal cerebral microstructure in premature neonates with congenital heart disease. AJNR Am J Neuroradiol. 2013;34:2026–33.

Phillips AB, Nevin P, Shah A, Olshove V, Garg R, Zahn EM. Development of a novel hybrid strategy for transcatheter pulmonary valve placement in patients following transannular patch repair of tetralogy of Fallot. Catheter Cardiovasc Interv. 2016;87:403–10.

Pulver AF, Puchalski MD, Bradley DJ, Minich LL, Su JT, Saarel EV, Whitaker P, Etheridge SP. Safety and imaging quality of MRI in pediatric and adult congenital heart disease patients with pacemakers. Pacing Clin Electrophysiol. 2009;32:450–6.

Rajput RS, Das S, Makhija N, Airan B. Efficacy of dexmedetomidine for the control of junctional ectopic tachycardia after repair of tetralogy of Fallot. Ann Pediatr Cardiol. 2014;7:167–72.

Reddy VY, Exner DV, Cantillon DJ, Doshi R, Bunch TJ, Tomassoni GF, Friedman PA, Estes NA, Ip J, Niazi I, Plunkitt K, Banker R, Porterfield J, Ip JE, Dukkipati SR, Leadless Ii Study Investigators. Percutaneous implantation of an entirely intracardiac leadless pacemaker. N Engl J Med. 2015;373:1125–35.

Reddy VY, Knops RE, Sperzel J, Miller MA, Petru J, Simon J, Sediva L, de Groot JR, Tjong FV, Jacobson P, Ostrosff A, Dukkipati SR, Koruth JS, Wilde AA, Kautzner J, Neuzil P. Permanent leadless cardiac pacing: results of the LEADLESS trial. Circulation. 2014;129:1466–71.

Redlin M, Kukucka M, Boettcher W, Schoenfeld H, Huebler M, Kuppe H, Habazettl H. Blood transfusion determines postoperative morbidity in pediatric cardiac surgery applying a comprehensive blood-sparing approach. J Thorac Cardiovasc Surg. 2013;146:537–42.

Reynolds D, Duray GZ, Omar R, Soejima K, Neuzil P, Zhang S, Narasimhan C, Steinwender C, Brugada J, Lloyd M, Roberts PR, Sagi V, Hummel J, Bongiorni MG, Knops RE, Ellis CR, Gornick CC, Bernabei MA, Laager V, Stromberg K, Williams ER, Hudnall JH, Ritter P, Micra Transcatheter Pacing Study Group. A leadless intracardiac transcatheter pacing system. N Engl J Med. 2016;374:533–41.

Ricci MF, Andersen JC, Joffe AR, Watt MJ, Moez EK, Dinu IA, Garcia Guerra G, Ross DB, Rebeyka IM, Robertson CM. Chronic neuromotor disability after complex cardiac surgery in early life. Pediatrics. 2015;136:e922–33.

Ritter P, Duray GZ, Steinwender C, Soejima K, Omar R, Mont L, Boersma LV, Knops RE, Chinitz L, Zhang S, Narasimhan C, Hummel J, Lloyd M, Simmers TA, Voigt A, Laager V, Stromberg K, Bonner MD, Sheldon TJ, Reynolds D, Micra Transcatheter Pacing Study G. Early performance of a miniaturized leadless cardiac pacemaker: the Micra Transcatheter Pacing Study. Eur Heart J. 2015;36:2510–9.

Roksund OD, Clemm H, Heimdal JH, Aukland SM, Sandvik L, Markestad T, Halvorsen T. Left vocal cord paralysis after extreme preterm birth, a new clinical scenario in adults. Pediatrics. 2010;126:e1569–77.

Romlin BS, Wahlander H, Berggren H, Synnergren M, Baghaei F, Nilsson K, Jeppsson A. Intraoperative thromboelastometry is associated with reduced transfusion prevalence in pediatric cardiac surgery. Anesth Analg. 2011;112:30–6.

Sarrechia I, Miatton M, De Wolf D, Francois K, Gewillig M, Meyns B, Vingerhoets G. Neurocognitive development and behaviour in school-aged children after surgery for uni-ventricular or biventricular congenital heart disease. Eur J Cardiothorac Surg. 2016;49:167–74.

Seghaye MC, Grabitz R, Alzen G, Trommer F, Hornchen H, Messmer BJ, von Bernuth G. Thoracic sequelae after surgical closure of the patent ductus arteriosus in premature infants. Acta Paediatr. 1997;86:213–6.

Society of Thoracic Surgeons Blood Conservation Guideline Task Force, Ferraris VA, Brown JR, Despotis GJ, Hammon JW, Reece TB, Saha SP, Song HK, Clough ER, Society of Cardiovascular Anesthesiologists Special Task Force on Blood Transfusion, Shore-Lesserson LJ, Goodnough LT, Mazer CD, Shander A, Stafford-Smith M, Waters J, International Consortium for Evidence Based Perfusion, Baker RA, Dickinson TA, FitzGerald DJ, Likosky DS, Shann KG. 2011 update to the Society of Thoracic Surgeons and the Society of Cardiovascular Anesthesiologists blood conservation clinical practice guidelines. Ann Thorac Surg. 2011;91:944–82.

Szekely A, Cserep Z, Sapi E, Breuer T, Nagy CA, Vargha P, Hartyanszky I, Szatmari A, Treszl A. Risks and predictors of blood transfusion in pediatric patients undergoing open heart operations. Ann Thorac Surg. 2009;87:187–97.

Toren P, Horesh N. Psychiatric morbidity in adolescents operated in childhood for congenital cyanotic heart disease. J Paediatr Child Health. 2007;43:662–6.

Travelli FC, Herrington CS, Ing FF. A novel hybrid technique for transcatheter pulmonary valve implantation within a dilated native right ventricular outflow tract. J Thorac Cardiovasc Surg. 2014;148:e145–6.

Vecoli C, Borghini A, Foffa I, Ait-Ali L, Picano E, Andreassi MG. Leukocyte telomere shortening in grown-up patients with congenital heart disease. Int J Cardiol. 2016;204:17–22.

Vergales JE, Wanchek T, Novicoff W, Kron IL, Lim DS. Cost-analysis of percutaneous pulmonary valve implantation compared to surgical pulmonary valve replacement. Catheter Cardiovasc Interv. 2013;82:1147–53.

Videbaek J, Laursen HB, Olsen M, Hofsten DE, Johnsen SP. Long-term nationwide follow-up study of simple congenital heart disease diagnosed in otherwise healthy children. Circulation. 2016;133:474–83.

Wang G, Bainbridge D, Martin J, Cheng D. The efficacy of an intraoperative cell saver during cardiac surgery: a meta-analysis of randomized trials. Anesth Analg. 2009;109:320–30.

Wilkoff BL, Bello D, Taborsky M, Vymazal J, Kanal E, Heuer H, Hecking K, Johnson WB, Young W, Ramza B, Akhtar N, Kuepper B, Hunold P, Luechinger R, Puererfellner H, Duru F, Gotte MJ, Sutton R, Sommer T, EnRhythm MRISPSSI. Magnetic resonance imaging in patients with a pacemaker system designed for the magnetic resonance environment. Heart Rhythm. 2011;8:65–73.

Wilson WM, Benson LN, Osten MD, Shah A, Horlick EM. Transcatheter pulmonary valve replacement with the Edwards sapien system: the Toronto experience. JACC Cardiovasc Interv. 2015;8:1819–27.

Yon TF, Amka P, Pildes RS, Tatooles CJ. Diaphragmatic paralysis after surgical ligation of patent ductus arteriosus. Lancet. 1977;2:461.

Zahn EM, Nevin P, Simmons C, Garg R. A novel technique for transcatheter patent ductus arteriosus closure in extremely preterm infants using commercially available technology. Catheter Cardiovasc Interv. 2015;85:240–8.

Zbar RI, Chen AH, Behrendt DM, Bell EF, Smith RJ. Incidence of vocal fold paralysis in infants undergoing ligation of patent ductus arteriosus. Ann Thorac Surg. 1996;61:814–6.

Chapter 16
Cardiopulmonary Bypass in Children and Infants

Filip De Somer

Introduction

Cardiac surgery can be considered one of most important medical advances of the twentieth century. John Gibbon performed the first successful cardiac operation with cardiopulmonary bypass (CPB) (Edmunds 2003). Initially, the technology was complex and unreliable and was therefore slow to develop. The introduction of better and more hemocompatible polymers in combination with better pumps and monitoring has led to extraordinary improvements over the years. These improvements were not only related to the equipment but also to a better understanding of the normal and pathological physiology.

The better design and improved conduct of pediatric cardiopulmonary bypass (CPB) are responsible for the fact that complex cardiac anomalies can nowadays be corrected earlier in life with low mortality and morbidity. Nevertheless, initiating CPB in a neonate remains a challenge because of child's low blood volume, its often immature organs, and abnormal anatomical structures.

In this chapter some of the improvements as well as some of the remaining problems will be discussed.

Components of CPB

Due to the heterogeneity of the pediatric population and the often abnormal anatomy, there is no such thing as a standard CPB circuit for neonatal and pediatric cardiac surgery. The most challenging components are vascular access, tubing, pump, and oxygenator choice.

F. De Somer, PhD
University Hospital Ghent, Heart Center 5IE-K12, De Pintelaan 185, B-9000 Ghent, Belgium
e-mail: Filip.DeSomer@UGent.be

© Springer International Publishing Switzerland 2017
A. Dabbagh et al. (eds.), *Congenital Heart Disease in Pediatric and Adult Patients*, DOI 10.1007/978-3-319-44691-2_16

Vascular Access

Since the start of CPB in the early 1950s of the last century, nonoptimal vascular access was known to have a direct impact on the hemodynamic support of a patient. From a physiological and anatomical point of view, the venous and arterial circulations are quite different. The arterial circulation is mainly a high-pressure low-compliance system, whereas the venous system is a low-pressure, high-compliance system. As a consequence, problems encountered in obtaining optimal arterial or venous access will be different.

Problems with arterial cannulation are mostly related to inappropriate sizing of the arterial cannula or to bleeding of the cannulation site. Undersizing of the cannula diameter leads to high shear stress and pressure drop over the cannula tip, which creates hemolysis and activates leukocytes and blood platelets. In addition, the high blood velocity inside the arterial cannula creates a jet inside the aorta causing selective perfusion, while the venturi effect might steal blood from the brain vessels. On the other hand, oversizing of the cannula will cause partial obstruction of the vessel lumen and increases the work load for the heart during weaning, when the heart has to eject against a high resistance. High resistance inside the cannula or arterial line is less of a problem as the cannula is located downstream of the arterial blood pump. In most centers sizing is done empirically based upon historical experience as most manufacturers only provide pressure-flow curves for their cannulas using water instead of with a blood analogue or blood. As water has a lower viscosity, this can lead to major bias. In order to overcome this problem, a simple technique has been proposed which is represented in Fig. 16.1 (De Wachter et al. 2002).

We can represent these data by a parabolic fit: $\Delta P_{water} = a \cdot Q_{water}^{2} + b \cdot Q_{water}$ In the example above, we obtain: $\Delta P_{water} = 166.98 \cdot Q_{water}^{2} + 23.64 \cdot Q_{water}$

In order to obtain the values for blood with a given hematocrit and temperature, we need to rescale the coefficients with ratios of density and dynamic viscosity:

$$a_{blood} = a_{water} \cdot \frac{\rho_{blood}}{\rho_{water}} \qquad b_{blood} = b_{water} \cdot \frac{\mu_{blood}}{\mu_{water}}$$

Calculate density and viscosity for water and blood

$$r_{water} = 997 \frac{kg}{m^{3}} \qquad \text{water density}$$

$$h_{water} = 0.001 \frac{kg}{m \cdot s} \qquad \text{water viscosity at } 20'C$$

Blood characteristics during cardiopulmonary bypass

$$Hct := 25\% \qquad \text{Hematocrit}\,[\%]$$

$$T_{blood} := 32 \qquad \text{Arterial blood temperature}\,['C]$$

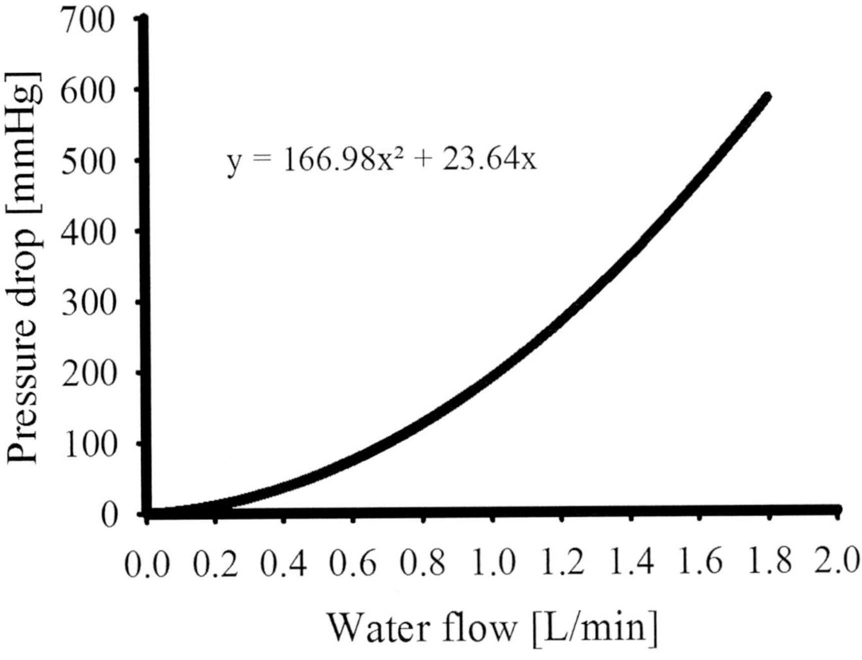

Fig. 16.1 Pressure flow curve (water) Medtronic DLP 77108 (Provided by the manufacturer)

$$\rho_{blood} = 1.09\,\frac{gm}{cm^3}\cdot Hct + 1.035\,\frac{gm}{cm^3}\cdot(1-Hct)$$

$$\rho_{blood} = 1.049\times10^3\,\frac{kg}{m^3}\qquad \text{Blood density during CPB}$$

$$\eta_{plasma} = \frac{\exp\left[-5.64+\dfrac{1800}{(T_{blood}+273)}\right]}{100}\cdot poise$$

$$\eta_{blood} = \eta_{plasma}\cdot\exp(2.31\cdot Hct)\qquad \eta_{blood} = 2.314\cdot cpoise$$

Calculate ratios

$$\rho_{ratio} = \frac{\rho_{blood}}{\rho_{water}} = 1.052\qquad \eta_{ratio} = \frac{\eta_{blood}}{\eta_{water}} = 2.314$$

What is the pressure drop over a 77108 DLP cannula during CPB at a blood flow of 0.8 L/min?

$$Q := 0.8 \quad \text{Flow in L/min}$$
$$\Delta P_{\text{water}} := 166.98 \cdot Q^2 + 23.64 \cdot Q = 126$$
$$\Delta P_{\text{blood}} := 166.98 \cdot \rho_{\text{ratio}} \cdot Q^2 + 23.64 \cdot \eta_{\text{ratio}} \cdot Q = 156$$

Assessing access of the venous side is more complex due to more stringent boundary conditions. In the normal circulation, venous return toward the heart is governed by the pressure difference between the mean circulatory filling pressure and the pressure in the right atrium.

This pressure difference is approximately 7 mmHg (Guyton et al. 1954, 1957, 1962). When venous access is established, the wide, low-resistance, collapsible blood vessels are connected with smaller-diameter, stiff, artificial conduits of known physical characteristics. Because of the smaller diameters of both the venous line and the venous cannula, higher pressure differences are needed to obtain optimal venous drainage (Galletti and Brecher 1962). The necessary pressure difference to achieve optimal drainage will depend on tubing diameter, tubing length, and blood viscosity (Ni et al. 2001). The latter in its turn will be dependent on both hematocrit and temperature. In order to overcome the combined pressure drop of both venous cannula and venous line, a negative pressure is applied by using gravity (siphon) or assisted venous drainage. When applying negative pressure, venous drainage will first increase linearly with the increase in negative pressure, while the resistance will remain more or less constant. However, at a certain point, a further increase in pressure will partially collapse the vein, with no further increase in blood flow, and, therefore, resistance will start to increase (Galletti and Brecher 1962). Correct choice of a venous cannula is critical as it will represent the smallest diameter and, thus, the highest resistance. Reducing the diameter by 50 % will reduce flow to 1/16th of the original flow. Also, the length of this smallest diameter is important, as doubling the length of the cannula will decrease flow by 50 %. Another point of interest is the ratio between the diameter of the vein and the cannula. According to Galetti, this ratio should be around 0.5 in order to avoid collapse of the vein around the side holes of the cannula (Galletti and Brecher 1962). Although the diameter ratio is important, also the design of the cannula and cannula tip (De Somer et al. 2002) will influence the drainage efficiency.

In children vacuum-assisted venous drainage (VAVD) is becoming more and more the standard. This technique applies vacuum on the venous reservoir in order to increase the pressure differential (Durandy and Hulin 2006; Durandy 2009a, b). However, it should not be used as a solution for correcting improper cannula position. If VAVD is used under such conditions, one mainly will increase resistance in the cannula. At the same time, a higher blood velocity will be generated over those openings of the cannula which are not blocked by the improper position. Finally, this will increase shear stress and lead to an increase in hemolysis. Before applying any form of assisted venous drainage, one should check proper cannula placement. After this check, one can use assisted venous drainage in cases where one wants to reduce priming volume by placing the oxygenator at the same height as the patient or by using a smaller-diameter venous line or by combining both strategies (Pappalardo et al. 2007).

Table 16.1 Impact of tubing diameter on venous line pressure drop

Tubing diameter [inch]	3/16	1/4
Blood flow [L/min]	1	1
Pressure difference [mmHg]	51	11
Velocity [cm/s]	94	53
Reynolds number	2019	1514
Wall shear stress [dynes/cm^2]	54	15

Data generated with:
Hematocrit, 25 %
Temperature, 32 °C
Tubing length, 150 cm

The reported vacuum that should be applied for optimal drainage lies between −30 and −80 mmHg. The absolute value will depend upon where this negative pressure is measured in the circuit. The purpose of measuring the pressure is to estimate the pressure at the cannula tip as this will give us information with respect to risk for vein collapse. Vein collapse will occur once the negative pressure at the cannula tip exceeds −4 mmHg. Unfortunately, the pressure at the cannula tip is difficult to obtain in clinical practice so most perfusionists measure the pressure somewhere between the cannula and the reservoir top. As a result, the obtained pressure value is the sum of the resistance in the cannula and the venous line between the measurement point and the cannula tip. The latter might explain the large differences in reported values. This is illustrated in Table 16.1, which shows the impact on blood velocity and required pressure difference when 3/16 in. tubing or 1/4 in. tubing is used for obtaining a venous drainage of 1 L/min.

In general, assisted venous drainage is helpful in all cases where siphon drainage alone is insufficient due to high resistances in the venous cannula and venous line and in cases where venous pressure remains high despite proper cannula position and in those cases where the operative field is not dry (Murai et al. 2005).

Optimizing arterial and venous vascular access is mandatory as it will determine the maximum blood flow that can be obtained and thus oxygen delivery to the organs. Malposition of a cannula can obstruct cerebral blood supply or cause a preferential flow into the descending aorta leading to an inappropriate oxygen supply to the brain. Alternatively obstruction of the superior vena caval cannula may decrease cerebral venous drainage and potentially lead to brain dysfunction. Nowadays, many of these problems can be detected early in time by routine use of cerebral oxygenation by near-infrared spectroscopy (NIRS) (Gottlieb et al. 2006; Ginther et al. 2011; Redlin et al. 2011).

Tubing

The tubing in the CPB circuit interconnects all of the main components of the circuit. A variety of polymers can be used for the manufacture of tubing, but most are made of PVC with exception of the tubing used in the pump boot which is often silicone. The length and size of the tubing will have a major impact on volume, shear

Table 16.2 Characteristics of different pediatric tubings

Tubing diameter [inch]	1/8	3/16	1/4	3/8
Volume [mL/m]	8	18	32	71
Pressure difference [mmHg/L]	234	54	15	5
Velocity [cm/s]	210	94	53	23
Reynolds number	3028	2019	1514	1009
Wall shear stress [dynes/cm^2]	247	54	15	6

Data generated with:
Hematocrit, 25 %
Temperature, 32°C
Tubing length, 150 cm
Blood flow, 1 LPM

stress, and pressure drop (Table 16.2), and the clinician will have to make a choice based upon the clinical conditions.

Blood Pumps

From an engineering perspective, pumps can be classified into two main categories: displacement pumps and rotary pumps. The energy in displacement pumps is characterized by periodic volumetric changes of a working space. A typical displacement pump is the roller pump. The principle of operation of this pump is that two rollers, placed opposite to each other, "roll" the blood through a piece of tubing. When the pump completely occludes the tubing, the pump is capable of generating both positive and negative pressures, and therefore it can be also used as blood aspirating pump. Because of its working principle, a roller pump is relatively independent of factors such as resistance and hydrostatic pressure head, which are encountered in the average CPB circuit. The output of an occlusive roller pump depends upon two main variables: the number of revolutions per minute of the pump head and the internal diameter and length of the tubing held in the pump head:

$$Q = \pi \cdot radius^2 \cdot length \cdot RPM$$

where RPM = revolutions per minute.

A disadvantage of roller pumps is spallation (Briceno and Runge 1992; Peek et al. 2000). Due to the continuous compression of the tubing by the roller, the polymer of the tubing starts to weaken and to erode, resulting in the generation of small particles (Briceno and Runge 1992; Kim and Yoon 1998; Peek et al. 2000). In order to control spallation, it is advocated to use a dynamic occlusion setting of the pump rollers (Tamari et al. 1997). Due to the high resistances encountered in neonatal and pediatric CPB circuits, roller pumps remain the first choice. In larger children or young adults, one might prefer a rotary pump and more specific a centrifugal pump. Centrifugal pumps operate on the principle of moving fluid by creating a pressure gradient between the inlet and the outlet of the pump. The pressure gradient results from the creation of a vortex by the rotation of the pump head. The rotating motion creates an area of low pressure in the center and an area of high pressure on the sides. The resulting rate of blood flow will depend upon the pressure gradient and the resistance at the outlet of the pump. The latter is a function of two variables: the CPB circuit (oxygenator, filter, tubing, arterial cannula) and the systemic vascular resistance of the patient. Because the flow produced by a centrifugal pump directly depends on the pressure that the centrifugal pump generates, a centrifugal pump is called a pressure pump. In contrast to a roller pump, a centrifugal pump is afterload dependent and thus influenced by changes in resistance in both the circuit and the patient. For this reason a centrifugal pump should always be used in conjunction with a flow meter. Although a centrifugal pump, due to its non-occlusive working principle, has no spallation, high resistances after the pump may lead to high shear stresses and hot spots inside the pump head (Araki et al. 1995a, b; Ganushchak et al. 2006).

Oxygenator

The oxygenator is without doubt the most important component in the CPB circuit. It is not only responsible for exchanging oxygen and carbon dioxide but also for the administration of volatile anesthetics. The oxygenator comprises an integrated heat exchanger that allows cooling and warming of the patient. A heat exchanger is indispensible as some extensive repairs may require hypothermia and/or deep hypothermic circulatory arrest (DHCA). Most recent oxygenators are now available with an integrated filter thus avoiding the need for a separate arterial line filter (Lin et al. 2012; Ginther et al. 2013). In pediatric surgery most centers use an open venous reservoir with integrated cardiotomy. The latter filters and defoams blood aspirated from the surgical field. The main reason for choosing open systems lays in the fact that open systems allow assisted venous drainage which is helpful in optimizing venous drainage and in reducing priming volume (Durandy 2013, 2015).

Nowadays, exclusively extraluminal hollow fiber membrane oxygenators are used. For neonatal and pediatric usage, several sizes are available. The final decision which to use is usually made based upon priming volume, surface area, rated blood flow, and available connections all in relation to the size of the patient and the type of surgical repair. Table 16.3 shows the characteristics of some neonatal and pediatric oxygenators. Originally the reference flow of a given oxygenator was defined by the Association for the Advancement of Medical Instrumentation (AAMI) as the flow rate at which normothermic whole blood having a hemoglobin content of 120 g/L, a base excess of 0, and a venous saturation of 65 % will increase its oxygen content by 45 mL oxygen per liter blood. This proposed value offered sufficient safety in acyanotic children but could pose a problem in cyanotic children that are often presented with much lower venous saturation. For this reason, contemporary pediatric oxygenators easily can have oxygen transfers up to 75 mL/L at the nominal maximum flow given by the manufacturer. As a result the reference flow (AAMI conditions) can be much higher (Table 16.3) than the recommended flow. Based upon this characteristic, one could use a smaller oxygenator, with the resulting lower hemodilution and contact activation, in selected cases (Durandy 2010a).

Table 16.3 Characteristics of contemporary neonatal and pediatric oxygenators

Oxygenator	Membrane surface area [m²]	Membrane material	Maximum blood flow [L/min]	Reference blood flow [L/min]	Heat exchanger surface area [m²]
Terumo FX05	0.5	PP	1.5	2.5	0.035
LivaNova D100[a]	0.22	PP	0.7	1	0.03
LivaNova D101[a]	0.61	PP	2.5	3.5	0.06
Maquet Neonatal Quadrox-i	0.38	PP	1.5	N/A	0.07
Maquet Pediatric Quadrox-i	0.8	PP	2.8	N/A	0.15
Medtronic Pixie[a]	0.67	PP	2	N/A	N/A
Medos Hilite 1000[a]	0.39	PP	1	N/A	0.074
Medos Hilite 2800[a]	0.8	PP	2.8	N/A	0.16

PP microporous polypropylene, *PET* polyethylene terephthalate, *N/A* not available
[a]No integrated filter

Priming and Hemodilution

The total priming volume of a CPB circuit is determined by the components selected (De Somer et al. 1996b). It is important to select a smaller oxygenator that will function close to its maximal capacity for flow rather than selecting a large oxygenator that will function toward its lower level. However, independent of the choice of oxygenator, its priming volume will be fixed. The priming volume taken by the tubing, on the other hand, is determined by its length and diameter and mainly controlled by the surgical team (Ni et al. 2001). The total amount of priming volume is important as it will determine the dilution of the blood components. However, also the composition of the priming fluid is a point of consideration. Excessive dilution of blood coagulation factors below 45 % should be prevented by using fresh frozen plasma in the priming solution (Brauer et al. 2013). This is especially important in cyanotic children as they have in general a lower plasma volume or in children with complex repairs (Pouard and Bojan 2013). As many institutions do not routinely screen coagulation factors before cardiac surgery, often fibrinogen concentration is used as a reference, keeping its concentration above 1 g/L. Huge differences in target hemoglobin during CPB are reported going from 50 to 100 g/dL (Nicolas et al. 1994; Gruber et al. 1999). Due to a lack of sufficient randomized prospective studies (Wilkinson et al. 2014), it is still unclear what is the optimal hemoglobin concentration during CPB. But one should not focus alone on hemoglobin concentration as final oxygen delivery (DO_2) will be dependent on both hemoglobin concentration and pump flow. As a consequence one can tolerate lower hemoglobin concentrations as long as vascular access allows for high pump flows, but when anatomical limitations restrict vascular access, a higher hemoglobin concentration might be desirable. This can be easily demonstrated by the following example: if we consider a minimum DO_2 of 300 mL/min/m² in a child with a body surface of 0.22 m², then the required blood flow would be 490 mL/min at a hemoglobin of 100 g/L, but we would need a blood flow of 1970 mL/min at a hemoglobin of 50 g/L to achieve the target DO_2. It is quite obvious that the latter is hardly obtainable.

Prophylactic use of both fresh frozen plasma and packed red cells without arguments is not recommended (Wilkinson et al. 2014; Desborough et al. 2015).

Beside the impact of the priming solution on blood coagulation and oxygen transport, its composition will also affect colloid oncotic pressure. There is evidence that priming with a high-colloid oncotic pressure, by adding albumin, results in less fluid overload by the end of CPB and is advantageous in neonates compared to a priming solution only containing crystalloids (Pouard and Bojan 2013).

Reflection on the composition of the priming volume and composition becomes even more important; now more and more centers prefer normothermic conditions even for complex repairs such as transposition of the great arteries (Durandy 2010b).

In the early days of cardiac surgery, hemodilution was seen as a huge benefit for the cardiac surgical population of that time as it could avoid blood prime. Despite this advantage it became obvious over the years, due to better monitoring techniques and extensive research, that hemodilution has its limits. Hemodilution will have a linear impact, when blood flow is constant, on total oxygen content. Hemodiluting a patient with a normal hematocrit of 40 % to a hematocrit of 20 % will thus decrease the oxygen content per liter blood by 50 %. When this happens in healthy patients, not on CPB bypass, this loss will be compensated by a compensatory increase in cardiac output which is facilitated by the reduced viscosity caused by the hemodilution. During CPB a fixed blood flow per square meter of body surface is used, typically between 2.2 and 3.0 L/min/m². Maintaining this fixed flow during excessive hemodilution might jeopardize oxygen delivery to the tissue as the physiological compensatory increase in flow is absent.

Another disadvantage of hemodilution is the decrease in viscosity and plasma proteins. The decrease in viscosity leads to a loss in density of capillaries in the microcirculation (Tsai et al. 1998). Research has shown that this negative effect can be in part attenuated by using fluids with a higher viscosity for hemodilution as increasing the viscosity of plasma is directly associated with increased perivascular nitric oxide concentration, an effect related to vasodilatation, and increased perfusion and capillary density compared with the same procedure using fluids with a lower viscosity (Tsai et al. 2005). Although the fluids used in this study had a viscosity much higher than those commercially available, it seems favorable to use priming solutions with a higher viscosity (Manduz et al. 2008). The decrease in plasma proteins will result in a decrease in plasma colloid oncotic pressure which may play an important role in the fluid accumulation often seen after CPB. Tissue edema is secondary to increased capillary permeability caused by the systemic inflammatory response induced by CPB. In neonates the combination of this increased capillary permeability and the decrease of the colloid oncotic pressure seems to worsen the situation (Jonas 2004). Maintaining colloid oncotic pressure during bypass has been linked to decreased myocardial edema (Foglia et al. 1986) and reduced fluid accumulation. The lower fluid accumulation was then associated with a shorter stay in intensive care and a lower mortality (Haneda et al. 1985).

Metabolism During CPB

The primary function of CPB is to maintain the circulation in order to prevent organ dysfunction during and after the surgical repair. Oxygen delivery is one of the most important variables in achieving this goal. Oxygen delivery will depend upon the hemoglobin concentration and the pump flow. In adults it has been demonstrated that there exist a close correlation between the lowest hematocrit on bypass and morbidity (Habib et al. 2003). However, it is questioned whether this is due to the low hematocrit by itself or due to a low DO_2 (Ranucci et al. 2005). Recent research showed that maintaining DO_2 above 280 mL/min/m^2 could reduce the incidence of acute kidney injury from 29.8 to 12.1 %. As this research was done in an adult population at temperatures above 32°C, one could question whether these findings could be extrapolated to a pediatric population. But it clearly demonstrates that when a low hematocrit is targeted during CPB, one will need to maintain higher blood flows. On the other hand, when anatomical limitations limit the size of the vascular access, one should keep the hematocrit higher during CPB.

The microcirculation is the ultimate destination of red blood cells (RBC) to transport oxygen to the tissue cells. Its success defines the primary function of the cardiovascular system. Inside the microcirculation there are two main determinants of oxygen transport to the tissue, convective transport of red blood cells to the capillaries and the passive diffusion of oxygen leaving the RBC to the mitochondria in the cells (Ince 2014). The convective transport is represented by:

$$DO_2 = \left[\left(cte \cdot Hb \cdot S \right) + \left(PO_2 \cdot k \right) \right] \cdot Q$$

where Q = blood flow [mL/min], Hb = hemoglobin concentration [g/mL], cte = [1.34 mL/g], S = amount of oxygen bound to hemoglobin[%], PO_2 = partial oxygen tension [mmHg], and k = oxygen solubility [mL/mL].

For a long time, it was considered sufficient to maintain blood flow in order to provide the tissue in the microcirculation with oxygen. However, an equal contribution to oxygen transport to tissue is governed by the ability of oxygen to reach the cells from the red blood cell by passive diffusion. The further away the tissue cell is from the oxygen-carrying RBC, for example, by excessive hemodilution (Atasever et al. 2011), or the less oxygen solubility of tissue cells (e.g., by edema), the more difficulty, even in the presence of sufficient flow in the filled capillaries, the oxygen will have in reaching these cells. The diffusive capacity of the microcirculation depends upon the functional capillary density (FCD), or the density of capillaries in a given volume of tissue, and is described by Fick's law as the product of the difference between the partial pressure of oxygen at the RBC minus that at the mitochondria times the diffusion constant divided by the distance between the RBC and the mitochondria (Boerma and Ince 2010; Ince 2014). Immediately after and during CPB, there will be a loss of FCD. The percentage loss will depend upon the degree of hemodilution, the viscosity, and the filling status of the microcirculation. As a consequence more cells will depend upon the oxygen supply by a single capillary (Krogh 1919). Just increasing cardiac output maybe insufficient to correct the resulting tissue hypoxemia, and microcirculatory recruitment procedures are needed. Potential treatment options besides increasing flow are increasing partial CO_2 tension, increasing mean arterial pressure, and maintaining a normal viscosity. In order to validate the efficiency of the different options, NIRS is extremely helpful as it helps to define the pressure range in which the autologous regulation is maintained (Moerman et al. 2013).

Special groups within the neonatal and pediatric CPB population are cyanotic children. There is quite a debate on what is the best oxygenation strategy in this group especially in the period before ischemia and during reperfusion of the myocardium after surgical repair. Maintaining high partial oxygen tensions in cyanotic patients at the beginning of CPB leads to reoxygenation injury with significant organ damage, including the myocardium, and triggers the systemic inflammatory response (del Nido et al. 1987; del Nido et al. 1988; Modi et al. 2002; Caputo et al. 2014; Kagawa et al. 2014). One of the strategies proposed to avoid reoxygenation injury is the use of controlled reoxygenation. This technique targets an arterial partial oxygen tension (PaO_2) similar to the patient's preoperative oxygen saturation when starting CPB. It has been shown to ameliorate reoxygenation injury in experimental models (Ihnken et al. 1995; Ihnken et al. 1998a), in adult patients (Ihnken et al. 1998b), and, more recently, in cyanotic pediatric patients with mixed pathologic features that are undergoing cardiac surgery (Caputo et al. 2009).

Another challenge is to define the best oxygenation strategy for children requiring deep hypothermia with circulatory arrest (DHCA) or hypothermia with low flow. Hypothermia will slow down the metabolism. The relationship between the cerebral metabolic rate for oxygen ($CMRO_2$) and temperature is best represented by a log-linear model (McCullough et al. 1999). However it should be noted that at a temperature of 20°C, the $CMRO_2$ is still 24% of baseline. For this reason it is extremely important to ensure uniform cerebral hypothermia as it is critical to the successful use of DHCA. At the same time, efforts should be made to increase oxygen availability to the cells. Hypothermia will shift the oxygen dissociation curve (ODC) to the left. The P50 value, partial oxygen tension at which the hemoglobin is 50% saturated, is around 26.6 mmHg at 37°C but will decrease to approximately 13 mmHg at 20°C, making it more difficult to release the hemoglobin-bound oxygen at the tissue level. During normothermia venous saturation can decrease to 30% before $CMRO_2$ will decrease to less than 90% of normal, but in infants at 17°C, venous saturation must be maintained at greater than 95% to maintain $CMRO_2$ at greater than 90 % of its temperature appropriate value (Dexter and Hindman 1995). Due to this increase in hemoglobin's affinity for oxygen at 19°C, 80 % of the $CMRO_2$ will be no longer primarily provided by hemoglobin-bound oxygen but by dissolved oxygen (Dexter et al. 1997). In order to improve oxygen availability during DHCA, many centers use a pH-stat acid-base strategy. This approach targets a pH of 7.4 at the real blood temperature, e.g., 20°C. The higher carbon dioxide content will shift the ODC more to the right, and P50 will increase from 13 to 15.3 mmHg. However, pH-stat by itself is insufficient as the shift to the right is limited and thus has to be accompanied with measures to improve the amount of dissolved oxygen. This can be done by using hyperoxia. It is important to notice that the definition of hyperoxia in this context means a venous partial oxygen tension of >400 mmHg (Pearl et al. 2000). Increasing oxygen tension from 125 to 525 mmHg will increase the amount of soluble oxygen from 4 to 18 mL/L and safe DHCA time by 20 min in a child at 16°C.

Because of the many variables involved, it remains a challenge to predict neurological outcome after DHCA or hypothermia with low flow. An impressive amount of research in this domain has been done at Children's Hospital in Boston looking at the impact of all variables discussed above. Based upon their research, the best approach for DHCA is the combination of hyperoxia with a higher hematocrit and pH-stat strategy. The hypothermia will decrease metabolic rate and thus increase the safe duration of DHCA, while the use of a higher hemoglobin and hyperoxia will allow for better hyperoxygenation of the brain before onset of DHCA. The efficiency of the hyperoxygenation and monitoring of remaining metabolism and oxygen consumption during DHCA can be done with NIRS. The better the hyperoxygenation and the lower the metabolic rate, the longer the period of declining saturation. Finally, a plateau will be reached with minimal oxygen extraction. The duration of this plateau period is a useful predictor of behavioral and histological evidence of injury after DHCA (Sakamoto et al. 2001).

Systemic Inflammation During CPB

Inflammation is the body's humoral and cellular protective response to injury (Davies and Hagen 1997). The systemic inflammatory reaction during cardiac surgery is multifactorial and triggered by almost every part of the procedure, starting with anesthesia (Gu et al. 2002), skin incision, and sternotomy. Subsequently, systemic inflammatory reaction syndrome (SIRS) is further triggered during CPB by contact activation between blood and foreign surface and later by the ischemia and reperfusion of the myocardium (Durandy 2014). Also hypothermia and blood transfusions are known to activate the inflammatory response (Laffey et al. 2002). The first descriptions of the systemic inflammatory response to CPB correctly identified multiple causal factors, including the activation of complement, coagulation, fibrinolysis, inflammatory cytokines, and cytodestructive mediators generated by white cells (Butler et al. 1993). Initially research mainly focused on systemic cytokines and failed to link other host response systems to adverse clinical events (Landis 2009). Despite decades of research, the clinical advances to attenuate SIRS have been disappointing.

Controlling the Host Response

Despite heparinization, factor XII is absorbed onto the foreign surface of the CPB within seconds after initiation, and thrombin will be generated in direct relation to CPB time (Boisclair et al. 1993; Brister et al. 1993). Under normal conditions the intrinsic coagulation will generate in response to injury and small amounts of thrombin. This thrombin is sufficient to initiate hemostasis but not enough to cause thrombus formation (Monroe et al. 2002). The signal becomes amplified when thrombin binds to platelets through its high-affinity thrombin receptor and protease-activated receptor-1 (PAR1) and initiates several positive feedback loops. At the end of this so-called amplification phase, the stage is set for the large burst of thrombin generation that is essential to stable clot formation. Uncontrolled thrombin generation in the bypass circuit may create a prothrombotic risk to the grafted vessel but as well a risk for systemic bleeding. The systemic bleeding risk is caused by the consumption of clotting factors and the unwanted activation of the platelet PAR1 receptor by thrombin in the bypass circuit (Ferraris et al. 1998; Landis 2009). Desensitization of platelets by thrombin is the main cause of the clinical platelet deficit recognized in CPB surgery. Kallikrein and thrombin are also linked to proinflammatory activation of leukocytes and endothelial cells via bradykinin and PAR1 receptors expressed throughout the vasculature (Kamiya et al. 1993; Kaplanski et al. 1997, 1998). The proinflammatory pathways activated by kallikrein and thrombin may explain some of the febrile and capillary leak symptoms seen in CPB (Wachtfogel et al. 1995; Lidington et al. 2000; Landis 2009). Proinflammatory activation of platelets and endothelial cells can be inhibited by agents that antagonize proteolytic activation of PAR1 (Poullis et al. 2000; Day et al. 2006). The benefit of this approach was demonstrated in neonates with hypoplastic left heart syndrome, where the use of aprotinin improved survival after stage 1 repair (Tweddell et al. 2002).

The complement system is activated via classical pathway of C3, secondary to IgM and IgG antibody absorption by the CPB circuit. (Landis et al. 2008). Many attempts have been done to control complement activation. Introduction of closed systems and smaller circuits and coating of all foreign surface with a bioactive or biopassive coating all showed a small attenuation in complement and cytokine generation, but none of these measures could demonstrate major clinical improvements (De Somer et al. 2000; Eisses et al. 2007).

Proinflammatory cytokines such as TNF-α, IL6, and IL8 are activated early during CPB, typically after 5–120 min. This initial proinflammatory phase is triggered by direct contact with foreign material. About 2–24 h after initiation of CPB, this initial release is followed by second anti-inflammatory phase, releasing anti-inflammatory markers such as IL1 and IL10. The anti-inflammatory phase is mainly governed by the body (McBride et al. 1995).

Leukocytes may also contribute to the systemic host response through the elaboration of reactive oxidant species. Neutrophils and monocytes will express their complement receptor CR3 which will mediate leukocyte adhesion to polymers. The adhered cells will try to phagocytose the polymer which the will trigger the same cytodestructive inflammatory cytokine, protease, and reactive oxygen pathways as occurs during genuine phagocytosis (Shappell et al. 1990; Rothlein et al. 1994). Another important source of oxidative stress is intravascular hemolysis, due to local areas of high shear stress in the CPB circuit (De Somer et al. 1996a). This shear stress will lead to the formation of free plasma hemoglobin.

Free plasma hemoglobin in the bloodstream can abrogate vasoprotective responses due to nitric oxide and may accumulate in the proximal tubules, causing direct renal injury, especially in patients with diabetes (Minneci et al. 2005). Peak oxidative stress due to hemolysis occurs at the time of cross clamp release, earlier than the first detectable inflammatory cytokine generation (Christen et al. 2005). A significant contribution to the "systemic inflammatory response" may therefore be due to oxidative stress and loss of vascular nitric oxide responses secondary to hemolysis. Especially aspiration of blood from the surgical field can contain high amounts of free plasma hemoglobin and activated blood platelets. Separating this blood from the systemic blood has shown to improve outcome (Aldea et al. 2002).

From the above it is clear that we should replace the terminology systemic inflammatory response by a definition that is emphasizing on the multisystemic etiology of this disorder such as systemic "host" response to surgery. Interventions should be focused to target on multiple effector pathways simultaneously. In order to increase knowledge, we should better report the observed systemic host response. A consensus paper looking at the published research pointed out that better reporting should comprise of (1) minimal CPB and perfusion criteria that may affect outcomes, (2) causal inflammatory markers that link exposures to outcomes, and (3) markers of organ injury that are practical to measure yet clinically meaningful (Landis et al. 2008).

Conclusions

Instituting CPB in a neonate or child for correction of congenital heart disease remains a challenge. Future research should focus on:

- Further miniaturization of the CPB circuit
- Improved vascular access
- Better strategies to control inflammation
- Better understanding of fluid homeostasis during and after CPB

References

Aldea GS, Soltow LO, Chandler WL, Triggs CM, Vocelka CR, Crockett GI, Shin YT, Curtis WE, Verrier ED. Limitation of thrombin generation, platelet activation, and inflammation by elimination of cardiotomy suction in patients undergoing coronary artery bypass grafting treated with heparin-bonded circuits. J Thorac Cardiovasc Surg. 2002;123:742–55.

Araki K, Taenaka Y, Masuzawa T, Tatsumi E, Wakisaka Y, Watari M, Nakatani T, Akagi H, Baba Y, Anai H, et al. Hemolysis and heat generation in six different types of centrifugal blood pumps. Artif Organs. 1995a;19:928–32.

Araki K, Taenaka Y, Wakisaka Y, Masuzawa T, Tatsumi E, Nakatani T, Baba Y, Yagura A, Eya K, Toda K, et al. Heat generation and hemolysis at the shaft seal in centrifugal blood pumps. ASAIO J. 1995b;41:M284–7.

Atasever B, Boer C, Goedhart P, Biervliet J, Seyffert J, Speekenbrink R, Schwarte L, de Mol B, Ince C. Distinct alterations in sublingual microcirculatory blood flow and hemoglobin oxygenation in on-pump and off-pump coronary artery bypass graft surgery. J Cardiothorac Vasc Anesth. 2011;25:784–90.

Boerma EC, Ince C. The role of vasoactive agents in the resuscitation of microvascular perfusion and tissue oxygenation in critically ill patients. Intensive Care Med. 2010;36:2004–18.

Boisclair MD, Lane DA, Philippou H, Sheikh S, Hunt B. Thrombin production, inactivation and expression during open heart surgery measured by assays for activation fragments including a new ELISA for prothrombin fragment F1 + 2. Thromb Haemost. 1993;70:253–8.

Brauer SD, Applegate 2nd RL, Jameson JJ, Hay KL, Lauer RE, Herrmann PC, Bull BS. Association of plasma dilution with cardiopulmonary bypass-associated bleeding and morbidity. J Cardiothorac Vasc Anesth. 2013;27:845–52.

Briceno JC, Runge TM. Tubing spallation in extracorporeal circuits. An in vitro study using an electronic particle counter. Int J Artif Organs. 1992;15:222–8.

Brister SJ, Ofosu FA, Buchanan MR. Thrombin generation during cardiac surgery: is heparin the ideal anticoagulant? Thromb Haemost. 1993;70:259–62.

Butler J, Rocker GM, Westaby S. Inflammatory response to cardiopulmonary bypass. Ann Thorac Surg. 1993;55:552–9.

Caputo M, Mokhtari A, Rogers CA, Panayiotou N, Chen Q, Ghorbel MT, Angelini GD, Parry AJ. The effects of normoxic versus hyperoxic cardiopulmonary bypass on oxidative stress and inflammatory response in cyanotic pediatric patients undergoing open cardiac surgery: a randomized controlled trial. J Thorac Cardiovasc Surg. 2009;138:206–14.

Caputo M, Mokhtari A, Miceli A, Ghorbel MT, Angelini GD, Parry AJ, Suleiman SM. Controlled reoxygenation during cardiopulmonary bypass decreases markers of organ damage, inflammation, and oxidative stress in single-ventricle patients undergoing pediatric heart surgery. J Thorac Cardiovasc Surg. 2014;148:792–801.e798; discussion 800–791.

Christen S, Finckh B, Lykkesfeldt J, Gessler P, Frese-Schaper M, Nielsen P, Schmid ER, Schmitt B. Oxidative stress precedes peak systemic inflammatory response in pediatric patients undergoing cardiopulmonary bypass operation. Free Radic Biol Med. 2005;38:1323–32.

Davies MG, Hagen PO. Systemic inflammatory response syndrome. Br J Surg. 1997;84:920–35.

Day JR, Taylor KM, Lidington EA, Mason JC, Haskard DO, Randi AM, Landis RC. Aprotinin inhibits proinflammatory activation of endothelial cells by thrombin through the protease-activated receptor 1. J Thorac Cardiovasc Surg. 2006;131:21–7.

De Somer D, Foubert L, Vanackere M, Dujardin D, Delanghe J, Van Nooten G. Impact of oxygenator design on hemolysis, shear stress, and white blood cell and platelet counts. J Cardiothorac Vasc Anesth. 1996a;10:884–9.

De Somer F, Foubert L, Poelaert J, Dujardin D, Van Nooten G, Francois K. Low extracorporeal priming volumes for infants: a benefit? Perfusion. 1996b;11:455–60.

De Somer F, Francois K, van Oeveren W, Poelaert J, De Wolf D, Ebels T, Van Nooten G. Phosphorylcholine coating of extracorporeal circuits provides natural protection against blood activation by the material surface. Eur J Cardiothorac Surg. 2000;18:602–6.

De Somer F, De Wachter D, Verdonck P, Van Nooten G, Ebels T. Evaluation of different paediatric venous cannulae using gravity drainage and VAVD: an in vitro study. Perfusion. 2002;17:321–6.

De Wachter D, De Somer F, Verdonck P. Hemodynamic comparison of two different pediatric aortic cannulas. Int J Artif Organs. 2002;25:867–74.

del Nido PJ, Benson LN, Mickle DA, Kielmanowicz S, Coles JG, Wilson GJ. Impaired left ventricular postischemic function and metabolism in chronic right ventricular hypertrophy. Circulation. 1987;76:V168–73.

del Nido PJ, Mickle DA, Wilson GJ, Benson LN, Weisel RD, Coles JG, Trusler GA, Williams WG. Inadequate myocardial protection with cold cardioplegic arrest during repair of tetralogy of Fallot. J Thorac Cardiovasc Surg. 1988;95:223–9.

Desborough M, Sandu R, Brunskill SJ, Doree C, Trivella M, Montedori A, Abraha I, Stanworth S. 2015. Fresh frozen plasma for cardiovascular surgery. Cochrane Database Syst Rev. (7):CD007614.

Dexter F, Hindman BJ. Theoretical analysis of cerebral venous blood hemoglobin oxygen saturation as an index of cerebral oxygenation during hypothermic cardiopulmonary bypass. A counterproposal to the "luxury perfusion" hypothesis. Anesthesiology. 1995;83:405–12.

Dexter F, Kern FH, Hindman BJ, Greeley WJ. The brain uses mostly dissolved oxygen during profoundly hypothermic cardiopulmonary bypass. Ann Thorac Surg. 1997;63:1725–9.

Durandy Y. The impact of vacuum-assisted venous drainage and miniaturized bypass circuits on blood transfusion in pediatric cardiac surgery. ASAIO J. 2009a;55:117–20.

Durandy YD. Pediatric cardiac surgery: effect of a miniaturized bypass circuit in reducing homologous blood transfusion. J Thorac Cardiovasc Surg. 2009b;138:1454; author reply 1454–1455.

Durandy Y. Perfusionist strategies for blood conservation in pediatric cardiac surgery. World J Cardiol. 2010a;2:27–33.

Durandy Y. Warm pediatric cardiac surgery: European experience. Asian Cardiovasc Thorac Ann. 2010b;18:386–95.

Durandy Y. Vacuum-assisted venous drainage, angel or demon: PRO? J Extra Corpor Technol. 2013;45:122–7.

Durandy Y. Minimizing systemic inflammation during cardiopulmonary bypass in the pediatric population. Artif Organs. 2014;38:11–8.

Durandy Y. Use of blood products in pediatric cardiac surgery. Artif Organs. 2015;39:21–7.

Durandy YD, Hulin SH. Normothermic bypass in pediatric surgery: technical aspect and clinical experience with 1400 cases. ASAIO J. 2006;52:539–42.

Edmunds Jr LH. Advances in the heart-lung machine after John and Mary Gibbon. Ann Thorac Surg. 2003;76:S2220–3.

Eisses MJ, Geiduschek JM, Jonmarker C, Cohen GA, Chandler WL. Effect of polymer coating (poly 2-methoxyethylacrylate) of the oxygenator on hemostatic markers during cardiopulmonary bypass in children. J Cardiothorac Vasc Anesth. 2007;21:28–34.

Ferraris VA, Ferraris SP, Singh A, Fuhr W, Koppel D, McKenna D, Rodriguez E, Reich H. The platelet thrombin receptor and postoperative bleeding. Ann Thorac Surg. 1998;65:352–8.

Foglia RP, Partington MT, Buckberg GD, Leaf J. Iatrogenic myocardial edema with crystalloid primes. Effects on left ventricular compliance, performance, and perfusion. Curr Stud Hematol Blood Transfus. 1986:53–63.

Galletti PM, Brecher GA. Heart-Lung bypass principles and techniques of extracorporeal circulation. New York: Grune & Stratton; 1962. p. 171–93.

Ganushchak Y, van Marken LW, van der Nagel T, de Jong DS. Hydrodynamic performance and heat generation by centrifugal pumps. Perfusion. 2006;21:373–9.

Ginther R, Sebastian VA, Huang R, Leonard SR, Gorney R, Guleserian KJ, Forbess JM. Cerebral near-infrared spectroscopy during cardiopulmonary bypass predicts superior vena cava oxygen saturation. J Thorac Cardiovasc Surg. 2011;142:359–65.

Ginther Jr RM, Gorney R, Cruz R. A clinical evaluation of the Maquet Quadrox-i Neonatal oxygenator with integrated arterial filter. Perfusion. 2013;28:194–9.

Gottlieb EA, Fraser Jr CD, Andropoulos DB, Diaz LK. Bilateral monitoring of cerebral oxygen saturation results in recognition of aortic cannula malposition during pediatric congenital heart surgery. Paediatr Anaesth. 2006;16:787–9.

Gruber EM, Jonas RA, Newburger JW, Zurakowski D, Hansen DD, Laussen PC. The effect of hematocrit on cerebral blood flow velocity in neonates and infants undergoing deep hypothermic cardiopulmonary bypass. Anesth Analg. 1999;89:322–7.

Gu YJ, Schoen P, Tigchelaar I, Loef BG, Ebels T, Rankin AJ, van Oeveren W. Increased neutrophil priming and sensitization before commencing cardiopulmonary bypass in cardiac surgical patients. Ann Thorac Surg. 2002;74:1173–9.

Guyton AC, Polizo D, Armstrong GG. Mean circulatory filling pressure measured immediately after cessation of heart pumping. Am J Physiol. 1954;179:261–7.

Guyton AC, Lindsey AW, Abernathy B, Richardson T. Venous return at various right atrial pressures and the normal venous return curve. Am J Physiol. 1957;189:609–15.

Guyton AC, Langston JB, Carrier Jr O. Decrease of venous return caused by right atrial pulsation. Circ Res. 1962;10:188–96.

Habib RH, Zacharias A, Schwann TA, Riordan CJ, Durham SJ, Shah A. Adverse effects of low hematocrit during cardiopulmonary bypass in the adult: should current practice be changed? J Thorac Cardiovasc Surg. 2003;125:1438–50.

Haneda K, Sato S, Ishizawa E, Horiuchi T. The importance of colloid osmotic pressure during open heart surgery in infants. Tohoku J Exp Med. 1985;147:65–71.

Ihnken K, Morita K, Buckberg GD, Ignarro LJ, Beyersdorf F. Reduction of reoxygenation injury and nitric oxide production in the cyanotic immature heart by controlling pO2. Eur J Cardiothorac Surg. 1995;9:410–8.

Ihnken K, Morita K, Buckberg GD. Delayed cardioplegic reoxygenation reduces reoxygenation injury in cyanotic immature hearts. Ann Thorac Surg. 1998a;66:177–82.

Ihnken K, Winkler A, Schlensak C, Sarai K, Neidhart G, Unkelbach U, Mulsch A, Sewell A. Normoxic cardiopulmonary bypass reduces oxidative myocardial damage and nitric oxide during cardiac operations in the adult. J Thorac Cardiovasc Surg. 1998b;116:327–34.

Ince C. The rationale for microcirculatory guided fluid therapy. Curr Opin Crit Care. 2014;20:301–8.

Jonas RA, editor. Comprehensive surgical management of congenital heart disease. London: Arnold; 2004.

Kagawa H, Morita K, Uno Y, Ko Y, Matsumura Y, Kinouchi K, Hashimoto K. Inflammatory response to hyperoxemic and normoxemic cardiopulmonary bypass in acyanotic pediatric patients. World J Pediatr Congenit Heart Surg. 2014;5:541–5.

Kamiya T, Katayama Y, Kashiwagi F, Terashi A. The role of bradykinin in mediating ischemic brain edema in rats. Stroke. 1993;24:571–5; discussion 575–6.

Kaplanski G, Fabrigoule M, Boulay V, Dinarello CA, Bongrand P, Kaplanski S, Farnarier C. Thrombin induces endothelial type II activation in vitro: IL-1 and TNF-alpha-independent IL-8 secretion and E-selectin expression. J Immunol. 1997;158:5435–41.

Kaplanski G, Marin V, Fabrigoule M, Boulay V, Benoliel AM, Bongrand P, Kaplanski S, Farnarier C. Thrombin-activated human endothelial cells support monocyte adhesion in vitro following expression of intercellular adhesion molecule-1 (ICAM-1; CD54) and vascular cell adhesion molecule-1 (VCAM-1; CD106). Blood. 1998;92:1259–67.

Kim WG, Yoon CJ. Roller pump induced tubing wear of polyvinylchloride and silicone rubber tubing: phase contrast and scanning electron microscopic studies. Artif Organs. 1998;22:892–7.

Krogh A. The number and distribution of capillaries in muscles with calculations of the oxygen pressure head necessary for supplying the tissue. J Physiol. 1919;52:409–15.

Laffey JG, Boylan JF, Cheng DC. The systemic inflammatory response to cardiac surgery: implications for the anesthesiologist. Anesthesiology. 2002;97:215–52.

Landis RC. Redefining the systemic inflammatory response. Semin Cardiothorac Vasc Anesth. 2009;13:87–94.

Landis RC, Arrowsmith JE, Baker RA, de Somer F, Dobkowski WB, Fisher G, Jonas RA, Likosky DS, Murkin JM, Poullis M, Stump DA, Verrier ED. Consensus statement: defining minimal criteria for reporting the systemic inflammatory response to cardiopulmonary bypass. Heart Surg Forum. 2008;11:E316–22.

Lidington EA, Haskard DO, Mason JC. Induction of decay-accelerating factor by thrombin through a protease-activated receptor 1 and protein kinase C-dependent pathway protects vascular endothelial cells from complement-mediated injury. Blood. 2000;96:2784–92.

Lin J, Dogal NM, Mathis RK, Qiu F, Kunselman A, Undar A. Evaluation of Quadrox-i and Capiox FX neonatal oxygenators with integrated arterial filters in eliminating gaseous microemboli and retaining hemodynamic properties during simulated cardiopulmonary bypass. Perfusion. 2012;27:235–43.

Manduz S, Sapmaz I, Sanri US, Karahan O, Bascil H, Dogan K. The influence of priming solutions used in cardiopulmonary bypass on blood viscosity in hypothermic conditions. ASAIO J. 2008;54:275–7.

McBride WT, Armstrong MA, Crockard AD, McMurray TJ, Rea JM. Cytokine balance and immunosuppressive changes at cardiac surgery: contrasting response between patients and isolated CPB circuits. Br J Anaesth. 1995;75:724–33.

McCullough JN, Zhang N, Reich DL, Juvonen TS, Klein JJ, Spielvogel D, Ergin MA, Griepp RB. Cerebral metabolic suppression during hypothermic circulatory arrest in humans. Ann Thorac Surg. 1999;67:1895–9; discussion 1919–821.

Minneci PC, Deans KJ, Zhi H, Yuen PS, Star RA, Banks SM, Schechter AN, Natanson C, Gladwin MT, Solomon SB. Hemolysis-associated endothelial dysfunction mediated by accelerated NO inactivation by decompartmentalized oxyhemoglobin. J Clin Invest. 2005;115:3409–17.

Modi P, Imura H, Caputo M, Pawade A, Parry A, Angelini GD, Suleiman MS. Cardiopulmonary bypass-induced myocardial reoxygenation injury in pediatric patients with cyanosis. J Thorac Cardiovasc Surg. 2002;124:1035–6.

Moerman A, Denys W, De Somer F, Wouters PF, De Hert SG. Influence of variations in systemic blood flow and pressure on cerebral and systemic oxygen saturation in cardiopulmonary bypass patients. Br J Anaesth. 2013;111:619–26.

Monroe DM, Hoffman M, Roberts HR. Platelets and thrombin generation. Arterioscler Thromb Vasc Biol. 2002;22:1381–9.

Murai N, Cho M, Okada S, Chiba T, Saito M, Shioguchi S, Gon S, Hata I, Yamauchi N, Imazeki T. Venous drainage method for cardiopulmonary bypass in single-access minimally invasive cardiac surgery: siphon and vacuum-assisted drainage. J Artif Organs. 2005;8:91–4.

Ni YM, Leskosek B, Shi LP, Chen YL, Qian LF, Li RY, Tu ZL, von Segesser LK. Optimization of venous return tubing diameter for cardiopulmonary bypass. Eur J Cardiothorac Surg. 2001;20:614–20.

Nicolas F, Daniel JP, Bruniaux J, Serraf A, Lacour-Gayet F, Planche C. Conventional cardiopulmonary bypass in neonates. A physiological approach – 10 years of experience at Marie-Lannelongue Hospital. Perfusion. 1994;9:41–8.

Pappalardo F, Corno C, Franco A, Giardina G, Scandroglio AM, Landoni G, Crescenzi G, Zangrillo A. Reduction of hemodilution in small adults undergoing open heart surgery: a prospective, randomized trial. Perfusion. 2007;22:317–22.

Pearl JM, Thomas DW, Grist G, Duffy JY, Manning PB. Hyperoxia for management of acid-base status during deep hypothermia with circulatory arrest. Ann Thorac Surg. 2000;70:751–5.

Peek GJ, Thompson A, Killer HM, Firmin RK. Spallation performance of extracorporeal membrane oxygenation tubing. Perfusion. 2000;15:457–66.

Pouard P, Bojan M. Neonatal cardiopulmonary bypass. Semin Thorac Cardiovasc Surg Pediatr Card Surg Annu. 2013;16:59–61.

Poullis M, Manning R, Laffan M, Haskard DO, Taylor KM, Landis RC. The antithrombotic effect of aprotinin: actions mediated via the proteaseactivated receptor 1. J Thorac Cardiovasc Surg. 2000;120:370–8.

Ranucci M, Romitti F, Isgro G, Cotza M, Brozzi S, Boncilli A, Ditta A. Oxygen delivery during cardiopulmonary bypass and acute renal failure after coronary operations. Ann Thorac Surg. 2005;80:2213–20.

Redlin M, Huebler M, Boettcher W, Kuppe H, Hetzer R, Habazettl H. How near-infrared spectroscopy differentiates between lower body ischemia due to arterial occlusion versus venous outflow obstruction. Ann Thorac Surg. 2011;91:1274–6.

Rothlein R, Kishimoto TK, Mainolfi E. Cross-linking of ICAM-1 induces co-signaling of an oxidative burst from mononuclear leukocytes. J Immunol. 1994;152:2488–95.

Sakamoto T, Hatsuoka S, Stock UA, Duebener LF, Lidov HG, Holmes GL, Sperling JS, Munakata M, Laussen PC, Jonas RA. Prediction of safe duration of hypothermic circulatory arrest by near-infrared spectroscopy. J Thorac Cardiovasc Surg. 2001;122:339–50.

Shappell SB, Toman C, Anderson DC, Taylor AA, Entman ML, Smith CW. Mac-1 (CD11b/CD18) mediates adherence-dependent hydrogen peroxide production by human and canine neutrophils. J Immunol. 1990;144:2702–11.

Tamari Y, Lee-Sensiba K, Leonard EF, Tortolani AJ. A dynamic method for setting roller pumps nonocclusively reduces hemolysis and predicts retrograde flow. ASAIO J. 1997;43:39–52.

Tsai AG, Friesenecker B, McCarthy M, Sakai H, Intaglietta M. Plasma viscosity regulates capillary perfusion during extreme hemodilution in hamster skinfold model. Am J Physiol. 1998;275:H2170–80.

Tsai AG, Acero C, Nance PR, Cabrales P, Frangos JA, Buerk DG, Intaglietta M. Elevated plasma viscosity in extreme hemodilution increases perivascular nitric oxide concentration and microvascular perfusion. Am J Physiol. 2005;288:H1730–9.

Tweddell JS, Hoffman GM, Mussatto KA, Fedderly RT, Berger S, Jaquiss RD, Ghanayem NS, Frisbee SJ, Litwin SB. Improved survival of patients undergoing palliation of hypoplastic left heart syndrome: lessons learned from 115 consecutive patients. Circulation. 2002;106:I82–9.

Wachtfogel YT, Hack CE, Nuijens JH, Kettner C, Reilly TM, Knabb RM, Bischoff R, Tschesche H, Wenzel H, Kucich U, et al. Selective kallikrein inhibitors alter human neutrophil elastase release during extracorporeal circulation. Am J Physiol. 1995;268:H1352–7.

Wilkinson KL, Brunskill SJ, Doree C, Trivella M, Gill R, Murphy MF. 2014. Red cell transfusion management for patients undergoing cardiac surgery for congenital heart disease. Cochrane Database Syst Rev. (2):CD009752.

Chapter 17
Atrioventricular Septal Defect (AVSD)

Ali Dabbagh and Iki Adachi

Introduction

Atrioventricular septal defect (AVSD) is a collective term for a spectrum of congenital heart disorders that are characterized by a deficiency of myocardial tissue at the atrioventricular (AV) junction. This group of hearts is also described as:

- Atrioventricular canal defect
- Common atrioventricular orifice
- Endocardial cushion defect
- Ostium primum atrial septal defect

AVSD occurs in two out of every 10,000 live births (Calabro and Limongelli 2006).

Cardiac Anatomy and Embryology

Since congenital heart diseases result from abnormal development of the heart during fetal life, understanding in cardiac embryology helps to explain how various cardiac malformations have developed. Nonetheless, it must be noted that many of

A. Dabbagh, MD (✉)
Cardiac Anesthesiology Department, Anesthesiology Research Center,
Shahid Beheshti University of Medical Sciences, Tehran, Iran
e-mail: alidabbagh@yahoo.com; alidabbagh@sbmu.ac.ir

I. Adachi, MD
Division of Congenital Heart Surgery, Baylor College of Medicine, Houston, TX, USA

Mechanical Circulatory Support, Texas Children's Hospital, Houston, TX, USA
e-mail: ixadachi@texaschildrens.org; iadachi@bcm.edu

© Springer International Publishing Switzerland 2017
A. Dabbagh et al. (eds.), *Congenital Heart Disease in Pediatric
and Adult Patients*, DOI 10.1007/978-3-319-44691-2_17

the embryologic explanations remain speculative without concrete evidence. It may be safer, therefore, to use the knowledge in embryology as a tool for better understanding in cardiac anatomy, rather than to consider them as scientific facts. The main etiologic mechanism of AVSD is believed to be impaired development of the "endocardial cushions"; hence, the term "endocardial cushion defect" is applied. Some researchers consider the endocardial cushions as the "forerunners" of the AV valves (Gaussin et al. 2005).

AVSD occurs approximately at the fifth week of gestation, i.e., when the superior and inferior endocardial cushions are going to be created and appear over the primitive left ventricle (LV) (Ray and Niswander 2012). The cells that constitute the endocardial cushion tissues are primarily endocardial in origin; however, these endothelial cells migrate into the inner layers of the heart tube to create the primitive mesodermal tissue of this tube, which is located in the crux of the heart. This critical process in formation of cardiac cushions is called *endothelial to mesenchymal transition of endothelial cells* in cardiac cushions (Zhang et al. 2014; Davey and Rychik 2016).

A range of cellular and molecular factors play a role in the development of cardiac cushions; would any of them be impaired, it may lead to endocardial cushion defects as demonstrated in the previous animal models:

- Transforming growth factors (TGFs) and proteins (like bone morphogenetic protein (BMP))
- Intercellular signaling molecules and enzymes
- Transcription factors and mutations in their related genes, like GATA4 transcription factor, TGF beta, FOG factor, Smad4, Zic family member 3 (Zic3), NK2 homeobox 5 (Nkx2.5), and T-box protein 5 (Tbx5)
- Extracellular matrices (Yamagishi et al. 2009; Moskowitz et al. 2011; Ray and Niswander 2012; Garside et al. 2013; Liu et al. 2013; Kathiriya et al. 2015; Stefanovic and Christoffels 2015)

The abnormal development of the endocardial cushions results in the defect in the septum at the crux of the heart and the loss of normal development of the AV valves. Since the degree of abnormalities in the septum and the AV valves varies considerably, there are various different phenotypes within the spectrum of AVSD. Cardiac morphology and physiology of AVSD are more understandable if one takes the following pathologic features into account:

1. *The common atrioventricular junction*: in normally structured hearts, the AV junction is "8-shaped," with two separate junctions for the mitral and tricuspid valves. In hearts with AVSD, there is no separation of the two junctions, forming a common "oval-shaped" ring, also known as "common atrioventricular valvular junction" (with often but not always with five leaflets).
2. *The defect in the septal structure*: in virtually all of the hearts with AVSD, there is a defect in the septum at the crux of the heart. Depending on the relationship of the AV valves and the septal defect, the defect can be at the ventricular level, at the atrial level, or the combination of both. For example, when the AV valve

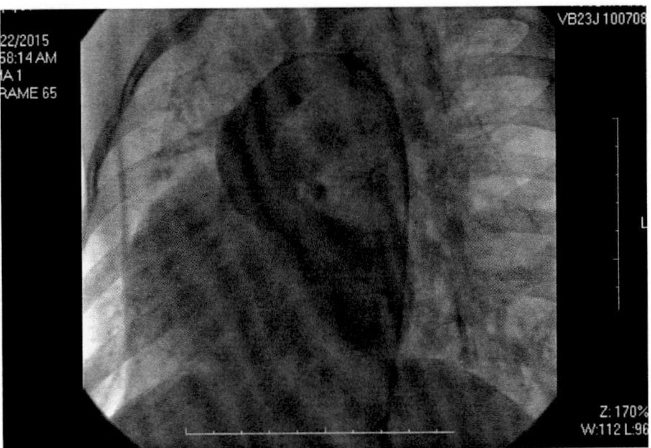

Fig. 17.1 Angiographic presentation of AVSD known as "goose neck deformity" before the start of systole

leaflets are completely adherent to the undersurface of the atrial septum, the resultant defect will limit the intracardiac shunting at the ventricular level (i.e., the so-called AV canal-type VSD). On the other hand, if the AV leaflets are completely adherent to the crest of the ventricular septum, the shunting will be only at the atrial level (i.e., ostium primum defect). In other forms, the leaflets of the common AV valve close neither, leaving the shunting at both the atrial and ventricular levels (i.e., complete AVSD) (Wenink and Zevallos 1988; Adachi et al. 2008, 2009a, b).

3. *Left ventricular outflow tract (LVOT)*: the pathologic feature of the AV valve junction (loss of normal the 8-shaped ring and resultant *oval-shaped ring*) impacts the morphology of the left ventricular outflow tract (LVOT). In normally structured hearts, the aorta is cradled in the waist of the 8-shaped AV junction. By contrast, the aorta is located more anteriorly in AVSD because of the loss of the "waist" at the AV junction due to the oval-shaped ring. Such an anterior location of the aorta will make the LVOT elongated, called *anterior scooping* of the aorta. In normal hearts, the LVOT length (i.e., the length from the cardiac apex to the aortic valve) is approximately equal to the LV inflow length (i.e., the length from the cardiac apex to the mitral valve). In AVSD, however, the LVOT length is increased relative to the inlet length. This anatomical feature is responsible for the typical angiographic appearance known as *goose neck deformity*; see Figs. 17.1, 17.2, and 17.3 (Craig 2006; Mahle et al. 2006; Adachi et al. 2008, 2009a, b, c; Shuhaiber et al. 2009).

Pathologic Findings and Associated Anomalies

The three main mechanisms described in the previous section lead to the pathologic findings seen in AVSD; all of them are the result of the main faulty developmental defect, i.e., *endocardial cushion defect*. The main pathologies found in patients with AVSD are the following (Craig 2006; Adachi et al. 2008):

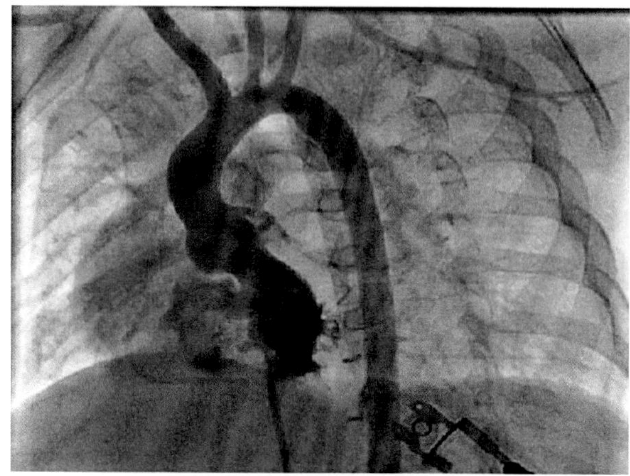

Fig. 17.2 Angiographic presentation of AVSD known as "goose neck deformity" in systole

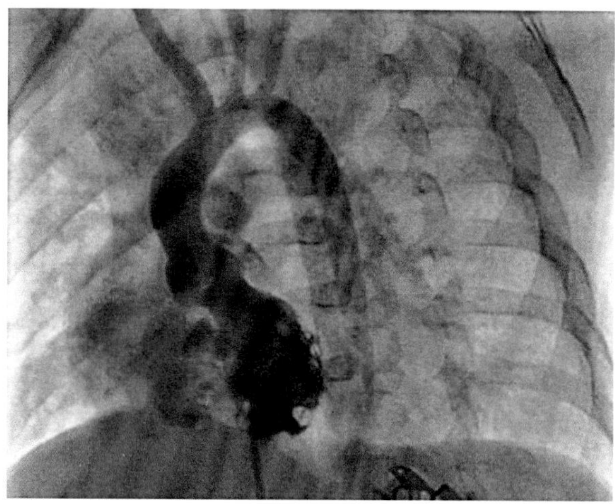

Fig. 17.3 Angiographic presentation of AVSD known as "goose neck deformity" in early systole

1. In normal hearts, each AV valve has a separate annular ring: one for the mitral valve and the other for the tricuspid valve. In hearts with AVSD, there exists *only one common valve ring*, i.e., just we could imagine that the AV junction failed to separate during fetal life, resulting in one common AV valve ring. This common annulus does not follow the normal figure of eight seen in normal AV valves; instead one ovale ring exits for connecting between atria and ventricles.

2. Normal mitral and tricuspid leaflets are not seen anymore; instead, a special anatomic configuration exists in these leaflets often described under the *Rastelli classification*. The common AV valve typically, but not always, has 5-leaflet configuration with common AV valve annulus (i.e., complete AVSD). Occasionally, there are two AV valve annuli within the common AV valve junction if a piece of tissue "band" divides the common AV valve to two separate orifices (i.e., partial

AVSD). The two orifices create separate right and left passages for blood. Despite having two AV valve annuli, however, these hearts still have a common AV valve junction, which is the fundamental feature of AVSD.

3. The pathologic annulus (i.e., oval-shaped common AV valve junction) decreases the space needed for the LVOT and aorta to emerge from the left ventricle; so, there is an anterior deviation and tendency for the aorta and LVOT named as *anterior scooping* of the aorta; see Figs. 17.1, 17.2, and 17.3 (Adachi et al. 2009a, b).

4. The anterior scooping of the aorta lengthens the course of blood movement from the LV through LVOT; in the normal hearts, the distance from the mitral valve till the LV apex (i.e., the LV inlet) is approximately equivalent to the distance from the LV apex to the aortic valve (i.e., LV outlet) causing the LV outlet/inlet ratio of 1/1. In AVSD, however, this ratio is increased due to anterior scooping of LVOT.

5. Orientation of the papillary muscles is different in hearts with AVSD. For example, the papillary muscles of the left AV valve in AVSD have more or less *superior-inferior orientation*, while the papillary muscles of the normal mitral valve have oblique orientation.

6. Defects in the interatrial septum with resultant shunting at the atrial level (*ASD primum*) are seen often in hearts with AVSD. There exist hearts with AVSD but not having primum ASD. This rare subset is called "AVSD with only ventricular component" (Adachi et al. 2009c). This rare form of AVSD is not often seen in clinical setting in part because this anatomy is considered as "AV canal-type VSD" or "inlet VSD." However, it must be remembered that what differentiates hearts with AVSD from VSD is the presence of common AV valve junction. Regardless of the level of intracardiac shunting, the hearts should be categorized under the spectrum of AVSD if there is a common AV junction.

7. Defects in the caudal and posterior section of the ventricular septum create shunting at the ventricular level as seen in *intermediate* and *complete* types of AVSD. As mentioned above, the ventricular-level defect is often called *inlet-type VSD*. However, care must be taken to use this terminology since "VSD" implies there is normal separation of the AV valve junctions.

8. The common AV valve typically has 5-leaflet configuration:

   - Superior bridging leaflets, *SBL* (also named anterior bridging leaflet).
   - Inferior bridging leaflets, *IBL* (also named posterior bridging leaflet); both SBL and IBL cross over the interventricular septum; also, each of these two leaflets is attached to both the right ventricle and left ventricle through chordae tendineae, though the chordae and their anatomic arrangement are different from normal.
   - Right anterolateral leaflet.
   - Right mural leaflet.
   - Left mural leaflet.

Classification of AVSD

In general, hearts with AVSD are classified into three subtypes based on the level of intracardiac shunting (Jacobs et al. 2000; Craig 2006; Adachi et al. 2008, 2009c; Shuhaiber et al. 2009; Buratto et al. 2014; Xie et al. 2014):

- *Complete AVSD* (both atrial- and ventricular-level shunting with a common AV valve). Complete AVSD is further subdivided to "Rastelli type A," "Rastelli type B," and "Rastelli type C" depending on the status of the superior bridging leaflet relative to the crest of the ventricular septum; detailed description of the Rastelli classification could be found in selected references.
- *Partial AVSD* (the so-called ostium primum ASD plus *cleft mitral valve*) in which a tongue of tissue attaches the two SB leaflet and IB leaflet to create two separate orifices in the common AV valve; however, these two orifices are never true valves because they do not have real structure of separate and complete annulus, and their leaflets have minimal resemblance to the leaflets of the normal hearts.
- *AVSD with only ventricular component* (typically described as *AV canal-type VSD*). This subtype of AVSD represents the mildest form of hearts with AVSD within the spectrum of AVSD. It is the least common form of the disease.

Associated Cardiac Anomalies

At times, AVSD is accompanied with some other cardiac malformations which complicate perioperative management and surgical procedure. The following cardiac anomalies may accompany AVSD (Craig 2006; Tchervenkov et al. 2006; Mitchell et al. 2007; Shuhaiber et al. 2009; Karl et al. 2010):

- Tetralogy of Fallot (TOF) (which associated with complete AVSD and its combination results in RVOTO in AVSD)
- Left ventricular outflow tract obstruction (congenital LVOTO) overlying AVCD
- Subaortic stenosis
- Double outlet right ventricle (DORV)
- Truncus arteriosus (or common arterial trunk)
- Common AV valve with single ventricle pathology
- Ventricular hypoplasia
- Left AV valve with double orifice
- Unbalanced complete AVCD
- Transposition of great arteries (TGA)
- Atrial isomerism (left or right type of isomerism)

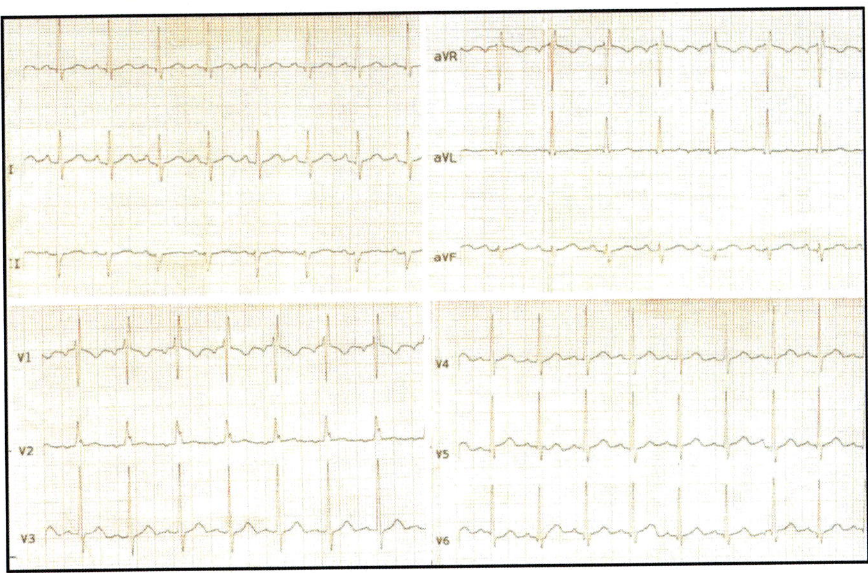

Fig. 17.4 Complete AVSD with left axis deviation, incomplete RBBB, and biventricular hypertrophy (Courtesy of Dr. Majid Haghjoo and Dr. Mohammad Rafie Khorgami)

Clinical Presentation and Diagnosis of the Disease

The clinical findings in AVSD usually present with signs and symptoms of heart failure and failure to thrive, both of them with varying degrees. Also, cyanosis is usually either mild or absent. The findings related to pulmonary hypertension or pulmonary overflow like tachypnea and reduced activity may be seen.

ECG findings are the result of anatomic abnormalities in the interventricular septum (Fig. 17.4):

- P wave abnormalities including superior P wave axis are seen in patients with left atrial isomerism; superior axis deviation is considered as one of the most characteristic findings in AVSD patients.
- AV node displacement from its normal position, leading to an enlarged bundle which paves its course alongside the ventricular septum.
- Axis is deviated from −40 to −150.
- Prolongation of the PR interval is due to intra-atrial conduction delay and may be seen in about 50 % of patients (first-degree AV block).
- Right bundle branch block (RBBB) (usually partial block).
- RVH pattern is always seen; however, LVH may be observed.
- *The most characteristic finding* in AVSD is superior orientation of the frontal QRS wave, i.e., superiorly oriented counterclockwise QRS loop; this loop

resembles "a figure-of-eight QRS loop" which lies on the upper part of the iso-electric line in the frontal plane; QRS is usually rSr´ or rsR´; also, QRS has moderate-to-severe left axis deviation (Feldt et al. 1970; Craig 2006; Khairy and Marelli 2007).

Echocardiography

Transthoracic echocardiography is the method of choice for preoperative diagnostic assessment. Intraoperative transesophageal echocardiography (TEE) provides even more detailed information necessary for surgical repair. These findings can be seen in intraoperative TEE (Craig 2006; Cohen and Stevenson 2007):

- Right ventricular (RV) hypertrophy.
- Right atrial (RA) hypertrophy.
- ASD.
- VSD: its severity depends on the subtype of disease.
- Different degrees of tricuspid regurgitation (TR) which would depend on the structure of the right side of the AV valve and also the severity of pulmonary hypertension.
- Pulmonary artery dilation especially when overflow of the pulmonary system is a marked finding.
- Subvalvular aortic stenosis (due to the effects of mitral chordae and scooped aorta) though not a common finding could be seen in some patients and mandates sophisticated TEE assessments following surgical correction immediately after weaning from bypass.

Surgical Repair

A number of factors impact the outcome of surgical repair for AVSD, which includes the repair technique, underlying chromosomal abnormalities, severity of the disease and its subtypes seen in each patient, other associated cardiac anomalies, severity of regurgitation in common AV valve, age-matched z scores, and a number of other factors (Craig 2006; Halit et al. 2008; Karl et al. 2010; Ong et al. 2012).

The first successful repair of AVSD was performed in 1954 on a 17-month-old girl by Lillehei et al. Since then, various different approaches have been used for repair of AVSD (Wilcox et al. 1997; Nicholson et al. 1999; Backer et al. 2007; Nunn 2007; Halit et al. 2008; Shuhaiber et al. 2009; Jonas and Mora 2010):

1 *Traditional single-patch technique* which utilizes one patch for closure of both ASD and VSD. The AV valves are divided into the right and left components and sutured to the single patch through a right atriotomy.

2 *Standard two-patch technique* which uses two separate patches for ASD and VSD, usually the pericardium for ASD and one "pericardium, PTFE, or the Dacron patch" for VSD.

3 *Modified single-patch technique* or the *Australian technique* described by Nicholson and Nunn in 1999 uses primary suture for VSD closure; i.e., as they described, they used "direct suturing of the common AV valve leaflets to the crest of the ventricular septum without using any material." The fundamental feature of this technique is a conversion of complete AVSD anatomy into "ostium primum ASD" anatomy, by suturing down the AV valve tissue directly on the crest of the ventricular septum. Owing to its simplicity, this technique has been gaining more popularity over the last decade. Some believe that this technique is best appropriate for younger patients (with an ideal age of 4 months). This technique results in significantly shorter bypass time and cross clamp time (Nicholson et al. 1999). Care must be taken, however, that this technique can result in distortion of the AV valve if the VSD component is very deep or asymmetrical (Adachi et al. 2009b).

4 *No-patch technique* which uses the common AV valve tissue for closing ASD and VSD.

Often, in these methods of repair, a right atriotomy is used, a number of maneuvers are done for preservation of the His bundle, the AV valve is repaired to prevent excessive postoperative regurgitation (sometimes annuloplasty is added to further correct the valves), and a left atrial catheter (LAC) is placed and fixed as the final step before weaning from bypass by the surgeon.

Intraoperative Management of Anesthesia

Table 17.1 demonstrates in brief the main challenges in anesthetic management of AVSD patients (Craig 2006; Shuhaiber et al. 2009).

There are a number of modalities used for the management of pulmonary hypertension before, during, and after CPB including (Craig 2006; Shuhaiber et al. 2009):

- Sophisticated multimodal cardiac monitoring including invasive blood pressure, TEE, NIRS, left atrial pressure, cardiac output monitoring, and other modes of monitoring which should be tailored for each patient

Table 17.1 Main challenges in anesthetic management of AVSD

Degree of left-to-right shunting
Management of pulmonary hypertension and RV failure
LV dysfunction and low cardiac output state (LCOS)
AV valve regurgitation (mitral regurgitation and/or tricuspid insufficiency)
AV conduction block and/or arrhythmias
Defects in surgical repair and/or residual shunt
Airway management which could be a real challenge especially when considering the large size of the tongue in trisomy 21 patients

- A combination of inotropes and vasopressors to augment hemodynamics adjusted by the use of monitoring data
- The use of inhaled nitric oxide (NO)
- Management of ventilation parameters to prevent overt PEEP and/or hyperventilation
- Controlling depth of anesthesia using enough analgesics
- Prevention of hypothermia

On the other hand, elevated filling pressures should be avoided in ventricles to prevent annular dilation of the AV valves and hence prevent AV regurgitation; left atrial pressure catheter is a useful monitor; LA pressure in the range of less than 10 mmHg is considered appropriate for weaning from cardiopulmonary bypass.

Postoperative Care for AVSD

The patients are not often extubated early; this might be longer in trisomy 21 with AVSD. Again, invasive blood pressure monitoring, NIRS, adequate pain management, management of blood pressure using inotropes and/or vasopressors, prevention of pulmonary hypertension using adequate analgesics, and pulmonary vasodilator strategies are among the main therapeutic methods used for postoperative care of these patients.

Reoperation

Early reoperation: Early reoperation is necessary especially when there is residual gap or any other suboptimal results of surgery, including severe AV valve regurgitation, LVOTO, or RVOT; the latter is usually seen when AVSD and TOF are superimposed (Shuhaiber et al. 2009; Bianchi et al. 2011; Raisky et al. 2014). Careful assessment with TEE after weaning from cardiopulmonary bypass should eliminate the need for early reoperation.

Reoperation in adults: Based on the ACC/AHA 2008 Guidelines, the following are the main indications for reoperation in adults (Warnes et al. 2008)

- Left AV valve regurgitation and stenosis which are symptomatic or cause arrhythmias (atrial or ventricular) or lead to progressive increase in dimensions of LV or deterioration of LV function; these need either valve repair or valve replacement.
- LVOT obstruction which has a mean gradient more than 50 mmHg or a peak instantaneous gradient more than 70 mmHg or LVOTO with a gradient less than 50 mmHg but associated with significant mitral regurgitation or aortic regurgitation.
- Residual and/or recurrent ASD or VSD which is associated with significant left-to-right shunt.

Outcome

The overall mortality rate for AVSD repair in experienced centers is in the range of 1–3 %. This is, however, largely dependent on the presence or absence of other factors such as prematurity, chronic lung disease, and chromosomal abnormalities. Mortality doubles with associated lesions especially if there are ≥2 major noncardiac anomalies. The best outcome is gained if repair is performed before the patient develops significant pulmonary disease. Approximately, the age of 3–6 months would be considered appropriate for surgical repair. The outcome of the patients does not seem to be overly influenced by the presence of trisomy 21, though some believe AVSD patients with trisomy 21 may have a better outcome. Anecdotally, patients without trisomy 21 tend to have more complex and dysmorphic AV valve morphology. Occurrence of left AV valve incompetency as well as LVOT obstruction is potential complications in the intermediate to long term. It remains to be seen which surgical technique (i.e., single-patch, modified single-patch, or two-patch techniques) would provide superior outcome in the long term (Tchervenkov et al. 2006; Shuhaiber et al. 2009; Miller et al. 2010; Atz et al. 2011; Bianchi et al. 2011; Raisky et al. 2014; Xie et al. 2014; Calkoen et al. 2016).

References

Adachi I, Uemura H, McCarthy KP, Ho SY. Surgical anatomy of atrioventricular septal defect. Asian Cardiovasc Thorac Ann. 2008;16:497–502.

Adachi I, Ho SY, Bartelings MM, McCarthy KP, Seale A, Uemura H. Common arterial trunk with atrioventricular septal defect: new observations pertinent to repair. Ann Thorac Surg. 2009a;87:1495–9.

Adachi I, Ho SY, McCarthy KP, Uemura H. Ventricular scoop in atrioventricular septal defect: relevance to simplified single-patch method. Ann Thorac Surg. 2009b;87:198–203.

Adachi I, Uemura H, McCarthy KP, Ho SY. Morphologic features of atrioventricular septal defect with only ventricular component: further observations pertinent to surgical repair. J Thorac Cardiovasc Surg. 2009c;137:132–8. 138 e131-132.

Atz AM, Hawkins JA, Lu M, Cohen MS, Colan SD, Jaggers J, Lacro RV, McCrindle BW, Margossian R, Mosca RS, Sleeper LA, Minich LL. Surgical management of complete atrioventricular septal defect: associations with surgical technique, age, and trisomy 21. J Thorac Cardiovasc Surg. 2011;141:1371–9.

Backer CL, Stewart RD, Mavroudis C. What is the best technique for repair of complete atrioventricular canal? Semin Thorac Cardiovasc Surg. 2007;19:249–57.

Bianchi G, Bevilacqua S, Solinas M, Glauber M. In adult patients undergoing redo surgery for left atrioventricular valve regurgitation after atrioventricular septal defect correction, is replacement superior to repair? Interact Cardiovasc Thorac Surg. 2011;12:1033–9.

Buratto E, McCrossan B, Galati JC, Bullock A, Kelly A, d'Udekem Y, Brizard CP, Konstantinov IE. Repair of partial atrioventricular septal defect: a 37-year experience. Eur J Cardiothorac Surg. 2015;47(5):796–802.

Calabro R, Limongelli G. Complete atrioventricular canal. Orphanet J Rare Dis. 2006;1:8.

Calkoen EE, Hazekamp MG, Blom NA, Elders BB, Gittenberger-de Groot AC, Haak MC, Bartelings MM, Roest AA, Jongbloed MR. Atrioventricular septal defect: From embryonic development to long-term follow-up. Int J Cardiol. 2016;202:784–95.

Cohen GA, Stevenson JG. Intraoperative echocardiography for atrioventricular canal: decision-making for surgeons. Semin Thorac Cardiovasc Surg Pediatr Card Surg Annu. 2007;10(1):47–50.

Craig B. Atrioventricular septal defect: from fetus to adult. Heart. 2006;92:1879–85.

Davey BT, Rychik J. The Natural History of Atrioventricular Valve Regurgitation Throughout Fetal Life in Patients with Atrioventricular Canal Defects. Pediatr Cardiol. 2016;37:50–4.

Feldt RH, DuShane JW, Titus JL. The atrioventricular conduction system in persistent common atrioventricular canal defect: correlations with electrocardiogram. Circulation. 1970;42:437–44.

Garside VC, Chang AC, Karsan A, Hoodless PA. Co-ordinating Notch, BMP, and TGF-beta signaling during heart valve development. Cell Mol Life Sci. 2013;70:2899–917.

Gaussin V, Morley GE, Cox L, Zwijsen A, Vance KM, Emile L, Tian Y, Liu J, Hong C, Myers D, Conway SJ, Depre C, Mishina Y, Behringer RR, Hanks MC, Schneider MD, Huylebroeck D, Fishman GI, Burch JB, Vatner SF. Alk3/Bmpr1a receptor is required for development of the atrioventricular canal into valves and annulus fibrosus. Circ Res. 2005;97:219–26.

Halit V, Oktar GL, Imren VY, Iriz E, Erer D, Kula S, Tunaoglu FS, Gokgoz L, Olgunturk R. Traditional single patch versus the "Australian" technique for repair of complete atrioventricular canal defects. Surg Today. 2008;38:999–1003.

Jacobs JP, Burke RP, Quintessenza JA, Mavroudis C. Congenital Heart Surgery Nomenclature and Database Project: atrioventricular canal defect. Ann Thorac Surg. 2000;69:S36–43.

Jonas RA, Mora B. Individualized approach to repair of complete atrioventricular canal: selective use of the traditional single-patch technique versus the Australian technique. World J Pediatr Congenit Heart Surg. 2010;1:78–86.

Karl TR, Provenzano SC, Nunn GR, Anderson RH. The current surgical perspective to repair of atrioventricular septal defect with common atrioventricular junction. Cardiol Young. 2010;20 Suppl 3:120–7.

Kathiriya IS, Nora EP, Bruneau BG. Investigating the transcriptional control of cardiovascular development. Circ Res. 2015;116:700–14.

Khairy P, Marelli AJ. Clinical use of electrocardiography in adults with congenital heart disease. Circulation. 2007;116:2734–46.

Liu Y, Lu X, Xiang FL, Lu M, Feng Q. Nitric oxide synthase-3 promotes embryonic development of atrioventricular valves. PLoS One. 2013;8, e77611.

Mahle WT, Shirali GS, Anderson RH. Echo-morphological correlates in patients with atrioventricular septal defect and common atrioventricular junction. Cardiol Young. 2006;16 Suppl 3:43–51.

Miller A, Siffel C, Lu C, Riehle-Colarusso T, Frias JL, Correa A. Long-term survival of infants with atrioventricular septal defects. J Pediatr. 2010;156:994–1000.

Mitchell ME, Litwin SB, Tweddell JS. Complex atrioventricular canal. Semin Thorac Cardiovasc Surg Pediatr Card Surg Annu. 2007;10(1):32–41.

Moskowitz IP, Wang J, Peterson MA, Pu WT, Mackinnon AC, Oxburgh L, Chu GC, Sarkar M, Berul C, Smoot L, Robertson EJ, Schwartz R, Seidman JG, Seidman CE. Transcription factor genes Smad4 and Gata4 cooperatively regulate cardiac valve development. [corrected]. Proc Natl Acad Sci U S A. 2011;108:4006–11.

Nicholson IA, Nunn GR, Sholler GF, Hawker RE, Cooper SG, Lau KC, Cohn SL. Simplified single patch technique for the repair of atrioventricular septal defect. J Thorac Cardiovasc Surg. 1999;118:642–6.

Nunn GR. Atrioventricular canal: modified single patch technique. Semin Thorac Cardiovasc Surg Pediatr Card Surg Annu. 2007;10(1):28–31.

Ong J, Brizard CP, d'Udekem Y, Weintraub R, Robertson T, Cheung M, Konstantinov IE. Repair of atrioventricular septal defect associated with tetralogy of Fallot or double-outlet right ventricle: 30 years of experience. Ann Thorac Surg. 2012;94:172–8.

Raisky O, Gerelli S, Murtuza B, Vouhe P. Repair of complete atrioventricular septal defect: close to the moon? From giant leap for the medical community to small steps for our patients. Eur J Cardiothorac Surg. 2014;45:618–9.

Ray HJ, Niswander L. Mechanisms of tissue fusion during development. Development. 2012;139:1701–11.

Shuhaiber JH, Ho SY, Rigby M, Sethia B. Current options and outcomes for the management of atrioventricular septal defect. Eur J Cardiothorac Surg. 2009;35:891–900.

Stefanovic S, Christoffels VM. GATA-dependent transcriptional and epigenetic control of cardiac lineage specification and differentiation. Cell Mol Life Sci. 2015;72:3871–81.

Tchervenkov CI, Hill S, Del Duca D, Korkola S. Surgical repair of atrioventricular septal defect with common atrioventricular junction when associated with tetralogy of Fallot or double outlet right ventricle. Cardiol Young. 2006;16 Suppl 3:59–64.

Warnes CA, Williams RG, Bashore TM, Child JS, Connolly HM, Dearani JA, Del Nido P, Fasules JW, Graham Jr TP, Hijazi ZM, Hunt SA, King ME, Landzberg MJ, Miner PD, Radford MJ, Walsh EP, Webb GD. ACC/AHA 2008 Guidelines for the Management of Adults with Congenital Heart Disease: Executive Summary: a report of the American College of Cardiology/American Heart Association Task Force on Practice Guidelines (writing committee to develop guidelines for the management of adults with congenital heart disease). Circulation. 2008;118:2395–451.

Wenink AC, Zevallos JC. Developmental aspects of atrioventricular septal defects. Int J Cardiol. 1988;18:65–78.

Wilcox BR, Jones DR, Frantz EG, Brink LW, Henry GW, Mill MR, Anderson RH. Anatomically sound, simplified approach to repair of "complete" atrioventricular septal defect. Ann Thorac Surg. 1997;64:487–93. discussion 493–484.

Xie O, Brizard CP, d'Udekem Y, Galati JC, Kelly A, Yong MS, Weintraub RG, Konstantinov IE. Outcomes of repair of complete atrioventricular septal defect in the current era. Eur J Cardiothorac Surg. 2014;45:610–7.

Yamagishi T, Ando K, Nakamura H. Roles of TGFbeta and BMP during valvulo-septal endocardial cushion formation. Anat Sci Int. 2009;84:77–87.

Zhang H, von Gise A, Liu Q, Hu T, Tian X, He L, Pu W, Huang X, He L, Cai CL, Camargo FD, Pu WT, Zhou B. Yap1 is required for endothelial to mesenchymal transition of the atrioventricular cushion. J Biol Chem. 2014;289:18681–92.

Chapter 18
Atrial Septal Defect and Ventricular Septal Defect

Ali Dabbagh

Atrial Septal Defect

Introduction

Atrial septal defect (ASD) is the general name for a number of diseases which their etiology is mainly a congenital defect in the interatrial septum. ASD, after bicuspid aortic valve and mitral valve prolapse, is the third most common congenital heart disease; also, it is much more frequent in women than men (McCarthy et al. 2003; Geva et al. 2014).

Embryology

Detailed discussions on the embryology of ASD could be found in Chap. 2 – Cardiovascular System Embryology and Its Development – however, a brief discussion is presented here.

The septation process is an embryologic stage leading to chamber formation; this process in the common atrium starts at the beginning of the fifth week and includes the following steps (McCarthy et al. 2003; Gittenberger-de Groot et al. 2005; Sukernik and Bennett-Guerrero 2007; Asrress et al. 2015; Calkoen et al. 2016):

1. A sickle-formed crest comes down from the roof of the common atrium, which makes *septum primum.*
2. Septum primum develops caudally toward endocardial cushion in the atrioventricular canal.

A. Dabbagh, MD
Cardiac Anesthesiology Department, Anesthesiology Research Center,
Shahid Beheshti University of Medical Sciences, Tehran, Iran
e-mail: alidabbagh@yahoo.com; alidabbagh@sbmu.ac.ir

© Springer International Publishing Switzerland 2017
A. Dabbagh et al. (eds.), *Congenital Heart Disease in Pediatric and Adult Patients*, DOI 10.1007/978-3-319-44691-2_18

3. Now, *ostium primum* is in the common atrium, allowing interatrial blood flow.
4. Superior parts of septum primum are fenestrated by apoptosis; so *ostium secundum* is created, allowing right-to-left shunt in the fetal circulation; the obliterated superior part of the septum primum will be completed by *septum secundum*.
5. From the common atrial wall roof, a crescent muscular mass grows downward on the right side of the septum primum, producing the superior parts of interatrial septum; it covers the main part of the *ostium secundum* and is called *septum secundum*.
6. Now, we nearly have the future interatrial septum which is composed of two merging septa: *septum primum* and *septum secundum*.
7. There is a defect in the septum secundum called *fossa ovalis* which is usually compensated by *septum primum*; however, a wide range of defects may affect fossa ovalis and, hence, create gaps or deficiencies in the flap valve.
8. Also, there is *foramen ovale*, a defect in the borders of septum primum and septum secundum, which is an obliquely elongated cleft in the interatrial septum; it will be open as long as fetal circulation persists; after birth, due to transition from fetal circulation to normal circulation, pressure in the left cardiac chambers increases and foramen ovale is closed, at first physiologically and after a while anatomically.
9. Pulmonary veins are relocated from the right atrium to the left atrium.
10. *Sinus venosus* is the part of tissue separating right pulmonary veins from the SVC from the posterior and inferior aspects of the free wall of the right atrium; *coronary sinus septum* is the part of myocardial tissue separating the coronary sinus from the left atrium; also, the left venous valves and the septum spurium merge with the right side of the septum secundum (Anderson et al. 2003; Geva et al. 2014; Asrress et al. 2015; Calkoen et al. 2016).

Classification

Let's review the classification of the most common types of ASD based on the above embryological sequence of events, which is presented in detail in Table 18.1 (Kerut et al. 2001; Sukernik et al. 2001; Oliver et al. 2002; McCarthy et al. 2003; Van Praagh et al. 2003; Ashley 2004; Sukernik and Bennett-Guerrero 2007; John et al. 2011; Briggs et al. 2012; Asrress et al. 2015).

Pathophysiology of ASD

Due to ASD, during the early course of the disease, oxygenated blood flows from left to right, leading to the following events (Oliver et al. 2002; Azarbal et al. 2005; Tobis and Azarbal 2005; Warnes et al. 2008; Geva et al. 2014; Zvaigzne et al. 2014):

Table 18.1 Classification of ASD lesions

Type of ASD	Mechanism of ASD	Occurrence of the lesion/ clinical outcome	Associated lesions
ASD secundum (ASD II)	Failure in pulling down of the septum primum and deficient septum secundum	The most common type of ASD: 70 % of all ASDs are ASD II; 65–70 % of ASD II are female; about half of them are closed spontaneously; chance of spontaneous closure is more in smaller-size defects and in less than 1 year of age; increasing age and larger defects, less chance for spontaneous closure	Mitral valve prolapse Mitral valve stenosis Pulmonary stenosis
ASD primum (ASD I)	If the ostium primum is not closed by the septum primum, ASD I results; ASD I is located close to the atrioventricular valves and is often associated with an atrioventricular septal defect discussed in Chap. 18 – AV Septal Defects	50 % of ASD I patients are female; usually, surgical treatment is often mandatory for closure of ASD I, because there is very little chance for spontaneous closure	Cleft mitral valve (always) Inlet ventricular septal defect Septal aneurysms
Sinus venosus type ASD (SVASD)	SVASD is an unusual type of ASD, with two common locations: If located superiorly, it is near the entry of SVC If located inferiorly, it is near the entry of IVC It is often associated with anomalous attachment of venae cavae and pulmonary veins Often, due to these anatomic locations, it is discussed under partial anomalous pulmonary venous drainage	40–50 % of SVASD patients are female. There is usually no spontaneous closure; surgical treatment is often mandatory	Partial anomalous venous return Overriding superior vena cava
Coronary sinus septal defect (CSSD)	CSSD occurs if the delicate tissue separating the coronary sinus from the left atrium is not completed; the result is blood shunting through the defect and the orifice of the coronary sinus	Uncommon type of ASD	Unroofed coronary sinus Left superior vena cava persistence Partial/total anomalous venous return

(continued)

Table 18.1 (continued)

Type of ASD	Mechanism of ASD	Occurrence of the lesion/ clinical outcome	Associated lesions
Persistent foramen ovale (PFO)	The pathologic defect is the same as the pathology if fetal circulation persists (persistent fetal circulation, PFC) which is associated with increased pressure in the right side which overcomes the left side	PFO, as an independent lesion, is present in as much as 25 % of general population; so, its occurrence should be considered independently from defects in the interatrial septum	Similar to PFO

- In nearly all of the ASD patients, there are varying degrees of interatrial shunt; if the pressure is higher in one side, the blood would be shunted from that side to the either side.
- Often, there is a *left-to-right shunt* in ASD patients; the severity of the shunt and its direction depends on two main factors: *size of the defect* in the interatrial septum and *left and right atrial pressures* and the relationship between them.
- In ASD secundum, if the defect is less than *10 mm*, the amount of shunt is usually negligible, and the severity of right heart overload and pulmonary hypertension is very low.
- If the defect is large enough to induce considerable shunt flow, then, the lungs are overflowed due to *recirculation of oxygenated blood* to the lungs.
- Increased blood volume load to the lungs often leads to *enlargement of the right heart chambers* (right atrium and ventricle) often associated with impaired function of the right atrium; also, the pulmonary and right heart vascular system (both arteries and veins) are enlarged, due to pulmonary overflow.
- Over time, pulmonary overflow, pulmonary vascular bed remodeling, ventricular remodeling, and trophic changes in the right and left ventricles lead to *pulmonary hypertension* with different severities; the incidence of right heart failure and pulmonary vascular disease is more in female patients compared with male patients and, also, in untreated adults.
- Meanwhile, decreased blood flow through the left heart leads to shrinkage or compromised growth of the left ventricle and aorta; the final result could be diminished systemic output and, finally, *left ventricular systolic dysfunction*.
- If pulmonary hypertension persists and, also, the process of shrinkage in the aorta and left ventricle continues, the final poor event, which is *Eisenmenger syndrome*, ensues presented as increased pulmonary pressure over the systemic pressure accompanied with different degrees of right heart failure; a full discussion of right heart failure could be found in Chap. 33 – Right Heart Failure.
- Often, in the course of the disease, *exercise intolerance* occurs due to impaired hemodynamics, though it is not a common event during the early stages of the disease; however, with advanced age, intolerance increases insidiously.
- Often, enlargement of the right heart, especially the right atrium, is associated with a range of *arrhythmias* which are discussed more in Chap. 37 – Arrhythmias and Their Management.

- For prevention of the disastrous final outcomes, *treatment is necessary*: smaller ASDs impose less burden on the heart and might be closed spontaneously; however, larger ASDs cause significant burden on the heart leading to unwanted consequences which mandate treatment.
- Some *neurologic complications* might occur during the process of the disease due to the abnormal shunts; for example, paradoxical emboli or rare desaturation episodes may lead to aura, migraine headaches, or even transient ischemic events in the central nervous system.

Diagnosis of ASD

In ASD patients, the process of diagnostic workup should aim mainly the following:

- Presence of ASD
- Size of ASD
- Location of ASD
- The effect of ASD shunt on the left and right ventricular function
- The effect of ASD shunt on pulmonary circulation
- Any possible associated lesions

Clinical Diagnosis of ASD

Clinical presentation and the course of the disease The majority of the patients are asymptomatic during neonatal and early childhood. Any of the following findings like slow weight gain, tachypnea, or recurrent respiratory infections during infancy should raise suspicion. Most of them are acyanotic; however, very rarely, mild transient cyanosis may happen in the newborn which is due to right-to-left shunt. In physical examination, the precordium is hyperdynamic. Fixed splitting of the second heart sound is heard through respiratory cycles; the severity of pulmonary component of second heart sound (P2) corresponds with the severity of pulmonary hypertension only if it is present. So, the diagnosis in this time domain is usually an incidental finding by echo during routine clinical or paraclinical assessment like looking for the origin of an incidental heart murmur or anything abnormal found in chest X-ray or other studies. Untreated adults have more symptoms and signs, especially related to potential pulmonary hypertension. More explanation regarding adult patients with ASD could be found in Chap. 14 – Anesthetic Management of Adults with Congenital Heart Disease (Andrews et al. 2002; Lammers et al. 2005; Geva et al. 2014; Zvaigzne et al. 2014).

In a considerable number of patients with *ASD secundum*, the chance of spontaneous closure is high; in fact, the chance of spontaneous closure is higher in those patients with smaller-size defects and in less than 1 year of age; but, increasing age and larger defects are not in favor of spontaneous defect closure. On the other site, *sinus venosus ASD* and *ASD primum* nearly always need surgical treatment and have significant hemodynamic consequences. Interestingly, *more than one-fourth* of all adult patients with congenital heart defects are ASD cases, and among them, about *75 % are ASD secundum* (Warnes et al. 2008; Vasquez and Lasala 2013).

Exercise intolerance This is an uncommon finding in young ASD patients. However, with increasing age, in those who have been untreated, the frequency of exercise intolerance increases surreptitiously due to aggravation of pulmonary vascular function. If ASD secundum remains unrepaired, exercise capacity will decrease as much as 50–60 % of the predicted values (Geva et al. 2014).

Pulmonary hypertension It is not a common finding in neonates and young children; but may be much more frequent in untreated adults. Increasing age and female gender are two main predisposing factors for the occurrence of pulmonary hypertension in untreated ASD; Down syndrome, sleep apnea, and pulmonary vascular embolic events are other risk factors. Eisenmenger syndrome is seen in 5–10 % of untreated adults (Rosas and Attie 2007; Warnes et al. 2008).

Electrocardiography

The main ECG findings include:

- Tall P wave due to right atrial enlargement; inverted P waves in inferior leads suggest sinus venosus ASD.
- First-degree AV block may be seen; also, right bundle branch block (usually incomplete form) may be seen especially in untreated adults.
- Right axis deviation – if leftward or left superior QRS axis deviation is seen, one should sought for ASD primum.
- Rhythms other than sinus rhythm are not common; however, atrial fibrillation or flutter may occur in adult patients with prolonged disease leading to right atrium enlargement, often occurring after 40 years.
- Hypertrophy of the right ventricle (presented in ECG by RSR' pattern in right precordial leads) may be seen due to pulmonary hypertension (Webb and Gatzoulis 2006; Lam and Friedman 2011; Geva et al. 2014; Zvaigzne et al. 2014) (Fig. 18.1).

CXR

CXR is often abnormal in ASD; however, normal CXR does not rule out ASD. These are the most common findings in CXR of ASD patients:

- Cardiomegaly, which is mainly due to dilation of right-sided chambers, best seen in lateral views; however, in ASD primum, dilation of left-sided chambers may lead to cardiomegaly which may be better seen in lateral views.
- Pulmonary artery trunk and its perfusion domain are enlarged and plethoric; however, a discordance between the main pulmonary artery body and lung fields,

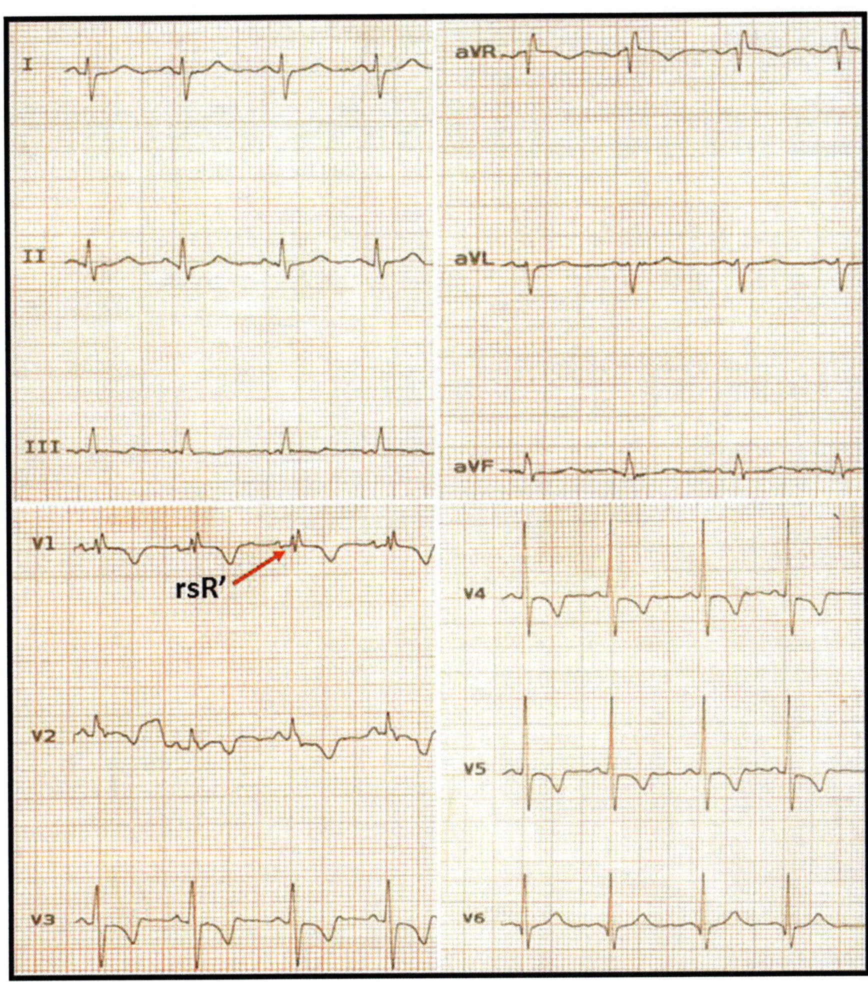

Fig. 18.1 Atrial septal defect. The RSR' pattern in lead V1 and right axis deviation are typical characteristics (Courtesy of Dr Majid Haghjoo and Dr Mohammadrafie Khorgami)

leading to a normal appearance of lung fields in the presence of enlarged pulmonary artery trunk, may be indicative of pulmonary vascular obstructive lesion.
- Small aortic knuckle due to shrinkage of left heart chambers (Webb and Gatzoulis 2006; Geva et al. 2014; Zvaigzne et al. 2014).

Imaging Techniques in Diagnosis of ASD

Diagnosis of ASD should be done and/or confirmed through imaging techniques in such a way to demonstrate shunting across the interatrial septal defect; also, any possible right ventricle overload or associated diseases should be detected and diagnosed. These techniques include mainly echocardiography and, also, cardiac CT, cardiac MR, and catheterization (Warnes et al. 2008).

Echocardiography

There is no doubt that two-dimensional transthoracic echocardiography with Doppler is considered as the cornerstone for evaluation of ASD, though not all ASDs can be visualized with transthoracic echocardiography. Echocardiography is the most common diagnostic modality used for all types of ASD both during primary assessment of the defect and during follow-up visits (Kharouf et al. 2008). The main elements that should be considered in a comprehensive echocardiographic evaluation for ASD mainly include:

- Visualization of ASD, with definite characterization of its size (as much as possible)
- Determining the direction of interatrial flow
- Right heart examination
- Pulmonary artery pressure measurement
- Assessment and estimation of the pulmonary/systemic flow ratio
- Assessment of the associated abnormalities

Initial assessment of ASD during echocardiography should specifically include the following steps:

1. Assessment of the ASD defect including *location, size, number, shunting, gradient (peak/mean)*, and *rims*
2. Right ventricle size and function
3. Right ventricle systolic pressure
4. Pulmonary artery pressure
5. Septal motion/curvature
6. Pulmonary veins
7. Pulmonary valve
8. Possible mitral valve prolapse (MVP)
9. Left ventricle size and function
10. Left atrium size
11. Possibility of aortic regurgitation and pulmonary insufficiency

Post-intervention assessment of ASD should focus on the following steps:

1. Any possible residual leak
2. Right ventricle size/function
3. Septal motion/curvature
4. LV size/function
5. Possible mitral valve prolapse (MVP)
6. Pulmonary valve
7. Right ventricle systolic pressure
8. Pulmonary artery pressure
9. Pericardial effusion

Common views for detection of ASD:

- Apical four-chamber view.
- Parasternal short axis view.

- Subcostal views.
- Also, note that not all ASDs can be detected with transthoracic echocardiography.

Other Imaging Studies

Cardiac MR It allows both anatomic assessment and, also, the hemodynamic effects of interatrial defects, and it has a great application in sinus venosus ASD. Also, cardiac MR is considered the *gold standard* in the assessment of RV volume and function and, also, the pulmonary artery and veins. Cardiac MR is the most accurate and the fastest data acquisition modality. However, this technology is not usually used before treatment of ASD secundum and has limited application before treatment of ASD primum (Webb and Gatzoulis 2006; Kharouf et al. 2008; Warnes et al. 2008; Geva et al. 2014).

Cardiac CT Especially when using high-resolution cardiac CT, many great data could be acquired; however, the data gained from cardiac CT are not significantly more than the data gained from cardiac MR; also, the risk of radiation in cardiac CT should be considered.

Catheterization studies It is not usually indicated to use cardiac catheterization in ASD unless one of the following three (Warnes et al. 2008; Geva et al. 2014):

- In ASDs which are going to be closed with percutaneous devices, i.e., ASD secundum
- To assess any associated anomaly not diagnosed with other noninvasive imaging modalities
- For adult ASD to assessment of the coronary system

Treatment

Regardless of age, ASD closure leads to *improvements in the course* of the disease, both the patient symptoms and improvement in pulmonary vascular disease, pulmonary arterial pressure, ventricular remodeling, and chamber size. *Time of repair* depends mainly on the type and size of defect, age of the patient, associated symptoms, associated anomalies, and a number of other concomitant factors; however, if treatment is delayed, clinical parameters aggravate; so, the sooner treatment is done, the better the general outcome and life expectancy will be. Also, surgical closure, if performed before 25 years old, usually leads to normal life span. On the other side, if ASD leads to severe irreversible PAH and no evidence of a left-to-right shunt, there is no evidence in favor of ASD closure (Rosas and Attie 2007; Engelfriet et al. 2008; Warnes et al. 2008; Yalonetsky and Lorber 2009; Humenberger et al. 2011; Geva et al. 2014).

Percutaneous closure of *ASD secundum* with sufficient rims is the preferred approach; cardiac MR or cardiac catheterization is used for full assessment of *ASD secundum* and any potential associated anomaly before repair. However, *surgical closure* is the only treatment in ASD primum and sinus venosus ASDs. Also, surgical closure of ASD secundum is considered when surgical repair/replacement of a tricuspid valve is planned concomitantly or the anatomy of ASD secundum is not appropriate for deploying a percutaneous device (Warnes et al. 2008). In patients with a diagnosis of ASD primum or sinus venosus ASD (confirmed by echocardiography), no more sophisticated imaging modality is usually needed before surgery (Rigatelli et al. 2007; Kharouf et al. 2008; Warnes et al. 2008; Yalonetsky and Lorber 2009; Humenberger et al. 2011; Geva et al. 2014).

According to the "ACC/AHA 2008 Guidelines for the Management of Adults with Congenital Heart Disease," ASD closure in adults (percutaneously or surgically) may be considered if the patient meets the following criteria (*Level of Evidence: C*):

- Net left-to-right shunting.
- Pulmonary artery pressure two-thirds of the systemic pressure or less than that.
- Pulmonary vascular resistance less than two-thirds of the systemic vascular resistance or it responds to pulmonary vasodilator therapy or test occlusion of the defect (Warnes et al. 2008).

Anesthesia for ASD Treatment

Anesthesia for surgical treatment Using anesthetic drugs with both hemodynamic stability and, also, the capacity to do fast-track extubation seems logic. Also, it is recommended to have an arterial line, a central venous line, and TEE monitoring. Usually, pulmonary artery catheter is not recommended, since it does not increase any data more than TEE. Antibiotic prophylaxis should be considered; Chap. 4 describes fully the antibiotic regime.

Anesthesia for interventional treatment (device closure of ASD): although sedation could be used, often general anesthesia and tracheal intubation are preferred since TEE is almost always used for defining the correct deployment of the device and ruling out any residual defect.

Ventricular Septal Defect

Introduction

Ventricular septal defect usually named "VSD" is among the most common congenital heart diseases; in fact, it is the most common congenital defect at birth. If those defects that are part of other complex congenital heart disease are taken into account, VSD includes up to 40 % of all congenital heart diseases (Hoffman 1995; Roguin et al. 1995; Hoffman et al. 2004; Penny and Vick 2011; Jortveit et al. 2016). It involves the interventricular septum (IVS) and is often an isolated defect; however, it might be associated with other congenital disease(s) or as a component part of a complex congenital heart disease like:

- The conotruncal defects (tetralogy of Fallot, transposition of great arteries, congenitally corrected transposition, DORV, DOLV)
- Left-sided obstructive lesions like subaortic stenosis, aortic coarctation, and interrupted aortic arch (Warnes et al. 2008)

IVS which is the main site of the lesion is composed of two parts:

- The inferior segment which is muscular
- The superior segment which is membranous

In the majority of the cases, blood flows through the left ventricle to the right ventricle, leading to pulmonary overflow, but systemic desaturation is either absent or minimal. Most of the small VSDs are closed spontaneously during the first year of life (Hoffman 1995; Roguin et al. 1995), while the larger ones or "multiple VSD" cases usually need intervention; if they remain untreated, the resulting pulmonary overflow causes sustained increase in pulmonary vascular resistance (PVR), pulmonary hypertension, and, finally, shunt reversal; as a result, systemic desaturation ensues. Although spontaneous closure is a common phenomenon in infancy and childhood, it is a less frequent phenomenon in adulthood.

Embryology and Classification of VSD

At the beginning of the fifth week, the primeval ventricles start expanding, leading to the development of the apical parts of the future ventricles from the primary heart tube. This phenomenon has a crucial role in the development of IVS, with its two main parts:

- *Muscular IVS* which is developed from the bulboventricular flange; the majority of VSDs are located in this muscular component of IVS.
- *Membranous IVS* which connects the upper margin of the bulboventricular flange to the anterior and posterior endocardial cushions; in the "developed" heart, membranous IVS is the smaller part of the septum, at the base of the heart, located between "inlet" and "outlet" parts of the muscular IVS and beneath the right cusp and the noncoronary cusp of the aortic valve; the membranous septum is divided by the tricuspid valve into two parts known as the pars atrioventricularis and the pars interventricularis; the membranous IVS comprises a small portion of IVS; however, it forms an important boundary between the right-sided chambers and the aortic root (Soto et al. 1980; Minette and Sahn 2006; Anderson et al. 2014).

The development of these two parts of IVS is discussed in Chap. 2 – Cardiovascular System Embryology and Development – in detail; however, a brief discussion is presented here:

1. Creation of a median ridge known as the muscular IVS, located near the apex of the ventricular floor; the edge of muscular IVS is concave and free.
2. Height of IVS is achieved by expansion of the ventricles on each side.
3. IVS myoblasts start active proliferation and increasing size.
4. Completion of the conal septum as a result of tissue extension, starting from the inferior part of endocardial cushion up to the top of muscular IVS; finally, these tissues merge with neighboring portion of the conus septum.
5. Three sources of tissue take part in the closure of interventricular opening and formation of membranous IVS: the *left* bulbar ridge, the *right* bulbar ridge, and the endocardial cushions.
6. The final step is the closure of the opening above the muscular IVS: with development of the membranous IVS, interventricular foramen closes completely.

The *primary ventricular septum* or *primary ventricular fold* is produced following the trabeculation of the ventral part of the muscular IVS. However, there is a smooth part on the dorsal wall of IVS, named the *inlet septum*; this nomenclature is used because it is located nearby the AV canals. The *moderator band* or *septomarginal trabecula* is located on the right wall of muscular IVS, between the primary trabeculated fold and the inlet septum. This structure is a firm connection between the muscular septum and the anterior papillary muscle. When the right ventricular chamber expands, the moderator band is formed nearby the AV canal and dorsal muscular IVS. Eventually, a large part of the mature right ventricular chamber is formed by this expansion. However, if this anatomic area expands incompletely, the developing tricuspid part of the atrioventricular canal remains attached to the interventricular foramen, leading to tricuspid atresia and/or other tricuspid valve anomalies (Lamers and Moorman 2002; Gittenberger-de Groot et al. 2005; Togi et al. 2006; Lin et al. 2012; Spicer et al. 2013; Poelmann et al. 2014; Spicer et al. 2014).

Embryologically speaking, a VSD could occur due to one of the following mechanisms:

- Incomplete development of the proximal conotruncal swellings
- Failure in fusion of the muscular and membranous ventricular septa
- Fusion in merging of the ventral and dorsal endocardial cushions (deficiency in atrioventricular septal)
- Deficiency in the development of the interventricular muscular septum

According to Jacobs et al., VSD is described under four basic subtitles presented in Table 18.2; this classification is based on both embryologic development of IVS and anatomic features of VSD (Jacobs et al. 2000; Penny and Vick 2011).

Pathophysiology

The main determinants of the disease and its pathophysiologic course are:

- The *amount* and the *direction* of interventricular shunt (determined by VSD size, severity of increase in PVR, and the balance between systemic and pulmonary pressures)
- The degree of *volume loading* imposed to each cardiac chamber (Tweddell et al. 2006; Aguilar and Eugenio, 2009; Penny and Vick 2011)

Table 18.2 Classification of VSD

Type of VSD	Mechanism of VSD	Occurrence of the lesion/clinical outcome	Associated lesions
Nonmuscular VSDs including three groups:			
1. Perimembranous			
2. Outlet type			
3. Inlet type			
1. *Perimembranous VSD (also known as paramembranous VSD, conotruncal VSD)*	Involves the membranous part of IVS and lies in the outflow tract of the left ventricle immediately beneath the aortic valve	The most common type of VSD, approximately 80 % of all VSDs	Usually extends into muscular, inlet, or outlet portion of ventricular septum
1.1. *Superior border perimembranous VSD; also known as conoventricular VSD* Extends until below the aorta or pulmonary artery or both			
1.2. *Posterior border perimembranous VSD* Involves tricuspid valve or its annulus			
1.3. *Inferior border perimembranous VSD* Passes over the conduction bundle			
2. *Outlet type VSD (also known as subpulmonary VSD, juxta-arterial VSD, supracristal VSD, infundibular VSD, subarterial VSD, doubly committed)*	*Mechanism and location*: the fibrous continuity that is between aortic and pulmonary valves borders the VSD; so, the VSD is located immediately below the pulmonary valve, just inferior to the center of the right coronary cusp	*Occurrence*: accounts for 6 % of all VSDs; more common in oriental population than western countries (about 30 % in oriental compared to 6 % in western populations)	*Associated lesions*: risk of aortic valve regurgitation due to the location of defect just below the right coronary cusp The risk of heart block is really low due to far location from his bundle
3. *Inlet type VSD (atrioventricular canal type)*	Located just below the septal leaflet of the tricuspid valve	Accounts for 5–8 % of all the VSDs	Straddling AV valve chordae

(continued)

Table 18.2 (continued)

Type of VSD	Mechanism of VSD	Occurrence of the lesion/clinical outcome	Associated lesions
4. *Muscular VSDs*			
4.1. *Apical muscular*	Located in the apical muscular part of IVS with multiple apparent channels on right ventricular side and single defect on the left ventricular side	*All muscular VSDs account for 5–20 % of all the VSDs*	
4.2. *Mid-muscular or central muscular*	Located in the *mid-muscular* segment of IVS with multiple apparent channels on right ventricular side and single defect on the left ventricular side		
4.3. *High muscular*	Located in the upper part of the muscular IVS with multiple apparent channels on right ventricular side and single defect on the left ventricular side		
4.4. *Swiss cheese muscular*	Multiple defects in muscular IVS		

However, there are a number of secondary factors which could also affect the pathophysiology of the disease; they are not universal in all VSD patients; however, they occur in some patients and include:

- Presence and degree of prolapse in aortic valve
- Presence and degree of obstruction in blood flow through pulmonary outflow tract or systemic outflow tract (Tweddell et al. 2006; Spicer et al. 2014)

During the early days after birth, the degree of shunt is not severe even in large-size VSDs, since pulmonary vascular resistance is relatively high in early days of neonatal life; however, after normalization of the pulmonary vascular system and resulting drop in PVR, the degree of shunt increases, leading to clinical symptoms and signs including those related to pulmonary overflow and left ventricular hypertrophy. In the minority of the neonates, PVR does not drop after birth due to VSD leading to sustained neonatal pulmonary pressure; however, this is not the typical clinical history of VSD; as a matter of fact, PVR remains low until late childhood or early adulthood in most of the cases. However, the effect of long-term pulmonary overflow would be increased work of the left ventricle and dilation of the left ventricle, and, if untreated, it will lead to left ventricular failure; added to this problem are the chronic effects of pulmonary overflow and the resulting pulmonary hypertension. The final clinical picture is a change in shunt direction from left-to-right shunt to usually irreversible right-to-left shunt pattern. If the disease is still ignored, the effects of long-term increased PVR result in right heart failure leading to final stage biventricular failure associated with irreversible pulmonary hypertension (Tweddell et al. 2006; Penny and Vick 2011; Spicer et al. 2013, 2014).

Diagnosis

Clinical findings Usually signs and symptoms are absent in early life; however, they start to appear after 4–8 weeks and somewhat earlier in premature neonates. The main clinical findings in VSD patients mainly include the following (Penny and Vick 2011; Spicer et al. 2014):

General Findings

- Growth retardation which is due to a number of factors including increased blood flow to the pulmonary vascular bed leading to increased breathing work and, also, decreased oxygen delivery to the systemic organs, since larger amounts of blood flow are directed toward the lungs instead of systemic vascular bed and other organs than the lungs.

Respiratory Findings

- The effects of increased pulmonary vascular blood flow on large airways may be seen as some degrees of pressure on tracheobronchial tree, leading to signs and symptoms of large airway disease.
- In addition, increased pulmonary vascular blood flow in the microvascular system is associated with decreased free space for small airways in the peripheral lung fields, leading to signs and symptoms of smaller airway diseases like tachypnea, wheeze, and respiratory distress; these clinical findings due to pulmonary vascular occlusive disease may be seen even as early as 6–12 months of life, especially in patients having unrestrictive VSD.

Cardiovascular Findings

- Left ventricular hypertrophy, if occurred, is associated with cardiac apex lateral displacement; also, hyperactive precordium is a common clinical finding in patients with volume or pressure overload.
- In auscultation of the heart, a pansystolic murmur is often found which is usually inversely related with the size of VSD.

- In severe pulmonary hypertension (Eisenmenger syndrome), the patient maybe cyanotic, associated with clubbing; usually the pansystolic murmur vanishes, and instead, a loud P2 is auscultated due to contraction of the right ventricle against high-pressure pulmonary vascular system; usually, the clinical findings related to Eisenmenger syndrome do not develop until the teenage years.
- Irregular pulses may be seen in a minority of patients having underlying arrhythmias.

Chest X-ray Some general findings are seen in CXR of VSD patients and mostly include:

- Cardiomegaly – usually showing left ventricle hypertrophy; in addition, right ventricular hypertrophy is seen in a considerable number of the patients.
- Increased vascular markings of the lung fields; however, in patients with Eisenmenger syndrome, the vascular markings fade off the lungs.
- Hyperaeration of the lung fields in patients with increased pulmonary blood flow and the resulting effect on small airways, leading to hyperinflation of the peripheral lung fields (Minette and Sahn 2006; Penny and Vick 2011; Spicer et al. 2014).

Electrocardiography There is no specific sign in small VSDs especially in early neonates; however, there are signs of left ventricular hypertrophy after a while; in addition, signs of right axis deviation and right ventricular hypertrophy are seen especially in patients with pulmonary overcirculation or pulmonary hypertension. A minority of VSD patients may have right bundle branch block (RBBB). Complete heart block may be seen in some (Minette and Sahn 2006; Penny and Vick 2011; Bai et al. 2012; Spicer et al. 2014) (Fig. 18.2).

Cardiac catheterization The main objective is to assess pressures over the chambers and in vascular beds, especially pulmonary system, since closure of VSD in a patient with suprasystemic pulmonary pressure (Eisenmenger syndrome) leads to deteriorating pulmonary hypertension and very poor outcome. Also, the complexity and number of "defects" could be assessed more accurately. In addition, any associated anomalies like concomitant aortic regurgitation can be evaluated, especially in patients with a subpulmonary (supracristal) VSD (Minette and Sahn 2006; Tweddell et al. 2006; Warnes et al. 2008; Penny and Vick 2011).

Echocardiography It is considered as the base of all diagnostic modalities, both in decision-making and in conduction of treatment; the *initial assessment* of VSD patients should focus mainly on the following aspects, preferably in the following order of assessment (Cao et al. 2011; Penny and Vick 2011; Spicer et al. 2014).

First of all, the defect in the septum should be assessed regarding the following items:

- Morphology of the defect
- Malalignment of the defect in relation to IVS
- Size and number of the defect(s)
- Location(s) of the defect(s)
- Gradient across the defect

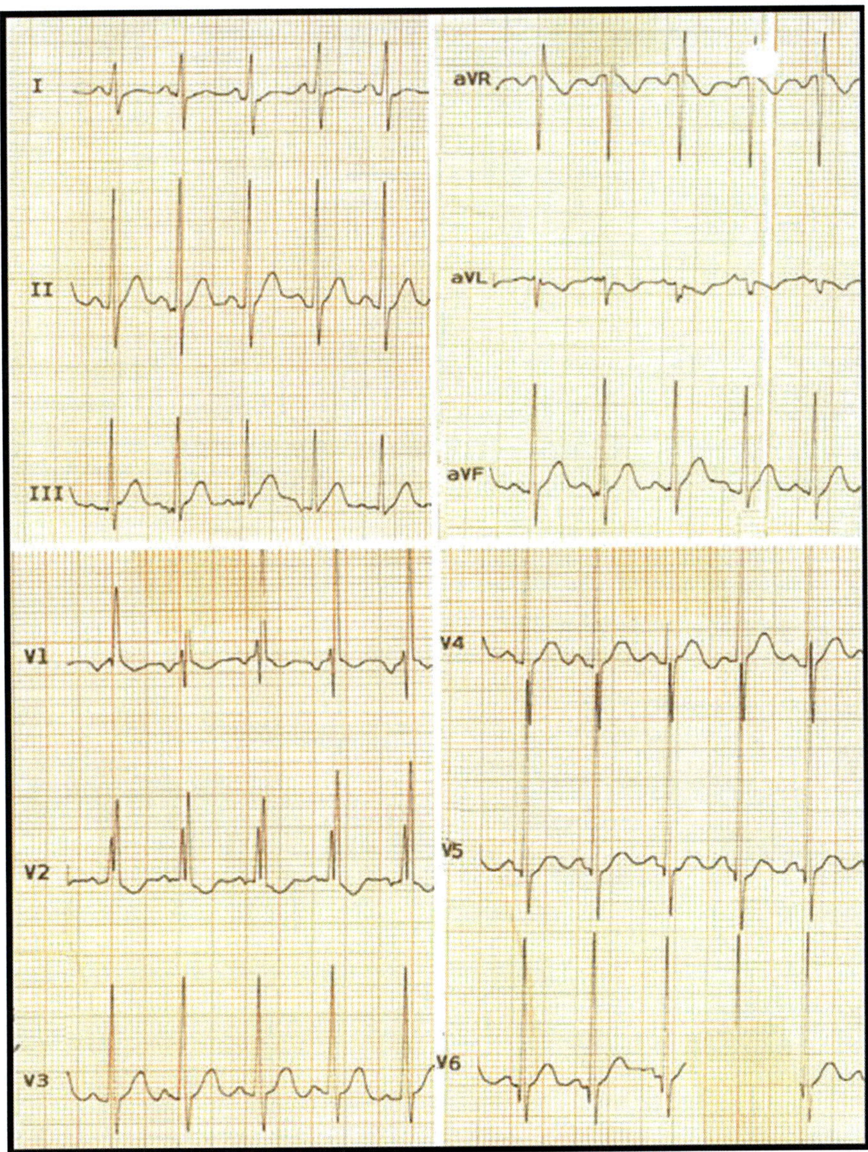

Fig. 18.2 Ventricular septal defect with pulmonary vascular disease. This ECG shows biventricular hypertrophy and left atrial abnormality (Courtesy of Dr Majid Haghjoo and Dr Mohammadrafie Khorgami)

Then, the tricuspid valve should be assessed with special focus on the following items:

- Morphology of the tricuspid valve
- Redundant/aneurysmal tissue in the tricuspid valve
- Possibility of tricuspid regurgitation

Right ventricular outflow tract (RVOT) with special concerns regarding:

- Hypertrophy of the right ventricle
- Pulmonary stenosis (PS)

Left ventricular outflow tract (LVOT) with special concerns regarding:

- Subaortic ridge
- Prolapse of the coronary cusps
- AS/AI

Mitral valve with special concerns regarding:

- Supra-mitral ring
- MS/MR

Also, the following aspects should be assessed:

- LV size/function
- LA size
- Checking for the presence of PDA
- Checking for the presence of aortic coarctation
- RV systolic pressure and pulmonary artery pressure

In *postoperative/post-bypass echocardiographic assessment*, the most important post-cardiopulmonary bypass or postoperative assessment should be any possible residual VSD or any possible VSD patch leak, which may lead to surgical reassessment of the defect for successful closure; also, the function of left and right sides of the heart and their adaptation with the new post-correction condition should be examined. Afterward, it is recommended to reassess the following parts:

- Left ventricular outflow tract (LVOT).
- Right ventricular outflow tract (RVOT).
- Mitral valve.
- Checking for the presence of PDA.
- Checking for the presence of aortic coarctation.
- LV size/function.
- LA size.
- RV systolic pressure and pulmonary artery pressure should be assessed (Roberson et al. 1991; Minette and Sahn 2006; Cao et al. 2011; Penny and Vick 2011; Bai et al. 2012; Spicer et al. 2014).

Treatment

The main approach in treatment is *surgical patch closure* of the defect using atrioventricular valve approach or semilunar valve approach; ventriculotomy is rarely recommended due to its major sequelae. For muscular defects especially those that are apical, *transcatheter closure* is used more than other types of VSD due to a very difficult surgical approach. Currently, transcatheter closure is not a routine practice for perimembranous VSDs, due to high rate of heart blocks due to atrioventricular dissociations in which its chance does not decrease over time; also, some degrees of impairments in adjacent valves may occur. Possibly, with invention of softer devices, this method will be used much more frequently for perimembranous defects. Also, in some of the smaller patients with very "difficult" apical VSDs, there is still room for using pulmonary artery banding, to prevent irreversible pulmonary hypertension in hope of future corrective surgery. The difficulties in closing muscular apical defects have led some centers to use hybrid approach inserting a device in the operating room after surgical exposure of the lesion through a sternotomy (Minette and Sahn 2006; Tweddell et al. 2006; Friesen and Williams 2008; Penny and Vick 2011; Spicer et al. 2014).

Anesthetic Management

Volatile agents or intravenous anesthetics are both used; no conclusive data in favor of any has been published yet. Pulmonary artery catheter is not indicated as a routine monitoring; however, invasive arterial line and central line are both used as a routine anesthetic practice in these patients. Pulmonary vascular resistance should be managed to prevent and increase or decrease in blood pressure; increased PVR leads to right-to-left shunting and desaturation, while decreased PVR leads to pulmonary overcirculation and increased left-to-right shunting. On table extubation is used in many centers, with attention to PVR and pulmonary arterial pressure; in patients with prolonged defects (especially the adults) or those with associated mixed anomalies, more sophisticated assessment should be done before early extubation, especially ruling out any residual defect. Also, RV function, LV function, and pulmonary artery pressure should be assessed after bypass using TEE. Appropriate postoperative management of pain is a basic need. In patients with previous history of PA banding, care should be given to control hemostasis in corrective redo surgeries. In patients undergoing device closure, general anesthesia is often the preferred approach especially when using TEE for detection of residual defects (Takeuchi et al. 2000; Galante 2011; Twite and Friesen 2014).

Outcome

The overall outcome of children with VSD is favorable; Jortveit et al. studied 3495 children with VSD; their overall mortality and/or morbidity rate was very low (Jortveit et al. 2016):

- Arrhythmias 4.6 %
- Aortic regurgitation 3.4 %
- Endocarditis 0.9 %
- Pulmonary hypertension 0.3 %

References

Aguilar NE, Eugenio LJ. Ventricular septal defects. Bol Asoc Med P R. 2009;101:23–9.

Anderson RH, Webb S, Brown NA, Lamers W, Moorman A. Development of the heart: (2) Septation of the atriums and ventricles. Heart. 2003;89:949–58.

Anderson RH, Sarwark AE, Spicer DE, Backer CL. Exercises in anatomy: holes between the ventricles. Multimed Man Cardiothorac Surg: MMCTS/European Assoc Cardio-Thorac Surg. 2014;2014.

Andrews R, Tulloh R, Magee A, Anderson D. Atrial septal defect with failure to thrive in infancy: hidden pulmonary vascular disease? Pediatr Cardiol. 2002;23:528–30.

Ashley EA, Niebauer J. Chapter 14, Adult congenital heart disease. In: Cardiology explained. London: Remedica; 2004.

Asrress KN, Marciniak M, Marciniak A, Rajani R, Clapp B. Patent foramen ovale: the current state of play. Heart. 2015;101:1916–25.

Azarbal B, Tobis J, Suh W, Chan V, Dao C, Gaster R. Association of interatrial shunts and migraine headaches: impact of transcatheter closure. J Am Coll Cardiol. 2005;45:489–92.

Bai W, An Q, Tang H. Application of transesophageal echocardiography in minimally invasive surgical closure of ventricular septal defects. Tex Heart Inst J. 2012;39:211–4.

Briggs LE, Kakarla J, Wessels A. The pathogenesis of atrial and atrioventricular septal defects with special emphasis on the role of the dorsal mesenchymal protrusion. Differentiation; Res Biol Divers. 2012;84:117–30.

Calkoen EE, Hazekamp MG, Blom NA, Elders BB, Gittenberger-de Groot AC, Haak MC, Bartelings MM, Roest AA, Jongbloed MR. Atrioventricular septal defect: from embryonic development to long-term follow-up. Int J Cardiol. 2016;202:784–95.

Cao H, Chen Q, Zhang GC, Chen LW, Li QZ, Qiu ZH. Intraoperative device closure of perimembranous ventricular septal defects in the young children under transthoracic echocardiographic guidance; initial experience. J Cardiothorac Surg. 2011;6:166.

Engelfriet P, Meijboom F, Boersma E, Tijssen J, Mulder B. Repaired and open atrial septal defects type II in adulthood: an epidemiological study of a large European cohort. Int J Cardiol. 2008;126:379–85.

Friesen RH, Williams GD. Anesthetic management of children with pulmonary arterial hypertension. Paediatr Anaesth. 2008;18:208–16.

Galante D. Intraoperative management of pulmonary arterial hypertension in infants and children – corrected and republished article. Curr Opin Anaesthesiol. 2011;24:468–71.

Geva T, Martins JD, Wald RM. Atrial septal defects. Lancet. 2014;383:1921–32.

Gittenberger-de Groot AC, Bartelings MM, Deruiter MC, Poelmann RE. Basics of cardiac development for the understanding of congenital heart malformations. Pediatr Res. 2005;57:169–76.

Hoffman JI. Incidence of congenital heart disease: I. Postnatal incidence. Pediatr Cardiol. 1995;16:103–13.

Hoffman JI, Kaplan S, Liberthson RR. Prevalence of congenital heart disease. Am Heart J. 2004;147:425–39.

Humenberger M, Rosenhek R, Gabriel H, Rader F, Heger M, Klaar U, Binder T, Probst P, Heinze G, Maurer G, Baumgartner H. Benefit of atrial septal defect closure in adults: impact of age. Eur Heart J. 2011;32:553–60.

Jacobs JP, Burke RP, Quintessenza JA, Mavroudis C. Congenital heart surgery nomenclature and database project: ventricular septal defect. Ann Thorac Surg. 2000;69:S25–35.

John J, Abrol S, Sadiq A, Shani J. Mixed atrial septal defect coexisting ostium secundum and sinus venosus atrial septal defect. J Am Coll Cardiol. 2011;58, e9.

Jortveit J, Leirgul E, Eskedal L, Greve G, Fomina T, Dohlen G, Tell GS, Birkeland S, Oyen N, Holmstrom H. Mortality and complications in 3495 children with isolated ventricular septal defects. Arch Dis Child. 2016;101(9):808–13.

Kerut EK, Norfleet WT, Plotnick GD, Giles TD. Patent foramen ovale: a review of associated conditions and the impact of physiological size. J Am Coll Cardiol. 2001;38:613–23.

Kharouf R, Luxenberg DM, Khalid O, Abdulla R. Atrial septal defect: spectrum of care. Pediatr Cardiol. 2008;29:271–80.

Lam W, Friedman RA. Electrophysiology issues in adult congenital heart disease. Methodist Debakey Cardiovasc J. 2011;7:13–7.

Lamers WH, Moorman AF. Cardiac septation: a late contribution of the embryonic primary myocardium to heart morphogenesis. Circ Res. 2002;91:93–103.

Lammers A, Hager A, Eicken A, Lange R, Hauser M, Hess J. Need for closure of secundum atrial septal defect in infancy. J Thorac Cardiovasc Surg. 2005;129:1353–7.

Lin CJ, Lin CY, Chen CH, Zhou B, Chang CP. Partitioning the heart: mechanisms of cardiac septation and valve development. Development. 2012;139:3277–99.

McCarthy K, Ho S, Anderson R. Defining the morphologic phenotypes of atrial septal defects and interatrial communications. Images Paediatr Cardiol. 2003;5:1–24.

Minette MS, Sahn DJ. Ventricular septal defects. Circulation. 2006;114:2190–7.

Oliver JM, Gallego P, Gonzalez A, Dominguez FJ, Aroca A, Mesa JM. Sinus venosus syndrome: atrial septal defect or anomalous venous connection? A multiplane transoesophageal approach. Heart. 2002;88:634–8.

Penny DJ, Vick 3rd GW. Ventricular septal defect. Lancet. 2011;377:1103–12.

Poelmann RE, Gittenberger-de Groot AC, Vicente-Steijn R, Wisse LJ, Bartelings MM, Everts S, Hoppenbrouwers T, Kruithof BP, Jensen B, de Bruin PW, Hirasawa T, Kuratani S, Vonk F, van de Put JM, de Bakker MA, Richardson MK. Evolution and development of ventricular septation in the amniote heart. PLoS One. 2014;9, e106569.

Rigatelli G, Cardaioli P, Hijazi ZM. Contemporary clinical management of atrial septal defects in the adult. Expert Rev Cardiovasc Ther. 2007;5:1135–46.

Roberson DA, Muhiudeen IA, Cahalan MK, Silverman NH, Haas G, Turley K. Intraoperative transesophageal echocardiography of ventricular septal defect. Echocardiography (Mount Kisco, NY). 1991;8:687–97.

Roguin N, Du ZD, Barak M, Nasser N, Hershkowitz S, Milgram E. High prevalence of muscular ventricular septal defect in neonates. J Am Coll Cardiol. 1995;26:1545–8.

Rosas M, Attie F. Atrial septal defect in adults. Timely Top Med Cardiovasc Dis. 2007;11, E34.

Soto B, Becker AE, Moulaert AJ, Lie JT, Anderson RH. Classification of ventricular septal defects. Br Heart J. 1980;43:332–43.

Spicer DE, Anderson RH, Backer CL. Clarifying the surgical morphology of inlet ventricular septal defects. Ann Thorac Surg. 2013;95:236–41.

Spicer DE, Hsu HH, Co-Vu J, Anderson RH, Fricker FJ. Ventricular septal defect. Orphanet J Rare Dis. 2014;9:144.

Sukernik MR, Bennett-Guerrero E. The incidental finding of a patent foramen ovale during cardiac surgery: should it always be repaired? A core review. Anesth Analg. 2007;105:602–10.

Sukernik MR, Mets B, Bennett-Guerrero E. Patent foramen ovale and its significance in the perioperative period. Anesth Analg. 2001;93:1137–46.

Takeuchi M, Kinouchi K, Fukumitsu K, Kishimoto H, Kitamura S. Postbypass pulmonary artery pressure influences respiratory system compliance after ventricular septal defect closure. Paediatr Anaesth. 2000;10:407–11.

Tobis MJ, Azarbal B. Does patent foramen ovale promote cryptogenic stroke and migraine headache? Tex Heart Inst J. 2005;32:362–5.

Togi K, Yoshida Y, Matsumae H, Nakashima Y, Kita T, Tanaka M. Essential role of Hand2 in interventricular septum formation and trabeculation during cardiac development. Biochem Biophys Res Commun. 2006;343:144–51.

Tweddell JS, Pelech AN, Frommelt PC. Ventricular septal defect and aortic valve regurgitation: pathophysiology and indications for surgery. Semin Thorac Cardiovasc Surg Pediatr Card Surg Annu. 2006;9(1):147–52.

Twite MD, Friesen RH. The anesthetic management of children with pulmonary hypertension in the cardiac catheterization laboratory. Anesthesiol Clin. 2014;32:157–73.

Van Praagh S, Geva T, Lock JE, Nido PJ, Vance MS, Van Praagh R. Biatrial or left atrial drainage of the right superior vena cava: anatomic, morphogenetic, and surgical considerations – report of three new cases and literature review. Pediatr Cardiol. 2003;24:350–63.

Vasquez AF, Lasala JM. Atrial septal defect closure. Cardiol Clin. 2013;31:385–400.

Warnes CA, Williams RG, Bashore TM, Child JS, Connolly HM, Dearani JA, Del Nido P, Fasules JW, Graham Jr TP, Hijazi ZM, Hunt SA, King ME, Landzberg MJ, Miner PD, Radford MJ, Walsh EP, Webb GD. ACC/AHA 2008 guidelines for the management of adults with congenital heart disease: executive summary: a report of the American College of Cardiology/American Heart Association Task Force on Practice Guidelines (writing committee to develop guidelines for the management of adults with congenital heart disease). Circulation. 2008;118:2395–451.

Webb G, Gatzoulis MA. Atrial septal defects in the adult: recent progress and overview. Circulation. 2006;114:1645–53.

Yalonetsky S, Lorber A. Comparative changes of pulmonary artery pressure values and tricuspid valve regurgitation following transcatheter atrial septal defect closure in adults and the elderly. Congenit Heart Dis. 2009;4:17–20.

Zvaigzne CG, Howarth AG, Patton DJ. Atrial shunts: presentation, investigation, and management, including recent advances in magnetic resonance imaging. Cardiol Young. 2014;24:403–16.

Chapter 19
Tetralogy of Fallot

Gerald A. Bushman

Introduction

As a knowledge base, congenital heart disease has only recently evolved within the expertise of the pediatric or cardiac anesthesiologist as pediatric cardiac anesthesiology has become recognized as a discrete subspecialty (DiNardo et al. 2010). Historical attempts to "simplify" the cardiac malformations that may be encountered typically ignored specific anatomic details in favor of slotting the lesions into broad categories such as "cyanotic" or "noncyanotic." Early textbooks on anesthesia for the congenital cardiac patient often divided cardiac anomalies in very general ways, pointing out specific memorable features associated with some lesions (Lake). Although useful in the era where most anesthesiologists did not have significant insight into this subspecialty of pediatric disease, rapid advances in the successful surgical treatment of congenital cardiac disease have been paralleled by accumulation of specific cognitive and technical skills by anesthesiologists dedicated to the care of such patients (DiNardo et al. 2010). Contemporary pediatric cardiac anesthesiologists share knowledge of congenital cardiac disease, echocardiography, and the physiologic challenges of catheterization lab procedures with the pediatric cardiologist; the details of surgical technique and management of cardiopulmonary bypass with the cardiac surgeon; and the management and expectations of preoperative care and postoperative convalescence (including the management of extracorporeal membrane oxygenation) with the pediatric cardiac intensive care physician. The assessment of a patient with congenital heart disease by the contemporary pediatric cardiac anesthesiologist is a complex synthesis of the anatomic details of a specific cardiac lesion, their implications on the baseline and expected physiology of the

G.A. Bushman, MD
Pediatric and Cardiac Anesthesiology, Anesthesia Critical Care Medicine,
Children's Hospital Los Angeles; Keck School of Medicine,
University of Southern California, Los Angeles, CA, USA
e-mail: GBushman@chla.usc.edu

© Springer International Publishing Switzerland 2017
A. Dabbagh et al. (eds.), *Congenital Heart Disease in Pediatric and Adult Patients*, DOI 10.1007/978-3-319-44691-2_19

patient, the patient's status within the natural history of the lesion, consideration of how anesthesia techniques and the operative environment will predictably intrude on the homeostasis of the patient's cardiac physiology, and how those risks might be tolerated and minimized. The author's goal for the next two chapters is not to present an encyclopedic review of the material with inarguable advice on anesthesia technique and management. Instead a contextual presentation including embryology and anatomy, physiology correlated with the anatomy, medical and surgical management, and the natural history of the disease is presented with the assumption that a well-informed practitioner can apply their enhanced knowledge of the cardiac disease in making informed choices regarding anesthesia management.

For the purposes of precisely delineating cyanotic congenital cardiac disease, it is useful to consider the physiologic substrate of cyanosis as it derives from cardiac (rather than pulmonary) etiologies. Cyanosis or systemic desaturation of arterial blood may be the result of an inadequate amount of pulmonary blood flow relative to systemic blood flow, that is, a pulmonary to systemic flow ratio (Qp/Qs) of less than one (Waldman and Wernly 1999). Alternatively, cyanosis may result from abnormal mixing within the cardiac chambers of fully saturated pulmonary venous blood with desaturated systemic venous blood and access of the desaturated admixture to the arterial circulation (Tharakan 2011). Desaturation of arterialized blood due to intracardiac mixing is largely independent of the pulmonary to systemic flow ratio, and the Qp/Qs of a mixing lesion may be greater than one if there are intracardiac septal defects and a suitably low pulmonary vascular resistance compared to systemic vascular resistance. The eponymous representatives of these different cyanotic anomalies are tetralogy of Fallot (TOF) and transposition of the great arteries (TGA). They are a part of the broader group of cardiac anomalies due to conotruncal malformation that also includes double outlet right ventricle and truncus arteriosus.

Case Presentation

A 6-month-old infant presents for surgical resection of a recently diagnosed intra-abdominal tumor believed to be a Wilms' tumor. The patient also has tetralogy of Fallot. Surgical correction of the cardiac defect has been deferred because the patient has had stable arterial saturations of about 92 % without overt hypercyanotic episodes.

What is TOF and when is it typically repaired? What affects the timing of repair?

Should this patient have definitive cardiac repair prior to laparotomy?

What are the cardiac findings to investigate prior to undertaking laparotomy? How are the cardiac findings relevant to the patient's perioperative course?

What are the management issues of the induction and maintenance of anesthesia for laparotomy?

What is the importance of preoperative or intraoperative beta-blockade?

What postoperative risks should be anticipated and how should they be minimized?

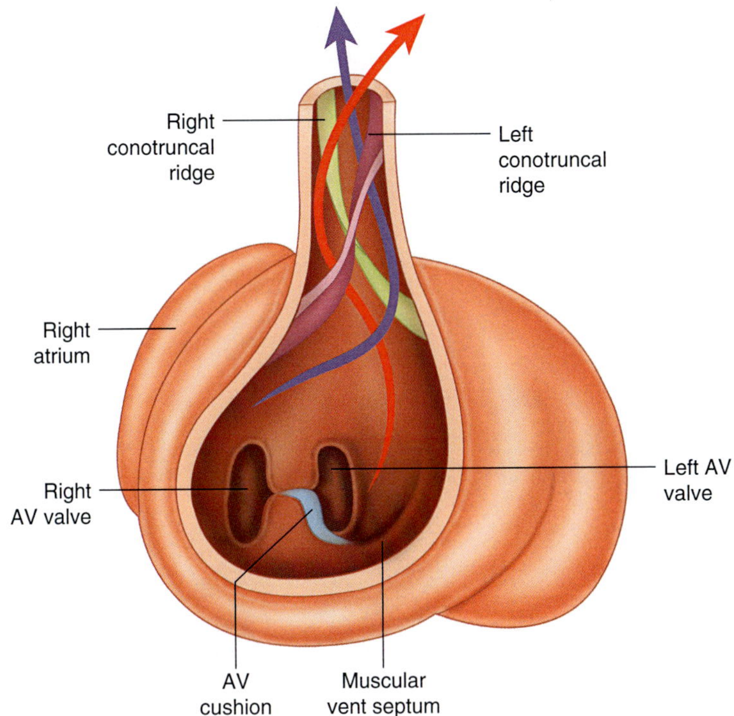

Fig. 19.1 Conotruncal spiraling

Embryology and Anatomy

The embryologic substrate of tetralogy of Fallot (TOF) is abnormal conotruncal development (Rudolph). Normally, fetal ventricular partitioning occurs as the muscular septum grows from the floor of the ventricular chamber and the membranous septum develops from the atrioventricular valve apparatus and the bulbar ridges. The bulbar ridges of the bulbus cordis and the truncal ridges of the truncus arteriosus grow toward each other in order to form the primitive aorticopulmonary trunk, which has a spiral septation (Fig. 19.1). The coordination of the further development of the bulbus cordis with normal spiraling and septation of the primitive truncus results in a right ventricular outflow tract in unobstructed continuity with the pulmonary artery, and the left ventricular outflow tract in unobstructed continuity with the aorta, with the membranous and muscular portions of the ventricular septum intact. In TOF, asymmetric fusion of the bulbar and truncal ridges during maturation causes anterior malalignment of the aorticopulmonary septum. Further abnormal conal rotation contributes to anterior malalignment of the ventricular septum and an aortic position that overrides the ventricular septal defect rather than being committed to the left ventricular outflow tract (Bartelings and Gittenberger-de Groot 1991). By week 7, the process is complete, and the anatomic substrate for

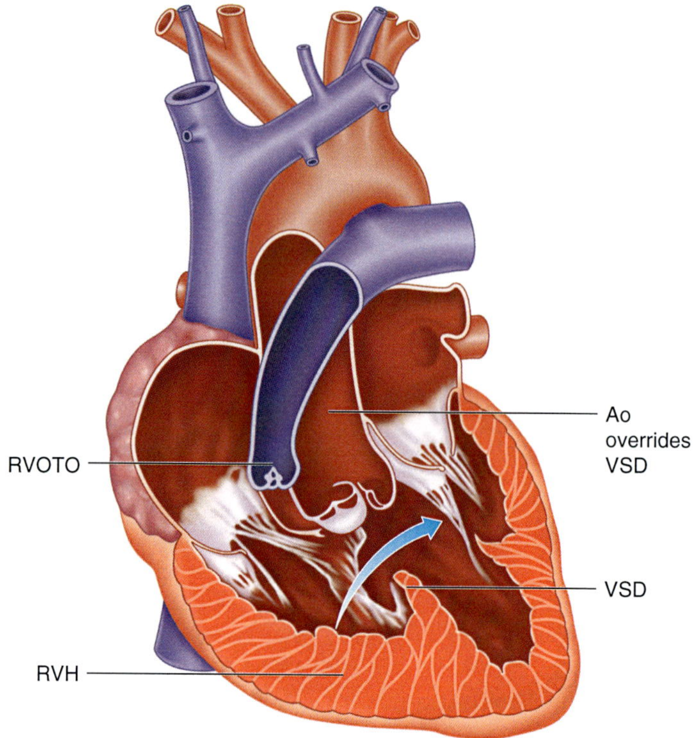

Fig. 19.2 Features of TOF

three of the four components of tetralogy of Fallot are present: hypoplasia of the right ventricular outflow tract with pulmonary valve stenosis, a ventricular septal defect (VSD), and an aortic position overriding the VSD. The development of right ventricular hypertrophy (RVH) is often a postnatal event and depends on the degree of fixed and dynamic obstruction of the right ventricular outflow tract (RVOT) and pulmonary valve (PV) (Allen) (Fig. 19.2).

Uncomplicated TOF

Presentation and Anatomic Correlation

A neonate born with TOF typically has three of the four important anatomic components: a perimembranous VSD, an anteriorly malaligned right ventricular outflow tract with stenosis or hypoplasia of the pulmonary valve or main pulmonary artery, and an overriding aorta that is positioned over the VSD rather than more posteriorly related to the left ventricular outflow tract (Anderson and Weinberg 2005). Often, depending on the degree of obstruction to pulmonary blood flow by the hypoplastic portions of the RVOT, a neonate demonstrates little or no cyanosis and may have chest X-ray evidence of cardiomegaly, consistent with the findings of a ventricular septal defect. This is especially true in the first few days of life when the ductus arteriosus is likely to be open. Any signs or symptoms referable to the VSD and pulmonary overcirculation regress over weeks to months, and the patient begins to develop the fourth component of TOF, right ventricular hypertrophy.

It is useful to consider the RVOT obstruction as having two physiologic components that correlate with the anatomic details present in the patient. The RVOT obstruction due to dysmorphology of the pulmonary valve or pulmonary artery has a "fixed" restrictive effect on pulmonary blood flow. That is, the obstruction does not significantly change with the loading or contractile conditions of the RV, the heart rate, or the systemic afterload. As the neonate grows, the restriction to pulmonary blood flow by the fixed obstruction becomes more important, and desaturation occurs as the Qp/Qs decreases below one.

Because of the small, anteriorly malaligned RVOT, the "dynamic" obstruction typically occurs at the infundibulum of the right ventricle (Little et al. 1963). Unlike the fixed obstruction that may be present at the pulmonary valve or pulmonary artery, the dynamic obstruction of the RVOT varies with the contractile state, the preload and afterload conditions of the right ventricle, and with the heart rate. While the fixed RVOT obstruction tends to worsen according to the degree of obstruction relative to the infant's size and decreases in arterial saturation are gradual, the dynamic obstruction at the infundibulum reflects progressive concentric hypertrophy and disorganization of the myofibrils of the infundibulum unrelated to the infant's growth (Geva et al. 1995). Dynamic RVOT obstruction worsens with time irrespective of growth (Soto et al. 1981). The hypercyanosis seen during a "Tet spell" is episodic and related to specific situations associated with tachycardia, decreased preload and/or afterload, and/or increased contractile performance of the RV.

Under quiet conditions, infants normally do not experience the decreases in preload or afterload that would precipitate a "Tet spell." However, crying is the behavior that most frequently causes the infant to become tachycardic with increased cardiac output (CO) precipitating hypercyanosis. Relative to the increased CO, the amount of blood that can traverse the RVOT is decreased, and the right-to-left shunt at the ventricular septal defect increases. The Qp/Qs during these episodes decreases, and the proportional decrease in arterial oxygen saturation (SaO_2) correlates with the relatively decreased pulmonary blood flow. In addition, the aortic valve overriding the VSD is in excellent position to receive systolic blood flow ejected from the right as well as the left ventricle as the impediment of RVOT obstruction (analogous to "mechanical" pulmonary vascular resistance) approaches systemic vascular resistance. The mainstay of medical management in such patients prior to operative repair is beta-blockade with propranolol, which reduces the incidence and severity of infundibular spasm (Thapar and Rao 1990).

As RVOT obstruction becomes important in infancy in TOF, failure to thrive is rarely seen, and if present, noncardiac causes should be considered. It is much more common for these infants to be in the upper percentile of weight for their length and age, as the usual reaction from parents to the hypercyanosis that occurs with crying is to placate the infant with additional feeding.

Historical Therapeutic Approaches and Outcomes

The concept of surgical palliation of TOF originated with the observation that patients with cyanotic heart disease who also had a patent ductus arteriosus (PDA) outlived cyanotic patients without a PDA. Beginning in 1944, a classic Blalock-Taussig shunt (BTS) was performed in selected toddlers and children to relieve cyanosis (Blalock and Taussig 1945). Smaller children with the most severe manifestations of TOF usually did not survive infancy to undergo palliation.

The classic BTS is an end-to-side anastomosis of the subclavian artery to the pulmonary artery allowing a stable source of pulmonary blood flow that grows with the patient (Fig. 19.3). Patients typically remained somewhat desaturated. Manifestations of chronic hypoxemia and polycythemia were increasingly seen in

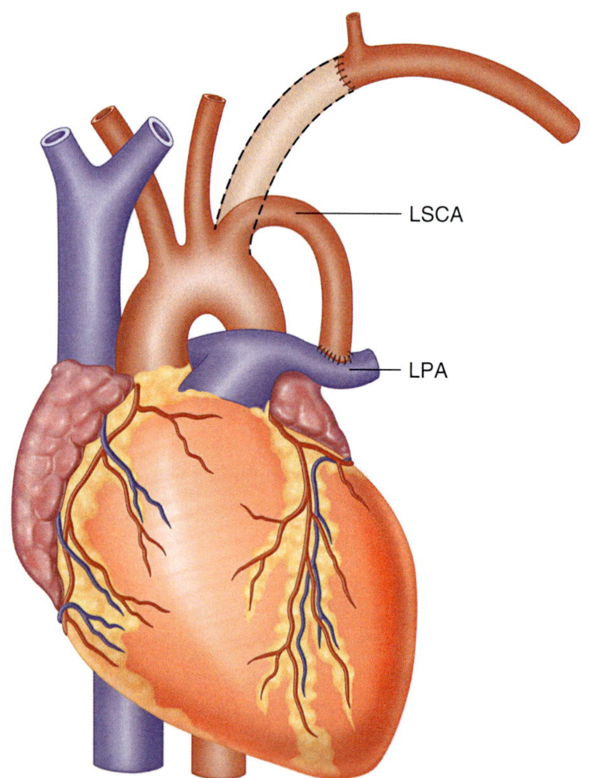

Fig. 19.3 Classic BT shunt

long-term survivors of initial palliative shunting; however, the paroxysms of hyper-cyanosis that the patient typically attempted to relieve by squatting were resolved (Hansen et al. 1995). In that era, complete surgical repair was not contemplated. Attempts at evolving the concept of a systemic-to-pulmonary shunt that would provide more durable relief of cyanosis resulted in the Waterston shunt, which created an aortopulmonary window from the ascending aorta to the right pulmonary artery, and the Potts shunt, which created a window from the descending aorta to the left pulmonary artery (Pickering et al. 1971; Levy and Blalock 1939) (Fig. 19.4). These shunts provided torrential, but often one-sided blood flow to the pulmonary circulation (Trucoone et al. 1974; Newfeld et al. 1977).

When Clarence Walton Lillehei initiated the era of complete repair of TOF in 1954, the VSD was closed, and the RVOT was reconstructed utilizing extracorporeal circulation (Lillehei et al. 1955, 1986) (Fig. 19.5). Many of the patients were survivors of Waterston and Potts shunts, and a high incidence of pulmonary artery distortion and pulmonary vascular disease (often in one lung) was appreciated (Trucoone et al. 1974). The potential of complete repair obviated the notion that the shunt was permanent palliation, and further modifications of the systemic-to-pulmonary artery shunt reflected the consideration that as a palliative strategy preceding complete repair, the temporary augmentation of pulmonary blood flow should be controlled rather than excessive, and the pulmonary artery architecture and growth potential should be undamaged by the shunt (Lamberti et al. 1984). The contemporary refinements of the early shunts are the modified Blalock-Taussig shunt (MBTS), a Gore-Tex tube from the right innominate or subclavian artery to the right pulmonary artery, and the central shunt, a Gore-Tex tube from the ascending aorta to the main pulmonary artery (Fig. 19.6). When palliation is required, a stable and predictable

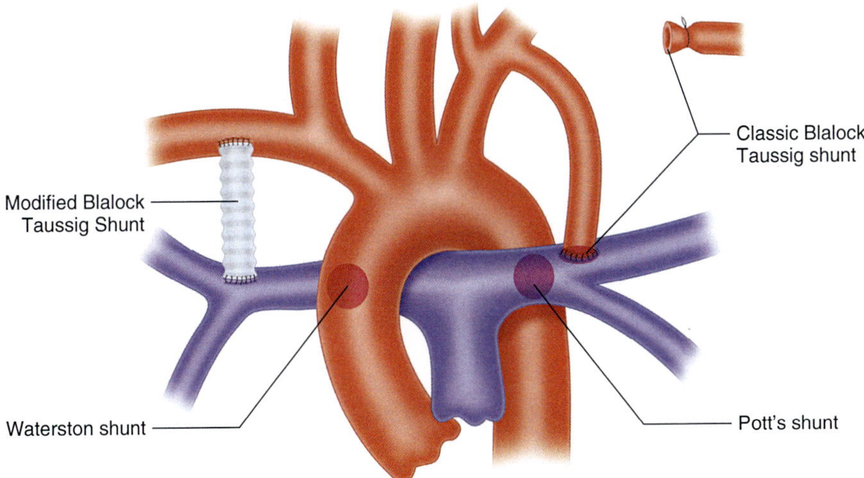

Fig. 19.4 Types of shunts

Fig. 19.5 TOF repair

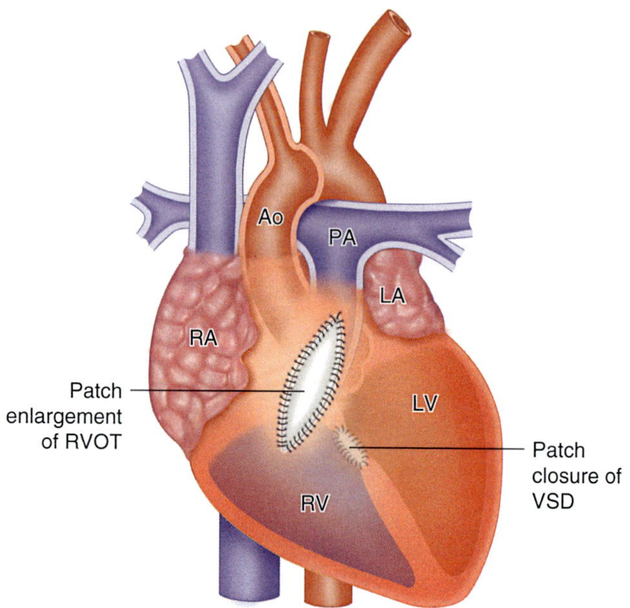

augmentation of pulmonary blood flow can be accomplished by choosing carefully the size of the shunt and the placement of the proximal anastomosis. The longevity of the shunt is less a concern as complete repair can now be undertaken at low risk on most patients during infancy (Stephenson et al. 1978).

Early outcome data from the first several decades of complete TOF repair showed the likelihood of survival, and an acceptable long-term result was closely related to how completely the right ventricular outflow tract obstruction was relieved (Bahnson 1982). Complete surgical excision of the pulmonary valve was common, and the right ventriculotomy was extended to the apex of the heart to fully resect the infundibulum and any prominent right ventricular muscle bands (Kirklin and Karp 1970). Acute pulmonary insufficiency associated with this approach is initially well tolerated in most patients. It took many decades for long-term outcome data to demonstrate that right ventricular dysfunction and failure (and the associated left ventricular dysfunction from septal shift), tricuspid valve insufficiency, and severe ventricular arrhythmias as a result of ventricular hypertrophy and dilation were the consequences of the aggressiveness in managing the RVOT in the original complete repair (Garson et al. 1979).

Nonetheless, despite the early application of surgical and anesthesia efforts and perfusion technology in the 1950s through the 1970s, there are many adult survivors of palliative shunting followed by complete repair of TOF. As the incidences of pulmonary vascular disease, branch pulmonary artery stenosis due to the shunt, right ventricular failure with occasional left ventricular failure, and chronic arrhythmias are now well defined in this adult cohort, contemporary surgical repair is aimed at not only excellent short-term survival but also intact and functional long-term survival, even at the expense of occasional late reintervention to optimize the RVOT (Myers et al. 2014; Cuypers et al. 2014).

Fig. 19.6 MBTS and central shunts

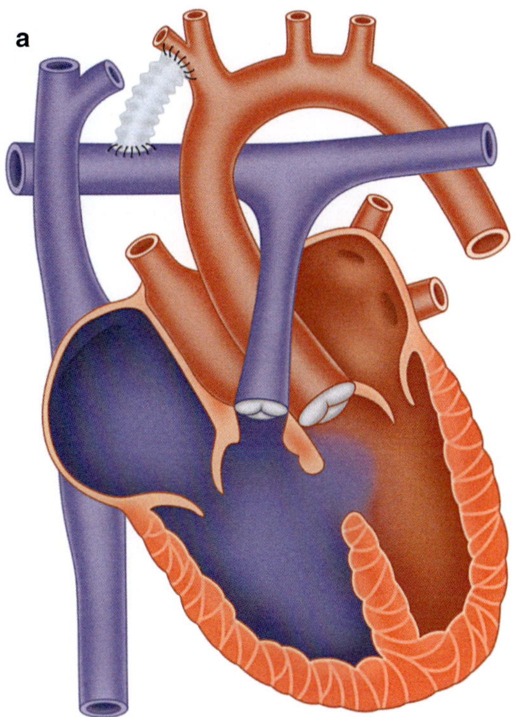

MBTS from RSCA to RPA

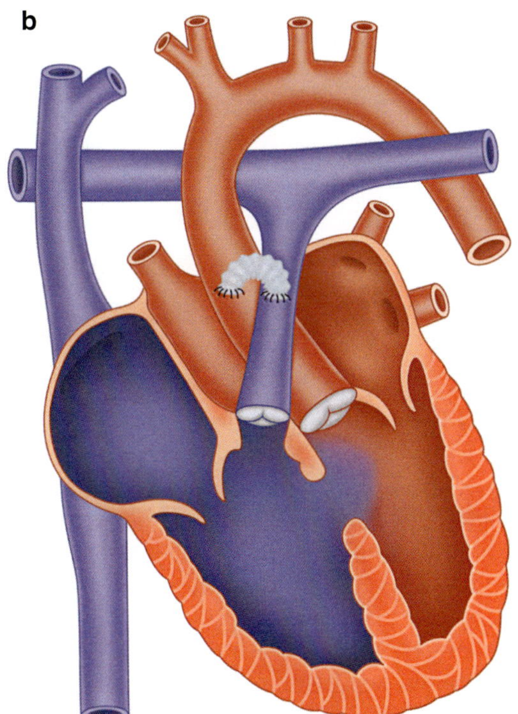

Central shunt from Asc Ao to MPA

Contemporary Surgical Management and Outcomes

Tetralogy of Fallot is typically diagnosed in the neonatal period or early infancy. Although prenatal diagnosis is possible, it is not common for the lesion to be identified before birth unless there is also pulmonary atresia or hypoplastic right heart syndrome. The presentation is related to the amount of fixed obstruction of the RVOT and cyanosis, and a crescendo/decrescendo systolic heart murmur with a diminished pulmonary component is common. Chest X-ray eventually shows the pathognomonic boot-shaped cardiac silhouette due to right ventricular hypertrophy, and an ECG shows RV hypertrophy and exaggerated right axis deviation for age during infancy (Allen). The anatomic diagnosis is confirmed by echocardiography, and only in the case of specific complex variations would catheterization and angiography be indicated.

Because of the common availability of echocardiography, infants are usually diagnosed early, before severe manifestations of infundibular hypertrophy and paroxysms of hypercyanosis are evident. As dynamic obstruction progresses, medical management with propranolol is frequently used to reduce hypercyanosis, while preparations for surgery are undertaken.

Timing of Surgery

The timing of surgery for uncomplicated TOF is somewhat controversial (Steiner et al. 2014; Barron 2013). Excellent results have been obtained in some centers by operative repair in the first few months of life prior to the development of significant cyanosis, justifying the approach with the argument that the time the infant is chronically and episodically hypoxemic is minimized by early repair (Tamesberger et al. 2008; Hirsch et al. 2000). Although fixed obstruction is reliably addressed in the neonate or young infant, hypertrophy of the disorganized myofibrils of the infundibulum may still occur after early repair and lead to early reintervention (Kaza et al. 2009). More commonly, repair is undertaken when cyanosis and hypercyanosis become more severe, typically at 6–12 months of age.

Surgical Technique

Closure of the VSD in TOF is usually straightforward, and the use of a pericardial or synthetic patch is standard. Contemporary surgical techniques of RVOT reconstruction have evolved over time and now reflect a refined understanding of the long-term consequences of previous efforts at completely relieving RVOT obstruction (Vida et al. 2014; Bacha 2012; Karl 2008). Although acute pulmonary insufficiency is well tolerated, the eccentric hypertrophy that occurs in the RV due to chronic volume loading often has clinically important long-term sequelae (Fraser 2015).

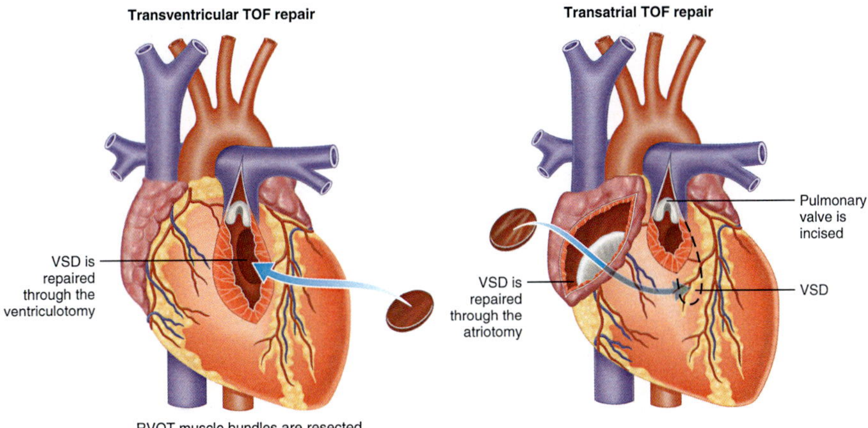

Fig. 19.7 Transventricular and transatrial repair

Because the regurgitant fraction of the RV decreases with increased heart rate associated with activity, the adverse impact of RV dilation on RV function may be clinically subtle until the RV is severely dysfunctional, especially if the tricuspid valve remains competent (Borowski et al. 2004). The most common late surgical reintervention in patients who have had previous repair of TOF is to place a functional valve into the pulmonary position to protect the RV from further long-term effects of pulmonary insufficiency (Babu-Narayan et al. 2014; Quail et al. 2012). Somewhat less common is reintervention to relieve RVOT obstruction resulting from recurrent infundibular hypertrophy or progression of native pulmonary valve stenosis (Yoo et al. 2012).

Institutional preferences for transatrial resection of the infundibulum in selected cases versus routine right ventriculotomy exist (Hoohenkerk et al. 2008) (Fig. 19.7). Bicaval cannulation and aortic occlusion are required for each. In either approach, care is taken by the surgical team to evaluate the RVOT, size of the pulmonary annulus and the morphology of the pulmonary valve, and the sizes of the main and proximal branch pulmonary arteries and create an individual surgical plan for each patient. If a ventriculotomy is required for infundibulectomy in a patient with an adequate pulmonary valve annulus, it is limited to the sub-annular infundibulum and not extended to the apex of the RV (Bacha 2012). Depending on the appearance of the pulmonary valve, one or two leaflets may be left intact if they are not severely dysplastic because some pulmonary valve competence (even if it is associated with mild obstruction) is of both short-term and long-term value in preserving RV function (Vida et al. 2014). If aggressive RVOT resection extending across the annulus with total resection of the pulmonary valve is required, a monocusp valve (usually homograft) may be incorporated into the RVOT patch leaving a nonautologous valve leaflet in the pulmonary position (Chiappini et al. 2007) (Fig. 19.8). This technique provides the RV with some protection by reducing pulmonary insufficiency in the postoperative period. Although the longevity of the homograft pulmonary monocusp is limited, its use seems to be associated with a more benign postoperative course. Some authors advocate creating the monocusp from Gore-Tex for increased durability (Turrentine et al. 2002) (Fig. 19.9).

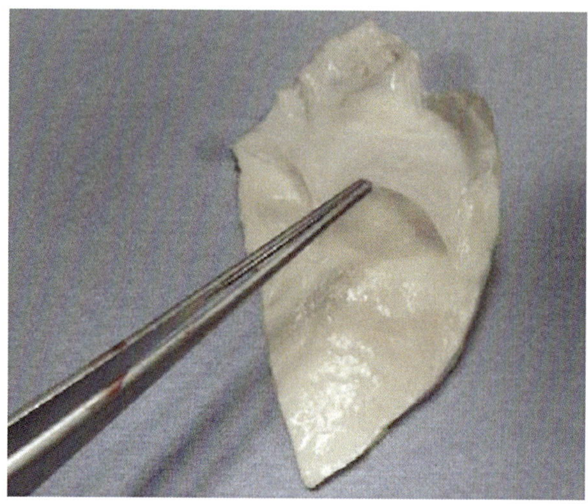

Fig. 19.8 Homograft monocusp (Mulinari et al. 2008)

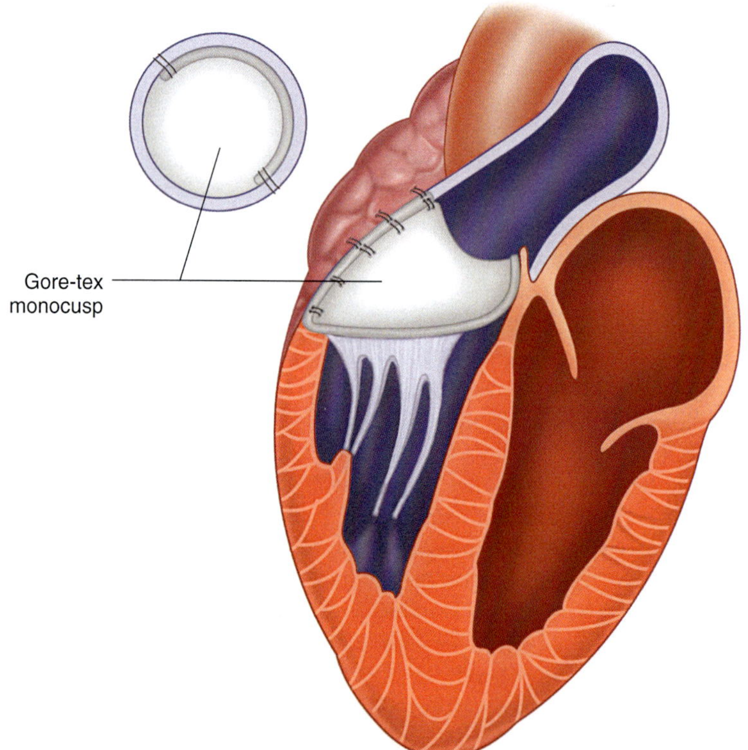

Fig. 19.9 Gore-Tex monocusp

Natural History of Operative Correction

The natural history of patients following TOF repair is primarily related to the outcome of the RVOT. With the improvement in the surgical techniques in the last 60 years, the incidences of left ventricular failure and pulmonary vascular disease have significantly decreased (Cuypers et al. 2014; Alexiou et al. 2001; Burchill et al. 2011; Lindsey et al. 2010). The VSD repair seems to not be a long-term issue. The typical ECG of a postoperative TOF patient often shows right bundle branch block or conduction delay from the placement of the VSD patch, but progression to heart block is rare. Ventricular arrhythmias, when they occur, may be suggestive of morphologic changes of the right ventricle late after repair and indicate the need to reexamine the patient's hemodynamics.

In the eccentrically hypertrophic dilated RV, arrhythmias are associated with a change in right ventricular geometry, but coronary perfusion and RV ischemia are not an issue. The normal preload/stroke volume relationships are maintained but at larger end-systolic and end-diastolic volumes. In contrast, in the concentrically hypertrophic RV, arrhythmias may be indicative of increases in RV wall thickness and stress that threaten coronary blood flow to the endocardium. In the normal low pressure RV, right coronary blood flow to the RV endocardium occurs in systole and diastole, but when the RV systolic pressure increases in response to obstruction, the coronary artery flow pattern occurs mainly in diastole (as in the normal left ventricle). The reduced compliance of the concentrically hypertrophic right ventricular chamber also increases the preload dependence of the right ventricle, that is, decreased end-diastolic volume is associated with severe decreases in stroke volume. Otherwise, the relationship between stroke volume and preload is flattened with increased end-diastolic volumes being associated with increased end-diastolic pressure, but not stroke volume (Fig. 19.10).

Pulmonary valve replacement is the most common surgical reintervention late after initial repair in patients with TOF (Burchill et al. 2011; Geva 2006). The indications are varied, but most relate to the protection of the right ventricle and limiting

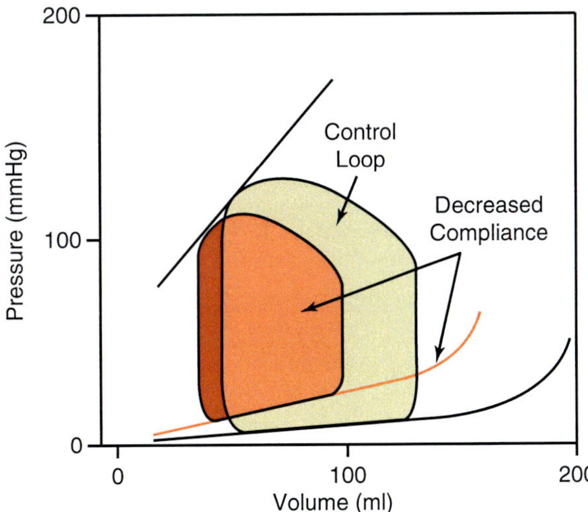

Fig. 19.10 Compliance curve

its exposure to chronic volume loading (or pressure loading) conditions. Prior to the deleterious late effects on right ventricular function, chronic eccentric dilation of the RV can lead to early tricuspid valve insufficiency if the valve annulus dilates and the valve leaflets fail to coapt. Protection of the tricuspid valve is important for the patient's long-term well-being in that prosthetic valve replacement of the tricuspid valve, although technically simple, is associated with its own unfavorable long-term outcomes (Cheng et al. 2012). Mechanical valves in the tricuspid position have a high incidence of failure from thrombus or pannus formation despite the use of anticoagulation. Biologic valves in the tricuspid position do not require anticoagulation but have limited durability, which is of concern in the pediatric population (Said et al. 2014).

Timing of pulmonary valve (PV) replacement may be difficult because symptoms of RV dysfunction, especially associated with pulmonary insufficiency, are subtle until the RV has overtly failed. MRI imaging may be useful in establishing volumetric measurements of cardiac chamber size and regurgitant volumes, and stress testing with echocardiography may reveal subtle presentations of RV dysfunction (Babu-Narayan et al. 2014). If PV replacement is delayed until RV function is significantly compromised, the recovery of RV function after valve replacement is not reliable (Hallbergson et al. 2014).

Although surgical PV replacement is low risk in the older child and teenager, there may be increased risk of repeat sternotomy, including complex surgical bleeding and accidental reentry complications violating the right ventricular outflow tract which is often adhered to the posterior sternal table. Increasing interest in the percutaneous placement of a catheter-delivered pulmonary valve into the right ventricular outflow tract by the interventional cardiologist has led to some promising early outcomes and technical success (Cuypers et al. 2014; Cheatham et al. 2015). (Recurrence of RVOT obstruction cannot currently be managed with a catheter technique.) However, the overall risk of surgical PV replacement utilizing cardiopulmonary bypass is very low, and the long-term history of such reconstruction is reliably favorable. It is premature to conclude that percutaneous PV replacement will accomplish the same safety profile and long-term outcomes, despite the attractiveness of avoiding a repeat sternotomy.

Comorbidities

Important comorbidities associated with tetralogy of Fallot include malformations of the multipotent neural crest cells. Derived from the ectoderm germ layer, these cells differentiate into neural cells, connective tissue, pharyngeal arches, parts of the cardiac septum and ultimate bulboventricular/truncal apparatus, and endocrine tissue of thyroid, parathyroid, and thymus glands. DiGeorge syndrome (22q11 deletion) and similar microdeletion syndromes account for some of the frequently observed anomalies seen in 20 % of patients with TOF (Lammer et al. 2009). Palatal anatomic abnormalities (such as clefts) and functional abnormalities (such as velopharyngeal incompetence) may be seen (Wyse et al. 1990). Disorders of parathyroid function, renal anomalies, laryngotracheal/esophageal anomalies, immune disorders from reduced T cell function, skeletal anomalies, and hearing and developmental disorders are frequently encountered in patients with these chromosome disorders. In addition to TOF, the other cardiac anomalies associated with these genetic conditions usually have a substrate of embryologic conotruncal malformation (e.g., ventricular septal defect, transposition of the great arteries, truncus arteriosus, and double outlet right ventricle). Therefore, the potential associations of VACTERL syndrome, DiGeorge syndrome, velocardiofacial syndrome, and CHARGE syndrome should specifically be considered when caring for a patient with TOF (Shprintzen et al. 1981).

Nonsyndromic comorbidities that are important are primarily related to the hematologic consequences of chronic hypoxemia (Tempe and Virmani 2002). A normal hematocrit is frequently seen in cyanotic patients when physiologic anemia is otherwise expected at 2–3 months of age because of increased erythropoiesis. If the infant is nutritionally competent, polycythemia develops over the following months.

The most important consequence of polycythemia in the cyanotic patient about to undergo surgery is platelet dysfunction (Zabala and Guzzetta 2015). Although the platelet count is usually normal, the function of the platelets is diminished. Platelet microparticles are overproduced in cyanotic conditions because of shear forces associated with hyperviscosity of the blood, and there is a higher concentration of circulating immature platelets that have already been activated. Functional stimulation testing of the patient's platelets to an ADP challenge is decreased and inversely proportional to the patient's baseline hematocrit.

Anesthesia Considerations

Most patients with TOF undergo corrective surgery as infants (Kirsch et al. 2009). Many of these patients have a chronic degree of cyanosis, and some also have hypercyanotic spells that may be treated with a beta-blocker. Correlating the parents' observation of cyanosis to the echocardiogram findings of fixed and dynamic obstruction is often useful in predicting how labile the patient's arterial saturation may be under anesthesia, although it is important to note that parents often underreport their infant's episodes of desaturation despite proactively and frequently feeding hoping to minimize the episodes of crying and cyanosis (Sharkey and Sharma 2012).

Although not routinely used by many anesthesiologists caring for infants, there are cogent reasons to consider a premedication in an infant with TOF. If an intravenous (IV) catheter is to be placed prior to induction, the use of a premedication may reduce the likelihood of a hypercyanotic spell during placement (Montero et al. 2015). If an inhalation induction is planned, a sedated infant who is not crying is less likely to "spell" during induction. Although there are some concerns about respiratory depression in a patient with cyanosis, it is the bias of the author that the benefits of a non-opioid premedication are preferable, and an inhalation induction of anesthesia is routinely performed deferring IV placement until the patient is anesthetized.

The hemodynamic goals during the administration of anesthesia relate to the dynamic portion of RVOT obstruction (Pierce et al. 2012). (There is little the anesthesiologist can do to significantly alter the fixed portion of RVOT obstruction.) In the infant's baseline state, crying and other activities that increase cardiac output are associated with relatively less pulmonary blood flow as more blood is shunted right to left across the VSD and right ventricular blood is ejected out of the aorta in the face of an increasingly obstructive infundibulum. Under anesthesia, the loading conditions of the RV and the patient's systemic afterload are also factors that can be altered by the choice and implementation of anesthesia medications and technique. Decreased venous preloading of the right ventricle can be associated with increased infundibular obstruction and right-to-left shunting. Therefore, dehydration is poorly tolerated, and if the patient does not have an IV preoperatively, the feeding schedule including the administration of clear liquids should be meticulously planned. Likewise, significant decreases in systemic afterload are associated with increased right-to-left shunting. High doses of volatile agents or the administration of vasodilating intravenous medications such as propofol may be associated with vasodilation and hypercyanosis. Suboptimal depth of anesthesia during important stimulation may be associated with a hyperdynamic response that leads to a "Tet spell."

A wide variety of anesthetic techniques and agents have been successfully used and are not contraindicated as long as the important physiologic goals are met (White 2011). It is of historical interest to note that until it became unavailable, the use of halothane carefully administered was similar to "inhalational beta-blockade" and accomplished the modest decrease in cardiac contractility and heart rate beneficial to TOF physiology (Greeley et al. 1986). The preferential dilation by halothane of the capacitance vessels prior to the resistance vessels could theoretically make the TOF patient unstable, but if the inspired concentration of halothane was carefully limited, hypercyanotic spells during induction were rare. Sevoflurane is successfully used and has significantly less cardiodepression and vasodilation than halothane; "inhalational beta-blockade" does not occur with Sevoflurane. Ketamine has the obvious advantage of maintaining systemic vascular resistance and preload, but the drawbacks of tachycardia and a hyperdynamic state are somewhat inconsistent with our goals of hemodynamic control. Etomidate maintains preload and afterload conditions well, but the lack of depression of cardiac contractile function and heart rate is a disadvantage when the patient is stimulated by endotracheal intubation, unless adjunctive medications are used to blunt the sympathetic response.

The choice of induction agent is not as important as it may seem; careful induction of anesthesia in a patient with TOF is associated with increased mixed venous oxygen levels as long as adequate cardiac output is maintained (Tug 2000). Therefore the SaO2 of the TOF patient increases during induction as long as preload and afterload are adequate, and heart rate does not significantly increase. The author's opinion is the most common reason for a TOF patient to decompensate during induction other than extreme hemodynamic intrusion is airway misadventure. Meticulous and skilled airway management during induction and intubation is as important as the nuances of selecting the optimal induction technique and medications. Beyond the direct effects of hypoxia occurring with poor airway management during (IV) induction, airway obstruction or laryngospasm during poorly managed stage 2 or stage 3 of an inhalation induction is associated with hemodynamic intrusions that are specifically deleterious to the TOF patient (Parker et al. 1999). The hemodynamic effects of acute airway obstruction and the maneuvers required to relieve it are associated with decreases in preload that can precipitate cyanosis. Laryngospasm should be promptly treated with succinylcholine as both high levels of CPAP and propofol can precipitate hypercyanosis. Interestingly, hypercarbia associated with airway compromise in the unrepaired TOF patient is deleterious only because it is associated with sympathetic cardiac activation. Hypercarbia-induced elevations in pulmonary vascular resistance are somewhat irrelevant to right-to-left shunting because the pulmonary vascular bed is distal to the mechanical obstruction of the RVOT.

If a TOF patient has severe desaturation despite a patent, instrumented airway, it must be assumed that pulmonary blood flow is critically decreased. Volume expansion to increase preload, vasoconstriction to increase afterload and decrease right-to-left shunting, and control of inotropic function and heart rate with beta-blockade are acceptable treatments. Alpha-mediated vasoconstrictors are commonly used as both bolus and infusion therapy for hypercyanosis during anesthesia, and although medications such as phenylephrine are effective at first, their effectiveness is limited (Tanaka et al. 2003). If the vasoconstriction also leads to decreased cardiac output as is commonly seen in an infusion of phenylephrine, the concomitant decrease in mixed venous oxygen saturation (SvO2) results in less impressive increases in SaO2 over a short time, mimicking "tachyphylaxis." Therefore, it is recommended that vasopressor use be considered as an effective temporizing measure, while the patient's intravascular volume status is optimized, and beta-blockade considered. Intraoperative beta-blockade in the patient already on propranolol requires caution, and the use of esmolol, which can be titrated to effect, is advisable (Britt et al. 2014). The ultimate treatment for a hypercyanotic spell refractory to these measures, especially if associated with surgical manipulation of the heart, is to institute cardiopulmonary bypass.

Surgical repair of TOF is considered a low to moderate risk procedure in most institutions, and convalescence is usually uncomplicated. Advances in myocardial protection have made severe left or right ventricular dysfunction after repair uncommon (Dyamenahalli et al. 2000). Postoperative function of the right ventricle is most related to the intrusion and extent of ventricular muscle resection required to adequately relieve obstruction of the RVOT, and whether it is feasible to leave a portion of the native pulmonary valve in place or alternatively reconstruct the RVOT with a monocusp-type patch (Wells et al. 2002). In contrast to LV function, RV diastolic compliance is often poor after repair, requiring remodeling to significantly improve (Fogel et al. 2012). Postoperative improvement over time in measures of concentric RV hypertrophy is associated with improved RV diastolic function. If RV function is anticipated to be poor postoperatively, some surgeons will leave a small ASD to provide a "right-to-left pop-off." Echocardiographic examination of the surgical repair is commonly done in the operating room to rule out important residual VSD patch leaks or inadequately relieved RVOT obstruction and to assess ventricular function.

Common postoperative considerations are straightforward. Modest inotropic and lusitropic support may be useful to optimize RV function. Heart block may be seen after repair as the sutures for the VSD patch are in proximity to the conduction system, but it is most commonly temporary unless the surgeon has significantly misplaced a patch stitch. Right bundle branch block usually occurs and is often permanent (Karadeniz et al. 2014). Although malignant ventricular arrhythmias are not common, the postoperative occurrence of junctional ectopic tachycardia (JET) is seen in some patients and may be associated with an exaggerated decrease in cardiac output because the postoperative RV diastolic function is so dependent on adequate loading conditions (Zampi et al. 2012). Interestingly these patients are more stable immediately after surgery and during the 6–10 h required for myocardial reperfusion edema to resolve than they are at 12–24 h when JET is typically seen (Andreasen et al. 2008). This underscores the hemodynamic intrusion of ventricular dysmorphology on diastolic function and the importance of paced synchronous or normal sinus rhythm. Temporary atrial and ventricular pacing wires are commonly placed prior to sternal closure to assist managing these conditions (Barker et al. 2013).

Anatomic Variants of TOF

The specific anatomic details of the lesion may determine the timing of surgery. While the degree of RVOT usually informs the timing of repair in uncomplicated TOF, other considerations such as size or unusual location of the VSD, additional anomalies such as ductus arteriosus-dependent lesions, severely hypoplastic pulmonary arteries or pulmonary atresia, endocardial cushion defects, coronary artery anomalies involving an anomalous coronary artery crossing the surgical ventriculotomy site, and important noncardiac comorbidities that require urgent surgical intervention may lead the surgical team to perform a palliative systemic-to-pulmonary shunt during early infancy and defer complete repair to a later time.

PDA-Dependent Lesions

Pulmonary Atresia and Critical Pulmonary Stenosis

Some patients with TOF also have atresia or critical stenosis of the pulmonary valve, rendering them PDA dependent for pulmonary blood flow after birth. Normal transition from fetal to neonatal circulation cannot occur, and after stabilization of the neonate with prostaglandin E (PgE), surgical or interventional catheterization treatment is undertaken.

Preoperative evaluation of such complex variants must also carefully assess the morphology of the right ventricle (Yoshimura et al. 2002; Alsoufi et al. 2015). A tripartite right ventricle with an inlet, body, and outlet component is likely to grow and be ultimately usable in a complete repair that includes closure of the VSD. Most centers would attempt to establish antegrade blood flow from the right ventricle to the pulmonary artery by valvotomy or valvectomy as early as possible in the neonate.

The timing and technique of neonatal surgical pulmonary valvotomy has evolved since the 1970s (Humpl et al. 2003). Originally performed in the neonate utilizing

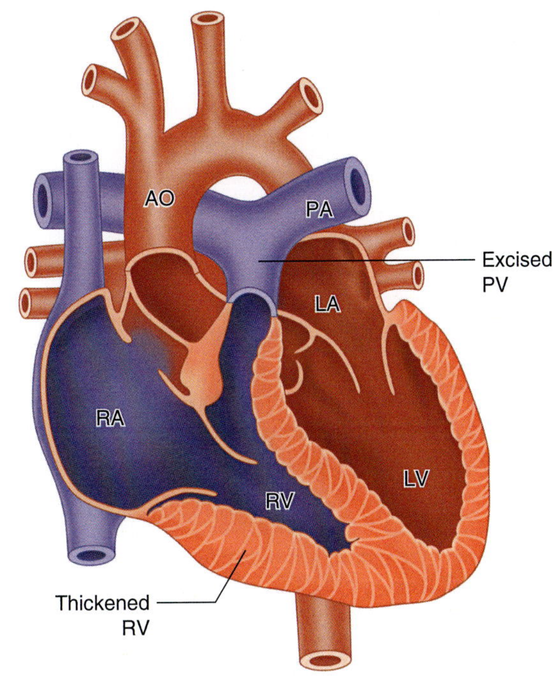

Fig. 19.11 Suicide RV and right-to-left atrial shunting

"inflow occlusion" or a brief period of cardiopulmonary bypass, the postoperative course of the patient was often stormy and unstable (Odegard et al. 2004). Now it is no longer undertaken as an emergency procedure in response to a neonate becoming cyanotic after delivery, presumably when the PDA constricts. PgE is routinely used to reopen the PDA to relieve cyanosis. Typically the caliber of an open PDA in a term neonate is 5 mm or larger, so persistent desaturation in the presence of a PDA demonstrated by echocardiography is indicative of moderate elevation of pulmonary vascular resistance. It is common to expectantly observe patients for several days after birth while on PgE in order to detect the beginnings of the normal decline in PVR that will manifest by the SaO_2 increasing to the 90s. At that time the chest X-ray should demonstrate nonoligemic lung fields and slight cardiomegaly. Surgical palliation is then undertaken under more stable conditions.

The surgical technique has also undergone refinement. An attempt is made to incise the commonly fused leaflets in an abnormal pulmonary valve, but simple relief of an obstructed valve does not immediately improve the neonate's physiology. The extreme concentric hypertrophy of the RVOT in these patients makes the postoperative convalescence difficult as the noncompliant RV leads to right-to-left shunting across a patent foramen ovale or atrial septal defect despite surgical relief of the obstruction at the pulmonary valve (Schwartz et al. 2013). Dynamic systolic obliteration of the RVOT often occurs even if it has no fixed obstruction and is sometimes referred to as "suicide right ventricle" (Fig. 19.11). In order to avoid severe cyanosis from this temporary condition, it is advisable to also place a modified Blalock-Taussig shunt that will provide additional pulmonary blood flow that is independent of RV loading and contractile dynamics. As the diastolic function of the RV improves after surgery, the amount of pulmonary blood flow provided by the shunt will be relatively less important as antegrade RV to PA blood flow increases.

It is also common for a neonate with critical pulmonary valve stenosis to undergo palliative balloon valvotomy in the cardiac catheterization laboratory as an alternative to surgery. Although it is technically successful most of the time to adequately open the valve by balloon dilation tearing fused valve leaflets, or even to puncture a pulmonary valve membrane with a wire and then dilate the dysmorphic valve, the possibility of "suicide RV" physiology is still pertinent. It is often necessary to leave the patient on PgE after the procedure until diastolic function improves enough to allow adequate antegrade pulmonary blood flow.

The advantage of an interventional catheterization procedure is that sternotomy is deferred. If however, after the PgE is weaned and discontinued, the estimation of the adequacy of the RV is incorrect or the infant's RVOT becomes severely obstructive prior to the planned surgical repair, the patient becomes very unstable since there is no auxiliary source of pulmonary blood flow. (In some centers a stent is placed in the PDA by the cardiologist at the time of pulmonary balloon valvotomy in an attempt to avoid that complication; however stent malposition and early failure are drawbacks to this approach that may adversely affect short-term outcome.) The advantage of neonatal surgical intervention is that both the valve and the RVOT can be addressed if needed, and a modified BT shunt placed which should be reliable in the event that the RVOT undergoes obstructive changes in the months prior to the planned corrective procedure. Good short-term results have been demonstrated with both strategies, and the prevalence of one approach is often an institutional preference.

Although the patient will for a time have two sources of pulmonary blood flow, heart failure is rarely seen since there are two ventricles to manage the volume load. Corrective surgical repair is often timed with regard to the type of RVOT reconstruction required, especially in the case of anticipated RV to pulmonary artery conduit implantation. Significant progression of cyanosis usually is not an issue as the patient receives pulmonary blood flow via the BTS and antegrade across the RV to the PA. Except under conditions of extreme hypotension, hypercyanotic episodes do not occur in TOF (or variants) palliated with a functioning BTS because the physiologic conditions that would normally precipitate the episode (increased CO) are also associated with increased BTS blood flow.

Non-PDA-Dependent Lesions

Absent Pulmonary Valve Syndrome

An uncommon TOF variant is absent pulmonary valve syndrome (Hraska 2005) (Fig. 19.12). When there is complete absence of pulmonary valve tissue, the proximal pulmonary artery undergoes aneurysmal dilation from the wide-open to-and-fro pulmonary blood flow. The resulting comorbidity is a combination of airway compression by the dilated pulmonary vasculature and tracheobronchomalacia

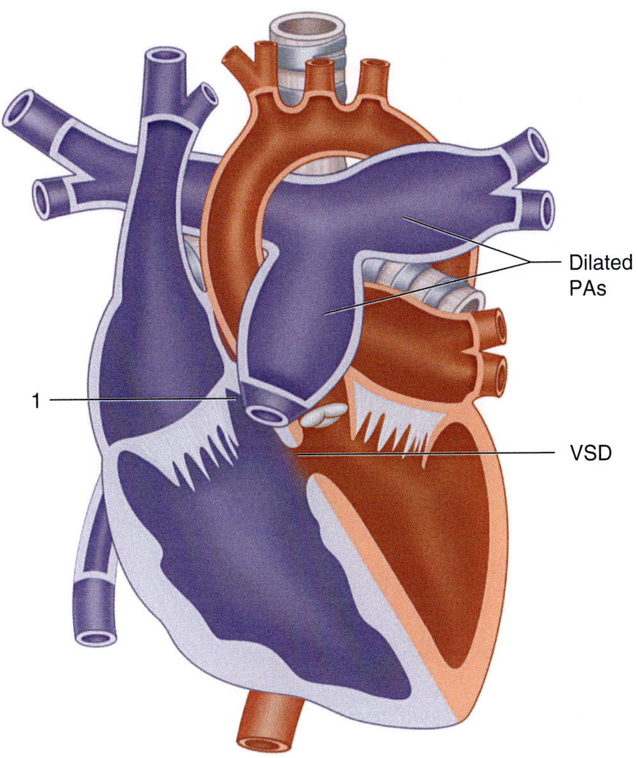

Fig. 19.12 Absent pulmonary valve syndrome. (*1*) absent pulmonary valve

from delayed maturation of the skeletal tracheobronchial tree. Neonates with this anomaly have notable respiratory distress and cyanosis with chest X-ray evidence of barotrauma and air trapping. Intubation and respiratory support prior to surgery are common, and often patients are on significant levels of PEEP or even ventilated in the prone position. Respiratory failure is an indication for neonatal complete repair, which includes the usual components of TOF repair as well as plication of the proximal dilated pulmonary artery. As with any patient with tracheomalacia, placement of a transesophageal echo probe may worsen airway obstruction. Persistent tracheobronchomalacia is relatively common and may delay ventilator weaning after surgery.

Coronary Artery Anomalies

Coronary artery anomalies present in up to 10 % of patients with TOF, and although they have no impact on the previously discussed physiology issues, they may pose serious implications for the surgeon in accomplishing reconstruction of the RVOT (Dabizzi et al. 1990). The most common abnormality is when the left anterior descending (LAD) coronary artery arises from the right coronary artery. If a transannular incision is required in the patient to relieve RVOT obstruction, the LAD may cross in the vicinity of the ventriculotomy site. As the artery cannot be sacrificed without significant damage to the left ventricle, the surgeon would modify his plan to reconstruct RVOT to PA continuity with a conduit, leaving the patient's native RVOT and epicardial coronary artery undisturbed. Although this can be easily done in the infant, the small size or the lack of durability of the conduit that might be used might lead the surgeon to alternatively palliate the patient with a modified BT shunt deferring corrective repair until the patient is larger. Therefore, in every case of TOF, echocardiographic interrogation of the proximal coronary arteries is routinely required for adequate surgical planning. Aortic root or selective coronary angiography to delineate the proximal coronary circulation when it cannot be discerned by echocardiography may be indicated.

Other Anomalies Requiring Palliative Shunting Prior to Complete Repair

Anatomic variants of TOF previously discussed have indicated either the need for a palliative intervention with or without a shunt procedure in the case of some types of critical pulmonary valve disease or have presented impediments to the usual surgical techniques of RVOT reconstruction in some cases of TOF with coronary anomalies. Two additional clinical situations might disturb the usual preoperative planning in a patient with TOF.

Additional Congenital Cardiac Anomaly

If there is a concomitant congenital cardiac lesion, consideration of the additional defect might alter the usual planning for TOF repair. A PDA-dependent lesion requiring ductal patency for systemic perfusion (e.g., coarctation/interrupted aortic arch) would require neonatal surgical intervention regardless of whether the specific anatomy of the TOF defect deserved immediate surgical attention. The risks and benefits of performing a palliative BTS versus complete TOF repair at the time of repairing another left heart obstructive lesion would be determined individually (Fraser et al. 2001). Most cardiac lesions with complex components of two more simple anomalies have a higher risk profile and worse short- and long-term outcome than either of the simpler anomalies separately considered. Additionally they are rarer, so the preoperative planning and judgments do not necessarily have the benefit of large previous experience or information in standard databases.

As previously discussed, TOF with PDA-dependent pulmonary circulation is a more frequently seen variant of TOF compared to left heart obstructive lesions. The alterations of surgical and palliative planning pertinent to those lesions are better understood. Placement of a modified or central shunt is an essential component of palliating these conditions and does not independently affect when the VSD repair and RVOT reconstruction might be done (Batra et al. 2005).

TOF in association with non-PDA-dependent anomalies such as atrioventricular canal has different considerations (Ong et al. 2012). Palliative shunting might be indicated if the clinical importance of cyanosis from the TOF component preceded the optimal time to undertake reconstruction of the endocardial cushion defect with regard to the maturity of the atrioventricular valve tissue. Whether undertaken separately or at the same time, the presence of two complex cardiac lesions usually complicates the surgical repair and adversely impacts the expected outcomes (Shuhaiber et al. 2012).

Additional Noncardiac Congenital Anomaly

TOF is frequently associated with a genetic syndrome (Gonzalez et al. 2009). In the most severe cases, consideration may be made for palliative shunting rather than complete repair if the extent or severity of the chromosome anomaly is not well defined in early infancy. Significant chromosome abnormalities are associated with a worse outcome for complete repair of TOF (Michielon et al. 2006).

Noncardiac conditions such as duodenal atresia, esophageal atresia with tracheo-esophageal fistula, meningomyelocele, diaphragmatic hernia, and others may require surgical intervention in the neonate prior to when TOF might be considered for complete repair. The preanesthesia cardiac screening strategy for neonates with congenital noncardiac anomalies is not clearly defined in the literature (White 2011; Walker et al. 2009). Midline defects are associated with a higher incidence of coexisting cardiac defects, and preoperative cardiac echocardiography in addition to pulse oximetry and a chest X-ray has been advocated (Ritter et al. 1999). Recently, the recommendation to include echocardiography has been challenged as unnecessary (in the case of duodenal atresia) if the neonate's pulse oximetry, chest X-ray, and cardiac exam are unremarkable and there is no associated Down syndrome (Short et al. 2014; Nasr et al. 2010; Keckler et al. 2008).

However the preanesthetic cardiac evaluation in the neonate presenting for urgent noncardiac repair should be directed at identifying lesions that might present unexpected instability under anesthesia. Although an unremarkable physical exam and pulse oximetry can be reassuring, the author opines that the most difficult anesthetic challenges could be presented by a neonate who has an undiagnosed PDA-dependent lesion that requires maintenance of the PDA for either systemic or pulmonary blood flow. Coarctation of the aorta, interrupted aortic arch, hypoplastic left heart syndrome, pulmonary atresia, and some other cardiac lesions are associated with fairly normal physical exams in the neonate when the ductus arteriosus is open. Pulse oximetry may appear unremarkable as a normal room air SaO2 in a newborn is often no higher than 95 %. In the author's opinion, identifying the presence of an occult cardiac lesion and preparing for a patient who would be critically affected by unstable ductal patency is the most important indication to proceed with cardiac echocardiography in these patients before urgent noncardiac surgery.

Physics and Physiology of Systemic Pulmonary Shunting

The use of the systemic-to-pulmonary arterial shunt has significantly advanced the palliative care of children with both single-ventricle cardiac lesions and children with two-ventricle anomalies where a temporary source of pulmonary blood flow is required pending corrective repair. The current use of a modified Blalock-Taussig shunt (MBTS) or a Gore-Tex central shunt from the aorta to the pulmonary artery has made previous versions such as the classic Blalock-Taussig shunt and the Waterston and Potts aortopulmonary window procedures obsolete.

In the neonate, usually a 3.5 or 4.0 mm Gore-Tex tube is used to create the shunt. The physiology of blood flow from the aorta through the shunt to the pulmonary circulation follows the principles of tube physics described by Poiseuille's law:

$$\text{Flow} = \pi\left(P_1 - P_2\right)\left(\text{radius}\right)^4 / 8\left(\text{viscosity}\right)\left(\text{length}\right)$$

In this model, flow through the tube is determined by both the physical characteristics of the tube (a multiplied direct effect of the radius and an inverse effect of length), the viscosity of the blood (an inverse effect), and physiologic variables that may be controlled to some degree by manipulation of the patient's hemodynamics. The driving pressure for the shunt is the patient's blood pressure (P1), and the resisting pressure (P2) is the pulmonary arterial pressure (Fig. 19.13).

It is a significant advantage of the MBTS that since the patient's blood pressure even during transition is higher than the pulmonary artery pressure; the shunt is usable even before pulmonary vascular resistance has lowered to the levels seen in older infants and toddlers. Given that the expected duration of time the shunt is required is only temporary (often only 3–6 months), the fact that it will not grow

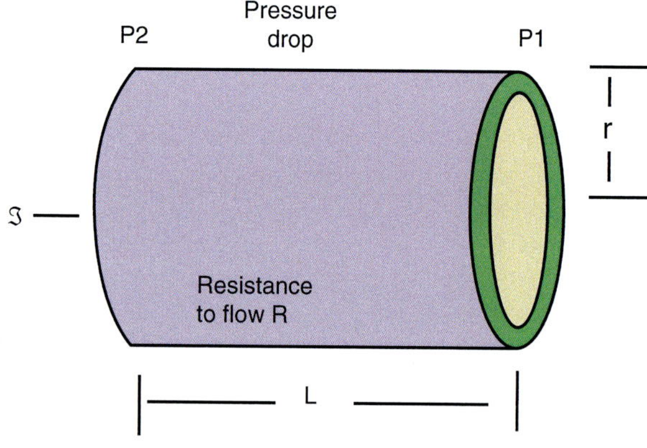

Fig. 19.13 Tube physics

with the patient is advantageous and allows the normal maturation of the pulmonary vascular bed to proceed with little chance of excessive shear stress causing damage to the pulmonary vasculature. The disadvantage of the MBTS is that it is an inefficient method of oxygenating the mixed venous blood because the gradient for oxygen uptake in the lung is narrow, and the result is that even with optimal function of the shunt, there is mild to moderate desaturation despite an elevated Qp/Qs ratio. Cardiomegaly and overcirculated lung fields on chest X-ray are common. This volume load can adversely affect the diastolic function of the ventricle, but this complication is more likely to be important in the single-ventricle model than in the two-ventricle model such as TOF.

The normal course of events in the infant who has undergone palliative shunting is that as the infant grows, the amount of pulmonary blood flow relative to the systemic cardiac output decreases, resulting in decreased saturations. Any clinical evidence of overcirculation such as failure to thrive or high-output cardiac failure resolves with growth. Chest X-ray evidence of cardiomegaly or overcirculated lung fields also resolves. In the presence of reduced pulmonary blood flow, the natural process of remodeling by regression of the medial muscular layer of the pulmonary vascular bed occurs. Although of historical interest in patients with Potts or Waterston shunts, pulmonary vascular resistance issues are not usually a feature of the TOF/MBTS patient about to have corrective surgery.

Anesthesia Issues of Systemic Pulmonary Shunting

The anesthesia management of a neonate who is undergoing placement of a palliative MBTS or central shunt is challenging. A detailed understanding of the surgical procedure and the effects of anesthetic technique, ventilation, and vasoactive medications on blood pressure (P1) and pulmonary vascular resistance (P2) are essential.

If the neonate is on a PgE infusion to maintain patency of the ductus arteriosus, arterial saturations should be in the 80s to mid-90s, depending on how effectively the pulmonary vascular resistance has fallen since delivery. In the presence of the PDA, the MBTS is often done with a median sternotomy incision so that the shunt can be completed and then the ductus arteriosus (DA) ligated through the same incision (Fig. 19.14). Cardiopulmonary bypass is typically available as a standby resource, but it is common to attempt to avoid it in order to avoid the hematologic intrusions on the neonate's coagulation system if possible. It is helpful to consider in siting the pulse oximeter probes, blood pressure cuff, and arterial catheter that part of the procedure will involve partial occlusion of the circulation to the right arm. Cerebral and somatic oximetries are also useful. The aorta, right innominate artery, and main and right pulmonary artery are dissected and mobilized. A small dose of heparin is administered according to institutional protocol. A side-biting C-clamp is positioned on the innominate (or subclavian) artery, and the proximal end of the 3.5–4.0 mm Gore-Tex shunt is anastomosed with a running suture. Typically the C-clamp occludes a significant portion of the radius of the artery and

Fig. 19.14 BTS creation

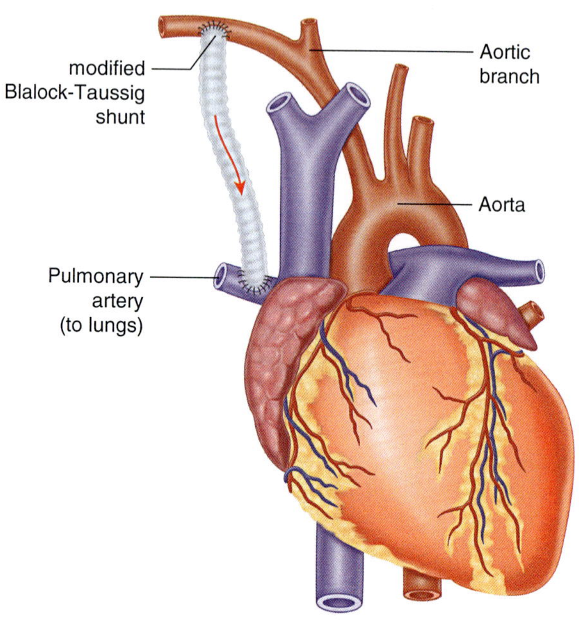

causes a decrease in systemic cardiac output by causing an elevation in "mechanical resistance" analogous to increased systemic vascular resistance. In the setting of a PDA, which mimics the physiology of the pending BTS, inotropic support to maintain an adequate blood pressure may be helpful during this stage to compensate the decrease in P1 caused by the partial occlusion clamp. Changes in ventilation are not usually necessary. As this anastomosis is completed, the shunt is filled with heparinized saline, and a bulldog-type clamp is used to occlude the open end to facilitate trimming to an appropriate length for the planned distal anastomosis. The C-clamp on the innominate artery is removed and normal hemodynamics restored. Attention is then turned to the pulmonary artery, and a C-clamp is placed on the right pulmonary artery. During this time, pulmonary blood flow will be diminished by nearly half, and as the PDA is providing blood flow from the distal transverse aorta to the left pulmonary artery, inotropic support of blood pressure (P1) will continue to be useful. Additional adjustments in FiO2 and minute ventilation in order to maintain arterial saturations in the 80s are often required. In theory, pulmonary artery hypertension should be avoided as an elevated P2 could compromise blood flow via the DA; however, the deleterious effects of hypocarbia on cerebral blood flow should also be considered in the neonate. The minimal benefit of lowering PVR with hyperventilation should be weighed against the intrusion on neonatal cerebral autoregulation associated with acute hypocarbia. When the shunt is complete, the C-clamp on the pulmonary artery and the occlusion clamp on the shunt are removed as the distal anastomosis is de-aired and the suture tightened. Since there is now pulmonary blood flow via the DA and the shunt, the SaO2 normally rises to or above the mid-90s. The FiO2 should be decreased to 30–40% during this time. The expected SaO2 in a term size neonate with a 3.5–4.0 shunt should be 80–90%. Attention is turned to the PDA, and after test occlusion with a clamp to verify the function of the MBTS is adequate to oxygenate the patient at 30–40% FiO2, the DA is ligated.

In the hemodynamic model of an unrepaired TOF patient without a PDA, the urgent or emergent placement of a MBTS is a more difficult exercise in hemodynamic manipulation. The order of the surgical procedure is as described above, but there is no safety margin of a DA supplying a cardiac output-dependent source of pulmonary blood flow during the procedure. Antegrade pulmonary blood flow relies on adequate RV filling, an adequately maintained systemic vascular resistance, and control of heart rate and contractile function to avoid a hyperdynamic cardiac state. Failure to accomplish these hemodynamic goals is associated with progressive and paroxysmal hypercyanosis. During creation of the MBTS, placement of the C-clamp on the innominate or carotid artery is usually well tolerated initially as it creates mechanical resistance to systemic cardiac output that reduces right-to-left shunting across the VSD similar to the administration of an alpha-adrenergic agent. In general, inotropic support during placement of the proximal end of the shunt is not required and may precipitate hypercyanosis by causing a hyperdynamic infundibulum to become more obstructive to RV blood flow into the pulmonary artery. In the absence of a PDA, when the pulmonary artery is partially occluded to complete the distal anastomosis of the shunt, SaO2 decreases markedly. Manipulations of ventilation and FiO2 are often only minimally successful. Attempts to augment cardiac output are counterproductive as the right-to-left shunt is worsened. Adequate volume loading and careful control of heart rate are the only manipulations available to the anesthesiologist. Careful communication between the surgeon and anesthesiologist is required when the patient experiences significant arterial desaturation to consider whether the patient is too unstable to complete the shunt without instituting cardiopulmonary bypass.

Troubleshooting the apparently failing shunt in the operating room is an exercise of collaboration and communication between the surgeon and anesthesiologist. After the shunt is completed, regardless of whether CPB was utilized, the physiologic model of TOF converts to the model described by the components of Poiseuille's law with P1 and P2 controllable by the anesthesiologist. Inotropic support to increase shunt flow is common for a short time after surgery when the patient is at risk for shunt thrombosis. The critical clinical dilemma in the operating room or the post-op intensive care unit is when the patient's saturations decline despite adequate hemodynamics. In the operating room, it is easy for the surgeon to palpate the shunt or verify flow by using a handheld Doppler. If the shunt is patent, decreased shunt flow is usually related to decreased P1 or blood pressure. To a lesser degree, elevations in P2 or pulmonary vascular pressures may also decrease shunt flow. The range of clinically observed variation of PVR is narrow compared to the absolute levels of SVR, and in the absence of hypotension, P2 issues are not as often associated with shunt malfunction. Appropriate management of cardiac output and pulmonary vascular resistance should result in predictably stable arterial saturations. If this cannot be accomplished in the operating room, it is necessary to verify that there is not a technical problem with the shunt causing decreased flow. It may be useful to connect a needle and pressure tubing to a transducer and directly measure the pulmonary artery pressure distal to the shunt. If it is low, shunt failure is the diagnosis and is due to a technical issue with one of the anastomoses, thrombosis, or both. If the pressure is high, the patient has pulmonary hypertension, and therapy with inhaled nitric oxide is indicated (Bushman 2009). Nitric oxide is preferred in this situation to systemic vasodilators or milrinone because systemic vasodilation that would lower P1 is avoided.

In the intensive care unit, troubleshooting an apparently failing shunt is more problematic because the sternotomy incision is usually closed. Optimization of hemodynamics and pulmonary resistance is accomplished. A decrease in the intensity or the absence of an audible shunt murmur is suggestive of shunt failure, and echocardiography should be utilized to visualize the shunt. If despite echo evidence of shunt patency and an adequate cardiac output, arterial saturations are still inadequate, a trial of nitric oxide for presumed pulmonary hypertension is indicated. If the patient continues to be desaturated, additional study in the cardiac catheterization suite may be needed to evaluate the patency of the shunt.

Anesthesia Issues of the Patient with a BTS for Complete Repair

After successful palliation with a MBTS, the TOF patient will present later for corrective repair as decreased saturations and hypercyanotic spells are mitigated by the shunt. The anesthetic considerations are primarily directed at maintaining the relationship between P1 and P2 without regard for intracardiac right-to-left shunting as determined by the dynamic determinants of infundibular obstruction. A TOF patient with a patent shunt cannot have a "Tet spell" provided blood pressure and cardiac output are maintained during the induction and maintenance of anesthesia. If a patient with a shunt is having hypercyanosis, the patency of the shunt should be considered suspect. Management is then directed at optimizing preload and afterload and controlling contractile state and heart rate in determining the patient's right-to-left shunting across the VSD and the resulting arterial saturation.

As with any patient with a PDA, a patient with a MBTS who is placed on cardiopulmonary bypass (CPB) has obligatory runoff through the shunt that decreases systemic perfusion from the aortic cannula. This is associated with decreased venous saturations on bypass that seem unrelated to the flow rates calculated for the patient's size. The initial maneuver performed by the surgeon after CPB is initiated is to ligate the shunt. Communication with the perfusionist regarding the presence of the shunt and when it is ligated is useful in interpreting the adequacy of calculated flows on CPB and the significance of mixed venous saturation monitoring from the venous circuit.

Conclusion

In approximately 80 years, TOF has benefited from an evolution of palliative and corrective procedures that optimized the natural history of patients with the disease. It is currently accepted that patients with TOF not only have a limited duration of hypoxemia as infants but also undergo surgical repair with an acceptably low mortality rate and excellent short- and midterm outcome. The late outcomes are also excellent even though for some patients there is procedural reintervention for issues related to the RVOT. The complications of pulmonary vascular disease, left ventricular dysfunction, and arrhythmias are now largely of historical interest. Reoperation to revise the RVOT and implant a pulmonary valve is of low risk and predictably good outcome. The functional status and life expectancy of most adult patients with TOF are normal or nearly normal.

TOF also serves the practitioner with an excellent model to consider the unique correlation of anatomy and physiology in unrepaired TOF as well as the considerations of the arterial shunt model in the two-ventricle cardiac lesion.

Bibliography

Alexiou C, Mahmoud H, Al-khaddour A, Gnanapragasam J, Salmon A, Keeton B, Monro J. Outcome after repair of tetralogy of fallot in the first year of life. Ann Thorac Surg. 2001;71(2):494–500.

Allen H, Driscoll D, Shaddy R, Feltes T. Moss & Adams' heart disease in infants, children, and adolescents: including the fetus and young adult. Lippincott Williams and Wilkins 8th ed. 2013, p. 969–89.

Alsoufi B, Mori M, McCracken C, Williams E, Samai C, Kogon B, Kanter K. Results of primary repair versus shunt palliation in ductal dependent infants with pulmonary atresia and ventricular septal defect. Ann Thorac Surg. 2015;100(2):639–46.

Anderson R, Weinberg P. The clinical anatomy of tetralogy of fallot. Cardiol Young. 2005;15:38–47.

Andreasen J, Jonhsen S, Ravn H. Junctional ectopic tachycardiac after surgery for congenital heart disease in children. Intensive Care Med. 2008;34:895–902.

Babu-Narayan S, Diller G, Gheta R, Bastin A, Karonis T, Li W, Shore D. Clinical outcomes of surgical pulmonary valve replacement after repair of tetralogy of fallot and potential prognostic value of preoperative cardiopulmonary exercise testing. Circulation. 2014;129(1):18–27.

Bacha E. Valve-sparing options in tetralogy of fallot surgery. Semin Thorac Cardiovasc Surg Pediatr Card Surg Annu. 2012;15(1):24–6.

Bahnson H. Surgical treatment of pulmonary stenosis: a retrospection. Ann Thorac Surg. 1982;33:96–8.

Barker GM, Affolter J, Saenz J, Cox CS, Forbess JM, Scott WA, Zeltser I. Temporary atrial pacing for cardiac output after pediatric cardiac surgery. Pediatr Cardiol. 2013;34(7):1605–11.

Barron DJ. Tetralogy of fallot: controversies in early management. World J Pediatr Congenital Heart Surg. 2013;4(2):186–91.

Bartelings M, Gittenberger-de Groot A. Morphogenetic considerations on congenital malformations of the outflow tract. Part 1: common arterial trunk and tetralogy of fallot. Int J Cardiol. 1991;32(2):213–30.

Batra A, Starnes V, Wells W. Does the site of insertion of a systemic-pulmonary shunt influence growth of the pulmonary arteries? Ann Thorac Surg. 2005;79(2):636–40.

Blalock A, Taussig H. The surgical treatment of malformations of the heart in which there is pulmonary stenosis or pulmonary atresia. JAMA. 1945;128:189–92.

Borowski A, Ghodsizad A, Litmathe J, Lawrenz W, Schmidt K, Gams E. Severe pulmonary regurgitation late after total repair of tetralogy of fallot : surgical considerations. Pediatr Cardiol. 2004;25(5):466–71.

Britt J, Moffett B, Bronicki R, Checchia P. Incidence of adverse events requiring intervention after initiation of oral beta-blocker in pediatric cardiac intensive care patients. Pediatr Cardiol. 2014;35(6):1062–6.

Burchill L, Wald R, Harris L, Colman J, Silversides C. Pulmonary valve replacement in adults with repaired tetralogy of fallot. Semin Thorac Cardiovasc Surg Pediatr Card Surg Annu. 2011;14(1):92–7.

Bushman G. Essentials of nitric oxide for the pediatric (cardiac) anesthesiologist. Semin Cardiothorac Vasc Anes. 2001;5(1):79–90.

Cheatham J, Hellenbrand W, Zahn E, Jones T, Berman D, Vincent J, McElhinney D. Clinical and hemodynamic outcomes up to 7 years after transcatheter pulmonary valve replacement in the US melody valve investigational device exemption trial. Circulation. 2015;131(22):1960–70.

Cheng J, Russell H, Stewart R, Thomas J, Backer C, Mavroudis C. The role of tricuspid valve surgery in the late management of tetralogy of fallot: collective review. World J Pediatr Congenital Heart Surg. 2012;3(4):492–8.

Chiappini B, Barrea C, Rubay J. Right ventricular outflow tract reconstruction with contegra monocuspid patch in tetralogy of fallot. Ann Thorac Surg. 2007;83(1):185–7.

Cuypers J, Menting E, Konings E, Opić P, et al. The unnatural history of tetralogy of fallot: prospective follow-up of 40 years after surgical correction. Circulation. 2014;130(22):1944–54.

Dabizzi RP, Teodori G, Barletta GA, Caprioli G, Baldrighi G, Baldrighi V. Associated coronary and cardiac anomalies in the tetralogy of fallot. An angiographic study. Eur Heart J. 1990;8:692–704.

DiNardo J, Andropoulos D, Baum V. Special article: a proposal for training in pediatric cardiac anesthesia. Anesth Analg. 2010;110(4):1121–5.

Dyamenahalli U, Mccrindle B, Barker G, Williams W, Freedom R, Bohn D. Influence of perioperative factors on outcomes in children younger than 18 months after repair of tetralogy of fallot. Ann Thorac Surg. 2000;2000(69):1236–42.

Fogel M, Sundareswaran K, de Zelicourt D, Dasi L, Pawlowski T, Rome J, Yoganathan A. Power loss and right ventricular efficiency in patients after tetralogy of fallot repair with pulmonary insufficiency: clinical implications. J Thorac Cardiovasc Surg. 2012;143:1279–85.

Fraser C. The ongoing quest for an ideal surgical repair for tetralogy of fallot: focus on the pulmonary valve. J Thorac Cardiovasc Surg. 2015;149(5):1364.

Fraser CD, Mckenzie ED, Cooley DA. Tetralogy of fallot : surgical management individualized to the patient. Ann Thorac Surg. 2001;71(5):1556–61.

Garson A, Nihill M, McNamara D, Cooley D. Status of the adult and adolescent after repair of tetralogy of fallot. Circulation. 1979;59:1232–40.

Geva T. Indications and timing of pulmonary valve replacement after tetralogy of fallot repair. Semin Thorac Cardiovasc Surg. 2006;9(1):11–22.

Geva T, Ayres N, Pac F, Pignatelli R. Quantitative morphometric analysis of progressive infundibular obstruction in tetralogy of fallot: a prospective longitudinal echocardiographic study. Circulation. 1995;92:886–92.

Gonzalez J, Shirali G, Atz A, Taylor S, Forbus G, Zyblewski S, Hlavacek A. Universal screening for extracardiac abnormalities in neonates with congenital heart disease. Pediatr Cardiol. 2009;30(3):269–73.

Greeley W, Bushman G, Davis D, Reves J. Comparative effects of halothane and ketamine on systemic oxygen saturation in children with cyanotic heart disease. Anesthesiology. 1986;65:666.

Hallbergson A, Gauvreau K, Powell A. Right ventricular remodeling after pulmonary valve replacement : early gains, late losses. Ann Thorac Surg. 2014;99(2):660–6.

Hansen P, Slane P, Rueckert P, Clark S. Squatting revisited: comparison of haemodynamic responses in normal individuals and heart transplantation recipients. Br Heart J. 1995;74(2):154–8.

Hirsch J, Mosca R, Bove E. Complete repair of tetralogy of fallot in the neonate: results in the modern era. Ann Surg. 2000;232(4):508–14.

Hoohenkerk G, Schoof P, Bruggemans E, Rijlaarsdam M, Hazekamp M. 28 years' experience with transatrial-transpulmonary repair of atrioventricular septal defect with tetralogy of fallot. Ann Thorac Surg. 2008;85(5):1686–9.

Hraska V. Repair of tetralogy of fallot with absent pulmonary valve using a new approach. Semin Thorac Cardiovasc Surg Pediatr Card Surg Annu. 2005;8:132–4.

Humpl T, Söderberg B, Mccrindle BW, Nykanen DG, Freedom RM, Williams WG, Benson LN. Percutaneous balloon valvotomy in pulmonary atresia with intact ventricular septum. Circulation. 2003;108:826–32.

Karadeniz C, Atalay S, Demir F, Tutar E, et al. Does surgically induced right bundle branch block really effect ventricular function in children after ventricular septal defect closure? Pediatr Cardiol. 2014;36:481–8.

Karl T. Tetralogy of fallot: current surgical perspective. Ann Pediatr Cardiol. 2008;1(2):93–100.

Kaza A, Lim H, Dibardino D, Bautista-Hernandez V, Robinson J, Allan C, Pigula F. Long-term results of right ventricular outflow tract reconstruction in neonatal cardiac surgery: options and outcomes. J Thorac Cardiovasc Surg. 2009;138(4):911–6.

Keckler S, St Peter S, Spilde T, Ostlie D, Snyder C. The influence of trisomy 21 on the incidence and severity of congenital heart defects in patients with duodenal atresia. Pediatr Surg Int. 2008;24(8):921–3.

Kirklin J, Karp R. The tetralogy of fallot from a surgical viewpoint. Philadelphia: WB Saunders; 1970.

Kirsch R, Glatz A, Gaynor J, Nicolson S, Spray T, Wernovsky G, Bird G. Results of elective repair at 6 months or younger in 277 patients with tetralogy of fallot : a 14-year experience at a single center. J Thorac Cardiovasc Surg. 2009;147(2):713–7.

Lake C. Pediatric cardiac anesthesia. McGraw-Hill/Appleton and Lange. 2nd ed. 1993.

Lamberti J, Carlisle J, Waldman J, et al. Systemic-pulmonary shunts in infants and children. Early and late results. J Thorac Cardiovasc Surg. 1984;88(1):76–81.

Lammer E, Chak J, Iovannisci D, Schultz K, et al. Chromosomal abnormalities among children born with conotruncal cardiac defects. Birth Defects Res A Clin Mol Teratol. 2009;85(1):30–5.

Levy S, Blalock A. Experimental observations on the effects of connecting by suture the left main pulmonary artery to the systemic circulation. J Thorac Surg. 1939;8:525–30.

Lillehei C, Cohen M, Warden H, et al. Direct vision intracardiac correction of the tetralogy of fallot, pentalogy of fallot, and pulmonary atresia defects: report of first ten cases. Ann Surg. 1955;142(3):418–42.

Lillehei C, Varco R, Cohen M, Warden H, et al. The first open heart corrections of tetralogy of fallot: a 26–31 year follow-up of 106 patients. Ann Surg. 1986;204(4):490–502.

Lindsey C, Parks W, Kogon B, Sallee D, Mahle W. Pulmonary valve replacement after tetralogy of fallot repair in preadolescent patients. Ann Thorac Surg. 2010;89(1):147–51.

Little J, Lavender P, DeSanctis R. The narrow infundibulum in pulmonary valvar stenosis. Circulation. XXVIII August. 1963:182–9.

Michielon G, Marino B, Formigari R, Gargiulo G, Picchio F, Digilio M, Di Donato R. Genetic syndromes and outcome after surgical correction of tetralogy of fallot. Ann Thorac Surg. 2006;81(3):968–75.

Montero J, Nieto N, Vallejo I, Montero S. Intranasal midazolam for the emergency management of hypercyanotic spells in tetralogy of fallot. Pediatr Emerg Care. 2015;4:269–71.

Mulinari LA1, Navarro FB, Pimentel GK, Miyazaki SM, Binotto CN, Pelissari EC, Miyague NI, da Costa FD. The use and midium-term evaluation of decellularized allograft cusp in the surgical treatment of the tetralogy of fallot. Rev Bras Cir Cardiovasc. 2008; 23(2):197–203.

Myers J, Ghanayem N, Cao Y, et al. Outcomes of systemic to pulmonary artery shunts in patients weighing less than 3 kg : analysis of shunt type, size, and surgical approach. J Thorac Cardiovasc Surg. 2014;147(2):672–7.

Nasr A, McNamara PJ, Mertens L, Levin D, James A, Holtby H, Langer JC. Is routine preoperative 2-dimensional echocardiography necessary for infants with esophageal atresia, omphalocele, or anorectal malformations? J Pediatr Surg. 2010;45(5):876–9.

Newfeld E, Waldman D, et al. Pulmonary vascular disease after systemic-pulmonary arterial shunt operations. Am J Cardiol. 1977;39(5):715–20.

Odegard KC, Schure A, Saiki Y, Hansen DD, Jonas RA, Laussen PC. Anesthetic considerations during caval inflow occlusion in children with congenital heart disease. J Clin Ultrasound. 2004;18(2):144–7.

Ong J, Brizard C, d'Udekem Y, Weintraub R, Robertson T, Cheung M, Konstantinov I. Repair of atrioventricular septal defect associated with tetralogy of fallot or double-outlet right ventricle: 30 years of experience. Ann Thorac Surg. 2012;94(1):172–8.

Parker J, Brooks D, Kozar L, Render-Teixeira C, Horner R, et al. Acute and chronic effects of airway obstruction on canine left ventricular performance. Am J Respir Crit Care Med. 1999;160(6):1888–96.

Pickering D, Trusler G, Lipton I, Keith J. Waterston anastomosis: comparison of results of operation before and after age 6 months. Thorax. 1971;26:457–9.

Pierce J, Sharma S, Hunter C, Bhombal S, Fagan B, Corchado Y, Bushman G. Intraoperative hypercyanosis in a patient with pulmonary artery band: case report and review of the literature. J Clin Anesth. 2012;24(8):652–5.

Quail M, Frigiola A, Giardini A, Muthurangu V, Hughes M, Lurz P, Taylor A. Impact of pulmonary valve replacement in tetralogy of fallot with pulmonary regurgitation: a comparison of intervention and nonintervention. Ann Thorac Surg. 2012;94(5):1619–26.

Ritter S, Tany L, Shaddy R, Minich L. Are screening echocardiograms warranted for neonates with meningomyelocele? Arch Pediatr Adolesc Med. 1999;153(12):1264–6.

Rudolph A. Congenital diseases of the heart: clinical-physiological considerations. Wiley-Blackwell 3rd ed. 2009; p. 345–85.

Said S, Burkhart H, Schaff H, Johnson J, Connolly H, Dearani J. When should a mechanical tricuspid valve replacement be considered? J Thorac Cardiovasc Surg. 2014;148(2):603–8.

Schwartz MC, Glatz AC, Dori Y, Rome JJ, Gillespie MJ. Outcomes and predictors of reintervention in patients with pulmonary atresia and intact ventricular septum treated with radiofrequency perforation and balloon pulmonary valvuloplasty. Pediatr Cardiol. 2013;35(1):22–9.

Sharkey A, Sharma A. Tetralogy of fallot: anatomic variants and their impact on surgical management. Semin Cardiothorac Vasc Anesth. 2012;2:88–96.

Short S, Pierce J, Burke R, et al. Is routine preoperative screening echocardiogram indicated in all children with congenital duodenal obstruction? Pediatr Surg Int. 2014;6:609–14.

Shprintzen RJ, Goldberg RB, Young D, Wolford L. The velo-cardio-facial syndrome: a clinical and genetic analysis. Pediatrics. 1981;67:167–72.

Shuhaiber J, Robinson B, Gauvreau K, Breitbart R, Mayer J, Del Nido P, Pigula F. Outcome after repair of atrioventricular septal defect with tetralogy of fallot. J Thorac Cardiovasc Surg. 2012;143(2):338–43.

Soto B, Pacifico A, Ceballos R, Bargeron L. Tetralogy of fallot: an angiographic-pathologic correlative study. Circulation. 1981;64(3):558–66.

Steiner M, Tang X, Gossett J, Malik S, Prodhan P. Timing of complete repair of non-ductal-dependent tetralogy of fallot and short-term postoperative outcomes, a multicenter analysis. J Thorac Cardiovasc Surg. 2014;147(4):1299–305.

Stephenson L, Friedman S, Edmonds L. Staged surgical management in tetralogy of fallot in infants. Circulation. 1978;58(5):837–41.

Tamesberger M, Lechner E, Mair R, Hofer A, Sames-dolzer E, Tulzer G. Early primary repair of tetralogy of fallot in neonates and infants less than four months of age. Ann Thorac Surg. 2008;86(6):1928–35.

Tanaka K, Kitahata H, Kawahito S, Nozaki J, Tomiyama Y, Oshita S. Phenylephrine increases pulmonary blood flow in children with tetralogy of fallot. Can J Anaesth. 2003;50(9):926–9.

Tempe D, Virmani S. Coagulation abnormalities in patients with cyanotic congenital heart disease. J Cardiothorac Vasc Anesth. 2002;16(6):752–65.

Thapar M, Rao P. Use of propranolol for severe dynamic infundibular obstruction prior to balloon pulmonary valvuloplasty (a brief communication). Cathet Cardiovasc Diagn. 1990;4:240–1.

Tharakan J. Admixture lesions in congenital cyanotic heart disease. Ann Pediatr Cardiol. 2011;4(1):53–9.

Trucoone N, Bowman F, Malm J, Gersony W. Systemic to pulmonary artery shunts in the first year of life. Circulation. 1974;49:508–11.

Tug M. Ketamine infusion versus isoflurane for the maintenance of anesthesia in the prebypass period in children with tetralogy of fallot. Children. 2000;14(5):557–61.

Turrentine M, Mccarthy R, Vijay P, Mcconnell K, Brown J. PTFE monocusp valve reconstruction of the right ventricular outflow tract. Ann Thorac Surg. 2002;73(3):871–9.

Vida V, Guariento A, Castaldi B, et al. Evolving strategies for preserving the pulmonary valve during early repair of tetralogy of fallot : mid-term results. J Thorac Cardiovasc Surg. 2014;147(2):687–96.

Waldman J, Wernly J. Cyanotic congenital heart disease with decreased pulmonary blood flow in children. Pediatr Clin North Am. 1999;46(2):385–404.

Walker A, Stokes M, Moriarty A. Anesthesia for major general surgery in neonates with complex cardiac defects. Paediatr Anaesth. 2009;19:119–25.

Wells W, Arroyo H, Bremner R, Wood J, Starnes V. Homograft conduit failure in infants is not due to somatic outgrowth. J Thorac Cardiovasc Surg. 2002;124(1):88–96.

White M. Approach to managing children with heart disease for noncardiac surgery. Paediatr Anaesth. 2011;21(5):522–9.

Wyse R, Mars M, al-Mahdawi S, Russell-Eggitt IM, Blake KD. Congenital heart anomalies in patients with clefts of the lip and/or palate. Cleft Palate J. 1990;27(3):258–64.

Yoo B, Kim J, Kim Y, Choi J, Park H, Park Y, Sul J. Impact of pressure load caused by right ventricular outflow tract obstruction on right ventricular volume overload in patients with repaired tetralogy of fallot. J Thorac Cardiovasc Surg. 2012;143(6):1299–304.

Yoshimura N, Yamaguchi M, Ohashi H, Oshima Y, Oka S, Yoshida M, Tei T. Pulmonary atresia with intact ventricular septum: strategy based on right ventricular morphology. J Thorac Cardiovasc Surg. 2002;126(5):1417–26.

Zabala L, Guzzetta N. Cyanotic congenital heart disease (CCHD): focus on hypoxemia, secondary erythrocytosis, and coagulation alterations. Pediatr Anaesth. 2015;25(10):981–9.

Zampi JD, Hirsch JC, Gurney JG, Donohue JE, Yu S, Lapage MJ, Charpie JR. Junctional ectopic tachycardia after infant heart surgery: incidence and outcomes. Pediatr Cardiol. 2012;33(8):1362–9.

Chapter 20
Transposition of the Great Arteries

Gerald A. Bushman

Case Presentation

A 6-h-old male infant was delivered with Apgar scores of six and four at a community hospital. Initial SaO_2 was 78 % and it has decreased to 56 % despite endotracheal intubation and supplemental oxygen. The blood pressure is 40/22 with a heart rate of 188. There is a significant metabolic acidosis on an arterial blood gas.

What intervention should be done immediately? How is a fetal pattern of circulation restored in the neonate and of what value is it when the diagnosis of distress is undetermined?

After an echocardiogram reveals TGA with an intact ventricular septum, plans are made to perform an atrial septostomy at the bedside. Why is a septostomy required if the ductus arteriosus is open with prostaglandin E (PgE)?

How can the adequacy of resuscitation be assessed after septostomy?

When should corrective surgery be performed?

While coming off of cardiopulmonary bypass after arterial switch, the patient is hypotensive despite elevated CVP. How should this be assessed? What is the differential diagnosis?

One week after arterial switch procedure, the patient is feeding poorly and is scheduled for a gastrostomy tube. What considerations are important in planning anesthesia care?

G.A. Bushman, MD
Pediatric and Cardiac Anesthesiology, Anesthesia Critical Care Medicine,
Children's Hospital Los Angeles, Keck School of Medicine,
University of Southern California,
Los Angeles, CA, USA
e-mail: GBushman@chla.usc.edu

© Springer International Publishing Switzerland 2017
A. Dabbagh et al. (eds.), *Congenital Heart Disease in Pediatric and Adult Patients*, DOI 10.1007/978-3-319-44691-2_20

Embryology

TGA represents about 5% of all patients with congenital heart disease and approximately one-third of conotruncal defects with situs solitus (Ferencz et al. 1995) (Fig. 20.1). TGA does not represent an alternative model of fetal or neonatal blood flow with a clear morphogenic explanation, and early attempts to understand the anatomy and postulate the embryology relied on surveys of autopsy specimens. Because the lesion is lethal during early infancy, an abundance of cadaver material has been available through the years showing many variations and subtle anatomic nuances that are difficult to classify in a unifying embryologic theory (Samànek 2000).

Two main hypotheses are recognized (Marino et al. 2002). Gore and Edwards proposed that TGA was caused by the lack of the normal clockwise rotation of the aorta (AO) toward the left ventricle (LV), presumably due to the lack of maturation of the subpulmonary conus with persistence of the subaortic conus (Goor and Edwards 1973). ("Conus" specifically refers to the muscular cardiac segment between the atrioventricular valves and the semilunar valves as defined by Drs. Van Praagh and Van Praagh.) In this scenario, TGA is an extreme case of aortic malposition that is on the spectrum of defects that includes malalignment ventricular septal defects, tetralogy of Fallot, and double outlet right ventricle. This theory seems to adequately explain the morphologic differences seen in TGA related to variations of the right ventricular outflow tract (RVOT) or left ventricular outflow tract (LVOT) and the positions of the pulmonary artery and VSD, but the presentation of TGA with an intact ventricular septum is difficult to explain. A simpler theory by de la Cruz offers that linear rather than spiral septation of the truncus occurs and the

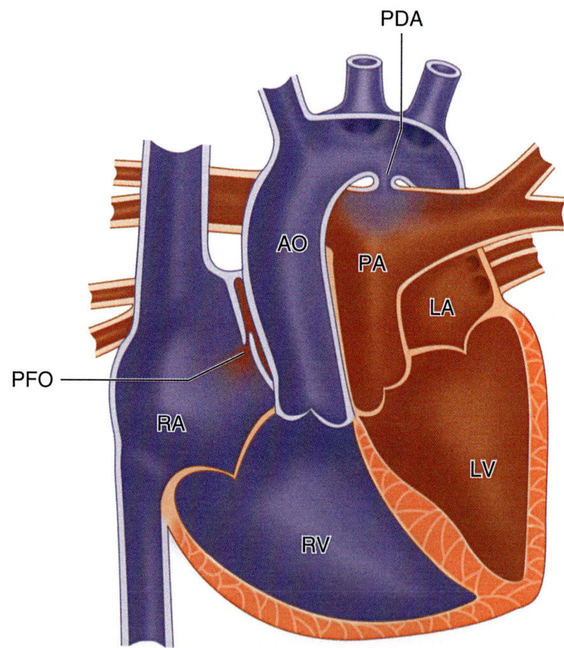

Fig. 20.1 Transposition of the great arteries

failure of the aortopulmonary septum to spiral leads the aorta to remain in continuity with the anterior conus of the right ventricle (De La Cruz and Da Rocha 1956). This explanation, however, fails to clarify the origin of the large variability of conal anatomy that presents in TGA.

Terminology and Anatomy

Historically, the basis for terminology describing a complex cardiac defect is derived from pathologic examinations of cardiac specimens and refined by clinical and physiologic correlation and ultimately an understanding and description of the failure of morphologic development. The absence of a unifying theory of the maldevelopment of the heart in TGA and the large variability of anatomic presentations related to the position of the great vessels relative to each other and observed outflow tract abnormalities have made consistent descriptive terminology problematic (Mair et al. 1971). A nomenclature report on TGA published in a review in 2000 provides details of widely accepted terminology that are beyond the scope of this chapter (Jaggers et al. 2000).

The classification suggested by Van Praagh describes morphology and forms the general basis for most imaging descriptions of the anatomic variables in TGA (Houyel et al. 1995; Van Praagh 1984; Van Praagh et al. 1975). This format is useful for conceptualizing the malformation and its variations. Cardiac position is left sided (levocardia), right sided (dextrocardia), or midline (mesocardia). The main cardiac segments are the atria, ventricles, and great arteries. The connecting cardiac segments are the atrioventricular (AV) canal complex between the atria and ventricles and the conus between the ventricles and the great arteries. Malpositions of the main segments may be described as solitus, inversus, or ambiguous. Additionally the visceral situs is described as situs solitus if the pulmonary (right) atrium is on the right and the right-sided abdominal organs (the liver, gall bladder) and the tri-lobe lung are also on the right and the pulmonary venous (left) atrium and the left-sided abdominal organs (the stomach, spleen) and the bilobe lung are on the left. Situs inversus is mirror image reversal of the normal situs solitus. Situs inversus is rare and not usually associated with medical issues. Diagnosis is usually incidental, while the patient is undergoing imaging for other conditions. Situs ambiguous refers to the random abnormal distribution of the abdominal organs and is highly associated with heterotaxy cardiac malformations, including single ventricle lesions.

The sequential segmental analysis usually reported by echocardiogram in TGA includes the cardiac position and direction of the apex, the position and morphology of the atria, the atrioventricular connections, the ventriculoarterial (VA) connections, and the positions of the great vessels. Atrioventricular connections are concordant when the systemic venous right atrium (RA) empties into the morphologic right ventricle and the pulmonary venous left atrium empties into the morphologic left ventricle. Discordance refers to when the systemic venous right atrium empties into the morphologic left ventricle and the pulmonary venous left atrium empties into the morphologic right ventricle. The discrete commitment of the atrioventricular apparatus to the ventricular inlet is also described. A double inlet ventricle has both AV valve apparatus committed to the ventricular inlet. Ventriculoarterial or outlet connections are referred to as concordant if the pulmonary artery is connected to the right ventricle and the aorta to the left ventricle and discordant if the pulmonary artery is connected to the left ventricle and the aorta to the right ventricle. Double outlet connections refer to one great vessel and more than 50 % of the other committed to either the right or the left ventricle. Note that the above classification describes the intrinsic connections of the main cardiac and connecting segments sequentially and does not describe the positions of the great arteries relative to each other.

Simple Transposition of the Great Arteries

Pathologic heart specimens showing an aorta arising from the right ventricle and the pulmonary artery from the left ventricle have been observed since the late 1700s (Leibman et al. 1969). Historically, more than half of infants presenting as neonates with severe cyanosis have the diagnosis of TGA (Farre 1814). TGA is associated with an intact ventricular septum 55 % of the time and with a VSD of variable size 45 % of the time. The age of the demise of such patients historically seemed related to the size of the atrial septal defect, with most not surviving infancy (Leibman et al. 1969). Contemporary analysis shows that TGA occurs approximately 1:3200 live births with a strong male predilection of 1.6–3.2:1 (Hoffman and Kaplan 2002). The segmental description of simple TGA is atrioventricular concordance with ventriculoarterial discordance (Van Praagh 1984; Allen et al. 2001a). The designation of the spatial relationship of the great vessels as "*D*" or "*L*" completes the anatomic description. D-TGA refers to the location of the right and left ventricles in their normal positions. The aorta is usually anterior and to the right of the pulmonary artery, although occasionally it may be directly anterior or anterior and to the left.

The hemodynamic derangement from TGA is derived from the two parallel loops of circulation created by the transposed great arteries (Ewer et al. 2012). One loop is:

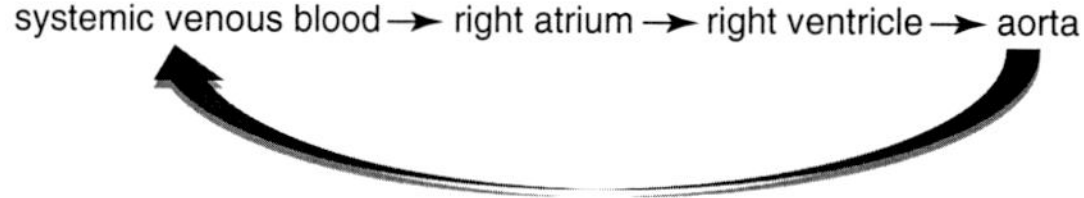

Likewise, the other loop is:

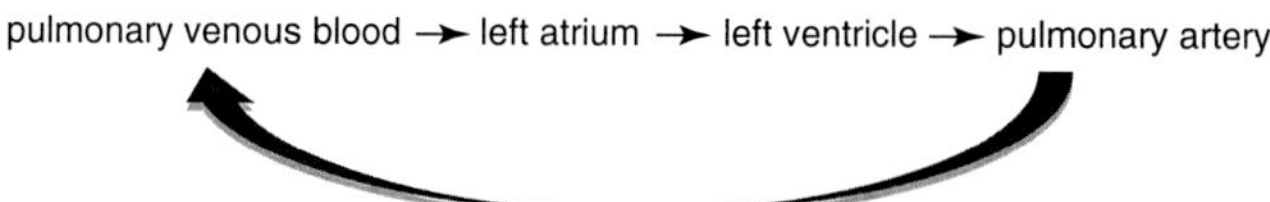

In the worst case, the highly oxygenated blood in the pulmonary venous loop never accesses the systemic circulation, and the systemic output from the aorta in the systemic venous loop never accesses the pulmonary vascular bed to allow

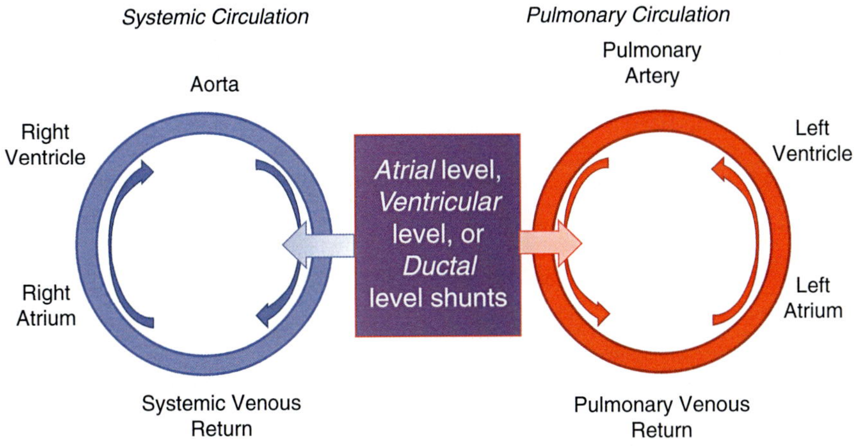

Fig. 20.2 Arterial and venous mixing in TGA

oxygenation and carbon dioxide exchange. Extrauterine survival requires a site of mixing such as an intracardiac shunt (ASD or VSD) or extracardiac shunt (PDA) (Fig. 20.2).

An additional hemodynamic issue important in the first few months of life is related to the pulmonary vascular bed being in connection with the left ventricle. In utero and during transition from fetal to neonatal circulation, the pulmonary vascular resistance (PVR) is high. At birth, the PVR decreases rapidly as the lungs are expanded and the vascular bed relaxes because of the effect of vasoactive mediators and oxygen (Fig. 20.3). In the weeks and months following birth under normal circumstances, the medial muscle layer of the pulmonary arteriole regresses and remodels. In this period the left ventricle will decondition as PVR decreases, unless there is a nonrestrictive VSD to allow the resistance circuit of the LV to include systemic circulation via the RV.

Although recent recommendations show screening of newborns routinely with pulse oximetry is effective in detecting cyanotic lesions such as TGA, this practice only benefits patients with TGA who have an adequate ASD to survive the early neonatal period (Ewer et al. 2011; Rasiah et al. 2006). Unfortunately, a routine obstetrical ultrasound may not carefully evaluate the outflow tracts and great vessels in the fetus, but a carefully performed fetal cardiac ultrasound that identifies TGA potentially allows the fetus to be delivered in a facility prepared for the expectant use of prostaglandin E (PgE) and transport availability for subspecialty cardiology care (Calderon et al. 2012). Prenatal diagnosis reduces the potential neurodevelopmental complications that may arise in a neonate with TGA when compared to patients whose diagnosis is delayed until severe cyanosis and cardiovascular collapse occur after birth because the patent foramen ovale is too small for adequate mixing and the ductus arteriosus closes (Blalock 1950).

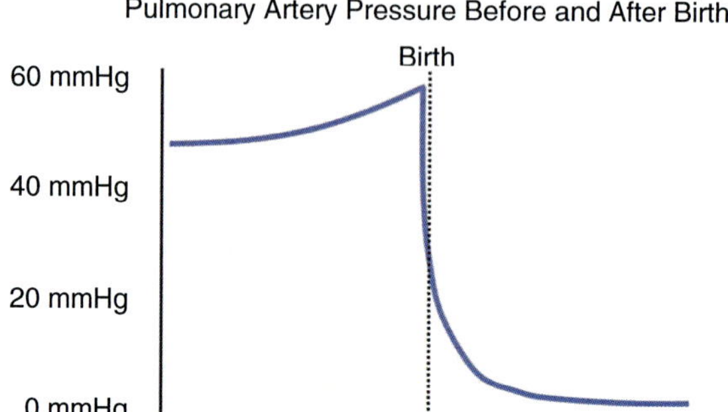

Fig. 20.3 PVR transition

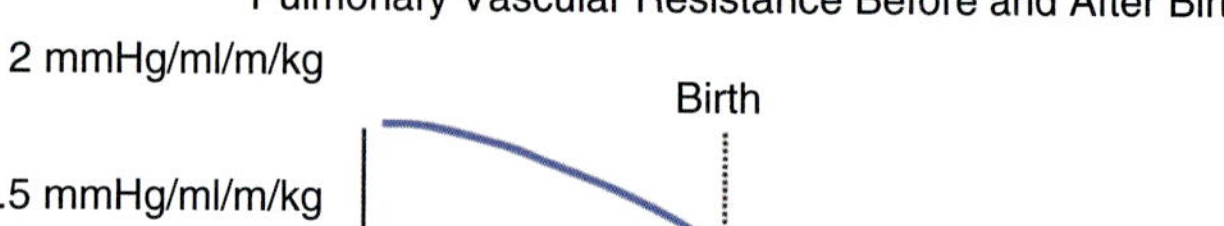

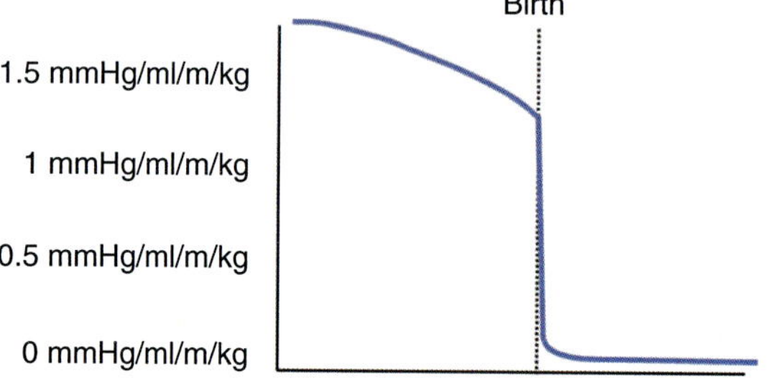

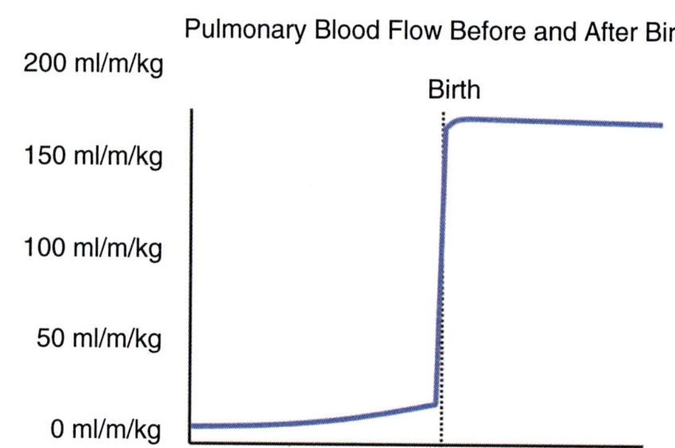

Clinical Presentation

The clinical presentation of neonates with TGA is variable. For survival there must be a shunt at the atrial level, the ventricular level, or a patent ductus arteriosus. If there is inadequate shunting, cyanosis is severe and cardiovascular collapse occurs rapidly. Although most neonatologists would institute PgE in the face of cyanosis without overt respiratory distress syndrome, a PDA is not as efficient as an atrial septal defect in providing mixing of systemic venous and pulmonary venous blood. For this reason after diagnosis by echocardiogram, emergency balloon septostomy is routinely performed either at the bedside with echocardiographic guidance, or in the catheterization lab if the septostomy is anticipated to be complex. The helpfulness of a ventricular septal defect, if present, is variable. Depending on the size of the VSD and in particular the morphology of the conal septum, the VSD may be either an effective source of mixing or ineffective because the streaming characteristics of blood ejected through the conal septum render the VSD inoperative as a site of mixing.

Patients with TGA who have large ASDs or VSDs may be more difficult to detect at birth. Their cyanosis may be mild to moderate and if overlooked, the other physical signs of TGA may not be impressive. As the PVR decreases in the days and weeks after birth, a normal infant demonstrates a modest increase in arterial saturation, but the infant with TGA will demonstrate progressive high-output heart failure and continued desaturation. Chest x-ray will show increased pulmonary vascular markings consistent with pulmonary overcirculation and cardiomegaly, especially if there is an unrestrictive VSD present. Symptoms and signs of a left-to-right shunt such as poor weight gain, diaphoresis, tachycardia, and a cardiac gallop may be present. Persistent cyanosis is a function of the intracardiac mixing that occurs despite an elevated Qp/Qs ratio.

Historical Therapeutic Approaches and Outcomes

Before discussing the details of contemporary surgical management of TGA, it is useful to review the advances in surgical technique and physiologic insight that led to the current application of the arterial switch. Early attempts to palliate TGA preceded the era of open-heart surgery. Autopsy specimens had led to the understanding that the age of a patient's demise was strongly related to the presence and size of an intra-atrial communication. The Blalock-Hanlon procedure was described in 1950 and represented the first palliative operation that seemed to be associated with improved survival in older infants compared to the natural history of the unrepaired lesion (Blalock 1950; Blalock and Hanlon 1948). Using a modified technique of inflow occlusion, a surgical ASD was created via a right thoracotomy. Increasingly surgery was performed in younger infants with an expected early survival over 85%, with most patients operated on from the 1940's to the 1970's experiencing improvements in percent arterial saturaion (Hermann et al. 1975). The midterm and late results were not nearly as good (Alexi-Meskishvili and Sharykin 1984). Mortality in the weeks after surgery was still substantial, but survivors of the first few months tended to have prolonged survival to 10 years or more. Nonetheless it was clear that a more definitive approach to palliation was required.

Early attempts to repair the lesion by arterial switch were largely unsuccessful because of the technical difficulty in transferring the coronary arteries to the neoaorta (Yacoub and Radley-Smith 1978; Senning 1959; Bailey et al. 1954). Animal experiments by Alfred Blalock and C. Rollins demonstrated in a canine model the feasibility of connecting the pulmonary veins to the superior vena cava (SVC) and the right atrium (RA) and hypothesized that a similar approach might be made in infant patients with TGA (Blalock and Hanlon 1948). This introduced consideration that instead of reversing the aorta and pulmonary artery, the pulmonary and systemic venous pathways might be reconstructed, obviating the need for coronary reconstruction inherent to the arterial switch. In 1952 Walton Lillehei attempted an extracardiac "venous switch" by connecting the right pulmonary veins to the right atrium and the inferior vena cava (IVA) to the left atrium (Lillehei and Varco 1953). Further modifications by Thomas Baffes and Willis Potts in 1956 were described and as these procedures were done without cardiopulmonary bypass, they were commonly used for the next 10 years with increasing short-term success (Baffes 1956). In 1954 Harold Albert published the use of an intra-atrial flap to redirect systemic and pulmonary venous flow to the contralateral atrioventricular valve in dogs (Albert 1954). William Mustard and others advanced the technique that became the Mustard procedure, which used a prosthetic patch to create the intra-atrial baffle on cardiopulmonary bypass, diverting pulmonary venous blood to the tricuspid valve and systemic venous blood (SVB) to the mitral valve (Mustard et al. 1964). Also in the late 1950s, Ake Senning demonstrated the atrial switch could be done with autologous material (pericardium), although the procedure seemed more difficult (Senning 1959) (Fig. 20.4). Initially in the 1960s Senning's procedure was largely abandoned in small infants because the technical challenges of creating the patch reduced the size of the atrial chambers, and low cardiac output after surgery was common (Mustard et al. 1964). The Mustard procedure was more successful in most surgeons' hands and its survival statistics continued to improve. However by 1975, the midterm shortcomings of the Mustard

Fig. 20.4 Mustard/Senning intracardiac blood flow

Systemic venous blood is baffled (SVB) through the ASD to the mitral orifice, enters the LV and is ejected out the MPA.
Pulmonary venous (PV) blood is baffled through the ASD to the tricuspid valve, enters the RV and is ejected out the aorta.

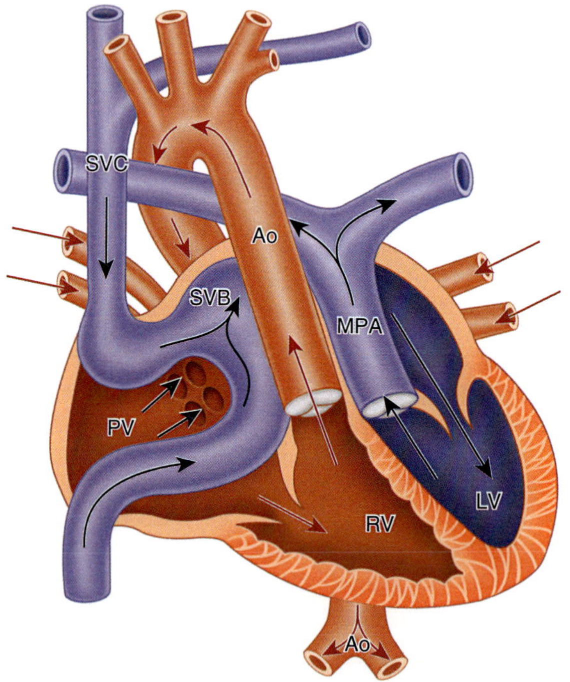

procedure were becoming more obvious as older survivors presented with right- and left-sided venous obstruction as they grew (Quaegebeur et al. 1977). Arrhythmias and heart block were also increasingly common by 10 years after a Mustard procedure. Resurgent interest in Senning's procedure, which avoids nonautologous materials, and the increasingly successful technical application of the technique in small infants, made it the most common palliative procedure performed for TGA through the 1980s (Senning 1959). Baffle obstruction due to patient growth in the first 10 years was reduced compared to the Mustard procedure and cardiac surgeons better managed the technical complexities of the baffle in infants. In many centers, infant survival of the Senning and Mustard procedures was equivalent and the midrange outlook for the patients with Senning baffles somewhat better (Williams et al. 2003).

In institutions performing Senning and Mustard procedures for TGA, care of the neonate and young infant was focused on expedient cardiac diagnosis and resuscitation of hypoxemia and low cardiac output. Atrial septostomy during stabilization was essential and was performed by balloon or blade, usually in the catheterization laboratory. As adequate atrial mixing was established, vasopressor and PgE infusions could usually be weaned and discontinued. Oxygen and ventilator therapy were also weaned and discontinued. In many instances, the stabilized infant was observed to make sure that atrial mixing remained adequate and that pulmonary vascular resistance was falling and then discharged home with careful follow-up.

In the 1980s the mortality for complex cardiac surgery in neonates was higher than contemporary survival data, partly because other than extracorporeal membrane oxygenation, reliably effective medical therapy for pulmonary hypertension was not available. (Nitric oxide by inhalation became available in the early 1990s in some institutions, and in that decade the management of persistent pulmonary hypertension in pediatric cardiac patients who were still in transition when undergoing surgery became more effective.) It was common to defer when possible repair of TGA for at least a few weeks to months. When the infant was observed to have overcirculation of the lungs and mild high-output heart failure, an atrial switch procedure was performed electively. Most institutions felt that the intra-atrial baffle part of the procedure was technically easier on an infant who was 4 kg rather than on a neonate, and surgery better tolerated when PVR had fallen. With regard to intraoperative management of inspired oxygen (FiO$_2$), minute ventilation, and expected arterial saturations (SaO$_2$), cardiac anesthesiologists in that era learned from the neonatal care of infants with TGA that although increases in pulmonary to systemic flow ratios (Qp/Qs) could be accomplished with ventilator maneuvers and increased FiO$_2$, in the presence of adequate atrial level mixing, the changes in Qp/Qs are not reflected in major improvements in arterial saturation.

As survival data from patients with TGA from the 1950s onward accumulated, it became obvious that although atrial switch palliation was superior to atrial septectomy in improving survival through infancy and childhood, there were still long-term challenges for the 84% who survived 10 years and the 77–80% who survived 20–30 years (Williams et al. 2003). Event-free incidence in survivors over three decades was less than 20% (Cuypers et al. 2014). Events were described as late failures of the operative procedure (reoperation required for baffle-related obstruction of systemic or pulmonary venous flow). Events could also be natural history issues such as arrhythmias and heart block, and late heart failure due to systolic dysfunction and tricuspid regurgitation as the inability of the right ventricle and tricuspid valve (physiologic "mitral valve") to function as systemic pumping structures over a lifetime became more obvious (el-Said et al. 1972; Culbert et al. 2003; Martin et al. 1990).

Contemporary Management and Interventions Prior to Surgery

Medical stabilization of the newborn diagnosed with TGA involves managing acidosis and hypoxemia that occurs when the intracardiac shunts are insufficient to allow adequate mixing and the ductus arteriosus closes. In any newborn patient with cyanosis of cardiac origin, PgE is administered to reconstitute ductal patency and allows blood flow into the lungs from the aorta (Fig. 20.5). Although in TGA, this maneuver increases pulmonary blood flow, unless there is an adequate amount of intracardiac mixing, the improvement in cyanosis may be negligible. Therefore, in the absence of a large ASD or VSD, balloon or blade atrial septostomy is usually required to improve atrial level mixing (Fig. 20.6). Successful enlargement of the atrial level shunt should result in immediate improvement in arterial saturation (SaO_2) as measured by pulse oximetry.

Some neonates and infants who have adequate mixing after an atrial septostomy may fail to improve their oxygen saturations if they also have pulmonary hypertension (Newfeld et al. 1974). Pulmonary hypertension as a transitional problem in neonates with cardiac disease is common, usually transient, and may be managed with nitric oxide by inhalation. Additionally, TGA patients are known to occasionally present

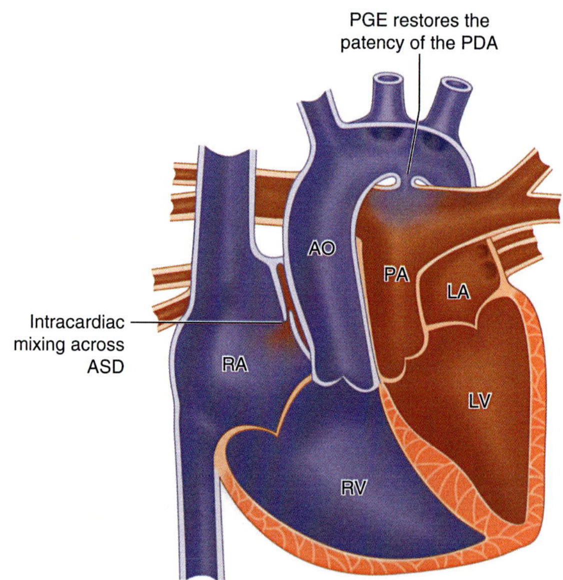

Fig. 20.5 TGA/PDA

Fig. 20.6 Atrial septostomy

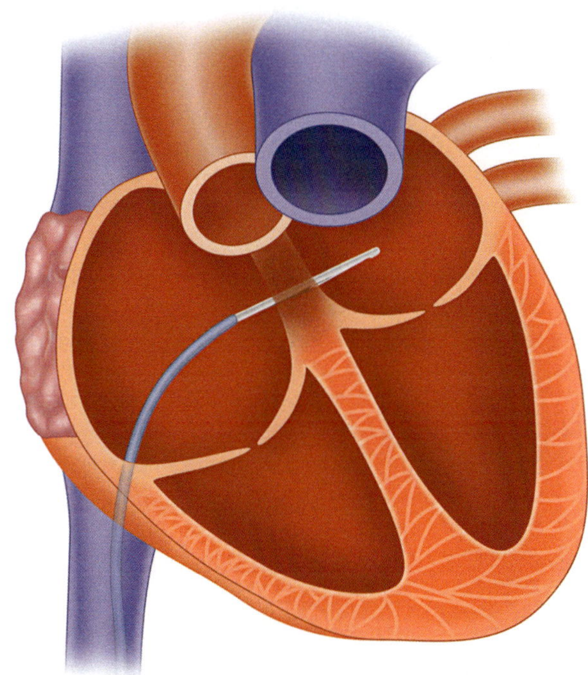

with persistent pulmonary vascular disease that seems out of proportion to the duration of time they experience physiology that predisposes them to pulmonary over-circulation (Roofthooft et al. 2007). In this small subset of TGA patients, pulmonary hypertension may be less reactive, and careful hemodynamic assessment is required before surgical correction is undertaken to rule out other lesions that may have put the pulmonary vascular bed at risk by elevating pulmonary venous pressure.

An unresolved issue is the contribution of atrial septostomy to the ultimate development of brain injury due to embolic stroke or intracerebral hemorrhage. Although the Rashkind septostomy has been performed since the 1960s, the issue of optimizing neurodevelopmental outcome was less relevant in the era where surgical outcomes were not as successful (Rashkind and Miller 1966). As surgical palliation with the Senning and Mustard procedures was replaced in most centers with surgical correction by the arterial switch, survival outcomes continued to improve through the 1990s until today. Much research is now devoted to optimizing functional outcomes, including neurodevelopmental achievement and long-term freedom from reoperation. When imaged with MRI, patients with TGA (like many cardiac anomalies), have a higher incidence of structural brain anomalies and peri-ventricular leukomalacia than infants without cardiac defects. Although there is literature indicting the septostomy procedure as an additional risk for brain injury by provoking embolic phenomena, the clinical context of hypoxia and decreased cardiac output may play a contributory role (McQuillen et al. 2006; Petit et al. 2009). The independent relation of the septostomy in causing neurologic injury has been both confirmed and discarded by conflicting studies.

The presence of a VSD is an unreliable site of mixing in many cases because of streaming of pulmonary and systemic venous blood past the septal defect into the respective great vessels. Nonetheless, a VSD does have implications on the hemodynamic modeling of left ventricular systolic performance prior to surgery in that if the VSD is large enough, the LV does not decondition as the PVR drops. In TGA with an intact ventricular septum, the normal fall in pulmonary vascular resistance that occurs the first few weeks of life is associated with reduced systolic pressure in the left ventricle. In the era of atrial switch palliation where the left ventricle remained the pulmonary ventricle, this was not a relevant issue. But the current application of the arterial switch procedure that restores the left ventricle as the systemic ventricle makes it an important consideration (Adhyapak et al. 2007). The arterial switch procedure is usually performed the first few weeks of life in order to avoid imposing systemic workload on a deconditioned left ventricle. Performing the procedure while the LV is still conditioned to perform at "systemic" pressures is associated with improved outcomes and reduced need for prolonged vasopressor support or extracorporeal support for ventricular failure.

Contemporary Surgical Management and Outcomes

In the 1970s when most infants were undergoing Mustard and Senning procedures for TGA, it was identified that patients with TGA/VSD continued to have poor outcomes despite early good results in TGA with intact ventricular septum. The arterial switch procedure was therefore applied to these patients with poor but improving short-term outcomes. Unlike the Norwood procedure for hypoplastic left heart syndrome where the "transfer of technology" was very slow and widespread improvement in outcomes delayed, the technical details associated with success of the arterial switch were widely adopted, and by the mid-1980s most neonates with TGA with or without a VSD underwent arterial switch, accomplishing anatomic correction.

The arterial switch procedure was described by Jatene in 1976 and has undergone modifications, including those proposed by Lecompte in order to improve the technical performance of the great vessel reconstruction, and improvements in techniques of coronary reimplantation especially when there are variations from the normal origination of the coronary ostia. Although there are institutional variations in technique, the common elements are:

1. Median sternotomy is performed with harvesting of pericardium for patch augmentation of the neopulmonary artery or septal defect closure.
2. The coronary artery anatomy is inspected to identify coronary anomalies and plan reimplantation sites.
3. The great vessels, branch pulmonary arteries, and patent ductus arteriosus are mobilized.
4. Heparin is administered and cardiopulmonary bypass initiated with bicaval or single atrial venous cannulation. The PDA is ligated as bypass is initiated. Temperature and perfusion techniques vary among institutions, but deep hypothermic circulatory arrest is rarely indicated.

5. Venting of the left ventricle is accomplished by a pulmonary venous catheter or through the ASD.
6. Aortic occlusion and cardioplegia administration are routine.
7. Patch closure of any septal defects is done.
8. The aorta is transected above the sinotubular junction and the coronary arteries are disconnected with a button of aortic tissue.
9. The main pulmonary artery (MPA) is transected.
10. Coronary button reimplantation to the neoaorta and anastomosis of the ascending aorta to the proximal neoaorta is performed.
11. Relocation of the pulmonary artery bifurcation to the neopulmonary artery with patch augmentation as needed is done.
12. Ultrafiltration is commonly utilized (Fig. 20.7)

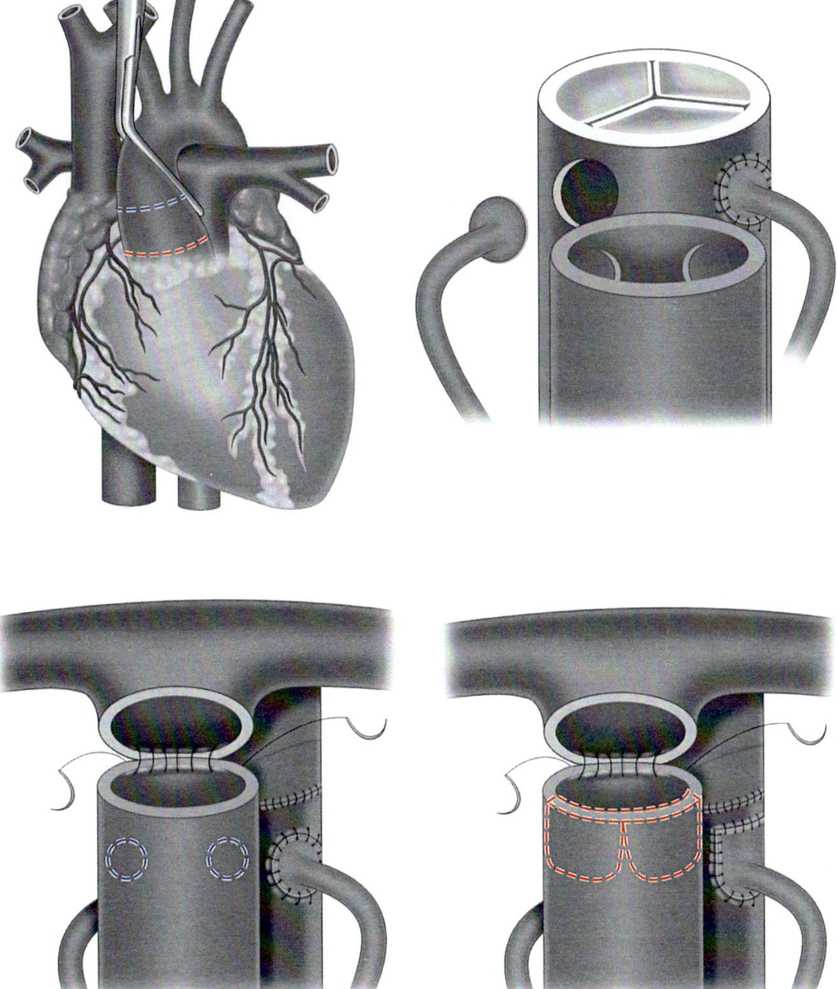

Fig. 20.7 Arterial switch

De-airing of the heart and reperfusion after removal of the aortic cross clamp begins the period where the reconstruction is critically assessed. Coronary perfusion should be immediately obvious and myocardial recovery rapid as evidenced by the return of a normal electrocardiogram. During reperfusion, echocardiographic evidence of adequate systolic ventricular function should be verified with particular assessment for wall motion abnormalities of the left ventricle that might indicate a technical problem with coronary reimplantation. Usually coronary issues result in overt ventricular dysfunction in the distribution of the left main or right coronary artery, and this assessment is straightforward when the aortic occlusion time is not excessive and myocardial protection meticulously performed. However in the event of a prolonged cross-clamp time or technical issues that interfere with adequate cardioplegia administration, the differential diagnosis of ventricular systolic dysfunction is more problematic (coronary issue versus myocardial stunning). Direct inspection of the coronary arteries and their perfusion as well as the epicardial appearance of well-perfused myocardium is essential.

The issue of LV reconditioning after repair in the TGA patient manifests even after successful surgery. (The fragility under stress of apparently "normal" ventricular function may be especially important in infants whose convalescence after surgery is complex, necessitating additional operative procedures or imaging studies requiring anesthetics.) The only patients who (intraoperatively) retain systolic LV performance adequate to easily assume systemic workload are the TGA patients who have a large VSD. All others can be assumed to have some intolerance to the requirement that they accomplish a "normal" systolic pressure after repair. This may persist for days to weeks after repair.

Additionally the issue of poor ventricular diastolic function makes intraoperative management of the patient's hemodynamics challenging. The conduct of reperfusion after removal of the aortic cross clamp is critical. The LV after arterial switch is extremely noncompliant and easily distends with small volume overload. The release of the vena cava tapes and filling of the heart on bypass require great care and are just as critical as when weaning from bypass in order to avoid distending the LV. Ventricular distension causes longitudinal stretch of the coronary arteries leading to further ventricular dysfunction due to myocardial ischemia. The author's preference is preemptive inotropic support with dopamine or low-dose epinephrine and lusitropic support with milrinone in order to optimize systolic and diastolic function with a small left ventricular end-diastolic volume. The value of nitroglycerin to prevent coronary spasm in neonates is controversial. Potent vasodilators such as nitroprusside are difficult to use in neonates with poor diastolic function because the margin between effective afterload reduction and overt hypotension may be small. If cardiac distension occurs after weaning from bypass, rapid removal of intravascular volume may be necessary or return to cardiopulmonary bypass may be required.

Additional echocardiographic examination to discover residual lesions such as intracardiac defects or valve problems should be performed during reperfusion. As the cardiac chambers are gently filled during bypass, evidence of pulmonary hypertension should be evaluated by examining the amplitude of the Doppler jet of tricuspid insufficiency. Overt right ventricular failure is rare even in the presence of pulmonary hypertension, but leftward ventricular septal shift may compromise left ventricular function. The right and left ventricular outflow tracts and proximal great vessels should be interrogated for evidence of turbulence indicating problems with a VSD patch or arterial reconstruction. The pulmonary artery branches should be visually inspected to make sure they are not under tension. The great artery reconstruction usually places the main pulmonary artery anterior to the aorta with the branch pulmonary arteries draping to either side making recannulation of the aorta somewhat more difficult if needed after cannula removal. Complete examination of the anatomic adequacy of repair should be performed prior to decannulation.

Postoperative intensive care is typical of any neonate having complex cardiac surgery. Control of the inflammatory effects of cardiopulmonary bypass and the resulting coagulopathy and capillary leak, optimization of cardiac output especially in the first eight hours after reperfusion when myocardial energy stores are being normalized, and careful hemodynamic monitoring and intervention are required. Monitoring acid-base status is often supplemented by determinations of lactate levels, mixed venous oxygen saturation, and cerebral and somatic near-infrared spectrometry to assess cardiac output (De 2008; Kreeger et al. 2012; Weiss et al. 2005; Ranucci et al. 2010; Chakravarti et al. 2009). Injury currents on the electrocardiogram are abnormal and should prompt consideration of coronary insufficiency that is likely technical in origin. Temporary renal insufficiency is often seen and meticulous attention to fluid management, electrolytes, and diuresis is required. Glucose management is controversial, and although insulin is often required postoperatively for hyperglycemia, the unconfirmed benefits of "tight control" must be weighed against the risk of iatrogenic hypoglycemia to the neonatal brain (Falcao et al. 2008; Scohy et al. 2011). For some centers, leaving the sternum open for a brief time postoperatively is an institutional preference. Ventilator support is typically provided until hemodynamic stability is accomplished and sedation weaned. Although narcotics and minor tranquilizers are commonly used for postoperative sedation, emerging strategies, such as dexmedetomidine, an alpha 2 agonist, are accumulating an increasing evidence basis for use (Chrysostomou et al. 2009; Obayah 2006; Jones 2013). The use of propofol for postoperative sedation is problematic because of its deleterious effects on hemodynamic function and the rare possibility of lactic acidosis. Muscle relaxants may be used intermittently if needed in the intubated patient, but their routine or prolonged use may lead to increased incidents of failed or delayed weaning from ventilator support. Neonates who have been given muscle relaxants must be carefully assessed prior to extubation, ideally with a nerve stimulator. Residual weakness is common and the duration of action of even intermediate acting agents is prolonged when given repeatedly or as an infusion, especially in the neonate and small infant whose pharmacokinetic processes are not mature.

As initial application of the arterial switch procedure progressed as an alternative to a Senning or Mustard procedure in the patient with TGA/VSD in the 1970s to its increasing application as the standard of care in the 1980s, the surgical mortality declined significantly (Cohen and Wernovsky 2006). Institutional mortality rates for simple TGA with either intact interventricular septum or with a VSD vary between 2 and 11 % and often are used to benchmark the performance of a pediatric cardiac surgery program (Rudra et al. 2011). Known risk factors for increased mortality include low birth weight or prematurity, complex coronary anomalies or intramural coronary artery, concomitant LV obstruction at the conal septum or aortic arch (in patients with a VSD), and late presentation and diagnosis beyond the neonatal period. Institutional experience of the operating team, including the surgeon, anesthesiologist, and perfusionist, seems to also be related to success (Hirsch et al. 2008).

Not only are the expected short-term outcomes excellent, the long-term outcomes are much better than those seen in patients who have had a Mustard or Senning procedure (Dibardino et al. 2004). Late survival of over 90 % is expected, mostly intervention free (Ruys et al. 2013). Arrhythmias, heart block, and ventricular dysfunction are rare, and most patients have a normal functional class (American Heart Association) and exercise tolerance. Late follow-up of these patients is focused on the long-term fate of the main pulmonary artery and its branches and the aortic valve. Late stenosis of the pulmonary artery branches and dilation of the pulmonary artery or aortic root are described and are the focus of technical modifications of the surgical technique. Occasional reoperations to revise the aortic root or replace the aortic valve are reported (Cohen and Wernovsky 2006). There are a small number of postoperative patients (up to 10 %) who have silent coronary insufficiency detected on myocardial perfusion imaging that has prompted preemptive stent intervention in the catheterization lab. These coronary problems may be related to ostial injury, late fibrosis or reactive injury to the artery, or late kinking from epicardial scarring, and their natural history is unknown (Bonnet et al. 1996). The oldest survivors of successful arterial switch have not yet commonly undergone coronary revascularization.

Comorbidities

TGA is rarely associated with genetic syndromes (e.g., Turner, Noonan, Williams, Marfan, or Down syndromes), chromosome abnormalities such as trisomy 8 and 18, or anomalies involving the same embryologic substrate as the cardiac tube or branchial arches (e.g., VACTERL and CHARGE syndromes) (Ferencz et al. 1995, 1997; Bonnet et al. 1996; Marino 1996). There is an occasional infrequent association with chromosome deletion 22q11 and DiGeorge syndrome (Melchionda et al. 1995; Van Mierop and Kutsche 1986). Heterotaxy and isomerism syndromes are the only genetic syndromes highly associated with TGA (Ferencz et al. 1995).

Additional Anesthetic Considerations

The preanesthesia evaluation should focus on defining the patient's anatomic findings and the physiologic impact of those findings. Adequacy of neonatal resuscitation in patients who presented with severe cyanosis and shock should include the recovery of end organ performance such as cardiac function, renal and liver function, and assessment of any neurologic injury. The adequacy of mixing after septostomy by echocardiogram and the patient's pulse oximetry should help identify patients who have pulmonary hypertension and are significantly desaturated despite imaging evidence of an adequate ASD. This should prompt consideration of whether the expected transitional change in PVR is delayed or alternatively if an unappreciated cardiac anomaly exists that threatens the pulmonary vascular bed. If PgE is being administered, the presence of apnea or other complications of its use such as fever, hypotension, or reduced gastrointestinal perfusion pressures should be considered. In the patient with a large, widely patent ductus arteriosus and a VSD, the possibility that there is also an unrecognized coarctation of the aorta should be considered. This disastrous finding would present when the PDA is ligated at the onset of bypass as elevated resistance to flow and delayed lower body cooling on cardiopulmonary bypass and venous desaturation and metabolic acidosis despite adequate perfusion flows.

Anatomic variants that will complicate or prolong the surgical procedure or perfusion technique should be identified and considered in preoperative planning (e.g., malaligned VSD with outflow tract obstruction, aortic arch hypoplasia, or coarctation of the aorta.) Coronary artery patterns are variable in TGA and identifying the origins of the left and right coronary ostia should be done in preoperative imaging if possible. Although early literature seemed to indicate the coronary pattern was a risk factor, as surgical techniques for location and reimplantation of the coronary ostia evolved and the early mortality of the procedure improved, coronary anatomy is believed to not have an important impact on survival unless there is single ostial origin of both main arteries or an intramural coronary artery. Noncardiac anomalies are infrequent in TGA (except L-TGA is often associated with heterotaxy), but neonates who are premature or small for gestational age are at increased risk. Patients who were inadequately resuscitated after an unstable presentation are at increased risk. Infants who were diagnosed late, especially if they have an intact ventricular septum are especially at risk for LV dysfunction postoperatively. Persistent pulmonary hypertension is an infrequent condition, but if present it increases the likelihood of ECMO support or inhaled nitric oxide being required after repair.

The anesthesiologist who has experience with infants several months old coming to the operating room for an atrial switch is often comfortable with an inhalation induction of anesthesia in patients with TGA. Also, the concept that FiO_2 and PCO_2 management may affect Qp/Qs but do not significantly change SaO_2 is reassuring when the patient's arterial saturation does not change much with induction of anesthesia. In neonates, intravenous access is usually available, and it is common to perform induction with an opioid or ketamine. The author's preference for airway management is nasotracheal intubation because fixation of the endotracheal tube is more secure, and it is more difficult for the patient to be inadvertently extubated with the manipulation of a transesophageal echo probe. Invasive monitoring catheters are routine for hemodynamic monitoring, blood sampling, and vasopressor administration. (See the "Addendum" at the end of this chapter.) Transesophageal echo probe placement is routine, and as neonatal patients are particularly susceptible to laryngeal or esophageal trauma, airway compression, and left atrial compression and hemodynamic changes from the probe, vigilance is highly encouraged. The use of antifibrinolytic agents, perfusion protocols, and preferences for inotropic medication are largely institutional preferences and their discussion in this chapter will not be undertaken.

Complex TGA

As previously discussed, simple D-TGA with and without a VSD represents the majority of cases presenting with this cardiac diagnosis, but there are specific anomalies that represent variations in anatomy that require modifications in surgical planning and procedure. These complex forms of TGA also have a short-term survival profile somewhat worse than simple transposition, and a natural history arc that is defined by more interventions and a worse long-term outcome.

TGA with Aortic Coarctation

Although TGA is rarely associated with coarctation of the aorta (4%), when a coarctation is present in a patient with TGA, it is usually in association with a VSD (Williams et al. 2003). Aortic arch hypoplasia and right ventricular outflow tract obstruction are occasionally seen. As in any patient with aortic arch obstruction, restoring the patency of the ductus arteriosus is required after birth in order to accomplish systemic perfusion. Interestingly, in TGA with a coarctation, when the ductus is reopened with PgE, the oxygen saturation of blood perfusing the lower extremities is higher than that of the right upper extremity, which is the opposite of what is seen in coarctation of the aorta with normally related great vessels (Aziz et al. 1968) (Fig. 20.8).

Repair of TGA with a coarctation of the aorta and a VSD is straightforward if there is no malalignment of the VSD resulting in conal septal outflow tract obstruction of the RV or the LV. An arterial switch and VSD repair are performed as previously described, and the aortic issue is addressed at the same time usually utilizing a brief period of deep hypothermic circulatory arrest.

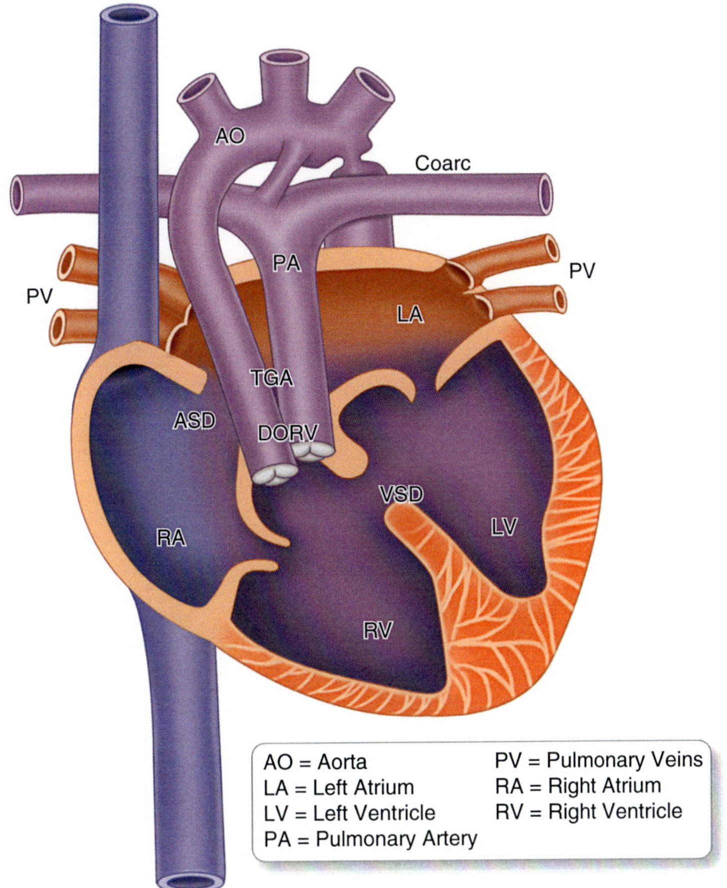

Fig. 20.8 TGA/coarctation of the aorta

TGA with Conal Septal Deviation

Although about a third of the 45 % of all TGA patients who have a VSD do not have significant conal septal deviation, the remainder does. Therefore about 25 % of TGA/VSD patients have outflow tract obstruction of either the left or right ventricle. Malalignment of the conal septum is also occasionally associated with hypoplasia of a ventricular chamber and malformation or malposition of the tricuspid or mitral valve. Preoperative surgical planning carefully considers ventricular chamber sizes, the annulus Z-scores and morphology of the AV and semilunar valves, and the location and the size of the VSD.

Conal Septal Deviation-TGA/VSD and LVOT Obstruction

Patients with TGA and a VSD who also have anatomic left ventricular outflow tract obstruction represent less than 10 % of all patients with TGA (Williams et al. 2003). The obstruction may be related to posterior deviation of the conal septum, a discrete membrane or diffuse fibromuscular tunnel of the LVOT, straddling tricuspid valve apparatus protruding into the left ventricular outflow tract through the VSD, or complex obstruction from anomalous attachments of the mitral valve (Fig. 20.9).

This anatomy complicates the neonatal presentation of TGA, as physiology more consistent with critically decreased pulmonary blood flow is present if the obstruction is severe, similar to patients with critical pulmonary stenosis or pulmonary atresia. Restoration of ductal patency is crucial to provide pulmonary blood flow. In cases of less severe obstruction, the typical TGA mixing physiology may be more obvious.

Palliative placement of a systemic to pulmonary shunt in the neonatal period allows delay of further surgical correction until the patient is an older infant. The most common surgical options for repair are the Rastelli procedure and the Nikaidoh reconstruction.

Rastelli palliation involves enlarging the VSD and patching it so that LV blood is ejected into the aorta. The potential for developing late subaortic stenosis exists if the intraventricular tunnel to the aorta is not adequately large, and with the patient's growth, this becomes an increasing reason for reoperation. Optimal creation of the tunnel may be hampered by a small VSD, especially in the inlet position, or if atrioventricular valve tissue from either side straddles the VSD. The main pulmonary artery trunk is divided, the proximal stump oversewn, and a conduit is placed to

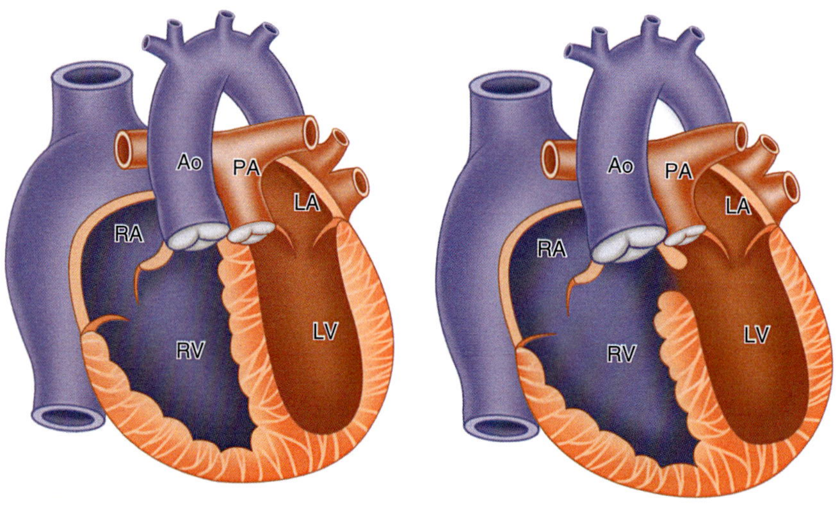

Fig. 20.9 TGA with LVOTO. Isolated form has no VSD. Complex form has VSD and atrioventricular valve tissue straddling the VSD

create right ventricular to pulmonary artery continuity (Fig. 20.10). This also is a common cause of reintervention as the patient grows. As the RV to PA conduit functionally reduces the size of the RV, a hypoplastic RV is a relative contraindication to the procedure. Additionally, if there is an anomalous coronary artery crossing the RVOT, it may preclude placement of the conduit.

The outcome of a successful Rastelli procedure is still somewhat unsatisfying (Emani et al. 2009). The mortality of the initial procedure is as high as 7%, and the long-term freedom from reoperation poor (Mandell et al. 1990). Conduit failure occurs in 21% of patients by 15 years, and LVOT or LV tunnel obstruction is seen in 10%. The 20-year survival is as low as 59% (Dearani et al. 2001). (Fig. 20.11).

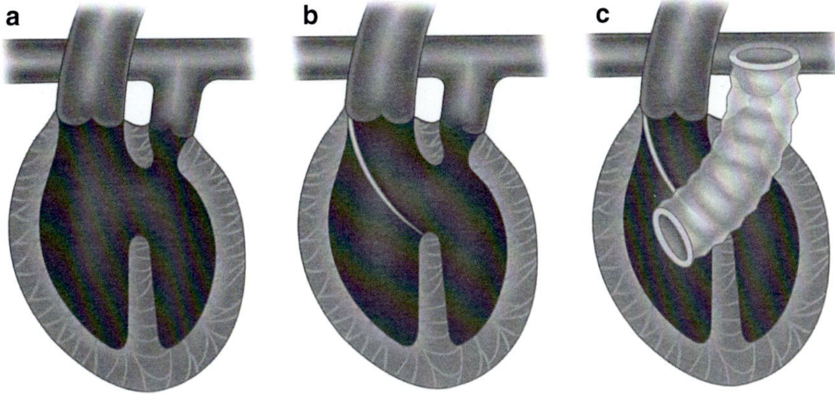

Fig. 20.10 (**a–c**) Rastelli repair of TGA/VSD/LVOTO

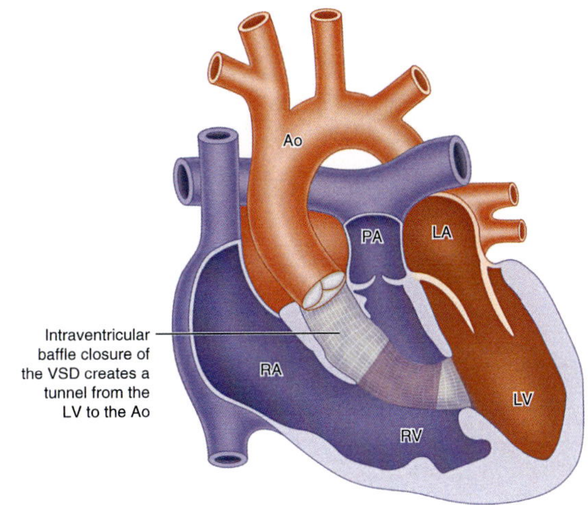

Fig. 20.11 VSD baffle in Rastelli repair

The Nikaidoh procedure translocates the aortic root from the right ventricle to the left ventricle and reconstructs both the left and right bulboventricular outflow tracts (Nikaidoh 1984). This technically demanding operation restores a nearly anatomically correct repair and avoids the use of a conduit to connect RV to PA (Morell et al. 2005). Although not widely applied, a mortality rate of 5 % is reported for this operation from a few centers. Freedom from reoperation is excellent (Yeh et al. 2007). (Fig. 20.10, 20.11, and 20.12).

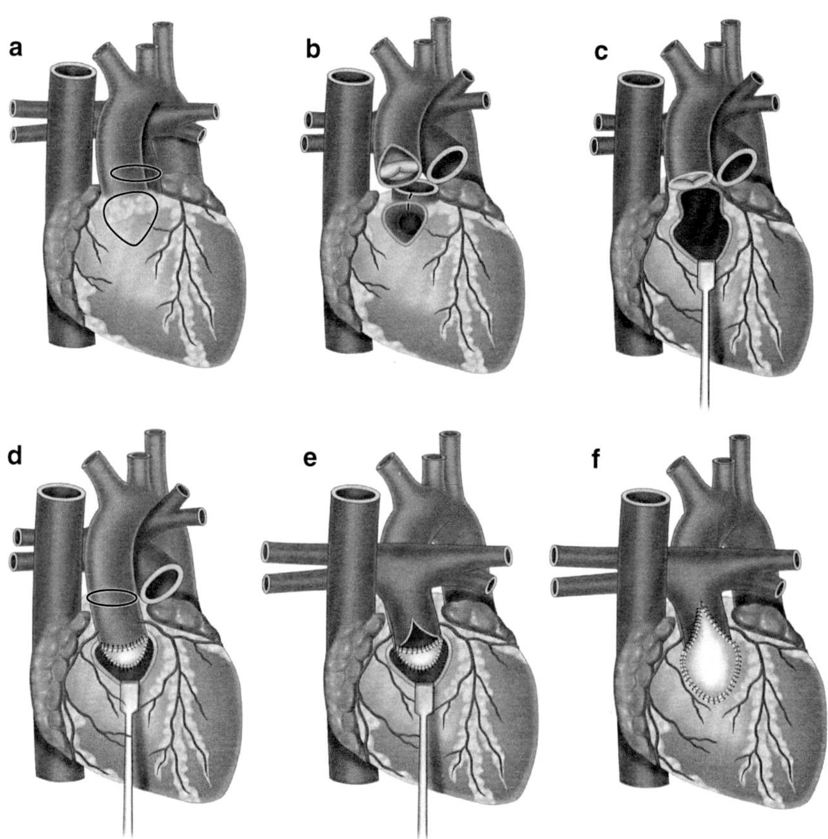

Fig. 20.12 (a–f) Nikaidoh procedure

Conal Septal Deviation-Taussig Bing Anomaly

Double outlet right ventricle has several anatomic variants where the specific position of the VSD defines distinct physiology. For example, when the VSD is subaortic, the patient is typically overcirculated and in high-output heart failure, and arterial saturations are nearly normal. When the VSD is subpulmonic and the aortic and pulmonary annuli are in a side-by-side arrangement, it is called the Taussig-Bing anomaly (Fig. 20.13). The physiology is similar to that of transposition of the great vessels and is defined by mixing of oxygenated blood from the LV streaming through the VSD into the pulmonary artery, while desaturated blood streams into the aorta. Often the streaming patterns preclude adequate mixing and saturations are typically very low despite adequate pulmonary blood flow and an anatomically large VSD.

In contrast to simple TGA where the additional presence of a coarctation is rare, in the setting of right ventricular outflow tract obstruction and Taussig-Bing anomaly, aortic arch obstruction is seen in 53 % of patients (Comas et al. 1996). Ductal closure after birth is not tolerated and restoring ductal patency in anticipation of neonatal repair is required.

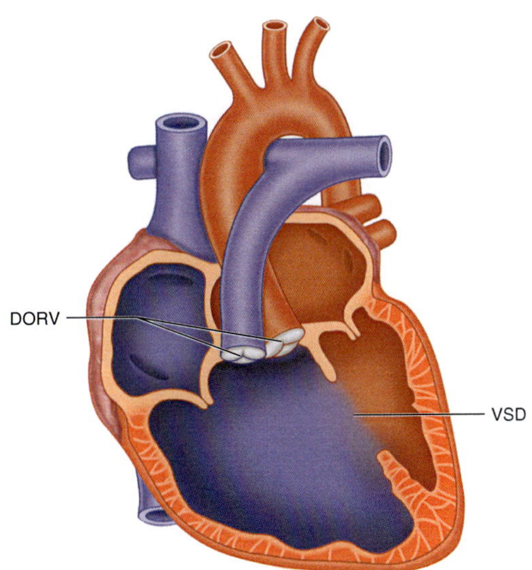

Fig. 20.13 DORV

Fig. 20.14 DORV/arterial switch

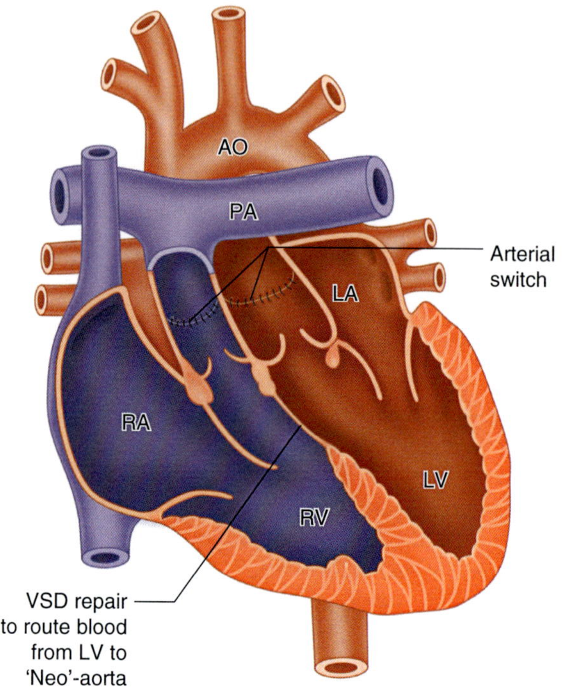

The intracardiac defect in Taussig-Bing anomaly is repaired by creating an intraventricular tunnel from the LV to the aorta if the location of the aorta in relation to the interventricular septum is favorable or by arterial switch operation if the distance between the LV and the aorta is remote (Fig. 20.14). The arterial switch has been used successfully in patients with side-by-side and anterior-posterior relationships of the aorta and pulmonary artery (Rodefeld et al. 2007). It is also combined with aortic arch reconstruction when arch obstruction is present. The short-term survival is 90 %, and although the 15-year survival is 85–89 %, there are a small number of patients who require reoperation for residual aortic arch obstruction or recurrent RVOT obstruction (Alsoufi et al. 2008).

Corrected Transposition of the Great Arteries

Corrected transposition is a rare type of TGA with atrioventricular discordance and ventriculoarterial discordance (Allen et al. 2001b) (Fig. 20.15). The atria are usually situs solitus, and the atrioventricular valve apparatus is inverted making the outlet for the right atrium a morphologic mitral valve, while the outlet for the left atrium is a morphologic tricuspid valve. There is ventricular inversion, so the left-sided tricuspid valve empties into a morphologic right ventricle and the left ventricle is on the right side. The outlet for the left-sided right ventricle is the aorta and the

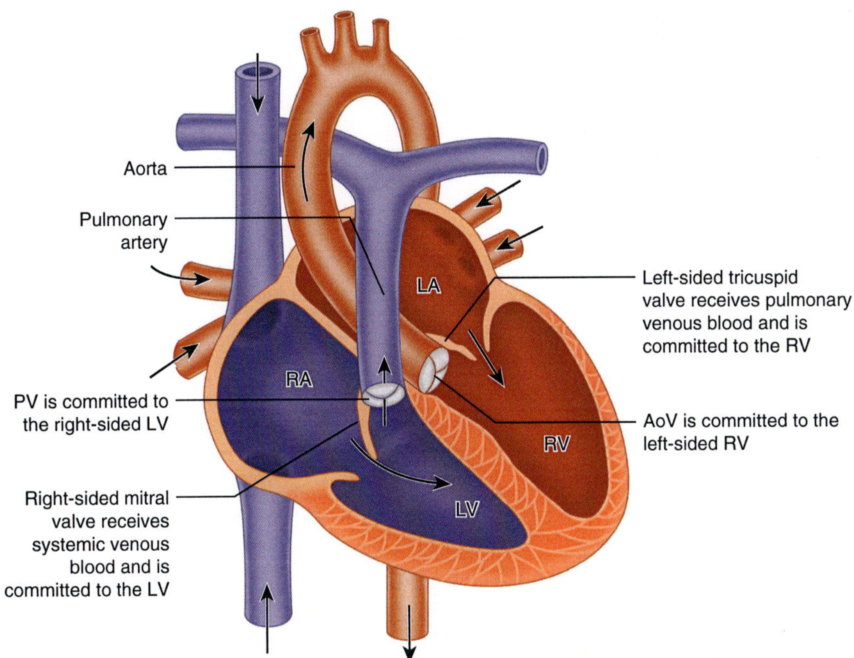

Fig. 20.15 Corrected TGA

pulmonary artery arises from the right-sided left ventricle. There are no specific symptoms referable to the defects in segmental arrangement in the infant unless there are additional cardiac anomalies. As a result, the defect may not present until adulthood.

Cardiac variations of corrected TGA are common. Most patients (60–80 %) have a large perimembranous VSD associated with a large left-to-right shunt. Many patients (30–50 %) have obstruction to pulmonary blood flow from fibro-muscular LVOT obstruction (LVOTO). If LVOT obstruction and a VSD are both present, there is cyanosis with right-to-left shunting similar to tetralogy of Fallot. The tricuspid valve is morphologically abnormal in 90 % of corrected TGA, but far fewer patients have early disturbances of tricuspid valve function (Freedom 1999). When it occurs it is often a severe Ebstein's type malformation with inferior displacement of the valve into the right ventricle associated with valve regurgitation or alternatively tricuspid stenosis from valve dysplasia (Gladman et al. 1996). This is associated with heart failure in the young patient.

Abnormalities of atrioventricular conduction are also seen (Wallis et al. 2011). The location of the SA node is normal in these hearts just lateral to the junction where the superior vena cava enters the right atrium, but the AV node is positioned beneath the right atrial appendage instead of the posterior inferior area of the inter-atrial septum near the coronary sinus. The course of the long bundle that divides the right bundle branch leftward to the morphologic right ventricle and the left bundle to the right-sided left ventricle is markedly abnormal. Patients with corrected TGA have a 10% incidence of complete heart block at birth. Even if they have normal conduction, heart block is still gradually progressive (Anderson et al. 1974). By adolescence up to 15% have heart block, and by 45 years of age, 30–50% of patients have heart block (Anderson et al. 1973; Huhta et al. 1983).

Presentation of patients with corrected TGA is related to the presence or severity of the above associated cardiac lesions. In the absence of these, most infants and young children are not symptomatic (Presbitero et al. 1995). Patients usually come to early diagnosis if they have a large VSD and acyanotic heart failure, a VSD with LVOTO to pulmonary blood flow with cyanosis, or heart failure in association with tricuspid valve regurgitation. Likewise, early diagnosis is facilitated in the neonate if there is a PDA-dependent lesion such as severe coarctation of the aorta.

Surgical repair of septal defects, resection of outflow tract obstruction in the right-sided left ventricle, and pacing interventions are often done in children with corrected transposition, although the surgical outcome is worse with higher operative mortality and lower 10-year survival estimates than similar repairs in otherwise normal hearts. Surgical injury to the abnormally located conduction tissue is common (De Leval et al. 1979).

With or without concomitant cardiac lesions, the long-term survival of patients with corrected transposition is most related to the inevitable progression of tricuspid valve dysfunction and systolic failure of the left-sided right ventricle. The predictable failure of the anatomy of corrected transposition is a manifestation of the lack of durability of right heart structures when located in the systemic rather than the pulmonary circuit (Peterson et al. 1988). Although tricuspid valve replacement is occasionally performed, the only surgical therapy in the setting of end-stage congestive cardiomyopathy is cardiac replacement. Theoretically, conversion to single ventricle physiology with total extracardiac cavopulmonary shunt is possible, but insufficient data exists to anticipate a likely outcome (Karl 2011).

The preemptive treatment of corrected transposition has been investigated and indications for surgical intervention are evolving. The argument that the natural history of the failing left-sided AV valve and ventricle leads to early death or cardiac transplantation is a compelling reason to consider alternative surgical therapies that might avoid those endpoints. Anatomic correction can be accomplished by an arterial switch procedure combined with a Senning atrial switch (ASO/Senning) (Brawn 2005) (Fig. 20.16). This restores the morphologic left ventricle and mitral valve on the right side of the heart to function as systemic structures and the morphologic right ventricle and tricuspid valve on the left side of the heart to function as pulmonary structures.

Many advocate ASO/Senning as indicated in the younger child who is having symptoms from RV failure or tricuspid valve insufficiency (Jahangiri et al. 2001). Unlike the patient with no symptoms and no associated cardiac lesions, the short-term outcome for these patients without intervention is immediately poor. Regardless of whether an ASO/Senning is performed on a symptomatic or an asymptomatic patient, it is unknown at this time whether this extends the life expectancy of the patient or simply changes the problems occurring in the natural arc of

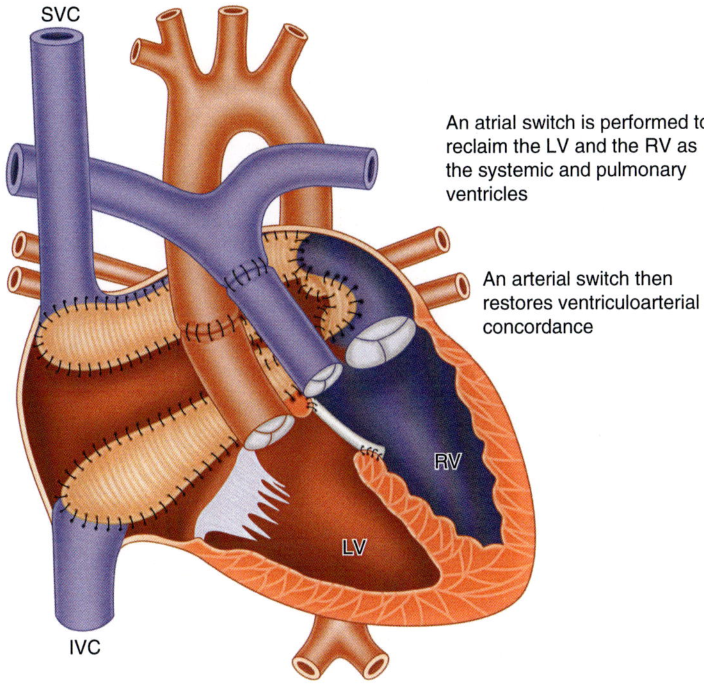

Fig. 20.16 Arterial switch/Senning for corrected TGA

their cardiac disease. Answering these questions is difficult because of the rarity of the condition compared to other cardiac anomalies. Also confounding the analysis is the problem that prior to an ASO/Senning, the right-sided left ventricle must be reconditioned, and although this may be accomplished with a pulmonary artery band (PAB), the process of increasing LV myocardial muscle mass over time is unpredictable. Another variable is that the older the patient, the more ineffective LV remodeling may be (Quinn et al. 2008). In a neonate or young infant, retraining as evidenced by MRI estimation of LV muscle mass, LV wall thickness, and LV pressures may occur in a few months; in the older child, the time required is less predictable. Not all patients survive PAB preparation of the LV or demonstrate an appropriate response to the procedure to further undergo ASO/Senning repair (Winlaw et al. 2005). Although some centers report a 90 % 10-year survival for small series of patients who undergo PAB and then ASO/Senning, identifiable risk factors for poor outcome are preoperative RV failure or tricuspid insufficiency. These promising results may be misleading in that this survival group is favorably selected because patients who failed to successfully endure LV retraining are not included. Late ventricular dysfunction is known to occur after apparently successful ASO/Senning resulting in far less successful long-term outcomes.

Current trends in the application of the ASO/Senning strategy for avoiding cardiac failure in patients with corrected transposition support doing the procedure prior to the onset of tricuspid insufficiency and ventricular dysfunction. Unfortunately many of these patients are not yet diagnosed. Even when there is a diagnosis, the procedure is inherently risky with a 10 % mortality rate and this may not be acceptable to asymptomatic patients. Comparing the 90 % survival reported by a few centers to a cohort of like patients who are asymptomatic and do not undergo surgery is difficult because the cardiac defect is rare (Sano et al. 1995; Gaies et al. 2009). When endpoints such as persistent tricuspid valve problems, need for atrial baffle revision, need for reoperation on the pulmonary valve or pulmonary artery, neoaortic valve incompetence, and impaired LV function are considered, it becomes obvious that the ASO/Senning type anatomic correction is applicable to a complex set of patients who continue to have difficult issues after surgery and frequently require reoperation (Voskuil et al. 1999). It seems that the important natural history issues of tricuspid insufficiency and heart failure are not resolved and are replaced by an even longer list of adverse potential problems. Therefore anticipation that the "double-switch" procedure is predictably successful for symptomatic or asymptomatic patients is speculative and not supported by large data sets at this time.

Addendum on Invasive Monitoring Catheter Insertion: Author's Opinion

As many of the cardiac lesions discussed such as TOF and TOGV require operative repair while the patient is a neonate or infant, the subject of invasive monitoring catheter placement is pertinent. Invasive arterial and central venous monitoring catheters have long been an expected skill of the pediatric cardiac anesthesiologist, and the literature guiding their use and various insertion practices is varied and controversial. The topic is important because a busy pediatric cardiac anesthesiologist may insert as many as 15–20,000 arterial catheters and a similar number of central venous catheters in a 30-year career. The author's bias based on literature and personal experience is that success rate and complication profile of arterial and central venous catheter insertion improves with operator experience and "procedural self-awareness". The exception to this caveat is the infrequent but disastrous ischemic complication of a lower extremity due to femoral artery catheterization in an infant or small toddler, where ischemic events seem to be unpredictable and episodic, mainly related to the patient's size. Serious ischemic injury due to a femoral artery catheter in an infant or small toddler occurs more frequently than when peripheral arterial sites are used; therefore, it seems reasonable to use the femoral artery as infrequently as possible in these patients.

Ultrasound for CVL Placement and Arterial Cannulation

Ultrasound has provided an anecdotal but not evidence-based impact on the incidence of some complications. When ultrasound first became widely used in central catheter placement in the 1990s, it appeared that its greatest benefit was to the low-volume proceduralist and that compared to an operator with a high volume of experience, the differences were difficult to demonstrate. Emerging data over the subsequent decades may evolve differently because the number of practitioners with high-volume experience without the use of ultrasound has decreased. Trainees taught CVL cannulation with ultrasound often do not have a nuanced appreciation of the relevant surface landmarks.

Ultrasound used to visualize puncture of a central vein or to verify wire placement after puncture seems intuitively useful. However, ultrasound does not reduce to zero complications such as inadvertent arterial puncture. Hand-eye-brain coordination plays an important role in how effective ultrasound is in enhancing an individual practitioner's procedural success. Placement of central catheters into the arterial circulation still occurs, and the complete loss of control of the Seldinger guidewire into the catheterized vessel is still occasionally seen as a complication of lack of operator attention to detail.

The evolving use of ultrasound in arterial cannulation also has not reduced to zero the complications of insertion. Wire disruption of the arterial intima with failed cannulation of the artery seems to be related to operator skill and is independent of ultrasound visualization. In the most extreme case, avulsion of the artery during wire removal can occur if the wire remains captured by the intima, and in the lesser case, arterial thrombosis due to trauma often occurs in the setting of failed cannulation. These complications occur despite the use of ultrasound. The use of the ultrasound to visualize an artery that is small and cannot be palpated may paradoxically lead to an ischemic complication that wouldn't have occurred had a larger artery been chosen.

Based on his large personal procedural experience, the author recommends the reader adopt certain guiding principles of practice to minimize potential exposure to the most major complications (limb ischemia from an arterial catheter) and reduce the incidence of the more minor complications (e.g., malposition of the catheter, pneumothorax, inadvertent arterial placement of a guidewire, and failed attempt requiring a second site to be used). Line placement remains a tactile skill irrespective of the advantages of ultrasound visualization of the vessel. Some of the author's guiding principles (opinions) are presented:

1. Arterial site selection should preferably be a peripheral artery with collateral circulation, especially in the infant. Allen tests are difficult to interpret in an infant. In the upper and lower extremity, the radial artery is usually larger than the ulnar artery, and the posterior tibial artery is larger than the dorsal pedal artery. In a

premature infant, the posterior tibial artery is larger than the radial artery. Post-catheterization thrombosis is related to how atraumatically the catheter is inserted, the size of the catheter related to the size of the artery, and the duration of cannulation. Thrombosis after use in infants is common but of little consequence as long as the collateral artery is intact. Unfortunately, atraumatic insertion is difficult for the inexperienced practitioner; the author's strong bias is that cutdown technique (without ligation of the artery) in the infant is preferable and more successful than percutaneous technique. The goal over many thousands of placements is to reduce the number of unsuccessful attempts as much as possible and make successful cannulations with as little trauma as feasible. Failed cannulations often damage the artery making a subsequent attempt at cannulation more likely to be complicated. Placement of the catheter in the artery under direct vision rarely requires a guidewire and in the author's opinion is the least traumatic way to cannulate the artery in an infant. Fellows and attending faculty in the author's cardiac training program have successfully acquired the skill of radial and posterior tibial artery cutdown when carefully mentored. The additional benefit of a small scar from previous cutdown is that the site is identified as having been previously used and can be avoided in the future. If a percutaneous approach to a peripheral artery is undertaken (with or without ultrasound), the use of an IV catheter in a through-and-through puncture and slow withdrawal of the catheter until arterial pulsations are observed, and then careful placement of a small straight guidewire prior to advancing the catheter is associated with a high success rate.

2. Once a peripheral site in an infant has been used or attempted, it should not be reused. Neither should the collateral artery to the same limb be used/attempted.

3. The femoral artery should be avoided when possible in infants and small toddlers as the incidence of major ischemic injury is much higher prior to the age of 2–3 years and is unpredictably related to how uneventful insertion was performed or how well the catheter is functioning. The incidence of minor complications such as late presentation of leg length discrepancy due to ischemia of the femoral growth plate is increased and unappreciated at the time of catheterization. When the femoral artery is cannulated, the size of the catheter is important, and an atraumatic insertion technique is essential. If an ischemic complication with potential tissue loss occurs, an algorithmic approach to diagnosis and treatment is required. It is unclear that the use of ultrasound changes the complication profile of femoral arterial catheters in infants, although it may improve the likelihood of insertion. Therefore my concern is that the use of ultrasound to facilitate successful cannulation of small femoral arteries may paradoxically lead to more ischemic complications. A primary consideration by the author is to have minimized the use of femoral arterial catheters in infants (over the span of a career), utilizing radial and posterior tibial artery sites whenever possible. In patients over the age of 3 years, the careful use of the femoral artery is associated with a much safer complication profile.

The difficulty that the above recommendation obviously poses is that many pediatric anesthesiologists are not experienced enough to perform peripheral artery cannulation in an infant with a high success rate, and the decision to cannulate the femoral artery is made because it is technically more feasible. The operator who only occasionally places arterial lines in infants may not appreciate the increased risk of the technique because of their low volume of procedures, nonetheless, the risk is still high. Skill at peripheral cannulation with ultrasound guidance if needed or with cutdown technique is strongly encouraged if the profile of the anesthesiologist's practice is complex.

4. Novel arterial sites such as the brachial artery or axillary artery are reported as routine by some institutions that also cite low complication rates. However these approaches put the limb at risk due to the unknown amount of collateral circulation, and have the further disadvantage of both being close to neural structures. The frequent use of these techniques is outside of the author's experience.

5. The Seldinger technique is just as valuable for percutaneous arterial cannulation as it is essential for central venous catheterization. But if the wire doesn't advance very easily, there's a problem to be solved. (Withdrawing a guidewire through an insertion needle may shear the wire; the wire and needle should be removed as a unit. If it has been introduced via an IV catheter, removal is usually uneventful.) Forcefully advancing the wire is hazardous. If the tip of the wire is intra-intimal, the vessel may be damaged by further advancement or avulsed if the wire is forcibly removed.

6. There are separate complication profiles for internal jugular versus subclavian approaches to central venous cannulation and the author is convinced that both are successful in experienced hands. Subclavian catheters require care in insertion in patients having median sternotomy to avoid kinking the catheter; a common technical problem is to puncture the costoclavicular ligament during insertion. The insertion site should be lateral to the ligament and caudad enough to avoid the catheter kinking under the clavicle when the sternal retractor is in place. Left subclavian cannulation in infants is easier as the path of the guidewire into the SVC is more gradual than if approached from the right. In cardiac procedures, the occasional inadvertent violation of the pleura is rarely consequential as it is easily identified after median sternotomy. The occasional malposition of the subclavian catheter into a jugular vein may be suspected by resistance to the wire passing beyond the distance from the insertion site to the jugular bulb and the failure to elicit an arrhythmia with the wire. If the catheter is placed in the jugular instead of central circulation, the pressure recorded is higher than expected and external compression of the jugular vein in the sternocleidomastoid triangle at the base of the neck causes it to rise further. The optimal position of the tip of the catheter in the SVC or the right atrium is largely situation dependent and is easily adjusted by the surgeon trimming the catheter after right atriotomy.

7. Wire placement during CVL placement should be very easy and it may be useful to elicit an arrhythmia (except in high-risk conditions where ventricular fibrillation is likely), confirming venous placement. It is very difficult to cross the aortic valve retrograde with the guidewire in the event of inadvertent arterial puncture. (Likewise, although it is possible to place a guidewire into an artery, it is actually difficult to place a dilator over the wire into the artery because the tip of the dilator is sharp but soft. Difficulty in passing a dilator should alert the operator to troubleshoot the insertion, not push harder.) Wire position is reliably determined by ultrasound if needed. Dilator placement should be only so far as to enlarge the puncture hole of the vein and should meticulously follow the path of the wire

without distorting the path or else the wire can be easily bent. (A bent wire should be exchanged through an IV catheter.) Except when cannulating the femoral vein or right internal jugular vein, there is substantial risk of caval perforation by advancing the dilator too far.

8. In infants the risk of severe thrombosis of the great vein is increased and is related to many factors. It is likely that cannulation of the right internal jugular vein puts less of the upper extremity venous system at risk compared to the left internal jugular or either subclavian vein.

9. If there is a known persistent left superior vena cava (LSVC), there may be some merit in avoiding cannulation of the left subclavian or jugular veins. The course on the chest x-ray of a CVL catheter in the LSVC appears "arterial," and the cava often ends in the coronary sinus, so a thrombotic complication has severe implications for coronary circulation. An unsuspected LSVC encountered while attempting a left subclavian access has a different tactile feel as the guidewire makes a caudad turn just proximal to the left sternal border. If the operator doesn't recognize this and advances the dilator too aggressively, the cava may be perforated.

Despite the increasing use of ultrasound to improve the success and safety of arterial and venous access procedures, it seems likely that the operator's experience, attention to detail, accumulative learning, and "procedural awareness" skills remain the most important considerations to minimizing the likelihood of the most major complications of invasive monitoring catheters and reducing the incidences of minor complications and failed attempts.

Bibliography

Adhyapak S, Mahala B, et al. Impact of left ventricular function on early outcomes after arterial switch for D-transposition of the great arteries with intact ventricular septum. Indian Heart J. 2007;59(2):137–41.

Albert HM. Surgical correction of transposition of the great vessels. Surg Forum. 1954;5:74–7.

Alexi-Meskishvili V, Sharykin A. Blalock-Hanlon operation in transposition of great vessels of the heart in patients under 3 months of age. Grudn Khir. 1984;5:5–8.

Allen H, Driscoll D, Shaddy R, Feltes T. Moss & Adams' heart disease in infants, children, and adolescents: including the fetus and young adult. 8th ed. Philadelphia: Lippincott Williams and Wilkins; 2001a. p. 1097–146.

Allen H, Driscoll D, Shaddy R, Feltes T. Moss & Adams' heart disease in infants, children, and adolescents: including the fetus and young adult. 8th ed. Philadelphia: Lippincott Williams and Wilkins; 2001b. p. 1146–60.

Alsoufi B, Cai S, Williams W, Coles J, Caldarone C, Redington A, VanArsdell G. Improved results with single-stage total correction of Taussig- Bing anomaly. Eur J Cardiothorac Surg. 2008; 33(2):244–50.

Anderson R, Arnold R, Wilkinson J. The conducting system in congenitally corrected transposition. Lancet. 1973;1:1286–8.

Anderson R, Becker A, Arnold R, Wilkinson J. The conducting tissues in congenitally corrected transposition. Circulation. 1974;50:911–24.

Aziz K, Sanyal S, Goldblatt E. Reversed differential cyanosis. Br Heart J. 1968;30:288–90.

Baffes TG. A new method for surgical correction of transposition of the aorta and pulmonary artery. Surg Gynecol Obstet. 1956;102:227–33.

Bailey C, Cookson B, Downing D, Neptune W. Cardiac surgery under hypothermia. J Thorac Surg. 1954;27:73–91.

Blalock AH. The surgical treatment of complete transposition of the aorta and pulmonary artery. Surg Gynecol Obstet. 1950;90:1.

Blalock A, Hanlon C. Interatrial septal defect—its experimental production under direct vision without interruption of the circulation. Surg Gynecol Obstet. 1948;128:183–7.

Bonnet D, Bonhoeffer P, Piechaud JF, et al. Long-term fate of the coronary arteries after the arterial switch operation in newborns with transposition of the great arteries. Heart. 1996;76:274–9.

Brawn W. The double switch for atrioventricular discordance. Semin Thorac Cardiovasc Surg Pediatr Card Surg Annu. 2005;8:51–6.

Calderon J, Angeard N, et al. Outcomes in children with transposition of the great arteries. J Pediatr. 2012;161(1):94–8.

Chakravarti S, Mittnacht A, Katz J, Nguyen K, Joashi U, Srivastava S. Multisite near-infrared spectroscopy predicts elevated blood lactate level in children after cardiac surgery. J Cardiothorac Vasc Anesth. 2009;23(5):663–7.

Chrysostomou C, Sanchez De Toledo J, Avolio T, et al. Dexmedetomidine use in a pediatric cardiac intensive care unit: can we use it in infants after cardiac surgery? Pediatr Crit Care Med. 2009;10(6):654–60.

Cohen M, Wernovsky G. Is the arterial switch operation as good over the long term as we thought it would be? Cardiol Young. 2006;16 Suppl 3:117–24.

Comas J, Mignosa C, Cochrane A, Wilkinson J, Karl T. Taussig-Bing anomaly and arterial switch: aortic arch obstruction does not influence out- come. Eur J Cardiothorac Surg. 1996;10:1114–9.

Culbert E, Ashburn D, Cullen-Dean G, et al. Quality of life of children after repair of transposition of the great arteries. Circulation. 2003;108:857–62.

Cuypers J, Eindhoven J, Slager M, et al. The natural and unnatural history of the Mustard procedure: long-term outcome up to 40 years. Eur Heart J. 2014;35:1666–74.

De T. Near-infrared spectroscopy correlates with continuous superior vena cava oxygen saturation in pediatric cardiac surgery patients. Paediatr Anaesth. 2008;18:1163–9.

De La Cruz D, Da Rocha J. An onto-genetic theory for the explanation of congenital malformations involving the truncus and conus. Am Heart J. 1956;51:782.

De Leval M, Basto P, Stark J, et al. Surgical technique to reduce the risks of heart block following closure of ventricular septal defect in atrioventricular discordance. J Thorac Cardiovasc Surg. 1979;78:515–26.

Dearani J, Danielson G, Puga F, Mair D, Schleck C. Late results of the Rastelli operation for transposition of the great arteries. Semin Thorac Cardiovasc Surg Pediatr Card Surg. 2001;4:3–15.

Dibardino D, Allison A, et al. Current expectations for newborns undergoing the arterial switch operation. Ann Surg. 2004;239(5):588–98.

el-Said G, Rosenberg HS, et al. Dysrhythmias after mustard's operation for transposition of the great arteries. Am J Cardiol. 1972;30:526–32.

Emani S, Beroukhim R, Zurakowski D, et al. Outcomes after anatomic repair for D-transposition of the great arteries with left ventricular outflow tract obstruction. Circulation. 2009;120 suppl 1:S53–8.

Ewer A, Middleton L, Furmston A, et al. Pulse oximetry screening for congenital heart defects in newborn infants (pulse ox): a test accuracy study. Lancet. 2011;378(9793):785–94.

Ewer A, Furmston A, Middleton L, et al. Pulse oximetry as a screening test for congenital heart defects in newborn infants: a test accuracy study with evaluation of acceptability and cost-effectiveness. Health Technol Assess. 2012;16:2.

Falcao G, Ulate K, et al. Impact of postoperative hyperglycemia following surgical repair of congenital cardiac defects. Pediatr Cardiol. 2008;29(3):628–36.

Farre J. On malformations of the human heart. London: Longman, Hurst, Rees, Orme, and Brown; 1814.

Ferencz C, Brenner J, Loffredo C, Kappetein A, Wilson P. Transposition of great arteries: etiologic distinctions of out-flow tract defects in a case-control study of risk factors. In: Clark EB,

Markwald RD, Takao A, editors. Developmental mechanism of heart disease. Armonk: Futura Publishing; 1995. p. 639–53.

Ferencz C, Loffredo CA, Correa- Villasenor A, Wilson PD. Genetic and environmental risk factors of major cardiovascular malformations: the Baltimore-Washington Infant Study, 1981–89. In: Ferencz C, Loffredo CA, Correa-Villasenor A, Wilson P, editors. Perspectives in pediatric cardiology, vol. 5. 1st ed. Armonk: Futura Publishing Co. Inc; 1997. p. 867–8.

Freedom R. Congenitally corrected transposition of the great arteries: definitions and pathologic anatomy. Prog Pediat Cardiol. 1999;10(1):3–16.

Gaies M, Goldberg C, Ohye R, Devaney E, Hirsch J, Bove E. Early and intermediate outcome after anatomic repair of congenitally corrected transposition of the great arteries. Ann Thorac Surg. 2009;88:1952–60.

Gladman G, Casey F, Adatia I. Supravalvular stenosing tricuspid ring in congenitally corrected transposition. Cardiol Young. 1996;6:174–6.

Goor D, Edwards J. The spectrum of transposition of the great arteries with specific reference to developmental anatomy of the conus. Circulation. 1973;48(2):406–15.

Hermann V, Laks H, Kaiser G, et al. The Blalock-Hanlon procedure. Simple transposition of the great arteries. Arch Surg. 1975;110(11):1387–90.

Hirsch J, Gurney J, et al. Hospital mortality for Norwood and arterial switch operations as a function of institutional volume. Pediatr Cardiol. 2008;29(4):713–7.

Hoffman J, Kaplan S. The incidence of congenital heart disease. J Am Coll Cardiol. 2002;39:1890–900.

Houyel L, Van Praagh R, Lacour-Gayet F, et al. Transposition of the great arteries (20122012) pathologic anatomy, diagnosis, and surgical management of a newly recognized complex. J Thorac Cardiovasc Surg. 1995;110:613–24.

Huhta J, Maloney J, Ritter D, Ilstrup D, Feldt R. Complete atrioventricular block in patients with atrioventricular discordance. Circulation. 1983;183:1374.

Jaggers J, Cameron D, Herlong JR, Ungerleider R. Congenital heart surgery nomenclature and database project: transposition of the great arteries. Ann Thorac Surg. 2000;69:S205–35.

Jahangiri M, Redington A, Elliott M, Stark J, Tsang V, de Leval M. A case for anatomic correction in atrioventricular discordance? Effects of surgery on tricuspid valve function. J Thorac Cardiovasc Surg. 2001;121:1040–5.

Jones C. Perioperative uses of dexmedetomidine. Int Anesthesiol Clin. 2013;51(2):81–96.

Karl TR. The role of the Fontan operation in the treatment of congenitally corrected transposition of the great arteries. Ann Pediatr Cardiol. 2011;4:103–10.

Kreeger R, Ramamoorthy C, Nicolson S, et al. Evaluation of pediatric near-infrared cerebral oximeter for cardiac disease. Anna Thoracic Surg. 2012;94(5):1527–33.

Leibman J, Cullum L, et al. Natural history of transposition of the great arteries. Anatomy and birth and death characteristics. Circulation. 1969;40:237–62.

Lillehei CW, Varco RL. Certain physiological, pathological and surgical features of complete transposition of the great vessels. Surgery. 1953;34(3):376–400.

Mair D, Ritter D, Ongley P, Helmholz H. Hemodynamics and evaluation for surgery of patients with complete transposition of the great arteries and ventricular septal defect. Am J Cardiol. 1971;28:632–40.

Mandell V, Lock J, Parness I, Kulick T. The "laid-back" aortogram: an improved angiographic view for demonstration of coronary arteries in trans- position of the great arteries. Am J Cardiol. 1990;65(20):1379–83.

Marino B. Patterns of congenital heart disease and associated cardiac anomalies in children with Down syndrome. In: Marino B, Pueschel S, editors. Heart disease in persons with Down Syndrome. Baltimore: Paul H Brookes Publishing; 1996. p. 133–40.

Marino B, Digilio M, Versacci P, Anaclerio S, Dallapiccola B. Transposition of great arteries. Understanding its pathogenesis. Ital Heart J Supp. 2002;2:154–60.

Martin R, Qureshi S, et al. An evaluation of right and left ventricular function after anatomical correction and intra-atrial repair operations for complete transposition of the great arteries. Circulation. 1990;82:808–16.

McQuillen P, Hamrick S, et al. Balloon atrial septostomy is associated with preoperative stroke in neonates with transposition of the great arteries. Circulation. 2006;113(2):280–5.

Melchionda S, Digilio M, Mingarelli R, Novelli G, Scambler P, Marino B, et al. Transposition of the great arteries associated with deletion of chromosome 22q11. Am J Cardiol. 1995; 75(1):95–8.

Morell V, Jacobs J, Quintessenza J. Aortic translocation in the management of transposition of the great arteries with ventricular septal defect and pulmonary stenosis: results and follow-up. Ann Thorac Surg. 2005;79:2089–93.

Mustard WT, Keith JD, Trusler GA, Fowler R, Kidd L. The surgical management of transposition of the great vessels. J Thorac Cadiovasc Surg. 1964;48:953–8.

Newfeld E, Paul M, et al. Pulmonary vascular disease in complete transposition of the great arteries: a study of 200 patients. Am J Cardiol. 1974;34(1):75–82.

Nikaidoh H. Aortic translocation and biventricular outflow tract reconstruction. A new surgical repair for transposition of the great arteries associated with ventricular septal defect and pulmonary stenosis. J Thorac Cardiovasc Surg. 1984;88:365.

Obayah E. The use of dexmedetomidine in pediatric cardiac surgery. Blood. 2006;103(1):52–6.

Peterson R, Franch R, Fajman W, Jones R. Comparison of cardiac function in surgically corrected and congenitally corrected transposition of the great arteries. J Thorac Cardiovasc Surg. 1988;96:227–39.

Petit C, Rome J, et al. Preoperative brain injury in transposition of the great arteries is associated with oxygenation and time of surgery, not balloon atrial septostomy. Circulation. 2009;119(5): 709–16.

Presbitero P, Somerville J, Rabajoli F, Stone S, Conte M. Corrected transposition of the great arteries without associated defects in adult patients: clinical profile and follow up. Br Heart J. 1995;74:57–9.

Quaegebeur JM, Rohmer J, Brom AG. Revival of the senning operation in the treatment of transposition of the great arteries. Thorax. 1977;32:517–24.

Quinn D, McGuirk S, Metha C, et al. The morphologic left ventricle that requires training by means of pulmonary artery banding before the double-switch procedure for congenitally corrected transposition of the great arteries is at risk of late dysfunction. JTCVS. 2008;135(5):1137–44.

Ranucci M, Isgrò G, Carlucci C, De La Torre T, Enginoli S, Frigiola A. Central venous oxygen saturation and blood lactate levels during cardiopulmonary bypass are associated with outcome after pediatric cardiac surgery. Crit Care. 2010;14(4):R149.

Rashkind WJ, Miller WW. Creation of an atrial septal defect without thoracotomy. A palliative approach to complete transposition of the great arteries. JAMA. 1966;196:991.

Rasiah S, Publicover M, et al. A systematic review of the accuracy of first-trimester ultrasound examination for detecting major congenital heart disease. Ultrasound Obstet Gynecol. 2006;28(1):110–6.

Rodefeld MD, Ruzmetov M, Vijay P, Fiore AC, Turrentine MW, Brown JW. Surgical results of arterial switch operation for Taussig-Bing anomaly: is position of the great arteries a risk factor? Ann Thorac Surg. 2007;83(4):1451–7.

Roofthooft M, Bergman K, et al. Persistent pulmonary hypertension of the newborn with transposition of the great arteries. Ann Thorac Surg. 2007;83:1446–50.

Rudra H, Mavroudis C, et al. The arterial switch operation: 25-year experience with 258 patients. Ann Thorac Surg. 2011;92(5):1742–6.

Ruys T, van der Bosch A, Cuypers J, et al. Long-term outcome and quality of life after arterial switch operation: a prospective study with a historical comparison. Congenit Heart Dis. 2013;8(3):203–10.

Samànek M. Congenital heart malformations: prevalence, severity, survival, and quality of life. Cardiol Young. 2000;10:179–85.

Sano T, Riesenfield T, Karl TR, et al. Intermediate term outcome after intracardiac repair of associated cardiac defects in patients with atrioventricular and ventriculoarterial discordance. Circulation. 1995;92:II-272.

Scohy T, Golab H, Egal M, Takkenberg J, Bogers A. Intraoperative glycemic control without insulin infusion during pediatric cardiac surgery for congenital heart disease. Paediatr Anaesth. 2011;21(8):872–9.

Senning A. Surgical correction of transposition of the great vessels. Surgery. 1959;45:966–80.

Van Mierop L, Kutsche L. Cardiovascular anomalies in DiGeorge syndrome and importance of neural crest as a possible pathogenetic factor. Am J Cardiol. 1986;58:133–8.

Van Praagh R. Diagnosis of complex congenital heart disease: morphologic-anatomic method and terminology. Cardiovasc Intervent Radiol. 1984;7:115–20.

Van Praagh R, Weinberg P, et al. The transposition complexes, how many are there? Henry Ford Hospital International Symposium on Cardiac Surgery. East Norwalk/Conn: Appleton & Lange; 1975. p. 207–13.

Voskuil M, Hazenkamp M, Kroft L, et al. Postsurgical course for patients with congenitally corrected transposition of the great arteries. J Am Coll Cardiol. 1999;83:558.

Wallis G, Debich-Spicer D, Anderson R. Congenitally corrected transposition. Orphanet J Rare Dis. 2011;6:22.

Weiss M, Dullenkopf A, Kolarova A, et al. Near-infrared spectroscopic cerebral oxygenation reading in neonates and infants is associated with central venous oxygen saturation. Pediatric Anesth. 2005;15(2):102–9.

Williams W, McCrindle B, Ashburn D, Jonas R, Mavroudis C, Blackstone E. Outcomes of 829 neonates with complete transposition of the great arteries 12-17 years after repair. Eur J Cardiothorac Surg. 2003;24:1–10.

Winlaw D, McGuirk S, Balmer C, et al. Intention-to- treat analysis of pulmonary artery banding in conditions with a morphological right ventricle in the systemic circulation with a view to anatomic biventricular repair. Circulation. 2005;111:405–11.

Yacoub M, Radley-Smith R. Anatomy of the coronary arteries in transposition of the great arteries and methods for their transfer in anatomic correction. Thorax. 1978;33:418–24.

Yeh Jr T, Ramaciotti C, Leonard SR, Roy L, Nikaidoh H. The aortic translocation (Nikaidoh) procedure: midterm results superior to the Rastelli procedure. J Thorac Cardiovasc Surg. 2007;133:461–9.

Chapter 21
Right-Sided Obstructive Lesions

Robert Wong and Lorraine Lubin

Tetralogy of Fallot

Introduction

Tetralogy of Fallot (TOF) is one of the most common cyanotic cardiac defects, accounting for about 3–5 % of all congenital cardiac disease, with an estimated incidence of 0.2–0.8 per 100 live births (Apitz et al. 2009). Niels Stensen first described it in 1671 with its physiology refined later by Etienne-Louis Fallot in 1888. In 1924, Maude Abbott coined the term tetralogy of Fallot based on the four classic lesions that make up the disease

1. Ventricular septal defect (VSD)
2. Right ventricular outflow tract (RVOT) obstruction
3. Overriding aorta
4. Right ventricular hypertrophy (Stensen 1671–1672)

Today we know that TOF is a family of disease with similar intracardiac anatomy that can be highly variable in terms of pulmonary artery, RVOT, and pulmonary valve anatomy. Due to its involvement with pulmonary artery and valve and the

R. Wong, MD
Cedars Sinai Medical Center, Department of Anesthesiology,
8700 Beverly Blvd, Rm 4209, West Hollywood, CA 90048, USA

Cedars Sinai Medical Center, Department of Anesthesiology, Los Angeles, CA 90048, USA
e-mail: robert.wong@cshs.org

L. Lubin, MD (✉)
Director, Congenital Cardiac Anesthesiology, Operative Transesophageal Echocardiography,
Cedars Sinai Medical Center, Department of Anesthesiology,
8700 Beverly Blvd, Suite 8211, Los Angeles, CA 90048, USA
e-mail: Lorraine.Lubin@cshs.org

© Springer International Publishing Switzerland 2017
A. Dabbagh et al. (eds.), *Congenital Heart Disease in Pediatric and Adult Patients*, DOI 10.1007/978-3-319-44691-2_21

RVOT, it is discussed here in brief; a full discussion is presented in Chap. 19, Tetralogy of Fallot.

TOF is also commonly associated with other cardiac anomalies such as anomalous coronary arteries, right aortic arch, and atrioventricular valve defects.

Although the exact cause of the disease is still unknown, recent studies have shown certain genetic predisposition to the disease. In one study of patients with TOF, 25 % were found to have microdeletion of q11 region in chromosome 22. TOF is also commonly found in patients with 22q11 deletions such as in Di George syndrome and velocardiofacial syndrome. In those without any overt syndromes, the prevalence of deletions has been estimated at 6 % (Apitz et al. 2009).

Anatomy

The physiology of TOF is largely dependent on the severity of the right outflow tract obstruction. The ventricular defect found in TOF is usually large with unrestricted flow between the two ventricular chambers. As a result of this, right ventricular pressure is reflective of left ventricular pressure, and blood flow across the septal defect follows the path of least resistance. If the right outflow tract obstruction is higher than the resistance of blood going through the aorta, then blood flow will preferentially shunt right to left resulting in decreased pulmonary blood flow and desaturated blood entering the systemic circulation resulting in cyanosis. If left ventricular pressure is higher than right ventricular pressure, then blood flow will preferentially shunt left to right with saturated blood diverted away from the systemic circulation and into the pulmonary vasculature resulting in decreased cardiac output.

Presentation

Clinical presentation can vary depending on severity of anatomical right outflow tract obstruction and degree of shunting across the septal defect. Newborn with severe right outflow obstruction will present with cyanosis secondary to decreased pulmonary blood flow and increased mixing of desaturated blood. Those with moderate to mild right outflow obstruction are usually asymptomatic unless agitated in which cyanosis can ensue. Many with mild obstruction are diagnosed incidentally with auscultation of a harsh systolic murmur on exam. Those with mild obstruction can have pulmonary overcirculation and develop heart failure. Although most TOF are symptomatic and cyanotic to a certain degree, there are some who remain well saturated without any cyanosis for a period of time (pink tets).

Majority are asymptomatic when comfortable and at rest. However agitation and crying can worsen the right outflow tract obstruction resulting in cyanosis best seen in the lips and nail beds. As mentioned before a systolic murmur is usually present from the right outflow tract obstruction. Classically, it is described as a crescendo-decrescendo murmur heard best at the left mid-upper sternal border. As RVOT obstruction increases, so does the flow across the septal defect and the turbulent flow through the RVOT and the severity of the murmur. During severe "tet spells" when all blood is diverted across the septal defect, the systolic murmur may become absent.

Physical exam along with EKG and chest X-ray can be used for diagnosis, but echocardiography is used to confirm the disease. EKG will usually demonstrate signs of right axis deviation from increased right ventricular pressure, while chest X-ray may demonstrate the classic boot-shaped heart secondary to right ventricular hypertrophy. Using 2-D echocardiography, multiple components of TOF can be evaluated for preparation of surgical correction. The location and number of VSD should be noted. Both the degree of aortic override and extent of the septal defect can be evaluated via the parasternal and apical view. As mentioned before, the degree of right outflow tract obstruction can vary with location and severity and must be delineated prior to surgical correction. The parasternal short axis and subcostal coronal and sagittal views are best used to evaluate the pulmonary valve and right outflow tract. The pulmonary annulus should be assessed to determine if a transannular patch is needed during surgical correction. The pulmonary artery along with its branches should also be evaluated in the parasternal short axis, looking at size and anatomy. The coronary arteries should also be assessed with the parasternal short axis and long axis view looking for aberrant anatomy, specifically where the left anterior descending coronary originates from. This is important because anterior crossing coronary vessels may complicate surgical repair of right outflow tract obstruction. The aorta should also be assessed using the parasternal notch short and long axis view looking for anatomy and potential aortopulmonary collaterals and a PDA. Echocardiography can also be used to assess the degree of outflow tract obstruction by assessing blood flow via color Doppler and gradient calculation using the modified Bernoulli equation.

Treatment

Surgical repair of TOF usually occurs within the first year of life, usually before 6 months of age. It can be staged if the infant is too small to tolerate cardiopulmonary bypass, and time is needed for the infant to grow or completely repaired shortly after birth. Early repair for appropriate infants is currently the preferred route given the excellent outcomes. Studies have shown that minimizing right ventricular exposure to high pressure prevents irreversible remodeling of the right ventricle, specifically right ventricular hypertrophy and right ventricular failure (Al Habib et al. 2010). Goals of surgical repair are to relive the RVOT obstruction and separate the systemic circulation from the pulmonary circulation by closing off the VSD.

Most full infants undergo complete repair shortly after birth via an intra-atrial or intraventricular approach. Most prefer the intra-atrial approach so as to minimize scarring and injury to the ventricle, which can lead to impaired function and conduction abnormities postoperatively. Using either approach, the surgeon can relieve pulmonary stenosis, resect infundibular and subinfundibular muscle bundles, or create a transannular patch to open up the RVOT obstruction and patch up the VSD (Morales et al. 2009). In addition to minimizing damage to the ventricle, many surgeons attempt to maintain pulmonary valve competency by using a "valve sparring approach" whenever possible. This technique is applied to individuals with adequate pulmonary valve annulus size, as they do not need a transannular patch, unlike individuals with small or borderline annulus who usually require a transannular patch (Airan et al. 2006; Karamlou et al. 2006). Although a transannular patch opens up the RVOT obstruction, it also makes the pulmonary valve incompetent resulting in pulmonary insufficiency.

An alternative surgical approach is to create a valve conduit between the RV and the PA. Valve incompetency, regurgitation, and conduit stenosis are all complications that can occur overtime with a conduit.

Small and premature infants usually require a staged approach to correction due to high mortality associated with going on bypass. As a result they usually undergo a central shunt or BT shunt placed temporarily to provide an adequate source of pulmonary blood flow while they grow to an adequate size to tolerate a complete intracardiac repair on bypass. Once the child is of adequate size, the palliative pulmonary shunt is taken down, and the right outflow tract obstruction opened to allow for adequate pulmonary blood flow. At the same time, the VSD is closed off so to avoid shunting at the ventricular level.

Anesthetic Considerations

Anesthetic management of individuals with TOF should be to promote forward blood flow from the RV to the lungs and limiting right to left shunting of deoxygenated blood through the VSD. As mentioned before, the pathophysiology of TOF is decreased antegrade flow to the lungs secondary to the RVOT obstruction with shunting across the VSD resulting in cyanosis.

Depending on the severity of the obstruction, individuals may require supplemental oxygen therapy. Agitation to the infant should be avoided when possible as crying can increase pulmonary pressures and further decrease pulmonary perfusion and increase the amount of deoxygenated blood shunted systemically through the VSD. Premedication with oral midazolam (0.5 mg/kg) prior to inhalation induction can minimize the amount of stress and agitation and thus minimize "tet spells" that may result in severe cyanosis. Ketamine (1–4 mg/kg) and fentanyl can be used for induction if intravenous access is available. Adequate ventilation and oxygenation is important in these individuals as hypoxemia and hypercarbia can both increase pulmonary vascular resistance and result in overall increased right-sided pressures and obstruction. Tet spells with severe cyanosis benefit from Neo-Synephrine (5–10 mcg/kg) to increase the SVR. The alpha1 agonist results in direct vasoconstriction with increased left ventricle pressures, reversing the right to left shunt through the VSD and limiting deoxygenated blood into the systemic system. Another benefit of Neo-Synephrine is that it has no inotropic effects on the heart, which is beneficial as increased cardiac contractility and tachycardia can further impede pulmonary blood flow if the RVOT obstruction is dynamic such as in infundibular spasm. Increasing the depth of anesthesia with volatile agents can also be used for negative inotropic effects. Although this may help with infundibular spasm, it can also result in vasodilatation and drop in SVR, which can worsen shunting through the VSD. Volume infusion and maintaining adequate preload will help by increasing right heart filling pressure and increase overall blood pressure.

Arterial line should be placed opposite side of planned BT shunt if a stage procedure is being done, as the shunt can cause a steal effect resulting in an artificially lower blood pressure reading. Central line placement should be considered for volume replacement and vasoactive drug infusions post bypass.

Postoperatively, it is not uncommon to see decreased RV function or even RV failure as their RVs have been exposed to high pressures. This, coupled with injury to the ventricles during surgical repair, can result in less than optimal RV function immediately after surgery and may require vasoactive drugs such as epinephrine and milrinone (0.25–05 mcg/kg/min) for hemodynamic support. Abnormal conduction is also a common occurrence postoperatively given the close proximity of the conduction pathway to the VSD repair. As a result, atrioventricular pacing capability should be available to maintain AV synchrony, which will help with the RV function and cardiac output.

Congenital Pulmonic Valve Stenosis

Introduction

The incidence of congenital pulmonic stenosis is approximately 0.6–0.8 per 1000 live births and accounts for about 10 % of all congenital cardiac disease (Hoffman and Kaplan 2002). Pulmonic stenosis is defined as right ventricular tract obstruction at the level of the pulmonary valve. Where along the pulmonary valve, the obstruction occurs can vary.

Anatomy

Classically, the stenosis is at the valve with fusion of the valvular tissue around a fixed orifice resulting in a dome-shaped deformity. Koretzyk described a subset of pulmonary valve dysplasia where instead of the classic fused valves, the valves are not adherent to each other. Instead, obstruction occurs from (1) thickened leaflets rendering them rigid and immobile and (2) occurrence of tissue in the sinuses that restrict lateral movement of leaflets during systole. It is important to delineate between the two, as pulmonary valve dysplasia is associated with higher failure rates with balloon valvuloplasty compared to pulmonary valve stenosis and is commonly seen in Noonan's syndrome (Koretzky et al. 1969). Less common is subvalvular obstruction from fibromuscular narrowing below the pulmonary valve, which is associated with other congenital cardiac lesions such as TOF. Subvalvular lesions can be dynamic where increased contractility of the ventricle causes increase obstruction. Supravalvular stenosis can also occur with narrowing of the pulmonary artery above the pulmonary valve.

The underlying cause of pulmonic stenosis is unknown. During the fifth week of gestation, the conotruncus (bulbus cordis) divides into the ascending aorta and the main pulmonary artery. The pulmonary valve develops from the distal conotruncus, moving anterior and leftward of the aortic valve. Some have hypothesized that pulmonary stenosis occurs from maldevelopment of the distal conotruncus.

Presentation

Clinical presentation of congenital pulmonic stenosis can vary depending on the degree of stenosis. Those with trivial to mild pulmonary stenosis (gradient <40) are usually asymptomatic besides having a pulmonary ejection murmur at the second intercostal space. Multiple studies have shown those with mild pulmonic stenosis will usually have no progression of their disease and is generally considered benign (Drossner and Mahle 2008; Rowland et al. 1997).

Moderate pulmonary valve stenosis (gradient btw 40–60) can present with poor weight gain secondary to dyspnea and fatigue with feeding. Disease progression is somewhat variable with studies showing RVOT obstruction, decreased cardiac output, and increased right ventricular end-diastolic pressures later on in life (Hayes et al. 1993).

Those with severe stenosis (gradient >60) at birth can present with cyanosis from atrial shunting, heart failure from increased right ventricular end-diastolic pressure, and right ventricular hypertrophy and can lead to irreversible right ventricular dysfunction if not treated promptly (Krabill et al. 1985; Johnson 1962; Stone et al. 1974).

Critical pulmonic stenosis is the most severe with inadequate pulmonary blood flow through the RVOT. Because of this, it is paramount that the ductus arteriosus remains patent for pulmonary blood flow. Presentation is similar to severe pulmonic stenosis and if not treated in a timely manner may become life threatening (Freed et al. 1973).

Depending on the severity of the stenosis, patients may have enlarged right atrium and right ventricular hypertrophy manifesting radiographically as an enlarged cardiac silhouette and with right axis deviation on EKG.

Echocardiography is recommended to confirm the diagnosis of pulmonic stenosis given the relative ease at which the pulmonary valve and right heart can be visualized through transthoracic echocardiogram. Besides visualizing the amount of blood flow across the pulmonic valve, continuous wave Doppler can be used to estimate the gradient across the valve. A transvalvular gradient of <40 mmHg is considered mild stenosis, 40–60 mmHg moderate stenosis, and >60 mmHg severe stenosis.

Treatment

Balloon valvuloplasty is the first-line treatment for pulmonic stenosis confined to the valvular level. Those with critical pulmonic stenosis may require balloon valvuloplasty shortly after birth, whereas those with mild to moderate stenosis may have the valvuloplasty done electively at a later date with observation first. Balloon valvuloplasty is done through percutaneous access via the femoral vein, where a wire is advanced through the pulmonary valve. Once in position, a balloon is placed through the pulmonic valve and inflated to dilate the stenotic valve. It is not uncommon to see pulmonary regurgitation post balloon therapy. The amount of regurgitation can be limited by optimizing balloon size (Rao 2007). Right ventricular enlargement can develop overtime from the regurgitant flow. Currently there is no consensus regarding the timing of pulmonary valve replacement in those with severe pulmonary regurgitation post balloon valvuloplasty.

Those with typical pulmonic stenosis have excellent outcomes with balloon valvuloplasty with majority having gradients less than 20 mmHg post intervention. Potential complications with balloon valvuloplasty include perforation of the pulmonary valve, right ventricle, pulmonary artery, and damage to tricuspid valve resulting in regurgitant flow (Rao 2007; Stanger et al. 1990). Balloon valvuloplasty can also be used to treat dysplastic pulmonary valves, although outcomes are less favorable when compared to dome-shaped pulmonic stenosis and surgical correction may be required (Stanger et al. 1990; Tabatabaei et al. 1996).

Surgical repair is usually needed for dysplastic, supravalvular, and subvalvular pulmonary stenosis. With dysplastic pulmonary valve, surgical excision of the thickened leaflets and sometimes a transannular patch are needed to relive the obstructive lesion. Surgical correction is also recommended for supravalvular lesions due to the close proximity to the pulmonary artery, and most will require a transannular patch. Subvalvular lesions usually have a muscular component to the obstruction making balloon valvuloplasty an ineffective treatment option.

Anesthetic Considerations

The anesthetic goal for individuals with pulmonic stenosis is to promote forward blood flow from the RV to the pulmonary artery and to ensure adequate pulmonary perfusion. Individuals with severe stenosis and cyanosis may require supplemental oxygenation and prostaglandin therapy to ensure adequate oxygenation. For surgical repairs, arterial line should be placed for close blood pressure monitoring. Central access should be obtained for volume replacement and vasoactive drug infusion. Depending on the severity of the disease and preexisting RV function, inotropic support may be needed immediately after the surgical repair. Those with severe pulmonic stenosis may have dysfunctional RV and require inotropic agents such as milrinone (0.25–0.5 mcg/kg/min) and dobutamine (1–5 mcg/kg/min) to maintain cardiac output. Inotropic support should be used cautiously for individuals with subvalvular stenosis, as there is usually a dynamic component to the stenosis and the increased contractility and tachycardia can worsen the obstruction. Volume infusion and adequate preload can help with RV filling pressure and promote forward flow from the RV. However careful titration of volume should be considered for those with borderline RV function as too much preload can add additional stress to the ventricle and result in worsening function and decrease cardiac output. Adequate ventilation strategy is also important as hypercarbia and hypoxemia can both increase PVR and add additional strain to the already dysfunctional RV.

Pulmonary Atresia with Intact Ventricular Septum

Introduction

In pulmonary atresia with intact ventricular septum (PA/IVS), there is atresia of the pulmonary valve resulting in absent connection between the right ventricular outflow tract and the pulmonary artery. In addition, there is no communication between the two ventricles because of the intact septum and thus no way of mixing, making this a fatal structural cardiac defect unless surgically corrected.

PA/IVS accounts for approximately 3 % of all congenital cardiac defects with an estimated incidence of 4–8 per 100,000 live births (Hanley et al. 1993; Ekman Joelsson et al. 2001; Ashburn et al. 2004).Unlike pulmonary atresia with VSD, the cause of the PA/IVS is currently not known. There does not appear to be any associated genetic syndrome associated with the defect. There are hypotheses that it is an acquired defect in utero secondary to viral or inflammatory disease causing pulmonary valve atresia and abnormal fetal blood flow ultimately leading to PA/IVS (Kutsche and Van Mierop 1983).

Because of the wide range of anatomical defects found in PA/IVS, there is now a uniform reporting system defining PA/IVS as a congenital malformation with right ventricular outflow obstruction that is ductal dependent and can include pulmonary atresia, variable degree of tricuspid and right ventricular hypoplasia, and aberrant coronary anatomy (Lacour-Gayet 2000).

Anatomy

The pulmonary atresia in PA/IVS can be either muscular or membranous with majority being membranous. In membranous pulmonary atresia, the pulmonary valve annulus is small with fused leaflets resulting in RVOT obstruction. The right ventricle and infundibulum are usually well formed in membranous pulmonary atresia. Muscular pulmonary atresia occurs in about 25 % of PA/IVS and is associated with poor outcome secondary to severe right ventricular hypoplasia and anomalous coronary arteries (Dyamenahalli et al. 2004; Daubeney et al. 2002; Kipps et al. 2011). In muscular pulmonary atresia, the muscular infundibulum is obliterated resulting in complete obstruction of the RVOT.

The anatomy of the right ventricle in PA/IVS can vary widely from a dilated thin-walled ventricle to a severely hypoplastic hypertrophied ventricle. Normally the RV is divided into three parts or tripartite, the (1) inlet, (2) body, and (3) outlet. Those with a tripartite RV will allow for a biventricular repair, whereas bipartite or unipartite, with absent body and/or outlet, will need univentricular repair due to the inability to support full pulmonary blood flow (Dyamenahalli et al. 2004; Daubeney et al. 2002).

The tricuspid valve (TV) can also vary from small to dysplastic with stenotic or regurgitant flow. The size of the tricuspid valve has been found to correlate with the anatomy of the RV. A TV with a Z score of −4 will usually have a unipartite RV making biventricular repair unlikely, whereas a TV Z score of −2 to 0 is associated with a tripartite ventricle, making biventricular repair possible (Ashburn et al. 2004).

Coronary anatomy can also vary in PA/IVS from absent aortocoronary connection to stenosis and abnormal left to right coronary connections. Normally coronary perfusion is dependent on diastolic pressure and diastolic flow. However in PA/IVS, fistulae can form between the RV and coronary arteries. This combined with absent aortocoronary connections makes coronary perfusion dependent on retrograde flow from the RV during systole or right ventricle-dependent coronary circulation (RVDCC). Recognition of RVDCC is important to note as these patients are dependent on elevated RV pressures providing coronary perfusion via the fistulae between the RV and coronaries, and relieving the RVOT obstruction will decompress the right ventricle resulting in inadequate coronary perfusion, ischemia, infarction, and sudden cardiac death (Calder et al. 2007; Giglia et al. 1992). Because of this, it is important to delineate the anatomy of the RV, TV, and coronary circulation, as all three play a role in determining if the child will have a biventricular, 1½, or univentricular surgical repair.

Unlike PA/VSD, PA/IVS usually has normal anatomy distal to the pulmonary valve. Majority will have normal confluent branches coming off the main pulmonary artery with a left ductus supplying pulmonary blood flow. In some there are abnormal pulmonary artery with arterial connections between the aorta and pulmonary artery called major aortopulmonary collaterals (MAPCA).

In PA/IVS, there is RVOT obstruction from the pulmonary atresia and no blood flow from the RVOT to the pulmonary artery. Instead pulmonary blood flow depends on regurgitant flow into the right atrium where it can cross over to the left atrium via a patent foramen ovale and supply blood to the lungs via the ductus arteriosus. Because of this, all newborns with PA/IVS must have a patent ductus arteriosus in order to survive, as that is the only means of pulmonary blood flow. Those with PA/IVS will usually have a smaller PDA compared to normal infants due to decreased pulmonary blood flow through the ductus in utero. RV pressures in these patients are determined by the extent of RV egress. Those with severe tricuspid regurgitation may have normal RV pressures as blood flows freely back into the right atrium and is shunted to the left atrium via the patent foramen ovale. However in those with limited tricuspid regurgitation, RV pressure can become suprasystemic as the blood cannot move forward or backward. If RV sinusoids exist, blood can flow through these channels into the systemic circulation via the coronary circulation.

Presentation

Infants with PA/IVS will usually present with cyanosis secondary to right to left shunting at the atrial level and complete RVOT obstruction. Most neonates with PA/IVS will have normal fetal and birth history with tachypnea and hyperpnea during the newborn period. However if untreated, PA/IVS is ultimately fatal with approximately 50 % dying within 2 weeks and 85 % dying within 6 months (Leonard et al. 2000). As mentioned before, those with PA/IVS are dependent on a PDA for pulmonary blood supply and survival. Closure of the ductus arteriosus will lead to rapid deterioration including acidosis, hypoxia, cardiogenic shock, and ultimately death. There have been rare reports of PA/IVS surviving on aortopulmonary collaterals once the ductus arteritis closes off (McArthur et al. 1971). Depending on the anatomy, a variety of murmurs can be appreciated on auscultation. Those with severe tricuspid regurgitation will have a systolic murmur, while a continuous murmur might be heard secondary to the PDA. Similarly, chest X-ray in those with PA/IVS can be normal or have an enlarged cardiac silhouette if they have severe tricuspid regurgitation resulting in enlarged right atrium and ventricle. EKG will usually show left axis deviation secondary to absent or hypoplastic RV.

PA/IVS can be diagnosed via fetal ultrasound starting at the second trimester. Using the four-chamber view, one can look for an atretic pulmonary valve and hypoplastic tricuspid valve and right ventricle. Evaluating the anatomy of flow across the PDA can also help with diagnosing PA/IVS. In normal fetus, flow across the PDA is usually pulmonary to the aorta with the ductus in a horizontal position. However in PA/IVS the ductus is usually vertically oriented with flow across the PDA reversed, from aorta to pulmonary given the lack of communication between the RVOT and pulmonary artery (Sandor et al. 2002; Emmel et al. 2004).

Postnatally, diagnosis of PA/IVS is usually done with echocardiographic imaging and pulse wave Doppler showing atretic pulmonary valve and absent pulmonary blood flow. It is important to differentiate between PA/IVS and critical pulmonic stenosis as both can have similar findings echocardiographically. Besides diagnosis of PA/IVS, echocardiography can be used to evaluate the anatomy of these patients, which can vary widely as mentioned before. Right ventricle function and size should be measured as well as tricuspid annulus size as both play a role in determining the kind of surgical repair. Intracardiac mixing should also be assessed across the foramen ovale and ductus arteriosus to determine adequate pulmonary blood flow. Although angiography is the gold standard, as much of the coronary circulation and anatomy should be delineated by echocardiography to determine any aberrant coronary circulation and the possibility of sinusoids or fistulae between the RV and coronary circulation.

Cardiac catheterization is key in delineating coronary anatomy and circulation in PA/IVS. As mentioned before, PA/IVS is associated with an abnormal coronary circulation, from stenotic coronary vessels, anomalous or absent aortocoronary origins, and sinusoids and fistulae between the RV and coronary circulation. With cardiac catheterization, contrast is injected at the aorta to visualize the presence or absence of aortocoronary vessels and their individual intracardiac course. Contrast can also be injected into the RV to look for any communications between the RV and coronary circulation. It is essential to rule out RVDCC as decompression of the RV in these patients can lead to coronary steal, ischemia, infarction, and even death. In addition to the coronary anatomy, angiography can also be used to determine TV and RV size and morphology.

Treatment

Initial treatment of newborn with PA/IVS should be stabilization, ensuring adequate cardiopulmonary support. As pulmonary flow is supplied solely by the PDA, prostaglandin infusion is usually initiated to keep the PDA open. Supplemental oxygen and mechanical ventilation should be considered if there is marked cyanosis, hypoxia, or increased work of breathing. Inotropic support may also be needed for those with hypoperfusion and increasing metabolic acidosis. The amount of shunting across the atrial septum may also be inadequate due to a small PFO which will result in decreased cardiac output where by balloon atrial septostomy can be performed to increase mixing and the cardiac output. Almost all newborn with PA/IVS will have adequate shunting across the PFO as those with small or absent atrial communication usually undergo fetal demise.

There is currently no uniform approach to surgical repair in neonates with PA/IVS given the wide variety of anatomical difference found in the disease.

After initial stabilization, the focus should be on assessing the anatomy of the individual, including RV and TV size and coronary anatomy so as to decide on the appropriate surgical repair. Currently the surgical options include biventricular repair, palliative univentricular, or 1½ ventricular repair. Rarely cardiac transplantation is required when none of the three repairs are feasible. In biventricular repair, the pulmonary and system circulation are separated with two pumping ventricles providing blood flow to each. This usually requires a well-formed right ventricle and tricuspid valve without RVDCC to support adequate pulmonary blood flow. Univentricular repair is a palliative procedure where the pulmonary and systemic circulation is separated but with only one ventricle. The univentricular approach is reserved for those with small or hypoplastic RV that cannot provide adequate support for pulmonary blood flow. In the 1½ ventricle repair, the pulmonary and system circulation are separated with the left ventricle acting as the systemic pump and the right ventricle acting as the pulmonary pump partially. The 1½ ventricle repair is usually done when the RV or TV size is borderline and there is uncertainty regarding the RV's ability to support the entire pulmonary blood flow. As a result, a Glenn procedure is done where the RV only has to support half the pulmonary blood flow, whereas the other half from the SVC flows passively into the pulmonary artery. The benefit of this approach is that it preserves a two pumping ventricle system, and as the right ventricle is rehabilitated with improved size and function, it may eventually be able to support the entire pulmonary circulation. Cardiac transplantation is usually reserved for PA/IVS with aortocoronary atresia as they have extremely high mortality rates even with palliative repairs (Odim et al. 2006).

Anesthetic Considerations

Anesthetic goals and management for PA/IVS vary depending on the anatomy of the disease and the planned repair. Arterial line should be placed for close blood pressure monitoring and central access obtained for vasoactive drug infusion and volume replacement. Management of those undergoing a palliative shunt rests on balancing the pulmonary circulation with the systemic circulation. Ventilation should be aimed toward normocarbia and adequate oxygenation as hyperventilation can cause overcirculation of the pulmonary vasculature resulting in hypotension from a steal phenomenon from the systemic circulation.

Individuals undergoing a biventricular repair have hypertensive RV and can have RV dysfunction after surgical repair of the pulmonary atresia. Pulmonary hypertension is not uncommon postoperatively from the sudden increase in pulmonary blood flow to an unadjusted pulmonary vascular bed. Inotropic support along with adequate filling pressures is important in these patients in order to promote forward blood flow and to prevent collapse of the RV. Using nitric oxide to decrease the PVR and off-load the strained RV postoperatively can be beneficial in these patients. Mechanical ventilation strategy should be aimed toward lowering PVR and maintaining adequate oxygenation. Pulmonary edema from the acute increase in pulmonary flow postoperatively is also common and can cause difficulties in oxygenation. Because of this, care should be taken when considering early extubation for these patients even though mechanical positive ventilation can increase PVR and work against the dysfunctional RV.

Anesthetic goals of individuals undergoing the 1½ ventricle repair rest on adequate passive pulmonary blood flow and supporting forward blood flow from a partially unloaded RV. Maintaining adequate preload helps with passive pulmonary perfusion along with RV filling pressures for cardiac output. Ventilation strategy to prevent hypercarbia and hypoxemia should be employed to avoid increase in PVR and to promote passive pulmonary blood flow. Inotropic support may be needed to support RV dysfunction and the work of breathing. Early extubation if possible is preferred, as positive pressure mechanical ventilation increases intrathoracic pressure and can impede pulmonary blood flow.

Pulmonary Atresia with VSD

Introduction

Pulmonary atresia with VSD (PA/VSD) is a relatively rare congenital disease and is secondary to pulmonary atresia with a VSD and major aortopulmonary collateral arteries (MAPCA) supplying the pulmonary circulation. There is an estimated incidence of about 0.7 per 10,000 live births with approximately one-fifth of all TOF being PA/VSD variant (Malformations of the cardiac outflow tract in genetic and environmental risk factors of major cardiovascular malformations 1981). Just like TOF, there appears to be a genetic component to the disease with 22q11.2 deletion and 1q21.1 deletion both associated with PA/VSD (Carotti et al. 2010; van Engelen et al. 2010; Silversides et al. 2012).

Anatomy

Like TOF, PA/VSD consists of an anteriorly maligned ventral septal defect and overriding aorta, but instead of varying degree of RVOT obstruction, the pulmonary valve is atretic with complete obstruction of the RVOT. Like PA/IVS, the atretic pulmonary valve can be at the valvular level (membranous) or occur at the subpulmonary infundibulum (muscular). Because of the atretic pulmonary valve, there is no antegrade pulmonary blood flow from the RVOT during fetal growth, resulting in abnormal development of structures distal to the pulmonary valve such as small or atretic pulmonary artery and its branches. If a ductus arteriosus is present, pulmonary blood flow can originate from the ductus, resulting in confluent pulmonary arteries of varying size. If there is no ductus arteriosus, MAPCAs develop and provide pulmonary blood supply. MAPCAs originate from the splanchnic plexus in utero and eventually form tortuous connections between the aorta and various branches of the pulmonary artery (Liao et al. 1985). The number and size of the MAPCAs can vary with areas of stenosis commonly found more distally. The arborization patterns of the MAPCA are also variable and many times incomplete, leaving certain lung segments overperfused and others underperfused and becoming more narrow overtime. It is important to delineate the pulmonary artery anatomy and presence of MAPCAs in PA/VSD as they play an important role in determining management of the disease.

Presentation

Clinical presentation in those with PA/VSD can vary depending on the degree of intracardiac shunting and amount of pulmonary flow to the lungs. Those with a PDA will usually have some degree of cyanosis as most will lack any MAPCAs and are dependent on the PDA for pulmonary blood. These individuals require prostaglandins to keep their ductus open before their surgical treatment. Those without a ductus arteriosus will develop MAPCAs and depending on the amount of flow through the MAPCAs may be cyanotic or normally saturated. Those with small or restrictive MAPCAs will have insufficient pulmonary blood flow and present with cyanosis, whereas those with large and unrestricted MAPCAs will have normal saturations, but also overcirculation of the pulmonary vascular bed and left ventricle and over time developing pulmonary hypertension and heart failure.

PA/VSD can be diagnosed during the second trimester via fetal ultrasound, looking for pulmonary atresia in utero (Seale et al. 2009). Postnatally, the diagnosis of PA/VSD is confirmed with echocardiography. EKG is usually unremarkable with normal sinus rhythm with right axis deviation from right ventricular hypertrophy. Chest X-ray will show the characteristic boot-shaped heart from RV hypertrophy with hypoperfused lung fields if MAPCAs are restrictive or pulmonary edema if MAPCAs are unrestrictive. Echocardiography will show the typical anterior maligned VSD with an overriding aorta along with pulmonary atresia with no blood flow from the RV to the pulmonary artery. Presence of MAPCAs should also be sought out via continuous blood flow patterns. Because echocardiography will not be able to delineate all MAPCAs, cardiac catheterization and angiography are needed to investigate the entire pulmonary vasculature anatomy along with all supplying MAPCAs. MRA and CT angiography can be used to look at the pulmonary vasculature anatomy, but because it does not provide hemodynamic information and has less refined imaging, they are not routinely utilized (Lin et al. 2012).

With cardiac catheterization, diagnostic angiography can be used to look at all sources of pulmonary blood flow along with detailed images of the native pulmonary artery anatomy. In addition to identifying all MAPCAs supplying the pulmonary vasculature, it is important to note what lung segments are supplied by MAPCAs and/or native pulmonary artery and if any of the vessels are restrictive or stenotic. Furthermore, hemodynamic information can be obtained such as pressures and areas of stenosis in each MAPCA, along with pressures in the pulmonary vasculature. All of this information is important in an individual in PA/VSD when deciding how to surgically repair the disease.

Treatment

Initial treatment in neonates with PA/VSD should be to stabilize the patient ensuring adequate cardiopulmonary support. Given the complexity and spectrum of the disease, initial treatment can vary. For those with cyanosis, therapy should be aimed at increasing pulmonary blood flow. If a PDA exists, prostaglandin should be initiated to keep the ductus open to maintain pulmonary circulation. Supplemental oxygen may be needed if the ductus or MAPCAs are too restrictive and not providing adequate pulmonary blood flow resulting in marked cyanosis.

Those with pulmonary overcirculation from unrestricted MAPCAs will have normal oxygen saturations but will also have signs of pulmonary congestion and can lead to heart failure. Mechanical ventilation should be considered for those with pulmonary edema as they can tire out easily from the increased work of breathing. Diuretic therapy should be started to off-load the heart and treat the pulmonary edema.

After the patient is stabilized, the surgical correction can be planned. As mentioned above, PA/VSD can present with a spectrum of pulmonary artery anatomy and MAPCAs. Because of this, the surgical approach can vary depending on the individual's anatomy, but the goals are always to (1) relieve the RVOT obstruction so that adequate blood flow can occur between the RV and the lungs, (2) ensure that the pulmonary arteries are of adequate size either through reconstruction or rehabilitation of the vessels, (3) reattach the collaterals from the aorta to the pulmonary arteries (unifocalization), and (4) close the VSD.

Surgical repair should aim to lower RV pressures as studies have shown PA/VSD with elevated RV pressure postoperatively are associated with higher mortality (Kirklin et al. 1983). To achieve this, any RVOT obstruction is relived so that there is no impedance of flow from the RV to the PA. Total cross-sectional area of the pulmonary vasculature is maximized by recruiting as many lung segments as possible and correcting any stenotic vessels. It is also important to promote as much antegrade pulmonary blood flow so as to allow for continued growth of the hypoplastic pulmonary arteries.

In the best-case scenario where an individual has large collaterals with normal-caliber pulmonary vessels, a single-stage repair can be done where collaterals are unifocalized, the RVOT obstruction corrected, and the VSD closed off.

Unifocalization can be done as a staged approach if the pulmonary arteries are too small or if there are multiple segmental stenoses. For these individuals, a central shunt between the aorta and the hypoplastic pulmonary artery is created without unifocalization of the collaterals, to allow for maximal pulmonary artery growth. After 3–6 months, a cardiac catheterization is done to evaluate the growth and caliber of the pulmonary arteries to see if unifocalization is possible. If there is adequate pulmonary artery growth with low pulmonary pressures, unifocalization of the collaterals can occur with relief of the RVOT obstruction and repair of the VSD. The risks of undergoing unifocalization early on in life with small pulmonary arteries are thrombosed vessels, development of stenosis, and lack of collateral vessel growth (Liava'a et al. 2012; Fouilloux et al. 2012; D'udekem et al. 2005; Duncan et al. 2003). Individuals with small-caliber pulmonary arteries without severe segmental level stenosis can undergo collateral unifocalization in a single approach. Again a central shunt is created to promote pulmonary artery growth and development followed by collateral reanastomosis from the aorta to the native pulmonary arteries. However, the VSD and RVOT are left uncorrected until a later time when there is evidence that there is sufficient pulmonary artery growth and an adequate pulmonary vascular bed for the RV to supply the entire pulmonary blood flow. If the VSD is closed prior to creation of an adequate pulmonary vascular bed, RV dysfunction may ensue from increased pulmonary afterload, and without the VSD acting as a pop-off valve, it can lead to RV failure. Another option is to close the VSD, and if it appears that the RV cannot support the full pulmonary perfusion, a fenestration can be made at the VSD repair to off-load the RV. Once it is evident that the RV can support the full pulmonary circulation, the fenestration can be closed via transcatheter approach.

Anesthetic Considerations

As mentioned before, PA/VSD is essentially an extreme form of TOF, and thus anesthetic management is similar. Adequate ventilation should be used to decrease PVR and promote pulmonary perfusion. Major blood loss should be anticipated secondary to multiple suture lines from unifocalization of MAPCAs. Central access or large bore intravenous access should be available to replace volume loss along with arterial line for close hemodynamic monitoring.

RV dysfunction is not uncommon post CPB secondary to increased afterload from inadequate pulmonary vascular bed. Strategies to decrease PVR should be employed such as adequate ventilation and nitric oxide therapy, while inotropic support with milrinone, dobutamine, and epinephrine is used for inotropic support RV function. Patients with PA/VSD are not candidates for early extubation as unifocalization can result in lung reperfusion injury resulting in pulmonary edema, making ventilation and oxygenation difficult. Intrapulmonary bleeding from multiple vascular suture lines can also impede adequate ventilation. Frequent bronchial suctioning should be used with the support of PEEP to maintain adequate ventilation. Aggressive pain control should also be implemented to minimize systemic and pulmonary hypertension, which can cause bleeding from the multiple vascular suture line.

Ebstein's Anomaly

Introduction

Ebstein's anomaly is a rare congenital defect of the tricuspid valve and the right ventricle, with varying anatomic morphology. It accounts for less than 1 % of all congenital heart disease with an estimated incidence of 1 in 200,000 live births, affecting males and females equally (Lupo et al. 2011; Correa-Villaseñor et al. 1994). Studies have shown a heterogeneous genetic predisposition to the disease, while other studies have shown a correlation between lithium intake during pregnancy and Epstein's anomaly (Allan et al. 1982; Attenhofer Jost et al. 2007).

Anatomy

The tricuspid valve divides the right atrium from the right ventricle and normally consists of three leaflets (anterior, septal, and posterior) that are attached to the tricuspid valve annulus. In Ebstein's anomaly, the tricuspid leaflets are malformed secondary to failure to split during embryological development, with one or more leaflets attached to the right ventricle endocardium. The anterior leaflet is the largest of the three leaflets and usually remains attached to the tricuspid annulus, while the septal and posterior leaflets are usually absent or fused if present, with abnormal attachment to the right ventricle endocardium. This results in a dilated annulus with posterior downward displacement of the leaflets toward the RVOT creating a funnel-shaped tricuspid valve that is incompetent with varying degrees of regurgitation. In Ebstein's anomaly, the right ventricle is also divided into two chambers due to the abnormal attachment of the tricuspid valve onto the right ventricle endocardium. The proximal RV is known as the atrialized chamber due to apical displacement of the leaflets resulting in a continuous communication with the right atrium, while the distal chamber is the actual ventricle consisting of the trabecular and outlet portion of the RV.

Ebstein's anomaly is classified based on Carpentier's classification of the tricuspid valve, which provides important information about whether the tricuspid valve can be repaired or needs to be replaced. In type A, the true RV volume is adequate; type B, the anterior leaflet of the tricuspid valve moves freely with a large atrialized portion of the RV; type C, the anterior leaflet movement is severely restricted with possible RVOT obstruction; and type D, almost complete atrialization of the RV with some infundibulum present (Dearani and Danielson 2000). Another classification system is through echocardiographic description of the disease as mild, moderate, or severe, with descriptions of the amount of displacement of the valves and the degree of RV dilation (Allan et al. 1982). This method is not as descriptive and precise as Carpentier's classification but is much more simple.

Ebstein's anomaly has a high association with other cardiac defects such as bicuspid or atretic aortic valves, pulmonary atresia or hypoplastic pulmonary artery, subaortic stenosis, coarctation, mitral valve prolapse, accessory mitral valve tissue or muscle bands of the left ventricle, VSDs, and pulmonary stenosis.

Pathophysiology of Ebstein's anomaly is regurgitation of the blood flow through the tricuspid valve from the abnormal leaflets and functional impairment of the RV secondary to the partially atrialized RV. With the increased regurgitant flow and atrialized RV, the right atrium becomes enlarged overtime causing further increase a dilatation of the tricuspid valve annulus. With worsening regurgitant flow, the RV goes into failure, increasing right-sided pressures and resulting in interatrial shunt and cyanosis.

Presentation

Clinical presentation and symptoms can vary from asymptomatic to severe cyanosis and RV failure depending on the anatomic severity and age of onset of the disease and other coexisting cardiac defects. Newborns with severe forms of Ebstein's anomaly can present with cyanosis, cardiomegaly, and heart failure. Those with mild regurgitation and limited atrialization of the RV can present without any symptoms as a newborn and remain asymptomatic until late teens or well into adulthood. Once symptomatic, these individuals can have arrhythmias from the dilated right atrium and fatigue and cyanosis from the increased regurgitant flow and failing RV. Although rare, there have been cases of anatomical defect so severe that cardiomegaly, hydrops, and heart failure occur in utero leading to death.

Physical exam will vary depending on severity of disease. Newborns with severe forms of Ebstein's anomaly will present with severe cyanosis from increased right atrial pressures and interatrial shunting and signs of heart failure such as cardiomegaly and enlarged liver. Those with mild disease are usually asymptomatic and may present with only a systolic murmur with mid-diastolic murmur from the increased regurgitant flow across the tricuspid valve. Despite the severe regurgitant flow, V waves are often missing in jugular venous pulse secondary to the large right atrium absorbing the increased backflow volume. Chest X-ray can show a globular silhouette with normal or decreased pulmonary vascularity. EKG is usually abnormal in Ebstein's anomaly with most displaying a tall P wave from the enlarged right atrium along with a right bundle branch block. Ebstein's anomaly is also associated with AV conduction and arrhythmias secondary to AV node compression and abnormal central fibrous body formation. Although complete heart block is rare, it is estimated that up to 42 % can present with first-degree AV block (Attenjofer et al. 2005).

Diagnosis is usually with echocardiography, using the four-chamber view to evaluate the degree of apical displacement of the tricuspid valve along with the function of the right ventricle and any other intracardiac defects that might be present. The apical displacement of the septal leaflets of the tricuspid valve should be at least 8 mm/m^2 body surface area from the attachment of the anterior leaflet of the mitral valve. The individual tricuspid leaflets should be evaluated, looking for signs of failure of delamination and accessory attachments. The size of both the right atrium and right ventricle should be measured. The degree and location of the regurgitant flow and size of the annulus should be assessed for feasibility of a tricuspid valve repair versus replacement.

Treatment

Treatment of individuals with Ebstein's anomaly depends on the severity of the anatomical defect and its associated symptoms. Many with mild disease are asymptomatic and only require frequent follow-up with a cardiologist. Prostaglandin therapy should be started on newborns with severe cyanosis in order to maintain pulmonary perfusion via the ductus arteriosus. Nitric oxide may also be helpful in decreasing pulmonary pressures and promoting forward flow from the RV to the pulmonary vascular bed. Signs of heart failure should be treated with diuretics and digoxin. Individuals with Ebstein's anomaly are at high risk for thromboembolism, especially older patients with atrial fibrillation or unrepaired atrial shunts. It is recommended that these individuals undergo anticoagulation therapy (Warnes et al. 2008).

Surgical repair of Ebstein's anomaly should be delayed as long as possible due to the high mortality associated with surgical repair in the newborn period (Knott-Craig et al. 2007; Starnes et al. 1991). Surgery should be considered in adults with paradoxical emboli, signs of cyanosis, or signs of deteriorations from worsening heart failure such as cardiomegaly, decreased ventricular function, or progressive right ventricular dilatation. Presences of premature ventricular contractions or atrial tachyarrhythmia are also indications for surgical correction as they can be early indicators of increased stress on the right ventricle and are associated with higher surgical mortality (Attenjofer et al. 2005).

Surgical repair of Ebstein's anomaly in the neonate can vary depending on the severity of the anatomy and associated intracardiac defect. Biventricular repair is done when there is good delamination of the anterior valve with good mobility and adequate RV size and function. Single ventricle repair is reserved for those with a severely dysplastic anterior leaflet with small RV and pulmonary artery atresia. Those with good delamination of the anterior leaflet but with poor RV function or dilated RV can undergo 1 1/2 ventricle repair where a bidirectional cavalpulmonary shunt is created to decrease the systemic venous volume load on the RV. Whenever appropriate, valve repair is preferred over replacement given lower complications and mortality (Augustin et al. 1997; Vargas et al. 1998). Although there does not appear to be any difference in rate of reoperation with bioprosthetic valve versus mechanical valve, most will replace with a bioprosthetic valve given the high incidence of thrombosis with mechanical valve and the need for lifetime anticoagulation therapy with mechanical valve. The valve is usually placed in an interatrial position with possible complications including coronary compression and injury to the conduction tissue resulting in complete AV conduction block.

Anesthetic Considerations

Given the wide spectrum in presentation of Ebstein's anomaly, all individuals should have a complete assessment of the severity of their disease including symptoms such as exercise tolerance and presence of cyanosis. Those with cyanosis may require prostaglandin therapy to keep their PDA open for adequate pulmonary circulation. Individuals with Ebstein's will also benefit from decreased pulmonary vascular resistance. Nitric oxide can be used to lower PVR to promote pulmonary blood flow, along with adequate ventilation strategies to prevent hypercarbia and hypoxemia. Ketamine (1–4 mg/kg) or etomidate (0.2–0.3 mg/kg) can be used for intravenous induction. Those without intravenous access can be induced via a smooth inhalation induction with oral versed (0.5 mg/kg) for anxiolysis to minimize agitation as crying can increase PVR and worsen cyanosis. Arterial line should be placed for close blood pressure monitoring. If undergoing a single ventricle repair, the arterial line should be placed opposite side of the planned shunt placement. Central access should also be considered for vasoactive drug infusions and volume replacement both intraoperatively and postoperatively. Given the high risk for embolic events, all lines should be cleared of air bubbles, and filters should be placed in all intravenous lines. Depending on the severity of the disease, individuals may benefit from inotropic support postoperatively with milrinone (0.25–0.5 mcg/kg/min) or dobutamine (1–5 mcg/kg/min), especially those with preexisting RV dysfunction. Adequate preload may also help hemodynamically in those with poor functioning RV. Nitric oxide can also be beneficial in off-loading the right ventricle if dysfunction is present postoperatively. Dysrhythmias such as supraventricular tachycardia, functional rhythm, and AV block are common postoperatively given the proximity of the repair to the intracardiac conduction pathway, and temporary pacing wires should be considered.

References

Airan B, Choudhary SK, Kumar HV, et al. Total transatrial correction of tetralogy of Fallot: no outflow patch technique. Ann Thorac Surg. 2006;82:1316.

Al Habib HF, Jacobs JP, Mavroudis C, et al. Contemporary patterns of management of tetralogy of Fallot: data from the society of thoracic surgeons database. Ann Thorac Surg. 2010;90:813.

Allan LD, Desai G, Tynan MJ. Prenatal echocardiographic screening for Ebstein's anomaly for mothers on lithium therapy. Lancet. 1982;2:875.

Apitz C, Webb GD, Rdington AN. Lancet. 2009;374:1462–71.

Ashburn DA, Blackstone EH, Wells WJ, et al. Determinants of mortality and type of repair in neonates with pulmonary atresia and intact ventricular septum. J Thorac Cardiovasc Surg. 2004;127:1000.

Attenhofer Jost CH, Connolly HM, Dearani JA, et al. Ebstein's anomaly. Circulation. 2007;115:277.

Attenjofer CH, Connolly HM, Edwards WD, Hayes D, Warnes CA, Danielson GK. Ebstein's anomaly-review of a multifaceted congenital cardiac condition. Swiss Med Wkly. 2005;135:269–81.

Augustin N, Schmidt-Habelmann P, Wottke M, et al. Results after surgical repair of Ebstein's anomaly. Ann Thorac Surg. 1997;63:1650.

Calder AL, Peebles CR, Occleshaw CJ. The prevalence of coronary arterial abnormalities in pulmonary atresia with intact ventricular septum and their influence on surgical results. Cardiol Young. 2007;17:387.

Carotti A, Albanese SB, Filippelli S, et al. Determinants of outcome after surgical treatment of pulmonary atresia with ventricular septal defect and major aortopulmonary collateral arteries. J Thorac Cardiovasc Surg. 2010;140:1092.

Correa-Villaseñor A, Ferencz C, Neill CA, et al. Ebstein's malformation of the tricuspid valve: genetic and environmental factors. The Baltimore-Washington Infant Study Group. Teratol. 1994;50:137.

D'udekem Y, Alphonso N, Nogaard MA, Cochrane AD, Grigg LE, Wilkinson JL, Brizard CP. Pulmonary atresia with ventricular septal defects and major aortopulmonary collateral arteries: unifocalization brings no long-term benefits. J Thorac Cardiovasc Surg. 2005;130:1496–502.

Daubeney PE, Delany DJ, Anderson RH, et al. Pulmonary atresia with intact ventricular septum: range of morphology in a population-based study. J Am Coll Cardiol. 2002;39:1670.

Dearani JA, Danielson GK. Congenital heart surgery nomenclature and database project: Ebstein's anomaly and tricuspid valve disease. Ann Thorac Surg. 2000;69:S106.

Drossner DM, Mahle WT. A management strategy for mild valvar pulmonary stenosis. Pediatr Cardiol. 2008;29:649.

Duncan BW, Mee RBB, Prieto LR, Rosenthal GL, Mesia CI, Qureshi A, Tucker OP, Rhodes JF, Latson LA. Staged repair of tetralogy of Fallot with pulmonary atresia and major aortopulmonary collateral arteries. J Thorac Cardiovasc Surg. 2003;126:694–702.

Dyamenahalli U, McCrindle BW, McDonald C, et al. Pulmonary atresia with intact ventricular septum: management of, and outcomes for, a cohort of 210 consecutive patients. Cardiol Young. 2004;14:299.

Ekman Joelsson BM, Sunnegårdh J, Hanseus K, et al. The outcome of children born with pulmonary atresia and intact ventricular septum in Sweden from 1980 to 1999. Scand Cardiovasc J. 2001;35:192.

Emmel M, Bald R, Brockmeier K. Pulmonary atresia with intact ventricular septum and right coronary artery to right ventricle fistula detected in utero. Heart. 2004;90:94.

Fouilloux V, Bonello B, Kammache I, Fraisse A, Mace L, Kreitmann B. Management of patients with pulmonary atresia, ventricular septal defect, hypoplastic pulmonary arteries and major aorto-pulmonary collaterals: focus on the strategy of rehabilitation of the native pulmonary arteries. Archives Cardiovascular Dis. 2012;105:666–75.

Freed MD, Rosenthal A, Bernhard WF, et al. Critical pulmonary stenosis with a diminutive right ventricle in neonates. Circulation. 1973;48:875.

Giglia TM, Mandell VS, Connor AR, et al. Diagnosis and management of right ventricle-dependent coronary circulation in pulmonary atresia with intact ventricular septum. Circulation. 1992;86:1516.

Hanley FL, Sade RM, Blackstone EH, et al. Outcomes in neonatal pulmonary atresia with intact ventricular septum. A multiinstitutional study. J Thorac Cardiovasc Surg. 1993;105:406.

Hayes CJ, Gersony WM, Driscoll DJ, et al. Second natural history study of congenital heart defects. Results of treatment of patients with pulmonary valvar stenosis. Circulation. 1993;87:I28.

Hoffman JI, Kaplan S. The incidence of congenital heart disease. J Am Coll Cardiol. 2002;39:1890.

Johnson AM. Impaired exercise response and other residua of pulmonary stenosis after valvotomy. Br Heart J. 1962;24:375.

Karamlou T, McCrindle BW, Williams WG. Surgery insight: late complications following repair of tetralogy of Fallot and related surgical strategies for management. Nat Clin Pract Cardiovasc Med. 2006;3:611.

Kipps AK, Powell AJ, Levine JC. Muscular infundibular atresia is associated with coronary ostial atresia in pulmonary atresia with intact ventricular septum. Congenit Heart Dis. 2011;6:444.

Kirklin JW, Blackstone EH, Kirklin JK, et al. Surgical results and protocols in the spectrum of tetralogy of Fallot. Ann Surg. 1983;198:251.

Knott-Craig CJ, Goldberg SP, Overholt ED, et al. Repair of neonates and young infants with Ebstein's anomaly and related disorders. Ann Thorac Surg. 2007;84:587.

Koretzky ED, Mller JH, Korns ME, Schwartz CJ, Edwards JE. Congenital pulmonary stenosis resulting from dysplasia of valve. Circulation. 1969;40:43–53.

Krabill KA, Wang Y, Einzig S, Moller JH. Rest and exercise hemodynamics in pulmonary stenosis: comparison of children and adults. Am J Cardiol. 1985;56:360.

Kutsche LM, Van Mierop LH. Pulmonary atresia with and without ventricular septal defect: a different etiology and pathogenesis for the atresia in the 2 types? Am J Cardiol. 1983;51:932.

Lacour-Gayet F. Congenital heart surgery nomenclature and database project: right ventricular outflow tract obstruction-intact ventricular septum. Ann Thorac Surg. 2000;69:S83.

Leonard H, Derrick G, O'Sullivan J, Wren C. Natural and unnatural history of pulmonary atresia. Heart. 2000;84:499.

Liao PK, Edwards WD, Julsrud PR, et al. Pulmonary blood supply in patients with pulmonary atresia and ventricular septal defect. J Am Call Cardiol. 1985;6:13–43.

Liava'a M, Brizard CP, Konstantinov IE, Robertson T, Cheung MM, Weintraub R, d'Udekem Y. Pulmonary atresia, ventricular septal defect, and major aortopulmonary collaterals: neonatal pulmonary artery rehabilitation without unifocalization. Ann Thorac Surg. 2012;93:185–92.

Lin MT, Wang JK, Chen YS, et al. Detection of pulmonary arterial morphology in tetralogy of Fallot with pulmonary atresia by computed tomography: 12 years of experience. Eur J Pediatr. 2012;171:579.

Lupo PJ, Langlois PH, Mitchell LE. Epidemiology of Ebstein anomaly: prevalence and patterns in Texas, 1999–2005. Am J Med Genet A. 2011;155A:1007.

Malformations of the cardiac outflow tract in genetic and environmental risk factors of major cardiovascular malformations. In: Ferencz CLC, Correa-Villasenor A, et al, editors. The Baltimore-Washington Infant Study 1981–1989. Armonk: Futura Publishing; 1997.

McArthur JD, Munsi SC, Sukumar IP, Cherian G. Pulmonary valve atresia with intact ventricular septum. Report of a case with long survival and pulmonary blood supply from an anomalous coronary artery. Circulation. 1971;44:740.

Morales D, Zara F, Fraser C. Tetralogy of Fallot repair: the right ventricle infundibulum sparing (RVIS) strategy. Semin Thorac Cardiovasc Surg Pediatr Card Surg Ann. 2009;12:54–5.

Odim J, Laks H, Tung T. Risk factors for early death and reoperation following biventricular repair of pulmonary atresia with intact ventricular septum. Eur J Cardiothorac Surg. 2006;29:659.

Rao PS. Percutaneous balloon pulmonary valvuloplasty: state of the art. Catheter Cardiovasc Interv. 2007;69:747.

Rowland DG, Hammill WW, Allen HD, Gutgesell HP. Natural course of isolated pulmonary valve stenosis in infants and children utilizing Doppler echocardiography. Am J Cardiol. 1997;79:344.

Sandor GG, Cook AC, Sharland GK, et al. Coronary arterial abnormalities in pulmonary atresia with intact ventricular septum diagnosed during fetal life. Cardiol Young. 2002;12:436.

Seale AN, Ho SY, Shinebourne EA, Carvalho JS. Prenatal identification of the pulmonary arterial supply in tetralogy of Fallot with pulmonary atresia. Cardiol Young. 2009;19:185.

Silversides CK, Lionel AC, Costain G, et al. Rare copy number variations in adults with tetralogy of Fallot implicate novel risk gene pathways. PLoS Genet. 2012;8:e1002843.

Stanger P, Cassidy SC, Girod DA, et al. Balloon pulmonary valvuloplasty: results of the valvuloplasty and angioplasty of congenital anomalies registry. Am J Cardiol. 1990;65:775.

Starnes VA, Pitlick PT, Bernstein D, et al. Ebstein's anomaly appearing in the neonate. A new surgical approach. J Thorac Cardiovasc Surg. 1991;101:1082.

Stensen N. Embrio monstro affinis parisiis dissectum. Acta Med Philos Hafniensa. 1671–1672;1:202–03.

Stone FM, Bessinger Jr FB, Lucas Jr RV, Moller JH. Pre- and postoperative rest and exercise hemodynamics in children with pulmonary stenosis. Circulation. 1974;49:1102.

Tabatabaei H, Boutin C, Nykanen DG, et al. Morphologic and hemodynamic consequences after percutaneous balloon valvotomy for neonatal pulmonary stenosis: medium-term follow-up. J Am Coll Cardiol. 1996;27:473.

van Engelen K, Topf A, Keavney BD, et al. 22q11.2 deletion syndrome is under-recognised in adult patients with tetralogy of Fallot and pulmonary atresia. Heart. 2010;96:621.

Vargas FJ, Mengo G, Granja MA, et al. Tricuspid annuloplasty and ventricular plication for Ebstein's malformation. Ann Thorac Surg. 1998;65:1755.

Warnes CA, Williams RG, Bashore TM, et al. ACC/AHA 2008 guidelines for the management of adults with congenital heart disease: a report of the American College of Cardiology/American Heart Association Task Force on Practice Guidelines (writing committee to develop guidelines on the management of adults with congenital heart disease). Circulation. 2008;118:e714.

Chapter 22
Congenital Mitral Valve Anomalies

Shahzad G. Raja and I. Gavin Wright

Introduction

Congenital anomalies of the mitral valve represent a broad spectrum of lesions that are often associated with other congenital heart anomalies. The reported incidence of congenital anomalies of the mitral valve in an echocardiographic study of 13,400 subjects was 0.5 % (Banerjee et al. 1995). These lesions affect valve function in a variable manner. When indicated, surgical intervention results in good long-term results (Hoashi et al. 2010; Lee et al. 2010; Serraf et al. 2000). In the last few years, enhanced knowledge of the functional as well as anatomical aspects of these lesions accompanied by concomitant significant advances in the diagnosis as well as anesthetic and surgical management has contributed to improved outcomes. This chapter provides an overview of the different congenital malformations that can affect the mitral valve excluding mitral valve anomalies in atrioventricular septal defects (AVSD) and univentricular hearts and focuses on the anesthetic and surgical management of these congenital mitral anomalies.

Embryology

The embryology of the mitral valve is complex and its knowledge is crucial for understanding the various anomalies that can affect it. Mitral valve formation begins during the fourth week of gestation. During the sixth week, fusion of the

S.G. Raja, BSc, MBBS (Hons.), MRCS, FRCS (C-Th) (✉)
Harefield Hospital, London, UK
e-mail: drrajashahzad@hotmail.com

I.G. Wright, MB ChB, FCA (SA)
Royal Brompton and Harefield NHS Foundation Trust, London, UK

© Springer International Publishing Switzerland 2017
A. Dabbagh et al. (eds.), *Congenital Heart Disease in Pediatric
and Adult Patients*, DOI 10.1007/978-3-319-44691-2_22

endocardial cushions partitions the atrioventricular canal into right and left atrioventricular junctions (Kanani et al. 2005). Failure of fusion of the superior and inferior cushions, presumably secondary to a deficiency of the vestibular spine, is responsible for producing atrioventricular septal defects. Normally, the lateral cushion forms the posterior mitral leaflet, while the anterior leaflet derives from the union of the left part of the superior and inferior cushions. During the eighth week, the shape of the mitral orifice looks like a crescent, the two ends of which are connected to compacting columns in the trabecular muscle of the left ventricle. These columns form a muscular ridge, the anterior and posterior parts of which become the papillary muscles (Oosthoek et al. 1998). The metamorphosis of the ridge into the papillary muscles implies a gradual loosening of muscle, which is called delamination. The abnormal compaction of the ventricular trabecular myocardium is responsible for producing mitral valve prolapse. Simultaneously, as for the tricuspid valve, the cushion tissue loses contact with the myocardium of the ridge, except at the insertion of the future tendinous cords. The very rare Ebstein's malformation of the mitral valve results from a failure of excavation of the posterior leaflet from the parietal ventricular wall. The chordae can be demarcated between the eleventh and thirteenth week of development by the appearance of defects in the cushion tissue at the place where the tips of the papillary muscles are attached to the leaflets. Both leaflets and chordae originate from the cushion tissue as verified by their similar immunohistochemical characteristics (Oosthoek et al. 1998). In contrast, papillary muscles are derived from the ventricular myocardium. A lack of evolution of the tendinous cords results in hammock or arcade mitral valve. The more severe anomaly of the leaflet is represented by the imperforate mitral valve. Finally, as each stage of this embryological development may be abnormal, the different malformations of the mitral valve can be either isolated or associated.

Classification of Congenital Mitral Valve Anomalies

The published literature to date reports seven classification systems of congenital mitral valve lesions (in the setting of concordant atrioventricular and ventricle-atrial connections with the exclusion of atrioventricular canal defects and hypoplastic left heart syndrome) that are outlined in Table 22.1.

Anatomical Classification Systems

Davachi and colleagues, in 1971, were one of the first to systematically assess and classify congenitally malformed mitral valves based on postmortem assessment (Davachi et al. 1971). They used a segmental classification according to whether the lesion affected the leaflets, commissures, tendinous chords, or papillary muscle arrangements. In 1977, Collins-Nakai et al. critiqued this segmental classification as

Table 22.1 Classification systems of congenital mitral valve anomalies

Author	Year	Basis of Classification	MV Lesions	Classification System
Davachi et al. (1971)	1971	Anatomical	MS and MR	Segmental classification of MR and (surgical + autopsy) MS based on predominant lesion: 1. Leaflet 2. Commissures 3. Chords 4. Papillary muscles
Carpentier et al. (1976), Chauvaud et al. (1998)	1976 1998[a]	Surgical Surgical	MS and MR MR only	Classification based on predominant Lesion: MR: Type 1: normal leaflet motion Type 2: leaflet prolapsed Type 3: restricted leaflet motion A: normal papillary muscle B: abnormal papillary muscle MS: A: predominant valvular lesion with normal papillary muscle B: predominant valvular lesion with abnormal papillary muscle
Collins-Nakai et al. (1977)	1977	Anatomical	MS only	Based on associated lesions: (surgical + autopsy + echo) 1. Isolated MV disease 2. Supramitral ring ± other cardiac defects 3. MS and other left-sided lesions or atrial shunt 4. MS and tetralogy of Fallot
Ruckman and van Praagh et al. (1978)	1978	Autopsy	MS only	1. Typical congenital MS 2. Hypoplastic congenital MS 3. Parachute mitral valve 4. Supramitral ring 5. Double orifice mitral valve
Moore et al. (1994)	1994	Echo + surgical	MS only	1. Typical hypoplastic MV symmetrical papillary muscles 2. Atypical hypoplastic MV – asymmetrical papillary muscles 3. Parachute mitral valve 4. Supramitral ring 5. Double orifice mitral valve
Mitruka and Lamberti et al. (2000)[b]	2000	Descriptive	MR and MS	1. Hemodynamic: MR, MS, or mixed 2. Segmental: (i) Supravalvular ii. Valvar (A) and annular (B) leaflet (iii) Subvalvular (A) and chordal (B) papillary muscle (iv) Mixed

(continued)

Table 22.1 (continued)

Author	Year	Basis of Classification	MV Lesions	Classification System
Oppido et al. (2008)	2008	Surgical	MR and MS	1. Hemodynamic: (i) Predominant MR (ii) Predominant MS 2. Functional: (i) Normal leaflet motion (ii) Prolapsed leaflet (iii) Restricted leaflet 3. Segmental: (i) Annulus/leaflets (ii) Chords (iii) Papillary muscles (iv) Mixed 4. Leaflet tissue: (i) Dysplastic (ii) Non-dysplastic

MR mitral regurgitation, *MS* mitral stenosis, *MV* mitral valve

[a]Revised in 1998

[b]Congenital heart surgery nomenclature and database project

they noted 97 % (37 out of 38) of their patients with congenital mitral stenosis had more than one segment of the mitral valve apparatus affected (Collins-Nakai et al. 1977). They concluded that it was misleading to classify patients based on one anatomic segment of the mitral valve (Collins-Nakai et al. 1977). They proposed a classification based on associated cardiac defects (e.g., associated left-sided lesion, tetralogy of Fallot, or no associated defects) (Table 22.1).

In 1978, Ruckman and van Praagh focused their attention on stenotic mitral valve defects and noted that typically congenital mitral stenosis affected multiple valve segments (Ruckman and van Praagh 1978). Commonly, the leaflet margins were thickened, tendinous chords appeared shortened, interchordal spaces were obliterated, and the two papillary muscles were underdeveloped and closely spaced. They coined the term "typical congenital mitral valve stenosis" to describe this most common defect with two distinct papillary muscle arrangements. The remainder of stenotic mitral valve defects were classified as "parachute mitral valve" (a single papillary muscle variant), "hypoplastic mitral valve" (miniature valve as seen in hypoplastic left heart syndrome), "double orifice mitral valve," and "supramitral ring." "Supramitral ring" earned a category of its own even though from their work it was clear that it was rarely an isolated defect. As a result, by necessity, some patients were classified into multiple categories based on this system. In 1994, Moore et al. (1994) expanded van Praagh's classification by adding "atypical congenital mitral stenosis" to differentiate between groups with symmetrical (typical mitral stenosis) and asymmetrical (atypical mitral stenosis) papillary muscle arrangements. His description of "atypical congenital mitral stenosis" resembled Oosthoek's (Oosthoek et al. 1997) description of "parachute-like asymmetrical valve" (see complex mitral valve lesions).

Surgical Classification

In 1976, Carpentier et al. (1976) introduced a surgical classification system to specifically facilitate the development of tailored techniques for congenital mitral valve repair. It was based on the "predominant lesion," as he also observed that multisegment pathology was the most prevalent. His description and classification was based on observations at surgery made via the left atrium. Prior to this all classifications were based on the pathologists' view of the defect. The Carpentier classification was based on leaflet motion: normal, restricted, or prolapsed. In addition it considered the predominant anatomic and hemodynamic effects (Table 22.1). This description of congenital mitral valve defects was widely accepted and utilized over the next three decades (Serraf et al. 2000; Carpentier et al. 1976; Chauvaud et al. 1998; Oppido et al. 2008; Uva et al. 1995; McCarthy et al. 1996; Prifti et al. 2002; Stellin et al. 2010; Wood et al. 2005; Zias et al. 1998). His team dramatically expanded the repertoire of operative techniques and in doing so popularized mitral valve repair for congenital defects. In 2008, Oppido and colleagues (Oppido et al. 2008) further refined the classification system by adding a further level to Carpentier's classification, the quality of leaflet tissue: normal or dysplastic. In their surgical series, dysplastic leaflets were associated with less favorable and less durable repairs.

Complex Congenital MV Lesions

Anatomical pathologists and cardiac surgeons introduced descriptive terms for what they perceived as very distinct congenital mitral valve lesions. However, many have argued that the majority of cases do not fit the classic morphologic pattern but are the incomplete forms or the so-called forme fruste (Rosenquist 1974; Mitruka and Lamberti 2000). As a result these descriptive terms are not stand-alone terms and require further clarification to facilitate effective communication.

"Parachute mitral valve" refers to an anomaly of the mitral valve apparatus where all tendinous cords insert into one papillary muscle as noted by Edwards in 1963 (Schiebler et al. 1961). The other papillary muscle is either absent or severely hypoplastic. As a pathologist, he observed the mitral valve through the incised left ventricle and noted that the anomaly had a parachute-like appearance. Others later observed that in the setting of isolated papillary muscle, the tendinous chords are often short and fused with interchordal spaces partially or completely obliterated (Hoashi et al. 2010; Davachi et al. 1971; Chauvaud et al. 1998; Shone et al. 1963). Commissures are frequently underdeveloped and the leaflets may be dysplastic or deficient. The combination of these lesions can give rise to a funnel rather than a parachute-like appearance. It is frequently associated with a "supramitral ring" (Davachi et al. 1971; Ruckman and van Praagh 1978) that is often an integral part of the mitral valve leaflets (Banerjee et al. 1995; Asante-Korang et al. 2006). It is a membranous or fibrous shelf that arises from the atrial side of the anterior mitral valve leaflet and posteriorly attaches to the leaflet, annulus, or the left atrial wall below the level of the left atrial appendage (Banerjee et al. 1995). Parachute mitral valve is commonly classified as a malformation of the papillary muscles. However, that is too simplistic. It is often the associated lesions of other valve segments (e.g., commissural underdevelopment, dysplastic leaflets, and shortened and fused tendinous chords) that determine the severity of valvar dysfunction (stenosis and regurgitation) and hence the need for cardiac intervention.

In addition to a supramitral ring, parachute mitral valves are frequently associated with subaortic obstruction and coarctation of the aorta. When obstruction at all four levels is present, it is then referred to as Shone's complex (Shone et al. 1963).

Parachute-like asymmetrical valve was described by Oosthoek et al. (1997) in 1997 as an anomaly that is an incomplete form of the true parachute valve with two papillary muscles: one hypoplastic and the other dominant receiving the majority of tendinous chords. He further described that one of the papillary muscles was often elongated, located higher in the left ventricle with its tip reaching to the annulus, and attached at both its base and lateral side to the left ventricular wall. The valve leaflets could be directly attached to the hypoplastic papillary muscle. Parachute-like asymmetrical valves formed a spectrum of anomalies, rather than a well-defined entity. Only one out of Oosthoek's 29 cases could be described as a "true" parachute valve (Oosthoek et al. 1997). Two decades earlier Rosenquist also demonstrated that most papillary muscle anomalies were often mild or incomplete forms (which were common among patients with coarctation) and that the "true" parachute anomaly, with a single papillary muscle, was rare (Rosenquist 1974).

Anomalous mitral arcade was first described by Layman and Edwards in 1967 as "an anomaly of the mitral valve that consisted of connection of the left ventricular papillary muscles to the anterior mitral valve leaflet, either directly or through the interposition of unusually short tendinous chords" (Layman and Edwards 1967). When viewed from the left ventricle, the two papillary muscles resembled two pillars, and the bridging fibrous tissue in-between the papillary muscles resembles the arch of an arcade.

Hammock mitral valve was first described in 1976 by Carpentier et al. (1976), and it referred specifically to the appearance of the mitral valve apparatus from its left atrial aspect as viewed at cardiac surgery. The hammock appearance arose when the valvar orifice was at least partially obstructed by intermixed tendinous chords that attached to abnormal papillary muscles implanted just beneath the posterior leaflet (Carpentier and Brizard 2006).

Double orifice mitral valve is a rare anomaly (0.05 % of congenital cardiac abnormalities) that is usually found incidentally or in combination with other abnormalities, most commonly AV canal defects. In itself, it is rarely a cause of significant regurgitation or stenosis (Zalzstein et al. 2004).

Although it is not a true mitral valve lesion, it is convenient to include cor triatriatum (heart with three atria) in the discussion. It is rare – 0.5 % of congenital cardiac defects – and may be associated with other defects including ASD (see below), anomalous pulmonary venous drainage, VSD, bicuspid aortic valve, coarctation of the aorta, Fallot's tetralogy, DORV, common AV canal, persistent left SVC with unroofed coronary sinus, and hypoplastic mitral valve.

Both right (very rare) and left atrial forms occur, but the left atrial type, or *cor triatriatum sinister*, is of concern here. A membrane dividing the left atrium into an upper and a lower chamber exists, and its presentation is similar to that of mitral stenosis, though if the orifice is large enough, it may be asymptomatic, and only discovered incidentally or in later years when it fibroses or calcifies or when investigating the onset of atrial fibrillation. The membrane lies above the level of the left atrial appendage, whereas a mitral ring lies below it. In its simplest form (20 % of cases), there is a membrane with a single or multiple (10 %) orifices in it. The majority of the remainder (about 70 %) are associated with an ASD, either above the membrane or below it, with the direction of the shunt through the ASD being determined by the relevant pressure gradients at the time, usually left to right in the former (e.g., though right to left if associated with Fallot's tetralogy) and right to left in the latter.

Clinical Features

The nature and severity of symptoms in patients with congenital mitral valve anomalies relate to etiology, rate of onset and progression, left ventricle function, pulmonary artery pressure, and the presence of coexisting valvular or myocardial diseases.

Congenital Mitral Stenosis

Patients with severe mitral stenosis may present with respiratory distress from pulmonary edema shortly after birth if a significant atrial septal communication is not present. The presence of an atrial septal defect decompresses the left atrium, resulting in a clinical picture of pulmonary over circulation and decreased systemic cardiac output.

Patients with mild-to-moderate mitral stenosis present after the neonatal period with signs of low cardiac output and right heart failure such as pulmonary infections, failure to gain weight, exhaustion and diaphoresis with feeding, tachypnea, and chronic cough.

Children with mitral stenosis may present with the insidious onset of exercise limitation and other clinical signs.

Pulmonary congestion is evidenced by increasing severity of dyspnea (depending on the degree of mitral stenosis) that may range from dyspnea during exercise to paroxysmal nocturnal dyspnea, orthopnea, or even frank pulmonary edema. Dyspnea may be precipitated or worsened by an increase in blood flow across the stenotic mitral valve (e.g., pregnancy, exercise) or by a reduction in diastolic filling time achieved by increasing the heart rate (e.g., emotional stress, fever, respiratory infection, atrial fibrillation with rapid ventricular rate).

Signs of right heart failure, including peripheral edema and fatigue, may be present.

Patients with mitral stenosis, including those previously without symptoms, may develop atrial fibrillation, although this is an uncommon event in childhood. It results from chronic distension of the left atrium. Atrial fibrillation may cause loss of the atrial kick to left ventricle filling that reduces systemic output; this may precipitate or exacerbate congestive heart failure. Thromboembolic events (seeding of systemic emboli) occur in 10–20 % of patients with mitral stenosis. Many of these emboli lodge in the brain, causing a stroke. Infective endocarditis (a rare event) should be suspected when embolization occurs during sinus rhythm.

Hemoptysis may be caused by rupture of dilated bronchial veins. Pink frothy sputum may be a manifestation of frank pulmonary edema. Both are associated with end-stage severe mitral stenosis but rarely occur in pediatric patients.

Chest pain occurs in approximately 15 % of patients with mitral stenosis.

Dysphagia can be produced by compression of the esophagus as a result of a dilated left atrium. It rarely occurs in children.

Hoarseness can occur if the dilated left atrium impinges on the recurrent laryngeal nerve. It is a rare manifestation of severe mitral stenosis, especially in childhood.

Congenital Mitral Regurgitation

Children with minor degrees of mitral regurgitation are usually asymptomatic. With increased amounts of mitral regurgitation, fatigue may be reported, but children can tolerate severe mitral regurgitation surprisingly better than adults can. Once pulmonary hypertension develops, complaints such as tachypnea and dyspnea with light activity become more prominent. With the most severe mitral regurgitation, children may experience limited growth and failure to thrive. Hemoptysis can develop during the later stages. Children may remain asymptomatic with no complications of mitral regurgitation until the second or third decade of life. An indolent course of mitral regurgitation may be deceptive because of the ability of the heart to compensate for the altered hemodynamics. This occurs because of changes in cardiac pump loading such that increased diastolic filling increases preload, whereas left ventricular ejection, in part into the left atrium, reduces afterload. By the time symptoms become apparent, serious and irreversible LV dysfunction may have developed.

Vital signs are usually normal in mild regurgitation. With increasing mitral regurgitation, heart and respiratory rates may be increased. In patients with severe mitral regurgitation, arterial pulse has been characterized as having a small volume with a sharp upstroke. Rarely, irregular pulse may be indicative of associated atrial fibrillation.

A left atrial lift is a second impulse resulting from the increased volume that is displaced into the left atrium during systole. The second impulse should be felt near the time of the second heart sound. This sign is most helpful in thin children and young adults because their chest diameters are smaller and their hearts are closer to the chest wall. The cardiac impulse may be displaced to the left, and, in more advanced disease, a double impulse is felt.

Upon auscultation, the first heart sound is usually slightly diminished, whereas the second heart sound is usually split. With more severe mitral regurgitation, a third heart sound and a mid-diastolic low-frequency murmur may be present, caused by increased ventricular filling. When pulmonary hypertension develops, the pulmonary component of the second heart sound becomes louder and occurs earlier (as long as right ventricular function is not significantly impaired), reducing the splitting interval. Ejection systolic click may be present due to mitral valve prolapse.

Patients with mild mitral regurgitation may reveal no signs other than a characteristic apical systolic murmur. The mitral regurgitation murmur is characterized as blowing and high pitched, and it is loudest over the apex with radiation to the left axilla. The murmur is often pansystolic, beginning immediately after the first heart sound, and may continue beyond the aortic component of the second heart sound, thus obscuring the second heart sound. This murmur increases with increased afterload (squatting) and decreases with decreased preload (standing). Occasionally, radiation toward the sternum occurs when posterior leaflet abnormalities are present. Little correlation is noted between intensity of the murmur and severity of mitral regurgitation. The murmur occasionally may be confined to late systole only. The degree of mitral regurgitation in these patients is usually mild.

Congestive heart failure with pulmonary edema can occur with significant mitral regurgitation and pulmonary findings may be consistent with it. Compression of left main bronchus due to left atrial enlargement can cause ipsilateral wheezing and lung collapse. Significant and sustained mitral regurgitation can be associated with endocarditis and thromboembolism and have associated findings.

Diagnosis

The diagnosis of congenital mitral valve anomaly relies on the clinical findings, the chest radiography, the electrocardiogram (ECG), and most importantly the echocardiographic assessment. The positive diagnosis can often be made before the echocardiographic evaluation in the presence of an isolated mitral valve anomaly.

Congenital Mitral Stenosis

Electrocardiography

Electrocardiography findings may be normal in patients with mild mitral stenosis. Hemodynamically significant stenosis results in ECG findings of left atrial or biatrial enlargement and right ventricular enlargement in proportion to the severity of the obstruction.

Chest Radiography

Chest radiographic findings may include left atrial dilation, posteroanterior dilation secondary to high pulmonary vascular pressure and resistance, pulmonary venous congestion, and right ventricular enlargement.

Echocardiography

Echocardiography is the most important diagnostic tool to evaluate patients with mitral stenosis. This noninvasive imaging modality provides excellent anatomic and hemodynamic assessment of mitral stenosis.

Echocardiography provides the following:

- Direct anatomic data, such as visualization of valve leaflet morphology and motility as well as measurement of valve orifice dimensions
- Evaluation of left atrial size and detection of left atrial thrombi
- Indirect physiologic data (i.e., estimation of pressure gradients across the mitral valve and right ventricular systolic pressure), which may be measured using Doppler echocardiography

Transesophageal Echocardiography

Transesophageal echocardiography is used when transthoracic echocardiographic pictures are inadequate. It may also be used to guide intervention and assess results in the operating room and cardiac catheterization laboratory.

Dynamic Three-Dimensional (3D) Transthoracic and Transesophageal Echocardiography

These techniques can provide good insight into valvular motion and help preoperative planning in situations in which valve reconstruction is considered (Kutty et al. 2014). However, the accuracy of these techniques is currently limited by the quality of the original two-dimensional (2D) echocardiographic cross-sectional images, which can be adversely affected by patient motion, breathing, and cardiac arrhythmia such as atrial fibrillation.

Congenital Mitral Regurgitation

Chest Radiography

With mild mitral regurgitation, the heart size is normal. With increasing mitral regurgitation, cardiomegaly may develop, and left atrial enlargement becomes apparent. Left ventricle enlargement and pulmonary congestion may also be present. In cases of acute mitral regurgitation, pulmonary venous vascular markings may be increased and pulmonary edema may be seen without signs of left atrial enlargement. Left lung atelectasis and hyperinflation may be visible due to compression of the left main bronchus by enlarged left atrium.

Electrocardiography

The 12-lead ECG is likely to show normal results in children with mild mitral regurgitation. In more chronic mitral regurgitation, ECG findings demonstrate left atrial and left ventricle enlargement. When pulmonary hypertension is present, ECG may also demonstrate right ventricular hypertrophy. Rhythm changes, such as atrial fibrillation, are often observed in adults but are rare in children.

Transthoracic Echocardiography

Echocardiography is the most valuable technique used to evaluate mitral regurgitation. Echocardiography is usually readily available and portable. Knowledge of mitral valve apparatus, including the labeling of the scallops of each of the two valve leaflets, is essential. An understanding of the anatomy from surgeon's perspective is needed to explain the findings.

Two-dimensional (2D) echocardiography allows depiction of the size of the chambers and assessment of ventricular systolic function, as well as determination of the morphology of the mitral valve leaflets, the annulus, chordal tissue, and papillary muscles. The parasternal long axis view may provide the best images of mitral valve prolapse, whereas the parasternal short axis view is better for depicting papillary muscle anatomy and leaflet cleft.

M-Mode assessment of cardiac function is extremely important. Cardiac function should be carefully evaluated in mitral regurgitation, and one can use different techniques, including 2D, three-dimensional (3D), tissue Doppler, and strain imaging to assess the left ventricle function. The left ventricular ejection fraction should be hypernormal, indicating a preserved myocardial function with mitral regurgitation. In the presence of normal or mildly depressed function, one should expect myocardial failure postoperatively. Scalloping of mitral leaflets can occur in mitral valve prolapse and can be seen using M-Mode. In addition, ventricular dimensions should be measured and followed for left ventricle enlargement. Left ventricular hypertrophy can also be determined and may be present in hypertrophic cardiomyopathy with mitral regurgitation.

Color-flow Doppler echocardiography demonstrates width and direction of the regurgitant flow (Little et al. 2008). The degree of regurgitation may be underestimated if the jet hugs the walls of the atrium. Furthermore, because the structures are 3D, multiple views and scans must be performed with optimal transducer frequency and gain to determine the entire regurgitant jet.

Spectral Doppler imaging demonstrates a high-velocity signal across the mitral valve in systole entering retrograde into the left atrium. Mitral regurgitation can be seen and evaluated best in the apical four-chamber and parasternal long views. Concomitant mitral stenosis should also be determined. The peak velocity of mitral regurgitation can be used to calculate several other parameters, including left ventricle dP/dT.

Visualizing mitral regurgitation is not as difficult as classifying the severity. In adults, many echocardiographic methods are used with varying results. The grading of mitral regurgitation in the pediatric population as mild, moderate, and severe is based on the size and extent of the color-flow Doppler signal (jet area) into the left atrium (left atrial area).

Other factors to consider include left atrium and ventricular size and function. In mild mitral regurgitation, the signal is located in the proximal third of the left atrium near the mitral valve. The left atrium is usually not enlarged, and the ventricular function is normal. In moderate mitral regurgitation, the signal extends to the mid cavity, with left atrial dilation and increased ventricular function. With severe mitral regurgitation, the signal reaches the posterior third of the left atrium and the pulmonary veins, and the left atrium and ventricle are usually enlarged, with increased ventricular shortening fraction. Other techniques useful in quantification include measurement of vena contracta, proximal isovelocity surface area, systolic pulmonary vein flow reversal, and regurgitant fraction.

Transesophageal Echocardiography (TEE)

This may be required if further detailed anatomic information is needed. Transesophageal echocardiography views correlate better with angiographic grading than transthoracic views. In addition, intraoperative transesophageal echocardiography is absolutely essential in guiding mitral valve surgery and assessing the result.

3D Echocardiography

This provides an excellent anatomical evaluation of mitral valve and helps with decisions regarding therapy and possible surgical intervention.

Cardiac Magnetic Resonance Imaging

Cardiac MRI is a newer modality. Cardiac MRI provides 3D imaging of the heart and great vessels and does not depend on acoustic windows, as echocardiography does. Cardiac MRI provides more accurate evaluation of both left and right ventricular size and function. The degree of mitral regurgitation determined by cardiac MRI has not been adequately evaluated. However, velocity flow imaging may potentially provide additional information.

Table 22.2 Estimation of mitral regurgitation using angiography

Regurgitation grade	Description
Grade of 1+	Trace amounts of contrast are seen in the left atrium, but the amount is insufficient to outline the left atrium
Grade of 2+	The contrast opacifies the entire left atrium but less than that of the LV. The contrast clears quickly (within 2–3 beats)
Grade of 3+	The contrast opacifies the left atrium and LV equally
Grade of 4+	The contrast opacifies the left atrium more than the LV and progresses to the pulmonary veins

LV left ventricle

Cardiac Catheterization

Evaluation of mitral regurgitation in children usually does not require cardiac catheterization. Some pediatric patients undergo catheterization to evaluate other cardiac defects that may be present, or anomalous left coronary from the pulmonary artery (ALCAPA) is suspected, as this can cause mitral regurgitation secondary to myocardial ischemia or infarction.

Mitral regurgitation is best evaluated using angiography obtained in the right anterior oblique view. Retrograde flow of injected dye demonstrates the degree of mitral regurgitation, which is quantitatively graded (grades I–IV) depending on the level of left atrial opacification (Table 22.2). Left ventricular injections obtained via the retrograde approach are preferred to an anterograde approach to prevent the catheter from holding the mitral valve open and creating artifactual mitral regurgitation.

To quantitate mitral regurgitation, a combination of angiography and cardiac output measurements must be used. Either thermodilution or the Fick principle helps measure forward cardiac output, while angiography allows determination of total left ventricular output. Keep in mind that tricuspid regurgitation can invalidate the thermodilution method (Calafiore et al. 2009).

Subtracting the forward output from total left ventricular output yields the regurgitant fraction. A regurgitant fraction of 0.5 or greater is generally considered clinically significant.

The left ventricular ejection fraction may be increased initially; however, as the left ventricle decompensates, the ejection fraction decreases to normal or subnormal values, signifying left ventricular failure. As left ventricular failure develops, left ventricular end-diastolic pressure increases, resulting in an increase in left atrial and pulmonary venous pressure. Increased pulmonary venous pressure is manifested as an increase in pulmonary capillary wedge pressure. At catheterization, the wedge pressure a wave amplitude is increased along with a rapid rise of the v wave. The latter occurs when left ventricular compliance decreases.

Cardiac catheterization should be used when noninvasive data are discordant, limited, or differ from the clinical status of the patient. Ventriculography may add new information if more complex congenital cardiac problems are present.

Management of Congenital Mitral Valve Anomalies

In the past decade, the surgical approach to congenital mitral valve disease has significantly evolved as successive midterm and long-term series have been reported (Serraf et al. 2000; Chauvaud et al. 1998; Oppido et al. 2008; Uva et al. 1995; Prifti et al. 2002). Pediatric patients can derive the same benefits from mitral valve repair as adults with regard to preservation of valvular tissue, subvalvular apparatus, and ventricular geometry, leading to optimal valve and ventricular function. Furthermore, avoidance of mechanical prostheses is especially desirable in young children, in whom annular growth should be fostered and who may have little physical space for the prosthesis in the heart.

After pediatric mitral valve replacement, mismatch between native annulus and mitral prosthesis has been shown to be a risk factor for both early and late death (Caldarone et al. 2001; Kojori et al. 2004; Günther et al. 2000). The probability of mitral valve prosthesis re-replacement was demonstrated to be inversely related to the absolute size of the prosthesis initially implanted (Raghuveer et al. 2003). Finally, the cumulative risk generated by a lifelong commitment to anticoagulation should be avoided whenever possible.

Diagnostic tools are evolving rapidly and allow superior anatomic diagnosis and monitoring of the surgical repair. The range of surgical techniques modified from adult surgery into pediatric practice or specially developed for pediatric patients is large and allows tailoring of the surgical techniques to anatomic requirements.

Congenital mitral valve disease is rare and frequently associated with other cardiac malformations. Because it is usually complex, intervention is ideally postponed to allow time for annular growth and tissue maturity (Kruithof et al. 2007). This is usually considered to be safe, because depressed systolic ventricular function has been shown to recover after successful mitral valve surgery in pediatric patients (Krishnan et al. 1997; Murakami et al. 1999). Severe congestive cardiac failure refractory to maximal medical therapy, however, can result in surgery being undertaken in the first months of life.

Timing of Surgery

Indications for surgery vary according to the etiology and anatomy, the age of the patient, the size of the mitral valve annulus, and the clinical status. Neonates and infants with severe mitral valve disease are only considered for operation if they have severe symptoms. No symptoms are necessary if the valve can be repaired simply without annuloplasty (cleft mitral valve); for more complex valves, symptoms are usually present at the time of surgery. Surgical indications for patients with predominant mitral stenosis are dictated by symptoms only. No specific threshold figure for either pulmonary arterial pressure or transmitral gradient triggers a surgical indication if few or no symptoms are present (Oppido et al. 2008). An intervention before the first year of life is rarely needed in cases of isolated regurgitation.

Anesthetic Management

Mitral valve stenosis and the lesions obstructing flow at left atrial level (cor triatriatum, supramitral ring) essentially have the same requirements with regard to anesthetic goals and techniques. The main areas of concern are management of preload and afterload, heart rate, and pulmonary artery pressure (PAP), bearing in mind coexisting cardiac abnormalities. Pure congenital mitral stenosis is uncommon, and it is usually associated with other lesions, particularly Shone's complex (Shone et al. 1963).

Hypovolemia reduces the pressure gradient and hence flow across the stenotic lesion, while excessive fluid (and the Trendelenburg position) risks pulmonary edema. Afterload needs to be sufficient for adequate coronary artery perfusion, as well as that of other organs. A slower heart rate allows a longer diastolic period for blood to cross the lesion, though too slow a rate reduces cardiac output. Tachycardia reduces diastolic time for flow through the lesion, and atrial fibrillation loses the invaluable atrial contraction propelling blood through it, as well as increasing heart rate. Rises in PAP reduce left-sided preload and can be caused by noxious stimuli – induction needs to be smooth, including intubation, and pain managed. Hypoxia, hypercarbia, and acidosis worsen pulmonary hypertension and should be controlled (allowing for any right to left cardiac shunts). A mild reduction of PCO_2 and rise in FiO_2 are allowed. Maneuvers to reduce pulmonary hypertension such as high FiO_2, hyperventilation to reduce PCO_2, inhaled nitric oxide, phosphodiesterase inhibitors such as milrinone (including inhaled milrinone, with less systemic vasodilator effect), prostacyclin infusion, and sildenafil can collectively expose the pulmonary capillaries to high flow in the presence of back pressure from the stenotic lesion, risking pulmonary congestion and edema, and are thus best utilized post repair, where they are invaluable in aiding right ventricular performance post bypass and reducing the risk of pulmonary hypertensive crises, including in the postoperative period. Sildenafil (intravenous infusion of enteral) significantly reduces the incidence of pulmonary hypertensive crises when added to nitric oxide and is useful in preventing rebound pulmonary hypertension when weaning nitric oxide (see also Chaps. 29 and 31). Nitric oxide is more effective in pulmonary hypertension caused by mitral stenosis in the child than in the adult. In Shone's syndrome, the anesthetic technique needs to target the predominant lesion, which can be difficult to determine. Maintenance of a patent ductus with a prostaglandin E2 infusion, if relevant, must be continued. Note that paracetamol is as effective in closing a PDA as ibuprofen (Cochrane Review 2015).

Premedication, while smoothing induction, requires caution. Benzodiazepines can cause unwanted vasodilatation, opiates respiratory depression and worsening of pulmonary hypertension, and anticholinergics a rise in heart rate. Unless the stenotic lesion is severe and provided dosages are modest, these effects are unlikely to be significant. Topical local anesthetic cream at the sites of potential venous cannulation is useful.

In the absence of pre-existing venous access, induction with inhaled sevoflurane and securing venous access for administration of opiate and muscle relaxant are usual. High percentages of sevoflurane are significantly myocardial depressant. Halothane can cause unwanted arrhythmias, particularly nodal rhythm. Nitrous oxide causes modest rises in pulmonary artery pressure and increases the size of any air emboli. Intravenous induction with propofol, with its vasodilator properties, may need compensatory vasoconstrictor administration. Alpha agonists are usually used (metaraminol, phenylephrine) and cause reflex slowing of the heart rate, which is useful unless profound. Intravenous midazolam can cause significant vasodilatation. Ketamine is theoretically contraindicated, though heart rate and pulmonary artery pressure rises were only of the order of 10 % in one study in children undergoing cardiac catheterization (Morray et al. 1984). Opiates such as fentanyl, sufentanil, and remifentanil can cause significant bradycardia, and pancuronium a tachycardia, the coadministration of both compensating for each other's effect, though unwanted tachycardia can predominate. Rocuronium and cisatracurium are acceptable muscle relaxants. Atracurium may be relatively contraindicated because of histamine release and consequent vasodilatation.

Monitoring is standard for cardiac surgery. PA catheters (5 F pediatric PA catheters are available) are controversial, potentially causing arrhythmias, thrombosis, pulmonary infarcts, and PA damage. Wedge readings are not reliable LAP estimates in the presence of pulmonary hypertension. PA and LA lines can be placed by the surgeon intraoperatively if deemed necessary. Transesophageal echocardiography (TEE) is vital to confirm the diagnosis, as a monitor of hemodynamics, to aid de-airing at the end of bypass and to assess the adequacy of surgical repair. 3D echocardiography when feasible is superior in mitral valve assessment. Small 3D TEE probes are not yet available, but existing 3D probes are usable in larger children.

Maintenance with an opiate bias and low-dose inhalation agent is suitable. Post-cardiopulmonary bypass, measures to reduce pulmonary hypertension are applied, the purpose being to aid right ventricular function in the early postoperative period and help prevent pulmonary hypertensive crises. A PDE3 inhibitor, e.g., milrinone, is the usual initial inotrope. Levosimendan is as effective (Lechner et al. 2012), also lowers PAP, and has the advantage of having an active metabolite with a long duration of action post infusion, typically 7 days.

Mitral valve surgery carries the risk of damage to the AV node, requiring AV pacing. The circumflex coronary artery can be compressed by annuloplasty material or prosthetic valve rings or occluded by encircling sutures (Azakie et al. 2003). This will manifest on the TEE with lateral LV wall hypokinesia. The circumflex artery can be visualized with multiplane TEE – at a transducer angle of about 105 degrees, follow the course of the left main stem coronary artery as it leaves the left coronary sinus and then the circumflex artery as the probe is rotated to the left. With color Doppler (set at a low frequency to enhance the signal, as flow is almost at right angles to the ultrasound beam), flow can be qualitatively assessed – turbulence for narrowing and cessation for occlusion. Care must be taken to follow the artery carefully, so as not to confuse it with the adjacent coronary sinus (Ender et al. 2010).

The PAP may return to normal or only partially fall immediately post repair. It may take weeks to months to normalize and may never become normal. Attempts to normalize pulmonary artery pressures postoperatively may result in unnecessary prolongation of ventilation and stay in the intensive care unit.

Mitral Regurgitation

Pure congenital mitral regurgitation is rare. It is associated with other pathologies such as LV dilatation of whatever cause, including cardiomyopathy, ALCAPA, or connective tissue disorders causing prolapse such as Marfan's syndrome and Ehlers-Danlos syndrome.

The main hemodynamic goals during anesthesia are a reduction in afterload, which decreases regurgitant flow in favor of forward flow and a mildly raised heart rate – bradycardia raises LVEDV, increasing mitral regurgitation. Patients are usually on an ACE inhibitor preoperatively to cause afterload reduction. These patients are frequently on diuretic therapy and may be hypovolemic as a consequence, with resultant reduction in LV filling. This should be judiciously corrected. PAP may be elevated, and increases must be avoided as for mitral stenosis.

Induction with sevoflurane is tolerated. Care is needed if ventricular function is poor. Pancuronium usefully increases the heart rate, but other muscle relaxants are acceptable. Maintenance with sevoflurane or isoflurane (which also increases heart rate) combined with opiates as per mitral stenosis above is well tolerated.

Monitoring is as for mitral stenosis above. Again, TEE is invaluable. Left ventricular function expressed as ejection fraction is misleading, since this is flattered by ejection into the low-pressure left atrium. Thus, in the presence of moderate or severe mitral regurgitation, an ejection fraction of less than 60 % is likely to indicate LV dysfunction. This becomes apparent when the ejection fraction is reduced post repair. Inodilators such as milrinone or levosimendan are preferred over catecholamines, which raise afterload, and are also appropriate post-cardiopulmonary bypass.

Mitral regurgitation may coexist with mitral stenosis, in which case the anesthetic strategy favors the dominant lesion.

Surgical Techniques

Continuous cardiopulmonary bypass is established with bicaval and ascending aortic cannulation at mild hypothermia of 32 °C and pump flows of 150–200 mL/kg/min.

Intermittent antegrade cold blood cardioplegia is delivered every 20–30 min. Neither profound hypothermia nor circulatory arrest is required for isolated mitral valve surgery.

Through a midline sternotomy, access to the mitral valve is gained either by a left atriotomy in the interatrial groove, transseptally, or with a combined approach. Exposure is optimized by cannulating the superior vena cava at a distance from the cavoatrial junction and the inferior vena cava adjacent to the cavoatrial junction. A self-retaining mitral valve retractor adapted to the size of the patient is used throughout. Visualization of the valve is further enhanced by mattress sutures in the posterior annulus and pulling the inferior vena cava more snugly up and to the left. The valve is then methodically inspected, and findings are integrated with the

Table 22.3 Techniques for repair of congenital mitral valve anomalies

Resection of supravalvular stenosing ring
Valve
Resection of accessory mitral valve tissue
Closure of cleft/post-AVSD correction suture dehiscence
Patch closure of leaflet perforation
Leaflet resection
Sliding technique
Plication of redundant leaflet
Commissurotomy
Alfieri stitch
Annulus
De Vaga suture annuloplasty
Ring annuloplasty
Posterior pericardial annuloplasty
Anterior pericardial annuloplasty
Bilateral pericardial annuloplasty
Commissure plication annuloplasty
Chordae
Chordal shortening
Chordal transfer
Artificial chordate
Chordae prolongation
Chordae fenestration
Papillary muscle
Papillary muscle shortening: split and tuck in
Papillary muscle splitting

AVSD atrioventricular septal defect

preoperative investigations, with care to note the following: the presence of a supravalvular mitral ring; annular diameter; leaflet texture and size; number, distribution, and morphologic characteristics of chordae and papillary muscles; nature of commissural tissue; and, finally, the presence of any accessory mitral valve tissue or tag in the interchordal spaces. The valve orifice is measured with Hegar dilators before and after repair, and the value is compared to predicted normal values indexed to the body surface area according to a modification of the sizes originally described by Kirklin and Barrat-Boyes (Kirklin and Barrat-Boyes 1993). Surgical techniques are tailored to the anatomy and mechanism of dysfunction (Table 22.3).

Surgical Outcomes

The outcomes reported in the surgical literature in this group of patients are quite varied. Many authors have reported a significant incidence of poor outcomes, probably for a variety of reasons including complex mitral valve anatomy, frequent association with other heart defects, and a relative paucity of patients with these lesions, with consequently less experience with reconstructive techniques (Chauvaud et al. 1998; Uva et al. 1995; McCarthy et al. 1996). Other authors reported excellent results with a very low postoperative mortality and morbidity among patients undergoing mitral valve surgery (Prifti et al. 2002; Stellin et al. 2010; Yoshimura et al. 1999).

Most authors have reported a significantly higher mortality rate – higher than 30 % – among children undergoing mitral valve replacement (Zweng et al. 1989; Kadoba et al. 1990). However, other authors have reported acceptable early and long-term survival among children undergoing mitral valve replacement (Yoshimura et al. 1999).

In recent years, attempts to preserve the native mitral valve are preferred, especially in infants and young children. Mitral valve repair offers the advantages of avoiding thromboembolism, preserving chordal and subvalvular apparatus function, and potentially reducing the need for reoperation. Because of a wide spectrum of mitral valve lesions, which usually involve different sites of the valvular apparatus, multiple techniques of valve repair are required (Chauvaud et al. 1998; Uva et al. 1995; Prifti et al. 2002; Murakami et al. 1999; Aharon et al. 1994).

The need for ring annuloplasty procedure in the pediatric age group remains controversial. Chauvaud and associates (Chauvaud et al. 1998; Chauvaud et al. 1997) used ring annuloplasty in children over 2 years of age, whereas other groups have demonstrated that other types of annuloplasty techniques can be employed successfully in children and the prosthetic rings are not indispensable for achieving favorable results (Uva et al. 1995; McCarthy et al. 1996; Zias et al. 1998).

Surgical repair of congenital mitral valve stenosis has been typically associated with greater postoperative mortality and morbidity (Chauvaud et al. 1997; Moran et al. 2000) and a higher reoperation rate compared with mitral valve repair for insufficiency (Stellin et al. 2000). The hammock mitral valve is the most difficult malformation to correct owing to the considerable amount of muscle found beneath the mitral valve leaflet causing severe left ventricular inflow obstruction (Chauvaud et al. 1997; Stellin et al. 2000). The hammock mitral valve is defined as a very dysplastic mitral valve, without tendinous chordae, with the apex of the papillary muscles having direct continuity with the leaflet tissue (Layman and Edwards 1967). In parachute and hammock mitral valve, the single papillary muscle is split delicately at the midline in two halves (Carpentier et al. 1976; Chauvaud et al. 1998; Prifti et al. 2002), thus increasing the excursion of the mitral valve during diastolic phase. When necessary a commissurotomy procedure is also performed.

For pediatric patients undergoing surgery for congenital mitral valve anomalies, age less than 1 year, hammock mitral valve, cardiothoracic ratio greater than 0.6, and associated cardiac anomalies are recognized risk factors for death or reoperation (Prifti et al. 2002). Uva and associates (Uva et al. 1995) reported excellent results in children less than 1 year of age undergoing mitral valve surgery, with a 7-year actuarial survival of 94 %. On the other hand, Prifti and colleagues (Prifti et al. 2002) reported different results: 6 of 25 early deaths and 6 of 11 late deaths were patients less than 1 year old. In this series the correction of the associated heart defects also increased the operative risk, probably because of significantly longer cardiopulmonary and aortic cross-clamping times, more complex anatomy, and left ventricular hypertrophy and impaired left ventricular function, particularly in cases with left ventricular outflow tract obstruction and ventricular septal defect.

Conclusion

Management of congenital anomalies of the mitral valve in the pediatric age group remains a therapeutic challenge for the wide spectrum of the morphological abnormalities. Improvements in preoperative evaluation, anatomical analysis of valvular lesions, anesthetic management, and surgical techniques have made it possible to obtain good results. Mitral valve reconstructive procedures in infants and children with congenital mitral valve anomalies are effective and reliable with low mortality and low incidence of reoperation rate. Mitral valve repair should always be attempted, especially in infants, despite the frequent severity of mitral valve dysplasia, to avoid the drawbacks of the currently available prostheses.

References

Aharon AS, Laks H, Drinkwater DC, et al. Early and late results of mitral valve repair in children. J Thorac Cardiovasc Surg. 1994;107:1262–70.

Asante-Korang A, O'Leary PW, Anderson RH. Anatomy and echocardiography of the normal and abnormal mitral valve. Cardiol Young. 2006;16 (Suppl 3):27–34.

Azakie A, Russell J, McCrindle BW, Arsdell G, Benson L, Coles J, et al. Anatomic repair of anomalous left coronary artery from the pulmonary artery by aortic reimplantation: early survival, patterns of ventricular recovery and late outcome. Ann Thorac Surg. 2003;75:1535–41.

Banerjee A, Kohl T, Silverman NH. Echocardiographic evaluation of congenital mitral valve anomalies in children. Am J Cardiol. 1995;76:1284–91.

Calafiore AM, Gallina S, Iaco AL, et al. Mitral valve surgery for functional mitral regurgitation: should moderate-or-more tricuspid regurgitation be treated? A propensity score analysis. Ann Thorac Surg. 2009;87:698–703.

Caldarone CA, Raghuveer G, Hills CB, et al. Long-term survival after mitral valve replacement in children aged <5 years: a multi-institutional study. Circulation. 2001;104(12 Suppl 1):143–7.

Carpentier A, Brizard CP. Congenital malformations of the mitral valve. In: Stark J, de Leval M, Tsang V, editors. Surgery for congenital heart defects. London: Wiley; 2006. p. 573–90.

Carpentier A, Branchini B, Cour JC, Asfaou E, Villani M, Deloche A, et al. Congenital malformations of the mitral valve in children. Pathology and surgical treatment. J Thorac Cardiovasc Surg. 1976;72:854–66.

Chauvaud SM, Milhailenau SA, Gaer JAR, Carpentie AC. Surgical treatment of mitral valvar stenosis: "The Hospital Broussais" experience. Cardiol Young. 1997;7:5–14.

Chauvaud S, Fuzellier JF, Houel R, Berrebi A, Mihaileanu S, Carpentier A. Reconstructive surgery in congenital mitral valve insufficiency (Carpentier's techniques): long-term results. J Thorac Cardiovasc Surg. 1998;115:84–92.

Collins-Nakai RL, Rosenthal A, Castaneda AR, Bernhard WF, Nadas AS. Congenital mitral stenosis. A review of 20 years' experience. Circulation. 1977;56:1039–47.

Davachi F, Moller JH, Edwards JE. Diseases of the mitral valve in infancy. An anatomic analysis of 55 cases. Circulation. 1971;43:565–79.

Ender J, Selbach M, Borger MA, et al. Endocardiographic identification of iatrogenic injury of the circumflex coronary artery during minimally invasive mitral valve repair. Ann Thorac Surg. 2010;89:1866–72.

Günther T, Mazzitelli D, Schreiber C, et al. Mitral-valve replacement in children under 6 years of age. Eur J Cardiothorac Surg. 2000;17:426–30.

Hoashi T, Bove EL, Devaney EJ, et al. Mitral valve repair for congenital mitral valve stenosis in the pediatric population. Ann Thorac Surg. 2010;90:36–41.

Kadoba K, Jonas RA, Mayer JE, Castaneda AR. Mitral valve replacement in the first year of life. J Thorac Cardiovasc Surg. 1990;100:762–8.

Kanani M, Moorman AF, Cook AC, et al. Development of the atrioventricular valves: clinicomorphological correlations. Ann Thorac Surg. 2005;79:1797–804.

Kirklin KW, Barrat-Boyes BS. Anatomy, dimension and terminology. In: Kirklin KW, Barrat-Boyes BS, editors. Cardiac surgery. 2nd ed. London: Churchill Livingstone; 1993. p. 3–60.

Kojori F, Chen R, Caldarone CA, et al. Outcomes of mitral valve replacement in children: a competing-risks analysis. J Thorac Cardiovasc Surg. 2004;128:703–9.

Krishnan US, Gersony WM, Berman-Rosenzweig E, Apfel HD. Late left ventricular function after surgery for children with chronic symptomatic mitral regurgitation. Circulation. 1997;96:4280–5.

Kruithof BP, Krawitz SA, Gaussin V. Atrioventricular valve development during late embryonic and postnatal stages involves condensation and extracellular matrix remodeling. Dev Biol. 2007;302:208–17.

Kutty S, Colen TM, Smallhorn JF. Three-dimensional echocardiography in the assessment of congenital mitral valve disease. J Am Soc Echocardiogr. 2014;27:142–54.

Layman TE, Edwards JE. Anomalous mitral arcade. A type of congenital mitral insufficiency. Circulation. 1967;35:389–95.

Lechner E, Hofer A, Leitner-Peneder G, et al. Levosimendan versus milrinone in neonates and infants after corrective open-heart surgery: a pilot study. Pediatr Crit Care Med. 2012;13:542–8.

Lee C, Lee CH, Kwak JG, et al. Long-term results after mitral valve repair in children. Eur J Cardiothorac Surg. 2010;37:267–72.

Little SH, Pirat B, Kumar R, et al. Three-dimensional color doppler echocardiography for direct measurement of vena contracta area in mitral regurgitation: in vitro validation and clinical experience. JACC Cardiovasc Imaging. 2008;1:695–704.

McCarthy JF, Neligan MC, Wood AE. Ten years' experience of an aggressive reparative approach to congenital mitral valve anomalies. Eur J Cardiothorac Surg. 1996;10:534–9.

Mitruka SN, Lamberti JJ. Congenital heart surgery nomenclature and database project: Mitral valve disease. Ann Thorac Surg. 2000;69(4 Suppl):S132–46.

Moore P, Adatia I, Spevak PJ, Keane JF, Perry SB, Castaneda AR, et al. Severe congenital mitral stenosis in infants. Circulation. 1994;89:2099–106.

Moran AM, Daebritz S, Keane JF, Mayer JE. Surgical management of mitral regurgitation after repair of endocardial cushion defects: early and midterm results. Circulation. 2000;102(19 Suppl 3):III160–5.

Morray JP, Lynn AM, Hendon PS, et al. Hemodynamic effects of ketamine in children with congenital heart disease. Anesth Analg. 1984;895–9.

Murakami T, Nakazawa M, Nakanishi T, Momma K. Prediction of postoperative left ventricular pump function in congenital mitral regurgitation. Pediatr Cardiol. 1999;20:418–21.

Ohlsson A, Shah PS. Paracetamol (acetaminophen) for patent ductus arteriosus in preterm or low-birth-weight infants. Cochrane Database Syst Rev. 2015;(3):CD010061.

Oosthoek PW, Wenink AC, Macedo AJ, Gittenberger-de Groot AC. The parachute-like asymmetric mitral valve and its two papillary muscles. J Thorac Cardiovasc Surg. 1997;114:9–15.

Oosthoek PW, Wenink AC, Wisse LJ, et al. Development of the papillary muscles of the mitral valve: morphogenetic background of parachute-like asymmetric mitral valves and other mitral valve anomalies. J Thorac Cardiovasc Surg. 1998;116:36–46.

Oppido G, Davies B, McMullan DM, Cochrane AD, Cheung MM, d'Udekem Y, et al. Surgical treatment of congenital mitral valve disease: Midterm results of a repair-oriented policy. J Thorac Cardiovasc Surg. 2008;135:1313–20.

Prifti E, Vanini V, Bonacchi M, Frati G, Bernabei M, Giunti G, et al. Repair of congenital malformations of the mitral valve: early and midterm results. Ann Thorac Surg. 2002;73:614–21.

Raghuveer G, Caldarone CA, Hills CB, Atkins DL, Belmont JM, Moller JH. Predictors of prosthesis survival, growth, and functional status following mechanical mitral valve replacement in children aged <5 years, a multi-institutional study. Circulation. 2003;108 Suppl 1:II174–9.

Rosenquist GC. Congenital mitral valve disease associated with coarctation of the aorta: a spectrum that includes parachute deformity of the mitral valve. Circulation. 1974;49:985–93.

Ruckman RN, van Praagh R. Anatomic types of congenital mitral stenosis: report of 49 autopsy cases with consideration of diagnosis and surgical implications. Am J Cardiol. 1978;42:592–601.

Schiebler GL, Edwards JE, Burchell HB, DuShane JW, Ongley PA, Wood EH. Congenital corrected transposition of the great vessels: a study of 33 cases. Pediatrics. 1961;27(Suppl):849–88.

Serraf A, Zoghbi J, Belli E, et al. Congenital mitral stenosis with or without associated defects: an evolving surgical strategy. Circulation. 2000;102:III166–71.

Shone JD, Sellers RD, Anderson RC, Adams Jr P, Lillehei CW, Edwards JE. The developmental complex of "parachute mitral valve," supravalvular ring of left atrium, subaortic stenosis, and coarctation of aorta. Am J Cardiol. 1963;11:714–25.

Stellin G, Padalino M, Milanesi O, et al. Repair of congenital mitral valve dysplasia in infants and children: is it always possible? Eur J Cardiothorac Surg. 2000;18:74–82.

Stellin G, Padalino MA, Vida VL, Boccuzzo G, Orrù E, Biffanti R, et al. Surgical repair of congenital mitral valve malformations in infancy and childhood: a single-center 36-year experience. J Thorac Cardiovasc Surg. 2010;140:1238–44.

Uva MS, Galletti L, Gayet FL, Piot D, Serraf A, Bruniaux J, et al. Surgery for congenital mitral valve disease in the first year of life. J Thorac Cardiovasc Surg. 1995;109:164–74.

Wood AE, Healy DG, Nolke L, Duff D, Oslizlok P, Walsh K. Mitral valve reconstruction in a pediatric population: late clinical results and predictors of long-term outcome. J Thorac Cardiovasc Surg. 2005;130:66–73.

Yoshimura N, Yamaguchi M, Oshima Y, et al. Surgery for mitral valve disease in the pediatric age group. J Thorac Cardiovasc Surg. 1999;118:99–106.

Zalzstein E, Hamilton R, Zucker N, et al. Presentation, natural history, and outcome in children and adolescents with double orifice mitral valve. Am J Cardiol. 2004;93:1067–9.

Zias EA, Mavroudis C, Backer CL, Kohr LM, Gotteiner NL, Rocchini AP. Surgical repair of the congenitally malformed mitral valve in infants and children. Ann Thorac Surg. 1998;66:1551–9.

Zweng TN, Bluett MK, Mosca R, Callow LB, Bove EL. Mitral valve replacement in the first 5 years of life. Ann Thorac Surg. 1989;47:720–4.

Chapter 23
Congenital Anomalies of the Aortic Valve

Premal M. Trivedi

Case Scenario #1: Critical Aortic Stenosis of the Neonate

A 3.2-kg neonate with prenatally diagnosed valvular aortic stenosis (AS) is delivered at 37 weeks. Within minutes, the child is intubated for respiratory distress, and prostaglandin E1 is started to improve systemic perfusion. Cardiology is present at the bedside and performs a focused echocardiogram which reveals:

- Dysplastic and thickened aortic valve leaflets with minimal prograde flow: peak velocity across the valve of 4.5 m/s, peak gradient of 81 mmHg, and mean gradient of 40 mmHg
- No significant aortic insufficiency
- Moderately depressed biventricular function with moderate left ventricular dilation and endocardial fibroelastosis
- Poor coaptation of the mitral valve leaflets with severe central mitral regurgitation
- Mild hypoplasia of the aortic root, ascending aorta, and aortic arch
- Large patent ductus arteriosus with right-to-left shunting
- Patent foramen ovale with left-to-right shunting

As the left-sided cardiac structures are deemed to be of sufficient size to support the patient's cardiac output, the child is put forth for an emergent balloon aortic valvuloplasty. On arrival to the interventional cardiology suite, blood pressures measured via the umbilical arterial line are 40s/20s with a heart rate in the 150 s. Oxygenation and ventilation remain marginal in spite of the following ventilatory

P.M. Trivedi, MD
Baylor College of Medicine; Division of Pediatric Cardiovascular Anesthesiology;
Texas Children's Hospital, Houston, TX, USA
e-mail: pxtrived@texaschildrens.org

© Springer International Publishing Switzerland 2017
A. Dabbagh et al. (eds.), *Congenital Heart Disease in Pediatric
and Adult Patients*, DOI 10.1007/978-3-319-44691-2_23

parameters: FiO_2 of 1.0, peak inspiratory pressure (PIP) 35 cm H_2O, positive end-expiratory pressure (PEEP) 6 cm H_2O, and respiratory rate 30.

Prior to starting the procedure, pre- and post-ductal pulse oximetry probes are placed along with bilateral cerebral near-infrared spectroscopy (NIRS) monitors. Differential saturations are noted between the pre- and post-ductal probes, with pre-ductal saturations measuring 92 % versus 76 % post-ductally. An additional peripheral intravenous line is obtained to administer volume, while the indwelling umbilical venous line is set aside for infusions. Anesthesia is then induced and maintained using intermittent fentanyl dosing. To improve hemodynamics and provide a margin of safety during ballooning, epinephrine and calcium chloride infusions are also initiated. An arterial blood gas (ABG) obtained at this time shows a pH 7.23, pCO_2 66 mmHg, pO_2 47 mmHg, base deficit −7.1, and lactate 3.

Given the team's plans to approach the aortic valve through the right common carotid artery, a shoulder roll is placed to the extent the neck and the patient's head and endotracheal tube are turned to the left. Cerebral NIRS and ventilation are unchanged as the artery is accessed. Pressures subsequently obtained from the left ventricle and ascending aorta demonstrate a peak-to-peak gradient of 70 mmHg (peak systolic pressure in the left ventricle − peak systolic pressure in the aorta). With the severity of obstruction confirmed, the valve is then dilated with a 4 mm balloon catheter. This leads to a brief period of hypotension and desaturation that resolve with deflation and withdrawal of the balloon. On repeat measurement, the gradient is now reduced to 40 mmHg with only mild aortic insufficiency. Following a period of stabilization, the valve is ballooned once more using a larger 5 mm catheter. As before, hemodynamic instability ensues, but again resolves following removal of the catheter. A residual gradient of 30 mmHg is now present with unchanged aortic insufficiency.

An immediate improvement in left ventricular systolic function is noted, reflected by both echocardiography and an increase in oxygen saturation. Prograde flow is now observed through the aortic valve, and the extent of mitral regurgitation has decreased. Both factors have led to a decrease in left ventricular end-diastolic pressure and left atrial pressure, resulting in an increase in pulmonary blood flow and a decrease in right-to-left shunting across the ductus arteriosus. Pre-ductal oxygen saturations are now 100 % on a reduced FiO_2 of 0.5, and ventilation is also markedly improved. The post-valvuloplasty ABG is pH 7.29, pCO_2 36, pO_2 60, base deficit −6, and lactate 2.2. Of note, the patient's hematocrit which at the start of the case was 44 is now 25 secondary to hemodilution. Blood is thus transfused to increase oxygen delivery.

No further balloon dilations are planned given the marked clinical improvement observed and the risk of worsening the amount of aortic insufficiency. The patient is transferred to the cardiac intensive care unit stable but critically ill. Over the next 24 h, prostaglandin E1 will be slowly weaned in an attempt to increase left ventricular preload. Issues to be observed closely during this time include (i) the ability of the left ventricle to manage the entire cardiac output as the ductus arteriosus closes and (ii) any progression in the aortic valve insufficiency already present.

Case Scenario #2: The Ross Procedure

A 5-year-old child with a history of critical aortic stenosis status post balloon aortic valvuloplasty presents for aortic valve repair versus replacement. The patient was initially diagnosed on day 1 of life when a murmur was auscultated. Prior to valvuloplasty, the mean gradient across the aortic valve was ~50 mmHg. Following the procedure, the gradient was reduced to 18 mmHg, but moderate aortic insufficiency was noted to develop. Since that time, the patient has been followed with interval echocardiography which now demonstrates moderate aortic stenosis with a mean gradient of 37 mmHg and moderate-to-severe aortic insufficiency. Left ventricular function is preserved, but the ventricle is now severely dilated. Due to the presence of progressive aortic insufficiency in the setting of significant left ventricular dilation, surgical evaluation is requested. A Ross procedure is planned in the event that the valve cannot be repaired. The family questions the advantage of such a procedure over a bioprosthetic or mechanical valve replacement, but ultimately agrees to this plan.

On the day of surgery, the patient presents from home. His only medication is enalapril which was initiated to promote forward flow in the setting of aortic insufficiency. He is premedicated with oral midazolam and, following the placement of standard monitors, undergoes an uneventful inhalational induction with low-dose sevoflurane. Transesophageal echocardiography confirms the diagnosis and demonstrates a competent and adequately sized pulmonary valve. On the initiation of cardiopulmonary bypass, the aortic valve is determined to be irreparable, and so the Ross procedure is undertaken. The post-bypass period is significant only for bleeding requiring platelets, cryoprecipitate, and fresh frozen plasma. No neo-aortic regurgitation or stenosis is noted, and though biventricular function is mildly depressed, the patient is transferred to the intensive care unit on only low-dose epinephrine and milrinone infusions.

On postoperative day 1, however, ST depressions are noted in the inferior electrocardiogram leads along with the new finding of moderately depressed right ventricular function. Given the potential for myocardial ischemia induced by coronary reimplantation, cardiac catheterization with coronary angiography is performed. This reveals proximal right coronary stenosis due to an angulated anastomosis. The patient is thus transferred to the operating room where revision of the anastomosis is conducted. The postoperative course is subsequently uneventful with no further evidence of myocardial ischemia.

Valvular Aortic Stenosis

Congenital valvular aortic stenosis (AS) represents a continuum of anatomic lesions with equally broad clinical manifestations. Differences in the severity of valvular obstruction as well as the presence of associated lesions, such as hypoplasia of the left ventricle, mitral valve, or aortic arch, account for this variability. The most severe end of the spectrum is represented by hypoplastic left heart syndrome (HLHS); on the other end is the individual with mild isolated valvular stenosis with otherwise normal cardiac structures. Clinical presentation can thus range from the critically ill neonate who is ductal-dependent to the asymptomatic child or adolescent (Affolter and Ghanayem 2014). Treatment strategies mirror the diversity of this disease process. Both catheter-based and surgical therapies are employed with the goal of optimizing native valve function until replacement is indicated; often, each therapy is utilized at different points in the management of the same patient.

Anatomy

The normal aortic valve is composed of three equally sized and mobile cusps that coapt centrally (Fig. 23.1). This arrangement is altered in abnormal aortic valves, where cusp size and number may vary, and partial or complete fusion of cusps can

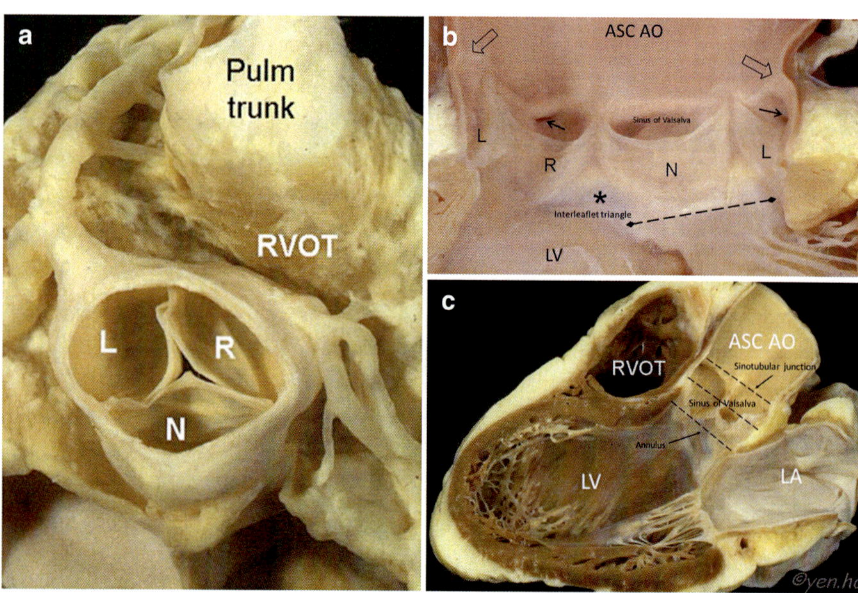

Fig. 23.1 (**a–c**): Anatomy of the aortic valve and root (**a**) Aortic valve in cross section. Each cusp is marked with (*L*), (*R*), and (*N*) representing the left, right, and noncoronary cusps, respectively. The left and right coronary arteries can be observed arising from their respective cusp. Note also how each cusp forms a pocket, termed the sinus of Valsalva. (**b**) Aortic valve viewed with the left cusp transected longitudinally. *Open arrows* note the level of the sinotubular junction, distal to which the ascending aorta (*ASC AO*) begins. Solid black arrows demonstrate the ostia of the right and left coronary arteries. (*R*), (*L*), and (*N*) mark the respective coronary cusps. The triangular space between each cusp is identified as the interleaflet triangle or trigone. The dotted line represents the area of fibrous continuity between the aortic and mitral valves. (**c**) Long-axis view of the left ventricular outflow tract, the aortic root, and the ascending aorta. The aortic root includes all structures between the annulus and the sinotubular junctions (the valve leaflets, their attachments, and the interleaflet triangles). The annulus of the aortic valve, the level of the sinuses of Valsalva, and the sinotubular junction are marked by *dotted lines* (Ho 2009)

occur (Maizza et al. 1993; Roberts 1973). The result is a valve that may feature a decreased orifice size, a compromised leaflet mobility, and an eccentric opening (Allen 2013). The sum of these characteristics determines the degree of stenosis observed. The most common among these abnormal morphologies is the bicuspid aortic valve (Allen 2013). Such a valve occurs in nearly 1.3 % of the general population and is characterized by the partial or complete fusion of two of the aortic valve cusps (Larson and Edwards 1984; Roberts 1970). The conjoined and non-conjoined cusps may be of equal or asymmetric size, and their commissures may be partially fused. Other anomalies of the aortic valve include a unicuspid valve in which two of the three commissures are fused, leaving only a single slit-like opening, and valves in which all three cusps are partially fused, creating a small central orifice. Occasionally, the valve leaflets defy characterization as either bicuspid or unicuspid and are simply described as immature and gelatinous (Elzenga and Gittenberger-de Groot 1985; Morris et al. 1990; Von Rueden et al. 1975). This tends to be true of the valves in neonates with critical aortic stenosis (Jonas and DiNardo 2004). Rarely, stenosis at the valvular level may result from a hypoplastic aortic annulus rather than any abnormality in the valve itself (Reeve and Robinson 1964).

Pathophysiology

Despite the immense variability in the anatomy and presentation of valvular AS, the pathology has a common element: increased left ventricular afterload that ultimately results in an imbalance between myocardial oxygen demand and coronary perfusion. In utero, the increased afterload can result in different phenotypes depending on the severity of the stenosis and the developmental stage at which it occurs (Marantz and Grinenco 2015). Those with lesser degrees of obstruction that develop late in gestation often maintain an adequate left ventricular size and function to accommodate a cardiac output in postnatal life (Allen 2013). Such individuals may present with failure to thrive or tachypnea as infants or may remain asymptomatic throughout childhood. Significant stenosis early in gestation, on the other hand, results in varying cardiac morphologies ranging from HLHS to severe left ventricular dilation (Affolter and Ghanayem 2014; Marantz and Grinenco 2015). The consequence of these more severe manifestations is a left ventricle that cannot manage the systemic circulation. Survival in postnatal life is then dependent on an atrial level shunt and a patent ductus arteriosus ("ductal-dependent" for systemic blood flow). The right ventricle in these cases accepts the bulk or all of the cardiac output and ejects not only to the pulmonary arteries but also systemically through the ductus arteriosus. Ductal closure invariably results in cardiovascular collapse and death.

In the child or adolescent with aortic stenosis, the pathophysiology is comparable to that observed in adults in that myocardial hypertrophy develops in response to the increased afterload (Opie 2004). By Laplace's law (wall stress = pressure × radius/2 × wall thickness), hypertrophy acts to reduce wall stress while maintaining stroke volume and cardiac output, but at the expense of an increased left ventricular end-diastolic pressure (LVEDP) and increased myocardial oxygen demand (Donner et al. and 1983). Coronary blood flow can thus be compromised as the gradient between aortic end-diastolic pressure and LVEDP diminishes. Conditions that decrease diastolic blood pressure or increase myocardial oxygen demand can thus predispose toward ischemia, myocardial dysfunction, and arrhythmias. At greatest risk is the subendocardium due to the high compressive forces at this location and distance from the epicardial coronary arteries (Allen 2013). In utero, marked elevations in intracavitary pressures and increased myocardial oxygen demand can result in endomyocardial fibroelastosis (EFE), which can further contribute to postnatal ventricular dysfunction (Alsoufi et al. and 2007). If untreated, aortic stenosis ultimately overwhelms the left ventricle's compensatory mechanisms and congestive heart failure ensues.

Critical Aortic Stenosis of the Neonate

Nearly 10 % of patients with congenital valvular AS present within the first year of life (Brown et al. 2003; Hastreiter et al. and 1963; McCrindle et al. 2001). Those who develop signs of failure as the ductus arteriosus closes are deemed to have critical aortic stenosis. Such neonates may present in cardiogenic shock as both systemic and coronary blood flow are compromised due to ductal closure. End-organ injury, myocardial ischemia, acidosis, and ultimately death result if untreated. Resuscitation entails the initiation of prostaglandin E1 to reopen the ductus and the use of inotropic and ventilatory support as needed to maximize oxygen delivery.

Definitive management is guided by the central decision of whether to employ a strategy of single-ventricle palliation versus biventricular repair (Alsoufi et al. 2007). Guiding this decision are factors such as the degree of left-sided hypoplasia observed and the presence of associated lesions like ventricular septal defects, arch hypoplasia, or coarctation of the aorta (Fig. 23.2). Those with severe hypoplasia of the left ventricle and mitral valve can proceed down the pathway of the Norwood procedure, the hybrid procedure, or heart transplantation depending on institutional preference and organ availability. Alternatively, if the neonate were to have only isolated critical AS with otherwise adequately sized structures, a strategy conducive to biventricular repair would be chosen. The "gray area" between these two extremes, however, presents a dilemma. Several studies have attempted to identify predictive factors to assist in the process of assessing the adequacy of the left ventricle to accommodate the systemic circulation (Hammon et al. 1988; Lofland et al. 2001; Rhodes et al. and 1991; Schwartz et al. 2001). Commonly referenced is the regression equation developed by the Congenital Heart Surgeons' Society that is used to predict 5-year survival probability with Norwood-type palliation versus a biventricular approach (Lofland et al. 2001). Parameters assessed included patient age, grade of endomyocardial fibroelastosis, z-score of the aortic valve and left ventricular length, ascending aorta diameter, and the presence of significant tricuspid

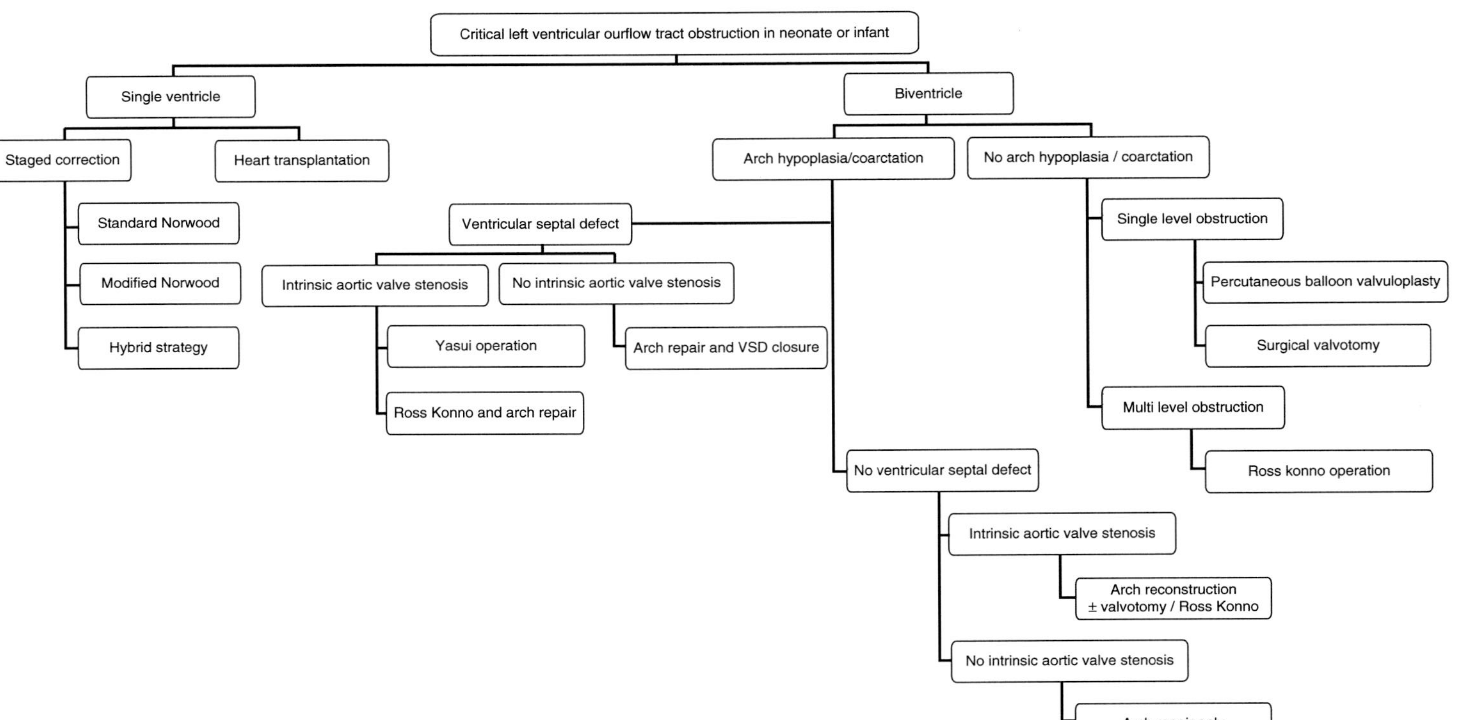

Fig. 23.2 Management options in neonates with critical left ventricular outflow tract obstruction (Alsoufi et al. 2007)

regurgitation. Underscoring the significance of appropriate initial therapy is data suggesting invariably worse outcomes when "crossover" between strategies is required (Rhodes et al. 1991).

For those neonates with isolated critical AS and adequate left heart structures, initial therapy entails either balloon or surgical valvuloplasty. No prospective randomized trials have compared outcomes between these techniques, and retrospective studies have yielded mixed data (McCrindle et al. 2001; Rehnstrom et al. 2007; Siddiqui et al. 2013). Confounding comparisons has been the evolution of both catheter-based and surgical techniques. Whereas surgical repair was once limited to rigid aortic valve dilation or blade commissurotomy, current techniques are more refined and include resection of nodular dysplasia and reconstruction of the aortic valve leaflets (Fig. 23.3) (Siddiqui et al. 2013). Such repairs, however, require cardiopulmonary bypass. Similar advances have been made in catheter

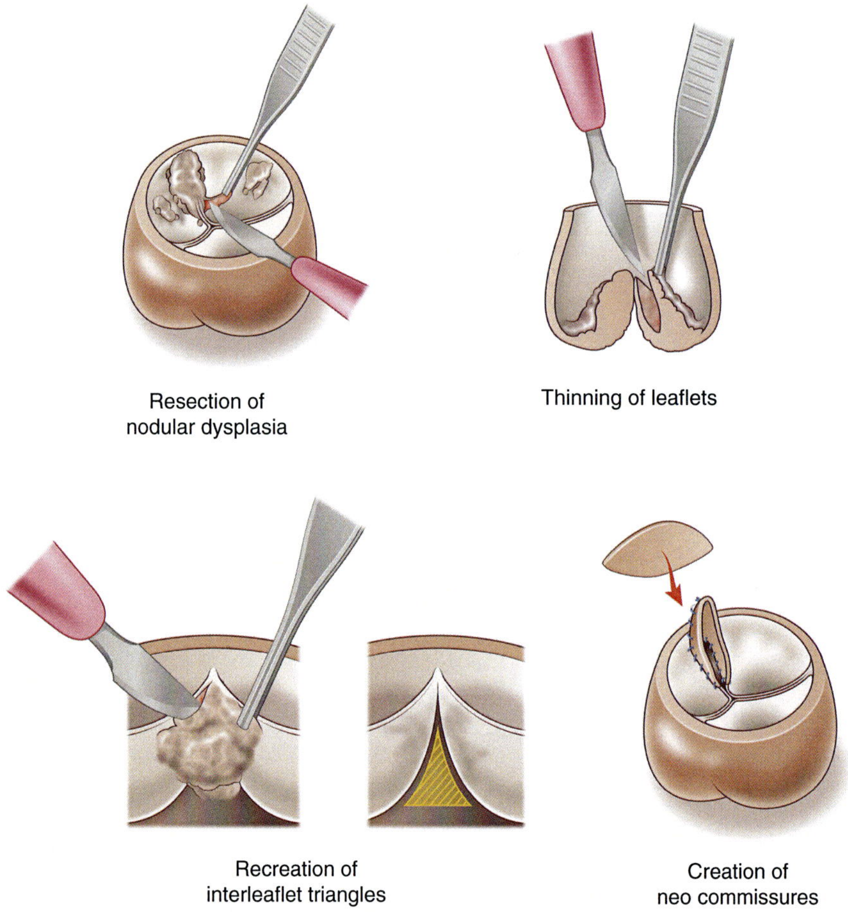

Fig. 23.3 Surgical techniques for the repair of critical aortic stenosis (Siddiqui et al. 2013)

technology, with improvements in the balloons and wires used in valvular dilation (Stapleton 2014).

Technical considerations of note in patients undergoing balloon valvuloplasty include the site of vascular access and potential use of rapid right ventricular pacing (Stapleton 2014). Either the femoral vessels or the right common carotid is commonly accessed. If the femoral vein is used, the aortic valve is approached antegrade; this route, however, is challenging as it requires passage across the atrial septum and through a potentially small left ventricle. The arrhythmias induced by catheter manipulation may exacerbate hemodynamic instability in an already tenuous patient. If the femoral artery is used, the aortic valve is approached retrograde. The most direct and expedient course to the aortic valve is achieved through the right common carotid. Long-term patency of this vessel does not appear to be affected (Borghi et al. 2001) if cannulated. If this approach is chosen, monitoring of cerebral oxygenation with cutaneous near-infrared spectroscopy probes may be useful to detect early signs of cerebral ischemia. Given the proximity of the catheters to the airway in this scenario, airway access may also be compromised. Vigilance is thus necessary to ensure that the endotracheal tube, if used, is not displaced or kinked. Rapid ventricular pacing is applied at the discretion of the interventional cardiologist at the time of balloon dilation. This serves to decrease left ventricular stroke volume, thereby minimizing the potential of balloon displacement during inflation with the associated risk of trauma to the aortic valve leaflets (Stapleton 2014).

While some degree of aortic insufficiency is expected following balloon dilation, the introduction of severe aortic insufficiency can be catastrophic. A recent series reported a 2% incidence of severe insufficiency immediately post-ballooning (Brown et al. 2010; Petit et al. 2012). The additional volume load imposed on the left ventricle by the regurgitant valve increases left ventricular end-diastolic pressure and, in concert with lower aortic end-diastolic pressure, may produce marked myocardial ischemia. Emergent valve repair or replacement is necessary in this circumstance to prevent myocardial infarction. Even in those who have only minimal insufficiency following initial ballooning, progression may occur over time such that one-third of patients have moderate-to-severe regurgitation at 10 years postprocedure (Stapleton 2014). As balloon valvuloplasty is a palliative therapy whose goal is not complete elimination but improvement of the stenosis, the need for reintervention is high. Over two-thirds of neonates undergoing balloon valvuloplasty require either repeat ballooning or surgical intervention at 10 years following the procedure (Brown et al. 2010; McElhinney et al. and 2005).

Rarely, aortic valve replacement is necessary in the neonate or infant with critical AS (Alsoufi et al. 2007). Indications include the presence of complex multilevel left ventricular obstruction, significant aortic regurgitation that develops during balloon valvuloplasty, or stenosis refractory to balloon valvuloplasty or surgical valvotomy. Options include the use of a mechanical valve, bioprosthetic valve, or the patient's own pulmonary valve. All such valves have drawbacks unique to the young and growing patient. Limitations common to bioprosthetic and mechanical valves include their lack of growth potential and subsequent need for frequent reoperation.

Bioprosthetic valves moreover undergo accelerated degeneration as early as 2 years after valve replacement (Gallo et al. 1988; Clarke et al. 1993; Mavroudis and Backer 2013). Mechanical valves, in contrast, are more durable but suffer from thromboembolic complications that require long-term warfarin anticoagulation (Allen 2013; Mazzitelli et al. 1998).

The Ross procedure may be offered as an alternative when the patient's pulmonary valve is of an adequate size and without stenosis or regurgitation (Al-Halees et al. 2002; Bansal et al. 2015; Kadner et al. 2008; Nelson et al. 2015; Ohye et al. 2001; Williams et al. 2005). This operation entails removing the stenotic aortic valve and replacing it with the patient's own pulmonary valve. A homograft is then used to reconstruct the right ventricular outflow tract. The advantage of this procedure is that the pulmonary valve maintains its potential for growth in the aortic position, is durable, and does not require anticoagulation. Concerns following the Ross procedure include (i) the need for interval replacement of the homograft used to reconstruct the right ventricular outflow tract, (ii) dilation of the neo-aortic root, and (iii) progressive neo-aortic regurgitation and stenosis (Nelson et al. 2015; Stulak et al. 2010). Due to the critically ill state in which neonates and infants who are in need of valve replacement present, mortality following this operation is high, ranging from 12 to 75 % (Brancaccio et al. 2014; Kadner et al. 2008; Kirkpatrick et al. 2008; Tan Tanny et al. 2013). The use of postoperative extracorporeal membrane oxygenation (ECMO) is occasionally needed (Mascio et al. 2014; Shinkawa et al. 2010).

Irrespective of the initial therapy chosen, principles of anesthetic management focus on supporting myocardial function, balancing systemic and pulmonary blood flow, and optimizing oxygen delivery. In the neonate presenting in cardiogenic shock, therapy consists of continuing or initiating prostaglandin E1, inotropic and/or vasopressor support, and mechanical ventilation (Affolter and Ghanayem 2014). Both epinephrine and dopamine appear to be effective inotropes in neonates (Barrington et al. 1995; Valverde et al. 2006). Vasopressor support, while useful in maintaining diastolic pressure, may also compromise splanchnic perfusion and worsen left ventricular function by increasing afterload. The benefits of such agents must be weighed against the potential for these risks. When choosing ventilatory settings, care should be taken to avoid increasing pulmonary blood flow at the expense of systemic and coronary perfusion. Increases in inspired oxygen or hyperventilation may decrease pulmonary vascular resistance, resulting in increased left-to-right shunting through the ductus in diastole. Diastolic hypotension and reduced pulmonary compliance may ensue. In the subgroup of neonates with significant lung injury, however, increased inspired oxygen and aggressive ventilation may be necessary to achieve even marginal gas exchange. The choice of anesthetic often includes a combination of opioids and benzodiazepines; most drugs can be utilized safely assuming that doses are titrated to maintain hemodynamics while providing analgesia and minimizing oxygen consumption. Given the potential for blood loss or hemodilution with intervention, blood should also be readily available.

The Child or Adolescent with Valvular Aortic Stenosis

In contrast to the neonate or infant with critical AS, older children and adolescents with valvular obstruction are commonly asymptomatic (Allen 2013). This reflects the milder degree of stenosis initially present in these individuals (Mavroudis and Backer 2013) as well as the relatively slow rate of stenotic progression (Allen 2013). On average, the transvalvular gradient increases by 1 mmHg per year (Davis et al. 2008); the exception occurs in children whose somatic growth greatly exceeds that of their stenotic aortic valve. When symptoms do occur, easy fatigability is most often reported (Ellison et al. 1976). Dyspnea on exertion, angina, and syncope can also occur as in adults, but are relatively uncommon even in those with severe stenosis (Wagner et al. 1977).

Clinical severity is assigned based on catheter-derived or Doppler-derived gradients (Table 23.1, (Maron and Zipes 2005)). Peak-to-peak pressure gradients are catheter-derived and reflect the difference between peak left ventricular and peak aortic pressures. Peak instantaneous gradients, on the other hand, are Doppler-derived and reflect the point in time in which the velocity of blood across the aortic valve is greatest. These pressure gradients thus provide different data points and should not be used interchangeably (Beekman et al. 1992).

Factors influencing the gradient beyond the extent of valvular stenosis include the patient's ventricular function and hemodynamic state at the time of measurement. Depressed ventricular function serves to underestimate one's gradient, whereas increased contractility and tachycardia may significantly increase the gradient recorded. Likewise, gradients obtained under deep sedation or anesthesia can underestimate the extent of obstruction present during normal activity. Such variables require consideration when determining the severity of valvular stenosis.

Timing of intervention is guided by an assessment of the measured gradient, ventricular function, symptoms, and the patient's level of activity (Allen 2013; Feltes et al. 2011). Those with peak-to-peak gradients >50 mmHg have an absolute indication for intervention even if asymptomatic given the increased and progressive risk of myocardial injury and sudden cardiac death. Individuals who wish to be active, have symptoms of angina or syncope, or have ischemic changes on exercise stress testing are directed toward intervention even with peak-to-peak gradients between 40 and 50 mmHg. Intervention is not recommended in the

Table 23.1 Categorizing severity of valvular aortic stenosis (Maron and Zipes 2005)

	Catheter-derived peak-to-peak gradient	Mean Doppler gradient	Peak instantaneous Doppler gradient
Mild	<30 mmHg	<25 mmHg	<40 mmHg
Moderate	30–50 mmHg	25–40 mmHg	40–70 mmHg
Severe	>50 mmHg	>40 mmHg	>70 mmHg

Assuming normal ventricular function and no shunting lesions asymptomatic patient with a peak-to-peak gradient <40 mmHg unless ventricular function is also depressed.

As with neonates and infants, management options in children and adolescents include balloon valvuloplasty and surgical valve repair or replacement. Both balloon valvuloplasty and surgical valve repair are palliative therapies whose goals include reducing ventricular afterload and delaying the need for valve replacement. When valve replacement is indicated due to either progressive regurgitation or recurrent stenosis refractory to ballooning, options include the use of a mechanical valve, bioprosthetic valve, or pulmonary valve autograft. None are ideal. Both mechanical and bioprosthetic valves commit the child to future valve replacement due to their inability to grow. Mechanical valves, moreover, require anticoagulation. The pulmonary autograft or Ross procedure, while providing a durable and functional neo-aortic valve, also requires subsequent reoperation. Compared to neonates and infants, reoperation on the neo-aortic valve is more common in children and adolescents undergoing the Ross procedure; reintervention on the right ventricular outflow tract, however, is less common (Nelson et al. 2015).

Anesthetic goals entail maintaining preload, afterload, and contractility while targeting a normal to low-normal heart rate. Extended periods without fluid intake or the use of agents that significantly diminish preload or afterload can place the patient at risk for hypotension with the induction of anesthesia. Minimizing the fasting period or placing a preoperative intravenous catheter to give fluids can help decrease this risk. In the individual with significant aortic stenosis, low diastolic pressures can quickly produce a sequence of myocardial ischemia, ventricular dysfunction, bradycardia, and cardiac arrest. Alternatively, significantly increased contractility and tachycardia due to an inadequate level of anesthesia can also cause subendocardial ischemia. Careful titration of drugs while monitoring hemodynamics is thus essential to balance myocardial oxygen demand and supply.

Case Scenario #3

A 13-month-old infant with Williams syndrome presents for repair of (i) supravalvular aortic stenosis (SVAS), (ii) supravalvular pulmonary stenosis, and (iii) bilateral branch pulmonary stenosis. Preoperative evaluation with transthoracic echocardiography demonstrates:

- Severe "hourglass" narrowing of the supravalvular aortic area with a peak velocity of 4.6 m/s
- Mild narrowing at the level of the transverse aortic arch and isthmus
- Moderate supravalvular pulmonary stenosis
- Moderate-to-severe diffuse hypoplasia of the branch pulmonary arteries
- Normal biventricular systolic function with moderate biventricular hypertrophy

A cardiac computed tomography angiogram (CTA) is also obtained and reveals the additional findings of mild hooding of the coronary arteries and discrete stenosis just distal to the left coronary ostium. No evidence of renal artery stenosis was seen and no other end-organ anomalies were identified. The patient is asymptomatic. On airway evaluation, mild mandibular hypoplasia is observed.

On the evening prior to surgery, the patient is admitted so that intravenous fluids can be administered during the fasting period. Anesthetic consent, including a discussion of the high risk of cardiac arrest during the pre-bypass period, is obtained. The family asks if there were any contingency plans if such an arrest were to occur, and the possibilities of extracorporeal membrane oxygenation (ECMO) or emergent initiation of cardiopulmonary bypass are presented.

The next morning, the availability of additional anesthesia staff, the surgeon, and the perfusionist is confirmed prior to entering the operating room. Blood has been delivered and checked, and the perfusionist is in the process of priming the bypass circuit. Having ensured the presence of the necessary personnel and equipment, intravenous premedication with midazolam is given, and the patient is brought to the operating room.

Following the placement of monitors, the patient is induced with fentanyl and 2 % sevoflurane. The airway is secured after the onset of muscle relaxant. Shortly thereafter, marked ST depressions are noted on the EKG with sinus tachycardia at a rate of 160. The noninvasive blood pressure cuff measures 70/30. While confirming the presence of end-tidal CO_2 and bilateral breath sounds, boluses of phenylephrine and volume are given until the ST segments normalize. An infusion of vasopressin is initiated, and as help arrives, invasive arterial and central venous lines are obtained. The nursing team preps and drapes the patient, and the surgeon prepares for incision. Within 30 min, cardiopulmonary bypass is commenced.

The operation entails a (i) Doty pericardial patch repair of the supravalvular aortic and pulmonary stenoses and (ii) homograft enlargement of the branch pulmonary arteries. On direct inspection, neither coronary hooding nor left proximal coronary stenosis is observed.

Separation from bypass occurs uneventfully on milrinone and esmolol infusions. Postoperative echocardiography reveals no residual supravalvular or branch pulmonary obstruction and hyperdynamic biventricular function. Extubation is achieved on postoperative day 1, and the patient is discharged home on postoperative day 5.

Supravalvular Aortic Stenosis

While rare in the general population, supravalvular aortic stenosis (SVAS) occurs in nearly 45–75 % of those with Williams-Beuren (Williams) syndrome (Collins 2013; Eronen et al. 2002). Other familial or sporadic forms account for the remainder of SVAS cases observed. Though the obstruction generally occurs at the level of the sinotubular junction, all areas of the aortic root can be affected, including the coronary arteries and aortic valve leaflets. Such multilevel obstruction substantially increases the risk of myocardial ischemia and cardiac arrest during anesthesia (Burch et al. 2008; Matisoff et al. 2015). Given the underlying defect in the elastin gene (Nickerson et al. 1995), other large vessels can also be involved, including the descending aorta and pulmonary, brachiocephalic, mesenteric, and renal arteries (Burch et al. 2008; Pober et al. 2008). This variability in the structures affected and the subsequent risk imparted illustrate the complexity of this disease and the challenge in managing it.

Anatomy and Pathophysiology

Supravalvular aortic stenosis is classified as either diffuse or localized (Mavoroudis and Backer 2013). The majority have stenosis localized to the sinotubular junction, resulting in the characteristic hourglass appearance of the ascending aorta. Approximately 25 % of patients, however, have diffuse stenosis that can extend to the aortic arch (Kim et al. 1999; Stamm et al. 1997). Thickening at the sinotubular junction produces a narrowed aortic outflow that results in an increased afterload on the left ventricle, hypertension in the aortic root, and limited excursion of the aortic valve leaflets in systole (Mavroudis and Backer 2013). The valve cusps, moreover, can become adherent to the enlarging ridge (Flaker et al. 1983; Peterson et al. 1965). When this occurs, blood flow into the sinuses of Valsalva, and thus coronary blood flow, can be restricted. Compounding the potential for diminished coronary blood flow are anomalies of the coronary arteries themselves. Due to the severe hypertension in the aortic root, coronary artery disease can develop, with the most profound changes occurring proximally (Kim et al. 1999; Stamm et al. 1997). Moreover, the same process that leads to thickening of the aorta can also extend to and narrow the coronary ostia, further limiting coronary flow (Meairs et al. 1984).

Supravalvar pulmonary stenosis (SVPS) commonly occurs in combination with SVAS and is observed in nearly 83 % of those with Williams syndrome (Bruno et al. 2003; Collins 2013; Eronen et al. 2002). This stenosis tends to be peripheral and diffuse, but central or discrete focal stenosis can also occur. In contrast to SVAS which tends to progress with time, SVPS may spontaneously regress (Giddins et al. 1989; Wren et al. 1990).

Congenital abnormalities of the aortic valve are uncommon, but, as noted previously, can develop due to exposure to high systolic pressures and adherence of the valve cusps to the thickened sinotubular ridge. Both valvular stenosis and insufficiency can occur.

These changes, in sum, produce a patient with increased myocardial oxygen demand and diminished myocardial oxygen supply. As in the patient with valvular AS, left ventricular hypertrophy develops in response to the increased afterload. The patient with SVAS, however, may also have right ventricular hypertrophy due to supravalvular pulmonary stenosis. Both ventricles, then, can be at risk for ischemia. Compounding this problem are the multifactorial reductions in coronary blood flow. Decreases in diastolic blood pressure or increases in myocardial demand can thus lead to biventricular subendocardial ischemia, fibrosis, papillary muscle infarction, and sudden death.

Table 23.2 Characteristics associated with low-, moderate-, and high-risk patients with Williams syndrome

Low risk	Moderate risk	High risk
Normal EKG	Mild stenosis of a branch pulmonary artery	Severe SVAS (>40 mmHg)
Normal echocardiogram	Hypertension	Symptoms or EKG findings consistent with ischemia
Minimal extracardiac anomalies	Mild-to-moderate SVAS (< 40 mmHg)	Coronary disease demonstrated on imaging
	Other mild cardiac anomalies (e.g., ventricular septal defect)	Severe left ventricular hypertrophy
	Repaired SVAS or SVPS without residual gradients	Biventricular outflow tract disease
	Mild left ventricular hypertrophy	Prolonged QTc on EKG
	Mild-to-moderate SVPS in isolation	
	Significant extracardiac disease such as difficult airway or severe gastroesophageal reflux	

Adapted from Matisoff et al. (2015)

Anesthetic Risk Assessment

Although no prospective studies have evaluated risk factors for anesthesia in patients with SVAS, consensus opinion based on experience and known risk factors for myocardial ischemia can be offered (Matisoff et al. 2015). Those at greatest risk appear to be patients with (i) biventricular outflow tract obstruction, (ii) moderate-to-severe SVAS (>40 mmHg), (iii) documented coronary anomalies, and (iv) symptoms or electrocardiogram signs consistent with ischemia, such as QT prolongation or ST-T wave abnormalities (Table 23.2). While the majority of patients may be asymptomatic, symptoms including angina, syncope, dyspnea on exertion, and diaphoresis with feeds have been noted in those with severe disease.

Treatment

Surgery is the recommended therapy for SVAS. Balloon dilation and stenting have been reported (Jacob et al. 1993; Pinto et al. 1994), but have significant risk due to the proximity of both the coronaries and aortic valve to the supravalvular obstruction (Allen 2013). This modality is generally reserved for the management of isolated peripheral pulmonary stenosis (Mavroudis and Backer 2013). Indications for surgery include a Doppler-derived mean gradient of greater than 40–50 mmHg or the presence of symptoms (Mavroudis and Backer 2013). Given the progressive nature of this disease, early surgery is often recommended. Preoperative evaluation may include computed tomography, cardiac catheterization, or magnetic resonance imaging. The benefits of such procedures, though, must be weighed against the risks of anesthesia (if needed to complete these studies).

Preferred surgical techniques to address SVAS include enlarging the aorta using either an inverted bifurcated patch or three individual patches in each of the sinuses of Valsalva (Doty et al. 1977; Hazekamp et al. 1999). Resection of the stenosis with an end-to-end anastomosis has also been used in patients with discrete obstruction. If the stenosis is more diffuse, a combined ascending aorta and arch patch plasty may be needed (Mavroudis and Backer 2013). For those with simultaneous involvement of the coronary arteries and aortic valve, the Ross procedure can be offered. Given that all of these procedures are performed with cardiopulmonary bypass, any associated lesions such as supravalvular or peripheral pulmonary stenosis are also addressed at the time of aortic repair.

Anesthetic Management

As for any complex patient, multidisciplinary communication and planning are needed to optimize outcome. The patient with SVAS should be evaluated prior to the day of surgery, and contingency plans in the event of a cardiac arrest, including the deployment of extracorporeal membrane oxygenation (ECMO), should be discussed. An assessment of organ systems beyond the heart and vasculature may also yield pertinent findings. In Williams syndrome, evidence of gastrointestinal reflux, hypercalcemia, and hypothyroidism may be present (Matisoff et al. 2015). Mandibular hypoplasia and malocclusion can also be observed and predispose to a difficult tracheal intubation.

Hemodynamic goals focus on maintaining preload, afterload, and contractility while avoiding tachycardia. Ensuring adequate preoperative hydration is critical, and this can be achieved either through minimizing the period of fasting or obtaining intravenous access for fluid administration. Prior to induction, premedication with midazolam may reduce anxiety and thus decrease the risk of myocardial ischemia associated with tachycardia or hypertension. Counterintuitively, ketamine may also be used for this purpose or to facilitate obtaining intravenous access. Though ketamine has the potential to increase heart rate, it also maintains contractility and systemic vascular resistance (SVR). Low doses can thus be useful in the management of these patients. Induction of anesthesia can be achieved with either inhalational or intravenous agents (or a combination of the two); it should be noted, however, that in high-risk patients, cardiac arrest has occurred even with low and incremental dosing of sevoflurane (Burch et al. 2008). Options for intravenous induction agents include etomidate, ketamine, and fentanyl (Andrzejowski and Mundy 2000; Burch et al. 2008; Horowitz et al. 2002; Kohase et al. and 2007; Matisoff et al. 2015; Medley et al. 2005). Any number of agents can be used to maintain anesthesia, but a balanced anesthetic with volatile agent and narcotic that allows for the preservation of SVR and contractility may be ideal.

Because of the rapidity with which decompensation can occur, vigilance is needed to identify initial signs of myocardial ischemia, most commonly heralded by ST changes. Phenylephrine should be administered to increase SVR if ST changes are observed, and either a phenylephrine or vasopressin infusion can be initiated to maintain SVR. In the event of an impending or actual cardiac arrest, epinephrine (and other standard resuscitation drugs) should also be available along with blood for the priming of an ECMO or bypass circuit. Beyond the induction period, other times of risk that merit increased vigilance include emergence due to the potential for hypertension, tachycardia, hypercapnia, and hypoxemia.

Those with a history of SVAS or SVPS who present for noncardiac surgery following repair should be assessed for any residual gradients or persistent symptoms. Such patients, and particularly those with a history of diffuse SVAS, can remain at high risk even after aortic reconstruction. Preoperative planning for such patients should include not only a discussion of intraoperative strategy but also preoperative admission for hydration and postoperative disposition.

References

Affolter JT, Ghanayem NS. Preoperative management of the neonate with critical aortic valvar stenosis. Cardiol Young. 2014;24(6):1111–6. doi:10.1017/S1047951114002029.

Al-Halees Z, Pieters F, Qadoura F, Shahid M, Al-Amri M, Al-Fadley F. The Ross procedure is the procedure of choice for congenital aortic valve disease. J Thorac Cardiovasc Surg. 2002;123(3):437–41; discussion 441–432.

Allen HD. Moss and Adams heart disease in infants, children, and adolescents : including the fetus and young adult. 8th ed. Philadelphia: Wolters Kluwer Health/Lippincott Williams & Wilkins; 2013.

Alsoufi B, Karamlou T, McCrindle BW, Caldarone CA. Management options in neonates and infants with critical left ventricular outflow tract obstruction. Eur J Cardiothorac Surg. 2007;31(6):1013–21. doi:10.1016/j.ejcts.2007.03.015.

Andrzejowski J, Mundy J. Anaesthesia for MRI angiography in a patient with Williams syndrome. Anaesthesia. 2000;55(1):97–8.

Bansal N, Kumar SR, Baker CJ, Lemus R, Wells WJ, Starnes VA. Age-related outcomes of the ross procedure over 20 years. Ann Thorac Surg. 2015;99(6):2077–83. doi:10.1016/j.athoracsur.2015.02.066; discussion 2084–2075.

Barrington KJ, Finer NN, Chan WK. A blind, randomized comparison of the circulatory effects of dopamine and epinephrine infusions in the newborn piglet during normoxia and hypoxia. Crit Care Med. 1995;23(4):740–8.

Beekman RH, Rocchini AP, Gillon JH, Mancini GB. Hemodynamic determinants of the peak systolic left ventricular-aortic pressure gradient in children with valvar aortic stenosis. Am J Cardiol. 1992;69(8):813–5.

Borghi A, Agnoletti G, Poggiani C. Surgical cutdown of the right carotid artery for aortic balloon valvuloplasty in infancy: midterm follow-up. Pediatr Cardiol. 2001;22(3):194–7. doi:10.1007/s002460010202.

Brancaccio G, Polito A, Hoxha S, Gandolfo F, Giannico S, Amodeo A, Carotti A. The ross procedure in patients aged less than 18 years: the midterm results. J Thorac Cardiovasc Surg. 2014;147(1):383–8. doi:10.1016/j.jtcvs.2013.02.037.

Brown DW, Dipilato AE, Chong EC, Lock JE, McElhinney DB. Aortic valve reinterventions after balloon aortic valvuloplasty for congenital aortic stenosis intermediate and late follow-up. J Am Coll Cardiol. 2010;56(21):1740–9. doi:10.1016/j.jacc.2010.06.040.

Brown JW, Ruzmetov M, Vijay P, Rodefeld MD, Turrentine MW. Surgery for aortic stenosis in children: a 40-year experience. Ann Thorac Surg. 2003;76(5):1398–411.

Bruno E, Rossi N, Thuer O, Cordoba R, Alday LE. Cardiovascular findings, and clinical course, in patients with Williams syndrome. Cardiol Young. 2003;13(6):532–6.

Burch TM, McGowan Jr FX, Kussman BD, Powell AJ, DiNardo JA. Congenital supravalvular aortic stenosis and sudden death associated with anesthesia: what's the mystery? Anesth Analg. 2008;107(6):1848–54. doi:10.1213/ane.0b013e3181875a4d.

Clarke D, Campbell D, Hayward A, Bishop D. Degeneration of aortic valve allografts in young recipients. J Thorac Cardiovasc Surg. 1993;105(5):934–41.

Collins 2nd RT. Cardiovascular disease in Williams syndrome. Circulation. 2013;127(21):2125–34. doi:10.1161/CIRCULATIONAHA.112.000064.

Davis CK, Cummings MW, Gurka MJ, Gutgesell HP. Frequency and degree of change of peak transvalvular pressure gradient determined by two Doppler echocardiographic examinations in newborns and children with valvular congenital aortic stenosis. Am J Cardiol. 2008;101(3):393–5. doi:10.1016/j.amjcard.2007.08.044.

Donner R, Carabello BA, Black I, Spann JF. Left ventricular wall stress in compensated aortic stenosis in children. Am J Cardiol. 1983;51(6):946–51.

Doty DB, Polansky DB, Jenson CB. Supravalvular aortic stenosis. Repair by extended aortoplasty. J Thorac Cardiovasc Surg. 1977;74(3):362–71.

Ellison RC, Wagner HR, Weidman WH, Miettinen OS. Congenital valvular aortic stenosis: clinical detection of small pressure gradient. Prepared for the joint study on the joint study on the natural history of congenital heart defects. Am J Cardiol. 1976;37(5):757–61.

Elzenga NJ, Gittenberger-de Groot AC. Coarctation and related aortic arch anomalies in hypoplastic left heart syndrome. Int J Cardiol. 1985;8(4):379–93.

Eronen M, Peippo M, Hiippala A, Raatikka M, Arvio M, Johansson R, Kahkonen M. Cardiovascular manifestations in 75 patients with Williams syndrome. J Med Genet. 2002;39(8):554–8.

Feltes TF, Bacha E, Beekman RH, Cheatham JP, Feinstein JA, Gomes AS, Hijazi ZM, Ing FF, de Moor M, Morrow WR, Mullins CE, Taubert KA, Zahn EM, American Heart Association Congenital Cardiac Defects Committee of the Council on Cardiovascular Disease in the Young, Council on Clinical Cardiology, Council on Cardiovascular Radiology and Intervention, American Heart, A. Indications for cardiac catheterization and intervention in pediatric cardiac disease: a scientific statement from the American Heart Association. Circulation. 2011;123(22):2607–52. doi:10.1161/CIR.0b013e31821b1f10.

Flaker G, Teske D, Kilman J, Hosier D, Wooley C. Supravalvular aortic stenosis. A 20-year clinical perspective and experience with patch aortoplasty. Am J Cardiol. 1983;51(2):256–60.

Gallo I, Nistal F, Blasquez R, Arbe E, Artinano E. Incidence of primary tissue valve failure in porcine bioprosthetic heart valves. Ann Thorac Surg. 1988;45(1):66–70.

Giddins NG, Finley JP, Nanton MA, Roy DL. The natural course of supravalvar aortic stenosis and peripheral pulmonary artery stenosis in Williams's syndrome. Br Heart J. 1989;62(4):315–9.

Hammon Jr JW, Lupinetti FM, Maples MD, Merrill WH, First WH, Graham Jr TP, Bender Jr HW. Predictors of operative mortality in critical valvular aortic stenosis presenting in infancy. Ann Thorac Surg. 1988;45(5):537–40.

Hastreiter AR, Oshima M, Miller RA, Lev M, Paul MH. Congenital aortic stenosis syndrome in infancy. Circulation. 1963;28:1084–95.

Hazekamp MG, Kappetein AP, Schoof PH, Ottenkamp J, Witsenburg M, Huysmans HA, Bogers AJ. Brom's three-patch technique for repair of supravalvular aortic stenosis. J Thorac Cardiovasc Surg. 1999;118(2):252–8. doi:10.1016/S0022-5223(99)70215-1.

Ho SY. Structure and anatomy of the aortic root. Eur J Echocardiogr. 2009;10(1):i3–10. doi:10.1093/ejechocard/jen243.

Horowitz PE, Akhtar S, Wulff JA, Al Fadley F, Al Halees Z. Coronary artery disease and anesthesia-related death in children with Williams syndrome. J Cardiothorac Vasc Anesth. 2002;16(6):739–41. doi:10.1053/jcan.2002.128407.

Jacob JL, Coelho WM, Machado NC, Garzon SA. Initial experience with balloon dilatation of supravalvar aortic stenosis. Br Heart J. 1993;70(5):476–8.

Jonas RA, DiNardo JA. Comprehensive surgical management of congenital heart disease. London/New York: Arnold; Distributed in the United States of America by Oxford University Press; 2004.

Kadner A, Raisky O, Degandt A, Tamisier D, Bonnet D, Sidi D, Vouhe PR. The Ross procedure in infants and young children. Ann Thorac Surg. 2008;85(3):803–8. doi:10.1016/j.athoracsur.2007.07.047.

Kim YM, Yoo SJ, Choi JY, Kim SH, Bae EJ, Lee YT. Natural course of supravalvar aortic stenosis and peripheral pulmonary arterial stenosis in Williams' syndrome. Cardiol Young. 1999;9(1):37–41.

Kirkpatrick E, Hurwitz R, Brown J. A single center's experience with the Ross procedure in pediatrics. Pediatr Cardiol. 2008;29(5):894–900. doi:10.1007/s00246-008-9224-1.

Kohase H, Wakita R, Doi S, Umino M. General anesthesia for dental treatment in a Williams syndrome patient with severe aortic and pulmonary valve stenosis: suspected episode of postoperatively malignant hyperthermia. Oral Surg Oral Med Oral Pathol Oral Radiol Endod. 2007;104(4):e17–20. doi:10.1016/j.tripleo.2007.04.013.

Larson EW, Edwards WD. Risk factors for aortic dissection: a necropsy study of 161 cases. Am J Cardiol. 1984;53(6):849–55.

Lofland GK, McCrindle BW, Williams WG, Blackstone EH, Tchervenkov CI, Sittiwangkul R, Jonas RA. Critical aortic stenosis in the neonate: a multi-institutional study of management, outcomes, and risk factors. Congenital Heart Surgeons Society. J Thorac Cardiovasc Surg. 2001;121(1):10–27.

Maizza AF, Ho SY, Anderson RH. Obstruction of the left ventricular outflow tract: anatomical observations and surgical implications. J Heart Valve Dis. 1993;2(1):66–79.

Marantz P, Grinenco S. Fetal intervention for critical aortic stenosis: advances, research and postnatal follow-up. Curr Opin Cardiol. 2015;30(1):89–94. doi:10.1097/HCO.0000000000000128.

Maron BJ, Zipes DP. Introduction: eligibility recommendations for competitive athletes with cardiovascular abnormalities-general considerations. J Am Coll Cardiol. 2005;45(8):1318–21. doi:10.1016/j.jacc.2005.02.006.

Mascio CE, Austin 3rd EH, Jacobs JP, Jacobs ML, Wallace AS, He X, Pasquali SK. Perioperative mechanical circulatory support in children: an analysis of the Society of Thoracic Surgeons Congenital Heart Surgery Database. J Thorac Cardiovasc Surg. 2014;147(2):658–64. doi:10.1016/j.jtcvs.2013.09.075: discussion 664–655.

Matisoff AJ, Olivieri L, Schwartz JM, Deutsch N. Risk assessment and anesthetic management of patients with Williams syndrome: a comprehensive review. Paediatr Anaesth. 2015;25(12):1207–15. doi:10.1111/pan.12775.

Mazzitelli D, Guenther T, Schreiber C, Wottke M, Michel J, Meisner H. Aortic valve replacement in children: are we on the right track? Eur J Cardiothorac Surg. 1998;13(5):565–71.

McCrindle BW, Blackstone EH, Williams WG, Sittiwangkul R, Spray TL, Azakie A, Jonas RA. Are outcomes of surgical versus transcatheter balloon valvotomy equivalent in neonatal critical aortic stenosis? Circulation. 2001;104(12 Suppl 1):I152–8.

McElhinney DB, Lock JE, Keane JF, Moran AM, Colan SD. Left heart growth, function, and reintervention after balloon aortic valvuloplasty for neonatal aortic stenosis. Circulation. 2005;111(4):451–8. doi:10.1161/01.CIR.0000153809.88286.2E.

Meairs S, Weihe E, Mittmann U, Vetter H, Kohler U, Forssmann WG. Morphologic investigation of coronary arteries subjected to hypertension by experimental supravalvular aortic stenosis in dogs. Lab Invest. 1984;50(4):469–79.

Medley J, Russo P, Tobias JD. Perioperative care of the patient with Williams syndrome. Paediatr Anaesth. 2005;15(3):243–7. doi:10.1111/j.1460-9592.2004.01567.x.

Morris CD, Outcalt J, Menashe VD. Hypoplastic left heart syndrome: natural history in a geographically defined population. Pediatrics. 1990;85(6):977–83.

Nelson JS, Pasquali SK, Pratt CN, Yu S, Donohue JE, Loccoh E, Ohye RG, Bove EL, Hirsch-Romano JC. Long-term survival and reintervention after the Ross procedure across the pediatric age spectrum. Ann Thorac Surg. 2015;99(6):2086–94. doi:10.1016/j.athoracsur.2015.02.068; discussion 2094–2085.

Nickerson E, Greenberg F, Keating MT, McCaskill C, Shaffer LG. Deletions of the elastin gene at 7q11.23 occur in approximately 90% of patients with Williams syndrome. Am J Hum Genet. 1995;56(5):1156–61.

Ohye RG, Gomez CA, Ohye BJ, Goldberg CS, Bove EL. The Ross/Konno procedure in neonates and infants: intermediate-term survival and autograft function. Ann Thorac Surg. 2001;72(3):823–30.

Opie LH. Heart physiology: from cell to circulation. 4th ed. Philadelphia: Lippincott Williams & Wilkins; 2004.

Peterson TA, Todd DB, Edwards JE. Supravalvular aortic stenosis. J Thorac Cardiovasc Surg. 1965;50(5):734–41.

Petit CJ, Ing FF, Mattamal R, Pignatelli RH, Mullins CE, Justino H. Diminished left ventricular function is associated with poor mid-term outcomes in neonates after balloon aortic valvuloplasty. Catheter Cardiovasc Interv. 2012;80(7):1190–9. doi:10.1002/ccd.23500.

Pinto RJ, Loya Y, Bhagwat A, Sharma S. Balloon dilatation of supravalvular aortic stenosis: a report of two cases. Int J Cardiol. 1994;46(2):179–81.

Pober BR, Johnson M, Urban Z. Mechanisms and treatment of cardiovascular disease in Williams-Beuren syndrome. J Clin Invest. 2008;118(5):1606–15. doi:10.1172/JCI35309.

Reeve Jr R, Robinson SJ. Hypoplastic annulus--an unusual type of aortic stenosis: a report of three cases in children. Dis Chest. 1964;45:99–102.

Rehnstrom P, Malm T, Jogi P, Fernlund E, Winberg P, Johansson J, Johansson S. Outcome of surgical commissurotomy for aortic valve stenosis in early infancy. Ann Thorac Surg. 2007;84(2):594–8. doi:10.1016/j.athoracsur.2007.03.098.

Rhodes LA, Colan SD, Perry SB, Jonas RA, Sanders SP. Predictors of survival in neonates with critical aortic stenosis. Circulation. 1991;84(6):2325–35.

Roberts WC. The congenitally bicuspid aortic valve. A study of 85 autopsy cases. Am J Cardiol. 1970;26(1):72–83.

Roberts WC. Valvular, subvalvular and supravalvular aortic stenosis: morphologic features. Cardiovasc Clin. 1973;5(1):97–126.

Schwartz ML, Gauvreau K, Geva T. Predictors of outcome of biventricular repair in infants with multiple left heart obstructive lesions. Circulation. 2001;104(6):682–7.

Shinkawa T, Bove EL, Hirsch JC, Devaney EJ, Ohye RG. Intermediate-term results of the Ross procedure in neonates and infants. Ann Thorac Surg. 2010;89(6):1827–32. doi:10.1016/j.athoracsur.2010.02.107; discussion 1832.

Siddiqui J, Brizard CP, Galati JC, Iyengar AJ, Hutchinson D, Konstantinov IE, Wheaton GR, Ramsay JM, d'Udekem Y. Surgical valvotomy and repair for neonatal and infant congenital aortic stenosis achieves better results than interventional catheterization. J Am Coll Cardiol. 2013;62(22):2134–40. doi:10.1016/j.jacc.2013.07.052.

Stamm C, Li J, Ho SY, Redington AN, Anderson RH. The aortic root in supravalvular aortic stenosis: the potential surgical relevance of morphologic findings. J Thorac Cardiovasc Surg. 1997;114(1):16–24. doi:10.1016/S0022-5223(97)70112-0.

Stapleton GE. Transcatheter management of neonatal aortic stenosis. Cardiol Young. 2014;24(6):1117–20. doi:10.1017/S1047951114002030.

Stulak JM, Burkhart HM, Sundt 3rd TM, Connolly HM, Suri RM, Schaff HV, Dearani JA. Spectrum and outcome of reoperations after the Ross procedure. Circulation. 2010;122(12):1153–8. doi:10.1161/CIRCULATIONAHA.109.897538.

Tan Tanny SP, Yong MS, d'Udekem Y, Kowalski R, Wheaton G, D'Orsogna L, Galati JC, Brizard CP, Konstantinov IE. Ross procedure in children: 17-year experience at a single institution. J Am Heart Assoc. 2013;2(2):e000153. doi:10.1161/JAHA.113.000153.

Valverde E, Pellicer A, Madero R, Elorza D, Quero J, Cabanas F. Dopamine versus epinephrine for cardiovascular support in low birth weight infants: analysis of systemic effects and neonatal clinical outcomes. Pediatrics. 2006;117(6):e1213–22. doi:10.1542/peds.2005-2108.

Von Rueden TJ, Knight L, Moller JH, Ewards JE. Coarctation of the aorta associated with aortic valvular atresia. Circulation. 1975;52(5):951–4.

Wagner HR, Weidman WH, Ellison RC, Miettinen OS. Indirect assessment of severity in aortic stenosis. Circulation. 1977;56(1 Suppl):I20–3.

Williams IA, Quaegebeur JM, Hsu DT, Gersony WM, Bourlon F, Mosca RS, Gersony DR, Solowiejczyk DE. Ross procedure in infants and toddlers followed into childhood. Circulation. 2005;112(9 Suppl):I390–5. doi:10.1161/CIRCULATIONAHA.104.524975.

Wren C, Oslizlok P, Bull C. Natural history of supravalvular aortic stenosis and pulmonary artery stenosis. J Am Coll Cardiol. 1990;15(7):1625–30.

Chapter 24
Anomalies of the Aortic Arch: Aortic Coarctation and Interrupted Aortic Arch

Ali Dabbagh and Sri O. Rao

Coarctation of Aorta

Introduction and Background

Coarctation of the aorta (CoA) or aortic coarctation is one of the most common types of congenital heart diseases presenting itself as an obstructive lesion most often in the thoracic aorta. Its prevalence is 1 in 2500 births; consisting 5–8 % of all congenital heart defects and often, a number of cardiovascular abnormalities are associated with CoA. The disease is much more frequent in males than females. The frequency of CoA is higher in some disease states like Turner syndrome: 15–20 % of CoA cases are Turner syndrome patients (Torok et al. 2015).

CoA is usually known as a "discrete narrowing" of the aorta located at the junction of the ductus arteriosus with the aortic body; this point is just distal to the origin of the left subclavian artery; hence the term "juxta-ductal" type CoA is used for it; however, other anatomical sites for CoA are possible, and CoA could affect other locations on the aorta in a highly variable manner.

Historically, CoA was regarded "just" as a local anatomic "narrowing" in the aortic isthmus which could be *cured and healed with a surgical procedure*; however, this is just an oversimplification. In fact, it is the clinical presentation of a broader embryologic impairment and part of a larger and more diffuse systemic disease often involving multiple left-sided cardiac structures; this is discussed more under "embryologic features of the disease" in the later paragraphs.

A. Dabbagh, MD (✉)
Cardiac Anesthesiology Department, Anesthesiology Research Center,
Shahid Beheshti University of Medical Sciences, Tehran, Iran
e-mail: alidabbagh@yahoo.com; alidabbagh@sbmu.ac.ir

S.O. Rao, MD
Novick Cardiac Alliance, 1750 Madison Ave, Suite 500, Memphis, TN 38104-6492, USA
e-mail: sri.rao@cardiac-alliance.org

© Springer International Publishing Switzerland 2017
A. Dabbagh et al. (eds.), *Congenital Heart Disease in Pediatric and Adult Patients*, DOI 10.1007/978-3-319-44691-2_24

Being part of a diffuse vasculopathy, CoA may not be totally resolved even after complete surgical resection of the stricture, mandating lifelong follow-up and continuous surveillance; a *bicuspid aortic valve* (BAV) is seen in up to 80 % of all CoA patients; male dominance is seen both in CoA and bicuspid aortic valve; also, there are a number of more challenging issues affecting the fate of the disease and our clinical practice:

- As mentioned, bicuspid aortic valve is the most common associated cardiac anomaly (up to 80 % of patients), while intracerebral berry aneurysm is the most common *noncardiac* anomaly (10 % of patients); both are in favor of an "underlying disease of the arterial system," possibly due to impairment of the neural crest tissue with a resulting "medial degeneration, aortic root disease, and cerebral aneurysm."
- The anatomic and pathologic features of CoA determine the existence or absence of the "hypoplastic aortic arch," nature of the disease being "simple CoA" or "mixed CoA" having concomitant associated cardiac abnormalities (e.g., ventricular septal defect, bicuspid aortic valve, subaortic stenosis, complex congenital heart defects, and other types of left-sided cardiac lesions).
- Treatment and prognosis depend on the clinical state of disease: age, clinical feature of the disease, associated anomalies, "simple CoA" or "mixed CoA", concomitant arch hypoplasia, hypertension, cerebral vascular involvement, etc.
- Prenatal and intrauterine diagnostic approaches for CoA are difficult and imprecise due to the presence of a large fetal patent ductus arteriosus.
- Serial echocardiography should be done after birth in patients with suspicious clinical findings to quickly treat cases of CoA and other obstructive left heart lesions.
- Anesthesia for coarctation of the aorta mandates an appropriate understanding of the pathology, which is more than simply a local narrowing; however, arteriopathy accompanied with possibility of left-sided heart disease in the younger patients and the extent of the distal collaterals in the older ones are among the main concerns; some cases are redo patients, and one should always care for perioperative treatment of hypertension and extracardiac comorbidities (Campbell 1970; Hornberger et al. 1994; Sharland et al. 1994; Franklin et al. 2002; Miyague et al. 2003; Warnes 2003; Paladini et al. 2004; Azakie et al. 2005; Head et al. 2005; Rosenthal 2005; Kanter 2007; Hijazi and Awad 2008; Tomar and Radhakrishanan 2008; Axt-Fliedner et al. 2009; Vohra et al. 2009; Kenny and Hijazi 2011; Pedersen et al. 2011; Keshavarz-Motamed et al. 2012; Pedersen 2012).

Embryology and Anatomic Features

The role of embryological maldevelopment leading to CoA clarifies the associated anomalies of the disease. Embryological neural crest cells constitute the main origin of many cardiac and noncardiac structures:

- The heart
- Outflow tracts of the heart
- Great vessels including the arch of the aorta
- Conotruncal structures
- The outflow endocardial cushions (which are the precursors of the semilunar valves)

Impaired development of the neural crest could lead to a number of congenital anomalies, both cardiac and noncardiac; the following are the main cardiac defects related to impaired development of the neural crest:

- CoA
- Bicuspid aortic valve
- Hypoplasia of the mitral valve
- Anomalies of the conotruncal structures
- Hypoplasia of the left ventricle
- Anomalies of the cardiac outflow tract (including hypoplasia of the left outflow tract)
- Interrupted aortic arch and hypoplasia of the aortic arch

However, these are the main noncardiac disorders associated with impaired development of the neural crest:

- DiGeorge syndrome
- Head and neck anomalies (which could lead to difficult intubation)
- CNS developmental delay

Development involves the third, fourth, and sixth pharyngeal crests as well as the neural crest disorders; however, this process is part of greater embryologic interactions leading to development of heart, great vessels, head, and neck structures; the entire process of organogenesis is highly dependent on the appropriate migration of the neural crest cells; a detailed discussion on embryology of the disease is presented in Chap. 2 – *Cardiovascular system embryology and development* (Van Mierop and Kutsche 1984, 1986; Kappetein et al. 1991; Towbin and Belmont 2000; Brown and Baldwin 2006; Carroll et al. 2006; High et al. 2007; Jain et al. 2011; Keshavarz-Motamed et al. 2011a; Phillips et al. 2013).

Etiology and Mechanism of the Disease

Having a better understanding of the underlying causes and mechanisms of CoA could improve the quality of our therapeutic approaches. This is why having knowledge of the correct etiologic mechanisms of the disease has a great effect on clinical outcomes, e.g., why the result of balloon dilatation or imperfect resection of the isthmal strictures increases the likelihood for recurrence of CoA (Jimenez et al. 1999).

There are two main potential etiologies proposed as the causative mechanism for CoA, namely, "ductal theory or ductus tissue theory" and "hemodynamic theory or flow theory," described as follows:

- *Hemodynamic theory or flow theory*: more widely accepted, this theory states that during the fetal period, the development of the aortic arch (including the length and the diameter of the arch) depends on "the amount of blood flow which passes through the arch"; if this blood flow is impaired (regardless of the underlying pathology), it has unwanted effect on the normal development of the aortic arch, leading to a narrowed and/or hypoplastic aortic arch; known as "Rudolph theory," this phenomenon explains the following main features of CoA: (1) the "posterior shelf" which is the characteristic and localized lesion of CoA; (2) the "intracardiac defects" seen as concomitant embryologic lesions in CoA and an explanation of associated intracardiac pathologies decreasing blood flow from the left heart to the arch of the aorta are among the most important etiologies of CoA; (3) "tubular hypoplasia" as a distinct but often concomitant lesion of CoA usually seen as narrowing of the aortic isthmus; and (4) the right-sided obstructive lesions are very rarely associated with CoA possibly because of increased flow shift from the left heart structures to right heart structures.

- *Ductal theory or ductus tissue theory*: this theory is also known as "Skodaic hypothesis"; in this theory, it is assumed that "abnormal distribution or aberrant migration" of smooth muscle cells (SMC) from ductus arteriosus to the adjacent aortic tissue leads to CoA, i.e., ectopic ductal tissue in the aortic isthmus causes CoA, which in turn causes constriction, usually in the isthmus of the aorta (i.e., the junction of the aorta with ductus arteriosus); this theory justifies why most cases of CoA are juxta-ductal type; though some major controversies exist regarding this theory, there are still a number of clinicians and embryologists who are "enthusiasts" of this theory; those who believe in this theory attribute the cellular and structural similarity between intimal function in CoA and the process of "ductus arteriosus closure" occurring after birth preceded by aggregation of smooth muscle cells in the intimal layer of the aorta at the site of CoA (Krediet 1965; Gillman and Burton 1966; Hutchins 1971; Heymann and Rudolph 1972; Rudolph et al. 1972; Shinebourne and Elseed 1974; Moore and Hutchins 1978; Ho and Anderson 1979; Momma et al. 1982; Van Meurs-Van Woezik and Krediet 1982; Russell et al. 1991; Jimenez et al. 1999; Liberman et al. 2004; Carroll et al. 2006; Kenny and Hijazi 2011).

Pathologic Findings

The main pathologic finding being the *hallmark of CoA* is the "posterior infolding" or "posterior shelf" of the aortic wall just opposite the site of ductus arteriosus attachment to the aorta; some authors have used the term "curtain lesion" to describe CoA. Usually, CoA is located posterolaterally, and the ductus arteriosus

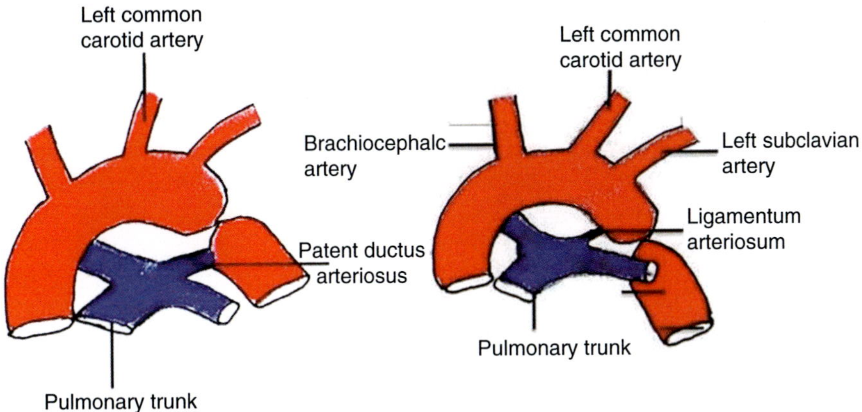

Fig. 24.1 Coarctation of the aorta; (**a**) pre-ductal type; (**b**) post-ductal type

is located on the anteromedial part of the aortic segment, both being on the same anatomic plane; this pattern is known as juxta-ductal CoA, though it is not always the only anatomical presentation of the disease. CoA is usually never seen with pulmonary atresia or pulmonary stenosis, while obstructive lesions of the aorta are a common feature seen in association with CoA. The anatomic relationships between the typical CoA and the adjacent vascular structures are presented in Fig. 24.1. Sometimes even circumferential CoA involving the whole lumen of the aorta is possible. Regarding the pattern of involvement in the lumen of the aorta, usually, CoA has a discrete pattern, though tortuous or segmented CoA is possible. CoA usually involves the aortic media, presenting itself as cystic medial necrosis which is the dominant pathologic feature of the disease; however, at times, cystic medial necrosis implicates the whole aortic lumen as an "entire circumferential lesion" with remnants of the ductus arteriosus found in the coarctation tissue. This would imply that there is a presence of ductal tissue; however, the main pathologic features of the aortic tissue are categorized as "cystic medial necrosis" accompanied by *hyperplastic intimal thickening*. Then there is intimal *proliferation and disruption of elastic tissues* which occurs after the isthmus of CoA. Some authors believe that cystic medial necrosis associated with intimal proliferation and disruption of elastic tissues is the main pathologic feature responsible for post-balloon angioplasty aneurysm formation in CoA patients. On the other hand, it is hypothesized that the arterial tree is more rigid in the pre-coarctation segment than the post-coarctation segment. The baroreceptors in the pre-coarctation area are affected due to pre-coarctation hypertension; a finding consistent with postoperative hypertension is seen both early and late in repaired CoA patients. There are some pathologic features in common between CoA and congenital aortic stenosis. The pathologic findings seen in CoA include the elastic properties of the aortic tissue which are not entirely resolved even years after surgeries with excellent results but are not limited to a finite region of the aorta; as a matter of fact, surgical repair of CoA does not resolve the underlying "inborn" pathology of "aortopathy"; "impaired elastic property of the vascular system" is the main reason which could contribute to *hypertension* even after treatment. This in turn causes increased load on the left ventricle leading to increased left ventricular mass, systolic and/or diastolic dysfunction of the left ventricle, and, finally, their related morbidities. There are others who believe that widespread vasculopathy seen in CoA patients is primarily the effect of abnormal hemodynamic status due to isthmus narrowing of CoA which is nearly totally resolved after correction of the stricture (Hutchins 1971; Ho and Anderson 1979; Sehested et al. 1982; Van Meurs-Van Woezik and Krediet 1982; Elzenga et al. 1986; Isner et al. 1987; van Son et al. 1993; Xu et al. 2000; de Divitiis et al. 2001, 2003, 2005; Vogt et al. 2005; Kuhn et al. 2009; Kenny and Hijazi 2011; Pedersen 2012; Niwa 2013; Lee and d'Udekem 2014).

Clinical Features

In the current era, we could not consider CoA simply as a mechanical stricture of the aorta, which could be relieved by surgery or alternative interventional procedures in the catheterization lab. Neither the natural life span nor the normal hemodynamic status is entirely gained even after complete and successful resection/ removal of CoA. Up to 20 % of patients have arterial hypertension (usually systolic), arterial atherosclerosis, premature coronary artery disease, heart failure, sudden cardiac death, unwanted side effects of different methods of CoA repair like post dilatation aneurysm formation, etc. more than the normal range of the population. However, the age of correction is also among the determinant factors affecting the outcome, though even early correction in the neonatal age does not normalize all clinical findings and "wipe off" all the CoA-related clinical features (Cohen et al. 1989; Findlow and Doyle 1997; Turner and Gaines 2007; Pedersen et al. 2011; Pedersen 2012; Vergales et al. 2013).

The clinical features of CoA are age dependent; so, we could classify them under three main subtitles:

Prenatal Period (Fetal Period)

Prenatal diagnosis of CoA is extremely imprecise even with the most advanced imaging; the following points should be kept in mind to be able to differentiate CoA in the fetal period:

- First of all, we should always keep in mind that diagnosis of CoA during the fetal period is somehow a difficult task mandating high levels of suspicion and careful prenatal care; the main reason is that the continuous blood flow through the ductus arteriosus interferes highly with the diagnostic evaluations.
- "Quantitative hypoplasia of the isthmus and transverse arch" is the most commonly observed sign in fetal assessment, which could be observed during serial prenatal echocardiography.

- Mixed CoA which includes the most severe cases of CoA is associated with "hypoplasia of the structures of the left heart" accompanied with stenosis in the aortic isthmus in fetal period; hence the antenatal diagnosis in severe CoA is much easier in "mixed CoA," while prenatal diagnosis of "simple CoA" is not likely due to the presence of the ductus arteriosus.
- In all CoA patients, whether simple or mixed, prenatal diagnosis of the disease may lead to "improved survival and preoperative clinical condition."
- Within the fetal period, CoA is a significant diagnostic challenge, though the hypoplastic left heart should always be considered as a differential diagnosis during fetal echocardiography studies; milder grades of CoA would often reveal a "near-normal" pattern of fetal echocardiography, especially in late pregnancy which makes the differentiation between "normal right heart structures" and "CoA-associated right heart findings" of diagnostic challenges in fetal echocardiography, mandating sophisticated attention regarding potential false-positive or false-negative results.

During antenatal assessments, we should always consider the potential chance for hypoplasia of left heart structures accompanied with stenosis in the aortic isthmus in fetal period, mandating serial assessments especially using sequential echocardiography:

- First arch Z scores
- Serial isthmal Z scores (in suspected cases with normal outcomes, this score improved to >-2; however, this score remained <-2 in those requiring surveillance or surgery.)
- Isthmal to ductal diameter ratio
- Isthmal flow disturbance
- The presence of a coarctation shelf
- Hypoplastic aortic arch or interrupted aorta
- Decreased flow through the ascending aorta
- Dilation of the right ventricle and pulmonary artery

Some of the above echo findings are more easily diagnosed during early pregnancy especially when performed as serial Z scores; while in late pregnancy, the diagnosis is really much more difficult mandating serial assessments especially using sequential echocardiography (Allan et al. 1987, 1988, 1989; De Smedt et al. 1987; Hornberger et al. 1994; Sharland et al. 1994; Kaine et al. 1996; Eapen et al. 1998; Franklin et al. 2002; Dodge-Khatami et al. 2005; Head et al. 2005; Rosenthal 2005; Matsui et al. 2008; Axt-Fliedner et al. 2009; Weisse 2011).

Neonatal Period

The clinical presentation of the neonates with CoA includes the signs and symptoms of low cardiac output; if CoA is a severe type lesion, especially when superimposed by closure of ductus arteriosus, clinical presentation of shock could be seen;

these patients would be diagnosed as critical neonatal CoA due to a severe juxtaductal CoA, clinically presenting with *different features of heart failure* as the following findings:

- Increased left ventricular filling pressure
- Increased right ventricular filling pressure (i.e., persisting the fetal right heart circulation with high pressure)
- Cardiomegaly
- Impaired left ventricle emptying
- Tachypnea
- Pulmonary edema
- Respiratory distress
- Cardiogenic shock
- Ischemia distal to aortic narrowing leading to organ injury (end organ ischemia in the liver, kidney, GI tract, etc.)
- Diminished or weak distal pulses including the femoral artery (Rosenthal 2005; Kenny and Hijazi 2011)

Infancy Period

If the infant with CoA passes the critical neonatal CoA (i.e., the ductus is not closed, and the patients receive appropriate medical treatment), collateral flow may begin to develop; however, during later infancy, *nonspecific features* of failure to thrive could be the predominant clinical feature along with cachexia and poor feeding. In almost all situations, weak lower limb pulses could be added to the diagnostic criteria (Rosenthal 2005; Kenny and Hijazi 2011).

Older Childhood and Adolescence Period

Often, the more subtle forms of CoA might be undetected until later years of life; however, older children and adolescents with CoA usually present with these findings:

- Hypertension
- Headache
- Claudication of the lower limb
- Exercise intolerance which could be at times the only clinical feature of the disease
- Weak femoral pulses
- Blood pressure gradient between upper and lower limbs

If adequate collateral vessels form during the early years, the above signs and symptoms could be very subtle, and the only remaining feature would be increased blood pressure in the upper extremity which is two standard deviations above normal limit for sex and age accompanied with delayed femoral pulse compared with proximal arterial sites. Also, increased blood flow through the intercostal arteries as the main collaterals would affect the rib margins and result in a typical feature in chest X-ray (CXR) referred to as "rib notching." Another diagnostic characteristic in chest X-ray is the border of the constricted aorta in the isthmal aortic region called "reverse 3 sign"; it is clear that "rib notching" on CXR is the result of increased intercostal artery flow so it would not be seen in neonates and younger children. These findings are seen in older children and adults and confirmed by transthoracic echocardiography (TTE), CT scanning, MR imaging, MR angiography (MRA), and aortic angiography. Detailed imaging prior to surgical- or catheter-based intervention is mandatory (Gotzsche et al. 1994; Connolly et al. 2003; Matsunaga et al. 2003; Rosenthal 2005; Secchi et al. 2009; Akdemir et al. 2010; De Caro et al. 2010; Feltes et al. 2011; Kenny and Hijazi 2011; Pedersen et al. 2011; Baykan et al. 2014; Cook et al. 2013; Khavandi et al. 2013; Ringel et al. 2013; Vergales et al. 2013; Eckroth-Bernard et al. 2014; Lee and d'Udekem 2014; Tong et al. 2014).

Adult Features

If CoA is not diagnosed during the infancy period, the ductus would be closed by time, and the aorta would become enlarged enough to produce the large-sized aortic segment, typical of the adulthood CoA. However, in this underlying pathology, if undiagnosed and untreated, more than 80 % of patients die before the age of 50. Other associated anomalies seen in adult CoA could be somewhat similar to the lower age range, including the presence of BAV or very rarely left-sided obstructive lesions.

Currently, the adult CoA patient populations comprised of those who have undergone surgical repair, balloon angioplasty, stenting, or a combination of the three methods, with or without residual recurrence of CoA. However, even in those without residual CoA, the clinician should always be aware of the possibility of cardiovascular problems including but not limited to the following:

- Arterial hypertension (usually systolic)
- Systemic arterial atherosclerosis
- Premature coronary artery disease
- Exercise intolerance
- Sudden cardiac death
- Stroke
- Heart failure
- Unwanted side effects of different methods of CoA repair like post dilatation aneurysm formation
- Associated anomalies (discussed in the next section)

Echocardiography in CoA

When assessing CoA by echo, the assessment should include complete evaluation throughout the course of the aorta starting from the anatomic left ventricular outflow tract and ending in the descending thoracic aorta, in such a way that any comorbid defects would be diagnosed (Marelli et al. 1993; Aboulhosn and Child 2015).

The common finding of CoA in echocardiography is narrowing of the aortic arch including 2-D assessments, as well as the pressure gradient >3 mmHg by Doppler flow velocity. When measuring the pressure gradient across the aortic arch, Doppler flow velocity prior to the point of coarctation should be measured; otherwise, the pressure difference would be exaggerated during calculation of the pressure gradient. Normally, flow in the descending aorta has a rapid upstroke in systole and brief retrograde flow in early diastole, while in coarctation the systolic upstroke is reduced with continuous forward flow in diastole. In neonatal CoA, an aortic arch measurement less than 4 mm will produce such a gradient as defined by the pressure gradient of CoA.

Echocardiographic Views Used in CoA

In transthoracic echo (TTE), apical two-chamber view is used for assessment of the descending thoracic aorta, suprasternal view for assessment of the arch, plus the descending aorta and thoracic aorta, and, finally, subcostal view for abdominal aorta; however, in transesophageal echocardiography (TEE), the standard exam with emphasis on views demonstrating the left ventricular outflow tract and the course of the aorta until diaphragm should be used (Miller-Hance and Silverman 2000; Shively 2000; Garg et al. 2009; Aboulhosn and Child 2015).

Echo Protocol

In preoperative assessment, the following comments should be assessed:

- Descending aorta through pulsed Doppler at the level of diaphragm.
- Aortic arch.
- Aortic arch sides and its branching.
- Ascending arch, transverse arch, isthmus, and descending aorta, with special consideration on size and gradient.
- Left subclavian artery.
- Any potential PDA should be searched carefully.
- Left ventricle, regarding its size and function.
- Left atrial size.
- Left-sided obstructive lesions.
- Ruling out regurgitation at any of the four main valves (aortic, mitral, pulmonary, and tricuspid).
- Right ventricle systolic function.
- Pulmonary artery pressure.

Also, in postoperative assessment, the following comments should be assessed (or reassessed):

- Descending aorta (pulsed Doppler at the level of diaphragm)
- Aortic arch throughout its course
- Ascending arch, transverse arch, isthmus, and descending aorta (size and gradient)
- Any residual PDA
- Left ventricle, regarding its size and function and the effects of repair on it
- Left-sided obstructive lesions (reassessment)
- Ruling out regurgitation at any of the four main valves (aortic, mitral, pulmonary, and tricuspid; reassessment)
- Right ventricle systolic function (reassessment)
- Pulmonary artery pressure (reassessment)

Associated Anomalies of CoA

CoA is associated with a number of cardiac and noncardiac anomalies discussed here.

Associated Cardiac Anomalies of CoA

Shinebourne reported in 1974 that among 162 patients with CoA, 83 had an intracardiac anomaly "resulting in increased blood flow" and 21 had "left-sided lesions present from birth," while none had "diminished blood flow or right-sided obstructive lesions"; a considerable number of complementary studies were published afterward; based on them, *cardiac anomalies* associated with CoA could be classified as the following.

Aortic Valve Lesions

Different aortic valve lesions have been reported to accompany CoA:

- Bicuspid aortic valve (BAV)
- Aortic valve stenosis
- Discrete subaortic stenosis
- Valve atresia
- Valve obstruction

However, BAV has been reported as the most common aortic valve lesion in CoA patients, being prevalent in 40–80 % of the patients with CoA; the proposed mechanism of bicuspid aortic valve is possibly the embryological etiology of CoA, i.e., maldevelopment of the neural crest which is the embryologic origin of all these structures, discussed earlier in this chapter; interestingly, BAV is not just another "obstructive lesion" added to the primary CoA lesion; instead it *significantly* affects the following aspects of CoA:

- Severity of the primary pathology
- Harshness of the shearing forces in the aortic lumen
- Magnitude of the eccentric jet in the aortic lumen
- Turbulent flow inside the lumen
- Left ventricle (LV) workload
- Seriousness of the clinical presentation of disease
- Clinical outcome of the disease
- Final postsurgical outcome (Quaegebeur et al. 1994; Aboulhosn and Child 2006; De Mozzi et al. 2008; Perloff 2010; Kenny and Hijazi 2011; Keshavarz-Motamed et al. 2011a, b, 2012, 2013; Keshavarz-Motamed and Kadem 2011)

Hypoplasia of the Left Heart Structures

Hypoplasia of the left heart structures could be seen in the most severe forms of CoA; however, hypoplasia of the right heart structures is not a common associated anomaly of CoA. Within the fetal period, CoA is a real challenge in diagnosis; the hypoplastic left heart should always be considered as a differential diagnosis during fetal echocardiography studies. Also, other possible left heart obstructive lesions may be seen such as mitral atresia (Hutchins 1971; Shinebourne and Elseed 1974; Sharland et al. 1994; Agnoleti et al. 1999; Connolly et al. 2003; Axt-Fliedner et al. 2009; Stressig et al. 2011; Curtis et al. 2012; Hartge et al. 2012; Cook et al. 2013).

Hypoplasia of Aortic Arch

In the setting of CoA, hypoplasia of the aortic arch could be classified as one of these three:

- *Proximal arch segment*: located just after the ascending arch of the aorta, this segment involves part of the aorta in the distance between the innominate artery and left common carotid artery; this segment should be $\geq 60\%$ of the diameter of the ascending aorta otherwise is considered hypoplastic.
- *Distal arch segment*: this segment is between left common carotid and left subclavian arteries and should be $\geq 50\%$ of the diameter of the ascending aorta in order to be non-stenotic.
- *Isthmic segment*: this is the third segment of the aortic arch and is located between the left subclavian artery and the ligamentum arteriosum; it should be $\geq 40\%$ of the diameter of the ascending aorta otherwise considered stenotic (Morrow et al.

1986; Kaine et al. 1996; Van Son et al. 1997; Dodge-Khatami et al. 2005; Celik et al. 2006).

Ventricular Septal Defect (VSD)

Based on a large multi-institutional study, in CoA classification, roughly 30 % are simple CoA, 30 % are associated with VSD, and 40 % are categorized under "complex CoA" lesions; often VSD in CoA patients is conotruncal (Quaegebeur et al. 1994; Glen et al. 2004; Kanter 2007; Kenny and Hijazi 2011).

Patent Ductus Arteriosus (PDA)

In CoA patients, ductus arteriosus maybe the only patent passage for blood flow to the distal parts of the body after the aortic isthmus; so, it is not uncommon to have a PDA with CoA, even if it is possible to start intravenous prostaglandin infusion (PGE1) to prevent distal ischemia and to maintain ductal patency; interestingly, PGE1 could also relieve some degrees of narrowing at the coarctation site, besides keeping ductus patent through widening of coarctation area (Liberman et al. 2004; Rosenthal 2005; Carroll et al. 2006).

Atrial Septal Defect (ASD)

The increased pressure in the ascending aorta is transferred back to the left ventricle and then left atrium to keep the foramen ovale open and impose a secundum-type ASD for CoA patients; however, this is very common (Rosenthal 2005).

Bovine Aortic Arch

The rightward deviation of the left common carotid artery to merge with the brachiocephalic trunk and form a large arterial trunk (bovine trunk) may be seen in CoA (Van Son et al. 1997).

Other Cardiac Anomalies

The other possible defects associated with CoA are (rarely) pulmonary stenosis, anomalous pulmonary venous drainage, persistent left superior vena cava (persistent LSVC) which could affect the normal flow to and from the left ventricle, ductus venous persistence which would create a blood flow to the right heart, and atrioventricular canal. As previously mentioned, right-sided obstructive lesions are usually not a common finding with CoA.

Associated Noncardiac Anomalies of CoA

CNS

In patients with CoA, intracerebral aneurysms are five times more common likely especially in those patients between 30 and 50 years old. It is recommended that these patients have assessments of the cerebral vessels by computed tomography angiography (CTA) or magnetic resonance imaging as a routine practice.

Gastrointestinal System

Atresia of the esophagus, tracheoesophageal fistula, diaphragmatic hernia, and atresia of the anorectal area are the main GI co-findings in CoA (Paladini et al. 2004).

Urogenital System

Variant degrees of agenesis or hypogenesis in kidneys or the urinary tract may be seen in CoA as associated anomalies.

Skeletal Anomalies

Clubfoot, osteogenesis imperfecta, and a number of other skeletal anomalies in the lower limb are seen in CoA patients (Smith et al. 1995; Paladini et al. 2004; Lee et al. 2012b).

Chromosomal Anomalies

- *Turner syndrome*: up to 15 % of patients are reported to have Turner syndrome.
- *Shone syndrome*: first described by Shone in 1963, this rare congenital complex is composed of four left heart obstructive lesions: "parachute mitral valve, supravalvular mitral ring, subaortic stenosis, and CoA."
- *PHACE syndrome*: *P*osterior fossa malformation, *H*emangioma, *A*rterial anomalies, *C*oarctation of the aorta, *E*ye abnormalities; also, there is a newer modification, PHACE(S), to code for *S*ternal clefting and *S*upraumbilical raphe; during surgery for correction of CoA, these patients are at increased risk of CNS events and should be monitored carefully.
- *Kabuki syndrome*: multiple congenital anomalies including developmental delay, cleft palate, facial appearance of the patient, skeletal malformations, and congenital cardiac defects are the main specifications of this genetic syndrome; 25–30 % of these patients have CoA.

- Ehlers–Danlos syndrome.
- Marfan syndrome.
- Loeys–Dietz syndrome.
- Monosomy X.
- Trisomy 21.
- Trisomy 18 (Shone et al. 1963; Hughes and Davies 1994; Digilio et al. 2001; Gravholt 2002; Paladini et al. 2004; Kataoka et al. 2006; McMahon and Reardon 2006; Dulac et al. 2008; Perloff 2010; Puttgen and Lin 2010; Schimke et al. 2013; Yuan 2013; Imada et al. 2014).

Urogenital System

Variant degrees of agenesis or hypogenesis in kidneys or the urinary tract may be seen in CoA as associated anomalies.

Skeletal Anomalies

Clubfoot, osteogenesis imperfecta, and a number of other skeletal anomalies in lower limb have been reported in CoA patients (Smith et al. 1995; Paladini et al. 2004; Lee et al. 2012b; Imada et al. 2014) (Table 24.1).

Table 24.1 Associated anomalies in coarctation of the aorta

Associated cardiac anomalies
Aortic valve lesions: bicuspid aortic valve (BAV); aortic valve stenosis; discrete subaortic stenosis; valve atresia; valve obstruction
Hypoplasia of the left heart structures: hypoplastic left heart syndrome, mitral stenosis
Hypoplasia of the aortic arch: proximal arch segment hypoplasia; distal arch segment hypoplasia; isthmic segment hypoplasia
Ventricular septal defect (VSD)
Patent ductus arteriosus (PDA)
Atrial septal defect (ASD)
Bovine aortic arch
Other cardiac anomalies: pulmonary stenosis, anomalous pulmonary venous drainage, persistent LSVC, persistent ductus venosus, atrioventricular canal defect
Associated noncardiac anomalies
CNS
GI tract
Urogenital system
Skeletal anomalies
Chromosomal anomalies: *Turner syndrome*; *Shone syndrome*; *PHACE syndrome*; *Kabuki syndrome*; Ehlers–Danlos syndrome; Marfan syndrome; Loeys–Dietz syndrome; Monosomy X; Trisomy 21; Trisomy 18

Therapeutic Approaches

The main therapeutic approaches considered for treatment of CoA could be categorized under three main classifications; each of them has a number of sub-modalities based on the practical method:

- *Surgical correction*
- *Balloon angioplasty* or *balloon dilatation*
- *Stent dilatation*

The last two are usually considered as *percutaneous interventions* (Suarez de Lezo et al. 2005; Akdemir et al. 2010; Eckroth-Bernard et al. 2014; Hijazi and Kenny 2014).

Surgical Correction

In 1944 "the first surgical correction of CoA" was first reported. Often, surgical correction of CoA is performed through a posterolateral thoracotomy and has been regarded for many decades as "the gold standard treatment for CoA." However, in the current era of interventional treatments, there is an ever-growing controversy regarding "the best treatment for CoA" with alternative options (mainly interventional methods including balloon dilatation or stenting) becoming much more popular. As catheter and stent technologies have matured, more centers are choosing stenting or balloon angioplasty as the primary choice for treatment of CoA not only in recurrent CoA but in native CoA. In recent years, with the development of covered stents and smaller delivery systems, many centers have reported improved outcomes and fewer long-term complications as compared to surgical cohorts. Despite this, stenting has not yet become the standard first choice, and some controversies remain yet. In 2011, *the American Heart Association* released its scientific statement:

> for native coarctation of the aorta, surgical repair (extended resection with an end-to-end anastomosis) remains the gold standard" while "balloon angioplasty with or without stent implantation" is considered as an alternative option with less invasiveness; though it should be kept in mind that "transcatheter treatment *does not necessarily replace* surgical management

However, The *Cochrane Database* systematic review published in 2012 has declared that "there is insufficient evidence with regards to the best treatment for coarctation of the thoracic aorta" (Mahadevan and Mullen 2004; Forbes et al. 2007a; Turner and Gaines 2007; Botta et al. 2009; Egan and Holzer 2009; Holzer et al. 2010; Feltes et al. 2011; Forbes et al. 2011; Padua et al. 2012; Hijazi and Kenny 2014; Sohrabi et al. 2014).

Some clinical notes should be considered in patients undergoing surgical correction of CoA:

- The majority of "neonatal and infantile CoA cases" are presented as "arch hypoplasia."

- In patients with arch hypoplasia, surgical correction is the first option.
- Usually, *end-to-end anastomosis with extended resection* is the best approach during the first months of life.
- Other surgical approaches for CoA repair include "subclavian flap angioplasty," "patch angioplasty," and "interposition graft repair."
- In surgical correction of CoA, postoperative complications should be followed vigorously, including *re-CoA* (recurrence of stenosis), *aneurysm* formation, persistent *hypertension* (at rest or during exercise), *stroke*, and accelerated *coronary artery disease*.
- Some of these postoperative complications are lethal though they are infrequent (like rupture at the site of surgical repair).

The relatively high rate of postoperative events in CoA patients underscores pathologic basis of the disease: "surgical correction of CoA only resects the local anatomic isthmus but not the underlying vascular impairment generating the disease."

Though isolated repair of CoA is associated with favorable results, all surgical approaches are associated with a chance of restenosis, i.e., re-CoA (with a rate of about 20–40 %); advanced microsurgical techniques accompanied with vigorous and sophisticated approximation of the two ends of the anastomosis may decrease restenosis rate, while weight and age at the time of operation could affect the chance of re-CoA. Fortunately, restenosis is often nonlethal and could be treated by surgical approach or by catheter-based intervention; each of these two methods has their merits and risks (Connors et al. 1975; Backer et al. 1995; Bouchart et al. 2000; Azakie et al. 2005; Suarez de Lezo et al. 2005; Abbruzzese and Aidala 2007; Hijazi and Awad 2008; Kuroczynski et al. 2008; Botta et al. 2009; Vohra et al. 2009; Kische et al. 2010; Feltes et al. 2011; Luijendijk et al. 2012; Pedersen 2012).

Balloon Dilatation

For many years, surgical repair of CoA was considered the only available definitive therapy for CoA patients; however, in 1979 Sos et al. collected coarcted segments of the aorta from postmortem specimens and demonstrated the ability to dilate the tissue; this finding was the first step in application of definitive nonsurgical therapies (Sos et al. 1979). Afterward, Singer and colleagues reported successful dilatation of CoA in a 42-day-old infant; it is interesting that this first case of balloon dilatation was done after unsuccessful surgical repair leading to restenosis (Singer et al. 1982).

Indications for balloon dilatation of CoA are the same as surgical repair and include:

1. Systolic pressure gradient before the stenosis of CoA, more than 20 mmHg
2. Severe CoA demonstrated in angiography associated with extensive collaterals

However, based on the current evidence, the following could be considered as the main applications of balloon dilatation angioplasty for CoA patients:

- Discrete CoA
- Discrete recurrent CoA
- Restenosis after previous surgical repair of CoA (i.e., ineffective surgical repair)
- Residual coarctation after surgical repair (i.e., ineffective surgical repair)
- Infants above 1 month and below 6 months having discrete narrowing but no evidence of arch hypoplasia
- Native CoA beyond neonatal period (*controversial*), though some believe the minimum age for balloon dilatation and stenting is 3 months (Abbruzzese and Aidala 2007)

A considerable number of studies have demonstrated balloon dilatation angioplasty as a good alternative among the first line of corrective treatments in order to remove isthmal stricture in discrete CoA, neonates, adolescents, and adults, with excellent long-term outcome. Also, the results of balloon dilatation are safe and effective, even years after primary therapy, i.e., during later clinical follow-up. However, other studies have shown that balloon dilatation of CoA causes neointimal proliferation of undifferentiated smooth muscle cells into the aortic lumen, causing restenosis after primary balloon dilatation. One of the issues with balloon dilatation which has been controversial is its application for native CoA especially when compared with other methods regarding the risk of aneurysm formation. Current evidence has not clearly resolved this controversy (Fawzy et al. 1992, 1997, 1999, 2004, 2008, Takahashi et al. 2000; Hassan et al. 2007a, b; Hijazi and Awad 2008; Rothman et al. 2010; Feltes et al. 2011).

Complications of balloon angioplasty are similar to stent dilatation, discussed more in the next section under "stent dilatation"; they include the following in brief:

- "Aortic disruption" and "aortic dissection."
- Blood leakage.
- Injury to the femoral artery and the resulting impaired femoral pulse.
- *The most common complication* is aortic aneurysm formation after balloon dilatation distal to the site of angioplasty, especially but not limited to native CoA.
- Restenosis which may lead to re-CoA (Feltes et al. 2011).

Stenting

Stenting includes transcatheter insertion of stents in order to implant and dilate the stent at the location of the isthmal stricture; this method has been described for the first time in 1991 with good results and is now considered as a first-line therapy in most adolescents and adults and those with restenosis. Short-term results of stenting in CoA (i.e., decreasing the gradient across the isthmal stricture) and also long-term outcomes (especially the incidence of post dilatation aneurysm formation and restenosis) are promising. Improvements in stent technology have decreased the age of stenting to smaller patients to as young as 3 months with these patients requiring multiple re-dilations to accommodate a growing patient's aorta. Success rate of stenting in CoA patients is more than 95 % with an immediate drop in systolic blood pressure gradient and increase in aortic diameter. Stenting for CoA has been compared with both balloon dilatation and surgical repair of CoA. Stenting leads to favorable clinical outcomes regarding relief of hypertension especially after surgical correction of CoA. Interestingly, some patients with no arm–leg gradient at rest may develop a blood pressure gradient with exercise (the so-called posttreatment exercise-induced hypertension "EIH"); however, CoA patients treated with stenting do not often experience this problem. Also, covered stents have been introduced for CoA patients as safer devices in order to prevent unwanted complications of bare metal stents including aortic wall trauma, aneurysm formation, and migration of stent; however, the current available evidence is in favor of equal safety and efficiency of the two types of stents though most experienced operators opt for covered stents in high-risk patients. Those include patients including those with underlying aortic aneurysm, patients with nearly occluded aorta and aortic atresia, patients with age of 40 or more, and patients with Turner syndrome.

The complications of stenting in CoA patients are infrequent, i.e., the chance for acute complications, especially rupture of the aorta, is very low (about 2 %); while the rate of long-term complications is relatively less than other therapeutic options. The rate of aneurysm formation is 5–10 % and the rate of restenosis about 10 % or less than that; however, sophisticated care is needed to detect and, if necessary, treat any untoward complication; these include:

- "Aortic disruption" and "aortic dissection" which can be life-threatening complications mandating aggressive and prompt treatment by the medical team (*immediate*).
- Blood leakage, i.e., blood extravasation at the site of stent implantation (*immediate*).
- Impaired femoral pulses especially when it is due to femoral arterial thrombosis (*immediate*).
- Intimal layer growth and proliferation inside the lumen of the stent which could lead to restenosis, leading to re-CoA, especially at "early age" patients with small bore stents (*long-term complication*).
- Stent migration or stent malpositioning.
- *The most common complication* is aortic aneurysm (*long-term complication*); the incidence of aneurysm formation is less than balloon angioplasty alone. Aneurysm formation may occur even after application of covered stents; aneurysm formation continues to have a persistent risk for all CoA patients, whether they are treated surgically, by balloon dilatation or stent dilatation with a mortality rate between <1 and >90 %; this wide range shows the very remarkable differences in management and outcome of aortic aneurysms related to CoA treatment. These patients can often be treated using endovascular stent grafts (Suarez de Lezo et al. 1999, 2005; Cheatham 2001; Hijazi 2003; Varma et al.

2003; Kothari 2004; Mahadevan and Mullen 2004; Markham et al. 2004; Forbes et al. 2007a; Forbes et al. 2007b; Marcheix et al. 2007; Hijazi and Awad 2008; Botta et al. 2009; Egan and Holzer 2009; Akdemir et al. 2010; De Caro et al. 2010; Holzer et al. 2010; von Kodolitsch et al. 2010; Feltes et al. 2011; Forbes et al. 2011; Godart 2011; Hormann et al. 2011; Kenny et al. 2011; Kenny and Hijazi 2011; Kannan and Srinivasan 2012; Luijendijk et al. 2012; Padua et al. 2012; Baykan et al. 2014; Khavandi et al. 2013; Ringel et al. 2013; Hijazi and Kenny 2014; Sohrabi et al. 2014).

Anesthesia for CoA

Preoperative Evaluation

Preoperative care depends mainly on the age of diagnosis; if the patient is diagnosed in the neonatal or infantile period, the main goal in preoperative care would be to stabilize hemodynamic status, correct the acidotic milieu of the under-perfused organs, and improve the underlying failing heart as much as possible; while in adolescent and adult CoA patients, we mainly aim to control blood pressure especially in the upper trunk and upper extremity.

Preoperative Care in Neonatal and Infantile Period

These should be performed in this group of CoA patients:

- Insert a reliable intravenous line (e.g., central venous line or umbilical vein line).
- Continue intravenous prostaglandin infusion to maintain patency of the ductus arteriosus.
- Keep hemodynamics stable and compensate for underlying heart failure, with the help of inotropes, fluid optimization, and diuretics.
- Assist ventilation whenever the patient is in respiratory failure.
- Start monitoring especially hemodynamic and respiratory monitoring.
- An indwelling arterial line from the right hand is the preferred approach for invasive blood pressure monitoring.

Preoperative Care in Older Children and Adults

- Control of upper trunk hypertension which could be effectively controlled with beta-blockers; however, vigorous treatment and "normalization" of blood pressure in the upper trunk should be avoided to prevent the possibility of post-ductal ischemia
- Assessment of LV function to check the contractility and the undiagnosed associated cardiac defects.

- Long-term CNS effects of CoA and possible microaneurysms.
- Well-developed network of collaterals to the lower limb and the spinal cord.

Intraoperative Anesthesia Management

Anesthesia induction and maintenance

Either intravenous or inhalational anesthesia agents or a combination of them could be used for induction; however, *extreme caution* should be exerted to prevent blood pressure drop after induction in patients with ductal-dependent distal flow. Also, for maintenance of anesthesia, both intravenous and inhalational agents could be used. Thoracic paravertebral block could have benefit both for intraoperative and postoperative analgesia; however, there is always the risk for masking signs of early postoperative paraplegia by the block; the same could be correct for thoracic epidural analgesia (Turkoz et al. 2013)

Lung ventilation should be kept at normocapnia to prevent potential cerebral vasoconstriction and reduce the risk of cord ischemia. One lung ventilation management is another challenge for anesthesiologist especially in the very young patients.

Monitoring

Pre-ductal and post-ductal SpO$_2$ and noninvasive BP monitoring should be started at the first stages of patient arrival on the operating room table and should be continued after installation of invasive arterial blood pressure monitoring; their data are useful especially during the clamp interval. *Invasive blood pressure monitoring* through the right arm shows the pre-ductal arterial pressure, unless there are abnormal patterns of aortic anatomy or circulation from the aorta to the upper extremities. Distal extremity blood pressure control should be done, if not possible by invasive blood pressure control and if not, at least through noninvasive blood pressure cuff. *Central venous catheter* helps us both provide fluids and give vasoactive drugs and, at the same time, manage the loading status of the patient.

CNS Monitoring

There should be close CNS monitoring both for the brain and the spinal cord. One should always keep in mind the possibility of rapid changes in blood pressure, the risk of spinal cord ischemia during aortic clamp especially below 1 year, the preexisting CNS vascular abnormalities including the congenital anatomic aberrations (in younger patients), or the acquired defects (in older patients) due to chronic head and neck hypertension; all of them stress on the importance of special attention to CNS monitoring.

Somatosensory and motor evoked potentials (SSEP and MEP) are both sensitive indicators of distal perfusion and could alarm anesthesiologist in case of ischemia distal to the clamp (including the spinal cord).

NIRS has gained important attention during the last decade as a monitoring not only for CNS but also as an indicator for perfusion of other organs; the following are among the main benefits of NIRS monitoring during perioperative care of CoA:

- It is a sensitive, real-time, and noninvasive monitor indicating the oxygenation status of the tissue; NIRS has been demonstrated in many studies to be an important indicator of maintained tissue perfusion; both *cerebral* and *somatic* assessments of perfusion are useful in these patients (i.e., cerebral rSO_2 and renal rSO_2).
- Cerebral impairments in CNS perfusion due to blood pressure drops affecting the NIRS number should be treated promptly, especially after induction of anesthesia or after removal of the clamp; also, it may help us avoid hyperventilation-inducing cerebral vasoconstriction.
- Using multisite NIRS is especially important when considering the possibility of blood flow manipulations and cord ischemia; besides monitoring CNS O_2 content, NIRS could monitor the possibility of ischemia induced by aorta clamping, which would be demonstrated as a decline in NIRS number, especially when the drop is much more severe than the cerebral NIRS.
- NIRS could let us know whether the collaterals are well developed or not; in neonates and young infants below 1 year, rapid drop in somatic NIRS usually happens due to violations in blood pressure during the procedure, especially during the clamp, due to less developed collaterals; while in patients older than 1 year, there is no such a great drop in NIRS after clamping mainly due to improved collateral flow (Berens et al. 2006; Moerman et al. 2013; Neshat Vahid and Panisello 2014; Scott and Hoffman 2014).

Vasoactive Drugs

One of the most important tasks of an anesthesiologist during CoA operation is the management of blood pressure during clamp manipulations, i.e., *to control blood pressure during clamp and to treat the aftermath of clamp*. For this purpose, during clamp time, "partial" and not "total normalization of blood pressure" is a key component; a moderate degree of hypertension and avoiding vigorous treatment of higher blood pressures during clamp time helps us prevent profound pressure drop after clamp removal; always keep mean arterial pressure (MAP) over 45 mmHg; meanwhile, in older patients, hypertensive episodes during clamp time are really dangerous regarding the risk of vascular events involving CNS arterial system (Imada et al. 2014).

Nitroprusside has an important role: the patients have a major arterial disease, so, there is a need to control the arterial tree response using nitroprusside in order to control blood pressure; this is of utmost importance during the clamp of the aorta (Gelman 1995).

Nitroglycerin is used as an effective and reliable agent for controlling blood pressure proximal to the clamp; some believe that it is more beneficial to sodium nitroprusside for proximal pressure control (Moerman et al. 2013).

Phenylephrine when the aorta is repaired and the surgeon wants to remove the clamp, a number of preventive strategies should be used to overcome the sudden drop in blood pressure including the use of vasoconstrictors like phenylephrine; however, careful and titrated use of vasopressors should always be the practice to prevent abrupt hypertensive spikes.

In older children and adults, usually, long-term upper trunk hypertension is seen in these patients, so, there should be a great concern regarding prevention of any potential untoward CNS hazards and assessment of possible microaneurysms. However, during aortic clamp in these patients, blood pressure should be balanced in such a way to prevent both increased intracerebral hypertension and also postductal ischemia in the lower limb. Besides, the long-term effect of CoA is associated with a well-developed network of collaterals which perfuse the lower limb and the spinal cord; their role should be regarded as well. Spinal cord protection needs vigilance, taking the time appropriately and with sophisticated care, and prevention of cord ischemia during the surgery; *careful beat-to-beat monitoring during clamp time* is the cornerstone of all these strategies.

Spinal Cord Protection Strategies

All surgical attempts should be done in order to keep *cross clamp time* less than 20 min.

NIRS this is a sensitive, real-time, and noninvasive useful monitor monitoring the oxygenation status and the possibility of anaerobic metabolism in ischemic tissues.

SSEP and MEP are sensitive monitors for detection of any potential ischemia in the spinal cord.

Prevention of overtreatment of blood pressure and early compensation for any blood pressure drop after clamp removal is necessary for adequate perfusion of the cord.

Prevention of hyperventilation is among the other necessary strategies for prevention of spinal cord ischemia.

Mild hypothermia (as low as 34–35° of centigrade) could help protect the spinal cord tissue.

Surgeon should *avoid clamping collaterals* during clamp period.

Patient Positioning

Usually, the patients have a left-sided aortic arch which is the common pattern of the aorta; so, the usual position is right lateral decubitus, which is accompanied with the left lung collapsed during surgery; its related considerations should be kept in mind (Table 24.2).

Table 24.2 A summary of intraoperative anesthesia management for CoA

Induction of anesthesia	Caution for prevention of blood pressure drop in ductal-dependent patients
Monitoring	1. Pre-ductal and post-ductal SpO_2 and noninvasive BP
	2. Pre-ductal and if possible post-ductal invasive BP
	3. Central venous catheter for monitoring and drug infusion
	4. Somatosensory and motor evoked potentials (SSEP and MEP)
	5. NIRS
Vasoactive drugs	1. Careful beat-to-beat monitoring during clamp time avoids vigorous treatment of blood pressure during clamp
	2. Avoid profound blood pressure drop after clamp removal (MAP always >45 mmHg)
	3. Nitroprusside, nitroglycerine, and phenylephrine should be used cautiously
	4. In older patients, hypertensive episodes during clamp time are really dangerous for CNS arteries
Protection of the spinal cord	SSEP and MEP
	Cross clamp time not to exceed 20 min
	Avoid profound blood pressure drop after clamp removal
	Prevention of hyperventilation
	Mild hypothermia (34–35° of centigrade)
	Surgeon should avoid clamping collaterals during clamp period

Postoperative Care

There are a number of main topics that should be considered as the core postoperative care in CoA patients:

- It is mandatory to monitor *postoperative blood pressure* vigorously, since the prevalence of this event is considerable after correction of the lesion; postoperative sodium nitroprusside, infusion of beta-blockers like esmolol, and ACE inhibitors could be added to fix the problem; the prevalence of postoperative hypertension is especially higher in those with a diagnosis of "small or hypoplastic aortic arch" before the operation (O'Sullivan et al. 2002; Rouine-Rapp et al. 2003; Tabbutt et al. 2008; Lee et al. 2012a).
- *Postoperative pain control* is another main feature that should be considered to effectively control blood pressure.
- Whenever possible, the patients should be extubated at the end of surgery; appropriate postoperative hemodynamic, respiratory, and metabolic conditions are prerequisites for extubation.
- Checking for motor activity in the postoperative period is an essential part of care that should not be neglected at all, of course as soon as the patient is awake and gains full muscle force recovery.

Clinical Outcome

In the current era of congenital heart disease, CoA is no longer considered as a simple disease especially when considering that treatment of CoA, with any of the modalities discussed in previous parts, is rarely definitive. Total resolution of the patients is faced with chronic challenges including recurrence (re-CoA) and/or aneurysm. Without treatment, mortality rate is increased; and the mean age of death in CoA patients is 32–34 years. Also, without treatment, survival of CoA patients, when calculated from the birth time until 58 years, is about 90 %; this is why early treatment is essential. Early curative treatment decreases the rate of mortality; while recurrence of aneurysm despite successful repair still remains as a major risk factor for death. Finally, CoA is associated with higher mortality and lower outcome in patients with associated anomalies; often this is the case in neonates and younger children who have significant associated morbidities (Shinebourne et al. 1976; Suarez de Lezo et al. 1999; Celermajer and Greaves 2002; von Kodolitsch et al. 2002, 2010; Verheugt et al. 2008; Axt-Fliedner et al. 2009; Lee and d'Udekem 2014).

Despite the morbidity and mortality, CoA patients have relatively acceptable functional health state and are comparable with normal population. However, the following points should be considered as comorbidities associated with CoA even after repair:

- Cardiac disease, including decreased cardiac output, and also heart failure presenting as increased mass of the left ventricle, systolic and/or diastolic dysfunction of the left ventricle.
- Hypertension mandating antihypertensive treatment.
- Diseases of the aorta and the aortic trunk (including aneurysm formation, ectasia in the ascending aorta, regurgitation of the ascending aorta, etc.).
- Though surgical correction of CoA removes the anatomic narrowing, the underlying vascular disease and possible vasculopathy still remain.
- Recurrence of aortic stenosis (i.e., Re-CoA) which is a relatively frequent problem necessitating repetitive intervention(s) including surgical or nonsurgical modalities; however, some believe that re-CoA is more frequent in the complex CoA compared with simple CoA patients.
- Premature coronary artery disease and/or and cerebrovascular disease.
- Aneurysm formation: different studies across different centers have announced very different rates for aneurysm formation after repair of CoA, 1–51 %. This could be to some degrees due to the diagnostic criteria for aneurysm. The following could be considered as risk factors for aneurysm formation:

  1. Patch graft technique
  2. Late repair of CoA
  3. High preoperative gradient across CoA

4. Bicuspid aortic valve
5. Inherent properties of the aortic wall (i.e., wall weakness)

- Acute kidney injury (AKI) is among the perioperative problems that might be encountered during repair of CoA (O'Rourke and Cartmill 1971; Fawzy et al. 1997, 2004, 2008, Celermajer and Greaves 2002; O'Sullivan et al. 2002; von Kodolitsch et al. 2002, 2010; Hassan et al. 2007a; Vohra et al. 2009; Pedersen et al. 2011; Pedersen 2012; Jang et al. 2014; Tong et al. 2014).

Other Forms of Aortic Stenosis

- Supravalvular aortic stenosis is categorized under a group of diseases with some similar properties. Among this classification, Williams syndrome is just mentioned here; though a detailed discussion could be found in Chap. 26.
- In brief, Williams syndrome is a syndrome with cardiovascular involvements, a characteristic facial appearance, endocrine and connective tissue abnormalities, and mild cognitive abnormalities; usually the aorta has a thick texture due to tissue changes. Stenosis is most severe at the sinotubular junction, being corrected suing a "Doty patch" to increase the diameter of the aorta at sinotubular junction; usually the incision is done at the point between right and noncoronary sinuses just above the aortic valve (Matisoff et al. 2015).

Interrupted Aortic Arch (IAA)

IAA is a disease of total aortic absence; and unlike CoA, no remnants of the aorta exist; the most common anatomic location for IAA is between left common carotid and left subclavian artery.

Two main theories are suggested for IAA:

- Blood flow theory, which considers IAA with malalignment of VSD and subaortic stenosis.
- Ductal tissue theory; only in type B of IAA this theory might be proposed; otherwise, in type A, ductal tissue theory is not considered a possibility.

Classification of IAA

The classification of IAA was introduced in 1959 by Celoria and Patton; this classification affects the clinical outcome and also the surgical procedure (Celoria and Patton 1959; McCrindle et al. 2005). The three main types of IAA are:

- Type A: the lesion is anatomically located at the isthmus, i.e., near the ductus and before the origin of the left subclavian artery.

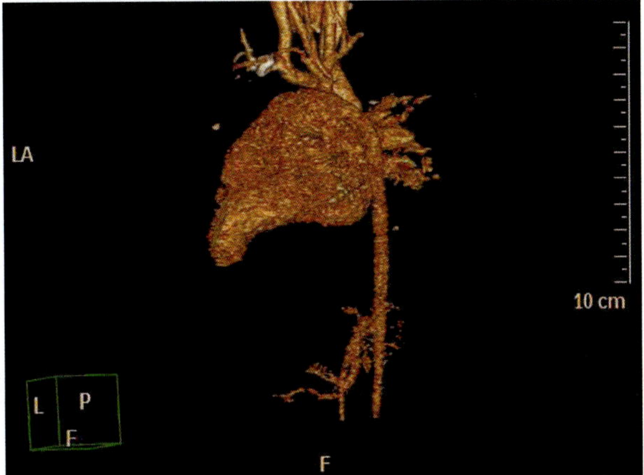

Fig. 24.2 Computer tomographic reconstruction of interrupted aortic arch type A. Note all the head, neck, and upper extremity vessels arise proximal to the ductus arteriosus. Distal blood flow beyond the aortic arch arises from the ductus arteriosus

- Type B: the lesion is located in the distal arch, i.e., between origin of left subclavian and left common carotid arteries; this is *the most common* type of IAA; in this type, the absence of the distal arch leads to impalpable pulses in both the left hand and femoral arteries, while the right hand has a palpable pulse. Also, there is strong association between type B and DiGeorge syndrome.
- Type C: the lesion is in the proximal arch, i.e., between origin of innominate and left common carotid arteries; this is an *extremely rare* form of IAA (Fig. 24.2).

Associated Anomalies

It has been demonstrated that nearly all of neonates with IAA have a coexisting congenital heart disease like (Patel et al. 2015):

- Ventricular septal defects (the most frequent associated cardiac anomaly)
- Truncus arteriosus
- Aorticopulmonary window
- Patent ductus arteriosus

Clinical Findings

Before birth, the clinical findings of the IAA patient are not critical since the blood flow to body's organs depends minimally on blood flow through the aorta. Distal blood flow is highly dependent on the patency of ductus arteriosus if IAA is diagnosed during fetal period; prostaglandin E1 infusion should be started promptly after birth to prevent ductal closure; otherwise, severe distal ischemia occurs with the following results:

- Hepatic ischemia leading to increased liver aminotransferases.
- Splanchnic and gut ischemia leading to necrotizing enterocolitis.
- Renal ischemia leading to anuria and severe kidney injury.
- In type B of IAA, there is risk of ischemia in those parts perfused by the left subclavian artery.
- Finally, distal ischemia leads to injury in all parts of the body and other organs, causing severe myocardial depression and low cardiac output.
- Impaired cerebral perfusion and acidosis lead to brain seizure.
- In brief, the prognosis of severe distal ischemia and systemic acidosis is poor (Oosterhof et al. 2004).

Diagnosis: IAA is usually diagnosed using echocardiography. Prenatal echocardiography could be of great help. Often, the majority of the patients need no further assessment including angiography; though in some cases with rare anatomic patterns of disease, magnetic resonance angiography (MRA) may be helpful to detect the lesion and concomitant anomalies much more precisely (Geva et al. 1993; Dillman et al. 2008). However, in echocardiography, the following are among the main items to be examined:

- The anatomic location of interruption (i.e., type of the disease).
- The length of interruption and discontinuity of the aorta.
- The diameter of the ascending aorta and the aortic valve.
- The narrowest portion of the left ventricular outflow tract (LVOT); an LVOT area is equal or less than 0.7 cm^2/m^2 and has been demonstrated as "a sensitive predictor" of post-repair LVOT obstruction (Geva et al. 1993).
- Other associated anomalies like VSD or ASD.
- The size and presence of the thymus for probability of DiGeorge syndrome.

The above items are to be compared with post-bypass exam findings in intraoperative TEE.

Infusion of intravenous prostaglandin in infants with IAA is an integral component of the treatment; so, in the minority of the cases that such a patient undergoes angiography, hemodynamic assessments are not so much useful except for the adequacy of LVOT which its measurement is not affected by prostaglandin infusion.

Treatment

IAA is a disease needing curative surgery to be treated. Prenatal diagnosis helps diagnose the disease and its types much earlier.

Surgical treatment the current method for treatment for IAA is single-stage repair of the aorta using direct anastomosis between the ascending and descending aorta. This procedure is done through median sternotomy and requires appropriate relief of both proximal and distal segments of the aorta before anastomosis. However, staged repair is used in some centers (Brown et al. 2006).

Although surgical approach for "native" IAA is considered as a curative method, IAA is a chronic disease, and subsequent treatments for relief of probable future restenosis are often part of the treatment protocol (Jegatheeswaran et al. 2010).

However, for the primary surgical relief, usually, hypothermic circulatory arrest cooling to 18 °C is used; however, a growing number of centers use selective antegrade cerebral perfusion for brain protection. Needless to say, neuromonitoring with both NIRS and Transcranial Doppler (TCD), hematocrit levels of 25 % or more, pH stat strategy, and especially, good experience of the surgeon to decrease the time of aortic clamp are the main determinants for good CNS outcome.

Usually no interventional treatment is considered as an option for native IAA, unless recurrence of stenosis after primary surgical repair; in some studies, the rate of restenosis needing interventional treatment is low; while some studies have claimed a relatively higher rate of restenosis needing relief of the stenotic site with balloon dilatation. However, as mentioned earlier, IAA is a chronic disease, so care should be given to detect any restenosis after primary successful surgical repair.

For the surgical operation to be done, sophisticated perioperative care is mandatory which begins with prenatal diagnosis, postpartum stabilization of the newborn using secure and safe intravenous lines, administering intravenous prostaglandin infusion with restoration of organ perfusion to prevent ischemia and acidosis, acid–base and respiratory therapy in order to normalize blood pH and keep PCO_2 between 40 and 50 torr, and other measures that are discussed under "anesthetic management."

Anesthetic management the perioperative care is discussed under three subtitles: preoperative, intraoperative, and postoperative period.

Preoperative management after birth, the following steps should be taken in before the surgical operation in order to prepare the patient for the procedure:

- *Intravenous prostaglandin* should be started as soon as possible through a safe and secure intravenous line; otherwise the patient will become severely acidotic due to closure of ductus arteriosus and the resulting lower limb ischemia; more than 40 years has passed from the first clinical experiments with intravenous prostaglandin infusion for prevention of ductal closure in ductal-dependent neonates; in all of these patents, including IAA, the administration of prostaglandin has given us the opportunity to prevent emergent and out of control surgical palliation (Freedom et al. 2000).
- *Inotropic support* is at times necessary; either infusions, dopamine or epinephrine, is an appropriate choice.
- *Treatment of acidosis* to reach to normal acid–base status; renal function should be restored to stable condition.
- *Other organs* should also function appropriately.
- *Oxygenation* status includes avoidance of excessive oxygen delivery leading to an unwanted drop in pulmonary vascular resistance (PVR); then, unnecessary decrease in PVR shifts the blood flow away from the systemic circulation toward the pulmonary vasculature; the final result would be aggravated ischemia of the distal limbs.

- *Ventilation* should be optimized: prevention of hyperventilation is necessary whether the infant has spontaneous ventilation or is intubated and mechanically ventilated; again, hyperventilation leads to unnecessary drop in PVR followed with a shift from systemic circulation to the pulmonary vasculature; PCO_2 between 40 and 40 torr is the target of ventilation.
- The patient should be prepared in the preoperative period for the course of operation.

Intraoperative Management

The same principles for preoperative period should be followed in the OR, including prostaglandin infusion, prevention of hyperventilation, and avoidance of unnecessary oxygen delivery. Also, the following should be considered:

- Arterial line should be established both pre- and post-interruption; for this purpose, often, the right radial artery is used for pre-interruption pressure, and the umbilical artery is used for the post-interruption pressure; the latter has two main uses, first for guaranteeing adequacy of perfusion in lower limbs and distal organs during cardiopulmonary bypass and second, for detection of any residual gradient between the ascending aorta and distal aorta after anastomosis just after weaning from bypass (i.e., inside the operating room).
- Prostaglandin infusion should be continued.
- The procedure is usually done through median sternotomy, with deep hypothermic arrest in 18 °C; however, some surgeons and centers prefer antegrade cerebral perfusion. So, adequacy of CNS protection should be monitored including the use of NIRS and TCD.
- At first, enough release of the ascending aorta and also the distal aorta is done; then, the ascending aorta is cannulated, and the patient is cooled until deep hypothermic arrest; proximal to distal anastomosis is done at this stage.
- Then, the patient is rewarmed up to 25 °C; in this stage, VSD is repaired, and finally, if there is an ASD, it is also repaired.
- Now, the patient is completely rewarmed and weaned from bypass.
- Often, an inotropic support is needed for weaning from bypass.
- Care should be given to treat any bleeding, including both packed cells, cryoprecipitate, and platelets; if there is leak through sutures of the anastomosis, the bleeding could be very severe and life-threatening.
- Intraoperative TEE is very helpful in detection of any underlying surgical defect, especially when its data are compared with preoperative echo findings.

Postoperative management if the procedure is done without complication, the inotropic support will be tapered up to 48 h after surgery. Pain management is an integral part of care. Then, the patient could be extubated. The following conditions could be the main reasons for unsuccessful weaning and extubation:

- *LVOT obstruction* (*LVOTO*): in patients with single-stage repair, the chance for LVOTO is less than other surgical approaches; also, in single-stage repair patients, would any stricture happen, it could be relieved much more easily with balloon dilatation; while in those having a conduit graft for primary surgical repair, any subsequent repair should be usually corrected using a new conduit graft; on the other hand, one of the most important predictive factors which could foresee the chance of LVOTO is the size of aortic annulus; when it is less than 4.5 mm, the chance for future LVOTO could be increased significantly.

- *Residual surgical defects* including mainly residual VSD and residual ASD.
- *Phrenic nerve* or *left recurrent* nerve palsy: this could be a source for complications like vocal cord paralysis and/or dysphagia which are at times difficult to treat and need both patience and frequent follow-up visits; at times, interventions like vocal fold medicalization or injection medialization laryngoplasty may be needed (Pham et al. 2014).

Usually, the above technical defects (especially the acute events) should be considered seriously especially by the surgeons as probable technical problems hindering weaning and extubation. Further evaluation and even, reoperation maybe needed.

However, a residual gradient between two sides of the anastomosis is considered negligible when it is less than 30 mmHg; however, higher gradients need more assessments by the surgeon.

References

Abbruzzese PA, Aidala E. Aortic coarctation: an overview. J Cardiovasc Med (Hagerstown). 2007;8:123–8.

Aboulhosn J, Child JS. Left ventricular outflow obstruction: subaortic stenosis, bicuspid aortic valve, supravalvar aortic stenosis, and coarctation of the aorta. Circulation. 2006;114:2412–22.

Aboulhosn J, Child JS. Echocardiographic evaluation of congenital left ventricular outflow obstruction. Echocardiography (Mount Kisco, NY). 2015;32 Suppl 2:S140–7.

Agnoleti G, Annecchino F, Preda L, Borghi A. Persistence of the left superior caval vein: can it potentiate obstructive lesions of the left ventricle? Cardiol Young. 1999;9:285–90.

Akdemir R, Agac MT, Acar Z. Aortic coarctation: angioplasty and stenting of a total occlusion. Acta Cardiol. 2010;65:467–70.

Allan LD, Chita SK, Al-Ghazali W, Crawford DC, Tynan M. Doppler echocardiographic evaluation of the normal human fetal heart. Br Heart J. 1987;57:528–33.

Allan LD, Chita SK, Anderson RH, Fagg N, Crawford DC, Tynan MJ. Coarctation of the aorta in prenatal life: an echocardiographic, anatomical, and functional study. Br Heart J. 1988;59:356–60.

Allan LD, Chita SK, Sharland GK, Fagg NL, Anderson RH, Crawford DC. The accuracy of fetal echocardiography in the diagnosis of congenital heart disease. Int J Cardiol. 1989;25:279–88.

Axt-Fliedner R, Hartge D, Krapp M, Berg C, Geipel A, Koester S, Noack F, Germer U, Gembruch U. Course and outcome of fetuses suspected of having coarctation of the aorta during gestation. Ultraschall Med. 2009;30:269–76.

Azakie A, Muse J, Gardner M, Skidmore KL, Miller SP, Karl TR, McQuillen PS. Cerebral oxygen balance is impaired during repair of aortic coarctation in infants and children. J Thorac Cardiovasc Surg. 2005;130:830–6.

Backer CL, Paape K, Zales VR, Weigel TJ, Mavroudis C. Coarctation of the aorta. Repair with polytetrafluoroethylene patch aortoplasty. Circulation. 1995;92:II132–6.

Baykan A, Narin N, Ozyurt A, Argun M, Pamukcu O, Mavili E, Sezer S, Onan SH, Uzum K. Cheatham platinum stent implantation in children with coarctation of the aorta: single-centre short-term, intermediate-term, and long-term results from Turkey. Cardiol Young. 2014;24:675–84.

Berens RJ, Stuth EA, Robertson FA, Jaquiss RD, Hoffman GM, Troshynski TJ, Staudt SR, Cava JR, Tweddell JS, Bert Litwin S. Near infrared spectroscopy monitoring during pediatric aortic coarctation repair. Paediatr Anaesth. 2006;16:777–81.

Botta L, Russo V, Oppido G, Rosati M, Massi F, Lovato L, Di Bartolomeo R, Fattori R. Role of endovascular repair in the management of late pseudo-aneurysms following open surgery for aortic coarctation. Eur J Cardiothorac Surg. 2009;36:670–4.

Bouchart F, Dubar A, Tabley A, Litzler PY, Haas-Hubscher C, Redonnet M, Bessou JP, Soyer R. Coarctation of the aorta in adults: surgical results and long-term follow-up. Ann Thorac Surg. 2000;70:1483–8; discussion 1488–1489.

Brown CB, Baldwin HS. Neural crest contribution to the cardiovascular system. Adv Exp Med Biol. 2006;589:134–54.

Brown JW, Ruzmetov M, Okada Y, Vijay P, Rodefeld MD, Turrentine MW. Outcomes in patients with interrupted aortic arch and associated anomalies: a 20-year experience. Eur J Cardiothorac Surg. 2006;29:666–73; discussion 673–664.

Campbell M. Natural history of coarctation of the aorta. Br Heart J. 1970;32:633–40.

Carroll SJ, Ferris A, Chen J, Liberman L. Efficacy of prostaglandin E1 in relieving obstruction in coarctation of a persistent fifth aortic arch without opening the ductus arteriosus. Pediatr Cardiol. 2006;27:766–8.

Celermajer DS, Greaves K. Survivors of coarctation repair: fixed but not cured. Heart. 2002;88:113–4.

Celik T, Kursaklioglu H, Iyisoy A, Turhan H, Amasyali B, Kocaoglu M, Isik E. Hypoplasia of the descending thoracic and abdominal aorta: a case report and review of literature. J Thorac Imaging. 2006;21:296–9.

Celoria GC, Patton RB. Congenital absence of the aortic arch. Am Heart J. 1959;58:407–13.

Cheatham JP. Stenting of coarctation of the aorta. Catheter Cardiovasc Interv Off J Soc Card Angiography Interv. 2001;54:112–25.

Cohen M, Fuster V, Steele PM, Driscoll D, McGoon DC. Coarctation of the aorta. Long-term follow-up and prediction of outcome after surgical correction. Circulation. 1989;80:840–5.

Connolly HM, Huston 3rd J, Brown Jr RD, Warnes CA, Ammash NM, Tajik AJ. Intracranial aneurysms in patients with coarctation of the aorta: a prospective magnetic resonance angiographic study of 100 patients. Mayo Clin Proc. 2003;78:1491–9.

Connors JP, Hartmann Jr AF, Weldon CS. Considerations in the surgical management of infantile coarctation of aorta. Am J Cardiol. 1975;36:489–92.

Cook SC, Hickey J, Maul TM, Zumberge N, Krieger EV, Valente AM, Zaidi AN, Daniels CJ. Assessment of the cerebral circulation in adults with coarctation of the aorta. Congenit Heart Dis. 2013;8:289–95.

Curtis SL, Bradley M, Wilde P, Aw J, Chakrabarti S, Hamilton M, Martin R, Turner M, Stuart AG. Results of screening for intracranial aneurysms in patients with coarctation of the aorta. AJNR Am J Neuroradiol. 2012;33:1182–6.

De Caro E, Spadoni I, Crepaz R, Saitta M, Trocchio G, Calevo MG, Pongiglione G. Stenting of aortic coarctation and exercise-induced hypertension in the young. Catheter Cardiovasc Interv Off J Soc Card Angiography Interv. 2010;75:256–61.

de Divitiis M, Pilla C, Kattenhorn M, Donald A, Zadinello M, Wallace S, Redington A, Deanfield J. Ambulatory blood pressure, left ventricular mass, and conduit artery function late after successful repair of coarctation of the aorta. J Am Coll Cardiol. 2003;41:2259–65.

de Divitiis M, Pilla C, Kattenhorn M, Zadinello M, Donald A, Leeson P, Wallace S, Redington A, Deanfield JE. Vascular dysfunction after repair of coarctation of the aorta: impact of early surgery. Circulation. 2001;104:I165–70.

de Divitiis M, Rubba P, Calabro R. Arterial hypertension and cardiovascular prognosis after successful repair of aortic coarctation: a clinical model for the study of vascular function. Nutr Metab Cardiovasc Dis. 2005;15:382–94.

De Mozzi P, Longo UG, Galanti G, Maffulli N. Bicuspid aortic valve: a literature review and its impact on sport activity. Br Med Bull. 2008;85:63–85.

De Smedt MC, Visser GH, Meijboom EJ. Fetal cardiac output estimated by Doppler echocardiography during mid- and late gestation. Am J Cardiol. 1987;60:338–42.

Digilio MC, Marino B, Toscano A, Giannotti A, Dallapiccola B. Congenital heart defects in Kabuki syndrome. Am J Med Genet. 2001;100:269–74.

Dillman JR, Yarram SG, D'Amico AR, Hernandez RJ. Interrupted aortic arch: spectrum of MRI findings. AJR Am J Roentgenol. 2008;190:1467–74.

Dodge-Khatami A, Ott S, Di Bernardo S, Berger F. Carotid-subclavian artery index: new echocardiographic index to detect coarctation in neonates and infants. Ann Thorac Surg. 2005;80:1652–7.

Dulac Y, Pienkowski C, Abadir S, Tauber M, Acar P. Cardiovascular abnormalities in Turner's syndrome: what prevention? Arch Cardiovasc Dis. 2008;101:485–90.

Eapen RS, Rowland DG, Franklin WH. Effect of prenatal diagnosis of critical left heart obstruction on perinatal morbidity and mortality. Am J Perinatol. 1998;15:237–42.

Eckroth-Bernard K, Yoon HR, Ryer EJ, Elmore JR. Percutaneous endovascular repair of adult aortic coarctation. J Vasc Surg. 2014;59:1120.

Egan M, Holzer RJ. Comparing balloon angioplasty, stenting and surgery in the treatment of aortic coarctation. Expert Rev Cardiovasc Ther. 2009;7:1401–12.

Elzenga NJ, Gittenberger-de Groot AC, Oppenheimer-Dekker A. Coarctation and other obstructive aortic arch anomalies: their relationship to the ductus arteriosus. Int J Cardiol. 1986;13:289–308.

Fawzy ME, Awad M, Hassan W, Al Kadhi Y, Shoukri M, Fadley F. Long-term outcome (up to 15 years) of balloon angioplasty of discrete native coarctation of the aorta in adolescents and adults. J Am Coll Cardiol. 2004;43:1062–7.

Fawzy ME, Dunn B, Galal O, Wilson N, Shaikh A, Sriram R, Duran CM. Balloon coarctation angioplasty in adolescents and adults: early and intermediate results. Am Heart J. 1992;124:167–71.

Fawzy ME, Fathala A, Osman A, Badr A, Mostafa MA, Mohamed G, Dunn B. Twenty-two years of follow-up results of balloon angioplasty for discreet native coarctation of the aorta in adolescents and adults. Am Heart J. 2008;156:910–7.

Fawzy ME, Sivanandam V, Galal O, Dunn B, Patel A, Rifai A, von Sinner W, Al Halees Z, Khan B. One- to ten-year follow-up results of balloon angioplasty of native coarctation of the aorta in adolescents and adults. J Am Coll Cardiol. 1997;30:1542–6.

Fawzy ME, Sivanandam V, Pieters F, Stefadouros MA, Galal O, Dunn B, Kinsara A, Khan B, Al-Halees Z. Long-term effects of balloon angioplasty on systemic hypertension in adolescent and adult patients with coarctation of the aorta. Eur Heart J. 1999;20:827–32.

Feltes TF, Bacha E, Beekman 3rd RH, Cheatham JP, Feinstein JA, Gomes AS, Hijazi ZM, Ing FF, de Moor M, Morrow WR, Mullins CE, Taubert KA, Zahn EM. Indications for cardiac catheterization and intervention in pediatric cardiac disease: a scientific statement from the American Heart Association. Circulation. 2011;123:2607–52.

Findlow D, Doyle E. Congenital heart disease in adults. Br J Anaesth. 1997;78:416–30.

Forbes TJ, Garekar S, Amin Z, Zahn EM, Nykanen D, Moore P, Qureshi SA, Cheatham JP, Ebeid MR, Hijazi ZM, Sandhu S, Hagler DJ, Sievert H, Fagan TE, Ringewald J, Du W, Tang L, Wax DF, Rhodes J, Johnston TA, Jones TK, Turner DR, Pedra CA, Hellenbrand WE. Procedural results and acute complications in stenting native and recurrent coarctation of the aorta in patients over 4 years of age: a multi-institutional study. Catheter Cardiovasc Interv Off J Soc Card Angiography Interv. 2007a;70:276–85.

Forbes TJ, Kim DW, Du W, Turner DR, Holzer R, Amin Z, Hijazi Z, Ghasemi A, Rome JJ, Nykanen D, Zahn E, Cowley C, Hoyer M, Waight D, Gruenstein D, Javois A, Foerster S, Kreutzer J, Sullivan N, Khan A, Owada C, Hagler D, Lim S, Canter J, Zellers T. Comparison of surgical, stent, and balloon angioplasty treatment of native coarctation of the aorta: an observational study by the CCISC (Congenital Cardiovascular Interventional Study Consortium). J Am Coll Cardiol. 2011;58:2664–74.

Forbes TJ, Moore P, Pedra CA, Zahn EM, Nykanen D, Amin Z, Garekar S, Teitel D, Qureshi SA, Cheatham JP, Ebeid MR, Hijazi ZM, Sandhu S, Hagler DJ, Sievert H, Fagan TE, Ringwald J, Du W, Tang L, Wax DF, Rhodes J, Johnston TA, Jones TK, Turner DR, Pass R, Torres A, Hellenbrand WE. Intermediate follow-up following intravascular stenting for treatment of coarctation of the aorta. Catheter Cardiovasc Interv Off J Soc Card Angiography Interv. 2007b;70:569–77.

Franklin O, Burch M, Manning N, Sleeman K, Gould S, Archer N. Prenatal diagnosis of coarctation of the aorta improves survival and reduces morbidity. Heart. 2002;87:67–9.

Freedom RM, Lock J, Bricker JT. Pediatric cardiology and cardiovascular surgery: 1950–2000. Circulation. 2000;102:Iv58–68.

Garg R, Murthy K, Rao S, Muralidhar K. Intra-operative trans-esophageal echocardiography in congenital heart disease. Ann Card Anaesth. 2009;12:166.

Gelman S. The pathophysiology of aortic cross-clamping and unclamping. Anesthesiology. 1995;82:1026–60.

Geva T, Hornberger LK, Sanders SP, Jonas RA, Ott DA, Colan SD. Echocardiographic predictors of left ventricular outflow tract obstruction after repair of interrupted aortic arch. J Am Coll Cardiol. 1993;22:1953–60.

Gillman RG, Burton AC. Constriction of the neonatal aorta by raised oxygen tension. Circ Res. 1966;19:755–65.

Glen S, Burns J, Bloomfield P. Prevalence and development of additional cardiac abnormalities in 1448 patients with congenital ventricular septal defects. Heart. 2004;90:1321–5.

Godart F. Intravascular stenting for the treatment of coarctation of the aorta in adolescent and adult patients. Arch Cardiovasc Dis. 2011;104:627–35.

Gotzsche CO, Krag-Olsen B, Nielsen J, Sorensen KE, Kristensen BO. Prevalence of cardiovascular malformations and association with karyotypes in Turner's syndrome. Arch Dis Child. 1994;71:433–6.

Gravholt CH. Turner syndrome and the heart: cardiovascular complications and treatment strategies. Am J Cardiovasc Drugs. 2002;2:401–13.

Hartge DR, Niemeyer L, Axt-Fliedner R, Krapp M, Gembruch U, Germer U, Weichert J. Prenatal detection and postnatal management of double outlet right ventricle (DORV) in 21 singleton pregnancies. J Matern Fetal Neonatal Med. 2012;25:58–63.

Hassan W, Awad M, Fawzy ME, Omrani AA, Malik S, Akhras N, Shoukri M. Long-term effects of balloon angioplasty on left ventricular hypertrophy in adolescent and adult patients with native coarctation of the aorta. Up to 18 years follow-up results. Catheter Cardiovasc Interv Off J Soc Card Angiography Interv. 2007a;70:881–6.

Hassan W, Malik S, Akhras N, Amri MA, Shoukri M, Fawzy ME. Long-term results (up to 18 years) of balloon angioplasty on systemic hypertension in adolescent and adult patients with coarctation of the aorta. Clin Cardiol. 2007b;30:75–80.

Head CE, Jowett VC, Sharland GK, Simpson JM. Timing of presentation and postnatal outcome of infants suspected of having coarctation of the aorta during fetal life. Heart. 2005;91:1070–4.

Heymann MA, Rudolph AM. Effects of congenital heart disease on fetal and neonatal circulations. Prog Cardiovasc Dis. 1972;15:115–43.

High FA, Zhang M, Proweller A, Tu L, Parmacek MS, Pear WS, Epstein JA. An essential role for Notch in neural crest during cardiovascular development and smooth muscle differentiation. J Clin Invest. 2007;117:353–63.

Hijazi ZM. Catheter intervention for adult aortic coarctation: be very careful! Catheter Cardiovasc Interv Off J Soc Card Angiography Interv. 2003;59:536–7.

Hijazi ZM, Awad SM. Pediatric cardiac interventions. JACC Cardiovasc Interv. 2008;1:603–11.

Hijazi ZM, Kenny DP. Covered stents for coarctation of the aorta: treating the interventionalist or the patient? JACC Cardiovasc Interv. 2014;7:424–5.

Ho SY, Anderson RH. Coarctation, tubular hypoplasia, and the ductus arteriosus. Histological study of 35 specimens. Br Heart J. 1979;41:268–74.

Holzer R, Qureshi S, Ghasemi A, Vincent J, Sievert H, Gruenstein D, Weber H, Alday L, Peirone A, Zellers T, Cheatham J, Slack M, Rome J. Stenting of aortic coarctation: acute, intermediate, and long-term results of a prospective multi-institutional registry--Congenital Cardiovascular Interventional Study Consortium (CCISC). Catheter Cardiovasc Interv Off J Soc Card Angiography Interv. 2010;76:553–63.

Hormann M, Pavlidis D, Brunkwall J, Gawenda M. Long-term results of endovascular aortic repair for thoracic pseudoaneurysms after previous surgical coarctation repair. Interact Cardiovasc Thorac Surg. 2011;13:401–4.

Hornberger LK, Sahn DJ, Kleinman CS, Copel J, Silverman NH. Antenatal diagnosis of coarctation of the aorta: a multicenter experience. J Am Coll Cardiol. 1994;23:417–23.

Hughes HE, Davies SJ. Coarctation of the aorta in Kabuki syndrome. Arch Dis Child. 1994;70:512–4.

Hutchins GM. Coarctation of the aorta explained as a branch-point of the ductus arteriosus. Am J Pathol. 1971;63:203–14.

Imada T, Okutani R, Oda Y. Anesthesia for aortic reconstruction in a child with PHACE syndrome. J Anesth. 2014;28:919–23.

Isner JM, Donaldson RF, Fulton D, Bhan I, Payne DD, Cleveland RJ. Cystic medial necrosis in coarctation of the aorta: a potential factor contributing to adverse consequences observed after percutaneous balloon angioplasty of coarctation sites. Circulation. 1987;75:689–95.

Jain R, Engleka KA, Rentschler SL, Manderfield LJ, Li L, Yuan L, Epstein JA. Cardiac neural crest orchestrates remodeling and functional maturation of mouse semilunar valves. J Clin Invest. 2011;121:422–30.

Jang WS, Kim WH, Choi K, Nam J, Jung JC, Kwon BS, Kim GB, Kang HG, Lee JR, Kim YJ. Incidence, risk factors and clinical outcomes for acute kidney injury after aortic arch repair in paediatric patients. Eur J Cardiothorac Surg. 2014;45:e208–14.

Jegatheeswaran A, McCrindle BW, Blackstone EH, Jacobs ML, Lofland GK, Austin 3rd EH, Yeh T, Morell V, Jacobs JP, Jonas RA, Cai S, Rajeswaran J, Ricci M, Williams WG, Caldarone CA, DeCampli WM. Persistent risk of subsequent procedures and mortality in patients after interrupted aortic arch repair: a Congenital Heart Surgeons' Society study. J Thorac Cardiovasc Surg. 2010;140:1059–1075.e1052.

Jimenez M, Daret D, Choussat A, Bonnet J. Immunohistological and ultrastructural analysis of the intimal thickening in coarctation of human aorta. Cardiovasc Res. 1999;41:737–45.

Kaine SF, Smith EO, Mott AR, Mullins CE, Geva T. Quantitative echocardiographic analysis of the aortic arch predicts outcome of balloon angioplasty of native coarctation of the aorta. Circulation. 1996;94:1056–62.

Kannan BR, Srinivasan M. Stent migration during transcatheter management of coarctation of aorta. Catheter Cardiovasc Interv Off J Soc Card Angiography Interv. 2012;79:408–13.

Kanter KR. Management of infants with coarctation and ventricular septal defect. Semin Thorac Cardiovasc Surg. 2007;19:264–8.

Kappetein AP, Gittenberger-de Groot AC, Zwinderman AH, Rohmer J, Poelmann RE, Huysmans HA. The neural crest as a possible pathogenetic factor in coarctation of the aorta and bicuspid aortic valve. J Thorac Cardiovasc Surg. 1991;102:830–6.

Kataoka K, Ozawa A, Inage A, Benson LN. Transcatheter repair of native coarctation in children with Turner syndrome: three case reports and literature review. Congenit Heart Dis. 2006;1:315–20.

Kenny D, Cao QL, Kavinsky C, Hijazi ZM. Innovative resource utilization to fashion individualized covered stents in the setting of aortic coarctation. Catheter Cardiovasc Interv Off J Soc Card Angiography Interv. 2011;78:413–8.

Kenny D, Hijazi ZM. Coarctation of the aorta: from fetal life to adulthood. Cardiol J. 2011;18:487–95.

Keshavarz-Motamed Z, Garcia J, Kadem L. Mathematical, numerical and experimental study in the human aorta with coexisting models of bicuspid aortic stenosis and coarctation of the aorta. Conf Proc IEEE Eng Med Biol Soc. 2011a;2011:182–5.

Keshavarz-Motamed Z, Garcia J, Kadem L. Fluid dynamics of coarctation of the aorta and effect of bicuspid aortic valve. PLoS One. 2013;8:e72394.

Keshavarz-Motamed Z, Garcia J, Maftoon N, Bedard E, Chetaille P, Kadem L. A new approach for the evaluation of the severity of coarctation of the aorta using Doppler velocity index and effective orifice area: in vitro validation and clinical implications. J Biomech. 2012;45:1239–45.

Keshavarz-Motamed Z, Garcia J, Pibarot P, Larose E, Kadem L. Modeling the impact of concomitant aortic stenosis and coarctation of the aorta on left ventricular workload. J Biomech. 2011b;44:2817–25.

Keshavarz-Motamed Z, Kadem L. 3D pulsatile flow in a curved tube with coexisting model of aortic stenosis and coarctation of the aorta. Med Eng Phys. 2011;33:315–24.

Khavandi A, Bentham J, Marlais M, Martin RP, Morgan GJ, Parry AJ, Brooks MJ, Manghat NE, Hamilton MC, Baumbach A, McPherson S, Thomson JD, Turner MS. Transcatheter and endovascular stent graft management of coarctation-related pseudoaneurysms. Heart. 2013;99:1275–81.

Kische S, Schneider H, Akin I, Ortak J, Rehders TC, Chatterjee T, Nienaber CA, Ince H. Technique of interventional repair in adult aortic coarctation. J Vasc Surg. 2010;51:1550–9.

Kothari SS. Dissection after stent dilatation for coarctation of aorta. Catheter Cardiovasc Interv Off J Soc Card Angiography Interv. 2004;62:421; author reply 421.

Krediet P. An hypothesis of the development of coarctation in man. Acta Morphol Neerl Scand. 1965;6:207–12.

Kuhn A, Baumgartner D, Baumgartner C, Horer J, Schreiber C, Hess J, Vogt M. Impaired elastic properties of the ascending aorta persist within the first 3 years after neonatal coarctation repair. Pediatr Cardiol. 2009;30:46–51.

Kuroczynski W, Hartert M, Pruefer D, Pitzer-Hartert K, Heinemann M, Vahl CF. Surgical treatment of aortic coarctation in adults: beneficial effect on arterial hypertension. Cardiol J. 2008;15:537–42.

Lee MG, d'Udekem Y. Coarctation of the aorta can no longer be considered a benign condition. Heart Lung Circ. 2014;23:297–8.

Lee MG, Kowalski R, Galati JC, Cheung MM, Jones B, Koleff J, d'Udekem Y. Twenty-four-hour ambulatory blood pressure monitoring detects a high prevalence of hypertension late after coarctation repair in patients with hypoplastic arches. J Thorac Cardiovasc Surg. 2012a;144:1110–6.

Lee SH, Kim JH, Lee JH, Kim SC. PHACE syndrome associated with club foot and thumb-in-palm deformity. J Dermatol. 2012b;39:1054–5.

Liberman L, Gersony WM, Flynn PA, Lamberti JJ, Cooper RS, Stare TJ. Effectiveness of prostaglandin E1 in relieving obstruction in coarctation of the aorta without opening the ductus arteriosus. Pediatr Cardiol. 2004;25:49–52.

Luijendijk P, Bouma BJ, Groenink M, Boekholdt M, Hazekamp MG, Blom NA, Koolbergen DR, de Winter RJ, Mulder BJ. Surgical versus percutaneous treatment of aortic coarctation: new standards in an era of transcatheter repair. Expert Rev Cardiovasc Ther. 2012;10:1517–31.

Mahadevan V, Mullen MJ. Endovascular management of aortic coarctation. Int J Cardiol. 2004;97 Suppl 1:75–8.

Marcheix B, Lamarche Y, Perrault P, Cartier R, Bouchard D, Carrier M, Perrault LP, Demers P. Endovascular management of pseudo-aneurysms after previous surgical repair of congenital aortic coarctation. Eur J Cardiothorac Surg. 2007;31:1004–7.

Marelli AJ, Child JS, Perloff JK. Transesophageal echocardiography in congenital heart disease in the adult. Cardiol Clin. 1993;11:505–20.

Markham LW, Knecht SK, Daniels SR, Mays WA, Khoury PR, Knilans TK. Development of exercise-induced arm-leg blood pressure gradient and abnormal arterial compliance in patients with repaired coarctation of the aorta. Am J Cardiol. 2004;94:1200–2.

Matisoff AJ, Olivieri L, Schwartz JM, Deutsch N. Risk assessment and anesthetic management of patients with Williams syndrome: a comprehensive review. Paediatr Anaesth. 2015;25:1207–15.

Matsui H, Mellander M, Roughton M, Jicinska H, Gardiner HM. Morphological and physiological predictors of fetal aortic coarctation. Circulation. 2008;118:1793–801.

Matsunaga N, Hayashi K, Okada M, Sakamoto I. Magnetic resonance imaging features of aortic diseases. Top Magn Reson Imaging. 2003;14:253–66.

McCrindle BW, Tchervenkov CI, Konstantinov IE, Williams WG, Neirotti RA, Jacobs ML, Blackstone EH. Risk factors associated with mortality and interventions in 472 neonates with interrupted aortic arch: a Congenital Heart Surgeons Society study. J Thorac Cardiovasc Surg. 2005;129:343–50.

McMahon CJ, Reardon W. The spectrum of congenital cardiac malformations encountered in six children with Kabuki syndrome. Cardiol Young. 2006;16:30–3.

Miller-Hance WC, Silverman NH. Transesophageal echocardiography (TEE) in congenital heart disease with focus on the adult. Cardiol Clin. 2000;18:861–92.

Miyague NI, Cardoso SM, Meyer F, Ultramari FT, Araujo FH, Rozkowisk I, Toschi AP. Epidemiological study of congenital heart defects in children and adolescents. Analysis of 4,538 cases. Arq Bras Cardiol. 2003;80:269–78.

Moerman A, Bove T, Francois K, Jacobs S, Deblaere I, Wouters P, De Hert S. Society of cardiovascular anesthesiologists: the effect of blood pressure regulation during aortic coarctation repair on brain, kidney, and muscle oxygen saturation measured by near-infrared spectroscopy: a randomized, clinical trial. Anesth Analg. 2013;116:760–6.

Momma K, Takao A, Ando M. Angiocardiographic study of coarctation of the aorta--morphology and morphogenesis. Jpn Circ J. 1982;46:174–83.

Moore GW, Hutchins GM. Association of interrupted aortic arch with malformations producing reduced blood flow to the fourth aortic arches. Am J Cardiol. 1978;42:467–72.

Morrow WR, Huhta JC, Murphy Jr DJ, McNamara DG. Quantitative morphology of the aortic arch in neonatal coarctation. J Am Coll Cardiol. 1986;8:616–20.

Neshat Vahid S, Panisello JM. The state of affairs of neurologic monitoring by near-infrared spectroscopy in pediatric cardiac critical care. Curr Opin Pediatr. 2014;26:299–303.

Niwa K. Aortopathy in congenital heart disease in adults: aortic dilatation with decreased aortic elasticity that impacts negatively on left ventricular function. Korean Circ J. 2013;43:215–20.

O'Rourke MF, Cartmill TB. Influence of aortic coarctation on pulsatile hemodynamics in the proximal aorta. Circulation. 1971;44:281–92.

O'Sullivan JJ, Derrick G, Darnell R. Prevalence of hypertension in children after early repair of coarctation of the aorta: a cohort study using casual and 24 hour blood pressure measurement. Heart. 2002;88:163–6.

Oosterhof T, Azakie A, Freedom RM, Williams WG, McCrindle BW. Associated factors and trends in outcomes of interrupted aortic arch. Ann Thorac Surg. 2004;78:1696–702.

Padua LM, Garcia LC, Rubira CJ, de Oliveira Carvalho PE (2012) Stent placement versus surgery for coarctation of the thoracic aorta. Cochrane Database Syst Rev 5:CD008204

Paladini D, Volpe P, Russo MG, Vassallo M, Sclavo G, Gentile M. Aortic coarctation: prognostic indicators of survival in the fetus. Heart. 2004;90:1348–9.

Patel DM, Maldjian PD, Lovoulos C. Interrupted aortic arch with post-interruption aneurysm and bicuspid aortic valve in an adult: a case report and literature review. Radiol Case Reports. 2015;10:5–8.

Pedersen TA. Late morbidity after repair of aortic coarctation. Dan Med J. 2012;59:B4436.

Pedersen TA, Munk K, Andersen NH, Lundorf E, Pedersen EB, Hjortdal VE, Emmertsen K. High long-term morbidity in repaired aortic coarctation: weak association with residual arch obstruction. Congenit Heart Dis. 2011;6:573–82.

Perloff JK. The variant associations of aortic isthmic coarctation. Am J Cardiol. 2010;106:1038–41.

Pham V, Connelly D, Wei JL, Sykes KJ, O'Brien J. Vocal cord paralysis and Dysphagia after aortic arch reconstruction and Norwood procedure. Otolaryngol Head Neck Surg Off J Am Acad Otolaryngol Head Neck Surg. 2014;150:827–33.

Phillips HM, Mahendran P, Singh E, Anderson RH, Chaudhry B, Henderson DJ. Neural crest cells are required for correct positioning of the developing outflow cushions and pattern the arterial valve leaflets. Cardiovasc Res. 2013;99:452–60.

Puttgen KB, Lin DD. Neurocutaneous vascular syndromes. Childs Nerv Syst ChNS Off J Int Soc Pediatr Neurosurg. 2010;26:1407–15.

Quaegebeur JM, Jonas RA, Weinberg AD, Blackstone EH, Kirklin JW. Outcomes in seriously ill neonates with coarctation of the aorta. A multiinstitutional study. J Thorac Cardiovasc Surg. 1994;108:841–51; discussion 852–844.

Ringel RE, Vincent J, Jenkins KJ, Gauvreau K, Moses H, Lofgren K, Usmani K. Acute outcome of stent therapy for coarctation of the aorta: results of the coarctation of the aorta stent trial. Catheter Cardiovasc Interv Off J Soc Card Angiography Interv. 2013;82:503–10.

Rosenthal E. Coarctation of the aorta from fetus to adult: curable condition or life long disease process? Heart. 2005;91:1495–502.

Rothman A, Galindo A, Evans WN, Collazos JC, Restrepo H. Effectiveness and safety of balloon dilation of native aortic coarctation in premature neonates weighing < or = 2,500 grams. Am J Cardiol. 2010;105:1176–80.

Rouine-Rapp K, Mello DM, Hanley FL, Mohan Reddy V, Soifer S. Effect of enalaprilat on post-operative hypertension after surgical repair of coarctation of the aorta. Pediatr Crit Care Med. 2003;4:327–32.

Rudolph AM, Heymann MA, Spitznas U. Hemodynamic considerations in the development of narrowing of the aorta. Am J Cardiol. 1972;30:514–25.

Russell GA, Berry PJ, Watterson K, Dhasmana JP, Wisheart JD. Patterns of ductal tissue in coarctation of the aorta in the first three months of life. J Thorac Cardiovasc Surg. 1991;102:596–601.

Schimke A, Majithia A, Baumgartner R, French A, Goldberg D, Kuvin J. Intervention and management of congenital left heart obstructive lesions. Curr Treat Options Cardiovasc Med. 2013;15:632–45.

Scott JP, Hoffman GM. Near-infrared spectroscopy: exposing the dark (venous) side of the circulation. Paediatr Anaesth. 2014;24:74–88.

Secchi F, Iozzelli A, Papini GD, Aliprandi A, Di Leo G, Sardanelli F. MR imaging of aortic coarctation. Radiol Med. 2009;114:524–37.

Sehested J, Baandrup U, Mikkelsen E. Different reactivity and structure of the prestenotic and poststenotic aorta in human coarctation. Implications for baroreceptor function. Circulation. 1982;65:1060–5.

Sharland GK, Chan KY, Allan LD. Coarctation of the aorta: difficulties in prenatal diagnosis. Br Heart J. 1994;71:70–5.

Shinebourne EA, Elseed AM. Relation between fetal flow patterns, coarctation of the aorta, and pulmonary blood flow. Br Heart J. 1974;36:492–8.

Shinebourne EA, Tam AS, Elseed AM, Paneth M, Lennox SC, Cleland WP. Coarctation of the aorta in infancy and childhood. Br Heart J. 1976;38:375–80.

Shively BK. Transesophageal echocardiographic (TEE) evaluation of the aortic valve, left ventricular outflow tract, and pulmonic valve. Cardiol Clin. 2000;18:711–29.

Shone JD, Sellers RD, Anderson RC, Adams Jr P, Lillehei CW, Edwards JE. The developmental complex of "parachute mitral valve," supravalvular ring of left atrium, subaortic stenosis, and coarctation of aorta. Am J Cardiol. 1963;11:714–25.

Singer MI, Rowen M, Dorsey TJ. Transluminal aortic balloon angioplasty for coarctation of the aorta in the newborn. Am Heart J. 1982;103:131–2.

Smith JC, Joransen JA, Heath B, Allen BC. Atypical aortic coarctation and innominate artery stenosis associated with clubfoot and lower leg ischemia in an infant. Teratology. 1995;52:357–60.

Sohrabi B, Jamshidi P, Yaghoubi A, Habibzadeh A, Hashemi-Aghdam Y, Moin A, Kazemi B, Ghaffari S, Abdolahzadeh Baghayi MR, Mahmoody K. Comparison between covered and bare Cheatham-Platinum stents for endovascular treatment of patients with native post-ductal aortic coarctation: immediate and intermediate-term results. JACC Cardiovasc Interv. 2014;7:416–23.

Sos T, Sniderman KW, Rettek-Sos B, Strupp A, Alonso DR. Percutaneous transluminal dilatation of coarctation of thoracic aorta post mortem. Lancet. 1979;2:970–1.

Stressig R, Axt-Fliedner R, Gembruch U, Kohl T. Preferential ductus venosus streaming toward the right heart is associated with left heart underdevelopment and aortic arch hypoplasia in human fetuses. Ultraschall Med. 2011;32 Suppl 2:E115–21.

Suarez de Lezo J, Pan M, Romero M, Medina A, Segura J, Lafuente M, Pavlovic D, Hernandez E, Melian F, Espada J. Immediate and follow-up findings after stent treatment for severe coarctation of aorta. Am J Cardiol. 1999;83:400–6.

Suarez de Lezo J, Pan M, Romero M, Segura J, Pavlovic D, Ojeda S, Algar J, Ribes R, Lafuente M, Lopez-Pujol J. Percutaneous interventions on severe coarctation of the aorta: a 21-year experience. Pediatr Cardiol. 2005;26:176–89.

Tabbutt S, Nicolson SC, Adamson PC, Zhang X, Hoffman ML, Wells W, Backer CL, McGowan FX, Tweddell JS, Bokesch P, Schreiner M. The safety, efficacy, and pharmacokinetics of esmolol for blood pressure control immediately after repair of coarctation of the aorta in infants and children: a multicenter, double-blind, randomized trial. J Thorac Cardiovasc Surg. 2008;136:321–8.

Takahashi K, Ino T, Ohkubo M, Akimoto K, Kishirou M. Restenosis after balloon angioplasty of coarctation: relationship with ductus arteriosus. Pediatr Int. 2000;42:658–67.

Tomar M, Radhakrishanan S. Coarctation of aorta--intervention from neonates to adult life. Indian Heart J. 2008;60:D22–33.

Tong F, Li ZQ, Li L, Chong M, Zhu YB, Su JW, Liu YL. The follow-up surgical results of coarctation of the aorta procedures in a cohort of Chinese children from a single institution. Heart Lung Circ. 2014;23:339–46.

Torok RD, Campbell MJ, Fleming GA, Hill KD. Coarctation of the aorta: management from infancy to adulthood. World J Cardiol. 2015;7:765–75.

Towbin JA, Belmont J. Molecular determinants of left and right outflow tract obstruction. Am J Med Genet. 2000;97:297–303.

Turkoz A, Balci ST, Can Guner M, Ulugol H, Vuran C, Ozker E, Turkoz R. Anesthesia management with single injection paravertebral block for aorta coarctation in infant. Paediatr Anaesth. 2013;23:1078–83.

Turner DR, Gaines PA. Endovascular management of coarctation of the aorta. Semin Interv Radiol. 2007;24:153–66.

Van Meurs-Van Woezik H, Krediet P. Changes after birth in the tunica media and in the internal diameter of the aortic isthmus in normal newborns. J Anat. 1982;134:573–81.

Van Mierop LH, Kutsche LM. Interruption of the aortic arch and coarctation of the aorta: pathogenetic relations. Am J Cardiol. 1984;54:829–34.

Van Mierop LH, Kutsche LM. Cardiovascular anomalies in DiGeorge syndrome and importance of neural crest as a possible pathogenetic factor. Am J Cardiol. 1986;58:133–7.

Van Son JA, Falk V, Schneider P, Smedts F, Mohr FW. Repair of coarctation of the aorta in neonates and young infants. J Card Surg. 1997;12:139–46.

van Son JA, Lacquet LK, Smedts F. Patterns of ductal tissue in coarctation of the aorta in early infancy. J Thorac Cardiovasc Surg. 1993;105:368–9.

Varma C, Benson LN, Butany J, McLaughlin PR. Aortic dissection after stent dilatation for coarctation of the aorta: a case report and literature review. Catheter Cardiovasc Interv Off J Soc Card Angiography Interv. 2003;59:528–35.

Vergales JE, Gangemi JJ, Rhueban KS, Lim DS. Coarctation of the aorta – the current state of surgical and transcatheter therapies. Curr Cardiol Rev. 2013;9:211–9.

Verheugt CL, Uiterwaal CS, Grobbee DE, Mulder BJ. Long-term prognosis of congenital heart defects: a systematic review. Int J Cardiol. 2008;131:25–32.

Vogt M, Kuhn A, Baumgartner D, Baumgartner C, Busch R, Kostolny M, Hess J. Impaired elastic properties of the ascending aorta in newborns before and early after successful coarctation repair: proof of a systemic vascular disease of the prestenotic arteries? Circulation. 2005;111:3269–73.

Vohra HA, Adamson L, Haw MP. Does surgical correction of coarctation of the aorta in adults reduce established hypertension? Interact Cardiovasc Thorac Surg. 2009;8:123–7.

von Kodolitsch Y, Aydin AM, Bernhardt AM, Habermann C, Treede H, Reichenspurner H, Meinertz T, Dodge-Khatami A. Aortic aneurysms after correction of aortic coarctation: a systematic review. Vasa. 2010;39:3–16.

von Kodolitsch Y, Aydin MA, Koschyk DH, Loose R, Schalwat I, Karck M, Cremer J, Haverich A, Berger J, Meinertz T, Nienaber CA. Predictors of aneurysmal formation after surgical correction of aortic coarctation. J Am Coll Cardiol. 2002;39:617–24.

Warnes CA. Bicuspid aortic valve and coarctation: two villains part of a diffuse problem. Heart. 2003;89:965–6.

Weisse AB. Cardiac surgery: a century of progress. Tex Heart Inst J. 2011;38:486–90.

Xu C, Zarins CK, Bassiouny HS, Briggs WH, Reardon C, Glagov S. Differential transmural distribution of gene expression for collagen types I and III proximal to aortic coarctation in the rabbit. J Vasc Res. 2000;37:170–82.

Yuan SM. Congenital heart defects in Kabuki syndrome. Cardiol J. 2013;20:121–4.

Chapter 25
Patent Ductus Arteriosus

Sthefano Atique Gabriel and Edmo Atique Gabriel

The ductus arteriosus consists in a fetal shunt vessel that, during prenatal life, diverts blood away from the pulmonary circulation into the systemic circulation toward the placenta. During normal postnatal adaptation, the main ductal shunt direction changes from left to right, carrying blood from aorta to the pulmonary artery. In healthy term and preterm newborn infants, hypoxia and decreased levels of systemic prostaglandins are considered the most important factors that stimulate the constriction of the ductus arteriosus. Recent studies, however, highlighted that vascular endothelial growth factor, transforming growth factor beta, and important inflammatory mediators as platelets and their paracrine effects also have a notorious role in the molecular mechanisms involved in definitive ductus arteriosus closure during the first postnatal days.

The failure of ductus arteriosus closure results in a left-to-right shunt that can lead to pulmonary vascular and left ventricular volume overload. Depending on the ductal diameter and the intensity of left-to-right shunt, the newborn may have many adverse clinical conditions including pulmonary edema, decreased lung compliance, pulmonary hemorrhage, bronchopulmonary dysplasia, prolonged ventilator dependence, and chronic lung disease. Important pathologies, such as necrotizing enterocolitis, myocardial dysfunction, systemic hypotension, altered intracerebral blood flow, and intracerebral and intraventricular hemorrhage, have been associated with failed ductal constriction.

According to Mitchell et al. (1971), patent ductus arteriosus accounts for 5–10 % of all congenital heart diseases with an incidence of 1 in 2,000 live births in children born at term. Diagnosis of patent ductus arteriosus in preterm neonates represents a challenge due to the nonspecific and possible late occurrence of clinical symptoms.

S.A. Gabriel, MD, PhD (✉)
Vascular and Endovascular Surgeon, Fellowship of Advanced Aortic Surgery,
Ospedale San Raffaele, Milan, Italy
e-mail: sthefanogabriel@yahoo.com.br

E.A. Gabriel, MD, PhD
Cardiac Surgeon, Coordinator and Professor of Medicine of União das Faculdades dos Grandes Lagos (Unilago), São José do Rio Preto, São Paulo, Brazil

© Springer International Publishing Switzerland 2017
A. Dabbagh et al. (eds.), *Congenital Heart Disease in Pediatric and Adult Patients*, DOI 10.1007/978-3-319-44691-2_25

However, the clinical and morphological aspects of the disease, the important radiologic and imaging information, the markers of hemodynamic significance, the specific and costly measurement of cerebral saturation by near-infrared spectroscopy, and the valuable use of urine and plasma biomarkers, such as natriuretic peptides, might help in identifying patients with compromised hemodynamic status.

Typical clinical signs of a patent ductus arteriosus are usually absent at early stages, and the exclusive use of clinical signs during the first week after birth has several limitations. Evans et al. (1992) considered that lower blood pressures are the only consistent clinical finding associated with a large patent ductus arteriosus on first day after birth. Instead of the existence of specific plasmatic measurements and the fact that patent ductus arteriosus diagnosis requires a combination of many diagnostic variables and a multidisciplinary effort, transthoracic echocardiography, as reported by Sallmon et al. (2016), remains the gold standard method for patent ductus arteriosus diagnosing. It allows direct visualization of the ductus; assessment of patent ductus arteriosus diameter and shunt pattern; determination of its size at the pulmonary and aortic end, shunt direction, and velocity; and a simultaneous evaluation of ventricular volumes, mass, and function. Transthoracic echocardiography also may precede clinical recognition of hemodynamically significant patent ductus arteriosus by 1.8 days.

Once the anatomic characteristics of the patent ductus arteriosus, specially its length and diameter, are quite variable, Krichenko et al. (1989) described these differences in children and adults based on findings from lateral aortography, classifying them into five types, A through E. Type A was represented by "conical" ductus, with well-defined aortic ampulla and constricted pulmonary artery end. Type B was represented by "window" ductus, with short-length, slightly constricted aortic end and wide pulmonary artery end. Type C was represented by "tubular" ductus, without any constrictions at the aortic end or the pulmonary artery end. Type D was represented by "saccular" ductus, with constricted aortic end and pulmonary artery end with a wide center. Type E was represented by "elongated" ductus, which is narrow with a constricted pulmonary artery end. The patent ductus arteriosus morphology of premature children that did not fit the Krichenko et al. classification was proposed by Philip et al. (2016) as type F ("fetal type") that was found exclusively in children born prematurely and was characterized as long, wide, and tortuous ductus.

Therapy options designed to close a patent ductus arteriosus in premature infants remain challenging for a dedicated medical team, and the decision of when to treat a patent ductus arteriosus in a preterm neonate and/or when not to treat is controversial. Previously, medical therapy with indomethacin or surgical ligation constituted the only two options for symptomatic patent ductus arteriosus. Indomethacin promotes ductal closure by inhibiting prostaglandin E_2. Nowadays, the use of paracetamol and the advent of smaller occlusion devices and transcatheter therapy have gained importance as alternative treatments of hemodynamically significant patent ductus arteriosus, with reports of even treating patients <1 kg.

Elhoff et al. (2016) reported that younger gestational age at birth is strongly correlated with increased likelihood of treatment failure with indomethacin. This author explains that the youngest neonates are often the most ill and most sensitive to the effects of a large left-to-right shunt and may benefit most from elimination, or at least reduction, of this shunt. Additionally, these patients may be most susceptible to cardiorespiratory instability following patent ductus arteriosus ligation. His research indicates a reasonable probability that timing of initiation of therapy influences likelihood of patent ductus arteriosus closure. Those deemed to have unsuccessful closure began treatment on day of life 4, as opposed to day of life 3 for those with treatment success. Those treated within the first 5 days of life were found to be significantly more likely to have documented closure of their patent ductus arteriosus than those treated on or after day of life 6.

Sallmon et al. (2016) highlighted that when treatment of a patent ductus arteriosus is considered clinically, three different general strategies have to be distinguished. First, a prophylactic treatment is initiated <24 h after birth to all infants. Second, a symptomatic treatment is initiated early, within 2–5 days, or late, up to 10–14 days in infants with signs of hemodynamically significant patent ductus arteriosus. The third option is early asymptomatic treatment that uses echocardiographic signs of failed ductal constriction in the absence of hemodynamic significance or clinical symptoms.

For prophylactic pharmacologic treatment or preterm newborn infants at risk for hemodynamically significant patent ductus arteriosus (6–24 h after birth), Sallmon et al. (2016) indicate the use of indomethacin at a dose of 0.1 mg/kg/dose IV every 12 h (three doses total). The last dose might be omitted if echocardiography suggests ductal constriction and the treatment should not be started within the first 6 h of life. The advantages of this clinical treatment include prevention of intraventricular hemorrhage and reduction in the risk of pulmonary hemorrhage.

For early pharmacologic treatment of asymptomatic preterm newborn infants with patent ductus arteriosus (<72 h after birth), Sallmon et al. (2016) indicate the use of indomethacin at a dose of 0.2 mg/kg/dose IV, followed by 0.1 mg/kg/dose every 12 h (three doses or more, total), or ibuprofen at a dose of 10 mg/kg/dose orally or intravenously, followed by 5 mg/kg at 24 and 48 h at the start of treatment. The last indomethacin dose might be omitted if echocardiography suggests pressure-restrictive patent ductus arteriosus. Ibuprofen orally should be followed by 2 mL/kg water or milk and is recommended not to use ibuprofen intravenously in the first 24 h of life. The advantages of this clinical strategy include reduction in the risk of pulmonary hemorrhage and in-hospital mortality.

For pharmacologic treatment in symptomatic preterm newborn infants with hemodynamically significant patent ductus arteriosus (>72 h after birth), Sallmon et al. (2016) indicate the use of ibuprofen at a dose of 10 mg/kg/dose orally or intravenously, followed by 5 mg/kg at 24 and 48 h at the start of treatment. The oral ibuprofen should be followed by 2 mL/kg water or milk (hyperosmolarity). This clinical treatment is designed only for infants with hemodynamically significant patent ductus arteriosus.

Hammerman et al. (2011) published the first case report of the use of paracetamol (15 mg/kg 6/6 h for 3 days), an inhibitor of the peroxidase component of prostaglandin-H_2 synthase, for the treatment of patent ductus arteriosus in a baby with patent ductus arteriosus who was given paracetamol for pain relief. Terrin et al. (2016), in a systematic and meta-analyzed review of the administration of paracetamol for the treatment of preterm neonates with patent ductus arteriosus, have observed a similar efficacy rate and safety profile of paracetamol and ibuprofen, but also have noted that further randomized control trials are necessary to support the use of paracetamol for patent ductus arteriosus in the current clinical practice and to elucidate the impact of paracetamol in the gestational age, birth weight, postnatal age, and the best modality of its administration. A reduced efficacy of paracetamol observed for extremely preterm neonates (gestational age <28 weeks) was explained by this author as result of a thin-walled ductus arteriosus that fails to develop extensive neointimal mounds.

The greater efficacy of paracetamol administered orally is observed when treatment is started in the first week of life which is elucidated by Terrin et al. (2016) as dependent of the circulating levels of prostaglandins, which are high in the first days of life and decrease as postnatal age increases.

An interesting result observed in this meta-analysis was an impaired efficacy if paracetamol was used after a previous treatment with COX inhibitor. On the other hand, when paracetamol was administered after COX inhibitor failure, the successful closure of patent ductus arteriosus maybe a result of an additive effect of the two drugs.

Dang et al. (2013) randomized 160 infants (gestational age ≤ 34 weeks) to oral ibuprofen ($n=80$) vs. oral paracetamol ($n=80$) in a non-blinded trial. Overall closure rates were similar at 79 % vs. 81 %, respectively, with less gastrointestinal bleeding and less jaundice in the paracetamol group. The 95 % confidence interval of the difference between these groups has demonstrated that the effectiveness of paracetamol treatment was not inferior to that of ibuprofen.

Oncel et al. (2016) highlighted that more neonates are managed conservatively, and the number of newborns receiving surgical ligation is declining. For this author, ibuprofen is the first choice in the clinical management of patent ductus arteriosus due to its higher safety profile and the fewer gastrointestinal and renal side effects when compared to indomethacin. Paracetamol is an emerging alternative in the management of patent ductus arteriosus with similar efficacy but lower side events than nonsteroidal anti-inflammatory drugs.

Portsman et al. (1967) introduced the first device for transcatheter closure of patent ductus arteriosus. Recently, Amplatzer Duct Occluder (St. Jude Medical, Plymouth, MN, USA) is the most frequently used device worldwide for patent ductus arteriosus closure. However, the percutaneous closure of the small patent ductus arteriosus using coil embolization became famous with the report of Cambier et al. (1992).

The patent ductus arteriosus closure with Amplatzer Duct Occluder is safe and effective, except for type B of Krishenko et al. (1989) due to short window type. The Amplatzer Duct Occluder has to be used with prudence in small children due to the possibility of aortic obstruction with the left retention disk.

For coil embolization of a patent ductus arteriosus, multiple coils are required; the surgical procedure becomes more technically challenging with prolonged procedure time and higher incidence of complications. Hooper et al. (2015), Hamrick and Hansmann (2010), Antonucci et al. (2010), Weber et al. (2008), Evans (2015), Heuchan and Clyman (2014), Jain and Shah (2015), Betham et al. (2011), Francis et al. (2010), Pacifici (2013), Oncel et al. (2013), Sinha et al. (2013), Van Overmeireet al. (2001), Tekgündüz et al. (2014) and Faella and Hijazi (2000).

References

Antonucci R, Bassareo P, Zaffanello M, et al. Patent ductus arteriosus in the pre- term infant: new insights into pathogenesis and clinical management. J Matern Fetal Neonatal Med. 2010;23(S3):34–7.

Betham J, Meur S, Hudsmith L, Archer N, Wilson N. Echocardiographically guided catheter closure of arterial ducts in small preterm infants on the neonatal intensive care unit. Catheter Cardiovasc Interv. 2011;77:40915.

Cambier PA, Kirby WC, Wortham DC, Moore JW. Percutaneous closure of the small (2.5 mm) patent ductus arteriosus using coil embolization. Am J Cardiol. 1992;69:815–6.

Dang D, Wang D, Zhang C, Zhou W, Zhou Q, Wu H. Comparison of oral paracetamol versus ibuprofen in premature infants with patent ductus arteriosus: a randomized controlled trial. PLoS One. 2013;8:e77888.

Elhoff JJ, Ebeling M, Hulsey TC, Atz AM. Potential unintended consequences of a conservative management strategy for patent ductus arteriosus. Congenit Heart Dis. 2016;11(1):52–7.

Evans N. Preterm patent ductus arteriosus: a continuing conundrum for the neonatologist? Semin Fetal Neonatal Med. 2015;20(4):272–7.

Evans N, Moorcraft J. Effect of patency of the ductus arteriosus on blood pressure in very preterm infants. Arch Dis Child. 1992;67(10, spec no):1169–73.

Faella HJ, Hijazi ZM. Closure of the patent ductus arteriosus with the amplatzer PDA device: immediate results of the international clinical trial. Catheter Cardiovasc Interv. 2000;51(1):50–4.

Francis E, Singhi AK, Lakshmivenkateshaiah S, Kumar RK. Transcatheter occlusion of patent ductus arteriosus in pre-term infants. JACC Cardiovasc Interv. 2010;3:550–5.

Hammerman C, Bin-Nun A, Markovitch E, et al. Ductal closure with paracetamol: a surprising new approach to patent ductus arteriosus treatment. Pediatrics. 2011;128:e1618–21.

Hamrick SE, Hansmann G. Patent ductus arteriosus of the preterm infant. Pediatrics. 2010;125: 1020–30.

Heuchan AM, Clyman RI. Managing the patent ductus arteriosus: current treatment options. Arch Dis Child Fetal Neonatal Ed. 2014;99:F431–6.

Hooper SB, Polglase GR, Roehr CC. Cardiopulmonary changes with aeration of the newborn lung. Paediatr Respir Rev. 2015;16(3):147–50.

Jain A, Shah PS. Diagnosis, evaluation, and management of patent ductus arteriosus in preterm neonates. JAMA Pediatr. 2015;169(9):863–72.

Krichenko A, Benson LN, Burrows P, Moes CA, McLaughlin P, Freedom RM. Angiographic classification of the isolated persistently patent ductus arteriosus and implication for percutaneous catheter occlusion. Am J Cardiol. 1989;63:877–80.

Mitchell SC, Korones SB, Berendes HW. Congenital heart disease in 56,109 births: incidence and natural history. Circulation. 1971;43:323–32.

Oncel MY, Erdeve O. Oral medications regarding their safety and efficacy in the management of patent ductus arteriosus. World J Clin Pediatr. 2016;5(1):75–81.

Oncel MY, Yurttutan S, Uras N, et al. An alternative drug (paracetamol) in the management of patent ductus arteriosus in ibuprofen-resistant or contraindicated preterm infants. Arch Dis Child Fetal Neonatal Ed. 2013;98:F94.

Pacifici GM. Clinical pharmacology of indomethacin in preterm infants: implications in patent ductus arteriosus closure. Paediatr Drugs. 2013;15(5):363–76.

Philip R, Rush Waller B, Agrawal V, Wright D, Arevalo A, Zurakowski D, Sathanandam S. Morphologic characterization of the patent ductus arteriosus in the premature infant and the choice of transcatheter occlusion device. Catheter Cardiovasc Interv. 2016;87(2):310–7.

Portsmann W, Wierny L, Warnke H. Closure of persistent ductus arteriosus without thoracotomy. Ger Med Mon. 1967;12:259–61.

Sallmon H, Koehne P, Hansmann G. Recent advances in the treatment of preterm newborn infants with patent ductus arteriosus. Clin Perinatol. 2016;43(1):113–29.

Sinha R, Negi V, Dalal SS. An interesting observation of PDA closure with oral paracetamol in preterm neonates. J Clin Neonatol. 2013;2:30–2.

Tekgündüz KS, Ceviz N, Caner I, et al. Intravenous paracetamol with a lower dose is also effective for the treatment of patent ductus arteriosus in pre-term infants. Cardiol Young. 2014;27:1–5.

Terrin G, Conte F, Oncel MY, et al. Paracetamol for the treatment of patent ductus arteriosus in preterm neonates: a systematic review and meta-analysis. Arch Dis Child Fetal Neonatal Ed. 2016;101(2):F127–36.

Van Overmeire B, Van de Broek H, Van Laer P, et al. Early versus late indomethacin treatment for patent ductus arteriosus in premature infants with respiratory distress syndrome. J Pediatr. 2001;138:205–11.

Weber SC, Rheinlaender C, Sarioglu N, et al. The expression of VEGF and its receptors in the human ductus arteriosus. Pediatr Res. 2008;64:340–5.

Chapter 26
Hypoplastic Left Heart Syndrome: Treatment Options

William M. Novick

Introduction

The publication by Norwood and colleagues from Boston Children's Hospital in 1983 represented a paradigm shift in the care of children with hypoplastic left heart syndrome (HLHS) (Norwood et al. 1983). Prior to this surgical innovation, children were given compassionate care only and survival without intervention was and remains zero at 1 year (Siffel et al. 2015). The focus of this chapter will be on the first-stage reconstruction, and interstage period of children with HLHS, bidirectional Glenn/Hemi-Fontan, and the modified Fontan are covered elsewhere. Early operative mortality for stage I reconstruction was significant, 34 % at 30 days, but has improved significantly in a number of centers (Murdison et al. 1990; Hraska et al. 2000; McGuirk et al. 2006). The initial operation has also changed significantly over time, from the central shunt originally described to modified Blalock-Taussig shunts with a tendency toward smaller shunt size. Although the Norwood operation provided children with HLHS an opportunity for surgical intervention, a number of children were still dying on the first postoperative day from acute cardiovascular collapse. Jobes and colleagues at Philadelphia Children's Hospital were able to demonstrate that the precise control of CO_2 levels would ameliorate the coronary steal and provide a more optimal postoperative course (Jobes et al. 1992). Despite this, discovery balance of the systemic and pulmonary circulations remained problematic and sudden cardiovascular collapse was not completely eliminated and mortality in the late 1990s remained in 15–20 %(Bartram et al. 1997).

W.M. Novick, MD
Surgery and International Child Health, University of Tennessee Health Science Center, Memphis, USA

William Novick Global Cardiac Alliance, Memphis, USA
e-mail: bill.novick@cardiac-alliance.org

© Springer International Publishing Switzerland 2017
A. Dabbagh et al. (eds.), *Congenital Heart Disease in Pediatric
and Adult Patients*, DOI 10.1007/978-3-319-44691-2_26

Concerns regarding coronary supply continued as interstage deaths following the stage I Norwood procedure persisted (Barron 2013). Sano and colleagues in 2003 published a sentinel paper reporting on the use of a right ventricular to pulmonary artery conduit utilizing a 5 mm Gore-Tex shunt as the source of pulmonary blood flow (Sano et al. 2003).

An alternative to immediate reconstruction in the newborn was reported in 2002; this "hybrid procedure" included bilateral pulmonary banding and insertion of a stent in the ductus arteriosus (Akintuerk et al. 2002). Subsequently a number of centers adopted the hybrid approach as the initial palliation for HLHS.

Pathology

The pathology of HLHS is typically subdivided into four different subtypes. Although there are other pathological configurations for which a stage I repair can be used, we will only focus on HLHS. The four subtypes are aortic atresia with mitral atresia, aortic atresia with mitral stenosis, aortic stenosis with mitral atresia, and aortic stenosis with mitral atresia. The ascending aorta is typically quite small between 2 and 4 mm, and this small size progresses into the transverse arch and isthmus before often ending in an area of coarctation. The spectrum atrial septal defects range from intact to a widely patent secundum defect. Left ventricular size can vary from diminutive to hypoplastic. Coronary ventricular fistulas can occur although they are rare. Mild forms of HLHS merge with the pathology of Shone's syndrome.

Diagnosis

Prenatal diagnosis is preferred as this allows the parents the opportunity to become educated about the options for treatment and for the local team to be aware and prepared for the subsequent birth of the child (Wolter et al. 2016). A fetal echocardiogram performed by an experienced individual will delineate the defect from other congenital cardiac malformations. Any newborn with a murmur should be considered for echocardiography before discharge as some children with heart disease do not display symptoms and in a few critical heart disease can exist (Al-Ammouri et al. 2016). Routine two-dimensional echocardiography with continuous and pulse Doppler analysis will fully define the intracardiac and aortic anatomy of the child with HLHS. Those children with highly restrictive atrial septal defects should either undergo balloon atrial septostomy or early operation as progressive deterioration can be expected if the restrictive defect is not addressed.

Preoperative Care

The birth of a neonate with HLHS that has received a prenatal diagnosis is attended by a pediatric critical care team that institutes the infusion of prostaglandins once vascular access is secured. Elective endotracheal intubation may be performed if transport times to the tertiary care center are prolonged. Supplemental oxygen is rarely needed and if required should prompt early assessment of the intra-atrial septum. Care of the child is directed toward preparation for operation, insuring optimal cardiopulmonary balance, absence of infection, complete assessment of cardiac, and any additional congenital or genetic disorders. The family should be thoroughly engaged during this time and discussions regarding options, prognosis, and potential complications reviewed.

Stage I Options

Modified Norwood Procedure

The cornerstones of providing a comprehensive stage I palliation for HLHS require:

1. Augmentation of the ascending aorta, arch, and isthmus and resection of the coarctation
2. Creation of a systemic to pulmonary artery shunt, typically from the innominate artery
3. Atrial septectomy

Augmentation is typically accomplished with a piece of pulmonary homograft, but other materials are possible. Complete autologous tissue augmentation can be performed utilizing the distal portion of the transected main pulmonary artery.

Sano Procedure

The Sano procedure was developed in order to eliminate the diastolic flow into the pulmonary circulation during diastole and thus raise the diastolic and thereby mean systemic pressure to improve coronary flow and hemodynamic stability following stage I correction of HLHS. The Sano procedure differs from the modified Norwood procedure primarily by the source of pulmonary blood flow. A right ventricular pulmonary artery conduit is used rather than a modified Blalock-Taussig shunt. No systemic diastolic flow occurs with this configuration for pulmonary blood flow.

Hybrid Procedure

The hybrid procedure was originally developed for those neonates that were premature; of low birth weight; having additional noncardiac defects, documented or presumed infection or presented late; and critically ill. Neonates with these issues were considered poor candidates for either a routine stage I reconstruction or Sano procedure. The hybrid procedure consists of insertion of a stent within the ductus arteriosus, bilateral branch pulmonary artery banding, and ± atrial septostomy. Ideally this is performed in a hybrid operating room suite, but if not available banding in the OR followed by immediate transfer to the catheterization laboratory for stenting and possible atrial septostomy can be performed. Stenting of the ductus can be supplanted by the administration of long-term intravenous or oral prostaglandins. A significant problem which has been noted is when coarctation develops proximal to the insertion of the ductus, thus compromising coronary and cerebral blood flow.

Transplantation

Cardiac transplantation for HLHS was initiated by Bailey in 1984 when he transplanted a baboon heart into a human female newborn (Al-Ammouri et al. 2016). Since that inauspicious beginning, cardiac transplantation became a viable option for the newborn with HLHS (Bailey 2004). Survival following transplantation is excellent, but pretransplant waiting continues to claim lives. The limiting factor is an adequate pool of neonatal or young infant donors (Bailey 2004; Carlo et al. 2016). Transplantation is now mostly reserved as a rescue procedure for heart failure after stage I reconstructions or hybrid procedures (Carlo et al. 2016).

Single Ventricle Reconstruction Trial

The Single Ventricle Reconstruction Trial was conceived and run by the Pediatric Heart Network investigators of North America between 2005 and 2008 (Bacha and del Nido 2012). A total of 555 patients were randomized to receive either a Blalock-Taussig shunt or RV to PA conduit as their source of pulmonary blood flow in the stage I reconstruction. Fifteen [15] centers participated in the study with the end points being either transplantation or survival to 12 months. Patients receiving the RV to PA conduit had a survival advantage, with 74 % surviving compared to 64 % of those receiving BT shunts [$p<0.01$] (Ohye et al. 2010). However, by 14 months there was no survival difference between the RV/PA or BT shunts. Centers with high volume tended to have better outcomes with the BT shunt, most likely a reflection of a greater experience and longer period of time to establish postoperative care protocols (Tabbutt et al. 2012). Another tendency which was observed but did not achieve statistical significance was for aortic atresia patients to do better with the

RV/PA shunt. Perhaps this reflects the improved systemic diastolic pressure and better coronary flow seen in the RV/PA shunt. Interstage mortality for the entire cohort was 12 %, and there was a significant difference between those with RV/PA conduits (6 %) and those receiving a modified BT shunt [18 %, $p < 0.001$] (Ghanayem et al. 2012). Children undergoing a hybrid procedure were not included in the Single Ventricle Reconstruction Trial randomization.

Hybrid Procedure

The hybrid procedure was initially reported in 2002. The quote from the Giessen group's initial publication of a series of children receiving the hybrid procedure describing their rationale for abandoning neonatal reconstruction was "The limited prognosis of patients with hypoplastic left heart (HLH) is caused by a still high mortality during stage I of the Norwood procedures. Additionally, a significant number of patients die in the period between the first and second step of the staged procedure" (Akintuerk et al. 2002). A later report by the Giessen group reported the results of 107 children who underwent the Hybrid procedure with an initial mortality of two patients (1.2 %) and an interstage mortality of 6.7 % (Schranz et al. 2015). The initial Giessen group's report resulted in a number of institutions attempting the Hybrid approach. Galantowicz and colleagues reported the results of their Hybrid program on the first 40 patients with HLHS (Galantowicz et al. 2008) and have more recently suggested that the Hybrid procedure should be considered as one of the initial procedures performed for HLHS (Galantowicz 2013). The Giessen group suggests that based upon their cumulative results since 1998 the Hybrid procedure should be an alternative choice for the first stage of palliation for HLHS (Galantowicz 2013). Subsequent reports have shown that RV size, systolic and diastolic function are comparable in Hybrid patients to classical Norwood reconstruction patients; the incidence for ECMO rescue is less after Hybrid than Norwood procedures and that surgically placed stents have less adverse events compared to percutaneous placement (Holzer et al. 2010; Bacha 2013; Mitchell et al. 2016).

Individualized Surgical Approach

Over the last two decades, a great deal has been learned about the surgical care of the child with HLHS. Twenty years ago there was only one option for reconstruction, the Norwood with a BT shunt, a second option for treatment was cardiac transplantation, and the final option for the families was compassionate care. Today there are three reconstructive options for these children and although survival has improved and much knowledge has been gained, we are still faced with an average 12-month survival of 64–74 %.

What do we know at this point about the surgical care of the child with HLHS (Pasquali et al. 2012)? Center and surgeon volume are important for improved survival (Bacha et al. 2008). These centers typically are those with the longest experience in the surgical treatment of children with HLHS. Patients with aortic atresia that receive a RV/PA shunt have significantly improved survival compared to those receiving BT shunts (Cua et al. 2006). Interstage mortality is significantly less for those patients receiving the RV/PA shunt (Tweddell et al. 2012). The subgroup that fares the best regardless of which shunt is used is the aortic stenosis/mitral stenosis group (Bacha and Hijazi 2005). The number of centers offering the hybrid procedure has increased steadily over the last decade (Honjo et al. 2009; Venugopal et al. 2010). Clearly improvement in mortality will require a more tailored approach to each child with HLHS, rather than making every child fit a particular surgical preference.

Summary

The surgical options for children with HLHS have greatly expanded over the last two decades. The knowledge gained has resulted in improved outcomes to the point where a number of centers are now reporting stage I mortality of less than 10 %. The refinement of which technique provides the optimal outcome is undoubtedly the way forward to continued improvement in mortality.

References

Akintuerk H, Michel-Behnke I, Valeske K, Mueller M, Thul J, Bauer J, Hagel KJ, Kreuder J, Vogt P, Schranz D. Stenting of the arterial duct and banding of the pulmonary arteries: basis for combined Norwood stage I and II repair in hypoplastic left heart. Circulation. 2002;105: 1099–103.

Al-Ammouri I, Ayoub F, Dababneh R. Is pre-discharge echocardiography indicated for asymptomatic neonates with a heart murmur? a retrospective analysis. Cardiol Young. 2016;26:1056–9.

Bacha EA. Individualized approach in the management of patients with hypoplastic left heart syndrome (HLHS). Semin Thorac Cardiovasc Surg Pediatr Card Surg Annu. 2013;16:3–6.

Bacha E, del Nido P. Introduction to the Single Ventricle Reconstruction trial. J Thorac Cardiovasc Surg. 2012;144:880–1.

Bacha EA, Hijazi ZM. Hybrid procedures in pediatric cardiac surgery. Semin Thorac Cardiovasc Surg Pediatr Card Surg Annu. 2005;8(1):78–85.

Bacha EA, Larrazabal LA, Pigula FA, Gauvreau K, Jenkins KJ, Colan SD, Fynn-Thompson F, Mayer Jr JE, del Nido PJ. Measurement of technical performance in surgery for congenital heart disease: the stage I Norwood procedure. J Thorac Cardiovasc Surg. 2008;136:993–7, 997. e991–92.

Bailey LL. Transplantation is the best treatment for hypoplastic left heart syndrome. Cardiol Young. 2004;14 Suppl 1:109–11; discussion 112–104.

Barron DJ. The Norwood procedure: in favor of the RV-PA conduit. Semin Thorac Cardiovasc Surg Pediatr Card Surg Annu. 2013;16:52–8.

Bartram U, Grunenfelder J, Van Praagh R. Causes of death after the modified Norwood procedure: a study of 122 postmortem cases. Ann Thorac Surg. 1997;64:1795–802.

Carlo WF, West SC, McCulloch M, Naftel DC, Pruitt E, Kirklin JK, Hubbard M, Molina KM, Gajarski R. Impact of initial Norwood shunt type on young hypoplastic left heart syndrome patients listed for heart transplant: a multi-institutional study. J Heart Lung Transplant Off Publ Int Soc Heart Transplant. 2016;35:301–5.

Cua CL, Thiagarajan RR, Gauvreau K, Lai L, Costello JM, Wessel DL, Del Nido PJ, Mayer Jr JE, Newburger JW, Laussen PC. Early postoperative outcomes in a series of infants with hypoplastic left heart syndrome undergoing stage I palliation operation with either modified Blalock-Taussig shunt or right ventricle to pulmonary artery conduit. Pediatr Crit Care Med. 2006;7:238–44.

Galantowicz M. In favor of the Hybrid Stage 1 as the initial palliation for hypoplastic left heart syndrome. Semin Thorac Cardiovasc Surg Pediatr Card Surg Annu. 2013;16:62–4.

Galantowicz MCJ, Phillips A, Cua CL, Hoffman TM, Hill SL, Rodeman R. Hybrid approach for hypoplastic left heart syndrome: intermediate results after the learning curve. Ann Thorac Surg. 2008;85:2063–70; discussion 2070–2061.

Ghanayem NS, Allen KR, Tabbutt S, Atz AM, Clabby ML, Cooper DS, Eghtesady P, Frommelt PC, Gruber PJ, Hill KD, Kaltman JR, Laussen PC, Lewis AB, Lurito KJ, Minich LL, Ohye RG, Schonbeck JV, Schwartz SM, Singh RK, Goldberg CS. Interstage mortality after the Norwood procedure: results of the multicenter Single Ventricle Reconstruction trial. J Thorac Cardiovasc Surg. 2012;144:896–906.

Grotenhuis HB, Ruijsink B, Chetan D, Dragulescu A, Friedberg MK, Kotani Y, Caldarone CA, Honjo O, Mertens LL. Impact of Norwood versus hybrid palliation on cardiac size and function in hypoplastic left heart syndrome. Heart. 2016;102:966–74.

Holzer R, Marshall A, Kreutzer J, Hirsch R, Chisolm J, Hill S, Galantowicz M, Phillips A, Cheatham J, Bergerson L. Hybrid procedures: adverse events and procedural characteristics – results of a multi-institutional registry. Congenit Heart Dis. 2010;5:233–42.

Honjo O, Benson LN, Mewhort HE, Predescu D, Holtby H, Van Arsdell GS, Caldarone CA. Clinical outcomes, program evolution, and pulmonary artery growth in single ventricle palliation using hybrid and Norwood palliative strategies. Ann Thorac Surg. 2009;87:1885–92; discussion 1892–1883.

Hraska V, Nosal M, Sykora P, Sojak V, Sagat M, Kunovsky P. Results of modified Norwood's operation for hypoplastic left heart syndrome. Eur J Cardiothorac Surg. 2000;18:214–9.

Jobes DR, Nicolson SC, Steven JM, Miller M, Jacobs ML, Norwood Jr WI. Carbon dioxide prevents pulmonary overcirculation in hypoplastic left heart syndrome. Ann Thorac Surg. 1992;54:150–1.

McGuirk SP, Stickley J, Griselli M, Stumper OF, Laker SJ, Barron DJ, Brawn WJ. Risk assessment and early outcome following the Norwood procedure for hypoplastic left heart syndrome. Eur J Cardiothorac Surg. 2006;29:675–81.

Mitchell EA, Gomez D, Joy BF, Fernandez RP, Cheatham JP, Galantowicz M, Cua CL. ECMO: incidence and outcomes of patients undergoing the hybrid procedure. Congenit Heart Dis. 2016;11:169–74.

Murdison KA, Baffa JM, Farrell Jr PE, Chang AC, Barber G, Norwood WI, Murphy JD. Hypoplastic left heart syndrome. Outcome after initial reconstruction and before modified Fontan procedure. Circulation. 1990;82:Iv199–207.

Norwood WI, Lang P, Hansen DD. Physiologic repair of aortic atresia-hypoplastic left heart syndrome. N Engl J Med. 1983;308:23–6.

Ohye RG, Sleeper LA, Mahony L, Newburger JW, Pearson GD, Lu M, Goldberg CS, Tabbutt S, Frommelt PC, Ghanayem NS, Laussen PC, Rhodes JF, Lewis AB, Mital S, Ravishankar C, Williams IA, Dunbar-Masterson C, Atz AM, Colan S, Minich LL, Pizarro C, Kanter KR, Jaggers J, Jacobs JP, Krawczeski CD, Pike N, McCrindle BW, Virzi L, Gaynor JW. Comparison of shunt types in the Norwood procedure for single-ventricle lesions. N Engl J Med. 2010;362:1980–92.

Pasquali SK, Jacobs JP, He X, Hornik CP, Jaquiss RD, Jacobs ML, O'Brien SM, Peterson ED, Li JS. The complex relationship between center volume and outcome in patients undergoing the Norwood operation. Ann Thorac Surg. 2012;93:1556–62.

Sano S, Ishino K, Kawada M, Arai S, Kasahara S, Asai T, Masuda Z, Takeuchi M, Ohtsuki S. Right ventricle-pulmonary artery shunt in first-stage palliation of hypoplastic left heart syndrome. J Thorac Cardiovasc Surg. 2003;126:504–9; discussion 509–510.

Schranz D, Bauer A, Reich B, Steinbrenner B, Recla S, Schmidt D, Apitz C, Thul J, Valeske K, Bauer J, Muller M, Jux C, Michel-Behnke I, Akinturk H. Fifteen-year single center experience with the "Giessen Hybrid" approach for hypoplastic left heart and variants: current strategies and outcomes. Pediatr Cardiol. 2015;36:365–73.

Siffel C, Riehle-Colarusso T, Oster ME, Correa A. Survival of children with hypoplastic left heart syndrome. Pediatrics. 2015;136:e864–70.

Tabbutt S, Ghanayem N, Ravishankar C, Sleeper LA, Cooper DS, Frank DU, Lu M, Pizarro C, Frommelt P, Goldberg CS, Graham EM, Krawczeski CD, Lai WW, Lewis A, Kirsh JA, Mahony L, Ohye RG, Simsic J, Lodge AJ, Spurrier E, Stylianou M, Laussen P. Risk factors for hospital morbidity and mortality after the Norwood procedure: a report from the Pediatric Heart Network Single Ventricle Reconstruction trial. J Thorac Cardiovasc Surg. 2012;144:882–95.

Tweddell JS, Sleeper LA, Ohye RG, Williams IA, Mahony L, Pizarro C, Pemberton VL, Frommelt PC, Bradley SM, Cnota JF, Hirsch J, Kirshbom PM, Li JS, Pike N, Puchalski M, Ravishankar C, Jacobs JP, Laussen PC, McCrindle BW. Intermediate-term mortality and cardiac transplantation in infants with single-ventricle lesions: risk factors and their interaction with shunt type. J Thorac Cardiovasc Surg. 2012;144:152–9.

Venugopal PS, Luna KP, Anderson DR, Austin CB, Rosenthal E, Krasemann T, Qureshi SA. Hybrid procedure as an alternative to surgical palliation of high-risk infants with hypoplastic left heart syndrome and its variants. J Thorac Cardiovasc Surg. 2010;139:1211–5.

Wolter A, Nosbusch S, Kawecki A, Degenhardt J, Enzensberger C, Graupner O, Vorisek C, Akinturk H, Yerebakan C, Khalil M, Schranz D, Ritgen J, Stressig R, Axt-Fliedner R. Prenatal diagnosis of functionally univentricular heart, associations and perinatal outcomes. Prenatal Diagn. 2016;36:545–54.

Yerebakan C, Valeske K, Elmontaser H, Yoruker U, Mueller M, Thul J, Mann V, Latus H, Villanueva A, Hofmann K, Schranz D, Akintuerk H. Hybrid therapy for hypoplastic left heart syndrome: myth, alternative, or standard? J Thorac Cardiovasc Surg. 2016;151:1112–23.e1115.

Chapter 27
Double-Outlet Right Ventricle

Zoel Augusto Quiñónez

Clinical Vignettes

Case 1

An ex-36-week, 3.1 kg, 6-week-old girl with a diagnosis of DORV and a subaortic VSD has been in the hospital for the duration of her life. The patient's respiratory status had worsened; her abdominal exam revealed a tense and distended belly and is now intubated. She had become increasingly difficult to ventilate, with peak pressures of 30 cmH$_2$O. Bloody stools prompted abdominal plain films that demonstrated portal venous gas. Her absolute neutrophil count (ANC) is 882 and she has increased bands of 20%. General surgery was consulted, and given her quick deterioration, they wish to take her to the operating room for an exploratory laparotomy and possible bowel resection for her necrotizing enterocolitis (NEC).

Vital signs: SpO$_2$ 92%, HR 148, RR 42, BP 68/22, and T 37.8 °C.

Her capillary refill is 5 s. Her urine output has been decreased at 0.5 ml/kg/h. Her transthoracic echo shows a subaortic VSD and greater than 50% override of the aorta and an atrial septal defect. Her remaining blood work shows a hemoglobin of 10.2 g/dl, a sodium of 130 meq/l, a blood urea nitrogen of 24 mg/dl, a blood creatinine of 0.9 mg/dl, a pH of 7.28, a base deficit of 3, and a lactate of 3.3 mmol/L. You will be managing her care in the operating room.

Z.A. Quiñónez, MD
Texas Children's Hospital, Baylor College of Medicine,
6621 Fannin Street, WT-17417, Houston, TX 77030, USA
e-mail: zoel.quinonez@bcm.edu; zaquinon@texaschildrens.org

© Springer International Publishing Switzerland 2017
A. Dabbagh et al. (eds.), *Congenital Heart Disease in Pediatric
and Adult Patients*, DOI 10.1007/978-3-319-44691-2_27

Case 2

A 4.1 kg, 3-month-old male with history of DORV and subaortic VSD presents for Stamm gastrostomy tube placement for failure to thrive. His past medical history is significant for 37-week normal spontaneous vaginal delivery. He takes propranolol at home because some of his desaturation is thought to be due to infundibular muscle spasm, although parents do not endorse discrete desaturations ("tet spells"), have no allergies, and have had no previous surgeries.

Vital signs: SpO_2 81 %, HR 122, RR 28, BP 80/36, and T 37 °C

On exam, he is a calm and thin-appearing infant with mild perioral cyanosis. His precordium is quiet; his capillary refill is 3 s. His transthoracic echo demonstrates a subaortic VSD and subvalvar pulmonic stenosis with a peak velocity of 4.1 m/s and a dynamic component; he has normal biventricular size and function. Blood work shows a hemoglobin of 11 g/dl. His chest x-ray shows clear lung fields bilaterally. Mother states that he does well with strangers.

Background

Double-outlet right ventricle is a complex lesion that accounts for many anatomic variants leading to different physiologic presentations and a varied number of surgical approaches. For the anesthesiologist caring for patients with this diagnosis, many of these anatomic factors will impact the patient's clinical presentation, the physiologic principles that will guide care, and expected difficulties that may arise during their perioperative management. Here we summarize the development of DORV, as well as the anatomic, physiologic, and surgical factors that may impact care of these patients.

Double-outlet ventricles (right or left) have been estimated to account for approximately 1 % of congenital heart disease, and double-outlet right ventricle (DORV) accounts for betwe en 3 and 9/100,000 births (Obler 2008). Vierordt, in 1898, described "partial transposition" for a lesion where only one great artery, the aorta, was transposed; but DORV was described as far back as 1703 by Mery (Obler 2008; Walters et al. 2000). In 1949, Taussig and Bing described transposition of the aorta with levoposition of the pulmonary artery and a subpulmonic ventricular septal defect (Taussig 1949). Subsequently, Lev and Volk termed this the "Taussig–Bing heart," part of the spectrum of DORV, when they reported a similar case in 1950 (Lev and Volk 1950). The first report of successful repair of DORV came from Kirklin and colleagues (1964), where an intraventricular tunnel repair was used to repair DORV with a subaortic VSD (Kirklin 1964).

Witham (1957) was the first to categorize "double-outlet right ventricle" as a diagnosis of congenital heart disease (Witham 1957); and Neufeld and colleagues (1962) were the first to classify the lesion (Neufeld 1962). But the foundation for our current classification system came from Lev in 1972, where he grounded categorization of DORV in the relationship of the VSD to the great arteries (Walters et al. 2000; Lev 1972a).

Embryology

One of the earliest references to an "infundibulum" came from Keith's (1909) description of "malformations of the heart" to the Royal College of Surgeons in England, in part to try to explain the development of a ventricular septal defect in the context of pulmonic stenosis (Keith 1909). Our current understanding on the development of double-outlet right ventricle still relies on theories of conotruncal development, particularly the segmentation and rotation, as well as growth and resorption of the conus, an embryologic structure that, in the normal heart, persists as the subpulmonic infundibulum (Jonas 2004a; Restivo et al. 2006).

During the fifth week of embryologic development, there is a partitioning of the truncus arteriosus and the conus arteriosus. The neural crest cells develop in a spiral pattern, ultimately leading to the development of outflow tracts and the great arteries. The pulmonary conus develops and becomes the infundibulum in the normal heart, separating the pulmonic valve from the atrioventricular valves with the muscular infundibulum. Resorption of the subaortic conus leaves the aortic valve in fibrous continuity with the atrioventricular valves. The two primary theories of the development of DORV are taken from Lev (1972) and Van Praagh et al. (1970) and differ in the process by which DORV forms (Lev 1972; Van Praagh et al. 1970).

In Lev's theory, failure of the spiral septation of the conotruncus leads to a parallel arrangement of the great arteries (transposition of the great arteries), and proper septation leads to the proper arrangement of the great arteries. Any intermediate arterial position along this spectrum (tetralogy of Fallot, DORV) occurs due to partial spiraling (Jonas 2004a; Van Praagh et al. 1970).

Van Praagh proposed that the development of tetralogy of Fallot (TOF) develops due to underdevelopment of the subpulmonic infundibulum (Jonas 2004a; VanPraagh 1970). In this theory, development of the conus during embryogenesis brings the pulmonary artery anteriorly toward the right ventricle and also raises it above the level of, and out of fibrous continuity with, the other three cardiac valves. Underdevelopment of the subpulmonic conus would leave the pulmonic valve in a more posterior and leftward position and the aorta more anterior and rightward. This also would cause malalignment of the conal septum with the ventricular septum, leading to obstruction from an anteriorly malaligned conal septum relative to the ventricular septum. From this theory, we can derive that DORV would involve further underdevelopment of the subpulmonic infundibulum and possibly overdevelopment or underabsorption of the subaortic infundibulum, leading to both arteries arising from the right ventricle. Here you would see bilateral coni with both semilunar valves separated from the fibrous continuity of the atrioventricular valves. The far end of this spectrum would be transposition of the great arteries (TGA), where a subaortic conus exists without a subpulmonic conus, and the pulmonic valve is over the left ventricle and in fibrous continuity with the atrioventricular valves, while the aortic valve is outside of fibrous continuity and has been pushed anteriorly by growth of the subaortic conus.

No one theory completely explains the spectrum of disease, leading to controversies over criteria for diagnosis of DORV. For instance, while pathologic assessment of hearts with a diagnosis of DORV seems to support Van Praagh's theory, only 9 of 24 (37.5%) of hearts with DORV studied by Howell et al. (1991) had bilateral coni, a criteria commonly used to distinguish DORV from either TOF or TGA (Howell et al. (1991)). These theories are, in any case, useful for conceptualization of the development of disease and for the categorization of these lesions. Whether certain features are regarded as strict "criteria" or simply as "descriptors" imply the stringency with which the diagnosis is judged.

Anatomy

About 86% of patients with double-outlet right ventricle have atrioventricular concordance (Walters et al. 2000); and between 55 and 77% of patients with double-outlet right ventricle are able to undergo a two-ventricle repair (Bradley 2007; Kleinert 1997). Patients in which a poorly formed ventricle, prohibitive atrioventricular valve anatomy, prohibitive papillary muscle or chordal configuration, or other complex anatomy precludes single-ventricle palliation will not be covered here. Single-ventricle palliation is discussed in other sections.

There are various classification systems for DORV. Lev (1972) initially categorized double-outlet right ventricle (DORV) based on the position of the ventricular septal defect (Lev 1972a). Kirklin and Barratt-Boyes (1993), as well as other authors, have asserted that this classification does not correlate to the surgical management required for repair, which makes sense when considering the multiple associated anomalies that can impact physiology, clinical presentation, and surgical repair (Kirklin 1993). A more clinically relevant classification of DORV for anesthesiologist is that proposed by the Society of Thoracic Surgeons and the European Society for Thoracic Surgery, which classifies DORV into five different subtypes (PS = pulmonic stenosis) (Spaeth 2014; Lacour-Gayet 2008):

1. VSD type: DORV with subaortic or doubly committed VSD (no PS)
2. TOF type: DORV with subaortic or doubly committed VSD and PS
3. TGA type: DORV with subpulmonary VSD (with or without PS)
4. Remote VSD type: DORV with a remote VSD (with or without PS)
5. DORV and AVSD

This classification allows for better conceptualization and understanding of physiologic and surgical goals.

1. VSD Type: DORV with Subaortic or Doubly Committed VSD (No PS)

Roughly 50% of those with DORV have a subaortic VSD (Walters et al. 2000). Generally, the subaortic VSD is perimembranous, and the defect is separated a variable distance from the aortic valve and can extend to the annulus of the tricuspid valve, which puts it in closer proximity to the conduction system (Walters et al. 2000).

In one autopsy series, 77% of those with a subaortic VSD had bilateral coni, with the remaining 23% having a subpulmonic conus only (Walters et al. 2000). This underscores the variability of conal configuration.

Another 10 % of those with DORV have a doubly committed VSD. Generally there is either a deficient conus bilaterally with a deficient conal septum or there can be a single conus under both great arteries (Walters et al. 2000). Some have dubbed this lesion "double-outlet both ventricles," as it may be difficult to distinguish between DORV and DOLV (double-outlet left ventricle) where a side-by-side arrangement of the great arteries overrides the VSD (Tchervenkov 2000).

2. TOF Type: DORV with Subaortic or Doubly Committed VSD and PS

In the series by Aoki et al. (1994), 48 % of those with a subaortic VSD, and 40 % of those with a doubly committed VSD, had PS (Aoki 1994). In their 20-year experience, Brown et al. (2001) also reported a 49 % and 33 % rate of PS in those with a subaortic and doubly committed VSD, respectively (Brown 2001). Most of the pulmonary outflow tract obstruction that occurs in DORV is subvalvar, highlighting its similarity to tetralogy of Fallot (TOF) (Spaeth 2014).

One of the controversies in the classification of DORV is its distinction from TOF (Spaeth 2014; Jonas 2004a; Mahle et al. 2008; Walters et al. 2000). Based on theories of the embryogenesis of DORV, the amount of aortic override and fibrous continuity between the aortic valve (AV) and the atrioventricular valves (AVV) has been used. Most authors advocate the use of the 50 % rule, where >50 % override of the aorta into the right ventricle is required for the diagnosis of DORV (Raju 2013; Bashore 2007; Walters et al. 2000; Kleinert 1997). But this may be difficult to distinguish both by echocardiography and by direct inspection by the surgeon and has little significance for management. With regard to fibrous continuity between the AV and the AVV, a significant percentage of patients with a subaortic VSD will have a subpulmonic conus only, preserving fibrous continuity between the AV and the AVV (Walters et al. 2000).

Nonetheless, DORV with a subaortic VSD and PS is part of the spectrum of DORV that poses similar management concerns to TOF for the anesthesiologist (Spaeth 2014).

3. TGA Type: DORV with Subpulmonary VSD (With or Without PS)

Subpulmonic VSD is present in roughly one-third of DORV cases (Walters et al. 2000; Aoki et al. 1994). Generally, the VSD is unrestrictive. The Taussig–Bing anomaly, as defined by Van Praagh et al. (1968), is a subset of DORV with a subpulmonic VSD in which there are bilateral coni with the semilunar valves at the same level (fibrous continuity between the semilunar and AVV), a side-by-side arrangement of the great arteries (L-malposed), and no PS (Van Praagh et al. 1968).

In the series by Aoki et al. (1994), of those with a subpulmonary VSD, 15 % had aortic outflow tract obstruction and 52 % had aortic arch obstruction of some kind, similar to the series by Soszyn et al. (2011), where incidence was 16 % and 51 %, respectively (Soszyn 2011; Aoki 1994). Arch hypoplasia is present in up to 78 % of DORV with subpulmonic VSD. Pulmonary outflow tract obstruction is very uncommon in TGA-type DORV (Soszyn 2011; Artrip 2006; Brown 2001; Walters et al. 2000; Aoki 1994).

Another controversy in the classification of DORV is its distinction from TGA (Jonas 2004a; Walters et al. 2000). Again, the amount of aortic override and fibrous continuity between the pulmonic valve (PV) and the atrioventricular valves (AVV) has been used (Jonas 2004a). As in distinguishing between DORV and TOF, most authors advocate the use of the 50% rule, where >50% override of the pulmonary artery into the right ventricle is required for the diagnosis of DORV (Jonas 2004a; Walters et al. 2000; Aoki 1994). But this may be difficult to distinguish and may not impact management. Additionally, some patients with a subpulmonic VSD will have a subaortic conus only, preserving fibrous continuity between the PV and the AVV (Walters et al. 2000; Kirklin 1993).

4. Remote VSD Type: DORV with a Remote VSD (With or Without PS)

DORV with remote (noncommitted) VSD represents 10–20% of the spectrum of DORV (Walters et al. 2000). This is defined as a lesion where the distance between the VSD and the great arteries is at least the diameter of the aortic valve (Lacour-Gayet 2008). The VSD tends to be either muscular or an inlet VSD, can be restrictive, and may be part of an associate AVSD (Spaeth 2014; Walters et al. 2000). Frequently, there are multiple VSDs, making surgical management difficult (Spaeth 2014; Lacour-Gayet 2008; Walters et al. 2000). While some authors suggest that these are predominantly single-ventricle lesions, at least one series by Artrip et al. (2006) reports that 70% underwent a two-ventricle repair (Artrip 2006).

5. DORV and AVSD

DORV with an atrioventricular septal defect is an uncommon lesion and usually requires single-ventricle palliation, as 86% of those requiring single-ventricle palliation in the series of TOF/DORV–AVSD by Raju et al. (2013) were diagnosed with DORV–AVSD (Raju 2013). A total of 52% of all patients with TOF/DORV–AVSD underwent palliation rather that two-ventricle repair. Seventy-four percent of all patients in the series had DORV–AVSD and 26% TOF–AVSD. A significant number or patients that underwent single-ventricle palliation had Rastelli C-type AVSD (76%), hypoplastic ventricle (61%), heterotaxy syndrome (42%), as well as TAPVR (29%) (Raju 2013).

Coronary Arteries

Typically with DORV, the coronary artery pattern tends to follow the rotation of the great arteries and mimic that of lesions with similar arterial position (Freire 2015). With an anteroposterior orientation of the great arteries (anterior aorta), TGA-type DORV, the coronary artery pattern is similar to that seen in TGA, with the right coronary artery arising from the posterior-facing sinus and the left coronary artery from the anterior-facing sinus (Freire 2015; Walters et al. 2000; Gordillo et al. 1993). In those with a rightward and posterior aorta, the coronary artery pattern presents similarly to those with TOF (Freire 2015). There is far more variability in coronary artery pattern in those with side-by-side arrangement of the great arteries (Lowry et al. 2013; Uemura et al. 1995; Gordillo et al. 1993). Position of the coronary arteries may preclude certain surgical repairs and should be considered before surgery (Jonas 2004a).

Clinical Presentation

Clinical signs and symptoms of DORV largely depend on which anatomic variant of the disease is present.

VSD-Type and TOF-Type DORV

Half of those carrying a diagnosis of DORV will present with a subaortic VSD and as many of those will present with pulmonary outflow tract obstruction (Walters et al. 2000). Most of the obstruction will be subvalvar and can present similar to that of TOF (Spaeth 2014; Walters et al. 2000). These patients may present with desaturation, whether continuous or intermittent ("tet spells"). Management is generally focused on maintaining adequate pulmonary blood flow, maintaining adequate preload, and preventing drops in systemic vascular resistance, all principles of management of TOF (Twite and Ing 2012).

In those with a subaortic or doubly committed VSD and little to no PS, the lesion relates more to an unrestricted VSD (Spaeth 2014; Lacour-Gayet 2008; Mahle et al. 2008). Children are usually mildly desaturated, but progress toward heart failure as their pulmonary vascular resistance falls over the first couple of months of life. If the patient is admitted after a late diagnosis, the patient may exhibit signs of significant overcirculation and heart failure (Spaeth 2014). These may include poor urine output, elevated blood urea nitrogen, elevated liver enzymes (alanine transferase, aspartate transferase), a lactic acidosis, as well as clinical signs of poor peripheral perfusion, such as decreased peripheral pulses or capillary refill (Dedieu and Burch 2013; Simmonds 2006). These patients may be receiving diuretics to decrease ventricular loading conditions or ACE inhibitors to reduce systemic afterload (Dedieu and Burch 2013; Simmonds 2006). Ventilation and oxygenation may be supported with positive airway pressure in those with respiratory insufficiency or failure due to substantial pulmonary overcirculation. Necrotizing enterocolitis has been reported in these children (Artrip 2006).

TGA-Type DORV

Variable amounts of intracardiac mixing are possible and will likely depend not only on the size of the VSD and the amount of override but the presence or absence of other anomalies, such as a patent ductus arteriosus (71.9%) or an atrial septal defect (68.4%), both of which are frequently present (Spaeth 2014). These children are generally cyanotic, and interventions designed to improve intracardiac mixing of blood may be initiated (Lacour-Gayet 2008; Artrip 2006). Prostaglandins are frequently initiated to maintain patency of their patent ductus arteriosus, especially in the setting of aortic arch obstruction. Balloon atrial septostomy may be required to achieve proper mixing (Jonas 2004a; Spaeth 2014).

DORV with Remote VSD

DORV with a remote, or noncommitted, VSD has a variable clinical presentation depending on the balance between the pulmonary and systemic circulations (Spaeth 2014; Artrip 2006). Clinical symptoms typically depends on the size of the septal defect(s) and the degree of POTO, as both a restrictive ventricular communication or POTO are not uncommon. (Spaeth 2014; Artrip et al. 2006) Early palliative interventions are designed to improve the physiologic state of patients with either limited pulmonary blood flow or pulmonary overcirculation, as definitive repairs are generally undertaken later in life (Spaeth 2014; Lacour-Gayet 2008).

DORV with AVSD

Presentation of patients depends on the balance between systemic and pulmonary blood flow. Brown et al. (2001) report that 25 % present with pulmonary outflow tract obstruction, which would limit pulmonary circulation (Brown 2001). These patients would likely require maneuvers to improve pulmonary blood flow, which include supplemental oxygen, adequate ventilation, appropriate acid–base status, and possibly the use of prostaglandins to maintain patency of a patent ductus arteriosus (Spaeth 2014). The presence of other lesions, such as heterotaxy syndrome, and total anomalous pulmonary venous return, will change the clinical picture (Spaeth 2014; Lacour-Gayet 2008). Please refer to chapters that address these specific lesions for clinical presentation.

Surgical Repair

Timing of surgery is usually early in life, with most advocating repair in the neonatal period, regardless of where in the spectrum of DORV the lesion lies (Jonas 2004a; Soszyn 2011; Lacour-Gayet 2008). For most cases of DORV, a biventricular repair is possible (Lacour-Gayet 2008; Brown 2001). As stated previously, DORV with a remote VSD, or that associated with an AVSD, is more likely to undergo single-ventricle palliation (Artrip 2006; Aoki 1994).

VSD-Type and TOF-Type DORV

Generally, DORV with a subaortic VSD, with or without PS, and those approaching the mid-spectrum of DORV can successfully undergo an intraventricular baffle repair (Spaeth 2014; Jonas 2004a; Walters et al. 2000). With an anatomy close to DORV, a patch closure is possible whether the diagnosis is DORV or TOF. As the distance between the aortic valve and the VSD widens, in the presence of a subaortic conus, a baffle is needed to direct blood from the left ventricle to the aorta (Spaeth 2014; Jonas 2004a; Mahle et al. 2008). In many of these cases, the VSD will need to be widened to achieve an adequate tunnel repair of caliber (Mahle et al. 2008). As the aortic valve moves further superiorly and away from the VSD, there is the pulmonic valve that is brought closer to the tricuspid valve. When this distance becomes narrower than the diameter of the aortic valve, the baffle is at risk for late development of restrictive flow (stenosis) of the tunnel (Jonas 2004a).

Mid-spectrum DORV or TGA-Type DORV with PS

As the distance between the pulmonary artery and the tricuspid valve becomes prohibitively close for an intraventricular repair, a Rastelli repair is typically used to create a biventricular repair (Jonas 2004a; Brown 2001). Here the main pulmonary artery (MPA) is divided and the proximal MPA stump is oversewn. An intraventricular baffle is created from the VSD that directs blood to the aortic valve; and subsequently a homograft conduit is used to direct blood from a right ventriculotomy to the distal divided segment of the MPA (Jonas 2004a; Mahle et al. 2008; Brown 2001).

An alternative, less common, repair is the REV repair, a pulmonary translocation to a right ventriculotomy with a Lecompte maneuver that requires division and reanastomosis of the ascending aorta (Jonas 2004a; Borromee 1988). Because there is a higher incidence of pulmonary regurgitation with this repair, it is usually reserved for patients with low preoperative pulmonary pressures (Jonas 2004a). Given that the pulmonary artery is usually under tension, care must be taken to avoid direct compression of an anterior coronary artery.

Lastly, aortic root translocation, or the Nikaidoh procedure, can be used for TGA-type DORV with PS (Jonas 2004a; Nikaidoh 1984). The aortic root translocation is accomplished by dividing the aorta with its valve and moving it posteriorly. This may involve coronary reimplantation. The pulmonary artery is also divided, the proximal stump oversewn, and a homograft used to connect the right ventricle to the MPA.

TGA-Type DORV

The arterial switch operation is the standard approach for DORV with a subpulmonic VSD and no PS (Taussig–Bing heart) (Jonas 2004a; Mahle et al. 2008; Brown 2001; Masuda et al. 1999). The operation proceeds in the same fashion as that for TGA.

Aortic Outflow Tract Obstruction and Aortic Arch Hypoplasia

Alternatively, Damus–Kaye–Stansel procedure with a right ventricle to pulmonary artery conduit may be used in cases of AOTO, including those with associated aortic arch narrowing or interruption (Spaeth 2014; Brown 2001).

Outcomes

In the 20-year experience of repair of DORV, Brown et al. (2001) report an early mortality of 4.8 %, with AVSD and aortic arch obstruction as risk factors for higher early mortality (Brown 2001). In this series, 63 % of high-risk patients underwent single-ventricle palliation with 90 % survival at 15 years, and patients from three different risk groups had a 95.8 % (low risk), 89.7 % (intermediate risk), and 89.5 % (high risk) survival at 15 years. Their freedom from reoperation at 15 years was 87 %, 72 %, and 100 % for these same risk categories. Artrip et al. (2006) reported surgical mortality rates of 0 % for VSD-type DORV repairs, 6 % for TOF-type repairs, 9 % for noncommitted VSD-type repairs, and 11 % for TGA-type repairs (Artrip 2006). This underscores an increased mortality for more complex repairs. In one of the largest series of 393 patients published, survival at the end of the study was 77 % and 79 %, respectively, with later surgery being associated with greater survival (Bradley 2007). In this study, Rastelli-type repair was associated with increased early reintervention and greater late mortality, whereas arterial switch operation was associated with greater early mortality, but improved long-term survival.

Anesthetic Management of Clinical Cases

Case 1

This patient's DORV is that of VSD type with unrestricted flow toward her lungs. This patient is 6 weeks old and likely presented with worsening heart failure and overcirculation as her pulmonary vascular resistance fell. And while NEC is less likely in full-term infants, it has been reported in at least one patient with DORV and an unrestricted VSD-type DORV (Artrip 2006). Her respiratory failure is likely a combination of her NEC and her significant pulmonary overcirculation (Spaeth 2014; Dedieu and Burch 2013; Hillier 2004). The patient is critically ill. With regard to the management of volume status in open abdominal surgery, she will require significant fluid resuscitation, as her metabolic demands and third-space losses can equal more than 10–15 ml/kg/h (Hillier 2004; Spaeth 1998). Her hemoglobin is low, and she is predisposed for diffuse intravascular coagulation. She is also hypotensive. With regard to her VSD-type DORV, her pulmonary overcirculation is preventing adequate oxygen delivery to her end organs, including her gut and her kidneys. Goals will include mitigating this left-to-right shunt while improving systemic oxygen delivery.

Given that she is already marginally hypotensive, she will require hemodynamic support, particularly because she will receive an anesthetic that may worsen her hypotension. Induction and maintenance may proceed with a volatile agent, as well as with titrated doses of opiate (fentanyl) along with muscle relaxant. Ventilation and oxygenation should maintain her baseline oxygen saturations with the understanding that full saturation and hyperventilation will increase the left-to-right shunt, which should be avoided (Spaeth 2014). This patient will need a central venous catheter and an arterial line for hemodynamic monitoring and inotropic support, as well as one or two peripheral venous catheters for resuscitation with blood products and intravenous fluid. An inotrope, such as dopamine or epinephrine, should be started to augment her systemic oxygen delivery. She is anemic for someone with a significant left-to-right shunt and hypoperfusion of vital organs. She will thus require ongoing transfusion with packed red blood cells along with plasma, and likely platelets.

Case 2

This represents a TOF-type DORV, per the STS and ESTS classification. In most of these, the obstruction is subvalvar and may have a dynamic component (Spaeth 2014; Walters et al. 2000). This patient is in stable condition, but desaturated. This desaturation is possibly attributable to intraventricular mixing, as well as to his dynamic obstruction. These children will likely not suffer from poor peripheral perfusion, because blood flow to the systemic circulation is not limited. And although parents report no intermittent desaturations, it is not uncommon for patients to experience these "tet spells" once exposed to the stress of induction, intubation, and surgical stimulus.

Although his mother reports that he does well with strangers, the stress of induction may cause stress, even if parental separation does not. A preoperative intravenous catheter is not always present for these children, in particular if they are coming to the hospital from home. Mask induction with 100 % oxygen is appropriate in those without venous access, as diminished pulmonary blood flow is a concern (Twite and Ing 2012). In case of infundibular spasm, volume, such as albumin or crystalloid fluid boluses, blood cells (useful here given his low hemoglobin level), phenylephrine, or femoral artery compression to increase afterload are first-line therapies to ameliorate infundibular spasm (Twite and Ing 2012). Beta-blockers, such as esmolol, may be useful, but not commonly necessary, as an infusion to mitigate the inotropic and chronotropic effects of sympathetic outflow on the myocardium and consequently infundibulum (Twite and Ing 2012). Avoiding light anesthesia and maintaining adequate preload are integral to preventing infundibular muscle spasm in TOF-like physiology (Twite and Ing 2012). Multiple anesthetic agents are acceptable for induction and maintenance of anesthesia. Midazolam and fentanyl are common at our institution to supplement a mask induction and maintenance of anesthesia with volatile agent. Ketamine has some benefit in increasing afterload and improving oxygen saturation in those with infundibular spasm, but may decrease PBF in those with the most severe pulmonary outflow tract obstruction (Jha et al. 2016).

Anesthetics should be geared toward tracheal extubation in those children in whom extubation is not contraindicated. For this reason, regional anesthetic techniques may be useful in providing the patient comfort and preventing response to stimulation, while minimizing the use of opiates intraoperatively. These include but are not limited to transversus abdominis plane block and caudal epidural anesthesia. Please see the Pain Medicine chapter for a full discussion.

References

Aoki M, Forbess JM, Jonas RA, Mayer JE, Castaneda AR. Result of biventricular repair for double-outlet right ventricle. J Thorac Cardiovasc Surg. 1994;107(2):338–49;discussion 349–50.

Artrip JH, Sauer H, Campbell DN, Mitchell MB, Haun C, Almodovar MC, Hraska V, Lacour-Gayet F. Biventricular repair in double outlet right ventricle: surgical results based on the STS-EACTS International Nomenclature classification. Eur J Cardiothorac Surg: Official J Eur Assoc Cardiothorac Surg. 2006;29(4):545–50.

Bashore TM. Adult congenital heart disease: right ventricular outflow tract lesions. Circulation. 2007;115(14):1933–47.

Beitzke A, Anderson RH, Wilkinson JL, Shinebourne EA. Two-chambered right ventricle: simulating two-chambered left ventricle. Br Heart J. 1979;42(1):22–6.

Borromee L, Lecompte Y, Batisse A et al. Anatomic repair of anomalies of ventriculoarterial connection associated with ventricular septal defect. J Thorac Cardiovasc Surg 1988; 95:96–102.

Bradley TJ, Karamlou T, Kulik A, Mitrovic B, Vigneswaran T, Jaffer S, Glasgow PD, Williams WG, Van Arsdell GS, McCrindle BW. Determinants of repair type, reintervention, and mortality in 393 children with double-outlet right ventricle. J Thorac Cardiovasc Surg. 2007;134(4):967–73. e6.

Brown JW, Ruzmetov M, Okada Y, Vijay P, Turrentine MW. Surgical results in patients with double outlet right ventricle: a 20-year experience. Ann Thorac Surg. 2001;72(5):1630–5.

Dedieu N, Burch M. Understanding and treating heart failure in children. Paediat Child Health. 2013;23(2):47–52.

Freire G, Miller MS. Echocardiographic evaluation of coronary arteries in congenital heart disease. Cardiol Young. 2015;25(8):1504–11.

Gordillo L, Faye-Petersen O, de la Cruz MV, Soto B. Coronary arterial patterns in double-outlet right ventricle. Am J Cardiol. 1993;71(12):1108–10.

Howell CE, Ho SY, Anderson RH, Elliott MJ. Fibrous skeleton and ventricular outflow tracts in double-outlet right ventricle. Ann Thorac Surg. 1991;51(3):394–400.

Jha AK, Gharde P, Chauhan S, Kiran U, Malhotra Kapoor P. Echocardiographic Assessment of the Alterations in Pulmonary Blood Flow Associated with Ketamine and Etomidate Administration in Children with Tetralogy of Fallot. Echocardiogr (Mount Kisco, NY). 2016;33(2):307–13.

Jonas RA. Double outlet right ventricle. In: Comprehensive surgical management of congenital heart disease. Boca Raton: CRC Press; 2004. p. 549–70.

Keith A. The Hunterian lectures on malformations of the heart. Lancet. 1909;174(4484):359–63.

Kirklin JW, Harp RA, McGoon DC. Surgical treatment of origin of both vessels from right ventricle, including cases of pulmonary stenosis. J Thorac Cardiovasc Surg. 1964;48:1026–36.

Kirklin JW, Pacifico AD, Blackstone EH, Kirklin JK, Bargeron LM. Current risks and protocols for operations for double-outlet right ventricle. Derivation from an 18 year experience. J Thorac Cardiovasc Surg. 1986;92(5):913–30.

Kirklin JK, Pacifico AD, Kirklin JW. Intraventricular tunnel repair of double outlet right ventricle. J Card Surg. 1987;2(2):231–45.

Kleinert S, Sano T, Weintraub RG, Mee RB, Karl TR, Wilkinson JL. Anatomic features and surgical strategies in double-outlet right ventricle. Circulation. 1997;96(4):1233–9.

Lacour-Gayet F. Biventricular repair of double outlet right ventricle with noncommitted ventricular septal defect, Semin Thorac Cardiovasc Surg Pediatr Card Surg Annu. 2002;5:163–72.

Lacour-Gayet F. Intracardiac repair of double outlet right ventricle. Seminars in thoracic and cardiovascular surgery. Pediatric cardiac surgery annual. 2008. p. 39–43.

Lacour-Gayet F. Management of older single functioning ventricles with outlet obstruction due to a restricted "VSD" in double inlet left ventricle and in complex double outlet right ventricle. Seminars in thoracic and cardiovascular surgery. Pediatric cardiac surgery annual. 2009. p. 130–2.

Lacour-Gayet F, Haun C, Ntalakoura K, Belli E, Houyel L, Marcsek P, Wagner F, Weil J. Biventricular repair of double outlet right ventricle with non-committed ventricular septal defect (VSD) by VSD rerouting to the pulmonary artery and arterial switch. Eur J Cardiothorac Surg Off J Eur Assoc Cardiothorac Surg. 2002;21(6):1042–8.

Lecompte Y, Batisse A, Di Carlo D. Double-outlet right ventricle: a surgical synthesis. Adv Card Surg. 1993;4:109–36.

Lev M. The conotruncus. I. Its normal inversion and conus absorption. Circulation. 1972a;46(3):634–6.

Lev M, Volk BW. The pathologic anatomy of the Taussig-Bing heart: riding pulmonary artery; report of a case. Bull Int Assoc Med Mus. 1950;31:54–64.

Lev M, Bharati S, Meng CC, Liberthson RR, Paul MH, Idriss F. A concept of double-outlet right ventricle. J Thorac Cardiovasc Surg. 1972b;64(2):271–81.

Lowry AW, Olabiyi OO, Adachi I, Moodie DS, Knudson JD. Coronary artery anatomy in congenital heart disease. Congenit Heart Dis. 2013;8(3):187–202.

Mahle WT, Martinez R, Silverman N, Cohen MS, Anderson RH. Anatomy, echocardiography, and surgical approach to double outlet right ventricle. Cardiol Young. 2008;18 Suppl 3:39–51.

Masuda M, Kado H, Shiokawa Y, Fukae K, Kanegae Y, Kawachi Y, Morita S, Yasui H. Clinical results of arterial switch operation for double-outlet right ventricle with subpulmonary VSD. Eur J Cardiothorac Surg: Off J Eur Assoc Cardiothorac Surg. 1999;15(3):283–8.

Neufeld HN, Lucas RV, Lester RG, Adams P, Anderson RC, Edwards JE. Origin of both great vessels from the right ventricle without pulmonary stenosis. Br Heart J. 1962;24:393–408.

Nikaidoh H. Aortic translocation and biventricular outflow tract reconstruction. J Thorac Cardiovasc Surg 1984;88:365–372.

Obler D, Juraszek AL, Smoot LB, Natowicz MR. Double outlet right ventricle: aetiologies and associations. J Med Genet. 2008;45(8):481–97.

Raju V, Burkhart HM, Rigelman Hedberg N, Eidem BW, Li Z, Connolly H, Schaff HV, Dearani JA. Surgical strategy for atrioventricular septal defect and tetralogy of Fallot or double-outlet right ventricle. Ann Thorac Surg. 2013;95(6):2079–84;discussion 2084–5.

Restivo A, Piacentini G, Placidi S, Saffirio C, Marino B. Cardiac outflow tract: a review of some embryogenetic aspects of the conotruncal region of the heart. Anat Rec A Discov Mol Cell Evol Biol. 2006;288(9):936–43.

Restivo A, Unolt M, Putotto C, Marino B. Double outlet right ventricle versus aortic dextroposition: morphologically distinct defects. Anat Rec. 2013;296(4):559–63.

Simmonds J, Franklin O, Burch M. Understanding the pathophysiology of paediatric heart failure and its treatment. Curr Pediatr 2006;16:398–405.

Soszyn N, Fricke TA, Wheaton GR, Ramsay JM, d'Udekem Y, Brizard CP, Konstantinov IE. Outcomes of the arterial switch operation in patients with Taussig-Bing anomaly. Ann Thorac Surg. 2011;92(2):673–9.

Spaeth JP. Perioperative Management of DORV. Semin Cardiothorac Vasc Anesth. 2014; 18(3):281–9.

Taussig HB, Bing RJ. Complete transposition of the aorta and a levoposition of the pulmonary artery; clinical, physiological, and pathological findings. Am Heart J. 1949;37(4):551–9.

Twite MD, Ing RJ. Tetralogy of Fallot: perioperative anesthetic management of children and adults. Semin Cardiothorac Vasc Anesth. 2012;16(2):97–105.

Uemura H, Yagihara T, Kawashima Y, Nishigaki K, Kamiya T, Ho SY, Anderson RH. Coronary arterial anatomy in double-outlet right ventricle with subpulmonary VSD. Ann Thorac Surg. 1995;59(3):591–7.

Van Praagh R. What is the Taussig-Bing malformation? Circulation. 1968;38(3):445–9.

Van Praagh R. Diagnosis of complex congenital heart disease: morphologic-anatomic method and terminology. Cardiovasc Intervent Radiol. 1984;7(3–4):115–20.

Van Praagh R, Van Praagh S, Nebesar RA, Muster AJ, Sinha SN, Paul MH. Tetralogy of Fallot: underdevelopment of the pulmonary infundibulum and its sequelae. Am J Cardiol. 1970;26(1):25–33.

Walters HL, Mavroudis C, Tchervenkov CI, Jacobs JP, Lacour-Gayet F, Jacobs ML. Congenital Heart Surgery Nomenclature and Database Project: double outlet right ventricle. Ann Thorac Surg. 2000;69(4 Suppl):S249–63.

Witham AC. Double outlet right ventricle; a partial transposition complex. Am Heart J. 1957;53(6):928–39.

Chapter 28
Double-Outlet Left Ventricle (DOLV)

Zoel Augusto Quiñónez and Jamie Wingate Sinton

Clinical Vignettes

Case 1

A 2-week-old 3.2 kg male with DOLV, subpulmonic VSD, and coarctation of the aorta presents for peripherally inserted central catheter (PICC) placement. The right arm is chosen for the PICC line as he has a persistent left superior vena cava without a bridging vein and his lower extremities are avoided because of possible partial obstruction to flow given his coarctation.

His past medical history is significant for full-term spontaneous vaginal delivery and the aforementioned unrepaired cardiac disease. He is currently on a continuous infusion of prostaglandin, but otherwise is not on any other medication and has no allergies or previous surgeries.

Vital signs: SpO2 (preductal) 93%, SpO2 (postductal) 84%, HR 146, RR 40, BP (right arm) 84/38, BP (left leg) 68/32, and T 36.4 C.

On exam, he is thin with a flat fontanel. He has a III/VI systolic murmur and radial to femoral delay on pulses; pulses are noted by Doppler only. His liver edge is palpable two centimeters below the costal margin. His echo confirms the anatomy of DOLV and a subpulmonic VSD with right to left flow in systole. His coarctation is juxtaductal with peak velocity 2 m/s, as well as normal biventricular size and function. Blood work is unremarkable, with a hemoglobin of 10.2 g/dl, a blood urea nitrogen of 11 mg/dl, a blood creatinine of 0.3 mg/dl, and a lactate of 1.1 mmol/L, and his chest X-ray shows bilateral hazy infiltrates.

Z.A. Quiñónez, MD (✉) • J.W. Sinton, MD
Division of Pediatric Cardiovascular Anesthesiology,
Texas Children's Hospital, Baylor College of Medicine,
6621 Fannin Street, WT-17417, Houston, TX 77030, USA
e-mail: zoel.quinonez@bcm.edu; zaquinon@texaschildrens.org; jrwingat@texaschildrens.org

© Springer International Publishing Switzerland 2017
A. Dabbagh et al. (eds.), *Congenital Heart Disease in Pediatric and Adult Patients*, DOI 10.1007/978-3-319-44691-2_28

Case 2

A 4.1 kg, 3-month-old male with history of DOLV and subaortic VSD presents for Stamm gastrostomy tube placement for failure to thrive. The surgeon plans a midline upper abdominal laparotomy with catheter brought out in the left hypochondrium. His past medical history is significant for a 35-week birth by induction of labor for preeclampsia and the aforementioned unrepaired cardiac disease. He takes propranolol at home because some of his desaturation is thought to be due to infundibular muscle spasm, although parents do not endorse discrete desaturations ("tet spells"), has no allergies, and has had no previous surgeries.

Vital signs: SpO2 82 %, HR 132, RR 32, BP 80/36, and T 37 C.

On exam, he is a thin-appearing infant with mild perioral cyanosis and dry mucus membranes. His precordium is quiet, his capillary refill is 3 s, and his liver edge is palpable less than one centimeter below costal margin. His echo confirms the anatomy of DOLV, subaortic VSD, PFO, and a 3.9 m/s peak velocity across his subpulmonic outflow tract with normal biventricular size and function. Blood work shows a hemoglobin of 10.6 g/dl. His chest X-ray shows clear lung fields bilaterally.

Background

Double-outlet ventricles (right or left) have been estimated to account for approximately one percent of congenital heart disease. Of the double-outlet ventricles, five percent of those are double-outlet left ventricles, with a reported incidence of one in 200,000 and with a male predominance (Van Praagh et al. 1989; Imai-Compton et al. 2010; Fukuda et al. 2004).

In actuality, until the mid-1960s, double-outlet left ventricle was seen as an embryologic impossibility (Grant 1962). When Fragoyannis (1962) first reported "transposition of the great vessels, both arising from the left ventricle," it was seen that both arteries actually arose from a posterior morphologic right ventricle (Fragoyannis and Kardalinos 1962). The first confirmed report of DOLV came from Sakakibara and colleagues' (1967) description of the first successful repair; but DOLV was first reported as early as 1819 (Coto et al. 1979). Given the rarity of DOLV, the vast majority of literature is limited to case reports and case series (Paul et al. 1970; Anderson et al. 1974; Conti et al. 1974; Brandt et al. 1976; Bharati et al. 1978; Stegmann et al. 1979; Coto et al. 1979; Sakamoto et al. 1997; Lopes et al. 2001; Alehan and Hallioglu 2003; Fukuda et al. 2004; Lilje et al. 2007; Sohn et al. 2008). Bharati and colleagues first classified the anatomic spectrum of this disease in 1978 (Bharati et al. 1978).

Embryology

Several theories have been proposed for the embryologic development of DOLV. Leftward shift of the conotruncus, conotruncal inversion, as well as differential conal growth or resorption have been implicated as mechanisms of development for DOLV (Paul et al. 1970; Anderson et al. 1974; Coto et al. 1979; Männer et al. 1997; Tchervenkov et al. 2000). Abnormalities of conotruncal or bulbar inversion create improper great arterial interrelations; and overzealous absorption of the conus leads to conal deficiencies. But, based on the theory of differential conal growth, it was long thought that bilateral absent conus was necessary for the diagnosis of DOLV (Tchervenkov et al. 2000). This was due to the idea that conal growth under a great artery pushes that artery anteriorly toward the right ventricle during development, whereby bilateral absent coni would be necessary for both arteries to overlie the posteriorly located left ventricle. Since the time this was originally proposed, all conal configurations have been identified in DOLV, making one unifying theory difficult to propose (Tchervenkov et al. 2000; Menon and Hagler 2008).

Anatomy

Levocardia and situs solitus may account for as much as 96 % of cases of DOLV (Gouton et al. 1996). In the largest of series by Van Praagh, most cases of DOLV have situs solitus and atrioventricular (AV) concordance (65 %) (Van Praagh et al. 1989; Menon and Hagler 2008). Those cases with tricuspid or mitral atresia and a hypoplastic right or left ventricle undergo single-ventricle palliation and will not be the focus of this discussion, as single-ventricle palliation is covered elsewhere.

Authors have categorized double-outlet left ventricle (DOLV) using various criteria, including the atrial situs, the concordance of the cardiac segments, the presence or absence of tricuspid valve anomalies, the position of the ventricular septal defect (VSD) relative to the great arteries, the relative positions of the great arteries to each other, and the presence of left- or right-sided obstructive lesions (Bharati et al. 1978; Tchervenkov et al. 2000; Menon and Hagler 2008). Given that, like double-outlet right ventricle (DORV), the pathophysiology of this lesion reflects a continuum that includes tetralogy of Fallot-type and transposition-type physiologies, this conceptualization may be useful. But maybe due to its scarcity and significant anatomic variations, DOLV is generally categorized by the position of the VSD as it relates to the great arteries and the presence or absence of obstructive lesions.

Ventricular Septal Defect

In the largest series, ventricular septal defects are almost always present in patients with DOLV and are generally subarterial (Van Praagh et al. 1989). Most of the cases of DOLV with situs solitus and AV concordance had a subaortic VSD (71 %), followed by a subpulmonic VSD (15 %), and doubly committed VSD (10 %) (Van Praagh et al. 1989). DOLV with a remote VSD or an intact septum is rare (Tchervenkov et al. 2000; Menon and Hagler 2008).

As with DORV, some controversy exists. To distinguish between DOLV with a subaortic VSD and transposition of the great arteries and between DOLV with a subaortic VSD and pulmonary stenosis and tetralogy of Fallot, again the imperfect

50% override rule is frequently used (Tchervenkov et al. 2000). It may be useful physiologically to think about the spectrum of disease in terms of similar lesions, but there is little utility from a surgical standpoint. Also, with respect to a doubly committed VSD in DOLV, it may be difficult to distinguish between DORV and DOLV where a side-by-side arrangement of the great arteries overrides the VSD. Some have called this "double-outlet both ventricles" (Kirklin and Barratt-Boyes 1993; Tchervenkov et al. 2000).

Right- and Left-Sided Obstructive Lesions

Almost universally (close to 90% in the series by Van Praagh), DOLV with subaortic VSD presents with pulmonary outflow obstruction (Van Praagh et al. 1989; Luciani et al. 2014). This pulmonary outflow tract obstruction (POTO) can be valvular or subvalvular (Tchervenkov et al. 2000). In comparison, only 20% of DOLV in the series by Van Praagh presented with a subpulmonic VSD. Similarly, almost 80% of DOLV with PA override presented with aortic outflow obstruction, with only a small percentage of DOLV with aortic override presenting with a left-sided obstructive lesion. Additionally, coarctation of the aorta or interrupted aortic arch frequently presents with aortic outflow tract obstruction in those with a subpulmonic VSD (Van Praagh et al. 1989).

Other Associated Anomalies

Many other associated anomalies have been reported with DOLV. A patent ductus arteriosus (79%) is present in a large majority of patients, as are atrial septal defects (74%). Left superior vena cava (26%) and right aortic arch (16%) were not uncommon in the series by (Imai-Compton et al. 2010). Ebstein's anomaly, heterotaxy syndrome, total anomalous pulmonary venous return, as well as a hypoplastic right ventricle may be present. In those with a single developed ventricle, both mitral and tricuspid atresia, as well as double-inlet left ventricle, pulmonic valve stenosis, and an unbalanced complete atrioventricular septal defect, have been seen as part of this single-ventricle anatomy (Tchervenkov et al. 2000). Again, our focus here is DOLV with two-ventricle anatomy.

Coronary Arteries

Coronary anatomy varies, with 38% of cases reviewed by Luciani and colleagues reporting coronary anomalies (Luciani et al. 2014). Among those, a single left coronary artery (LCA), two right coronary arteries (RCA), as well as a left anterior descending diagonal and two circumflex right coronary arteries have been described (Brandt et al. 1976; Luciani et al. 2014). Coronary anomalies may make certain repairs, such as pulmonary root translocation, prohibitive (Luciani et al. 2014).

Conduction System

The conduction system may be normal in DOLV. The atrioventricular node and bundle of His are normally positioned (assuming atrioventricular concordance) (Tchervenkov et al. 2000). The bundle of His may lie along the left side of the inferior margin of the subarterial VSD, in which case, if it is closed as in a perimembranous VSD, heart block can be avoided (Bharati et al. 1978).

Clinical Presentation

Clinical signs and symptoms of DOLV largely depend on which anatomic variant of the disease is present.

Subaortic VSD with or Without POTO

Given that the most common form of DOLV includes a subaortic VSD and pulmonary outflow tract obstruction (POTO), a large number of those diagnosed with DOLV will have physiology similar to tetralogy of Fallot (TOF) (Menon and Hagler 2008). In one series from the Hospital for Sick Children, Toronto, 4 of 19 (21 %) had a secondary diagnosis of TOF (Imai-Compton et al. 2010). These generally present with restricted flow to the pulmonary vasculature; and pulmonary blood flow (PBF) may be dependent on a patent ductus arteriosus. Persistent or intermittent desaturation may be present in these children; and the team or physician caring for the child may have implemented interventions designed to increase oxygenation and PBF (Twite and Ing 2012).

In those with a subaortic VSD and little to no POTO, the lesion relates more closely to transposition of the great arteries (TGA) with a VSD (Tchervenkov et al. 2000). Variable amounts of intracardiac mixing are possible and will likely depend not only on the size of the VSD and the amount of override but also the presence or absence of other anomalies, such as a PDA or an ASD, both of which are frequently present (Imai-Compton et al. 2010). With a significant amount of left-to-right shunt from a combination of a VSD, a PDA, and an ASD, symptoms of pulmonary overcirculation and heart failure may be present at the time of presentation, particularly toward the second month of life as pulmonary vascular resistance (PVR) falls (Latham et al. 2015). These patients may be on multiple diuretics as well as therapies designed to reduce afterload, such as ACE inhibitors, respectively (Dedieu and Burch 2013). Additionally, for patients with a decompensating respiratory status, maneuvers such as continuous or biphasic positive airway pressure may have been implemented to improve ventilation and oxygenation.

Subpulmonic VSD with or Without AOTO

In the largest series of DOLV to date, almost 80 % of those with a subpulmonic VSD presented with AOTO (Van Praagh et al. 1989). Not infrequently AOTO will also be accompanied by downstream obstruction, such as coarctation of the aorta or interrupted aortic arch (Tchervenkov et al. 2000). In many instances, children with a VSD and AOTO will be dependent on a patent ductus arteriosus for their systemic circulation, particularly if coarctation of the aorta or interrupted aortic arch is present, and may be acutely ill preoperatively (Tchervenkov et al. 2000; Gaynor 2001). If poor systemic perfusion exists, signs of end-organ hypoperfusion may be present. These may include poor urine output, elevated blood urea nitrogen, elevated liver enzymes (alanine transferase, aspartate transferase), lactic acidosis, as well as clinical signs of poor peripheral perfusion, such as decreased peripheral pulses or capillary refill. Depending on the degree of AOTO and systemic hypoperfusion, these children may be receiving prostaglandins to provide sufficient peripheral perfusion by maintaining patency of their ductus arteriosus.

DOLV with a subpulmonic VSD with no AOTO may present like a large VSD (Menon and Hagler 2008). These patients may have unrestricted pulmonary blood flow and be receiving therapy for heart failure symptoms, particularly as children grow and their PVR falls toward the second month of life. These patients may also be receiving diuretics to decrease ventricular loading conditions or ACE inhibitors to reduce systemic afterload (Dedieu and Burch 2013). Ventilation and oxygenation may be supported with positive airway pressure in those with respiratory insufficiency or failure due to substantial pulmonary overcirculation (Kato et al. 2014).

Supracristal and Remote VSD

DOLV with supracristal VSDs presents similar to DOLV with a subpulmonic VSD and no AOTO. There may be unrestricted PBF, and children may be receiving interventions for heart failure due to pulmonary overcirculation or depressed right ventricular function.

DOLV with a noncommitted, or remote, VSD is rare, with only a few authors reporting single cases (Pacifico et al. 1973; Bharati et al. 1978; Luciani et al. 2014). The clinical presentation will depend on the size of the septal defect as well as the presence of any right- or left-sided obstructive lesion.

Right Ventricular Dysfunction

Special consideration should be given to preoperative right ventricular dysfunction. In a series by Imai-Compton and colleagues (2010), all patients had some degree of right ventricular dysfunction on presentation (Imai-Compton et al. 2010). This is of particular importance for those patients receiving a right ventricular outflow patch in the setting of POTO or those receiving a right ventriculotomy either for pulmonary translocation or, more commonly, placement of a shunt. These patients will be at a higher risk of RV failure postoperatively (Luciani et al. 2014).

Surgical Repair

Broadly, the aim of surgical correction is to direct systemic venous blood toward the pulmonary artery and close the VSD, and many surgical approaches have been described based on anatomy (Stegmann et al. 1979; Tchervenkov et al. 2000).

Subaortic VSDs

For patients with subaortic VSDs, surgical treatment depends on great vessel anatomy. If the pulmonary stenosis is mild in the presence of a subaortic VSD, closure of the VSD with relief of pulmonic stenosis allows for preservation of native outflow tracts. Another option for outflow tract preservation is pulmonary root translocation; however, this is a technically challenging operation (Menon and Hagler 2008). If the aorta is rightward of the PA and pulmonic stenosis is present, a tetralogy of Fallot-type repair may proceed (Bharati et al. 1978; Menon and Hagler 2008). However, if the great vessels are d-malposed with an anterior aorta, relief of obstruction is difficult or impossible, and an RV-PA conduit (Rastelli) is often used (Brandt et al. 1976; Menon and Hagler 2008). When the great vessels are normally related and pulmonary atresia is present, an RV-PA conduit is used (Brandt et al. 1976). In general, if the VSD is near the tricuspid valve, the bundle of His is located along its inferior and posterior edges and is at risk for injury during repair (Tchervenkov et al. 2000).

Patent Pulmonary Outflow

If pulmonary stenosis is not present, ventricular septal defect closure often proceeds to connect the right ventricle to the pulmonary artery. This closure assumes adequate size of both ventricles (Brandt et al. 1976; Coto et al. 1979). In these cases, the VSD is usually subpulmonic or doubly committed and nonrestrictive (Coto et al. 1979).

Aortic Outflow Tract Obstruction

Alternatively, Damus-Kaye-Stansel procedure with a right ventricle to pulmonary artery conduit may be used in cases of AOTO, including those with associated aortic arch narrowing or interruption (Menon and Hagler 2008).

Single Ventricle

Single-ventricle palliation with a Fontan was previously quite rare and employed only in the case of atrioventricular valve atresia (Menon and Hagler 2008). Many children with functionally univentricular hearts are not Fontan candidates and may not even be candidates for surgical palliation (Sharratt et al. 1976; Sakamoto et al. 1997). More recently, single-ventricle palliation has been embraced especially for borderline cases in which a suboptimal biventricular repair may be associated with increased surgical mortality (Hickey et al. 2007; Imai-Compton et al. 2010).

Outcomes

Given that most reports of double-outlet left ventricle are case reports and case series, there is very little published outcome data (Imai-Compton et al. 2010; Luciani et al. 2014). In the 49-year experience from the Hospital for Sick Children, there was an equivalent 5-year survival for children undergoing single-ventricle or biventricular repair of 70–75%. Freedom from reintervention was 35% at 1 year, 21% at 2 years, and 0% at 7 years old. They also noted that children from earlier years underwent biventricular repair at a higher rate, whereas children from later years underwent univentricular repair. This is likely multifactorial (Imai-Compton et al. 2010). For those undergoing biventricular repair, Luciani and colleagues found a 92, 87, and 87% survival at 1, 5, and 10 years after corrective surgery in their case series and literature review (Luciani et al. 2014). Of note, all early deaths were attributed to right ventricular failure, and one patient had a late conversion to Fontan palliation due to right ventricular failure, again emphasizing right ventricular function as a concern in patients with DOLV undergoing corrective surgery. Surgery before 1992 and placement of a right ventricular outflow tract patch were associated with a higher degree of morbidity and mortality in this series of patients undergoing biventricular repair.

Summary of Clinical Cases

Case 1

As highlighted in the chapter, in those DOLV cases with a subpulmonic VSD, coarctation of the aorta is common. These children present with a physiology similar to a VSD with a coarctation and could be critically ill from pulmonary overcirculation and poor systemic perfusion. They may require prostaglandins to maintain a patent ductus arteriosus for perfusion of their lower body as well as vital organs, such as the kidneys, liver, and gut. While this child is stable, renal failure and hepatic injury and gut hypoperfusion may occur, represented as a lactic acidosis, transaminitis, elevated BUN/Cr, as well as with signs and symptoms of poor end-organ perfusion, such as decreased urine output. His preductal oxygen saturation of 92 % may be appropriate given his intraventricular mixing, but his chest X-ray indicates increased lung water from pulmonary overcirculation. His decreased postductal saturation indicates narrowing of his patent ductus arteriosus, necessitating prostaglandins. This is also represented by his radio-femoral pulse delay and the pressure gradient from his right arm to his left leg.

Anesthetic goals here include preventing additional pulmonary overcirculation and maintaining adequate perfusion pressure through the patent ductus arteriosus. Supplemental oxygen may increase the left-to-right shunt and exacerbate existing pulmonary overcirculation. While supplemental oxygen may be necessary after sedation has been administers, this must be balanced against the possibility of exacerbating the increased lung water this child has. Generally, at our institution, we provide minimal sedation for these cases; and in the case of a critically ill child, we may provide no sedation. Small, titrated doses of midazolam, fentanyl, or ketamine have been used successfully with a natural airway. Securing the arm by holding or taping it may be necessary to avoid oversedation. Local anesthetic infiltration at the insertion site, prior to PICC line placement, is extremely helpful.

Case 2

Very similar to TOF-type DORV, this case represents one end of the spectrum of disease in DOLV, which is that of a lesion physiologically similar to tetralogy of Fallot. Eerily similar to "Case 2" from the previous chapter, this patient is in stable condition, but desaturated. This patient has an oxygen saturation of 82 % and clear lung fields bilaterally, so the desaturation is likely due to a combination of intra-atrial and intraventricular mixing, as well as his significant dynamic POTO. These children will likely not suffer from poor peripheral perfusion, like the child in the previous case did, because blood flow to the systemic circulation is not limited. Desaturation from infundibular spasm seems possible based on the literature cited here. And, although parents report no intermittent desaturations, it is not uncommon for patients to experience these "tet spells" once exposed to the stress of induction, intubation, and surgical stimulus.

From here we proceed similarly to "Case 2" from the last chapter on DORV. Premedication may be useful in preventing infundibular spasm, even in a 3-month-old, to prevent agitation from undressing, placement of monitors, and mask induction. Mask induction with 100 % oxygen is appropriate in those without venous access, as diminished pulmonary blood flow is a concern. Beta-blockers, such as esmolol, may be useful as an infusion to mitigate the inotropic and chrono-tropic effects of sympathetic outflow on the infundibulum, but volume, blood, and increasing afterload are, again, the first-line therapies. Avoiding light anesthesia, but maintaining adequate preload, is integral to preventing infundibular muscle spasm in TOF-like physiology. Multiple anesthetic agents are acceptable for induction and maintenance of anesthesia. Midazolam and fentanyl are common at our institution to supplement a mask induction and maintenance of anesthesia with volatile agent. Ketamine has some benefit in increasing afterload and improving oxygen saturation in those with infundibular spasm, but may decrease PBF in those with the most severe POTO (Jha et al. 2016).

Anesthetics should be geared toward tracheal extubation in those children in whom extubation is not contraindicated. For this reason, regional anesthetic tech-niques may be useful in providing the patient comfort and preventing response to stimulation, while minimizing use of opiates intraoperatively. These include, but are not limited to, transversus abdominis plane block and caudal epidural anesthesia. Please see the Pain Medicine chapter for a full discussion.

References

Alehan D, Hallioglu O. Two-dimensional echocardiographic diagnosis of double outlet left ven-tricle with subaortic ventricular septal defect, pulmonary stenosis, and a hypoplastic left ven-tricle. J Am Soc Echocardiogr. 2003;16(1):91–3.

Anderson R, Galbraith R, Gibson R, Miller G. Double outlet left ventricle. Br Heart J. 1974; 36(6):554–8.

Bharati S, Lev M, Stewart R, McAllister HA, Kirklin JW. The morphologic spectrum of double outlet left ventricle and its surgical significance. Circulation. 1978;58(3 Pt 1):558–65.

Brandt PW, Calder AL, Barratt-Boyes BG, Neutze JM. Double outlet left ventricle. Morphology, cineangiocardiographic diagnosis and surgical treatment. Am J Cardiol. 1976;38(7):897–909.

Conti V, Adams F, Mulder DG. Double-outlet left ventricle. Ann Thorac Surg. 1974;18(4):402–10.

Coto EO, Jimenez MQ, Castaneda AR, Rufilanchas JJ, Deverall PB. Double outlet from chambers of left ventricular morphology. Br Heart J. 1979;42(1):15–21.

Dedieu N, Burch M. Understanding and treating heart failure in children. Paediatr Child Health. 2013;23(2):47–52.

Fragoyannis S, Kardalinos A. Transposition of the great vessels, both arising from the left ventricle (juxtaposition of pulmonary artery). Tricuspid atresia, atrial septal defect and ventricular septal defect. Am J Cardiol. 1962;10:601–4.

Fukuda T, Oku H, Nakamoto S, Mukobayashi M, Koike E. Successful pregnancy in a patient with double outlet left ventricle after a Rastelli operation using a prosthetic valve. Circulation J Off J Jpn Circulation Soc. 2004;68(5):501–3.

Gaynor JW. Management strategies for infants with coarctation and an associated ventricular septal defect. J Thorac Cardiovasc Surg. 2001;122(3):424–6.

Gouton M, Bozio A, Rey C, Sassolas F, Vaksmann G, Di Filippo S. [Double outlet left ventricle: a rare and unusual cardiopathy. Apropos of 7 new cases]. Arch des maladies du coeur et des vaisseaux. 1996;89(5):553–9.

Grant RP. The morphogenesis of transposition of the great vessels. Circulation. 1962;26:819–40.

Hickey EJ, Caldarone CA, Blackstone EH, Lofland GK, Yeh T, Pizarro C, Tchervenkov CI, Pigula F, Overman DM, Jacobs ML, McCrindle BW, Congenital Heart Surgeons' Society. Critical left ventricular outflow tract obstruction: the disproportionate impact of biventricular repair in borderline cases. J Thorac Cardiovasc Surg. 2007;134(6):1429–36; discussion 1436–7.

Imai-Compton C, Elmi M, Manlhiot C, Floh AA, Golding F, Williams WG, McCrindle BW. Characteristics and outcomes of double outlet left ventricle. Congenit Heart Dis. 2010;5(6): 532–6.

Jha AK, Gharde P, Chauhan S, Kiran U, Malhotra Kapoor P. Echocardiographic assessment of the alterations in pulmonary blood flow associated with ketamine and etomidate administration in children with tetralogy of fallot. Echocardiography (Mount Kisco, NY). 2016;33(2):307–13.

Kato T, Suda S, Kasai T. Positive airway pressure therapy for heart failure. World J Cardiol. 2014;6(11):1175–91.

Kirklin JW, Barratt-Boyes BG. Double outlet left ventricle. In: Kirklin JW, Barratt-Boyes BG, editors. Cardiac surgery: morphology, diagnostic criteria, natural history, techniques, results, and indications. New York, NY: Churchill-Livingston; 1993. p. 1501–9.

Latham GJ, Joffe DC, Eisses MJ, Richards MJ, Geiduschek JM. Anesthetic considerations and management of transposition of the great arteries. Semin Cardiothorac Vasc Anesth. 2015;19(3): 233–42.

Lilje C, Weiss F, Lacour-Gayet F, Rázek V, Ntalakoura K, Weil J, Lê TP. Images in cardiovascular medicine. Double-outlet left ventricle. Circulation. 2007;115(3):e36–7.

Lopes LM, Rangel PI, Soraggi AM, Furlanetto BH, Furlanetto G. Double-outlet left ventricle. Echocardiographic diagnosis. Arquivos Brasileiros Cardiologia. 2001;76(6):511–6.

Luciani GB, De Rita F, Lucchese G, Barozzi L, Rossetti L, Faggian G, Mazzucco A. Current management of double-outlet left ventricle: towards biventricular repair in infancy. J Cardiovasc Med (Hagerstown). 2014. doi: 10.2459/JCM.0000000000000101.

Männer J, Seidl W, Steding G. Embryological observations on the formal pathogenesis of double-outlet left ventricle with a right-ventricular infundibulum. Thorac Cardiovasc Surg. 1997;45(4):172–7.

Menon SC, Hagler DJ. Double-outlet left ventricle: diagnosis and management. Curr Treat Options Cardiovasc Med. 2008;10(5):448–52.

Pacifico AD, Kirklin JW, Bargeron LM, Soto B. Surgical treatment of double-outlet left ventricle. Report of four cases. Circulation. 1973;48(1 Suppl):III19–23.

Paul MH, Muster AJ, Sinha SN, Cole RB, Van Praagh R. Double-outlet left ventricle with an intact ventricular septum. Clinical and autopsy diagnosis and developmental implications. Circulation. 1970;41(1):129–39.

Sakamoto T, Imai Y, Takanashi Y, Hoshino S, Seo K, Terada M, Aoki M, Suetsugu F.[Surgical treatment of double outlet left ventricle], [Zasshi] [Journal]. Nihon Kyōbu Geka Gakkai. 1997;45(12):1922–30.

Sharratt GP, Sbokos CG, Johnson AM, Anderson RH, Monro JL. Surgical "correction" of solitus-concordant, double-outlet left ventricle with L-malposition and tricuspid stenosis with hypoplastic right ventricle. J Thorac Cardiovasc Surg. 1976;71(6):853–8.

Sohn S, Kim HS, Han JJ. Right ventricular outflow patch reconstruction for repair of double-outlet left ventricle. Pediatr Cardiol. 2008;29(2):452–4.

Stegmann T, Oster H, Bissenden J, Kallfelz HC, Oelert H. Surgical treatment of double-outlet left ventricle in 2 patients with D-position and L-position of the aorta. Ann Thorac Surg. 1979;27(2):121–9.

Tchervenkov CI, Walters HL, Chu VF. Congenital heart surgery nomenclature and database project: double outlet left ventricle. Ann Thorac Surg. 2000;69(4 Suppl):S264–9.

Twite MD, Ing RJ. Tetralogy of Fallot: perioperative anesthetic management of children and adults. Semin Cardiothorac Vasc Anesth. 2012;16(2):97–105.

Van Praagh R, Weinberg PM, Srebro J. Double-outlet left ventricle. In: Reimenschneider JA, Emmanouilides GC, Adams FH, editors. Moss' heart disease in Infants, children, and adolescents. Baltimore, MD: Williams & Wilkins; 1989. p. 461–85.

Chapter 29
Pulmonary Hypertension

Ali Dabbagh

Introduction

Pulmonary hypertension (PH) is a severe disease affecting significantly the outcomes of patients with a varying incidence in different studies: from 5 to 52 cases/one million population (Waxman and Zamanian 2013). PH affects many body organs including the heart and lungs and, also, affects growth and development especially in children and adolescents.

Definition PH is defined as the "progressive disease of the pulmonary vascular system, with a mean pulmonary artery pressure (mPAP) $\geq$25 mmHg at rest" or more than 30 mmHg on exercise; the values for mPAP $\geq$25 mmHg are the same in children above 3 months of age at sea level. For diagnosis of pulmonary arterial hypertension (PAH) in addition to mPAP $\geq$25 mmHg at rest, pulmonary arterial wedge pressure $\leq$15 mmHg and pulmonary vascular resistance (PVR) >3 Wood units/m^2 should be documented (Donti et al. 2007; Ryan et al. 2012; Twite and Friesen 2014; Abman et al. 2015; Low et al. 2015).

Classification

PH may be categorized based on the measured values of pulmonary pressure:

- Mild PH; mPAP = 25–40 mmHg
- Moderate PH; mPAP = 41–55 mmHg
- Severe PH; mPAP >55 mmHg (Forrest 2009)

A. Dabbagh, MD
Cardiac Anesthesiology Department, Anesthesiology Research Center,
Shahid Beheshti University of Medical Sciences, Tehran, Iran
e-mail: alidabbagh@yahoo.com; alidabbagh@sbmu.ac.ir

© Springer International Publishing Switzerland 2017
A. Dabbagh et al. (eds.), *Congenital Heart Disease in Pediatric and Adult Patients*, DOI 10.1007/978-3-319-44691-2_29

In addition, the World Health Organization has categorized PH under five major groups which are mentioned in Table 29.1, though there are some overlaps between these groups especially between the second and the third groups of PH (Friesen and Williams 2008; Ryan et al. 2012; Simonneau et al. 2013; Twite and Friesen 2014; Abman et al. 2015).

In addition, based on another classification, PH may be classified as precapillary PH and postcapillary PH; groups 1, 3, 4, and 5 are considered as precapillary PH and group 2 as postcapillary PH (Ivy et al. 2013; Pristera et al. 2016).

In adult patients, the most common frequencies of PH according to Anderson et al. are accordingly (Anderson and Nawarskas 2010):

- Idiopathic/familial PAH is the predominant etiology of PH (40–48%).
- Connective tissue disorders (15–30%).
- Congenital heart abnormalities (11%).
- Portal hypertension (7–10%).
- Anorexigens (3–10%).
- HIV infection (1–6%).

However, in *pediatric population*, though there are many similarities with adult PH, the frequency rates of PH etiologies differ from adults; pediatric PH is most commonly due to congenital heart disease (PH-CHD), idiopathic PH (also known as primary PH), and hereditary PH; neglected or poorly managed congenital heart diseases, especially when prolonged, are among the most common etiologies for pediatric PH (Donti et al. 2007; Kim et al. 2016).

Clinical Features

The main clinical signs and symptoms in PH-CHD include (Friesen and Williams 2008; McDonough et al. 2011; Monfredi et al. 2016):

- Shortness of breath (dyspnea)
- Early fatigability and exercise intolerance
- Chest pain
- Syncope or presyncope on exertion
- Right ventricular heave

Table 29.1 Classification of pulmonary hypertension

Classification	Definition/title	Pre- or postcapillary
Class 1	Pulmonary arterial hypertension (PAH)	Precapillary PH
Class 2	PH due to left heart disease	Postcapillary PH
Class 3	PH due to chronic obstructive lung disease (pulmonary disease)	Precapillary PH
Class 4	PH due to chronic thromboembolic (CTEPH)	Precapillary PH
Class 5	PH because of unclear multifactorial mechanisms	Precapillary PH

Beghetti (2006), Friesen and Williams (2008), Ryan et al. (2012), Ivy et al. (2013), Simonneau et al. (2013), Twite and Friesen (2014), Abman et al. (2015), Low et al. (2015), Pristera et al. (2016)

- Ejection click of pulmonary valve
- Split second heart sound with loud P2
- Systolic murmur in tricuspid valve due to tricuspid regurgitation
- Diastolic murmur due to pulmonary insufficiency
- Bulged jugular vein

Paraclinical Studies

Right heart catheterization and pulmonary angiography are the gold standard for hemodynamic assessment, definitive diagnosis, and assessment of vascular architecture in PH; however, a number of modern sensitive and specific noninvasive imaging modalities have been developed, and more are in progress with especial aim to replace these imaging tools instead of angiography for diagnosis, follow-up, and management of PH (Lang et al. 2010; Kreitner 2014; Gerges et al. 2015; Pristera et al. 2016).

Chest X-Ray

- Cardiomegaly mainly in the right-sided chambers
- Elevated cardiac apex due to RV enlargement and RV hypertrophy
- Enlargement of the pulmonary artery trunk especially in the outflow tract
- Decreased retrosternal border in lateral X-ray due to RV enlargement
- Shrinkage of distal branches of pulmonary arterial system leading to oligemic lung fields

Electrocardiography

- Right axis deviation
- Right ventricular hypertrophy presenting as R-to-S wave ratio > one in V1
- Right atrial enlargement presenting as amplitude of P wave especially in lead II
- Right bundle branch block (Fig. 29.1)

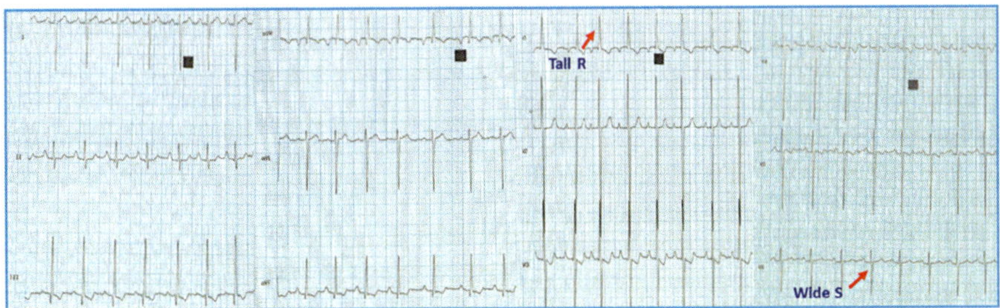

Fig. 29.1 Right ventricular hypertrophy. Typical ECG features are tall R wave in V1, deep S wave in V6, and right axis deviation (Courtesy of Dr Majid Haghjoo and Dr Mohammadrafie Khorgami)

Imaging Studies

Right heart *catheterization* and *pulmonary angiography* are the gold standard for hemodynamic assessment, definitive diagnosis, and assessment of vascular architecture in PH; however, a number of modern sensitive and specific noninvasive imaging modalities have been developed, and more are in progress in the next years with especial aim to replace the new imaging tools instead of angiography for diagnosis, follow-up, and management of PH (Lang et al. 2010; Kreitner 2014; Gerges et al. 2015; Pristera et al. 2016).

Echocardiography Signs of RV hypertrophy and some degrees of RV failure are seen; pulmonary insufficiency in diastole and tricuspid regurgitation in systole are seen in some of the patients.

Cardiac MR (CMR) and Multi-slice CT Scan Both of them are very important noninvasive imaging modalities and help us perform sophisticated and comprehensive assessments; according to "Expert consensus statement on the diagnosis and treatment of pediatric pulmonary hypertension" declared on May 2016 by "European Paediatric Pulmonary Vascular Disease Network, endorsed by ISHLT and DGPK," both CMR and CT have definitive role in pediatric PH; they let us gain noninvasive invaluable data regarding the right heart and the myocardium as well as the pulmonary vascular system hemodynamics; some believe that parenchymal and vascular assessment of the lungs may be more definitively assessed using CT (Gerges et al. 2015; Santos et al. 2015; Latus et al. 2016).

Radioisotope Ventilation/Perfusion Scan Demonstrates the vascular architecture of the lung demonstrating defects and gives structural information about the pathologies that could lead to PH or they can be due to PH (Latus et al. 2016).

Management

There are a number of major scopes in management of children congenital heart disease associated with PH (Kozlik-Feldmann et al. 2016):

- Definitive criteria should be used for operability and/or starting advanced therapies.
- Preoperative and postoperative management are really a great challenge.
- Management of Eisenmenger's syndrome needs sophisticated vigilance and advanced care.

Pharmacological Treatment

The pharmacology of PH for anesthesiologist involves two subclasses: pulmonary vascular system drugs and anesthetic drugs.

A full description of pharmacological agents used for the treatment of pulmonary hypertension could be found in Chap. 4 – Cardiovascular Pharmacology in Pediatric Patients with Congenital Heart Disease.

When using pharmacologic agents to treat PH, we should always consider that there are two distinct stages in treatment of PH:

- *Reversible* stage: in this stage, the changes in pulmonary vascular bed could be partially or near totally reversed using pharmacologic agents.
- *Irreversible* stage: if the disease progresses, the changes in pulmonary vascular system are fixed due to permanent vascular bed remodeling, and so, the pharmacologic agents are not usually effective.

Except for pharmacologic therapy, other treatment alternatives include "*heart and lung* transplantation" or "*lung transplant* with repair of the underlying cardiac defect"; however, they are not used in the majority of the patients (Suesaowalak et al. 2010).

The only FDA-approved pharmaceutical specifically for the treatment of pulmonary hypertension in children is inhaled nitric oxide (iNO) which is administered through the lungs. The other FDA-approved drugs for the treatment of pulmonary hypertension are used in adults and are often based on the pathways related to the endothelial cells, including prostacyclin analogues (epoprostenol, iloprost, treprostinil), phosphodiesterase 5 inhibitors (sildenafil and tadalafil), phosphodiesterase 3 inhibitors (mainly milrinone), endothelin receptor antagonist (bosentan, ambrisentan, and macitentan), and soluble guanylate cyclase stimulator (riociguat) (Benedict et al. 2007; Poor and Ventetuolo 2012; Ventetuolo and Klinger 2014; Abman et al. 2015; Jentzer and Mathier 2015; Liu and Jing 2015; Kim et al. 2016).

Currently available medications for pediatric PH follow one of the following pathways (Table 29.2):

1. *Nitric oxide*: the only FDA formally approved agent for treatment of PH in infants and neonates; the others are used in adults and in children; they are as off-label drugs; inhaled NO (iNO) increases cGMP, leading to smooth muscle relaxation and, subsequently, pulmonary vasodilation. iNO is transported very fast through the alveolar-capillary membranes and, then, rapidly metabolized by circulating erythrocytes, all in just a few seconds; so, iNO is an ideal drug; inhalation is the best targeted therapy in PH with the least systemic side effects. iNO dose starts from 2 to 5 ppm to a maximum of 40 ppm through endotracheal tube, face mask, or nasal cannula with specific delivery instruments; higher doses are both ineffective and may cause side effects like lung injury and/or increased methemoglobin levels; iNO should *not* be withdrawn abruptly, or there would be severe rebound PH (Latus et al. 2015; Kim et al. 2016; Moffett et al. 2016).
2. *Endothelin receptor antagonists*: effective in the treatment of *mild* to *moderate* PH; they include ambrisentan, bosentan, and macitentan; these agents counteract the effects of both endothelin receptors (ET_A and ET_B), leading to vasodilation in the pulmonary vascular system, and, also, inhibit vascular remodeling. Bosentan inhibits both ET_A and ET_B, lowering PAP and PVR, improving exercise tolerance. Bosentan is approved for use in children over 12 years in the USA and in children over 3 years in Canada. Hepatic function should be monitored seriously when administering ET-1 antagonists. Bosentan dose is:

   - 10–20 kg – initial: 31.25 mg once daily for 4 weeks; increase to maintenance dose of 31.25 mg twice daily

- >20–40 kg – initial: 31.25 mg twice daily for 4 weeks; increase to maintenance dose of 62.5 mg twice daily
- >40 kg – initial: 62.5 mg twice daily for 4 weeks; increase to maintenance dose of 125 mg twice daily (Allen et al. 2013; Liu et al. 2013)

3. *Prostacyclin system analogues* (epoprostenol, iloprost, beraprost, treprostinil "IV/subQ/inhaled/oral): these are effective in the treatment of *moderate* to *severe* PH; they cause pulmonary and systemic vasodilation through increasing cAMP; also, they have antiplatelet aggregation effects; they have very short onset of effect, so they act very rapidly and have short half-life. *Epoprostenol* is the most widely studied agent which is given through continuous IV infusion; for epoprostenol central venous line may be needed which should be cautious not to discontinue the infusion even during insertion of CV line. *Iloprost* is the inhaled analogue with clinical effectiveness similar to iNO. *Treprostinil* is the analogue which could be used subcutaneously or IV, and finally, *beraprost* is another analogue used orally (Friesen and Williams 2008; Twite and Friesen 2014; Kim et al. 2016; Moffett et al. 2016).

4. *Phosphodiesterase 5 (PDE-5) inhibitors*: mainly sildenafil and tadalafil and, at times, vardenafil; they lead to pulmonary vasodilation and inhibition of vascular remodeling. PDE 5 degrades cGMP, and when inhibited, accumulation of PDE 5 in smooth muscles of the pulmonary system leads to pulmonary vasodilation (both in acute and chronic PH). Sildenafil is available both as oral and intravenous forms but should be used with extreme caution to prevent life-threatening hypotension. In European Union, sildenafil has approval for patients between 1 and 17 years. However, in the USA, there are still some concerns, especially when iNO is available. The oral dose of sildenafil is 0.25–0.5 mg/Kg each 4–8 h, with a maximum dose of 2 mg/Kg each 4 h; titration of the dose should be based on clinical response; intravenous dose could be found in Table 29.2. These data are in large the same for tadalafil, except for its does which is found in Table 29.2 (Shah and Ohlsson 2011; Beghetti et al. 2014; Vorhies and Ivy 2014; Wang et al. 2014; Dodgen and Hill 2015; Perez and Laughon 2015; Lakshminrusimha et al. 2016).

5. *PDE-3 inhibitors*, mainly milrinone, have positive inotropy and arterial dilation effect with weak chronotropic effects so an *inodilator*. They inhibit PDE-3 isoenzyme in cardiomyocytes and vascular smooth muscle cells; so intracellular cAMP levels are peaked up which in turn leads to increased protein kinase A (PKA). With increased PKA, contractile elements of cardiomyocytes are activated. In smooth muscle cells of the arterial system, PKA leads to relaxation of the vessel wall. Dose and adverse effects are presented in Table 29.2 (Knight and Yan 2012; Ferrer-Barba et al. 2016).

6. *sGC stimulator* or soluble guanylate cyclase stimulator (riociguat): acts through stimulation of soluble guanylate cyclase causing pulmonary vasodilation and, also, inhibits vascular remodeling (Benedict et al. 2007; Suesaowalak et al. 2010; Poor and Ventetuolo 2012; Ventetuolo and Klinger 2014; Abman et al. 2015; Jentzer and Mathier 2015; Kim et al. 2016).

Table 29.2 Pharmacological agents used in the management of pulmonary hypertension

Drug	Recommended dose	Adverse effects	Clinical considerations
Inhaled nitric oxide (iNO): mechanism of action is increasing cGMP, leading to smooth muscle relaxation and, subsequently, pulmonary vasodilation			
iNO	2–5 ppm to a maximum of 40 ppm	Lung injury Increased methemoglobin levels Rebound severe pulmonary hypertension due to abrupt iNO withdrawal	The only FDA-approved agent for pediatric pulmonary hypertension Should not be over administered to prevent side effects Its cost may suggest to consider the drug as the last choice
Prostacyclin/prostacyclin analogues: their mechanism of action is pulmonary and systemic vasodilation through increasing cAMP; also, antiplatelet aggregation			
Epoprostenol	*Initial* infusion rate: 1–3 ng/Kg/min *Maintenance* infusion rate: 50–80 ng/Kg/min	Flushing, headache, nausea, diarrhea, jaw discomfort, rash, hypotension, and thrombocytopenia	Potential risk of hypotension and bleeding in children receiving drugs, such as anticoagulants, platelet inhibitors, or other vasodilators
Iloprost	*Initial* dose: 2.5 µg per inhalation; six times/day *Maintenance* dose: 5 µg per inhalation nine times/day	Cough, wheeze, headache, flushing, jaw pain, diarrhea, rash, and hypotension (at higher doses)	Potential risk of exacerbation of reactive airway disease
Treprostinil (IV/subcutaneous)	*Initial* infusion rate: 1.25–2 ng/Kg/min *Maintenance* infusion rate: 50–80 ng/Kg/min	Flushing, headache, nausea, diarrhea, musculoskeletal discomfort, rash, hypotension, thrombocytopenia, and pain at subcutaneous infusion site	Similar to epoprostenol
Treprostinil (inhaled)	*Initial* dose: three breaths (18 µg)/four times/day *Maintenance* dose: nine breaths (54 µg) four times/day	Cough, headache, nausea, dizziness, flushing, and throat irritation	Reactive airway symptoms and hypotension may occur at high doses
Treprostinil (oral)	*Initial* dose: 0.25 mg PO BID *Maintenance* dose: determined by tolerability	Headache, nausea, diarrhea, jaw pain, extremity pain, hypokalemia, abdominal discomfort, and flushing	If "twice daily" dosing is not tolerated, consider "three times daily" dosing

(continued)

Table 29.2 (continued)

Drug	Recommended dose	Adverse effects	Clinical considerations
PDE-5 inhibitors: inhibit phosphodiesterase-5, leading to pulmonary vasodilation and inhibition of vascular remodeling			
Sildenafil	*Oral* dose: 0.25–0.5 mg/Kg/q4–8 h *Intravenous* dose: loading dose 0.4 mg/Kg over 3 h Maintenance: continuous infusion of 1.5 mg/Kg/day	Headache, flushing, rhinitis, dizziness, hypotension, peripheral edema, dyspepsia, diarrhea, myalgia, and back pain	Coadministration of nitrates is contraindicated; sensorineural hearing loss and ischemic optic neuropathy have been reported
Tadalafil	Oral dose: 1 mg/Kg per day (single daily dose): preliminary studies	Similar to sildenafil No significant effect on vision	Similar to sildenafil
Antagonists of endothelin receptor: counteract with the effects of both endothelin receptors (ET$_A$ and ET$_B$), vasodilation of the pulmonary vascular system, and vascular remodeling inhibition			
Ambrisentan	Body weight <20 kg: 2.5–5 mg PO/four times daily Body weight >20 kg: 5–10 mg PO/four times daily	Peripheral edema, nasal congestion, headache, flushing, anemia, nausea, and decreased sperm count	Baseline liver enzymes and hemoglobin are needed Monitor based on clinical parameters
Bosentan	2 mg/Kg per dose PO, two times daily If body weight is 10–20 kg: 31.25 mg PO, two times daily If body weight is 20–40 kg: 62.5 mg PO, two times daily If body weight is >40 kg: 125 mg PO, two times daily	Pediatric abdominal pain, vomiting, extremity pain, fatigue, flushing, headache, lower limb edema, nasal congestion, hypotension, palpitations, dyspepsia, anemia, and decreased sperm count Potential risk of dose dependent increases in amino-transaminase levels	Liver enzymes and hemoglobin levels should be monitored; in patients with moderate or severe degrees of hepatic impairment , should be used cautiously Also, concomitant use of CYP3A4 inducers and inhibitors should be considered as important caution
Macitentan	10 mg PO, four times daily	Nasal congestion, headache, flushing, anemia, and decreased sperm count	The incidence of serum aminotransferase elevation is low Obtain baseline liver enzymes and hemoglobin and monitor as clinically indicated Teratogenicity REMS*

Table 29.2 (continued)

Drug	Recommended dose	Adverse effects	Clinical considerations
sGC stimulator: its action mechanism is stimulation of soluble guanylate cyclase leading to pulmonary vasodilation associated with inhibition of vascular remodeling			
Riociguat	*Initial* dose: 0.5–1 mg PO *Maintenance* dose: 2.5 mg PO, three times daily	Headache, dizziness, dyspepsia, nausea, diarrhea, hypotension, vomiting, anemia, gastroesophageal reflux, and constipation	Coadministration of nitrates and/or PDE-5 inhibitors is contraindicated In growing rats, effects on bone formation were observed Teratogenicity is a potential risk Visit www.adempasREMS.com
PDE-3 inhibitors: inhibit phosphodiesterase-3, leading to pulmonary and systemic vasodilation and improved myocardial function			
Milrinone	0.25–0.75 mcg/Kg/min Increase/decrease by minimum of 0.125 mcg/Kg/min at intervals no longer than Q 6 h *Parameters for titration of drug*: blood pressure; CO; CI	Arrhythmia, thrombocytopenia, myocardial ischemia, hypotension/vasodilation *No increase* in myocardial oxygen demand	May increase heart rate No risk of myocardial ischemia Increases cardiac output Risk of arrhythmia

Anderson and Nawarskas (2010), Ivy et al. (2013), Liu et al. (2013), Abman et al. (2015), Latus et al. (2015), Liu and Jing (2015), Hansmann et al. (2016), Kim et al. (2016), Moffett et al. (2016)

Anesthesia for Patients with Congenital Heart Disease and Pulmonary Hypertension

The anesthesiologists dealing with PH-CHD patients should keep in mind the ideal goals of the treatment which include preventing any unnecessary manipulations (e.g., avoiding pulmonary artery catheter insertion), preserving the function of the heart and preventing any imbalance in interventricular shunts, and, if possible, implementing pulmonary vasodilating strategies.

> **The Ideal Anesthesia Should Fulfill the Following Goals in Patients with PH-CHD**
> - Pulmonary vasodilating effect (i.e., decreasing PVR)
> - Preserving cardiac contractile function, cardiac function, and systemic vascular resistance (i.e., maintaining CO and SVR)
> - Short acting and easily titratable

Table 29.3 Alleviating and aggravating factors in PH

Provoking agents or aggravating factors	Alleviating measures
Hypoxia	100 % O2
Hypotension	Modulating cardiac output
Acidosis	Correction of hypotension and hypoxia
Pain	Hyperventilation to induce respiratory alkalosis
Forceful and/or harsh tracheal intubation	*Avoiding* extra pressure during ventilation, since it will overcome the "blood pushing pressure" in the pulmonary vascular system
Deep tracheal suctioning	Pulmonary vasodilators
Hypoventilation	Treatment of acidosis
Hypercarbia	Using appropriate and titrated anesthetic agents
	Using analgesics like fentanyl augmenting SVR to overcome PVR using vasodilators; there should be appropriate pulmonary/systemic pressure and any underlying right to left shunt be prevented; phenylephrine and epinephrine should be used if needed to augment SVR
	ECMO may be needed to support perfusion

The anesthesia management should be done with great caution with prevention of any provoking agent and administering alleviating measures which are integral part of treatment in PH especially during acute attacks; these counteracting measures are described briefly in Table 29.3 based on some of the international guidelines and reviews (Friesen and Williams 2008; Galante 2011; Ivy et al. 2013; Twite and Friesen 2014; Abman et al. 2015).

The anesthetic agents used for these patients are described in brief in Tables 29.4 and 29.5. In general, anesthetic regimen could include a selected combination of these agents (Friesen and Williams 2008; Galante 2011; Twite and Friesen 2014):

- Isoflurane and sevoflurane
- Fentanyl
- Midazolam
- Etomidate
- Propofol
- Ketamine (with major controversies for PH)

Table 29.4 Intravenous sedative and anesthetic agents

Medication	Mechanism of action	Dosing	Indication	Adverse events and specific clinical considerations
Propofol	Modulation of $GABA_A$ receptor complex	Bolus: 1–3 mg/Kg Infusion: 100–200 µg/Kg/min for procedural sedation	Procedural sedation	Do not use for prolonged sedation >4 h (risk of propofol infusion syndrome) Risk of cardiac output drop
Midazolam	Modulation of $GABA_A$ receptor complex	Infusion: 0.025–0.1 mg/Kg/h average: 0.05–0.1 mg/Kg/h	Amnesia, sedation, anxiolysis	Rapid tolerance with infusion Onset: 1–5 min Duration: 20–30 min
Lorazepam	Modulation of $GABA_A$ receptor complex	Bolus: 0.025–0.1 mg/Kg q 4 h Infusion:0.025 mg/Kg/h	Amnesia, sedation, anxiolysis	Risk of tolerance with infusion Onset: 1–5 min Duration: 20–30 min
Dexmedetomidine	Synthetic central α2 agonist (purely α2 vs clonidine)	0.3–0.7 µg/Kg/h	Sedation; some analgesia	For short-term ICU sedation; bradycardia and heart block in infants half-life: 6–12 min
Clonidine	α1 and α2 adrenoceptor agonist (90 % α2 with some α1 activity)	Infusion: 0.25–1 µg/Kg/h	Analgesia, sedation	Does not cause significant respiratory depression May lead to hypotension
Etomidate	Modulation of $GABA_A$ receptor complex	Children >10 years of age: 0.3 mg/Kg (0.2–0.6 mg/Kg).1	Sedation	Onset: 1 min Duration: 3–5 min
Ketamine	NMDA receptor antagonist	Bolus: 1.5–2 mg/Kg May administer incremental doses of 0.5–1 mg/Kg every 5–15 min as needed	Analgesia, sedation	Hallucinations Increased pulmonary pressure Dysphoria Excessive salivation Tachycardia Onset : 3–5 min Duration: 20–30 min

Table 29.5 Volatile anesthetics

Drug	MAC Value %	Comments
Isoflurane	1.6 (newborn) 1.87 (1–6 months) 1.8 (0.5–1 year) 1.6 (1–12 years)	Irritates the respiratory tract, which may lead to *laryngospasm* in children
Sevoflurane	3.3 (newborn) 3.1 (1–6 months) 2.7 (0.5–1 years) 2.55 (1–12 years)	A good choice for mask induction in pediatric anesthesia Decreases the chance of postoperative nausea and vomiting Shortened recovery time and more rapid recovery of perception, which might produce a state of restlessness
Desflurane	9.2 (newborn) 9.4 (1–6 months) 9.9 (0.5–1 years) 8.0–8.7 (1–12 years)	*Not suitable* for *mask* induction in pediatric anesthesia because of its pungent smell, respiratory tract irritation, apnea, and laryngospasm

MAC minimum alveolar concentration

References

Abman SH, Hansmann G, Archer SL, Ivy DD, Adatia I, Chung WK, Hanna BD, Rosenzweig EB, Raj JU, Cornfield D, Stenmark KR, Steinhorn R, Thebaud B, Fineman JR, Kuehne T, Feinstein JA, Friedberg MK, Earing M, Barst RJ, Keller RL, Kinsella JP, Mullen M, Deterding R, Kulik T, Mallory G, Humpl T, Wessel DL. Pediatric pulmonary hypertension: guidelines from the American Heart Association and American Thoracic Society. Circulation. 2015;132:2037–99.

Allen HD, Driscoll DJ, Shaddy RE, Feltes TF. Moss & adams' heart disease in infants, children, and adolescents: including the fetus and young adult. Philadelphia: Lippincott Williams & Wilkins; 2013.

Anderson JR, Nawarskas JJ. Pharmacotherapeutic management of pulmonary arterial hypertension. Cardiol Rev. 2010;18:148–62.

Beghetti M. Current treatment options in children with pulmonary arterial hypertension and experiences with oral bosentan. Eur J Clin Invest. 2006;36 Suppl 3:16–24.

Beghetti M, Wacker Bou Puigdefabregas J, Merali S. Sildenafil for the treatment of pulmonary hypertension in children. Expert Rev Cardiovasc Ther. 2014;12:1157–84.

Benedict N, Seybert A, Mathier MA. Evidence-based pharmacologic management of pulmonary arterial hypertension. Clin Ther. 2007;29:2134–53.

Dodgen AL, Hill KD. Safety and tolerability considerations in the use of sildenafil for children with pulmonary arterial hypertension. Drug Healthc Patient Saf. 2015;7:175–83.

Donti A, Formigari R, Ragni L, Manes A, Galie N, Picchio FM. Pulmonary arterial hypertension in the pediatric age. J Cardiovasc Med (Hagerstown). 2007;8:72–7.

Ferrer-Barba A, Gonzalez-Rivera I, Bautista-Hernandez V. Inodilators in the management of low cardiac output syndrome after pediatric cardiac surgery. Curr Vasc Pharmacol. 2016;14:48–57.

Forrest P. Anaesthesia and right ventricular failure. Anaesth Intensive Care. 2009;37:370–85.

Friesen RH, Williams GD. Anesthetic management of children with pulmonary arterial hypertension. Paediatr Anaesth. 2008;18:208–16.

Galante D. Intraoperative management of pulmonary arterial hypertension in infants and children – corrected and republished article. Curr Opin Anaesthesiol. 2011;24:468–71.

Gerges M, Gerges C, Lang IM. Advanced imaging tools rather than hemodynamics should be the primary approach for diagnosing, following, and managing pulmonary arterial hypertension. Can J Cardiol. 2015;31:521–8.

Hansmann G, Apitz C, Abdul-Khaliq H, Alastalo TP, Beerbaum P, Bonnet D, Dubowy KO, Gorenflo M, Hager A, Hilgendorff A, Kaestner M, Koestenberger M, Koskenvuo JW, Kozlik-Feldmann R, Kuehne T, Lammers AE, Latus H, Michel-Behnke I, Miera O, Moledina S, Muthurangu V, Pattathu J, Schranz D, Warnecke G, Zartner P. Executive summary. Expert consensus statement on the diagnosis and treatment of paediatric pulmonary hypertension. The European Paediatric Pulmonary Vascular Disease Network, endorsed by ISHLT and DGPK. Heart. 2016;102 Suppl 2:ii86–100.

Ivy DD, Abman SH, Barst RJ, Berger RM, Bonnet D, Fleming TR, Haworth SG, Raj JU, Rosenzweig EB, Schulze Neick I, Steinhorn RH, Beghetti M. Pediatric pulmonary hypertension. J Am Coll Cardiol. 2013;62:D117–26.

Jentzer JC, Mathier MA. Pulmonary hypertension in the intensive care unit. J Intensive Care Med. 2015;31:369–85.

Kim JS, McSweeney J, Lee J, Ivy D. Pediatric cardiac intensive care society 2014 consensus statement: pharmacotherapies in cardiac critical care pulmonary hypertension. Pediatr Crit Care Med. 2016;17:S89–100.

Knight WE, Yan C. Cardiac cyclic nucleotide phosphodiesterases: function, regulation, and therapeutic prospects. Horm Metab Res Horm Stoffwechselforschung Hormones Metabolisme. 2012;44:766–75.

Kozlik-Feldmann R, Hansmann G, Bonnet D, Schranz D, Apitz C, Michel-Behnke I. Pulmonary hypertension in children with congenital heart disease (PAH-CHD, PPHVD-CHD). Expert consensus statement on the diagnosis and treatment of paediatric pulmonary hypertension. The European Paediatric Pulmonary Vascular Disease Network, endorsed by ISHLT and DGPK. Heart. 2016;102 Suppl 2:ii42–8.

Kreitner KF. Noninvasive imaging of pulmonary hypertension. Semin Respir Crit Care Med. 2014;35:99–111.

Lakshminrusimha S, Mathew B, Leach CL. Pharmacologic strategies in neonatal pulmonary hypertension other than nitric oxide. Semin Perinatol. 2016;40:160–73.

Lang IM, Plank C, Sadushi-Kolici R, Jakowitsch J, Klepetko W, Maurer G. Imaging in pulmonary hypertension. JACC Cardiovasc Imaging. 2010;3:1287–95.

Latus H, Delhaas T, Schranz D, Apitz C. Treatment of pulmonary arterial hypertension in children. Nat Rev Cardiol. 2015;12:244–54.

Latus H, Kuehne T, Beerbaum P, Apitz C, Hansmann G, Muthurangu V, Moledina S. Cardiac MR and CT imaging in children with suspected or confirmed pulmonary hypertension/pulmonary hypertensive vascular disease. Expert consensus statement on the diagnosis and treatment of paediatric pulmonary hypertension. The European Paediatric Pulmonary Vascular Disease Network, endorsed by ISHLT and DGPK. Heart. 2016;102 Suppl 2:ii30–5.

Liu QQ, Jing ZC. The limits of oral therapy in pulmonary arterial hypertension management. Ther Clin Risk Manag. 2015;11:1731–41.

Liu C, Chen J, Gao Y, Deng B, Liu K. Endothelin receptor antagonists for pulmonary arterial hypertension. Cochrane Database Syst Rev. 2013(2):CD004434.

Low AT, Medford AR, Millar AB, Tulloh RM. Lung function in pulmonary hypertension. Respir Med. 2015;109:1244–9.

McDonough A, Matura LA, Carroll DL. Symptom experience of pulmonary arterial hypertension patients. Clin Nurs Res. 2011;20:120–34.

Moffett BS, Salvin JW, Kim JJ. Pediatric cardiac intensive care society 2014 consensus statement: pharmacotherapies in cardiac critical care antiarrhythmics. Pediatr Crit Care Med. 2016;17:S49–58.

Monfredi O, Heward E, Griffiths L, Condliffe R, Mahadevan VS. Effect of dual pulmonary vasodilator therapy in pulmonary arterial hypertension associated with congenital heart disease: a retrospective analysis. Open Heart. 2016;3:e000399.

Perez KM, Laughon M. Sildenafil in term and premature Infants: a systematic review. Clin Ther. 2015;37:2598–2607.e2591.

Poor HD, Ventetuolo CE. Pulmonary hypertension in the intensive care unit. Prog Cardiovasc Dis. 2012;55:187–98.

Pristera N, Musarra R, Schilz R, Hoit BD. The role of echocardiography in the evaluation of pulmonary arterial hypertension. Echocardiography (Mount Kisco, NY). 2016;33:105–16.

Ryan JJ, Thenappan T, Luo N, Ha T, Patel AR, Rich S, Archer SL. The WHO classification of pulmonary hypertension: a case-based imaging compendium. Pulm Circ. 2012;2:107–21.

Santos A, Fernandez-Friera L, Villalba M, Lopez-Melgar B, Espana S, Mateo J, Mota RA, Jimenez-Borreguero J, Ruiz-Cabello J. Cardiovascular imaging: what have we learned from animal models? Front Pharmacol. 2015;6:227.

Shah PS, Ohlsson A. Sildenafil for pulmonary hypertension in neonates. Cochrane Database Syst Rev. 2011;(8):CD005494.

Simonneau G, Gatzoulis MA, Adatia I, Celermajer D, Denton C, Ghofrani A, Gomez Sanchez MA, Krishna Kumar R, Landzberg M, Machado RF, Olschewski H, Robbins IM, Souza R. Updated clinical classification of pulmonary hypertension. J Am Coll Cardiol. 2013;62:D34–41.

Suesaowalak M, Cleary JP, Chang AC. Advances in diagnosis and treatment of pulmonary arterial hypertension in neonates and children with congenital heart disease. World J Pediatr WJP. 2010;6:13–31.

Twite MD, Friesen RH. The anesthetic management of children with pulmonary hypertension in the cardiac catheterization laboratory. Anesthesiol Clin. 2014;32:157–73.

Ventetuolo CE, Klinger JR. Management of acute right ventricular failure in the intensive care unit. Ann Am Thorac Soc. 2014;11:811–22.

Vorhies EE, Ivy DD. Drug treatment of pulmonary hypertension in children. Paediatr Drugs. 2014;16:43–65.

Wang RC, Jiang FM, Zheng QL, Li CT, Peng XY, He CY, Luo J, Liang ZA. Efficacy and safety of sildenafil treatment in pulmonary arterial hypertension: a systematic review. Respir Med. 2014;108:531–7.

Waxman AB, Zamanian RT. Pulmonary arterial hypertension: new insights into the optimal role of current and emerging prostacyclin therapies. Am J Cardiol. 2013;111:1A–6; quiz 17A–19A.

Chapter 30
Right Ventricular Failure

Yamile Muñoz and Renzo O. Cifuentes

Acronyms

AMP	Adenosine monophosphate
BP	Blood pressure
CO	Cardiac output
CVP	Central venous pressure
EDP	End-diastolic pressure
EDV	End-diastolic volume
EF	Ejection fraction
ESV	End-systolic volume
GMP	Guanosine monophosphate
ICU	Intensive care unit
iNO	Inhaled nitric oxide
LV	Left ventricle
PAOP	Pulmonary arterial occlusion pressure
PAP	Pulmonary artery pressure
PDE	3-Phosphodiesterase
PE	Pulmonary embolism
PVR	Pulmonary vascular resistance
RV	Right ventricle
RVOT	Right ventricular outflow tract

Y. Muñoz, MD (✉)
Cardiovascular and Thoracic Anesthesia, Novick Cardiac Alliance, Clínica Cardio VID,
Medellín, Colombia
e-mail: yamilemp@yahoo.com

R.O. Cifuentes, MD
Novick Cardiac Alliance, Universidad de Guayaquil, Guayaquil, Ecuador

© Springer International Publishing Switzerland 2017
A. Dabbagh et al. (eds.), *Congenital Heart Disease in Pediatric
and Adult Patients*, DOI 10.1007/978-3-319-44691-2_30

SV   Stroke volume
SVR   Systemic vascular resistance
TAPSE   Tricuspid annular plane systolic excursion
TAPSV   Tricuspid annular systolic velocity
TEE   Transesophageal echocardiography
TG   Transgastric
TR   Tricuspid regurgitation
TTE   Transthoracic echocardiography

Anatomy and Physiology of the Right Ventricle

Compared to the left ventricle (LV), the myocardium of the RV is thin, it is 1–3 mm thick, while its counterpart (LV) on its free wall is 10 mm. In a transverse cut, we can appreciate the complex geometrical shape of the RV, which has a crescent shape; the LV on the other hand has a circular shape. The free wall of the RV forms the anterior border of the heart, and the other half is part of the interventricular septum (Fig. 30.1a).

The right ventricular wall is made out of a superficial layer of oblique fibers that continue with the superficial myofibers of the LV and a deep layer of muscular fibers longitudinally aligned (Haddad et al. 2008b).

The normal contraction of the RV resembles a peristaltic movement that begins at the inflow tract, through the apical trabeculated portion and through the infundibulum. The normal ejection from the RV is due to the longitudinal shortening of the free wall as well as a reduction in the distance between the septum and the free wall causing a bellow effect. Under normal conditions, the LV contributes to 20–40 % of the RV contractile function.

RV perfusion happens in both systole and diastole, making it less susceptible to ischemia than the LV.

With this anatomical bases, we can see the relationship between the two ventricles and deduce that RV pathology can affect the LV and vice versa through a phenomenon called ventricular interdependence.

Furthermore the relationship volume over ventricular mass gives the RV a high compliance which allows it to manage greater volumes with minimal increase of the intracavitary pressure (Greyson 2008; Haddad et al. 2008b).

There are two fundamental aspects of the RV physiology. First is that it is characterized by a high compliance that can accommodate to large variations in venous return without a high impact in the end-diastolic pressure (EDP). We can make this assumption by observing a pressure–volume curve comparing the two ventricles, where we will see that the triangular shape of the RV is less steep during its diastolic phase than the LV's (Haddad et al. 2008a; Denault et al. 2013; Vandenheuvel et al. 2013).

Second is that the RV physiology is highly dependent on the afterload and slight elevations of the PVR lead to a marked reduction in its systolic function. In Fig. 30.2,

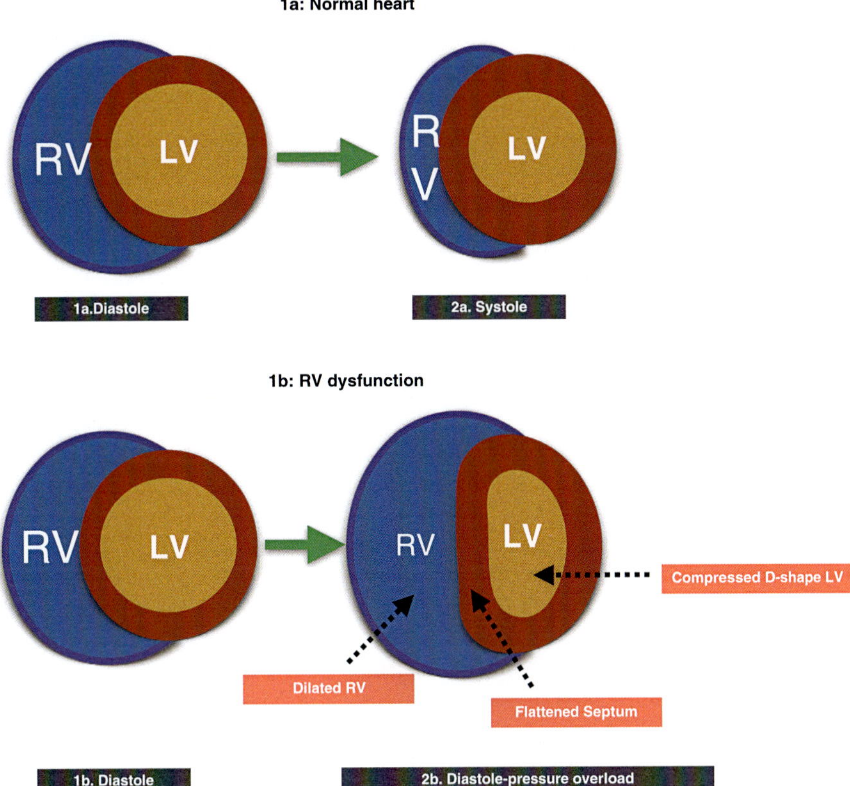

Fig. 30.1 *1a, 2a* represents the normal morphology of the RV and LV in systole and diastole. *1b, 2b* represents ventricular interdependence in RV dysfunction. There is dilation of the RV, flattening of the interventricular septum, and compression of the LV that resembles a D shape (D-shaped LV). This leads to a decrease in LV compliance leading to further increase in afterload

we can observe the effect of afterload on stroke volume (SV) compared on both RV and LV. For every increase in the afterload, the decrease in the SV is greater in the RV than in the LV (Haddad et al. 2008b).

The RV is attached to the pulmonary vascular bed that is a high-flow and low-resistance system; it is low resistance because the pulmonary arterioles have a thin media layer and few smooth muscle cells, making them very elastic, with a greater capacitance and capable of handling volume when recruited (Haddad et al. 2008a; Greyson 2012).

Even though the RV afterload is determined by many factors (pulmonary vascular resistance (PVR), distensibility of the pulmonary arterial system, and a dynamic component called inductance), PVR remains the most commonly used index to determine RV afterload (Price et al. 2010).

Pulmonary vascular tone is predominantly controlled by the vascular endothelium and by a balanced production of vasodilators (prostacyclin, nitric oxide) and

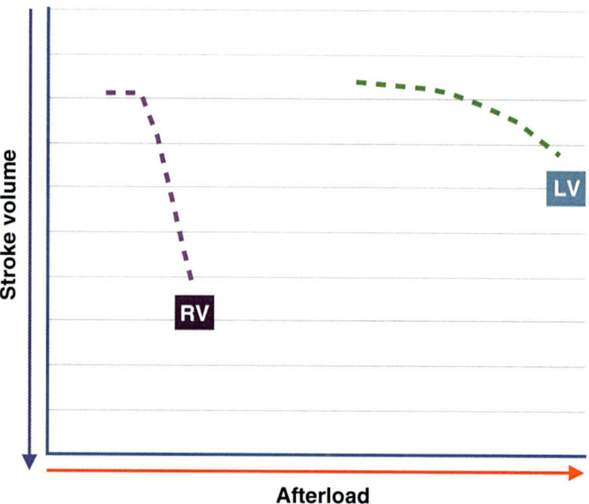

Fig. 30.2 Effect of afterload on stroke volume (SV) compared to both *RV* and *LV*

vasoconstrictors (endothelin 1, thromboxane A2, and serotonin). PVR is defined as the mean pulmonary arterial pressure (mPAP) minus pulmonary artery occlusion pressure (PAOP that provides an indirect measure of the left atrial pressure) divided by the cardiac output (CO). The normal range is 155–255 dyn/s/cm5:

$$PVR = 80 \times (mPAP - PAOP) / CO$$

This shows us very important details about the cardiac physiology:

1. PVR can be affected by an increase in the left atrial (LA) pressure; this can be due to diastolic, systolic, or mixed dysfunction of the LV and/or mitral disease (stenosis or regurgitation).
2. CO disorders can increase PVR; this is the case of congenital heart disease (CHD) with left to right shunt, fluid overload, or hyperdynamic states.
3. The lungs and the heart are linked together very closely, and their interaction is very important for the normal physiology. A disruption in the lungs can lead to an increase in PVR (e.g., interstitial lung disease, pulmonary embolism) (Zochios and Jones 2014).

Definition

RV failure is defined as a clinical syndrome resulting from the inability of the RV to maintain an adequate blood flow to the pulmonary circulation with a normal CVP and which progressively will lead to systemic hypoperfusion (Zarbock et al. 2014).

Etiology

It can be divided based on the pathophysiology (Vandenheuvel et al. 2013):

1. Volume overload
2. Altered contractility
3. Pressure overload

There are several perioperative factors that can alter these three elements of the cardiac output.

Volume Overload

The volume overload is caused by conditions such as tricuspid regurgitation (TR), atrial septal defects, and ventricular septal defects. A very important cause of volume overload in the perioperative setting is excessive administration of IV fluids. Based on what was discussed in reference to the anatomical and physiologic characteristics, the RV can accommodate more easily to volume overload with a relatively low increase in the wall tension. Therefore chronic volume overload is well tolerated but puts the patient at risk of acute decompensation, because a chronically overloaded RV has a limited capacity of increasing its contractility in the event of an acute increase of PVR.

Altered Contractility

The contractility can be affected by myocardial ischemia due to coronary artery disease or decrease in the perfusion pressure due to hypotension, arrhythmias, and intrinsic myocardial disease such as cardiomyopathies or cytokine-induced myocardial depression like sepsis. In observational studies, up to 40% of patients with sepsis have evidence of RV failure due predominantly to primary RV dysfunction (Itagaki et al. 2012).

Pressure Overload

The pressure overload is the most common cause of systolic dysfunction of the RV (Greyson 2012; Vandenheuvel et al. 2013).

PVR increases by perioperative factors like:

- Pulmonary vasoconstriction secondary to hypoxia, hypercapnia, and acidosis and cytokine release due to blood transfusion and protamine

- Reduction or compression of the pulmonary vascular bed induced by acute respiratory distress syndrome (ARDS), pulmonary embolism (PE), pneumothorax, and ventilation with large tidal volumes, high plateau pressures, and high positive end expiratory pressures (PEEP)
- Congestion of the pulmonary vascular bed in case of pulmonary hypertension secondary to valvular disease or chronic obstructive pulmonary disease (COPD) and LV failure that results in retrograde increase of pulmonary artery pressure (PAP)
- Mechanical obstruction like the one we see in pulmonary stenosis

RV dysfunction is present in many critically ill patients. ARDS is one of the most common conditions that challenges the right ventricle. The incidence of acute cor pulmonale in patients with ARDS is around 60 % without protective mechanical ventilation and 25 % with protective mechanical ventilation.

Postoperative RV failure is around 0.1 % in patients postcardiotomy, 2–3 % after a cardiac transplant, 25 % in CHD repair patients, and 30 % after the implantation of a ventricular assist device (VAD) (Greyson 2010; Krishnan and Schmidt 2015).

In patients with PE, the echocardiographic findings of RV dysfunction can be present in 29–56 % of the cases (Krishnan and Schmidt 2015).

The presence of RV failure is an independent predictor of mortality in any of the cases. Table 30.1 summarizes the causes of RV failure.

Pathophysiology

The initial response to acute RV overload is the increase in ventricular contractility. The rapid increase in contractile function in response to an increase in demand, called homeometric autoregulation or the Anrep effect, appears to be mediated through rapid alterations in calcium dynamics (Greyson 2008, 2010). As the pulmonary impedance increases, the sympathetic nervous system is activated releasing catecholamines which allow an increase in the pressures of the RV by increasing inotropy. If the PVR continues to increase, the RV dilates and the systolic volume is maintained by the Frank–Starling mechanism, since an increase of the end-diastolic volume (EDV) of the RV increases contractility (Simon 2010).

Once the ventricle reaches its limit of compensatory reserve, a greater increase in the afterload can induce a sudden hemodynamic collapse.

We must highlight three points in regard to a sudden hemodynamic collapse due to RV failure:

1. The decrease in cardiac output is a consequence of the ventricular interdependence; the dilation of the RV deviates the interventricular septum to the left decreasing LV compliance which in a retrograde fashion increases the RV's afterload furthermore (Fig. 30.1b).
2. The second element is the sustained increase in the PVR.
3. The third element of the hemodynamic collapse is the RV ischemia secondary to a decrease in the blood pressure (BP) which affects the contractility even more.

Table 30.1 RV dysfunction etiologies

Preload	*Low*	Hypovolemia (e.g., third spacing, copious urine output)
		Tamponade
	High	Fluid overload
		Left to right shunting (e.g., PFO, ASD, VSD, PDA)
		Valvular disease: tricuspid regurgitation, pulmonary regurgitation
Contractility	*Decreased inotropism*	Preexisting RV dysfunction due to CAD or valvular disease
		Myocardial stunning after cardiopulmonary bypass (CPB)
		Poorly protected myocardium
	Arrythmias	Atrial fibrilation, SVT, and VT
	Hypoperfusion	RCA occlusion
		RCA thromboembolism
		RCA air embolism
		Hypoperfusion secondary to LV dysfunction
		Mechanical obstruction or kinking of RCA or graft
Afterload	*Mechanical obstruction*	RVOT obstruction
		Pulmonary stenosis:
		Valvar
		Subvalvar
		Supravalvar
		Anastomotic stenosis
		Pulmonary veno-occlusive disease (PVOD)
	Pulmonary vasoconstriction	Hypoxia
		Hypercarbia
		Acidosis
		Blood transfusions
		Drugs: protamine
	Congestion of the pulmonary vascular bed	Preexisting PHTN due to valvular disease and COPD
		Postoperative LV dysfunction
	Compression and/or reduction of the pulmonary vascular bed	Pulmonary embolism
		Pneumothorax
		Acute lung injury or ARDS
		Positive pressure mechanical ventilation with high PEEP

PFO patent foramen ovale, *ASD* atrial septal defect, *VSD* ventricular septal defect, *PDA* patent ductus arteriosus, *LV* left ventricle, *RV* right ventricle, *CPB* cardiopulmonary bypass, *SVT* supraventricular tachycardia, *VT* ventricular tachycardia, *CAD* coronary artery disease, *RCA* right coronary artery, *RVOT* right ventricular outflow tract, *PVOD* pulmonary veno-occlusive disease, *PHTN* pulmonary hypertension, *COPD* chronic obstructive pulmonary disease, *ARDS* acute respiratory distress syndrome, *PEEP* positive end expiratory pressure

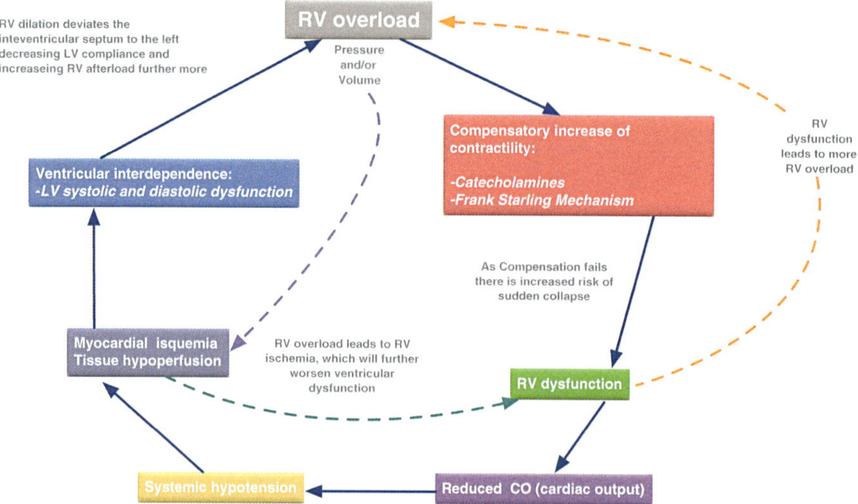

Fig. 30.3 Pathophysiology of RV failure. RV overload induces an initial compensation by increasing contractility (catecholamine release and the Frank–Starling mechanism). Compensation eventually fails and RV dysfunction will be established. RV dysfunction reduces CO, which will result in systemic hypotension that causes myocardial ischemia and tissue hypoperfusion. RV dysfunction itself will induce more RV overload. RV ischemia worsens RV dysfunction. RV failure causes RV dilation that will deviate the interventricular septum toward the left, decreasing LV compliance and increasing RV afterload furthermore; this is due to ventricular interdependence. LV systolic and diastolic dysfunction leads to more RV overload worsening RV failure

This is how we enter a vicious cycle in which the RV dysfunction per se generates more RV failure, and we go down a spiral of progressive ischemia, increased PVR, and shock (Fig. 30.3).

Diagnosis

As the clinical signs of RV failure in critically ill patients are nonspecific and share some similarities with other pathologies, the echocardiogram plays an important role in the diagnosis of RV dysfunction and any associated condition. Some authors even suggest that as the use of pulmonary artery catheter decreases, point-of-care echocardiography has become particularly important for detecting acute RV dysfunction both guiding specific therapies and monitoring the impact of supportive care, such as fluid therapy and mechanical ventilation (Yancy et al. 2013; Krishnan and Schmidt 2015).

At this point, it is important to mention that the measurement of CO using the method of thermodilution with a pulmonary artery catheter can be altered in the presence of TR secondary to dilation of the RV, making it difficult to assess the response to the medical management, though it remains the standard method to evaluate PAP and PVR. This is the reason why some authors recommended its use and to use echocardiography as a complementary study (Greyson 2012; Yancy et al. 2013).

Echocardiographic Evaluation of the RV

Visualization of the right ventricle can be challenging on transthoracic echocardiogram (TTE) because of its complex three-dimensional geometry and sonographic interference from the lungs. In the critically ill patient, transesophageal echocardiogram (TEE) gives us a better image quality compared to a TTE. The most commonly echocardiographic parameters used to assess the RV function are RV/LV area ratio, RV fractional area change (RVFAC), LV eccentricity index, tricuspid annular plane systolic excursion (TAPSE), and tricuspid annular systolic velocity (TAPSV) (King et al. 2014; Krishnan and Schmidt 2015):

1. RV/LV area ratio: is measured at the end of diastole by tracing the areas of the two chambers in the apical four-chamber view on TTE or the mid-esophageal four-chamber view on TEE. A ratio of 0.6 suggests moderate RV dilation, whereas a ratio of 1.0 indicates severe RV dilation.
2. RV fractional area change: is the ratio of the change in RV end-diastolic area to the RV end-systolic area ((RV ED area–ES area)/ED area). The trabeculations and papillary muscles should be included in the RV cavity when tracing the endocardial border. Normal values for RVFAC are ≥32 %, and RVFAC values <17 % represent severely decreased RV systolic function. It can be obtained on TEE in mid-esophageal four-chamber view and on TTE in the apical four-chamber view.
3. LV eccentricity index: normally, the interventricular septum is curved toward the right ventricle. The eccentricity index, a ratio of two perpendicular diameters of the LV cavity in the short-axis view (the anteroposterior and septolateral dimensions), is a quantitative measure of septal bowing that increases with RV volume and pressure overload. On TEE we obtain it in the TG mid-papillary short-axis view and on TTE parasternal short-axis view. It can be measured at the end of diastole and at the end of systole; its normal value is 1. If the relationship is greater than one (>1), it means that the RV is exposed to either a pressure or volume overload and shows a distorted interventricular septum and D-shaped LV (Krishnan and Schmidt 2015).
4. Tricuspid Annular Plane Systolic Excursion (TAPSE): is how far the tricuspid annulus moves from the end of diastole to the end of systole. TAPSE is usually acquired by placing an M-mode cursor through the tricuspid annulus and measuring the amount of longitudinal motion of the annulus at peak systole on an apical four-chamber view using TTE or by using TEE on deep TG of the RV trying to align the probe as vertically as possible to the apex of the heart. This measure is reproducible and has very low variability among the observers. A

Table 30.2 Echocardiographic parameters for RV function

Parameters	TTE	TEE	Abnormal values
1. RV:LV area ratio	Apical four chamber	ME four chamber	> 0.6
2. RV fractional area change	Apical four chamber	ME four chamber	< 35 %
3. LV eccentriciy index	Parasternal midpapillary short axis	TG midpapillary short axis	> 1
4. TAPSE[a]	Apical four chamber	Deep TG RV	< 16 mm
5. TAPSV[b]	Apical four chamber	Deep TG RV	< 10 cm/s

ME mid-esophageal, *TG* transgastric, *RV* right ventricle, *LV* left ventricle

[a]TAPSE: tricuspid annular plane systolic excursion

[b]TAPSV: tricuspid annular plane systolic velocity

TAPSE <16 mm is indicative of RV dysfunction (Zochios and Jones 2014; Krishnan and Schmidt 2015).

5. Tricuspid Annular Systolic Velocity (TAPSV): is the systolic velocity of the tricuspid annulus measured by tissue doppler imaging (TDI). On TEE we perform a deep TG of the RV; on TTE we use apical four-chamber view. The sample volume is placed at the tricuspid annulus or the middle of the basal segment of the RV free wall, and the peak systolic velocity (S') is determined. A value <10 cm/s is an indicator of RV dysfunction (Zochios and Jones 2014) (Table 30.2).

Management

How Do We Protect the RV?

We should identify the patient at risk of RV failure, particularly patients in which an acute increase in the afterload could lead to a decompensation. In these patients a non-pharmacological approach is proposed as a protective strategy that leads to avoiding factors that increase PVR. The intraoperative management of these patients must be directed to implement all the strategies to prevent an acute decompensation; this is accomplished by preventing hypoxia, hypercapnia, acidosis, hypothermia, and pain and to apply protective mechanical ventilation.

A proper management of the oxygenation and ventilation is needed in the prevention and treatment of RV failure (King et al. 2014).

The PVR is increased at both ends of the pulmonary volumes. In the poorly ventilated zones, the capillary vessels collapse due to the mechanism of pulmonary hypoxic vasoconstriction. In the zones of high PEEP and tidal volume, the distended alveoli compress the pulmonary vascular bed.

The principles of mechanical ventilation for these patients are:

1. Limit tidal volume (8 cc/Kg) and PEEP (<12 cmH$_2$O).
2. Keep plateau pressure moderated (<30 mmHg).

3. Avoid hypercapnia.
4. Maintain normoxia to prevent pulmonary hypoxic vasoconstriction.

These principles are potentially conflicting because limiting the tidal volume may produce hypercapnia.

Similarly, lower PEEP may leave alveoli collapsed, reducing their blood flow. Nevertheless, ventilator adjustment has the potential to significantly improve the circulation (Lahm et al. 2010; Krishnan and Schmidt 2015).

What to Do When the RV Is Failing?

When a patient is already on RV failure, the management goals should be:

1. Treat the underlying disease.
2. Ventilatory management: besides everything that has been mentioned, we should give a FiO2 of 100 %.
3. Hemodynamic management includes optimization of all the determinants of the CO (preload optimization, reduction of right ventricular afterload, improvement of right ventricular contractility, and increase in right coronary perfusion pressure).

Preload Optimization

Based on the studies of the physiology of the normal RV, the common practice has been to aggressively increase the intravascular volume. However more recent studies suggest a more conservative approach in regard to resuscitation with volume (King et al. 2014; Zochios and Jones 2014). The studies support the application of volume only to patients with low central venous pressure (CVP) and stable BP. However, the administration of volume can be deleterious if the preload reserve of the RV is depleted. In this stage, more volume expansion results in an increase in the EDP, worsening the TR and increasing the septal deviation to the left and initiating a vicious cycle of ventricular interdependence and ischemia which will lead to biventricular failure (Vlahakes 2012; Yancy et al. 2013; King et al. 2014; Zarbock et al. 2014; Zochios and Jones 2014; Krishnan and Schmidt 2015).

How to know on which side of Frank–Starling curve is our patient: The dynamic predictors of the response to fluids, such as variations in pulse pressure, stroke volume, arterial flow velocity, and LV outflow tract velocity-time integral, are based on the preload-related effects of ventilation (which dominate when RV function is normal). When beat-to-beat stroke volume also depends on changing RV afterload, as it typically is in RV failure, these dynamic indices may falsely signal preload dependency (Krishnan and Schmidt 2015). The respiratory variation of the pulse pressure or the systolic volume is used to predict the response to fluids in patients on mechanical ventilation; the studies show that these parameters are false positives in 34% of the patients with RV failure, leading to the unnecessary administration of IV fluids. Therefore, before administering fluids empirically to patients with known or suspected acute RV failure, echocardiography should be considered for measurement of baseline parameters (eccentricity index, degree of TR), to guide the therapeutic management and to evaluate the results. We could predict the results of fluid infusion by passive leg-raising maneuver, or diuresis with reverse Trendelenburg, and measure objectively the effects of the intervention with the echocardiographic parameters for RV function (Zochios and Jones 2014).

Unmonitored fluid challenges are inadvisable in any setting of RV failure. In patients with volume overload, the reduction of the intravascular volume (through diuresis or ultrafiltration) can improve the circulatory function (Price et al. 2010; Zarbock et al. 2014; Zochios and Jones 2014; Krishnan and Schmidt 2015).

Reduction of right ventricular afterload, improvement of right ventricular contractility, and increase in right coronary perfusion pressure:

The principles of the pharmacological management of RV failure are based on the use of different medications with different mechanisms of action to accomplish a decrease in the afterload due to their vasodilatory effect on the pulmonary vascular bed, to improve RV contractility because of their inotropic effect, to guarantee adequate arterial pressure, and to improve the coronary perfusion pressure of the RV (Price et al. 2010; Itagaki et al. 2012; King et al. 2014; Zarbock et al. 2014).

With regard to special symptomatic therapy, the fact whether RV dysfunction presents with a concomitant increase in PVR or whether PVR is within the normal range demands particular emphasis. If RV dysfunction presents with normal resistance values, positive inotropic substances are to be considered as first-line therapy. However, in the case of increased resistance, special therapy primarily requires the application of vasodilators (Zarbock et al. 2014).

There are two primary classes of positive inotropes: the sympathomimetic inotropes, which include dopamine, epinephrine, and dobutamine, and the inodilators, which include phosphodiesterase (PDE) three inhibitors and levosimendan.

RV systolic function can be improved with catecholamines that act by increasing intracellular cyclic AMP.

Among these we have dobutamine that exerts inotropic effects via the beta 1 receptor and variable vasodilatory effects through beta 2 receptor stimulation. The dose up to 10 mcg/Kg/min improves RV contractility and also vasodilates the pulmonary vascular bed. It may cause hypotension requiring concomitant use of vasopressors, due to beta 2-mediated systemic vasodilation.

Milrinone, a PDE-3 inhibitor (phosphodiesterase 3), increases inotropy and causes vasodilation of both the systemic and pulmonary vasculature. Milrinone increases LV contractility which results in increased RV systolic function through ventricular interdependence. One important issue with milrinone is its systemic vasodilator effect and, hence, its potential negative effect on the interventricular septal contribution to RV function. Thus, appropriate control of systemic vascular resistance must be incorporated into the plan selected for inotropic support of the RV free wall. If systemic hypotension develops, a vasopressor must also be given.

The combination of milrinone with vasopressin may be superior to norepinephrine in reducing the PVR-to-SVR ratio.

Levosimendan sensitizes troponin C to calcium and selectively inhibits PDE 3, improving diastolic function and myocardial contractility without increasing oxygen consumption. It is also a pulmonary and peripheral vasodilator through calcium desensitization, potassium channel opening, and PDE 3 inhibition.

This medication can also induce hypotension and requires concomitant administration with vasopressors.

The main disadvantage of the intravenous inodilators (dobutamine, milrinone, and levosimendan) is that they are not very selective and also that their decrease in the PVR is associated to a decrease of the systemic vascular resistance (SVR) as well, which decreases blood pressure, putting at risk perfusion to the coronaries and to other organs. Furthermore they can worsen the hypoxemia at the well-perfused but poorly ventilated areas, creating a right to left intrapulmonary shunt. The more specific pulmonary vasodilators can be useful to reduce the RV afterload as well as to manage pulmonary hypoxic vasoconstriction improving hypoxemia.

Inhaled nitric oxide (iNO) is a potent, rapidly acting, and selective pulmonary vasodilator. It decreases PVR by stimulating cyclic GMP release in smooth muscle cells. Rapid inactivation by hemoglobin in the pulmonary capillaries prevents systemic vasodilation. iNO has a short half-life, so it needs to be continuously delivered into the ventilator circuit. Because it is delivered as an inhalation agent, it only reaches ventilated regions of the lung, dilating those capillaries, resulting in better ventilation–perfusion matching and oxygenation while it prevents systemic hypotension. iNO treatment can lead to rebound pulmonary hypertension after rapid discontinuation.

PDE 5 inhibitors (sildenafil) increase downstream cyclic GMP signaling by blocking its degradation. Oral sildenafil has been shown to act synergistically with iNO and to decrease rebound pulmonary hypertension after iNO withdrawal.

Prostaglandin E1 and prostacyclin are both potent pulmonary vasodilators. Prostanoids promote vasodilation through activation of cyclic AMP. Like iNO, inhaled prostanoids improve ventilation–perfusion matching and do not cause systemic hypotension.

iNO, oral PDE 5 inhibitor sildenafil, and prostanoids result in a synergistic pulmonary vasodilation when given together.

Management with vasopressors is essential because as we have seen in the pathophysiology of RV failure, ischemia is the end result of the vicious cycle and perpetrates the downward spiral of the RV function. Also the effects of inodilators on the SVR cause a decrease in the arterial pressure.

Norepinephrine, a vasoconstrictor with strong alpha 1 and poor beta 1 effect, is a systemic pressor that can effectively be used in patients with acute RV dysfunction, because it improves the RV performance by increasing SVR and CO. In high doses it can have a deleterious effect by increasing PVR.

Dopamine increases the risk of tachyarrhythmias and is not recommended in cardiogenic shock.

Vasopressin is a non-sympathomimetic vasopressor that acts on the V1 receptor. Experimental studies have revealed vasodilating properties at low doses that include pulmonary vasodilatation through an NO-dependent mechanism via V1 receptors. This property manifests clinically as a reduction of the PVR and the relationship PVR/SVR. It also causes less tachyarrhythmias than norepinephrine. However, vasopressin can cause adverse effects to the myocardium; these effects are dose dependent: doses >0.4 U/min or even doses of 0.08 U/min in patients with cardiogenic shock which probably relate to direct myocardial effects, including coronary vasoconstriction (Itagaki et al. 2012).

RV Failure in the Pediatric Population

Low cardiac output (CO) is observed in approximately 25 % of all children undergoing cardiac surgery for congenital heart disease and may be related to left or right ventricular (RV) failure. RV failure is more common in the pediatric population than in the adult population and is associated with systemic hypotension and decreased coronary perfusion, which aggravates even further ventricular performance as we have already seen (Yancy et al. 2013; Hyldebrandt et al. 2014).

Although deviation in the interventricular septum is observed in adults with RV failure, this deviation might not occur in newborns because the myocardium of the newborns is relatively thicker and less compliant than the adult myocardium.

Indications for the use of inodilators, vasopressors, and pulmonary vasodilators are well described for the treatment of acute heart failure in adults. However, evidence for the choice of therapy in acute heart failure in children, especially neonates, is still very limited.

Summary

1. Perioperative RV failure and RV failure in the ICU are a complication associated with a significant increase of the morbidity and mortality of patients.
2. The knowledge of the complex anatomy and physiology of the RV is necessary to diagnose and to manage the syndrome.
3. Identifying RV dysfunction at early stages allows an adequate intervention and control of the precipitating events.
4. Echocardiography is not only a diagnostic tool, but it also allows us to evaluate the impact of the treatment on the RV.
5. The principles of mechanical ventilation for patients with acute RV failure consist of low tidal volumes and low PEEP with strict avoidance of hypercapnia and acidosis.
6. Volume overload worsen the RV dysfunction. All fluid changes should be followed closely monitored.
7. RV has increased sensitivity to changes in afterload. Reduction of RV afterload and optimization of RV preload and contractility form the principles of

management. Commonly it requires the combined use of inodilators, vasopressors, and pulmonary vasodilators.

8. It is essential to maintain adequate aortic root pressure to prevent the onset of RV ischemia. Vasopressors are useful in this setting.

References

Denault AY, Haddad F, Jacobsohn E, Deschamps A. Perioperative right ventricular dysfunction. Curr Opin Anaesthesiol. 2013;26:71–81.

Green EM, Givertz MM. Management of acute right ventricular failure in the intensive care unit. Curr Heart Fail Rep. 2012;9:228–35.

Greyson CR. Pathophysiology of right ventricular failure. Crit Care Med. 2008;36:S57–65.

Greyson CR. The right ventricle and pulmonary circulation: basic concepts. Rev Esp Cardiol. 2010;63:81–95.

Greyson CR. Right heart failure in the intensive care unit. Curr Opin Crit Care. 2012;18:424–31.

Haddad F, Doyle R, Murphy DJ, Hunt SA. Right ventricular function in cardiovascular disease, part II: pathophysiology, clinical importance, and management of right ventricular failure. Circulation. 2008a;117:1717–31.

Haddad F, Hunt SA, Rosenthal DN, Murphy DJ. Right ventricular function in cardiovascular disease, part I: anatomy, physiology, aging, and functional assessment of the right ventricle. Circulation. 2008b;117:1436–48.

Hyldebrandt JA, Frederiksen CA, Heiberg J, Rothmann S, Redington AN, Schmidt MR, Ravn HB. Inotropic therapy for right ventricular failure in newborn piglets: effect on contractility, hemodynamics, and interventricular interaction. Pediatr Crit Care Med. 2014;15:e327–33.

Itagaki S, Hosseinian L, Varghese R. Right ventricular failure after cardiac surgery: management strategies. Semin Thorac Cardiovasc Surg. 2012;24:188–94.

King C, May CW, Williams J, Shlobin OA. Management of right heart failure in the critically ill. Crit Care Clin. 2014;30:475–98.

Krishnan S, Schmidt GA. Acute right ventricular dysfunction: real-time management with echocardiography. Chest. 2015;147:835–46.

Lahm T, McCaslin CA, Wozniak TC, Ghumman W, Fadl YY, Obeidat OS, Schwab K, Meldrum DR. Medical and surgical treatment of acute right ventricular failure. J Am Coll Cardiol. 2010;56:1435–46.

Price LC, Wort SJ, Finney SJ, Marino PS, Brett SJ. Pulmonary vascular and right ventricular dysfunction in adult critical care: current and emerging options for management: a systematic literature review. Crit Care. 2010;14:R169.

Simon MA. Right ventricular adaptation to pressure overload. Curr Opin Crit Care. 2010;16:237–43.

Vandenheuvel MA, Bouchez S, Wouters PF, De Hert SG. A pathophysiological approach towards right ventricular function and failure. Eur J Anaesthesiol. 2013;30:386–94.

Vlahakes GJ. Right ventricular failure after cardiac surgery. Cardiol Clin. 2012;30:283–9.

Yancy CW, Jessup M, Bozkurt B, Butler J, Casey Jr DE, Drazner MH, Fonarow GC, Geraci SA, Horwich T, Januzzi JL, Johnson MR, Kasper EK, Levy WC, Masoudi FA, McBride PE, McMurray JJ, Mitchell JE, Peterson PN, Riegel B, Sam F, Stevenson LW, Tang WH, Tsai EJ, Wilkoff BL. 2013 ACCF/AHA guideline for the management of heart failure: a report of the American College of Cardiology Foundation/American Heart Association Task Force on Practice Guidelines. J Am Coll Cardiol. 2013;62:e147–239.

Zarbock A, Van Aken H, Schmidt C. Management of right ventricular dysfunction in the perioperative setting. Curr Opin Anaesthesiol. 2014;27:388–93.

Zochios V, Jones N. Acute right heart syndrome in the critically ill patient. Heart Lung Vessels. 2014;6:157–70.

Chapter 31
Coronary Artery Anomalies

P. Motta and J.E. Santoro

Introduction

Normal coronary arteries originate from the sinuses of Valsalva in the aortic root (Figs. 31.1 and 31.2a). The right coronary artery (RCA) takes off from the right coronary sinus, enters into the atrioventricular groove, gives branches to the infundibulum anteriorly, and takes an inferior direction to finish in the inferior interventricular groove.

After coming of the sinus of Valsalva, the left coronary artery (LCA) divides into the left anterior descending (LAD) and the circumflex (CX) arteries. The LAD artery runs within the interventricular groove to the apex of the heart. The CX extends to the left atrioventricular groove and occasionally (8 % of the cases left dominant system) gives off the inferior interventricular artery irrigating the diaphragmatic aspect of the right ventricle (RV). A balanced system is when both the CX and RCA provide a branch to the inferior interventricular groove (7 % of the population). Most of the time, just the RCA gives off a branch to the inferior interventricular groove (85 % right coronary dominance).

P. Motta (✉)
Department of Pediatric Cardiac Anesthesia,
Texas Children's Hospital – Baylor College of Medicine, Houston, TX, USA
e-mail: pxmotta@texaschildrens.org

J.E. Santoro
Yale University School of Medicine, Yale New Haven Children's Hospital, New Haven, USA
e-mail: jose.santoro@yale.edu

© Springer International Publishing Switzerland 2017
A. Dabbagh et al. (eds.), *Congenital Heart Disease in Pediatric and Adult Patients*, DOI 10.1007/978-3-319-44691-2_31

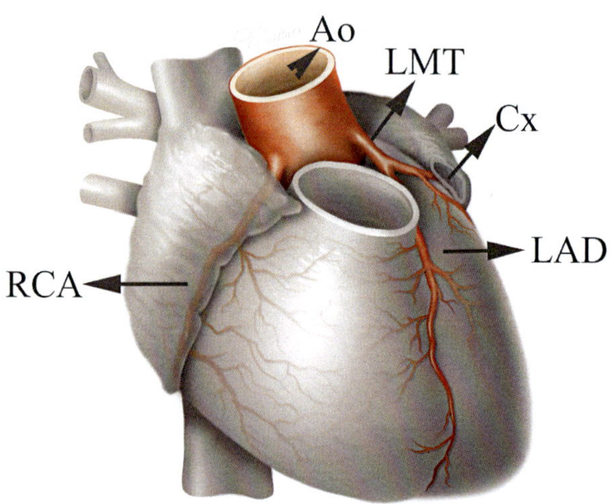

Fig. 31.1 Illustration of normal coronary anatomy showing the LMT arising from the left coronary sinus and the RCA off the right coronary sinus. The LMT after a short segment into the LAD who directs anteriorly and the CX extends to the left atrioventricular groove. Abbreviations: *LMT* left main trunk, *RCA* right coronary artery, *LAD* left anterior descending, and *CX* circumflex (2014 Texas Children's Hospital (Reprinted with permission); ©2013 Texas Children's Hospital)

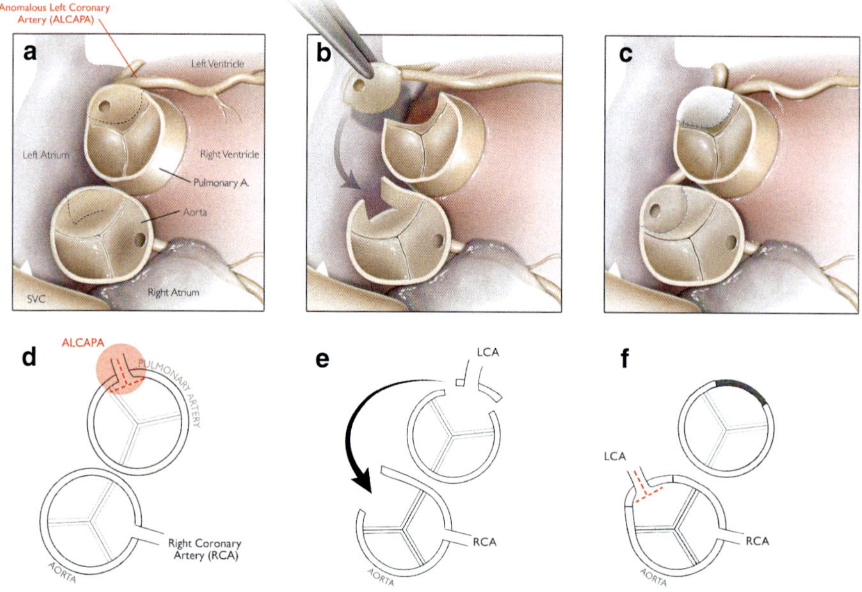

Fig. 31.2 Illustration showing the ALCAPA (**a, d**) left coronary artery arising from the left posterior sinus. (**b, e**) Harvest of the LCA of the PA. (**c, f**) Reimplantation of the LCA to the aorta and patch closure of the PA. Abbreviations: *ALCAPA* abnormal left coronary artery of the pulmonary artery, *LCA* left coronary artery (©2014 Texas Children's Hospital (Reprinted with permission); Copyright 2013 Texas Children's Hospital)

Embryology

The heart is the first functional organ during embryogenesis period. After initial formation of the ventricular loop, vascular formation is present and the myocardium is divided in trabeculations, where vascular beds will form. Subepicardial endothelial plexus eventually connects with endothelial sprouts in the walls of the aortic sinuses. The endothelial sprouts form a peritruncal ring, which invade the aortic wall from the outside. Of these sprouts, only two develop a lumen, producing orifices for the left and right coronaries. Cardiac function starts approximately 25 days after gestation. Coronary artery blood flow is not identified until the third trimester.

The failure of the development of the coronary sprout is responsible of CAA. In CAA only one branch develops causing a single coronary or both branches can develop from the same coronary sinus. In addition the pulmonary endothelial bud may develop from the LCA causing abnormal left coronary artery of the pulmonary artery (ALCAPA).

The low oxygen content increases coronary blood flow mediated by nitric oxide visible in fetal ultrasound. In pathologic fetal conditions such as hypoxemia, anemia, bradycardia, and intrauterine growth retardation, constriction of the arterial duct may affect the coronary blood flow. Flow that was evident earlier in fetal life will disappear with those conditions and return once the conditions are resolved.

Classification (Table 31.1)

There are several classifications of CAA. The CAA can be classified in terms of the origin, number, course, and ending, with or without hemodynamic compromise. The origin of the coronary arteries can be abnormal, such as ALCAPA arising from the PA or in abnormal aortic origin of the coronary arteries (AAOCA) arising from an abnormal site in the aorta (Figs. 31.2b, c). The AAOCA can present as single or multiple high take-off vessel/s with or without ostial stenosis, which originates from the contralateral sinus or the noncoronary sinus. When the origin of the left coronary artery originates from the pulmonary artery, the acronym changes to ALCAPA. The coronary artery course can also be anomalous such as retroaortic, intrerarterial, myocardial bridging, and septal have all been described. In addition, the coronary distal ending can be anomalous and classified as fistulous, arcade, or extracardiac. Finally it is of paramount importance for the clinician to know the hemodynamic consequences of the CAA (Oliveira et al. 2014; Angelini et al. 2002; Angelini 2007; Davis et al. 2001; Kim et al. 2006a).

Table 31.1 Classification of congenital coronary anomalies

Anatomic anomaly	Mechanism	Disease
Origin	High take-off Single coronary artery Multiple ostia Pulmonary origin Contralateral or noncoronary sinus origin	Either RCA or LCA Single LCA or RCA RCA and conus branch or LAD and CX different ostium ALCAPA ARCAPA ALCA-R ARCA-L ALAD
Course	Myocardial bridging Duplication	LAD (middle segment) Split LCA origin Split RCA origin
Distal ending	Fistula Arcade Extracardiac termination	Fistulas from RCA or LCA to RV, LV, SVC, or PA RVDCC Angiographic communication LAD-RCA LCA or LCA to extracardiac vessels (e.g., bronchial vessels, internal mammary, etc.)

Abbreviations: *RCA* right coronary artery, *LCA* left coronary artery, *LAD* left anterior descending artery, *CX* circumflex, *ALCAPA* abnormal left coronary artery off the pulmonary artery, *ARCAPA* abnormal right coronary artery off the pulmonary artery, *ALCA-R* abnormal left coronary artery off the right coronary sinus, *ARCA-L* abnormal right coronary artery off the left coronary sinus, *ALAD* abnormal left anterior descending artery, *RV* right ventricle, *LV* left ventricle, *SVC* superior vena cava, *PA* pulmonary artery, *RVDCC* right ventricle-dependent coronary circulation

Pathology

ALCAPA

ALCAPA is the most common causes of myocardial ischemia and infarction in children. The left coronary artery usually arises from the left posterior sinus of the pulmonary artery (Fig. 31.3). It is more frequently seen in males with a male-to-female ratio of 2.3:1 and an incidence of 1:300,000. This anomaly is rarely recognized in the neonatal period because the pulmonary pressures and oxygen saturation are similar to that of the systemic pressures and oxygenation. Thus, coronary ischemia does not manifest. After the neonatal period, the pulmonary pressure decreases progressively reducing coronary perfusion and eventually causing a reversal of flow to the pulmonary artery (PA) (coronary steal). The steal phenomenon not only decreases left ventricular (LV) function but also increases the end-diastolic pressure of the left ventricle. The decreased oxygen content of the blood originating from the PA aggravates LV ischemia. Unrepaired ALCAPA leads to dilation, infarction, or fibrosis of the LV. Fibrosis can lead to mitral

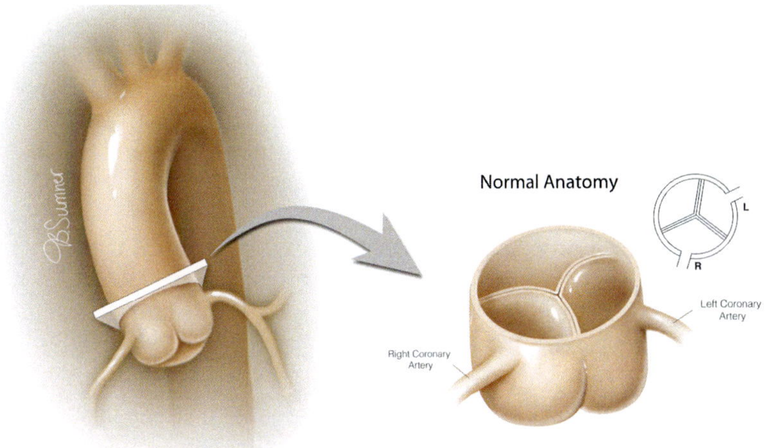

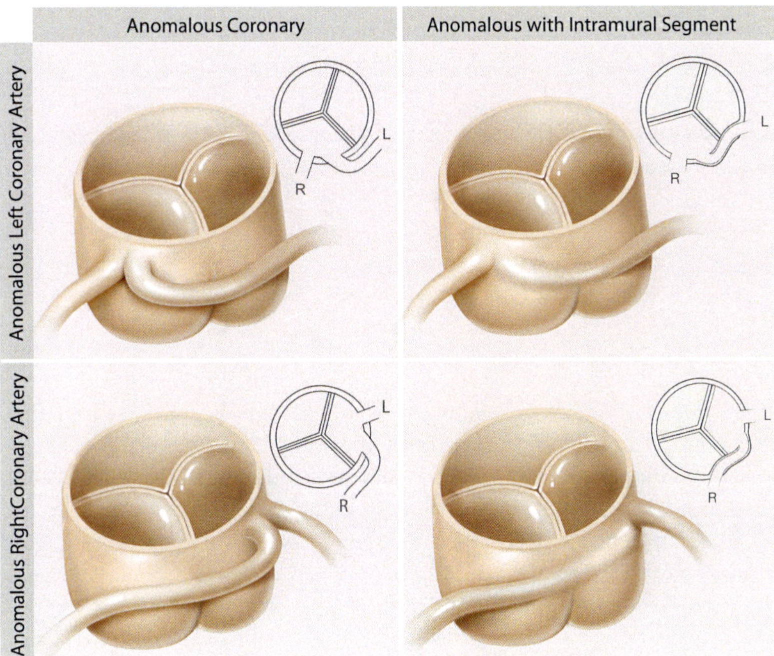

Fig. 31.3 Illustration showing the AAOCA A) normal coronary anatomy; B) abnormal left coronary from right aortic sinus; C) abnormal left coronary from right aortic sinus with intramural course; D) abnormal right coronary artery from left aortic sinus; E) abnormal right coronary artery from left aortic sinus with intramural course. ©2014 Texas Children's Hospital (reprinted with permission).

regurgitation. The RCA is usually enlarged, with a normal origin. Collateral circulation is crucial to compensate this disease. Collaterals run over the right ventricular outflow tract (RVOT) or through the interventricular septum and connect the two coronary arteries. Survival is related to the extent of collateral circulation from the RCA. About 10 % of patients with ALCAPA have good collateral flow and do not develop early myocardial ischemia as infants. The clinical presentation is delayed until adolescence or early adulthood. In neonates, the symptoms include interrupted crying, diaphoresis, and poor weight gain. In older children symptoms can range from shortness of breath to chest pain especially after any stress or Valsalva maneuver. Signs can be those of heart failure, tachycardia, angina, murmur, and cardiomegaly (Zheng et al. 2011).

Abnormal Right Coronary Artery of the Pulmonary Artery (ARCAPA)

ARCAPA is usually asymptomatic and is typically diagnosed when performing other cardiac surgeries or during autopsy. If the patient has a right dominant coronary system with lack of inter coronary system, ARCAPA may present as an infarction, often associated with other congenital anomalies like tetralogy of Fallot and aortopulmonary window (Vairo et al. 1992).

AAOCA

In AAOCA, the abnormal coronary originates opposite from the sinus of Valsalva (right or left). AAOCA is usually asymptomatic in infancy, and symptoms develop with exertion in adolescence and/or adulthood if there is a specific anatomic substrate. Risk factors for developing ischemia include an intramural segment, interarterial segment (between the aorta and pulmonary trunk), acute angle at take-off, and/or ostial stenosis. Early atherosclerosis can develop in these patients. There are several variants: the abnormal left coronary from the right aortic sinus (ALCA-R), abnormal right coronary artery from the left aortic sinus (ARCA-L), and abnormal left anterior descending from the right aortic sinus (ALAD) (Fig. 31.2b, c). In Davies et al. series of AAOCA, ALCA-R (58 %) was more common than ARCA-L (36 %). The abnormal vessel can take an interarterial (between the aorta and the pulmonary artery), retroaortic, prepulmonic, or septal (subpulmonic) course. The interarterial course though rare (5 %) is most frequently seen in patients with ALCA-R and has the highest risk for SCD during exercise. The mechanism for SCD involves coronary ostium stenosis and/or coronary artery compression leading to myocardial ischemia and ventricular tachycardia/ventricular fibrillation. During exercise the myocardial oxygen demand increases, but the supply cannot be met. The increased pressure in the cardiac chamber and/or the great vessels compresses the interarterial segment. Following the law of Laplace (tension = pressure × radius), smaller coronary vessels are at the highest risk of compression from the great vessels (Shriki et al. 2012; Erez et al. 2006; Davies et al. 2009).

Stenosis or Atresia of the Left Main Coronary Artery

This anomaly can present as a consequence in failure to develop or failure to canalize the left main trunk. Most of the time, this absence is compensated by collateral circulation from branches of the RCA.

Myocardial Bridges

Myocardial bridges are characterized by coronaries that run in the deeper layers of the myocardium producing ischemia, infarction, or arrhythmias.

Coronary Fistulas

These are abnormal connections between coronary arteries and abnormal connections between coronary arteries and cardiac chambers. Most of the time (>50%), these patients are asymptomatic, but a few can develop congestive heart failure, cardiac enlargement, arrhythmias, obstruction of veins in the right or left side of the heart, "steal" causing ischemia, angina, infective endocarditis, atherosclerosis or thrombosis, and embolization. Frequently patients with pulmonary atresia with an intact ventricular septum have fistulous communication (30–60%). In patients who associate coronary ostium stenosis, the coronary circulation depends on the RV pressures, and the entity is known as right ventricle-dependent coronary circulation (RVDCC). Patients with RVDCC are at the highest risk for cardiac arrest with induction of anesthesia, because of reduction on RV pressures, coronary perfusion is reduced (Powell et al. 2000; Brown et al. 2006).

Acquired Coronary Disease

Inflammatory Disease

Kawasaki disease presents in infancy and early childhood. More than 80% of the patient's initial presents less than 5 years of age. Kawasaki usually behaves as a self-limited vasculitis but can affect the coronary arteries leaving long-term damage. Clinical signs usually include skin rashes, conjunctivitis, lymphadenitis, and erythema of the palms and sole. There is no specific testing. During the acute phase, Kawasaki patient treatment focused on decreasing inflammation with high-dose aspirin and intravenous immunoglobulin therapy. With chronic treatment, anticoagulation might be indicated, particularly if there are coronary complications (e.g., coronary aneurysm). Rarely this patient would require surgery with coronary bypass grafting (CABG) (Urriola-Martinez and Molina-Mendez 2013).

Coronary Artery Allograft Vasculopathy (CAAV)

CAV is a multifactorial pathologic state mediated by immunologic, genetic, metabolic, and infectious factors that predisposes to the transplanted heart to CAAV. It is the most common cause of graft failure post heart transplantation in pediatrics. Younger children and infants have less incidence of CAAV, due to immaturity of the immune. Due to denervation, the patient will not feel chest pain, and sudden death could be the initial manifestation of this disease. Treatment is centered in optimizing the immunosuppression, but if it fails, re-transplantation is considered (Schumacher et al. 2012).

Diagnostic Tests

EKG

EKG is the initial test for patients with suspected CAA. Though EKG helps diagnosis of CAA, a normal EKG does not rule out the presence of CAA. In ALCAPA, the most common findings are abnormal Q waves with T wave inversion, in leads I, avL, and V4–V6 (see Fig. 31.4). In AAOCA, the EKG is usually normal at rest. In symptomatic patients, the EKG might be abnormal showing ST and T wave changes in the affected areas during an exercise stress test.

Echocardiography

For ALCAPA, echocardiogram is useful to diagnose the anatomic origin of the ALCAPA and to access the degree of LV impairment. Pulse and color flow Doppler can visualize the anomalous origin. A continuous low-velocity reverse flow in the posterior wall of the PA with a diastolic prominence is suggestive for ALCAPA. The myocardium has prominent fibrotic changes similar to endocardial fibroelastosis. The LV is dilated with decreased function, particularly at the anterolateral wall. In patients with later presentation, the RCA is dilated with abundant septal collaterals due to compensatory mechanisms. The ratio between the proximal RCA diameter to the aortic root diameter (RCA/AO) is usually >0.20 in ALCAPA, especially in older

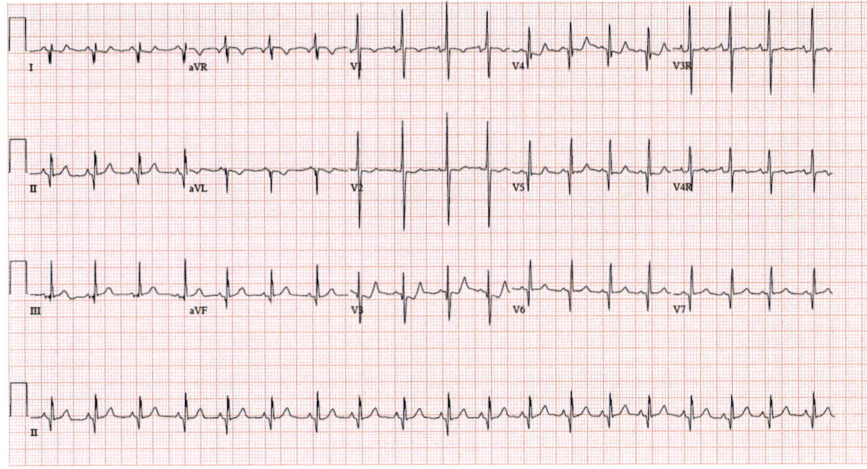

Fig. 31.4 EKG on an ALCAPA patient showing myocardial ischemia with Q waves and T wave inversion in leads I, avL, and V4–V6

patients who develop compensatory collateral circulation. The mitral valve needs to be assessed carefully because regurgitation is common due to papillary muscle ischemia and/or annular dilatation secondary to LV remodeling (Yang et al. 2007; Li et al. 2016; Estevez et al. 2008) (Fig. 31.5).

The use of transthoracic echocardiography (TTE) is equivocal in the diagnosis of AAOCA. Coronaries are not usually well visualized by TTE in older patients. If an abnormal coronary origin is detected by TTE, it may contribute to the diagnosis, but if the study is inconclusive, other studies should follow.

Due to the proximity of the esophagus to the aorta, transesophagic echocardiography (TEE) has better resolution to detect CAA. However, TEE is not often used as a diagnostic tool due to its invasive nature. TEE *is* useful in the intraoperative period of AAOCA repair (Fig. 31.6).

Chest Radiography

Infants who present with ALCAP usually have abnormal chest radiography. The more common findings include increased cardiothoracic ratio and pulmonary congestion due to LV failure (Fig. 31.7). AAOCA patients usually have normal chest radiography.

Stress Sestamibi Perfusion Scan

As previously mentioned, most of the AAOCA patients are asymptomatic at rest. Thus, triggering studies like stress sestamibi are necessary to elicit ischemia. Patients who have easily induced ischemia and large perfusion defects on stress testing are at increased risk for sudden death and may require early surgical approach.

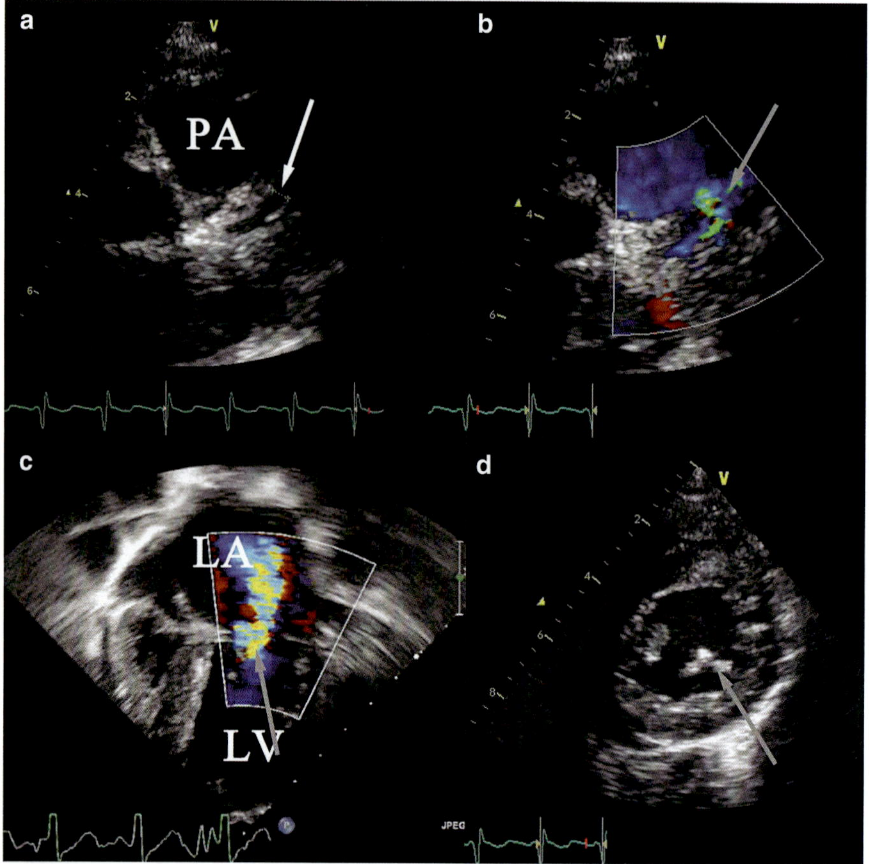

Fig. 31.5 Transthoracic echocardiography of an ALCAPA patient. (a) High parasternal view of the pulmonary artery (*PA*) with white arrow showing the ALCAPA. (b) Color flow Doppler in the previous window illustrating retrograde flow from the left coronary to the pulmonary artery (PA). (c) Apical four-chamber view showing severe mitral regurgitation flow from the left ventricle (*LV*) to the left atrium (LA). (d) Parasternal short axis view with arrow illustration of the calcified posteromedial papillary muscle

Computerized Tomographic Angiography (CTA)

New-generation imaging allows for EKG-gated CTA with three-dimensional post-processing reconstruction. This technique allows visualizing the coronary ostium, coronary morphology, and perfusion relationship to the cardiac cycle because the coronary compression may be dynamic (e.g., compression during systole). Early studies have found a good correlation of CTA findings and surgical anatomy with sensitivity for detection of significant CAA of 80–90 % (Kim et al. 2006a; Kim et al. 2006b).

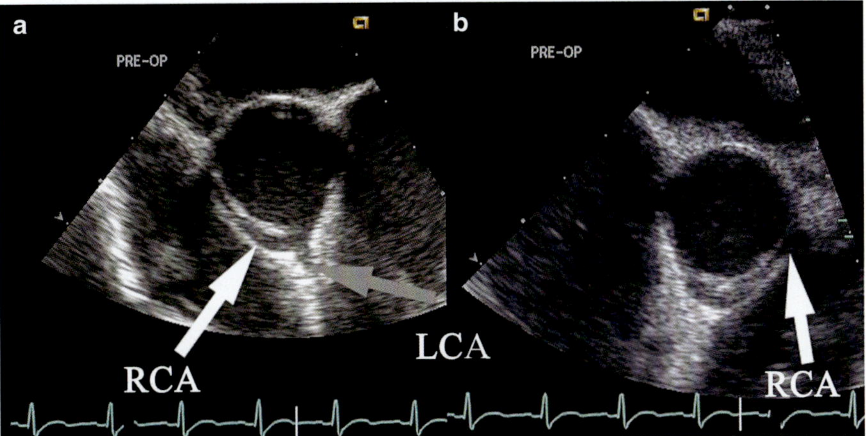

Fig. 31.6 Transesophageal echocardiography at the mid-esophagus aortic short axis view (**a**) abnormal left coronary artery (*LCA*) from the right aortic sinus (ALCA-R) gray arrow and normal right coronary artery (*RCA*); (**b**) abnormal right coronary artery from the left aortic sinus (ARCA-L) *white arrow*

Fig. 31.7 Chest radiography showed an increased cardiac silhouette and increased pulmonary vascularity

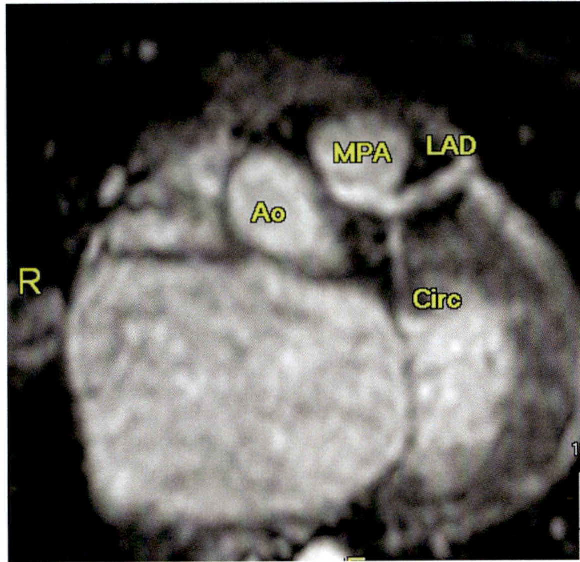

MRI

The use of MRI as a screening tool is secondary to CT because it is lengthy, and for most imaging, pediatric patients would require sedation. The advantage of MRI is that in addition to anatomical information, regarding coronaries arteries, the myocardial functions can be assessed (Fig. 31.8).

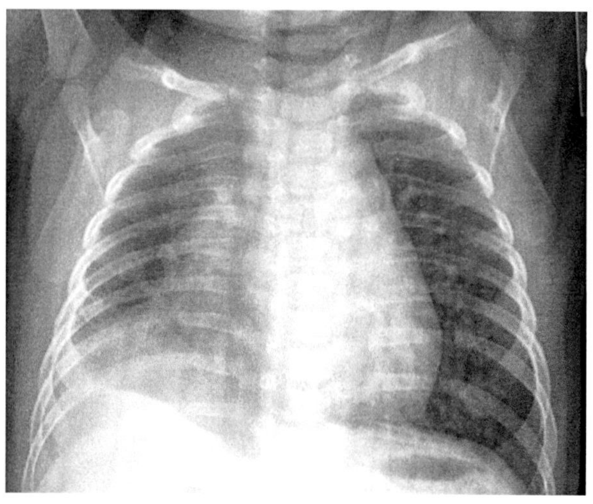

Fig. 31.8 MRI image showing the origin of the left coronary artery off the main pulmonary artery (MPA) and its bifurcation into the left anterior descending artery (directed anteriorly) and the circumflex (directed posteriorly). Abbreviation: *Ao* aorta

Catheterization Laboratory

The gold standard test is cardiac catheterization, but due to its invasive nature, it is left as the last resort and only performed in complex cases where echocardiography, CT, and MRI are inconclusive.

Management Algorithm

During the last few years, a multidisciplinary approach for CAA diagnosis and management at Texas Children's Hospital has been favored involving a team of cardiologists, surgeons, and anesthesiologists. The complete algorithm is presented in Fig. 31.9 (Mery et al. 2014).

Surgical Management

The surgical treatment for ALCAPA is direct coronary translocation and patch closure of the PA. Initial reports of LCA ligation have revealed a high mortality rate in infants. Mitral regurgitation usually regresses over time due to improved perfusion. Because of the severe heart failure, most of these patients may struggle in the initial postoperative period and require multiple inotropic support. The successful use of the left ventricular assist device (LVAD) has been reported in patients with ALCAPA who have failed weaning from CPB. Reoperation rates are higher in patients who require ECMO in the preoperative period. The most frequent indication for operation is residual mitral valve regurgitation. Patients who do not recover LV function

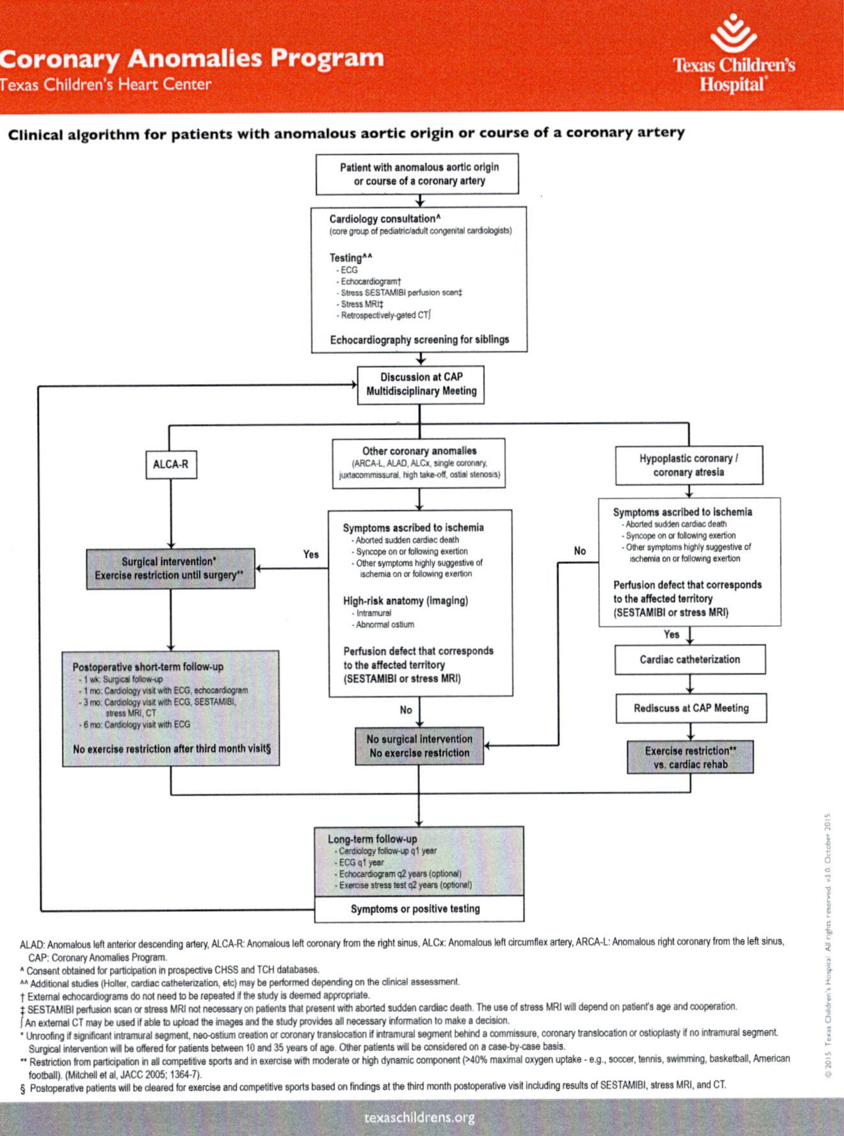

Fig. 31.9 Clinical algorithm used by the Texas Children's Hospital coronary anomalies program to evaluate and manage patients with AAOCA (©2013 Texas Children's Hospital (Reprinted with permission))

after coronary reimplantation may be listed for heart transplantation (Imamura et al. 2011; Cabrera et al. 2015).

Only AAOCA patients who are high risk for SCD require surgical repair. The initial repair entailed coronary artery bypass grafting (CABG), but there is

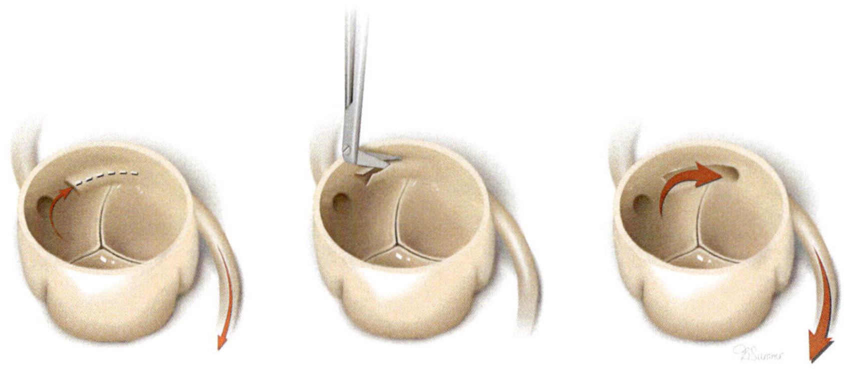

Fig. 31.10 Technique of coronary unroofing for treatment of AAOCA (©2014 Texas Children's Hospital (Reprinted with permission); ©2013 Texas Children's Hospital)

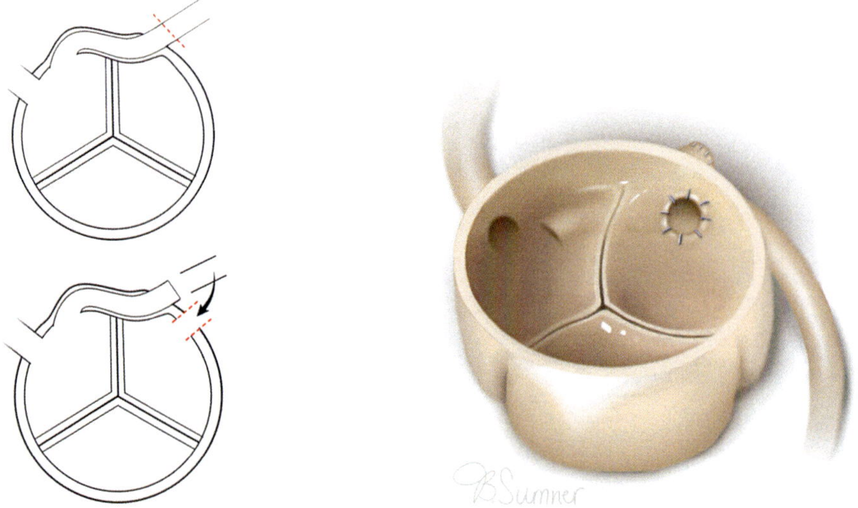

Fig. 31.11 Technique of coronary translocation for treatment of AAOCA (©2013, 2014 Texas Children's Hospital (Reprinted with permission); ©2013 Texas Children's Hospital)

concern of competitive flow from the abnormal coronary impeding maturation of the internal mammary graft. Currently, CABG is reserved for older patients who have concomitant atherosclerotic coronary disease or unusual anatomy that precludes translocation and/or unroofing. The present techniques used to treat AAOCA include coronary unroofing, coronary translocation, and neo-ostium creation (Figs. 31.10 and 31.11). All repairs are performed on CPB with mild hypothermia and aortic crossclamp through an aortotomy incision (Poynter et al. 2014; Mainwaring et al. 2014).

Anesthetic Considerations

The coronaries largely perfuse the cardiac chambers, while the heart is in diastole. The coronary perfusion pressure (CPP) is the aortic diastolic pressure minus the intracavitary pressure. The anesthetic goals should be tailored to maintain the CCP by increasing the oxygen supply and decreasing oxygen demand. During induction, it is vital to maintain the systemic vascular resistance and avoid tachycardia. A combination of vasopressors and beta-blockers should be considered to achieve hemodynamic goals.

Symptomatic patients with ALCAPA may have little cardiac reserve and significant ischemia. These patients usually require preoperative inotropic support, mechanical ventilation, and perhaps even preoperative ECMO for stabilization prior surgery. During induction of anesthesia of ALCAPA patients, it is important to avoid decreases in PA pressure with 100% FiO_2 and hyperventilation because this will aggravate ischemia due to the steal phenomenon. Significant inotropic support may be needed for weaning off CPB. Inotropic agents can improve cardiac function, but can also increase heart rate and myocardial oxygen consumption, which may worsen the ischemia. Nitroglycerin has been used to improve coronary perfusion. Cardiovascular depressant effects of volatile anesthetics are often poorly tolerated in infants with ALCAPA, and a high opioid technique may be preferred. Most patients are kept intubated and ventilated postoperatively to allow time for ventricular recovery.

TEE is a useful tool in the perioperative period. The best window to visualize the coronaries is the mid-esophagus short axis view. The TEE exam prior to CPB is important to confirm the preoperative diagnosis, examine for abnormal wall motion (AWM) abnormalities, and estimate the relationship of the defect with the aortic valve. The post CPB TEE exam is important to rule out new AWM abnormalities, to interrogate the aortic valve, which might be affected with the surgical procedure, and an examination of the coronary flow pattern (Fig. 31.5b).

AAOCA patients rarely develop vasospasm in the postoperative period so nitroglycerin is not routinely used prophylactically. Since surgical repair involves an aortotomy, the pressure should be managed within 20% of the baseline preoperative pressure to avoid bleeding from the suture line.

Outcome

More than ninety percent of undiagnosed or medically treated infants with ALCAPA will die within the first year of life. Sudden death frequently occurs in untreated older children and adults. Overall, the outcome of surgical repair of ALCAPA is good even though some patients will need temporary mechanical support. The late mortality of ALCAPA is commonly due to persistent LV dysfunction and/or arrhythmias.

AAOCA repair is very successful with little morbidity and mortality in most of the reported series. Typically patients are able to return to normal activity without limitations. Mainwaring reported a series of 50 patients with AAOCA over 5.7 years of postoperative follow-up, and only one patient required further treatment (transplantation). The rest of the population remained symptom-free (Mainwaring et al. 2011).

Case-based Contents

A 2-month-old, 5 kg boy was transferred to our institution for a second opinion regarding new findings of reported depressed heart function. On physical exam, he was well developed, well nourished, and in no distress. The S1 was normal and S2 was single and prominent. An II/VI systolic murmur at lower left and right sternal border was present. The echocardiogram indicated findings consistent with a LV infarct with echogenic papillary muscles, echogenic left lateral apical myocardium, severely depressed function, and moderate mitral regurgitation. ECG showed Q waves in leads I, AVL, V4, V5, and V6, but not acute ST segment changes (Fig. 31.3). Chest radiography showed an increased cardiac silhouette and increased pulmonary vascularity (Fig. 31.8). Unfortunately the echocardiography was inconclusive due to patient movement. MRI under sedation indicated a strong clinical suspicion of ALCAPA (Fig. 31.7). His first troponin was minimally elevated at 0.178 ng/mL. The patient was admitted to the telemetry floor for preoperative monitoring and was started on low-dose heparin drip and enalapril. The patient was scheduled for ALCAPA repair on CPB under general anesthesia. During surgery the diagnosis was confirmed upon visual inspection of the heart. The patient underwent repair of the ALCAPA with direct aortic implantation but was unable to wean of CPB due to poor LV function despite maximal doses of inotropes (milrinone and epinephrine). The patient was transitioned to a temporary LVAD (Rotaflow Centrifugal Pump®). Eventually, the LV function recovered, and the patient was weaned off LVAD on postoperative day 3 without further complications.

References

Angelini P. Coronary artery anomalies: an entity in search of an identity. Circulation. 2007;115:1296–305.

Angelini P, Velasco JA, Flamm S. Coronary anomalies: incidence, pathophysiology, and clinical relevance. Circulation. 2002;105:2449–54.

Brown TA, Emad M, Pablo M. Cardiac arrest at induction of anesthesia in a child with undiagnosed right-ventricular dependent coronary circulation: a case report. Paediatr Anaesth. 2006;16:1179–83.

Cabrera AG, Chen DW, Pignatelli RH, Khan MS, Jeewa A, Mery CM, McKenzie ED, Fraser Jr CD. Outcomes of anomalous left coronary artery from pulmonary artery repair: beyond normal function. Ann Thorac Surg. 2015;99:1342–7.

Davies JE, Burkhart HM, Dearani JA, Suri RM, Phillips SD, Warnes CA, Sundt 3rd TM, Schaff HV. Surgical management of anomalous aortic origin of a coronary artery. Ann Thorac Surg. 2009;88:844–7; discussion 847–848.

Davis JA, Cecchin F, Jones TK, Portman MA. Major coronary artery anomalies in a pediatric population: incidence and clinical importance. J Am Coll Cardiol. 2001;37:593–7.

Erez E, Tam VK, Doublin NA, Stakes J. Anomalous coronary artery with aortic origin and course between the great arteries: improved diagnosis, anatomic findings, and surgical treatment. Ann Thorac Surg. 2006;82:973–7.

Estevez R, Rueda F, Albert DC. Reverse flow in left coronary artery as the clue to diagnosis of an anomalous origin of the left coronary into pulmonary artery in an infant with dilated cardiomyopathy. Echocardiography. 2008;25:663–5.

Imamura M, Dossey AM, Jaquiss RD. Reoperation and mechanical circulatory support after repair of anomalous origin of the left coronary artery from the pulmonary artery: a twenty-year experience. Ann Thorac Surg. 2011;92:167–72; discussion 172–163.

Kim SY, Seo JB, Do KH, Heo JN, Lee JS, Song JW, Choe YH, Kim TH, Yong HS, Choi SI, Song KS, Lim TH. Coronary artery anomalies: classification and ECG-gated multi-detector row CT findings with angiographic correlation. Radiographics. 2006;26:317–33; discussion 333–314.

Li RJ, Sun Z, Yang J, Yang Y, Li YJ, Leng ZT, Liu GW, Pu LH. Diagnostic value of transthoracic echocardiography in patients with anomalous origin of the left coronary artery from the pulmonary artery. Med (Baltimore). 2016;95:e3401.

Mainwaring RD, Reddy VM, Reinhartz O, Petrossian E, MacDonald M, Nasirov T, Miyake CY, Hanley FL. Anomalous aortic origin of a coronary artery: medium-term results after surgical repair in 50 patients. Ann Thorac Surg. 2011;92:691–7.

Mainwaring RD, Reddy VM, Reinhartz O, Petrossian E, Punn R, Hanley FL. Surgical repair of anomalous aortic origin of a coronary artery. Eur J Cardiothorac Surg. 2014;46:20–6.

Maron BJ, Doerer JJ, Haas TS, Tierney DM, Mueller FO. Sudden deaths in young competitive athletes: analysis of 1866 deaths in the United States, 1980–2006. Circulation. 2009;119:1085–92.

Mery CM, Lawrence SM, Krishnamurthy R, Sexson-Tejtel SK, Carberry KE, McKenzie ED, Fraser Jr CD. Anomalous aortic origin of a coronary artery: toward a standardized approach. Semin Thorac Cardiovasc Surg. 2014;26:110–22.

Oliveira C, Mota P, Basso S, Catarino R. Congenital coronary variants and anomalies: prevalence in cardiovascular multislice computed tomography studies in a single center. Open J Radiol. 2014;4:163–72.

Powell AJ, Mayer JE, Lang P, Lock JE. Outcome in infants with pulmonary atresia, intact ventricular septum, and right ventricle-dependent coronary circulation. Am J Cardiol. 2000;86(1272–1274):A1279.

Poynter JA, Bondarenko I, Austin EH, DeCampli WM, Jacobs JP, Ziemer G, Kirshbom PM, Tchervenkov CI, Karamlou T, Blackstone EH, Walters 3rd HL, Gaynor JW, Mery CM, Pearl JM, Brothers JA, Caldarone CA, Williams WG, Jacobs ML, Mavroudis C, Congenital Heart Surgeons' Society AWG. Repair of anomalous aortic origin of a coronary artery in 113 patients: a Congenital Heart Surgeons' Society report. World J Pediatr Congenit Heart Surg. 2014;5:507–14.

Schumacher KR, Gajarski RJ, Urschel S. Pediatric coronary allograft vasculopathy – a review of pathogenesis and risk factors. Congenit Heart Dis. 2012;7:312–23.

Shriki JE, Shinbane JS, Rashid MA, Hindoyan A, Withey JG, DeFrance A, Cunningham M, Oliveira GR, Warren BH, Wilcox A. Identifying, characterizing, and classifying congenital anomalies of the coronary arteries. Radiographics. 2012;32:453–68.

Urriola-Martinez M, Molina-Mendez F. Anesthesia for coronary revascularization in patients with Kawasaki disease: case report. Arch Cardiol Mex. 2013;83:267–72.

Vairo U, Marino B, De Simone G, Marcelletti C. Early congestive heart failure due to origin of the right coronary artery from the pulmonary artery. Chest. 1992;102:1610–2.

Yang YL, Nanda NC, Wang XF, Xie MX, Lu Q, He L, Lu XF. Echocardiographic diagnosis of anomalous origin of the left coronary artery from the pulmonary artery. Echocardiography. 2007;24:405–11.

Zheng J, Ding W, Xiao Y, Jin M, Zhang G, Cheng P, Han L. Anomalous origin of the left coronary artery from the pulmonary artery in children: 15 years experience. Pediatr Cardiol. 2011;32:24–31.

Chapter 32
Heart Transplantation and Mechanical Circulatory Support in the Congenital Heart Patients

Alistair Phillips

Introduction

Congenital heart surgery was once believed to be uncorrectable, until the operation pioneered by Vivian Thomas and first performed in humans by Alfred Blalock, MD, on a patient of Helen Tausig, MD, showed that "blue babies could be helped" (Blalock and Taussig 1984). C. Walton Lillehei, MD, using cross circulation, then performed the first bypass procedures in 1955, when the advent of open heart surgery began (Warden et al. 1954). Dr. Christiaan Barnard performed the first heart transplant in 1967 (he trained under Dr. Lillehei at the University of Minnesota). Immunosuppression as we know it today began with the work of Drs. George Hitchings and Gertrude Elion with the development of 57–322 or Imuran (Hitchings and Elion 1985). Long-term heart allograft survival was not accomplished until the introduction of cyclosporine in the 1980s.

Congenital heart disease affects approximately 1 in every 4000 births with improved survival; it is estimated that over 90% of patients with congenital heart disease will live into adulthood. Unfortunately most of these patients will develop heart failure and will ultimately need a heart transplant, because their underlying heart condition can only be palliated. The main reasons for heart transplantation in congenital heart disease are (1) primary heart transplantation (newborn heart transplant for hypoplastic left heart syndrome or Ebstein's anomaly), (2) Eisenmenger syndrome with simple congenital heart disease with left-to-right shunting (acyanotic), (3) tetralogy of Fallot (repaired or palliated) and other complex CHD (cyanotic), (4) univentricular heart with and without Fontan circulation, and (5) systemic right ventricle

A. Phillips, MD
Co-Director Congenital Heart Program, The Heart Institute, Chief, Division of Congenital Heart Surgery, Division of Cardiothoracic Surgery, Department of Surgery, Cedars-Sinai Medical Center, Los Angeles, CA, USA
e-mail: Alistair.Phillips@cshs.org

© Springer International Publishing Switzerland 2017
A. Dabbagh et al. (eds.), *Congenital Heart Disease in Pediatric and Adult Patients*, DOI 10.1007/978-3-319-44691-2_32

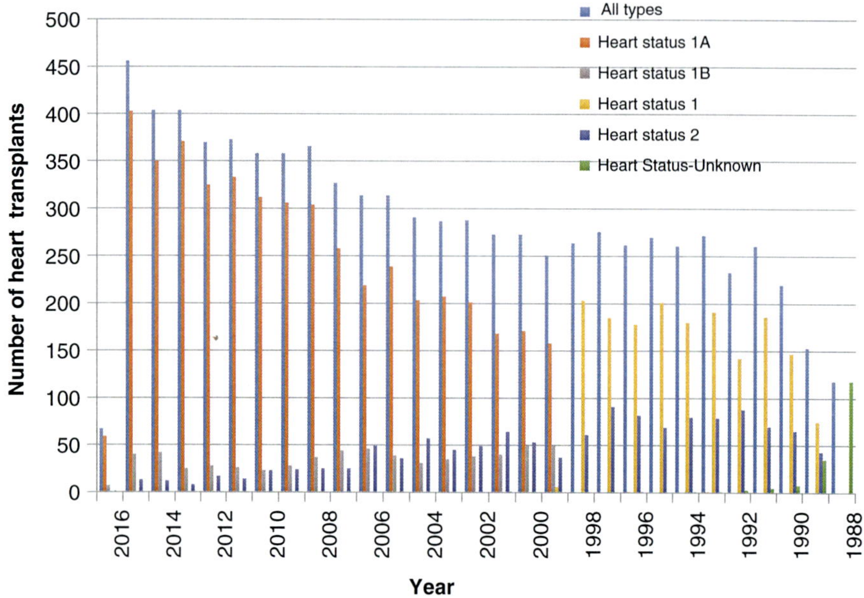

Fig. 32.1 Heart transplants per year and status at transplant from 1988 to May 2016 for pediatric patients 0 years to 18 years of age (From UNOS)

(congenitally corrected transposition of the great arteries (TGA) or TGA after atrial switch operation) (Attenhofer Jost et al. 2013).

Heart Transplantation for Congenital Heart Disease

Since 1988, from UNOS, there have been almost 8,500 pediatric (age 0–18 years of age) heart transplants; Fig. 32.1 shows the breakdown by year and status at time of transplant.

For May 2016, there are 41 patients waiting for a heart transplant less than 1 year old: 107 waiting, between 1 and 5 years of age: 74 waiting, between 6 and 10 years of age: and 106 waiting between 11 and 18 years of age. Between 2003 and 2004, the median wait times were 77 days for patients less than 1 year, 81 days for patients between 1 and 5 years of age, 63 days for patients between 6 and 10 years of age, and 62 days between 11 and 18 years of age (Kanter et al. 1999; Davies et al. 2008; Bailey et al. 2009; Saczkowski et al. 2010; Davies et al. 2011; Scully et al. 2011; Davies and Pizarro 2012; Jeewa et al. 2014; Karamlou et al. 2014; Alsoufi et al. 2016).

From UNOS, Fig. 32.2 shows the number of patients per year removed from the list secondary to death. It appears the number is reducing per year.

Congenital heart patients have worse 1-, 3-, and 5-year survival compared to patients with coronary artery disease and patients with cardiomyopathy (Fig. 32.3).

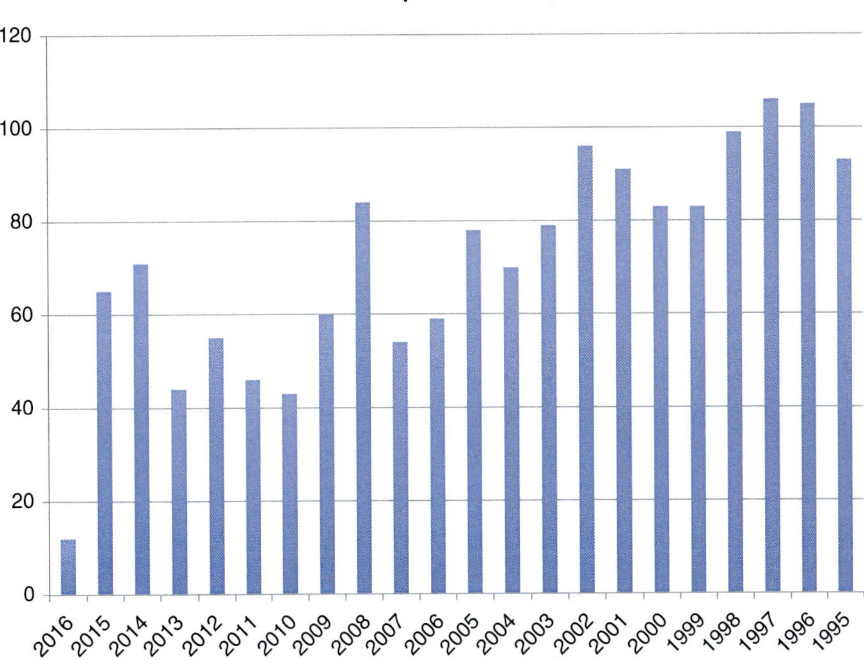

Fig. 32.2 Annual number of patients per year removed from UNOS list secondary to death

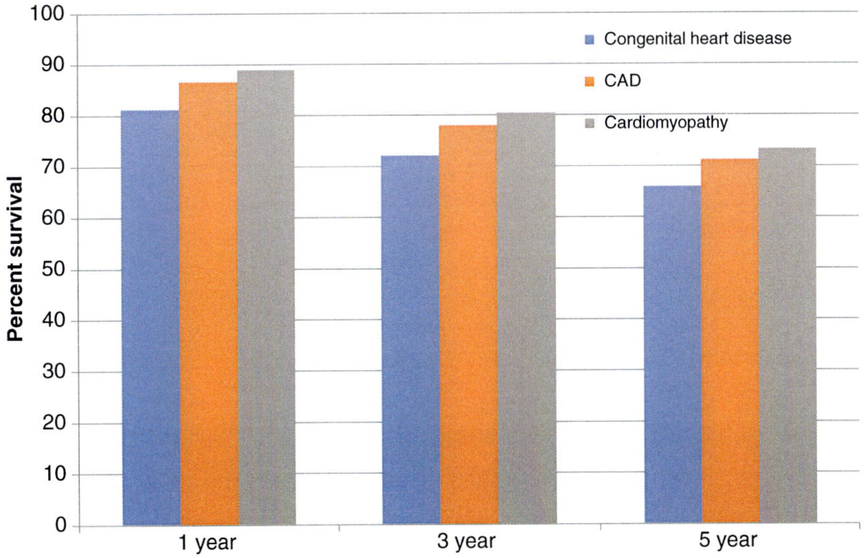

Fig. 32.3 1-, 3-, and 5-year survival in congenital heart patients compared to patients with coronary artery disease and patients with cardiomyopathy

It is difficult to determine why there are differences in survival because congenital heart patients are a very heterogeneous population. The most frequent diagnoses are listed in Table 32.1 (Lamour et al. 2009). Frequently they have had multiple previous operations. There surgeries are much more complicated given the pervious palliations and having to deal with arterial-to-pulmonary shunts, Glenn shunts (superior vena cava to pulmonary artery), or Fontan pathways (inferior vena cava to pulmonary artery). As result of the many operations and having foreign materials used in many of the repairs, patients are frequently sensitized with elevated plasma reactive antigens. Patients can also have other congenital abnormalities affecting other organ systems.

Lamour et al. found that patients with TGA had the best survival, 88%, and patients with atrioventricular canal had the worst survival, 62%, $p=0.02$. In the same report, the mean ischemic time was 228 min for patients with 1–2 previous sternotomies and 242 min for > 3 sternotomies (Bernstein et al. 2006). Fontan patients faired worse after a transplantation, with an actuarial 1-year survival of 75% compared to an 83% for other congenital heart diseases and 89% for patients without congenital heart disease (Hsu and Lamour 2015). Lamour et al. found that patients with Fontan had an increase in relative risk of death of 8.6, with 71% 1-year survival for Fontan patients and 83% for non-Fontan patients (Lamour et al. 2009). There is growing concern that Fontan circulation can lead to liver failure, which may explain the worse prognosis. From Lamour's paper, Table 32.2 shows the multivariable analysis for the risk factors for early- and constant-phase mortality.

Hsu and Lamour reviewed the causes of chronic heart failure in congenital heart disease patients (Table 32.3) (Almond et al. 2009).

These causes of chronic heart failure can be challenging to treat and for patients with Fontan circulation explain why they are twice as likely to die while waiting for a transplant if listed status 1 (Bernstein et al. 2006).

Mechanical Circulatory Support

With the complex congenital heart patients, many of which may have other organ involvement, long wait lists, and substantial numbers of patients dying on the wait list, mechanical circulatory support will help fill the void and may make some

Table 32.1 Major diagnostic categories for congenital heart disease patients undergoing heart transplantation

Diagnosis	n	% (of 488)
Single ventricle	176	36
d-Transposition of the great arteries	58	12
Right ventricular outflow tract lesions	49	10
Ventricular/atrial septal defect	38	8
Left ventricular outflow tract lesions	38	8
l-Transposition of the great arteries	39	8
Complete atrioventricular canal defect	37	8
Others	53	11
Total	488	100

Table 32.2 Causes of chronic heart failure in congenital heart disease

Systemic ventricular systolic or diastolic dysfunction
Single ventricle physiology
Left ventricular outflow tract obstruction
d-Transposition of the great arteries s/p atrial switch procedure
l-Transposition of the great arteries
Atrioventricular canal defect with chronic mitral regurgitation
Post-cardiopulmonary bypass
Pulmonary ventricular dysfunction
Tetralogy of Fallot with pulmonary or tricuspid insufficiency
Complications of the Fontan procedure
Protein-losing enteropathy
Intra-atrial reentrant tachycardia
Chronic effusions
Cyanosis

Table 32.3 Patient characteristics: VAD type

VAD	Total	LVAD	BiVAD
Long term	70		
Thoratec VAD (Thoratec Corp, Pleasanton, Calif)		29	24
Heartmate LVAS (Thoratec Corp, Pleasanton, Calif)		12	1
Novacor LVAS (WorldHeart Inc, Oakland, Calif)		3	…
EXCOR Pediatric (Berlin Heart AG, Berlin, Germany)		1	…
Short term	26		
BVS 5000 (Abiomed Inc, Danvers, Mass)		5	5
Bio-Pump (Medtronic, Minneapolis, Minn)		9	5
Bio-Pump (Medtronic, Minneapolis, Minn)		…	2
Total		59	37

Device unspecified, $n=3$
LVAD indicates left ventricular assist device, *BiVAD* biventricular assist device

patients better heart transplant candidates, for example, the Fontan failure patients. From January 20, 1999 to July 12, 2006, there were 3416 pediatric patients listed for heart transplant, 17 % died while waiting and 12 % remained on the list waiting (Blume et al. 2006).

The degree of invasive support, be it ECMO, mechanical ventilation, or inotropic support, has the biggest impact on wait list mortality (Almond et al. 2009).

ECMO was never a great bridge to transplantation with varying success with 35–58 % transplanted and discharged.

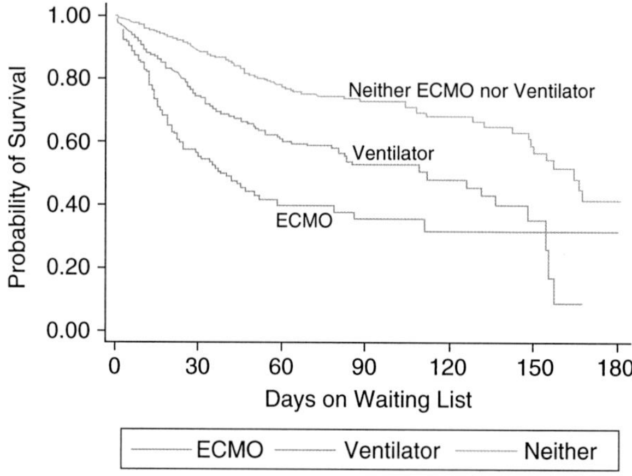

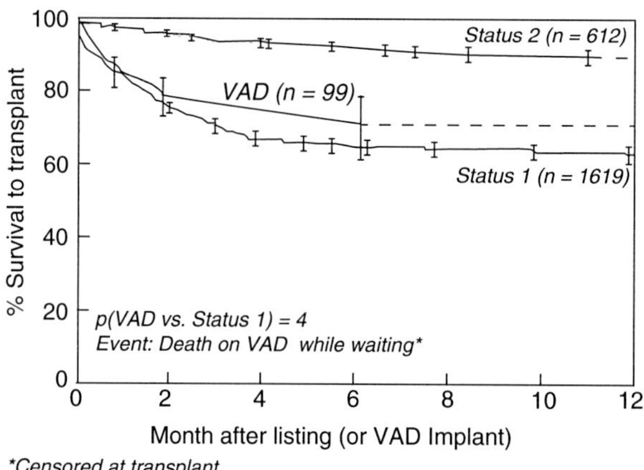

Fig. 32.4 Survival to transplantation of patients bridged to transplantation with VAD support versus other status 1 patients is not significantly different. Survival for status 2 patients also is shown

Between January 1, 1993 and December 31, 2003, 99 patients received a VAD of 2276 patients listed for transplant, 77 % of these patients were successfully transplanted (Zafar et al. 2015). In this report by Blume et al., there were varying degrees of VADs that were used to support these patients (Table 32.3), and there was no survival benefit compared to other status 1 patients (Fig. 32.4).

The three main risks identified from the study for death with VAD are (1) congenital origin, (2) female gender, and (3) year of implantation (Fig. 32.5) (Blume et al. 2006).

Fig. 32.5 Survival to transplantation of patients after VAD implantation stratified for (**a**) age at implantation and (**b**) congenital heart disease. Probability value is the unadjusted value

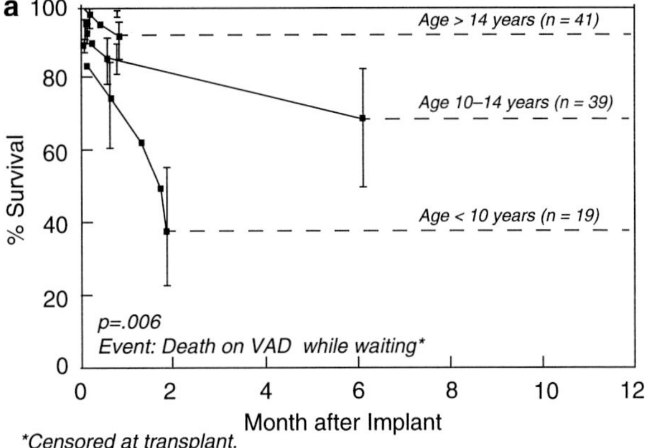

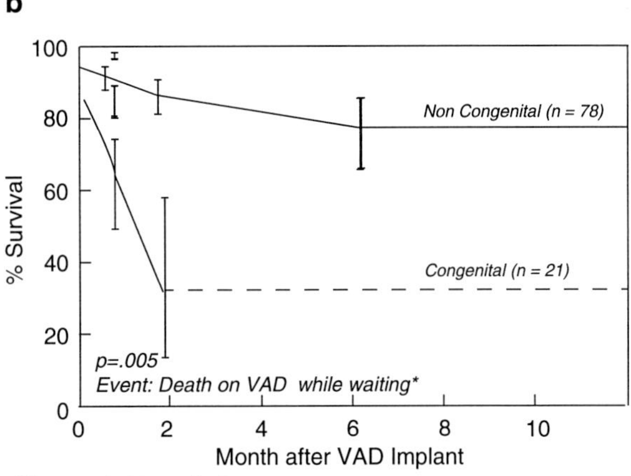

Using more durable devices that were designed for pediatric patients in particular, the Berlin Heart wait list mortality has improved (Berlin Heart 2013). In this review of the UNOS, data was reviewed and two populations were defined, ERA 1 (1999–2004) and ERA 2 (2005–2012); the authors also looked within each ERA VAD vs. non-VAD survival (Fig. 32.6) (Zafar et al. 2015).

The Berlin Heart is presently the only device FDA approved for use in pediatrics. It is still undergoing post-approval review. From 2000 to September 2013, there have been almost 600 Berlin hearts transplanted in the North America. From 2000 to 2008, there have been 144 implants in the USA at 37 institutions, mean time on support was 49 days, mean age was 4.1 years, and 60 % were for idiopathic dilated cardiomyopathy and 21 % complex congenital. Of these initial patients, 60 % were successfully transplanted, and 9 % were successfully weaned from support, with 25 % of patients dying on support (Berlin Heart 2013).

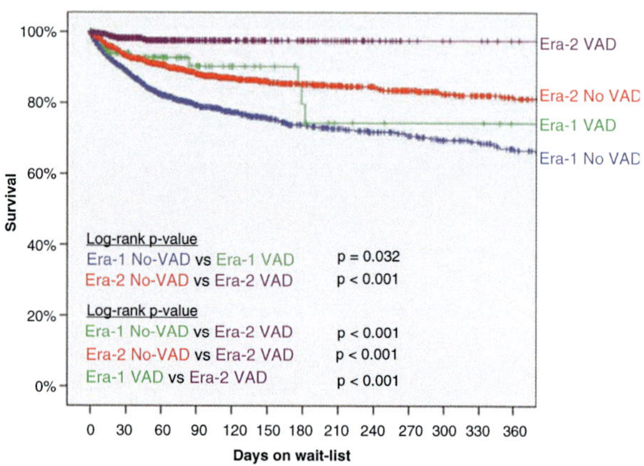

Fig. 32.6 Waiting list survival for different groups by era and ventricular assist device (VAD) use

10 months after getting a biventricular Berlin Heart

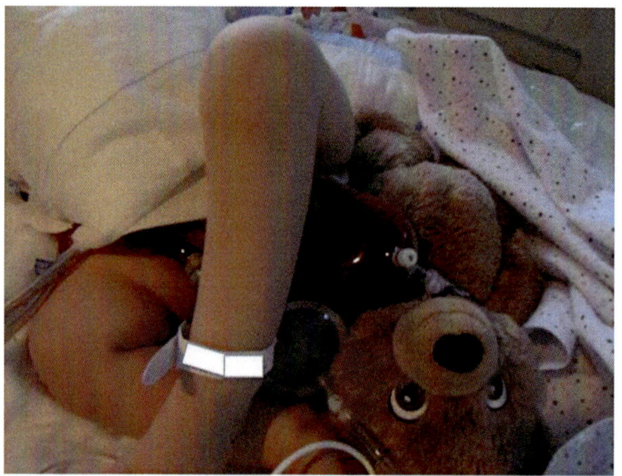

EXCOR® Pediatric

Overall Support time and outcomes

ERA	N	Median Days of support	Success Rate*
2000-2007 Pre IDE study	73	49	70% (51/73)
2007-2011 IDE Study	281	37	70% (198/281)
2011- 2013 Post Approval	140	47	78%** (89/114)

*Success rate calculated as those transplanted or weaned out of patients who met an endpoint

*114 of 140 patients have met endpoint in this group

EXCOR® Pediatric VAD

Serious Adverse Events

Patients with SAE	IDE Study N=109	Post-Approval Study N=15*
Major Bleeding	50 (45.9%)	4 (26.7%)
Major Infection	54 (49.5%)	4 (26.7%)
Neurological Dysfunction	33 (30.3%)	4 (26.7%)

New devices are being developed, and the NIH awarded $23.6 million for pre-clinical testing for devices for children, Pumps for Kids, Infants, and Neonates (PumpKIN). To date no new devices are on the horizon.

For our patients, we have developed an algorithm, especially for the single-ventricle patients, to determine the exact flow needed which can be difficult. In the single-ventricle patients, we use a temporary VAD, a centrifugal pump.

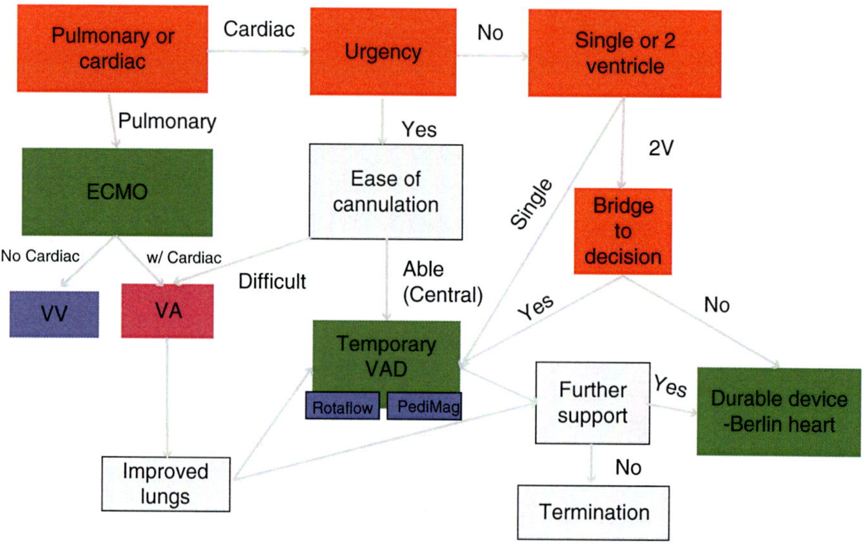

Conclusion

Since the land breaking work of Vivian Thomas, patients with congenital heart disease have been living longer with better quality of life. More patients are now living into adulthood. Many patients will require heart transplantation, and with low numbers of organs available, methods to bridge them are imperative.

References

Almond CS, Thiagarajan RR, Piercey GE, Gauvreau K, Blume ED, Bastardi HJ, Fynn-Thompson F, Singh TP. Waiting list mortality among children listed for heart transplantation in the United States. Circulation. 2009;119:717–27.

Alsoufi B, Mahle WT, Manlhiot C, Deshpande S, Kogon B, McCrindle BW, Kanter K. Outcomes of heart transplantation in children with hypoplastic left heart syndrome previously palliated with the Norwood procedure. J Thorac Cardiovasc Surg. 2016;151:167–74, 175.e161–162.

Attenhofer Jost CH, Schmidt D, Huebler M, Balmer C, Noll G, Caduff R, Greutmann M. Heart transplantation in congenital heart disease: in whom to consider and when? J Transplant. 2013;2013:376027.

Bailey LL, Razzouk AJ, Hasaniya NW, Chinnock RE. Pediatric transplantation using hearts refused on the basis of donor quality. Ann Thorac Surg. 2009;87:1902–8; discussion 1908–1909.

Berlin Heart I. Berlin Heart, Inc. Pediatric Advisory Committee. 20 Sept 2013.

Bernstein D, Naftel D, Chin C, Addonizio LJ, Gamberg P, Blume ED, Hsu D, Canter CE, Kirklin JK, Morrow WR. Outcome of listing for cardiac transplantation for failed Fontan: a multi-institutional study. Circulation. 2006;114:273–80.

Blalock A, Taussig HB. Landmark article May 19, 1945: the surgical treatment of malformations of the heart in which there is pulmonary stenosis or pulmonary atresia. By Alfred Blalock and Helen B. Taussig. JAMA. 1984;251:2123–38.

Blume ED, Naftel DC, Bastardi HJ, Duncan BW, Kirklin JK, Webber SA. Outcomes of children bridged to heart transplantation with ventricular assist devices: a multi-institutional study. Circulation. 2006;113:2313–9.

Davies RR, Pizarro C. Using the UNOS/SRTR and PHTS databases to improve quality in pediatric cardiac transplantation. World J Pediatr Congenit Heart Surg. 2012;3:421–32.

Davies RR, Russo MJ, Mital S, Martens TM, Sorabella RS, Hong KN, Gelijns AC, Moskowitz AJ, Quaegebeur JM, Mosca RS, Chen JM. Predicting survival among high-risk pediatric cardiac transplant recipients: an analysis of the United Network for Organ Sharing database. J Thorac Cardiovasc Surg. 2008;135:147–55, 155.e141–142.

Davies RR, Russo MJ, Hong KN, Mital S, Mosca RS, Quaegebeur JM, Chen JM. Increased short- and long-term mortality at low-volume pediatric heart transplant centers: should minimum standards be set? Retrospective data analysis. Ann Surg. 2011;253:393–401.

Hitchings GH, Elion GB. Layer on layer: the Bruce F Cain memorial Award lecture. Cancer Res. 1985;45:2415–20.

Hsu DT, Lamour JM. Changing indications for pediatric heart transplantation: complex congenital heart disease. Circulation. 2015;131:91–9.

Jeewa A, Manlhiot C, Kantor PF, Mital S, McCrindle BW, Dipchand AI. Risk factors for mortality or delisting of patients from the pediatric heart transplant waiting list. J Thorac Cardiovasc Surg. 2014;147:462–8.

Kanter KR, Tam VK, Vincent RN, Cuadrado AR, Raviele AA, Berg AM. Current results with pediatric heart transplantation. Ann Thorac Surg. 1999;68:527–30; discussion 530–521.

Karamlou T, Welke KF, McMullan DM, Cohen GA, Gelow J, Tibayan FA, Mudd JM, Slater MS, Song HK. Combined heart-kidney transplant improves post-transplant survival compared with isolated heart transplant in recipients with reduced glomerular filtration rate: analysis of 593 combined heart-kidney transplants from the United Network Organ Sharing Database. J Thorac Cardiovasc Surg. 2014;147:456–61.e451.

Lamour JM, Kanter KR, Naftel DC, Chrisant MR, Morrow WR, Clemson BS, Kirklin JK. The effect of age, diagnosis, and previous surgery in children and adults undergoing heart transplantation for congenital heart disease. J Am Coll Cardiol. 2009;54:160–5.

Saczkowski R, Dacey C, Bernier PL. Does ABO-incompatible and ABO-compatible neonatal heart transplant have equivalent survival? Interact Cardiovasc Thorac Surg. 2010;10:1026–33.

Scully BB, Zafar F, Schecter MG, Rossano JW, Mallory Jr GB, Heinle JS, Morales DL. Lung retransplantation in children: appropriate when selectively applied. Ann Thorac Surg. 2011;91:574–9.

Warden HE, Cohen M, Read RC, Lillehei CW. Controlled cross circulation for open intracardiac surgery: physiologic studies and results of creation and closure of ventricular septal defects. J Thorac Surg. 1954;28:331–41; discussion, 341–333.

Zafar F, Castleberry C, Khan MS, Mehta V, Bryant 3rd R, Lorts A, Wilmot I, Jefferies JL, Chin C, Morales DL. Pediatric heart transplant waiting list mortality in the era of ventricular assist devices. J Heart and Lung Transplant: Off Publ Int Soc Heart Transplant. 2015;34:82–8.

Part V
Postoperative Care

Chapter 33
Postoperative Cardiovascular and Hemodynamic Management in Pediatric Cardiac Surgery

Ramin Baghaei Tehrani

Introduction

Care of postoperative cardiac patients needs consideration of the patient as a whole. As a matter of fact, management of the cardiovascular system is the main duty of intensive care specialist.

Meticulous postoperative care requires comprehensive information of the preoperative diagnosis and condition as well as the details of surgical repair. In this regard, intensivist should have a close communication and collaboration with the operating room team.

In this chapter, we first review the important hemodynamic parameters measured by monitoring techniques and then describe some important postoperative complications related to cardiovascular system.

Transferring Patient from Operating Room

Postoperative care starts from the point when the operating room team decides to transfer the patient to the pediatric ICU. This is a very critical phase because various problems such as inadvertent alteration in rate of drug infusion, displacement of endotracheal tube, or hypothermia may result in deterioration of the patient condition.

The ICU team should be aware in advance of the hemodynamic state of the patient, medications, and the type and setting of the ventilator support (Mistry et al. 2008; Schlachta-Fairchild et al. 2008; Collins et al. 2011; Agha 2012).

R. Baghaei Tehrani, MD
Cardiac Surgery Department, Modarres Hospital, Faculty of Medicine, Shahid Beheshti
University of Medical Sciences, Tehran, Iran
e-mail: baghaei.ramin@gmail.com

© Springer International Publishing Switzerland 2017
A. Dabbagh et al. (eds.), *Congenital Heart Disease in Pediatric
and Adult Patients*, DOI 10.1007/978-3-319-44691-2_33

The handover of the surgical patient from the operating room staff to the ICU staff should be conducted by a standardized process. The handover is given usually by the anesthesiologist who discusses every related issue like airway and invasive lines, information about cardiopulmonary bypass, performed procedure, intraoperative echocardiographic findings, inotropes, etc. Obviously all staff should be present during the handoff process (Joy et al. 2011; Patil and Tailor 2013).

Monitoring Techniques

In order to manage the hemodynamic state, intensivist uses different monitoring techniques. The level of monitoring depends on the preoperative diagnosis and the type of surgical repair or palliation. There are some monitoring methods which are performed for all patients. These include continuous ECG, systemic arterial pressure, peripheral pulse oximetry, respiratory rate, and end-tidal CO_2.

Arterial oxygen saturation can be evaluated by pulse oximetry. Although pulse oximetry is an easy and noninvasive technique, it has important limitations. It works well only when there is good peripheral perfusion, and in the case of severe hypoxemia, it would not be accurate (Carter et al. 1998). In these conditions, PaO_2 and SpO_2 measured from an arterial blood gas sample are more reliable.

Near-infrared spectroscopy (NIRS), a marker of tissue oxygenation, is based on the arterial and predominantly venous oxygen saturation. NIRS is correlated with cardiac output and oxygen consumption (Hirsch et al. 2009). Today, this monitoring method is routinely used in most cardiac surgery centers worldwide.

Based on the underlying disease and the performed procedure, some invasive monitoring techniques are utilized. All of the parameters are achieved through the intracardiac lines.

Central venous catheter is routinely inserted for all cardiac surgeries, except for some simple palliative procedures. Central venous pressure (CVP), which is equal to the mean right atrial pressure (RAP), indicates the preload status. Bleeding, hypovolemia, or peripheral vasodilation would decrease CVP, and conversely, cardiac tamponade or right ventricular dysfunction would increase CVP. Oxygen saturation of blood sample drawn through central venous catheter could be very helpful for hemodynamic management. For example, any residual left to right shunt at the atrial level or anomalous pulmonary venous connection can abnormally rise right atrial oxygen saturation. Increased oxygen consumption due to low cardiac output or severe anemia cause reduced right atrial oxygen saturation.

Today, pulmonary artery (PA) catheter is inserted less frequently, but it remains useful in the management of patients with pulmonary arterial or venous hypertension. The mean PA pressure is elevated initially after weaning from cardiopulmonary bypass, but it should be less than 25 mmHg. In patients with pulmonary hypertension prior to surgery, mean PA pressure is usually more than 25 mmHg. The relationship of the PA pressure to the systemic pressure may be more helpful than the absolute values. If this ratio is greater than 50 %, a complete evaluation of various parameters such as ventricular function, cardiac output, systemic vascular resistance, and pulmonary vascular resistance should be performed. Finally, the same conditions that alter the oxygen saturation of the right atrium can influence the oxygen saturation of the pulmonary artery by the same manner.

Left atrial (LA) catheter is very useful in the management of mitral valve or left ventricular dysfunction. LA pressure is normally about 2 mmHg greater than CVP and demonstrates the preload status of the left ventricle (Kouchoukos et al. 1971). There are different causes of abnormally elevated LA pressure after cardiac surgery. Left ventricular dysfunction or hypertrophy, myocardial ischemia, mitral valve disease, large left to right shunt, and cardiac tamponade are among them (Wernovsky et al. 1995). It should be mentioned that alteration of LA oxygen saturation could indicate a serious problem. Reduced LA oxygen saturation can be the result of an atrial level right to left shunt or severe parenchymal lung disease with pulmonary venous desaturation.

Hemodynamic Complications

Low Cardiac Output

A significant percentage of patients experience low cardiac output (LCO) postoperatively that the number of which relates to the type of procedure and patient's condition. LCO usually occurs within 6–12 h after surgery (Wernovsky et al. 1995).

There are clinical signs or paraclinical parameters which help us to assess the cardiac output. These include the skin color and temperature, capillary refill, urine output, systemic arterial pressure, right and left atrial filling pressures, acid–base status, and peripheral O2 saturation measured by pulse oximetry (Kirklin et al. 1981).

In the early stages of decreased cardiac output, the changes are subtle. The skin temperature and capillary refill decrease, especially in the extremities. The urine output that should be at least 1 ml/kg/h diminishes to oliguric level. Metabolic acidosis with elevation of lactate level occurs. The pulse oximetry shows decreasing trend of O2 saturation level. The filling pressures of the right and left atrium may be decreased (excessive bleeding) or increased (myocardial dysfunction or tamponade). At last, the syndrome of LCO completes with the fall in systemic arterial pressure.

LCO may be caused by one or a combination of the following factors:

1 Residual intracardiac lesion
2 Factors related to the surgical procedure
3 Insufficient preload due to loss of intravascular volume
4 Excessive afterload due to vasoconstriction
5 Contractility dysfunction
6 Heart rate or rhythm changes

Residual Defects It is evident that any important residual defect can influence the postoperative course by its hemodynamic derangement. Residual lesions could be found by auscultation, intracardiac pressure, or arterial pressure monitoring and oxygen saturation data. For example, a wide pulse pressure and diastolic murmur may be due to significant aortic regurgitation following aortic valve repair. Further evaluation with echocardiography and/or cardiac catheterization should be performed in the case of compromising ventricular function.

Surgical-Related Factors These factors are classified in two general groups. The first group consists of factors related to surgical technique itself. For example, ventriculotomy could result in ventricular dysfunction postoperatively. Injury to the conduction system (sinoatrial or atrioventricular node) during surgery for VSD closure or repair of a sinus venosus ASD definitively influences the postoperative course. Ongoing bleeding after cardiac surgery may expose the patient not only to the risk of cardiac tamponade but also to the inflammatory response due to transfusion of blood products.

The second group consists of factors related to CPB and myocardial ischemia during cardiac surgery. The CPB with its unique exposure of blood components to the extracorporeal circuit may induce an immense systemic inflammatory response. This response, which is magnified in children due to the large bypass circuit, includes humoral and cellular reactions that finally result in the release of vasoactive substances and inflammatory mediators (Burrows et al. 1988).

Increased interstitial fluid and multiorgan failure (including the heart and lung) are the results of this systemic inflammatory response.

Myocardial injury may occur because of problems with cardioplegic protection, inadequate hypothermia, intracoronary air embolism, or insufficient coronary perfusion. Myocardial ischemia may present with a sudden onset fatal dysrhythmia or complete heart block rather than ECG changes in ST segment.

Preload The usual monitoring method to evaluate preload is the central venous pressure (CVP) or mean atrial pressure. Initially after surgery and CPB, the filling pressures are normal or slightly elevated. As the patient continues to rewarm and vasodilate, these pressures and consequently systemic blood pressure tend to be decreased. In this stage, intravascular volume infusion is necessary to maintain systemic pressure in the normal range (Friedman and George 1985).

Preload should be maintained higher in patients with noncompliant or hypertrophic ventricles and also in patients who are dependent on complete mixing at the atrial level.

Afterload Elevated afterload is frequently seen after cardiac surgery with CPB. It may occur in both systemic and pulmonary circulation. Increased afterload is caused by elevated systemic vascular resistance. This phenomenon results in decreased peripheral perfusion, which is manifested clinically by cool extremities and low urine output (Lehot et al. 1992).

High afterload is tolerated less well in neonates than in older infants and children, so they benefit from afterload reduction therapy. The clinician should recognize and improve conditions like pain and hypothermia which exacerbate vasoconstriction as well as utilizing a vasodilating agent. Phosphodiesterase inhibitors (e.g., Milrinone) and nitric compounds are used in combination with inotropic agents to reduce afterload and augment cardiac output (Stocker et al. 2007).

Contractility Dysfunction Cardiac contractility is the ability of the myocardium to generate force which is a load-independent property. Contractility dysfunction may be originated from preoperative, intraoperative, or postoperative factors. Pressure or volume overload, myocardial ischemia, anesthesia, hypoxia, acidosis, and various pharmacologic agents can depress cardiac contractility.

If low cardiac output persists after heart rate and preload and afterload are optimized, cardiac contractility should be reinforced by inotropic drugs. It seems that stating inotropic support in the operating room is better than waiting for the signs of low cardiac output to appear.

There are several inotropic agents and each has its own characteristic effects. The commonly used drugs in practice are dopamine, dobutamine, epinephrine, milrinone, isoproterenol, and norepinephrine.

Dopamine has effects on both α and β adrenergic receptors. The dose range of 2–5 μg/kg/min can increase renal blood flow by dilation of splanchnic vessels. Doses in the range of 5–10 μg/kg/min tend to enhance cardiac contractility by stimulation of myocardial β adrenergic receptors. Dopamine in the range of 10–20 μg/kg/min stimulates α receptors and cause peripheral and pulmonary vasoconstriction. It appears that the neonatal myocardium is less sensitive to the dopamine effect than that of older children (Driscoll et al. 1979).

Dobutamine is almost specific for cardiac β receptors. It can increase cardiac contractility without increasing systemic or pulmonary vascular resistance (Loeb et al. 1977). Its usual dose range is 2–10 μg/kg/min. Some patients respond to dobutamine with an extreme tachycardia. Dobutamine is contraindicated when there is systemic hypotension.

Isoproterenol is a strong inotropic and chronotropic agent. It acts as a selective β agonist. Isoproterenol cause peripheral and pulmonary vasodilation. Its usage is limited by tachycardia and oxygen consumption.

Epinephrine is usually utilized for patients with severe myocardial dysfunction. The dose range is 0.05–0.5 μg/kg/min. Epinephrine in lower doses cause increasing contractility and decreasing afterload by vasodilation (β agonist), while in higher doses cause severe peripheral vasoconstriction (α agonist). Epinephrine is not frequently used with doses higher than 0.2 μg/kg/min because of its adverse effect on renal perfusion. Norepinephrine is a potent α agonist so it has systemic vasoconstriction and moderate inotropism effects.

Milrinone is a phosphodiesterase inhibitor which acts mainly by afterload reduction. It has also positive inotropic effect. Milrinone is an ideal choice for patients with pulmonary hypertension because of its pulmonary vasodilatory effect (Stocker et al. 2007). Milrinone is contraindicated when there is systemic hypotension.

A combination of inotropic drugs should be considered in the management of patients with severe myocardial dysfunction or when side effects like systemic hypotension preclude continuation of medication.

Dysrhythmia ECG is an essential tool to identify whether the patient is in sinus rhythm postoperatively. It is obvious that sinus rhythm by providing the atrioventricular synchrony as well as contribution of atrial contraction is very important for maintaining cardiac output in the normal range, especially in the early postoperative period.

Sinus tachycardia must be differentiated from supraventricular, ventricular, or junctional tachycardia. Sinus tachycardia, which is a normal hemodynamic response, is usually related to an underlying condition like pain, anxiety, fever, or anemia. Some inotropic drugs like dopamine may induce severe tachycardia. Obviously, by relief of aggravating factors, heart rate would decrease.

Any of the tachyarrhythmia influence negatively on cardiac output (Hoffman et al. 2002b). They compromise diastolic filling of ventricles or diminish their systolic function. Treatment plan consists of lowering the inotrope dosage, if possible, and antiarrhythmic drugs. Sometimes inducing mild hypothermia and atrioventricular sequential pacing may be beneficial (Hoffman et al. 2002a).

Postoperative Bleeding and Cardiac Tamponade

Excessive postoperative bleeding occurs in very small percentage of patients. It is more frequent in deeply cyanotic patients, patients with preoperative severe ventricular dysfunction and reoperations (Gomes and McGoon 1970).

Cardiopulmonary bypass results in several alterations in the coagulation system. Thrombocytopenia and platelet dysfunction, dilution of coagulation factors, and fibrinolysis are among the factors that prevent normal hemostatic function. Both inadequate heparin neutralization and protamine overdose can cause coagulation disorder. Sometimes multiple factors lead to the syndrome of disseminated intravascular coagulation (DIC) which is very difficult to control (Guay and Rivard 1996).

Treatment of bleeding starts from the point that the surgeon incises the skin. Gentle handling of tissue, use of proper sutures and prosthetic materials, secure tensionless suture lines, and meticulous hemostasis are the basic surgical principles to prevent postoperative bleeding. In the ICU, management of bleeding consists of correction of underlying coagulation disorder by replacement of deficient factors. Platelet should be transfused if there is thrombocytopenia ($<50,000$ platelet/mm2). The use of fresh whole blood is very effective to reduce bleeding, especially in the neonatal population (Manno et al. 1991). If it is not available, combination of fresh frozen plasma, platelet concentrate, and cryoprecipitate will be useful.

Surgical re-exploration is indicated whenever the amount of chest tube drainage passes a critical level or the signs of tamponade occurs. In the absence of coagulopathy, hourly drainage more than 3 ml/kg for three consecutive hours or sudden drainage of more than 5 ml/kg in an hour are indications for re-exploration.

Some surgeons consider re-exploration if the blood loss exceeds 10 % of blood volume in 1 h or 20 % in 4 h.

Continuous postoperative bleeding not effectively drained by the chest tubes results in cardiac tamponade. This complication should be suspected when chest tube drainage stops in a patient with previous significant bleeding. Cardiac tamponade due to cardiac chambers compression by blood clots is manifested by elevated venous pressure, paradoxical pulse and then narrow pulse pressure, reduction of urine output, and systemic hypotension. Arterial pressure decreases with minimal or no response to volume loading or increased dosage of inotropes. Obviously, if not properly managed, tamponade quickly culminates in cardiac arrest.

Any patient suspected of having cardiac tamponade should be returned to the operating room. A rapidly deteriorating hemodynamic condition forces sternal opening to be done in the ICU. After removal of clots, all surgical sites should be meticulously examined for the source of bleeding. Decision about closing the sternum or leaving it open depends on the hemodynamic state, cardiac dilatation, and myocardial swelling.

It is necessary to discuss about two other forms of cardiac tamponade. The first, which is called dry tamponade, is seen in surgical patients with right ventricular dysfunction, frequently associated with pulmonary hypertension. Sudden increase in pulmonary arterial pressure leads to right ventricular dilatation which is already dysfunctional and compressed by the closed space of mediastinum. The signs of cardiac tamponade ensue and, if not relieved by sternal opening, can terminate in cardiac arrest. The second form is the delayed cardiac tamponade. It is a manifestation of post-pericardiotomy syndrome and occurs from several days to few weeks after cardiac surgery. When the pericardial effusion is sizable, with no response to anti-inflammatory drugs or corticosteroids, pericardial drainage by percutaneous or open methods is indicated (Horneffer et al. 1990).

Pulmonary Hypertension

Pulmonary hypertension after cardiac surgery is one of the challenging problems encountered in the postoperative period. Patients who have left to right shunt or pulmonary venous obstruction preoperatively are prone to develop postoperative pulmonary hypertension (Hoffman et al. 1981).

Elevated pulmonary arterial pressure can produce significant morbidity. Increased afterload of right ventricle leads to ventricular dysfunction and ultimately low cardiac output. Sometimes a sudden increase in pulmonary vascular resistance results in acute hemodynamic deterioration. This condition, which is termed pulmonary hypertensive crisis, could be a life-threatening problem and is manifested by the signs of low cardiac output, arterial desaturation, bradycardia, and cardiac arrest (Wheller et al. 1979). In patients with a communication between systemic and pulmonary circulation, increased pulmonary vascular resistance results in right to left shunt and hypoxemia. It should be mentioned that various factors such as acidosis, rise in PaCO2, respiratory infection, and endotracheal suctioning can precipitate pulmonary hypertensive crisis.

Treatment of postoperative pulmonary hypertension depends upon several factors including patient's age and diagnosis and cardiorespiratory function. Various pathophysiologic factors affect the pulmonary vascular resistance. Intensivist should seriously consider and manipulate these factors to control pulmonary artery pressure and prevent hypertensive crisis.

Increasing the depth of analgesia and sedation, especially before invasive procedures, is an important strategy to reduce pulmonary vascular resistance. As the decreased PaO2 and increased PaCO2 can constrict the pulmonary arteries, ventilator should be set up to achieve PaO2 > 100 mmHg and PaCO2 at 30–35 mmHg. Acidosis stimulates pulmonary hypertension, so PH should be kept at least 7.40 (Rudolph and Yuan 1966; Hoffman et al. 1981).

Regarding mechanical ventilation, both hypoinflation and hyperinflation of lungs should be avoided. Intrathoracic pressure should be kept as low as possible. Parenchymal lung abnormalities, like pneumonia and atelectasis, can also increase pulmonary arterial pressure. It is important to pay attention to chest radiographs and physical examination findings to detect and treat these problems.

Many of the inotropic drugs used after cardiac surgery have nonspecific vasoconstrictive effects when prescribed in high doses, so dose reduction of these drugs should be considered as a strategy to lower pulmonary vascular resistance. On the other hand, there are intravenous vasodilators which can treat pulmonary hypertension by different mechanisms. Nitric oxide donors like nitroprusside, milrinone, eicosanoid prostaglandins, gas nitric oxide, magnesium, isoproterenol, and dobutamine are among them. All of the abovementioned vasodilators, except for the nitric oxide, have nonspecific vasodilation, so systemic hypotension as a side effect can limit their usage (Atz and Wessel 1997). In chronic management, oral treatment with phosphodiesterase inhibitors (sildenafil) and endothelin receptor blocking agents (bosentan) is usually prescribed.

Conclusion

The improved results of cardiac surgery for congenital heart disease are attributed to the high quality of postoperative care in recent years. It is important to observe patients closely by repeated physical examination and to be vigilant for early signs of complications because anticipatory rather than reactive care leads to acceptable postoperative outcomes.

References

Agha RA. Handover in trauma and orthopaedic surgery – a human factors assessment. Ann Med Surg. 2012;1:25–9.

Atz AM, Wessel DL. Inhaled nitric oxide in the neonate with cardiac disease. Semin Perinatol. 1997;21:441–55.

Burrows FA, Williams WG, Teoh KH, Wood AE, Burns J, Edmonds J, Barker GA, Trusler GA, Weisel RD. Myocardial performance after repair of congenital cardiac defects in infants and children. Response to volume loading. J Thorac Cardiovasc Surg. 1988;96:548–56.

Carter BG, Carlin JB, Tibballs J, Mead H, Hochmann M, Osborne A. Accuracy of two pulse oximeters at low arterial hemoglobin-oxygen saturation. Crit Care Med. 1998;26:1128–33.

Collins SA, Stein DM, Vawdrey DK, Stetson PD, Bakken S. Content overlap in nurse and physician handoff artifacts and the potential role of electronic health records: a systematic review. J Biomed Inform. 2011;44:704–12.

Driscoll DJ, Gillette PC, Duff DF, McNamara DG. The hemodynamic effect of dopamine in children. J Thorac Cardiovasc Surg. 1979;78:765–8.

Friedman WF, George BL. Treatment of congestive heart failure by altering loading conditions of the heart. J Pediatr. 1985;106:697–706.

Gomes MM, McGoon DC. Bleeding patterns after open-heart surgery. J Thorac Cardiovasc Surg. 1970;60:87–97.

Guay J, Rivard GE. Mediastinal bleeding after cardiopulmonary bypass in pediatric patients. Ann Thorac Surg. 1996;62:1955–60.

Hirsch JC, Charpie JR, Ohye RG, Gurney JG. Near-infrared spectroscopy: what we know and what we need to know – a systematic review of the congenital heart disease literature. J Thorac Cardiovasc Surg. 2009;137(154-159):159e151–112.

Hoffman JI, Rudolph AM, Heymann MA. Pulmonary vascular disease with congenital heart lesions: pathologic features and causes. Circulation. 1981;64:873–7.

Hoffman TM, Bush DM, Wernovsky G, Cohen MI, Wieand TS, Gaynor JW, Spray TL, Rhodes LA. Postoperative junctional ectopic tachycardia in children: incidence, risk factors, and treatment. Ann Thorac Surg. 2002a;74:1607–11.

Hoffman TM, Wernovsky G, Wieand TS, Cohen MI, Jennings AC, Vetter VL, Godinez RI, Gaynor JW, Spray TL, Rhodes LA. The incidence of arrhythmias in a pediatric cardiac intensive care unit. Pediatr Cardiol. 2002b;23:598–604.

Horneffer PJ, Miller RH, Pearson TA, Rykiel MF, Reitz BA, Gardner TJ. The effective treatment of postpericardiotomy syndrome after cardiac operations. A randomized placebo-controlled trial. J Thorac Cardiovasc Surg. 1990;100:292–6.

Joy BF, Elliott E, Hardy C, Sullivan C, Backer CL, Kane JM. Standardized multidisciplinary protocol improves handover of cardiac surgery patients to the intensive care unit. Pediatr Crit Care Med. 2011;12:304–8.

Kirklin JK, Blackstone EH, Kirklin JW, McKay R, Pacifico AD, Bargeron Jr LM. Intracardiac surgery in infants under age 3 months: predictors of postoperative in-hospital cardiac death. Am J Cardiol. 1981;48:507–12.

Kouchoukos NT, Kirklin JW, Sheppard LC, Roe PA. Effect of left atrial pressure by blood infusion on stroke volume early after cardiac operations. Surg Forum. 1971;22:126–7.

Lehot JJ, Villard J, Piriz H, Philbin DM, Carry PY, Gauquelin G, Claustrat B, Sassolas G, Galliot J, Estanove S. Hemodynamic and hormonal responses to hypothermic and normothermic cardiopulmonary bypass. J Cardiothorac Vasc Anesth. 1992;6:132–9.

Loeb HS, Bredakis J, Gunner RM. Superiority of dobutamine over dopamine for augmentation of cardiac output in patients with chronic low output cardiac failure. Circulation. 1977;55:375–8.

Manno CS, Hedberg KW, Kim HC, Bunin GR, Nicolson S, Jobes D, Schwartz E, Norwood WI. Comparison of the hemostatic effects of fresh whole blood, stored whole blood, and components after open heart surgery in children. Blood. 1991;77:930–6.

Mistry KP, Jaggers J, Lodge AJ, Alton M, Mericle JM, Frush KS, Meliones JN. Advances in patient safety using six sigma(R) methodology to improve handoff communication in high-risk patients. In: Henriksen K, Battles JB, Keyes MA, Grady ML, editors. Advances in patient safety: new directions and alternative approaches (Vol. 3: performance and tools). Rockville: Agency for Healthcare Research and Quality (US); 2008.

Patil SS, Tailor K. Receiving patient from Operation Theater, assessment, preparation and handing-over process. In: Shah P, editor. Manual of pediatric cardiac intensive care. Bangladesh: Jaypee Brothers Medical Publishers; 2013.

Rudolph AM, Yuan S. Response of the pulmonary vasculature to hypoxia and H+ ion concentration changes. J Clin Invest. 1966;45:399–411.

Schlachta-Fairchild L, Elfrink V, Deickman A. Advances in patient safety patient safety, telenursing, and telehealth. In: Hughes RG, editor. Patient safety and quality: an evidence-based handbook for nurses. Rockville): Agency for Healthcare Research and Quality (US); 2008.

Stocker CF, Shekerdemian LS, Norgaard MA, Brizard CP, Mynard JP, Horton SB, Penny DJ. Mechanisms of a reduced cardiac output and the effects of milrinone and levosimendan in a model of infant cardiopulmonary bypass. Crit Care Med. 2007;35:252–9.

Wernovsky G, Wypij D, Jonas RA, Mayer Jr JE, Hanley FL, Hickey PR, Walsh AZ, Chang AC, Castaneda AR, Newburger JW, Wessel DL. Postoperative course and hemodynamic profile after the arterial switch operation in neonates and infants. A comparison of low-flow cardiopulmonary bypass and circulatory arrest. Circulation. 1995;92:2226–35.

Wheller J, George BL, Mulder DG, Jarmakani JM. Diagnosis and management of postoperative pulmonary hypertensive crisis. Circulation. 1979;60:1640–4.

Chapter 34
Postoperative Arrhythmias and Their Management

Majid Haghjoo and Mohammadrafie Khorgami

Early cardiac arrhythmias are well-known complications of pediatric cardiac surgery. Available data shows an incidence of 27–48 % (Rekawek et al. 2007). In early postoperative period of cardiac operations, arrhythmias are also a major cause of mortality and morbidity. Several reports have been published regarding late postoperative arrhythmias after cardiac surgeries such as the Mustard or Senning operation and Fontan procedures (Weber et al. 1666). Nevertheless, data related to the early postoperative period after cardiac surgery in children are limited. Arrhythmias that may be easily tolerated in normal heart can have a major influence on hearts with congenital defects (Triedman 2002).

Postoperative cardiac arrhythmias range from simple atrial or ventricular ectopies to major arrhythmias such as atrial flutter/fibrillation after Mustard/Senning or ventricular tachycardia after repair of tetralogy of Fallot (TOF). Other common arrhythmias are junctional ectopic tachycardia (JET) after repair of ventricular septal defect (VSD) or complete atrioventricular block (CHB) after any manipulation on conduction system (Delaney et al. 2006).

Several factors, including myocardial dysfunction, electrolyte disturbances, adrenergic stimulation, sutures in the myocardium, residual hemodynamic impairment, as well as pain and anxiety, have been implicated in the pathogenesis of early postoperative arrhythmias in children. The aim of this chapter is to present an overview of the common cardiac arrhythmias occurring in immediate postoperative period.

M. Haghjoo, MD, FESC, FACC (✉) • M. Khorgami, MD
Department of Cardiac Electrophysiology, Rajaie Cardiovascular Medical and Research
Center, Iran University of Medical Sciences, Tehran, Iran
e-mail: majid.haghjoo@gmail.com; rafikhorgami@gmail.com

© Springer International Publishing Switzerland 2017
A. Dabbagh et al. (eds.), *Congenital Heart Disease in Pediatric
and Adult Patients*, DOI 10.1007/978-3-319-44691-2_34

Postoperative Tachyarrhythmias

Postoperative tachycardias may be of atrial, junctional, or ventricular origins. The cause of these tachycardias is procedure-related injuries to the atria, conduction system, or ventricles and may be perpetuated by electrolyte disturbance, catecholamine stimulation, and hemodynamic disturbances. Supraventricular tachycardia is defined as arrhythmia originating from atria, atrioventricular node, and His bundle, whereas ventricular tachycardia originates from the structures located below His bundle including bundle branches, Purkinje system, and ventricular myocytes.

Supraventricular Tachycardias

In the evaluation of postoperative supraventricular tachycardia, we should first determine the mechanism of arrhythmia. Automatic tachycardias are the most common postoperative supraventricular tachycardias. Reentrant tachycardias are observed with lower frequency in early postoperative period.

Junctional Ectopic Tachycardia

Junctional ectopic tachycardia (JET) is the most common postoperative tachycardia in pediatric population (Zampi et al. 2012). The incidence of postoperative JET estimated to be between 3.6 and 10 % after repair of congenital heart defects and in some studies reported up to 27 % (Batra et al. 2006; Dodge-Khatami et al. 2002; Hoffman et al. 2002; Mildh and Hiippala 2011; Yildirim et al. 2008). This tachycardia is more common in infants. This tachycardia is characterized by ventricular rate of 140–220 bpm, atrioventricular (AV) dissociation, and less commonly 1:1 ventriculoatrial (VA) conduction (Fig. 34.1).

Although the majority of the postoperative JET spontaneously resolves after a few days, the period of sustained arrhythmia has devastating effect on the hemodynamic states that should be treated immediately and appropriately. At first step, the predisposing factors should be eliminated. These measures included body surface cooling to 34°C to 35°C, elimination of inotropes, correction of electrolyte abnormalities, and stabilization of hemodynamic condition (Lan et al. 2003). If the arrhythmias don't respond to these therapies, anti-arrhythmic drug is indicated and most experts begin with intravenous amiodarone. Compared with pre-amiodarone era, this drug markedly reduced postoperative mortality related to JET from 35 to 4 % (Probst et al. 2007). The conversion to sinus rhythm may be not possible in all patients with amiodarone; however, reducing the ventricular rate would be acceptable in these patients. Amiodarone is initiated with loading dose of 5 mg/kg intravenously during 1 h and then continued with infusion of 10–15 µg/kg/min (Perry et al. 1996; Kovacikova et al. 2009). Oral therapy should be started 1–2 days before

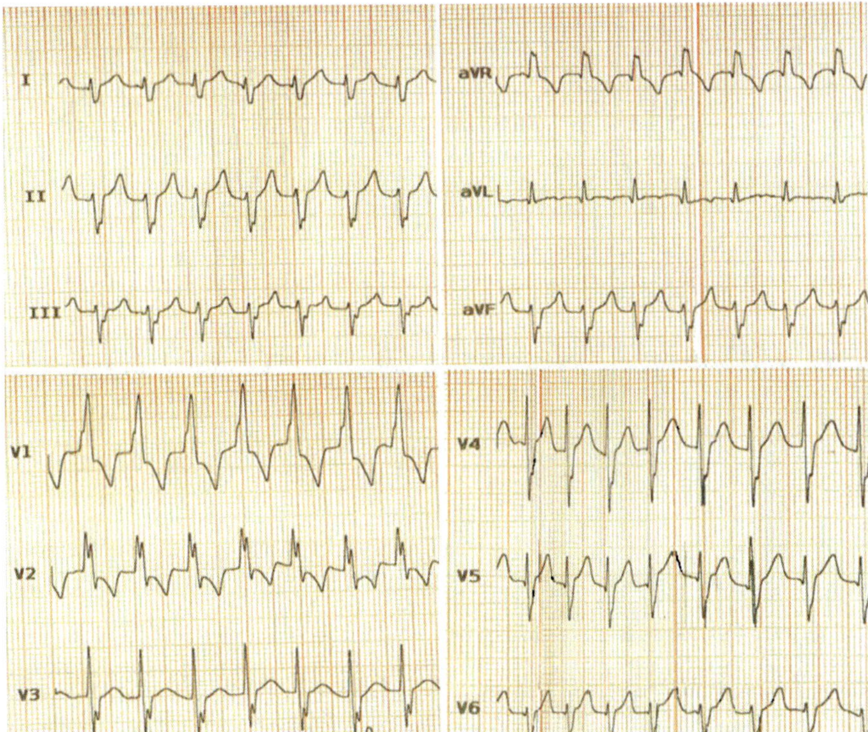

Fig. 34.1 Junctional ectopic tachycardia after complete atrioventricular septal defect repair. This ECG shows regular tachycardia with 1:1 ventriculoatrial conduction and right bundle branch block-type morphology

discontinuation of IV therapy. If the arrhythmia was refractory to amiodarone, beta-blocker, digoxin, or flecainide can be added to amiodarone regimen. Catheter ablation is rarely indicated in drug-refractory patients.

Atrial Tachycardia

Focal atrial tachycardia (AT) is the second postoperative tachycardia with automatic mechanism. This tachycardia is described as a narrow QRS tachycardia, ventricular rate of 150–250 bpm, warm up/cool down behavior, and variable atrial rate because of autonomic fluctuation (Walsh et al. 1992) (Fig. 34.2). Injury to atrial myocardium is one of the main pathologic factors. Vena caval cannulation during cardiac surgery and CV line insertion are other predisposing factors. Sinus node dysfunction is also a risk factor for AT. Automatic AT should be treated similar to JET.

Atrial flutter (AFL) and intra-atrial reentrant tachycardia (IART) are atrial arrhythmias with reentrant mechanism. These arrhythmias are recognized on an ECG by the presence of narrow QRS tachycardias and characteristic "sawtooth"

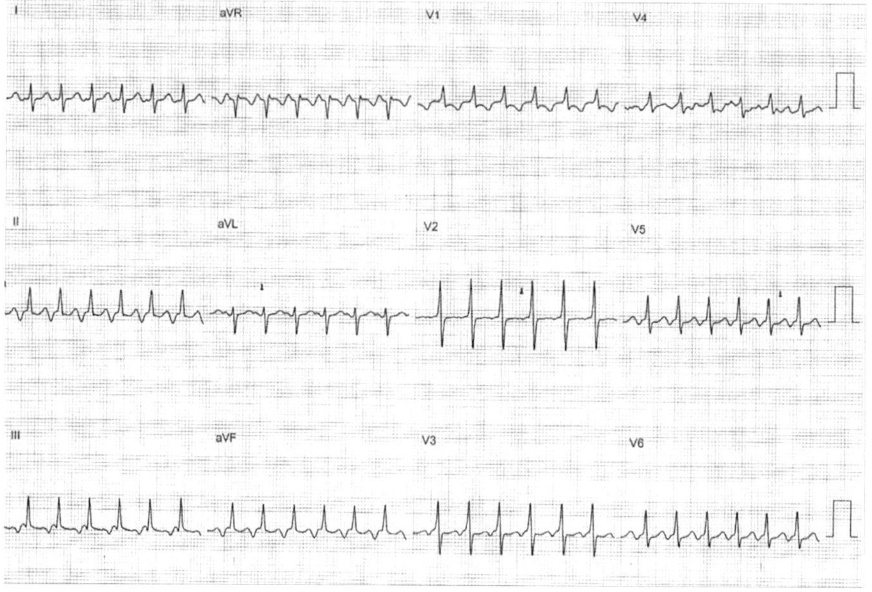

Fig. 34.2 Atrial tachycardia after Ebstein anomaly repair. Note that there is regular narrow QRS tachycardia with short PR and long RP interval, negative *P* waves in inferior leads, and positive *P* waves in leads I and aVL

wave in AFL or "isoelectric line" in IART at a regular rate of 240–440 bpm (Fig. 34.3). Ventricular rate depends on status of AV node (Fig. 34.4). Many factors predispose patients to AFL/IART. The most important factor is the degree of injury to atrial myocardium and region of scars and fibrotic tissue after atriotomy, incision, and suture lines. Other causes including the presence of atrial enlargement due to preexisting valvular disease and hemodynamic instability. Treatment should be focused on elimination of predisposing factors, rectification of residual defect as much as possible, and improvement of hemodynamic status. If the AFL/IAART are associated with acute hemodynamic instability, synchronized electrical cardioversion 0.5–1 J/kg should be done immediately. Success rate of cardioversion is reported up to 87 % (Texter et al. 2006). Anti-arrhythmic drug therapy is indicated if the arrhythmia persists. Class IC anti-arrhythmic drugs such as flecainide or propafenone are recommended for rhythm control in setting of preserved left ventricular function; however, amiodarone is the first choice drug in patients with reduced left ventricular function. Because of high incidence of amiodarone-related complications, careful patient follow-up is necessary. These assessments included ECG, chest X-ray, spirometry, and appropriate laboratory test including thyroid and liver function tests. If the rate control is planned, beta-blocker is the first line of therapy. Propranolol is usually well tolerated in children. In emergency setting, esmolol infusion with blood pressure monitoring is necessary. Most experts recommended the combination of class IC drugs with beta-blocker for prevention of 1:1 AV conduction after atrial rate reduction by class IC drugs.

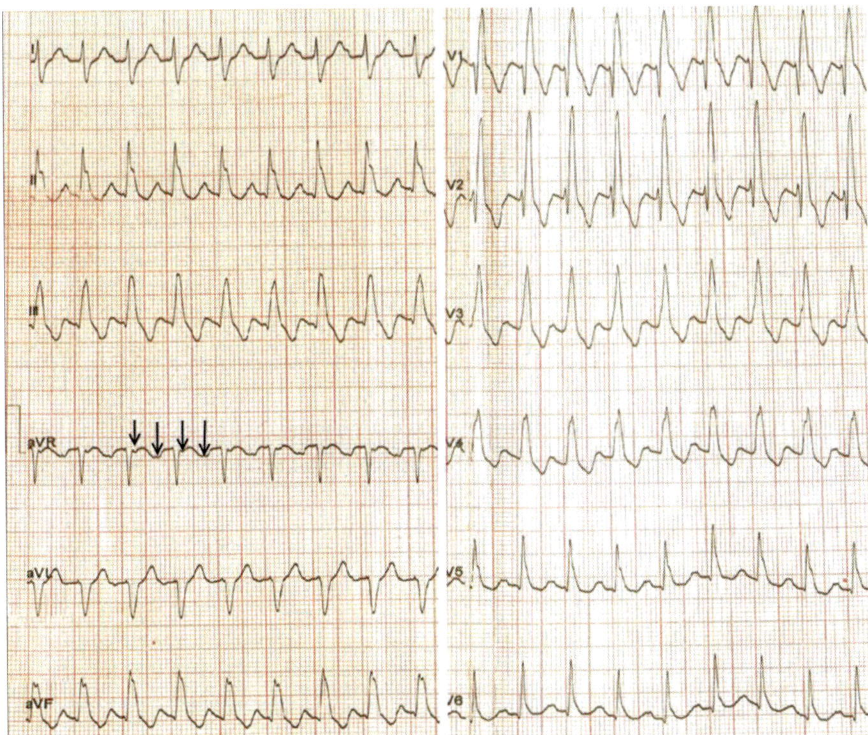

Fig. 34.3 Atrial flutter after atrial septal defect repair. This ECG shows regular wide QRS tachycardia with ventricular rate 150 beats/min and typical "sawtooth" pattern (*arrows*)

AV Nodal Reentrant Tachycardia and AV Reciprocating Tachycardia

AV reciprocating tachycardia (AVRT) and AV nodal reentrant tachycardia with reentrant mechanism are less common arrhythmia after cardiac operation. These arrhythmias are regular narrow QRS tachycardias with a heart rate of 150–250 bpm, paroxysmal initiation and termination, and P-wave deflection at the end of QRS or in the ST segment (Fig. 34.5). These arrhythmias may be controlled with vagal maneuvers but usually easily respond to intravenous adenosine. Treatment of underlying causes such as premature beats as a trigger, myocardial stress, and electrolyte disturbance has a critical role (Huang and Wood 2006).

Ventricular Tachycardias

Ventricular arrhythmia has been reported in 1–5 % of pediatric patients who have had palliative surgery for congenital heart disease; however, in Hoffman et al. study, incidence of non-sustained VT was 15.2 % (Delaney et al. 2006). VT refers

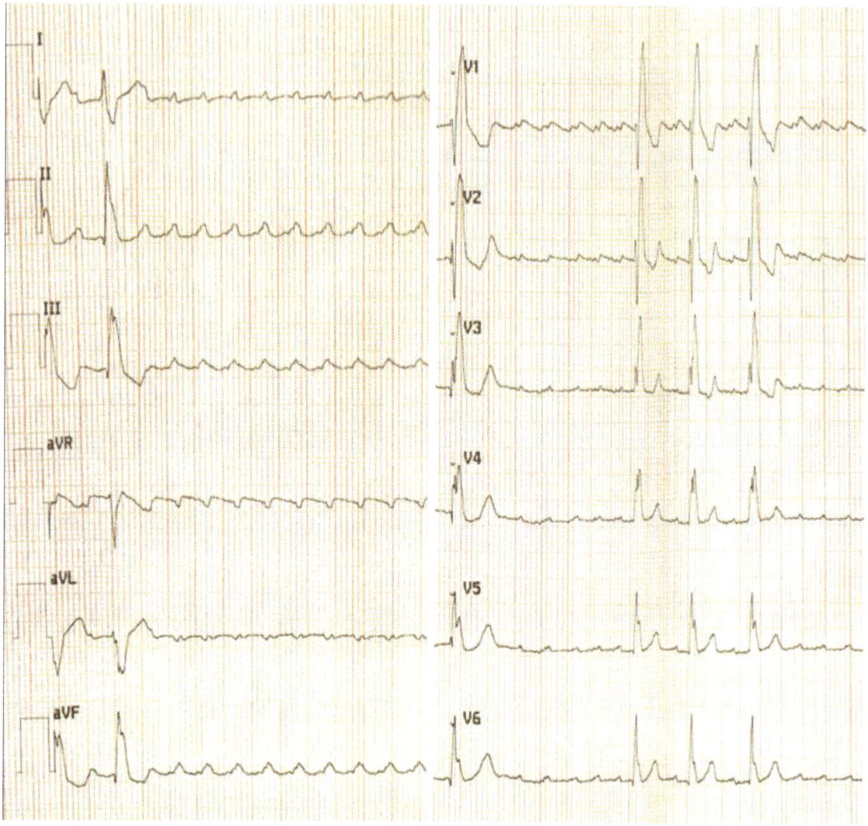

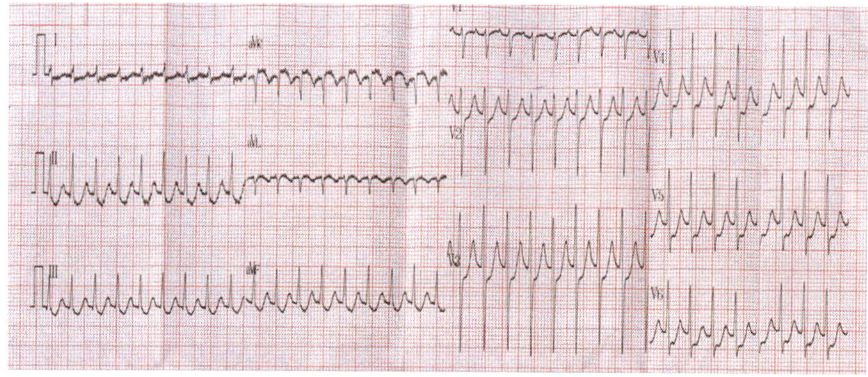

Fig. 34.4 Atrial flutter after adenosine injection. Typical "sawtooth" pattern is now clearly seen after adenosine-induced atrioventricular block

Fig. 34.5 Orthodromic atrioventricular tachycardia. Characteristic features are ST-segment depression in inferior and left precordial leads and ST-segment elevation in lead aVR

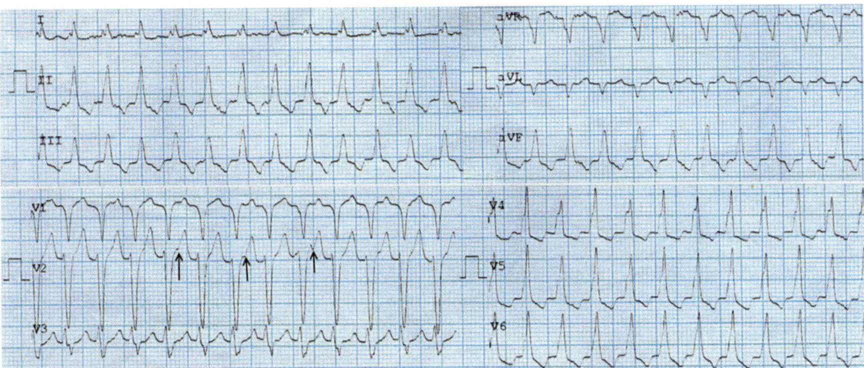

Fig. 34.6 Ventricular tachycardia after tetralogy of Fallot repair. There is atrioventricular dissociation (*arrows*), inferior axis, and left bundle branch block-type morphology (right ventricular outflow tract origin)

to wide QRS tachycardia with a heart rate ≥ 100 bpm, VA dissociation, and sometimes 1:1 VA conduction (Fig. 34.6). The SVT with aberrancy and antidromic AVRT also stay on the list of differential diagnosis of wide complex tachycardia. However, postoperative wide QRS tachycardia should be considered VT until proven otherwise.

Perioperative ischemic-reperfusion events after cardiopulmonary bypass with damage to myocardium are main predisposing factors. Measurement of myocardial biomarkers such as troponin I may be useful (Delaney et al. 2006; Pfammatter et al. 2002). Hypercathecolaminergic state, inotropes, and electrolyte and metabolic abnormalities may also predispose the pediatric patients to ventricular arrhythmias in early postoperative period (Peretto et al. 2014). Scar-related ventricular arrhythmia usually presents as monomorphic VT. This kind of arrhythmia has been observed both early and late after pediatric cardiac surgery. Some types of CHD like tetralogy of Fallot are more susceptible to this arrhythmia (Huehnergarth et al. 2008). The incidence of scar-related arrhythmia gradually increased with time, and the degree of damage to myocardium and extent of scar determine arrhythmia character and frequency (Zeppenfeld et al. 2007; Papagiannis 2005). Basically, all postoperative events that terminated to low cardiac output and decreased ventricular function could cause ventricular arrhythmia that itself could deteriorate the cardiac output that worsen the patient hemodynamic condition.

In most patients, postoperative premature ventricular complexes resolved spontaneously without serious complication. If the patient developed hemodynamically unstable VTs, immediate electrical cardioversion of 1–2 J/kg is indicated (Kleinman et al. 2010). In patients with stable sustained VT, intravenous amiodarone is the first-line therapy.

Postoperative Bradyarrhythmias

Sinus Node Dysfunction

Although sinus node dysfunction (SND) has been reported rarely in children with normal heart, it has been recognized with higher frequency in children with CHD especially after cardiac repair. SND may occur in the form of sinus arrest, sinoatrial (SA) exit block, marked sinus bradycardia, or brady-tachy syndrome. Majority of SNDs are a consequence of procedures associated with atrial tissue damage such as Mustard or Senning operation, Fontan procedure, secundum atrial septal defect (ASD) closure, and endocardial cushion defect repair (Walsh and Cecchin 2007). Only symptomatic patients require permanent pacing.

Atrioventricular Block

Despite the major progress in CHD management, atrioventricular block (AVB) continues to complicate 1–3 % of surgical repairs (Bonatti et al. 1998; Weindling et al. 1998). CHB is the most common type of conduction disturbance after CHD repair; however, second-degree and first-degree AVB may also occur. Most of postoperative CHBs are related to procedures involving the VSD closure; they usually occur early in the postoperative period; in few cases they also may occur several months or years after surgery. Early postoperative AVB can be temporary or permanent. Permanent pacing is not indicated in the former. In contrast, permanent pacing is necessary if second- or third-degree AVB persists at least 1 week after surgery, because the block is usually related to His bundle or trifascicular damage and this can be associated with risk of asystole and sudden cardiac death (Brugada et al. 2013).

Common Surgical Procedures Associated with Postoperative Arrhythmias

Atrial Septal Defect Closure

Supraventricular tachycardia is the most common arrhythmia after ASD surgical closure. The SA node dysfunction may also be observed due to surgical manipulation in the right atrium. Early postoperative arrhythmias are usually well tolerated because isolated ASD have benign course if treated in appropriate time and does not affect the cardiac reserve. Venous cannulations have a role in early arrhythmia and modification of surgical procedure decreased the incidence of arrhythmia (Bink-Boelkens et al. 1988).

In most studies, the main factor determining late postoperative arrhythmia is patient age at the time of ASD closure (Roos-Hesselinka et al. 2003; Murphy et al. 1990). Another important factor is the period of follow-up; an increased prevalence of arrhythmia was observed over the time. Patients with preoperative arrhythmia and sinus node disease have a greater chance for continuation of arrhythmia after surgery (Karpawich et al. 1965).

Ventricular Septal Defect Closure

VSD closure is the most common CHD surgical repair in pediatric group (Hoffman and Kaplan 2002). VSD type and location are the main factors in predicting conduction disorder and arrhythmia after surgery. Most of the VSDs are located in perimembranous area and less commonly in the muscular area. Understanding the anatomic course of conduction system and their relation with VSD is very important in avoiding injury to these structures. AV conduction system descends in posteroinferior rim of perimembranous VSD and left ventricular outflow tract, and therefore, this area is very susceptible to injury during surgical repair. In contrast to perimembranous VSD, AV conduction system runs at anterosuperior rim in inlet VSD and the risk of surgical damage is lower (Ho and Anderson 1985). In earlier reports, the incidence of AV block was as high as 25 %. Better knowledge of the AV conduction axis in different forms of CHD and improved surgical techniques decreased this risk to 1 % after perimembranous VSD closure (Andersen et al. 2006). Other important risk factors are Down syndrome, lower body weight, younger age, longer cardiopulmonary bypass time, higher surgical complexity, and residual defect (Tucker et al. 2007). The technique of repair has also a clear effect on postoperative arrhythmia; the prevalence of right bundle branch block (RBBB) and ventricular arrhythmias is higher in ventriculotomy approach than atriotomy (Houyel et al. 1990).

If third- or high-grade AV block persists more than 7–10 days after operation, permanent pacemaker is indicated (Brugada et al. 2013). Resolution of AV block has been observed in 9.6 % of the patients after permanent pacemaker implantation, but extraction of pacemaker in these patients is a controversial issue (Batra and Wells 2003). Sinus node dysfunction may be also observed due to venous cannulation. According to the guidelines, symptomatic SND may need pacemaker implantation (Roos-Hesselinka et al. 2006).

Atrioventricular Septal Defect Repair

Atrioventricular septal defect (AVSD) is an endocardial cushion defect that consists of a combination of ASD, VSD, and AV valve anomalies. There are two types of this anomaly: partial AVSD and complete AVSD.

Complexity of this defect makes complete surgical correction somewhat challenging. In this lesion, AV node shifted posteroinferiorly, and therefore, it may be damaged during repair. CHB is uncommon after partial AV canal repair, but complete AVSD is one of the most common settings for CHB after surgical repair. Younger age at operation, lower weight, and prolonged aortic cross clump are risk factors for CHB. Remaining residual septal defect and AV valve regurgitation predisposed patients to late postoperative arrhythmia.

Supraventricular tachyarrhythmias have been reported in 11.3 % after surgery (Chowdhury et al. 2009). Various forms of SVT including atrial flutter, atrial fibrillation, and focal atrial tachycardia were observed after surgical repair. The residual left to right shunts and AV valve regurgitation that usually progress with time and persistent of pulmonary hypertension are the risk factors for late postoperative SVT. The increased age at operation is another risk factor for SVT.

Tetralogy of Fallot Correction

The TOF correction includes VSD closure and repaired of RVOT stenosis with shaving, transannular patch, conduit, and homograft. Multiple factors are responsible for susceptibility to postoperative arrhythmias; right ventriculotomy, ventricular fibrosis, RV pressure/volume overload due to residual defects such as residual VSD, and pulmonary stenosis/regurgitation all are risk factors for developing ventricular. In addition, LV dysfunction, ventricular interaction, and mechanical dyssynchrony have a role in genesis of postoperative arrhythmias (Walsh and Cecchin 2007b).

Injury to conduction system during surgical repair results to RBBB in more than 90 % of patients. Pulmonary regurgitation effects on the PR interval and QRS duration and prolongation of these variables with time have prognostic value for the late postoperative arrhythmia.

In the study of Gatzoulis et al. (1995), QRS duration ≥ 180 ms and prolongation of QRS >5 ms/year over a 10-year period were predictors for ventricular tachycardia and late sudden death. Appropriate timing of TOF surgical correction and pulmonary valve replacement could significantly decrease the risk of ventricular arrhythmia in these patients. Late SCD is the well-recognized complication of TOF surgical correction. This complication has been reported in up to 4.6 % of patients. SCD is mainly related to ventricular arrhythmias and less commonly CHB (Chandar et al. 1990). To determine the risk of ventricular arrhythmia and SCD after surgical correction, a combination of various diagnostic modalities is necessary. These modalities include 24-h ambulatory ECG monitoring, exercise test, electrophysiologic study, signal averaging, echocardiography, and MRI (Steeds and Oakley 2004).

Ambulatory ECG monitoring is useful for evaluating PVC count and morphology. After TOF surgical correction, frequent PVCs have been reported in 20–40 % patients (Zimmermann et al. 1991; Kavey et al. 1982; Deanfield et al. 1984). Patient with PVCs and VT on resting ECG may benefit from exercise test (Garson et al. 1980). If PVCs and VT are still inducible during exercise test, patient has a significant cardiac dysfunction and may be at the risk of SCD. Suppression of PVCs during exercise testing may be associated with better prognosis, but PVC suppression does not necessarily indicate a benign prognosis.

The role of electrophysiologic study in predicting high-risk patient for sudden death still remained controversial. Chandar et al. (1990) reported that induction of sustained and non-sustained VT at EPS correlated with PVCs on ambulatory ECG monitoring and occurrence of syncope during follow-up. Two factors that associated with VT inducibility are older age at the time of repair and longer follow-up period after surgery (Dunnigan et al. 1984). Zimmermann et al. (1991) evaluated some variables that participate in ventricular arrhythmia after TOF repair. Thirty-two percent of the patients have late potentials. These patients are more likely to have inducible VT during EPS. The incidence of inducible VT during EPS in asymptomatic patients was 10 % in this study.

Surgical Repair of Univentricular Heart

Fontan procedure is a surgical technique in which blood from systemic venous return could access directly to pulmonary artery and bypass the heart. This procedure was done in congenital heart disease in which the subpulmonic ventricle or right heart is not properly formed. This surgical approach is done commonly in tricuspid atresia and pulmonary atresia. In classic Fontan, SVC is anastomosed to the right pulmonary artery and left atrial appendage to the left pulmonary artery. As a result, the right atrium is part of blood transmission pathway. There are two modifications of the original operation that are the most widely used today: In the *lateral atrial tunnel Fontan*, a baffle is placed in the right atrium to partition systemic from pulmonary venous blood, and in the *extracardiac conduit Fontan*, one end of a synthetic tube graft is connected to the inferior vena cava and the other end to the pulmonary artery confluence. Pressure and volume overload in the atria gradually provide necessary substrates for atrial arrhythmias and sinus node dysfunction. In addition, extensive atriotomy, suture lines, and injury to SA node and its blood supply are other important risk factors.

The postoperative arrhythmias have been reported in 14–50 % (Weber et al. 1666b; Porter et al. 1986; Girod et al. 1987). Atrial tachycardia is the most common arrhythmia after Fontan operation. Other arrhythmias such as JET and VT are observed less frequently. In Gelatt study (Gelatt et al. 1994), early atrial tachycardia after Fontan surgery was observed in 20 % of patients. This arrhythmia in addition to atriopulmonary connection and longer follow-up are independent risk factors for late arrhythmia. Loss of the sinus node dysfunction occurred in more than 50 % of patients during 10-year follow-up after Fontan procedure. Electrophysiologic study revealed abnormal sinus node dysfunction and intracardiac conduction delay in 60 % patients (Kurer et al. 1991). Bradyarrhythmias are usually better tolerated than tachyarrhythmia; however, SND predisposed patients to tachycardia-bradycardia syndrome. Similar to the tachyarrhythmias, early postoperative bradyarrhythmias are the predictors for late bradyarrhythmias. It appears that the incidence of early and late arrhythmias and SND is lower in *extracardiac conduit Fontan* compared with other surgical modalities (Nürnberg et al. 2004; Quinton et al. 2015).

Surgical Correction of Transposition of the Great Arteries

In transposition of great arteries (TGA), the left ventricle that received pulmonary venous return from LA is connected to the pulmonary artery, and the right ventricle that received venous return from RA is connected to the aorta. As a result, in case of inadequate mixing of right and left heart blood, severe cyanosis occurs.

Corrective surgeries include physiologic correction or atrial switch (Mustard and Senning operation) and anatomic repair or arterial switch. Anatomic LA is connected to subaortic ventricle (morphological RV) using pericardial tissue in Mustard operation and using atrial baffle in Senning operation. Also RA (received venous return) connected to subpulmonic ventricle (morphological LV). Redirecting systemic and pulmonary venous circulations in atrial switch is associated with extensive atriotomy and resultant injury to the SA node with subsequent risk of atrial tachyarrhythmia and SND.

Atrial flutter and ectopic atrial tachycardia are well-recognized arrhythmias after Mustard and Senning operation. The rate of these arrhythmias increased progressively with time along with loss of sinus rhythm and SA node function (Gillette et al. 1974; Khairy et al. 2004; Moons et al. 2004). Gelatt et al. (1997) reported sinus rhythm in 77 % patients in the first 5 years after operation that decreased to 40 % after 20 years. Predisposing factors were previous septectomy, postoperative bradycardia, and late atrial flutter. Such as Fontan operation, early postoperative arrhythmia is the risk factor for late arrhythmia and death. Anti-arrhythmic drugs are usually not effective in these patients. Pacemaker therapy is another treatment option for brady-tachy syndrome, syncope, symptomatic bradycardia, and ventricular dysfunction with bradycardia.

Arterial switch operation is associated with lesser manipulation of intracardiac structures. Therefore, atrial rhythm disturbance and arrhythmia are less common compared with atrial switch repair. Actually, corrected sinus node recovery times are normal in most patients. Furthermore, AH and HV intervals are preserved in most cases. In arterial switch, damage to AV node is uncommon and second- or third-degree AV blocks are limited to cases with VSD closure. RBBB is more common in TGA/VSD repair but also observed in TGA/IVS. Other complications after arterial switch are ventricular and atrial ectopies. Rhodes et al. (1995) reported PVCs in 70 % of patients in ambulatory ECG monitoring after operation that decreased to 30 % in mean 2.4-year follow-up. Obstruction of coronary artery during surgical anastomosis may result in myocardium ischemia/infarction and predisposed patients to ischemic ventricular arrhythmia. These patients may be asymptomatic and the presence of ventricular arrhythmia after arterial switch operation should arise suspicious to coronary artery obstruction (Mayer et al. 1990).

References

Andersen H, de Leval MR, Tsang V. Is complete heart block after surgical closure of ventricular septum defects still an issue? Ann Thorac Surg. 2006;82:948–57.

Batra AS, Wells WJ, Hinoki KW. Late recovery of atrioventricular conduction after pacemaker implantation for complete heart block associated with surgery for congenital heart disease. J Thorac Cardiovasc Surg. 2003;125:1291–3.

Batra AS, Chun DS, Johnson TR. A prospective analysis of the incidence and risk factors associated with junctional ectopic tachycardia following surgery for congenital heart disease. Pediatr Cardiol. 2006;27(1):51–5.

Bink-Boelkens MT, Meuzelaar KJ, Eygelaar A. Arrhythmias after repair of secundum atrial septal defect: the influence of surgical modification. Am Heart J. 1988;115(3):629–33.

Bonatti V, Agnetti A, Squarcia U. Early and late postoperative complete heart block in pediatric patients submitted to open-heart surgery for congenital heart disease. Pediatr Med Chir. 1998;20:181–6.

Brugada J, Blom N, Sarquella-Brugada G. Pharmacological and non-pharmacological therapy for arrhythmias in the pediatric population: EHRA and AEPC-Arrhythmia Working Group joint consensus statement. Europace. 2013;15:1337–82.

Chandar JS, Wolff GS, Garson Jr A. Ventricular arrhythmias in postoperative tetralogy of Fallot. Am J Cardiol. 1990;65(9):655–61.

Chowdhury UK, Diplomate NB, Airan B. Specific issues after surgical repair of partial atrioventricular septal: actuarial survival, freedom from reoperation, fate of the left atrioventricular valve, prevalence of left ventricular outflow tract obstruction, and other events. J Thorac Cardiovasc Surg. 2009;137:548–55.

Deanfield JE, McKenna WJ, Presbitero P. Ventricular arrhythmia in unrepaired and repaired tetralogy of Fallot. Relation to age, timing of repair, and hemodynamic status. Br Heart J. 1984;52:77–81.

Delaney J, Moltedo J, Dziura J. Early postoperative arrhythmias after pediatric cardiac surgery. J Thorac Cardiovasc Surg. 2006;131:1296–301.

Dodge-Khatami A, Miller OI, Anderson RH. Impact of junctional ectopic tachycardia on postoperative morbidity following repair of congenital heart defects. Eur J Cardiothorac Surg. 2002;21(2):255–9.

Dunnigan A, Pritzker MR, Benditt DL. Life threatening ventricular tachycardias in late survivors of surgically corrected tetralogy of Fallot. Br Heart J. 1984;52:198–206.

Garson A, Gillette PC, Gutgesell HP. Stress-Induced ventricular arrhythmia after repair of tetralogy of Fallot. Am J Cardiol. 1980;46(6):1006–12.

Gatzoulis MA, Till JA, Somerville J. Mechanoelectrical interaction in tetralogy of Fallot QRS prolongation relates to right ventricular size and predicts malignant ventricular arrhythmias and sudden death. Circulation. 1995;92:231–7.

Gelatt M, Hamilton RM, Mccrindle BW. Risk factors for atrial tachyarrhythmias after the Fontan Operation. J Am Coll Cardiol. 1994;24(7):1735–41.

Gelatt M, Hamilton RM, Mccrindle BW. Arrhythmia and mortality after the mustard procedure: a 30-year single-center experience. JACC. 1997;29(1):194–201.

Gillette PC, El-Said GM, Sivarajan N. Electrophysiological abnormalities after Mustard's operation for transposition of the great arteries. Br Heart J. 1974;36:186–91.

Girod DA, Fontan F, Deville C. Long term results after the Fontan operation for tricuspid atresia. Circulation. 1987;75:605–10.

Ho SY, Anderson RH. Conduction tissue in congenital heart surgery. World J Surg. 1985;9:550–67.

Hoffman JIE, Kaplan S. The incidence of congenital heart disease. J Am Coll Cardiol. 2002;39(12):1890–900.

Hoffman TM, Bush DM, Wernovsky G. Postoperative junctional ectopic tachycardia in children: incidence, risk factors, and treatment. Ann Thorac Surg. 2002;74(5):1607–1.

Houyel L, Vaksman NG, Fournier A. Ventricular arrhythmias after correction of ventricular septal defects: importance of surgical approach. J Am Coll Cardiol. 1990;16:1224.

Huang SK, Wood MA. Catheter ablation of cardiac arrhythmias. Philadelphia: W.B. Saunders; 2006.

Huehnergarth KV, Gurvitz M, Stout KK, Otto CM. Repaired tetralogy of Fallot in the adult: monitoring and management. Heart. 2008;94:1663–9.

Karpawich P, Antillon JR, Cappola PR. Pre- and Postoperative Electrophysiologic Assessment of Children with Secundum Atrial Septal Defect. Am J Cardiol. 1965;55:519–21.

Kavey RW, Blackman MS, Sondheimer HM. Incidence and severity of chronic ventricular arrhythmias after repair of tetralogy of Fallot. Am Heart J. 1982;103:342–50.

Khairy P, Landzberg MJ, Lambert J, et al. Long-term outcomes after the atrial switch for surgical correction of transposition: a meta-analysis comparing the Mustard and Senning procedures. Cardiol Young. 2004;14:284–92.

Kleinman ME, Chameides L, Schexnayder SM. Part 14: pediatric advanced life support 2010 American Heart Association Guidelines for cardiopulmonary resuscitation and emergency cardiovascular care. Circulation. 2010;122:S876–908.

Kovacikova L, Hakacova N, Dobos D. Amiodarone as a first-line therapy for postoperative junctional ectopic tachycardia. Ann Thorac Surg. 2009;88:616–22.

Kurer C, Tanner C, Vetter V. Electrophysiologic findings after Fontan repair of functional single ventricle. J Am Coll Cardiol. 1991;17:174–81.

Lan Y, Lee J, Wetzel G. Postoperative arrhythmia. Curr Opin Cardiol. 2003;18:73–8.

Mayer Jr JE, Sanders SP, Jonas RA, et al. Coronary artery pattern and outcome of arterial switch operation for transposition of the great arteries. Circulation. 1990;82:139–45.

Mildh L, Hiippala A. Rautiainen junctional ectopic tachycardia after surgery for congenital heart disease: incidence, risk factors and outcome. Eur J Cardiothorac Surg. 2011;39(1):75–80.

Moons P, Gewillig M, Sluysmans T, et al. Long term outcome up to 30 years after the Mustard or Senning operation: a nationwide multicenter study in Belgium. Heart. 2004;90:307–13.

Murphy JG, Gersh BJ, McGoon MD. Longterm outcome after surgical repair of isolated atrial septal defect: follow-up at 27 to 32 years. N Engl J Med. 1990;323:1645–50.

Nürnberg JH, Ovroutski S, Alexi-Meskishvili V. New onset arrhythmias after the extracardiac conduit Fontan Operation compared with the intra-atrial lateral tunnel procedure: early and midterm results. Ann Thorac Surg. 2004;78:1979–88.

Papagiannis J. Postoperative arrhythmias in tetralogy of Fallot. Hell J Cardiol. 2005;46:402–7.

Peretto G, Durante A, Limite LR. Postoperative arrhythmias after cardiac surgery: incidence, risk factors, and therapeutic management. Cardiol Res Pract. 2014;2014:15. Article ID 615987.

Perry J, Fenrich A, Edward HJ. Pediatric use of intravenous amiodarone: efficacy and safety in critically ill patients from a multicenter protocol. JACC. 1996;27(5):1246–50.

Pfammatter JP, Wagner B, Berdat P. Procedural factors associated with early postoperative arrhythmias after repair of congenital heart defects. J Thorac Cardiovasc Surg. 2002;123:258–62.

Porter CJ, Battiste LE, Humes RA. Risk factors for supraventricular tachyarrhythmias after Fontan procedure for tricuspid atresia (abstr). Am Heart J. 1986;112:645.

Probst V, Denjoy I, Meregalli PG. Clinical aspects and prognosis of Brugada syndrome in children. Circulation. 2007;115:2042–8.

Quinton E, Nightingale P, Hudsmith L. Prevalence of atrial tachyarrhythmia in adults after Fontan operation. Heart. 2015;101(20):1672–7. doi:10.1136/heartjnl-2015-307514.

Rekawek J, Kansy A, Miszczak-Knecht M. Risk factors for cardiac arrhythmias in children with congenital heart disease after surgical intervention in the early postoperative period. J Thorac Cardiovasc Surg. 2007;133:900–4.

Rhodes LA, Wernovsky G, Keane JF. Arrhythmias and intracardiac conduction after the arterial switch operation. J Thorac Cardiovasc Surg. 1995;109(2):303–10.

Roos-Hesselinka JW, Meijbooma FJ, Spitaelsa SEC. Excellent survival and low incidence of arrhythmias, stroke and heart failure long-term after surgical ASD closure at young age A prospective follow-up study of 21–33 years. Eur Heart J. 2003;24:190–7.

Roos-Hesselinka JW, Meijbooma FJ, Spitaelsa SEC. Outcome of patients after surgical closure of ventricular septal defect at young age follow-up of 22–34 years. Ann Thorac Surg. 2006;82:948–57.

Steeds RP, Oakley D. Predicting late sudden death from ventricular arrhythmia in adults following surgical repair of tetralogy of Fallot. Q J Med. 2004;97:7–13.

Texter KM, Kertesz NJ, Friedman RA. Atrial flutter in infants. J Am Coll Cardiol. 2006;48:1040–6.

Triedman JK. Arrhythmias in adults with congenital heart disease. Heart. 2002;87:383–9.

Tucker EM, Pyles LA, Bass JL. Permanent pacemaker for atrioventricular conduction block after operative repair of perimembranous ventricular septal defect. J Am Coll Cardiol. 2007;50(12):1196–200.

Walsh EP, Cecchin F. Arrhythmias in adult patients with congenital heart disease. Circulation. 2007;115:534–45.

Walsh EP, Saul JP, Hulse JE. Transcatheter ablation of ectopic atrial tachycardia in young patients using radiofrequency current. Circulation. 1992;86:1138–46.

Weber H, Hellenbrand W, Kleinman C. Predictors of rhythm disturbances and subsequent morbidity after the Fontan operation. Am J Cardiol. 1666;64:762–7.

Weindling SN, Saul JP, Gamble WJ, Mayer JE, Wessel D, Walsh EP. Duration of complete atrioventricular block after congenital heart disease surgery. Am J Cardiol. 1998;82:525–7.

Yildirim SV, Tokel K, Saygili B. The incidence and risk factors of arrhythmias in the early period after cardiac surgery in pediatric patients. Turk J Pediatr. 2008;50(6):549–53.

Zampi J, Hirsch J, Gurney J. Junctional ectopic tachycardia after infant heart surgery: incidence and outcomes. Pediatr Cardiol. 2012;33:1362–9.

Zeppenfeld K, Schalij MJ, Bartelings MM. Catheter ablation of ventricular tachycardia after repair of congenital heart disease: electroanatomic identification of the critical right ventricular isthmus. Circulation. 2007;116(20):2241–52.

Zimmermann M, Friedli B, Adamec R. Ventricular late potentials and induced ventricular arrhythmias after surgical repair of tetralogy of Fallot. Am J Cardiol. 1991;67:873–8.

Chapter 35
Postoperative Respiratory Management in Pediatric Cardiac Surgical Patients

Ali Dabbagh

How Does the Pediatric Patient Differ from the Adult Patient?

There are a number of main anatomic and physiologic differences between adult and children regarding airway and ventilation. These changes are most significant during neonatal period up to 1 year of age. Major differences are as follows (Dickison 1987; Adewale 2009; Walker and Ellwood 2009; Baker and Parico 2010; Heinrich et al. 2012; Sunder et al. 2012; Harless et al. 2014).

Anatomy

- The *occiput* is really protruding and the *head* is large enough to induce head flexion and major impediments in alignment of the airway for intubation.
- The *tongue* is larger compared with adults.
- Generally, the *airway* is smaller with a very small opening.
- More *cephalic location* of the airway located at the level of third and fourth cervical spines (C3 and C4); however, the airway moves more caudally as the child grows up, mainly as a result of cervical spine growth.
- The pediatric airway is *loose* compared with adults, since it has less cartilaginous tissue.
- The *epiglottis* is more edematous and floppy, having a "U"-shaped feature.
- Vocal cords do not conform a right angle with the larynx; instead, they have an anterior-inferior to posterior-superior angled fashion.

A. Dabbagh, MD
Cardiac Anesthesiology Department, Anesthesiology Research Center,
Shahid Beheshti University of Medical Sciences, Tehran, Iran
e-mail: alidabbagh@yahoo.com; alidabbagh@sbmu.ac.ir

© Springer International Publishing Switzerland 2017
A. Dabbagh et al. (eds.), *Congenital Heart Disease in Pediatric
and Adult Patients*, DOI 10.1007/978-3-319-44691-2_35

- Maybe the most practical point is that the *narrowest point* in pediatric airway is located distal to the vocal cords, while in adults, vocal cords are the narrowest part of airway; this is because of the shape of the larynx in pediatric patients which is *funnel shaped*, while larynx in adults is tunnel shaped.
- The *trachea* is smaller and shorter, increasing the chance for one lung intubation with the least neck movements.
- Adult difficult airway algorithms do not necessarily work for children and neonates, and pediatric difficult airway algorithms should be always available.

Physiology

There are a number of physiologic differences between adult and pediatric patients, mainly the following (Commare et al. 1994; Tripp and Bolton 1998; Ahmadpour-Kacho et al. 2011):

- The lung volume compared to weight is much smaller in children and neonates.
- The airway cross-sectional area is smaller creating higher resistance of airway.
- *Nasal ventilation* is the main route of ventilation especially in neonates.
- *Functional residual capacity* (FRC) compared to weight is less than adults leading to smaller reserve volumes which decompensates saturation much earlier during respiratory distress or induction of anesthesia or sedation for intubation.
- *Less cartilaginous structure* of the upper airway components and large lower airways leads to dynamic airway compression during forceful ventilation which is an early component of respiratory distress, since it induces more negative inspiratory pressure and more respiratory distress and finally, this would lead to aggravated ventilation and more respiratory distress in a vicious cycle.
- Smaller size of the *lower airways* leads to much more severe decrease in the total area of the airway due to a presumed airway edema compared to adults.
- The *main respiratory muscle* in neonates and adults is *diaphragm*; accessory muscles are neither efficient, nor they play a significant role in respiration; would there be any failure of diaphragm (e.g., due to paralysis of vagus nerve during the surgery), postoperative ventilation would be severely impaired; especially when considering that the respiratory muscles may even consume as much as 40 % of cardiac output and in a patient with underlying cardiac disease, it would be laboriously and rigorously tolerated.

On the other side, though there are many differences between adult and pediatric population, if pediatric acute respiratory distress syndrome happens, age is not considered as a criteria for definitive diagnosis (Pediatric Acute Lung Injury Consensus Conference Group 2015; Khemani et al. 2015).

Principals and Goals of Mechanical Ventilation

The history of mechanical ventilation has been attributed to decades ago; Galen has been cited as the first person to describe mechanical ventilation (Cheifetz 2003); however, there are a number of evidence available that demonstrate Avicenna, a Persian physician, has described tracheostomy, oropharyngeal intubation, and upper airway secretion clearing, all to treat stridor and respiratory distress (Aziz et al. 2000; Golzari et al. 2013; Dabbagh et al. 2014).

The main principle in mechanical ventilation is using life-support devices or respiratory assist maneuvers (or technologies) for supporting ventilation (partially or totally) in such a way that the physiologic compromise in respiratory function of the patient could be compensated for and/or improvements in patient comfort occurs (Villar et al. 2007; Pediatric Acute Lung Injury Consensus Conference Group 2015).

During the postoperative period of pediatric cardiac surgery, the time for post-bypass transition and subsiding of inflammatory response and edema is among the major time intervals that needs ventilatory support; it may be as positive pressure ventilation or could be as respiratory maneuvers used for assistance of ventilation. Also, there are minutes or hours that we should allow for observation of the respiratory status in controlled environment.

> Post-bypass transition and subsiding of inflammatory response and edema and also time interval needed for observation of respiratory status are critical events in pediatric cardiac surgery patients.

In general, the following have been considered as the main indications for utilization of mechanical ventilation:

- *Respiratory* indications: these include apnea, bradypnea, hypoventilation, chronic pulmonary lung disease, impaired oxygen and CO_2 transportation leading to respiratory failure, and respiratory exhaustion impending to arrest.
- *Cardiopulmonary support* and *cardiac indications* for installing mechanical ventilation: cardiopulmonary arrest and low cardiac output syndrome mandating removal of the work of breathing due to impaired ventricular function.
- *Neurologic* indications: especially when central drive of ventilation is impaired or when the level of consciousness is not appropriate enough leading to impaired protective reflexes and subsequent aspiration of the secretions and impaired pulmonary toilet.
- *Multiorgan disease* impairing many body systems including lungs.
- *Procedural-induced* disease processes like post-cardiopulmonary bypass.

Based on the above indications, the main goals of mechanical ventilation could be summarized as:

- Optimizing *gas exchange* through optimization of pulmonary mechanisms, removing underlying shunts or V/Q mismatches, optimization of airway protection, and installation of pulmonary toilet
- Providing *cardiopulmonary support* during post-bypass transition especially in low cardiac output, hemodynamic unstable patients, patients with inflammatory response, and patients with edema in lung tissues
- Improving *patient comfort* (which includes decreasing respiratory distress, alleviating the degree of upper and/or lower airway obstruction, decreasing the amount of oxygen consumption, and alleviating respiratory fatigue)
- Decreasing *work of breathing* imposed to patient
- Preventing any possible *ventilator-induced injury* to the respiratory system (mainly the lungs)
- Administering *inhaled pharmaceuticals*

Ventilation Considerations and Its Challenges Unique to the Congenital Heart Disease Patients

In congenital heart patients, a number of factors intervene with usual lung mechanics during artificial ventilation. These patients may have one or a number of the following especial items:

Mixing lesions and cardiac shunts These patients may have simultaneous hypoxemia (i.e., right to left shunts) or pulmonary volume overload and overcirculation (i.e., left to right shunts); the cyanotic patient needs care in order to prevent any increase in pulmonary vascular resistance; otherwise, the degree of cyanosis and the frequency and severity of cyanotic spells aggravate; measures must be taken to keep these patients pain-free, to prevent hypercarbia and/or hypoxia as much as possible, and to treat acidosis; in addition, the balance between pulmonary vascular resistance and systemic vascular resistance should be managed to prevent right to left shunting.

On the other hand, there are some patients who have *shunt-dependent pulmonary or systemic circulation*; sophisticated care should be taken to prevent shunt closure; otherwise, significant hemodynamic impairments happen; acidosis and/or organ ischemia occurs due to impaired perfusion distal to the shunt after its unplanned closure (e.g., patients with patent ductus arteriosus in whom perfusion distal to the shunt should be kept going to prevent distal body ischemia/necrosis).

Another major challenge in these patients is the process of weaning and extubation, though the general principles of extubation are discussed later in this chapter. However, infants who have shunt-dependent pulmonary blood flow and univentricular physiology are prone to high rate of extubation failure, mainly because cardiac and respiratory results of positive pressure ventilation are much more determining (Gupta et al. 2014).

Perioperative care of single ventricle physiology (including HLHS and Fontan procedure): during the recent years, with introduction of fast track anesthesia for congenital heart diseases, perioperative care of single ventricle patients has been moved toward early extubation or even "on the table" extubation since pain-free, spontaneous ventilation (i.e., negative-pressure ventilation) improves venous drainage after operation, leading to improved postoperative hemodynamics, decreased length of stay, and earlier ICU discharge. On the other hand, if underlying pulmonary hypertension persists and inhaled nitric oxide is going to be used, mechanical ventilation through endotracheal tube is the most favorable option, though iNO administration through nasal cannula or facemask is available; however, they are not the preferred route for iNO administration. Studies have shown that preoperative pulmonary hypertension is a risk factor for Fontan patients which may hinder earlier extubation; however, patients with univentricular physiology are prone to high rate of extubation failure (Lofland 2001; Fiorito and Checchia 2002; Morales et al. 2008; Gupta et al. 2014).

Right or left ventricular failure Usually, congenital heart surgeries are among the corrective procedures, and if managed properly, there is a little chance for right or left ventricular failure; however, there are a considerable number of patients who are at risk and mainly include those who have been neglected for a while, their treatment has been delayed, they have tolerated volume overload due to mixing lesions or pressure overload due to obstructive lesions, and now, the sequela of overload is presented as right or left ventricular failure or, even in worst cases, pulmonary hypertension. These patients need the most vigorous treatments including a long list of drugs, mechanical ventilation, a number of assist devices assisting right ventricle and left ventricle or biventricular assist devices, and, even at times, heart or heart and lung transplant. The impact of ventricular failure, especially left ventricle on the lungs is a real challenge. More sophisticated discussion on assist devices or transplant is reviewed in Chap. 33 – Heart Transplantation and Mechanical Circulatory Support in the Congenital Heart Patients (Pediatric Acute Lung Injury Consensus Conference Group 2015; Dalton and Macrae 2015; Emeriaud and Newth 2015; Essouri and Carroll 2015; Flori et al. 2015; Khemani et al. 2015; Quasney et al. 2015; Rimensberger and Cheifetz 2015; Sapru et al. 2015; Tamburro and Kneyber 2015; Valentine et al. 2015).

Fluid management is among the most important issues in postoperative management especially considering the effects of cardiopulmonary bypass and also varying degrees of underlying cardiac abnormalities; usually, fluid overload occurs early after cardiac surgical procedures; fluid overload leads to fewer ventilator-free days (VFDs), impaired oxygenation, impaired ventilation, lung edema, increased ICU stay, and impaired clinical condition, finally leading to worsening clinical outcome; of particular interest is prevention of *early* fluid overload which could significantly affect the clinical outcome (Arikan et al. 2012; Hassinger et al. 2014; Seguin et al. 2014; Khemani et al. 2015; Sinitsky et al. 2015; Ingelse et al. 2016).

Strategies for Ventilation and Ventilator Modes

Whatever the indication for using mechanical ventilation, these three main issues should always be kept in mind:

1. Mechanical ventilation *does not have a therapeutic role*; instead, it is a *supportive* measure.
2. The *process of weaning and extubation* should start at the first feasible and possible opportunity; in fact, whenever the pediatric patient can sustain his/her spontaneous breathing, weaning should start.
3. Mechanical ventilation always leads to *different degrees of lung lesions*; the endotracheal tube or other devices impose injuries and the patients are not easy, needing sedative agents; there is risk of infections and ventilator-associated pneumonia (VAP); cardiac-pulmonary interference may occur; however, the degree of lesion could be a wide range, from mild to severe, depending on the duration of ventilation and the technologies used for it (Villar et al. 2007; Newth et al. 2009; Bagheri et al. 2016).

Weaning, Readiness for Extubation, and Extubation Failure

Weaning Ventilator Support and Spontaneous Breathing Trials (SBTs)

The weaning process should be managed using the following maneuvers or ventilation criteria, in combination with a number of monitoring methods including respiratory and hemodynamic monitoring:

- Rate of mechanical ventilation
- Tidal volume (volume support ventilation weaning in volume-controlled modes)
- Pressure support (pressure support ventilation weaning in pressure-controlled modes)
- SBTs and CPAP (usually, infants intubated for more than 3 days need nasal CPAP and then nasal prongs after extubation)
- Extubation readiness test (ERT)

Considering these facts in mind, the general practice is in favor of keeping moderate amounts of ventilator support during weaning in such a way that the patient could have some respiratory muscle rest and perform daily ERT (Feldman 2015).

However, the current practice of pediatric mechanical ventilation and weaning is confronted with a lack of explicit ventilator protocols; as a matter of fact, this practice is a "selective adoption of adult mechanical ventilation principles"; however, many aspects of these adult protocols are associated with major challenges or at least doubts and dilemmas when "embraced" in pediatric critical care. Also, based on a recently published Cochrane systematic review by Wielenga et al., no evidence is available in supporting or rejecting "protocolled" over "non-protocolled" weaning on duration of mechanical ventilation with invasive ventilation modes in newborn infants (Schindler 2005; Khemani and Newth 2010; Bennett et al. 2014; Khemani et al. 2015; Wielenga et al. 2016).

Prediction Tests for Extubation Success

The clinical tests used for prediction of extubation were used first in research; however, they are now currently used in clinical practice. There are currently three tests used more commonly for prediction of extubation success; these include:

- *Rapid shallow breathing index* (RSBI = f/Vt): this index was first described by Yang and Tobin; it has a high sensitivity and low specificity which will be a reliable screening test for successful weaning; this index is a good practical predictor for extubation; higher RSBIs are predictive of extubation failure (Yang and Tobin 1991; Tobin and Jubran 2006; Newth et al. 2009).
- *Compliance, resistance, oxygenation, and pressure (CROP) index*: this index is another predictive measure for the assessment of adequacy of ventilation; CROP index is calculated with four variables:

$$CROP = Dynamic\,Compliance \times Maximal\,Negative\,Inspiratory\,Pressure \\ \times \left(PaO_2 \,/\, PAO_2\right) /\, Respiratory\,Rate$$

Lower CROP index values are predictive of extubation failure; especially with a CROP value of ≥ 0.15 ml/kg/breaths/min (Baumeister et al. 1997; Thiagarajan et al. 1999; Newth et al. 2009; Emeriaud and Newth 2015).

- *Volumetric capnography* draws the diagram of capnography considering concentration of CO_2 in airway gas versus volume of expiration. The slop of the diagram helps us calculate physiologic dead space which is the ratio of "dead space/tidal volume" or "V_D/V_T." If the V_D/V_T ratio is less than 0.05, extubation could be predicted successful; however, if the V_D/V_T ratio is more than 0.65, then extubation is predicted to be failed.

"Ready for Departure": Preparing for Extubation

Extubation criteria include a number of general clinical conditions and some measurable tests; clinical criteria for extubation are briefed in Table 38.1.

Table 38.1 Clinical criteria for extubation

CNS and muscular system	Wakefulness: the patient should be sufficiently awake
	The tone of muscles should be working completely in such a way to grasp firmly the objects like fingers of examiner or produce strong and forceful cough
Airway	Patent upper airway is mandatory which is tested through performing air leak test around the endotracheal tube
	Airway reflexes intact in such a way that could protect the lungs from aspiration
Cardiovascular system	Stable cardiovascular and hemodynamic parameters
	Minimal dose of inotropes
Respiratory system	Minimal respiratory secretions which will not create a clinical problem Normal range for breath sounds
	Ability to produce strong and forceful cough
	$SpO_2 > 94$ with minimal supplemental O_2 requirement (i.e., <30 %) Minimal need for pressure support (5–10 more than PEEP)
Water and electrolytes	No significant blood gas and/or electrolyte abnormalities
	Controlled water and loading status

Common tests used for assessment of extubation readiness include:

- Respiratory muscle strength demonstrated by negative inspiratory force (NIF)
- ETT "leak test" which assesses the leakage of air around the endotracheal tube and checks for upper airway patency; however, Wratney et al. demonstrated that an air leak pressure $\geq$ 30 cm H_2O in the non-paralyzed patient (either in the time before extubation or during the time of mechanical ventilation) cannot predict an increased risk for extubation failure (Wratney et al. 2008)

The "Extubation Procedure"

The following steps are basic steps in the extubation procedure:

- Ensuring adequacy of clinical criteria for extubation (Table 38.1).
- Sterile suctioning of the oropharynx, nostrils, and endotracheal tube.
- Emptying gastric contents through suctioning nasogastric tube.
- Having nasal prongs on the face before extubation and preparing oxygen face-mask, in order to decrease the chance of immediate hypoxia.
- Checking equipment for assisting ventilation devices including mask and bag attached to oxygen; devices for NIPPV or CPAP should be available.
- Checking for laryngoscope and different blades and blade sizes, different size tubes, and other ventilation devices to be available.
- Ventilator and related tubing should be ready.
- Checking for sedatives and muscle relaxants, adjusted by weight and including rapid sequence induction agents per needed.

- Checking for nebulizers including epinephrine and other agents to be available.
- Selected corticosteroids should be available as bolus and infusion doses to decrease any hoarseness or respiratory distress; also, diuretics should be available to treat volume overload and respiratory distress; of course, there is no proof that corticosteroids could prevent or treat post-extubation stridor in neonates or children (Khemani et al. 2009).
- Respiratory monitoring including arterial blood gases should be available.
- Describing the procedure for parents.

Predictors of Extubation Failure

Extubation failure (EF) is defined as *reintubation within 24–72 h*; based on pediatric studies, a failed extubation rate less than 10 % is accepted as the norm (Kurachek et al. 2003; Rothaar and Epstein 2003; Newth et al. 2009; Artime and Hagberg 2014; Saikia et al. 2015). Whatever the rate of EF, the trend of pediatric EF has significant differences with adults, including:

- The majority of pediatric patients weaned from mechanical ventilation in 2 days or less.
- RSBI, CROP, and volumetric capnography, though considered as criteria for prediction of extubation success, could be used as measures of prediction for EF.
- Protocols used in adult weaning with significant effect on extubation trend *do not have a significant effect* on time for weaning in pediatrics and neonates; in fact, there is paucity of evidence in supporting or rejecting the effects of "protocolled" over "non-protocolled" weaning regarding duration of mechanical ventilation.
- EF rate does not have significant difference between pressure support ventilation weaning, volume support ventilation weaning, and other methods.
- Obstruction of the upper airway is claimed as the most common etiologic factor for EF (Newth et al. 2009).
- The incidence of EF is higher in these patients:

1. Neonates and infants.
2. Patients with underlying cyanotic congenital heart disease.
3. Patients under prolonged mechanical ventilation.
4. Patients with increased RSBI, inadequate cough reflex, and thick unmanageable secretions could increase the chance for EF and could be used as predictive measures (Thiagarajan et al. 1999; Randolph et al. 2002; Rothaar and Epstein 2003; Newth et al. 2009; Khemani and Newth 2010; Artime and Hagberg 2014; Gupta et al. 2014; Saikia et al. 2015; Wielenga et al. 2016).

Noninvasive Ventilation

RAM Cannula

Nasal cannulas, nasal prongs, or often called RAM cannulas can deliver supplementary oxygen to the patient in relatively low amounts. They are mainly used when we decide to administer oxygen but the desired increase in FiO_2 is not so much high. FiO_2 increase by nasal prongs depends mainly on these factors:

- Oxygen flow
- The pattern of respiration of the patient

The following table demonstrates estimates of FiO_2 when applying nasal prongs:

Oxygen flow (liters per minute)	Highest achievable FiO_2 (%)
1	24
2	27
3	30
4 (*needs humidification*)	33
5 (*needs humidification*)	35
6 (*needs humidification*)	38

RAM cannula can induce CPAP when the nostrils are partially occluded by the cannula; some authors are in favor of this issue, while the others do not believe so (Iyer and Chatburn 2015; Nzegwu et al. 2015; Aktas et al. 2016; Gerdes et al. 2016).

nCPAP

Neonatal continuous positive airway pressure (nCPAP) is the special CPAP used for neonates aiming to use a noninvasive ventilation mode with the following goals:

- Improving oxygenation status
- Increasing functional residual capacity (FRC)
- Decreasing intrapulmonary shunts
- Decreasing the degree of alveolar collapse
- Decreasing ventilator-induced lung injury
- Decreasing the incidence of lung complications like VAP
- Decreasing the chance for reintubation
- Reducing the rate of readmission to critical care unit
- Decreasing mortality

More than 40 years has passed from invention of nCPAP; however, during the last years, great improvements have been made. According to Diblasi, the two most influential factors affecting outcome in neonates treated with nCPAP are "clinicians' abilities to perceive changes" which occur in pathophysiology of the infants who are under treatment with nCPAP and "quality of airway management"; also, other studies have demonstrated that careful selection of appropriate patient associated with the level of training and experience in ICU team affects the outcome. Although some believe that nCPAP and other noninvasive methods are good enough to prevent reintubation in neonates and infants after cardiac surgery, there is a significant difference between alternative modes of nCPAP and other noninvasive modes of ventilation; also, in neonates, risk of nasal injury and sternal dehiscence is real (Kurt et al. 2008; Diblasi 2009; Squires and Hyndman 2009; Zarbock et al. 2009; Boeken et al. 2010; Pelosi and Jaber 2010; Drevhammar et al. 2012; Bancalari and Claure 2013).

One of the Cochrane systematic reviews published in 2014 has compared noninvasive positive pressure ventilation (NIPPV) with nCPAP for preterm neonates after extubation (Lemyre et al. 2014) and has stated that:

- Clinical signs of extubation failure are significantly less common after using NIPPV compared with nCPAP.
- Reintubation within 2–7 days after extubation is less with NIPPV.
- These differences have no effect on chronic lung disease or mortality rate.
- Synchronization could have an important role in NIPPV.

High-Flow Nasal Cannula (HFNC)

HFNC has been extensively used in pediatric ICUs during the last 10 years, at times replacing nCPAP, due to its simple basics of function and excellent tolerance by the patients, especially because HFNC delivers humidified and warm air which is much better tolerated than cold air. HFNC delivers high flow rate of heated (34°C and 37°C) and humidified gas, often as much as 2 L/kg/min of blended air and oxygen which is heated and humidified. Some clinicians believe that it can improve the respiratory function in the following items (Manley et al. 2013; Yoder et al. 2013; Milesi et al. 2014; Wilkinson et al. 2016):

- Washout of dead space in the nasopharynx
- Improved gas exchange
- Clearance of the pulmonary mucociliary tract
- Lung oxygen delivery
- Humidification of delivered gases to the lungs
- Improved breathing pattern and decreased work of ventilation and breathing
- Post-extubation ventilatory support

There are some controversies about the efficacy of HFNCs. For example, two different Cochrane Database of Systematic Reviews published in 2014 have somewhat questioned (with different degrees of uncertainty) the efficacy of HFNC for infants with bronchiolitis and for children (Beggs et al. 2014; Mayfield et al. 2014).

On the other hand, a Cochrane Database of Systematic Reviews published in 2016 concluded that using HFNC could be useful as post-extubation support, with decreased chance of nasal trauma and pneumothorax in comparison with nasal CPAP (Wilkinson et al. 2016).

Miscellaneous Issues

Extracorporeal CO_2 Removal: $ECCO_2R$

$ECCO_2R$ implies partial respiratory support which can help remove carbon dioxide out of the blood using low levels of blood flow through an extracorporeal circuit with minimal effects on blood oxygenation. In patients under mechanical ventilation, there is always a chance for ventilator-induced lung injury (VILI); there are some ventilation modalities to counteract VILI; among them, ultra-protective ventilation strategies could be named which results in normal peak inspiratory pressure, very low tidal volumes, near normal lung oxygenation, and lower values for minute ventilation; this leads to nearly appropriate oxygenation, while hypercarbia remains a problem. $ECCO_2R$ is often used as part of ultra-protective ventilation strategies in order to remove CO_2 out of the body and compensate for CO_2 accumulation in ultra-protective ventilation strategies. In $ECCO_2R$, the amount of blood being perfused is very much lower than the amount of perfusion provided by ECMO. Also, $ECCO_2R$ is not a new modality; however, during the last years, its application in association with ultra-protective ventilation strategies has gained much more popularity (Habashi et al. 1995a; Habashi et al. 1995b; Kaushik et al. 2012; Camporota and Barrett 2016; Deniau et al. 2016).

HFV or HFOV

High-frequency ventilation or high-frequency oscillatory ventilation seems a superb protective measure in perioperative care of congenital heart disease children with injured lungs using very small and tiny tidal volumes and high rate of ventilation in order to keep airway pressure at the modest possible level. Though institution of HFV is delayed, there is a shift toward the early use of HFV during the last years. However, there is still paucity of evidence to demonstrate clearly the improved outcomes of early institution of HFV in respect to lung protection (Fessler et al. 2008; Khemani and Newth 2010).

Effect of HFV on outcome Based on the systematic review and meta-analysis performed by Duyndam et al., the available evidence scarcely supports that HFV can decrease mortality and length of stay in critically ill children beyond the newborn period (Duyndam et al. 2011). In addition, Henderson–Smart et al.

conducted a Cochrane Database of Systematic Reviews and showed that no controlled trial supports the use of HFOV in term or near-term infants with severe pulmonary dysfunction (Henderson-Smart et al. 2009).

Inhalational Routes of Drug Delivery

The list of drugs administered through inhalational route is an increasing list, especially with the application of newly designed targeted therapies, including nanostructured materials and nanostructured carriers (Dabbagh and Rajaei 2011). This is a list of drugs being used as inhalational therapies:

- Inhalational drugs used in treatment of *pulmonary hypertension* are very good and common examples; agents like iNO and treprostinil are used for treatment of pulmonary hypertension; they are fully discussed in Chap. 29– Pulmonary Hypertension.
- Inhaled insulin which is recently approved by FDA.
- Many antibiotics like inhalational ciprofloxacin encapsulated in liposomes or antituberculosis drugs which causes "massive reduction" of drug dose and decreased toxicity (Wood 1991; O'Callaghan 1994; Rastogi et al. 2006; Gupta and Ahsan 2010; Dabbagh and Rajaei 2011; Petkar et al. 2011; Stream and Bull 2012; Hamblin et al. 2014; Brashier et al. 2015).

Chest Physiotherapy

In patients undergoing congenital cardiac surgeries, using standard protocols for physiotherapy might improve pulmonary status; physiotherapy, especially aerobic exercise, could be useful in improving exercise capacity and also postoperative pulmonary function and cardiopulmonary fitness; however, this is a matter of controversy. In a systematic review, Pasquina et al. demonstrated that there is no proof for usefulness of prophylactic respiratory physiotherapy in prevention of pulmonary complications after cardiac surgery (Pasquina et al. 2003; Nagarajan et al. 2011; Kaminski et al. 2013; Duppen et al. 2015).

Chronic Respiratory Failure and Tracheostomy

Many years have passed since the first introduction of tracheostomy; even, many believe that it has been used in Medieval Islamic physicians, Avicenna to be named (Golzari et al. 2013; Dabbagh et al. 2014). The recently published analysis of the *Society of Thoracic Surgeons Congenital Heart Surgery Database* demonstrated an increasing rate of tracheostomy due to congenital heart surgery. The main indications were divided as preoperative indications (mainly prematurity, genetic anomalies, and preoperative mechanical ventilation) vs. postoperative ones (cardiac arrest, modes of extracorporeal support, injuries to the phrenic or laryngeal nerves, and neurologic insults); also, based on this report, the operative mortality was 25 % (Donnelly et al. 1996; Al-Samri et al. 2010; Mastropietro et al. 2016).

On the other hand, when speaking about different aspects of tracheostomy in congenital heart surgeries, the following items are still among the most controversial issues for tracheostomy, including pediatric surgery ICUs:

- *Timing* (i.e., early versus delayed): the only justified indication for early tracheostomy is patient comfort, i.e., when the patient suffers from pain due to endotracheal tube or other translaryngeal devices and tracheostomy is the preferred method for patient safety (Donnelly et al. 1996; Kremer et al. 2002; Al-Samri et al. 2010).
- *Indications*: prolonged ventilation is the most common indication in pediatric tracheostomy, though it has many controversial issues due to its risk/benefit assessments; this is followed by other less common indications like using aerosol treatments, nosocomial pneumonia, witnessed aspiration event needing emergent tracheostomy, and repeated reintubations (Donnelly et al. 1996; Kremer et al. 2002; Al-Samri et al. 2010).
- *Techniques*: unless there is a life-threatening emergency, pediatric tracheostomy is a procedure that should be done in the operating room while the patient is intubated; it is recommended to use a horizontal incision on the skin and then vertical tracheal incision; any tracheal resection is prohibited (Donnelly et al. 1996; Kremer et al. 2002; Fraga et al. 2009).
- *Risks/benefits*: benefits of tracheostomy include patient comfort, mobility and speech, oral ingestion, improved suctioning of the airway, decreased airway resistance and more secure airway, improved weaning process from mechanical ventilation, and decreased rate of VAP; none of them are yet proved to be correct; the main etiologies for *tracheostomy-related death* include cannula obstruction and accidental decannulation; however, the most frequent *early complications* are pneumomediastinum, pneumothorax, wound-related complications, and tracheostomy site bleedings; common *late complications* include tracheal stenosis and formation of granulation tissue (Donnelly et al. 1996; Kremer et al. 2002; Al-Samri et al. 2010; Mastropietro et al. 2016).

References

Adewale L. Anatomy and assessment of the pediatric airway. Paediatr Anaesth. 2009;19 Suppl 1:1–8.

Ahmadpour-Kacho M, Zahedpasha Y, Hadipoor A, Akbarian-Rad Z. Early surgical intervention for diaphragmatic paralysis in a neonate; report of a case and literature review. Iranian J Pediatr. 2011;21:116–20.

Aktas S, Unal S, Aksu M, Ozcan E, Ergenekon E, Turkyilmaz C, Hirfanoglu I, Atalay Y. Nasal HFOV with binasal cannula appears effective and feasible in ELBW newborns. J Trop Pediatr. 2016;62:165–8.

Al-Samri M, Mitchell I, Drummond DS, Bjornson C. Tracheostomy in children: a population-based experience over 17 years. Pediatr Pulmonol. 2010;45:487–93.

Arikan AA, Zappitelli M, Goldstein SL, Naipaul A, Jefferson LS, Loftis LL. Fluid overload is associated with impaired oxygenation and morbidity in critically ill children. Pediatr Crit Care Med. 2012;13:253–8.

Artime CA, Hagberg CA. Tracheal extubation. Respir Care. 2014;59:991–1002; discussion 1002–5.

Aziz E, Nathan B, McKeever J. Anesthetic and analgesic practices in Avicenna's canon of medicine. Am J Chin Med. 2000;28:147–51.

Bagheri B, Razavi S, Gohari A, Salarian S, Dabbagh A. Toll-like receptor 4 in ventilator-induced lung injuries: mechanism of disease. J Cell Mol Anesth. 2016;1:34–9.

Baker S, Parico L. Pathologic paediatric conditions associated with a compromised airway. Int J Paediatr Dent/The Br Paedodont Soc [and] Int Assoc Dent Children. 2010;20:102–11.

Bancalari E, Claure N. The evidence for non-invasive ventilation in the preterm infant. Arch Dis Child Fetal Neonatal Ed. 2013;98:F98–F102.

Baumeister BL, El-Khatib M, Smith PG, Blumer JL. Evaluation of predictors of weaning from mechanical ventilation in pediatric patients. Pediatr Pulmonol. 1997;24:344–52.

Beggs S, Wong ZH, Kaul S, Ogden KJ, Walters JA. High-flow nasal cannula therapy for infants with bronchiolitis. Cochrane Database Syst Rev. 2014;1:CD009609.

Bennett TD, Spaeder MC, Matos RI, Watson RS, Typpo KV, Khemani RG, Crow S, Benneyworth BD, Thiagarajan RR, Dean JM, Markovitz BP. Existing data analysis in pediatric critical care research. Front Pediatr. 2014;2:79.

Boeken U, Schurr P, Kurt M, Feindt P, Lichtenberg A. Early reintubation after cardiac operations: impact of nasal continuous positive airway pressure (nCPAP) and noninvasive positive pressure ventilation (NPPV). Thorac Cardiovasc Surg. 2010;58:398–402.

Brashier DB, Khadka A, Anantharamu T, Sharma AK, Gupta AK, Sharma S, Dahiya N. Inhaled insulin: a "puff" than a "shot" before meals. J Pharmacol Pharmacother. 2015;6:126–9.

Camporota L, Barrett N. Current applications for the use of extracorporeal carbon dioxide removal in critically ill patients. BioMed Res Int. 2016;2016:9781695.

Cheifetz IM. Invasive and noninvasive pediatric mechanical ventilation. Respir Care. 2003;48:442–53; discussion 453–48.

Commare MC, Kurstjens SP, Barois A. Diaphragmatic paralysis in children: a review of 11 cases. Pediatr Pulmonol. 1994;18:187–93.

Dabbagh A, Rajaei S. Halothane: is there still any place for using the gas as an anesthetic? Hepat Mon. 2011;11:511–2.

Dabbagh A, Rajaei S, Golzari SE. History of anesthesia and pain in old Iranian texts. Anesth Pain Med. 2014;4, e15363.

Dalton HJ, Macrae DJ. Extracorporeal support in children with pediatric acute respiratory distress syndrome: proceedings from the Pediatric Acute Lung Injury Consensus Conference. Pediatr Crit Care Med. 2015;16:S111–7.

Deniau B, Ricard JD, Messika J, Dreyfuss D, Gaudry S. Use of extracorporeal carbon dioxide removal (ECCO2R) in 239 intensive care units: results from a French national survey. Intensive Care Med. 2016;42:624–5.

Diblasi RM. Nasal continuous positive airway pressure (CPAP) for the respiratory care of the newborn infant. Respir Care. 2009;54:1209–35.

Dickison AE. The normal and abnormal pediatric upper airway. Recognition and management of obstruction. Clin Chest Med. 1987;8:583–96.

Donnelly MJ, Lacey PD, Maguire AJ. A twenty year (1971–1990) review of tracheostomies in a major paediatric hospital. Int J Pediatr Otorhinolaryngol. 1996;35:1–9.

Drevhammar T, Nilsson K, Zetterstrom H, Jonsson B. Comparison of seven infant continuous positive airway pressure systems using simulated neonatal breathing. Pediatr Crit Care Med. 2012;13:e113–9.

Duppen N, Etnel JR, Spaans L, Takken T, van den Berg-Emons RJ, Boersma E, Schokking M, Dulfer K, Utens EM, Helbing W, Hopman MT. Does exercise training improve cardiopulmonary fitness and daily physical activity in children and young adults with corrected tetralogy of Fallot or Fontan circulation? A randomized controlled trial. Am Heart J. 2015;170:606–14.

Duyndam A, Ista E, Houmes RJ, van Driel B, Reiss I, Tibboel D. Invasive ventilation modes in children: a systematic review and meta-analysis. Crit Care. 2011;15:R24.

Emeriaud G, Newth CJ. Monitoring of children with pediatric acute respiratory distress syndrome: proceedings from the Pediatric Acute Lung Injury Consensus Conference. Pediatr Crit Care Med. 2015;16:S86–101.

Essouri S, Carroll C. Noninvasive support and ventilation for pediatric acute respiratory distress syndrome: proceedings from the Pediatric Acute Lung Injury Consensus Conference. Pediatr Crit Care Med. 2015;16:S102–10.

Feldman JM. Optimal ventilation of the anesthetized pediatric patient. Anesth Analg. 2015;120:165–75.

Fessler HE, Hager DN, Brower RG. Feasibility of very high-frequency ventilation in adults with acute respiratory distress syndrome. Crit Care Med. 2008;36:1043–8.

Fiorito B, Checchia P. A review of mechanical ventilation strategies in children following the Fontan procedure. Im Paediatr Cardiol. 2002;4:4–11.

Flori H, Dahmer MK, Sapru A, Quasney MW. Comorbidities and assessment of severity of pediatric acute respiratory distress syndrome: proceedings from the Pediatric Acute Lung Injury Consensus Conference. Pediatr Crit Care Med. 2015;16:S41–50.

Fraga JC, Souza JC, Kruel J. Pediatric tracheostomy. J Pediatr (Rio J). 2009;85:97–103.

Gerdes JS, Sivieri EM, Abbasi S. Factors influencing delivered mean airway pressure during nasal CPAP with the RAM cannula. Pediatr Pulmonol. 2016;51:60–9.

Golzari SE, Khan ZH, Ghabili K, Hosseinzadeh H, Soleimanpour H, Azarfarin R, Mahmoodpoor A, Aslanabadi S, Ansarin K. Contributions of Medieval Islamic physicians to the history of tracheostomy. Anesth Analg. 2013;116:1123–32.

Gupta P, McDonald R, Goyal S, Gossett JM, Imamura M, Agarwal A, Butt W, Bhutta AT. Extubation failure in infants with shunt-dependent pulmonary blood flow and univentricular physiology. Cardiol Young. 2014;24:64–72.

Gupta V, Ahsan F. Inhalational therapy for pulmonary arterial hypertension: current status and future prospects. Crit Rev Ther Drug Carrier Syst. 2010;27:313–70.

Habashi NM, Borg UR, Reynolds HN. Low blood flow extracorporeal carbon dioxide removal (ECCO2R): a review of the concept and a case report. Intensive Care Med. 1995a;21:594–7.

Habashi NM, Reynolds HN, Borg U, Cowley RA. Randomized clinical trial of pressure-controlled inverse ration ventilation and extra corporeal CO2 removal for ARDS. Am J Respir Crit Care Med. 1995b;151:255–6.

Hamblin KA, Wong JP, Blanchard JD, Atkins HS. The potential of liposome-encapsulated ciprofloxacin as a tularemia therapy. Frontiers in Cellular and Infection Microbiology. 2014;4:79.

Harless J, Ramaiah R, Bhananker SM. Pediatric airway management. International Journal of Critical Illness and Injury Science. 2014;4:65–70.

Hassinger AB, Wald EL, Goodman DM. Early postoperative fluid overload precedes acute kidney injury and is associated with higher morbidity in pediatric cardiac surgery patients. Pediatr Crit Care Med. 2014;15:131–8.

Heinrich S, Birkholz T, Ihmsen H, Irouschek A, Ackermann A, Schmidt J. Incidence and predictors of difficult laryngoscopy in 11,219 pediatric anesthesia procedures. Paediatr Anaesth. 2012;22:729–36.

Henderson-Smart D, De Paoli A, Clark R, Bhuta T. High frequency oscillatory ventilation versus conventional ventilation for infants with severe pulmonary dysfunction born at or near term. Cochrane Database Syst Rev. 2009;2009, CD002974.

Ingelse SA, Wosten-van Asperen RM, Lemson J, Daams JG, Bem RA, van Woensel JB. Pediatric acute respiratory distress syndrome: fluid management in the PICU. Front Pediatr. 2016;4:21.

Iyer NP, Chatburn R. Evaluation of a nasal cannula in noninvasive ventilation using a lung simulator. Respir Care. 2015;60:508–12.

Kaminski PN, Forgiarini Jr LA, Andrade CF. Early respiratory therapy reduces postoperative atelectasis in children undergoing lung resection. Respir Care. 2013;58:805–9.

Kaushik M, Wojewodzka-Zelezniakowicz M, Cruz DN, Ferrer-Nadal A, Teixeira C, Iglesias E, Kim JC, Braschi A, Piccinni P, Ronco C. Extracorporeal carbon dioxide removal: the future of lung support lies in the history. Blood Purif. 2012;34:94–106.

Khemani RG, Newth CJ. The design of future pediatric mechanical ventilation trials for acute lung injury. Am J Respir Crit Care Med. 2010;182:1465–74.

Khemani RG, Randolph A, Markovitz B. Corticosteroids for the prevention and treatment of post-extubation stridor in neonates, children and adults. Cochrane Database Syst Rev. 2009;3:CD001000.

Khemani RG, Smith LS, Zimmerman JJ, Erickson S. Pediatric acute respiratory distress syndrome: definition, incidence, and epidemiology: proceedings from the Pediatric Acute Lung Injury Consensus Conference. Pediatr Crit Care Med. 2015;16:S23–40.

Kremer B, Botos-Kremer AI, Eckel HE, Schlondorff G. Indications, complications, and surgical techniques for pediatric tracheostomies – an update. J Pediatr Surg. 2002;37:1556–62.

Kurachek SC, Newth CJ, Quasney MW, Rice T, Sachdeva RC, Patel NR, Takano J, Easterling L, Scanlon M, Musa N, Brilli RJ, Wells D, Park GS, Penfil S, Bysani KG, Nares MA, Lowrie L, Billow M, Chiochetti E, Lindgren B. Extubation failure in pediatric intensive care: a multiple-center study of risk factors and outcomes. Crit Care Med. 2003;31:2657–64.

Kurt M, Boeken U, Litmathe J, Feindt P, Gams E. Oxygenation failure after cardiac surgery: early re-intubation versus treatment by nasal continuous positive airway pressure (NCPAP) or non-invasive positive pressure ventilation (NPPV). Monaldi Arch Chest Dis = Archivio Monaldi per le malattie del torace/Fondazione clinica del lavoro, IRCCS [and] Istituto di clinica tisiologica e malattie apparato respiratorio Universita di Napoli, Secondo ateneo. 2008;70:71–5.

Lemyre B, Davis PG, De Paoli AG, Kirpalani H. Nasal intermittent positive pressure ventilation (NIPPV) versus nasal continuous positive airway pressure (NCPAP) for preterm neonates after extubation. Cochrane Database Syst Rev. 2014;9:CD003212.

Lofland GK. The enhancement of hemodynamic performance in Fontan circulation using pain free spontaneous ventilation. Eur J Cardiothorac Surg. 2001;20:114–8; discussion 118–9.

Manley BJ, Owen LS, Doyle LW, Andersen CC, Cartwright DW, Pritchard MA, Donath SM, Davis PG. High-flow nasal cannulae in very preterm infants after extubation. N Engl J Med. 2013;369:1425–33.

Mastropietro CW, Benneyworth BD, Turrentine M, Wallace AS, Hornik CP, Jacobs JP, Jacobs ML. Tracheostomy after operations for congenital heart disease: an analysis of the Society of Thoracic Surgeons Congenital Heart Surgery Database. Ann Thorac Surg. 2016;101(6):2285–92.

Mayfield S, Jauncey-Cooke J, Hough JL, Schibler A, Gibbons K, Bogossian F. High-flow nasal cannula therapy for respiratory support in children. Cochrane Database Syst Rev. 2014;3:CD009850.

Milesi C, Boubal M, Jacquot A, Baleine J, Durand S, Odena MP, Cambonie G. High-flow nasal cannula: recommendations for daily practice in pediatrics. Ann Intensive Care. 2014;4:29.

Morales DL, Carberry KE, Heinle JS, McKenzie ED, Fraser Jr CD, Diaz LK. Extubation in the operating room after Fontan's procedure: effect on practice and outcomes. Ann Thorac Surg. 2008;86:576–81; discussion 581–72.

Nagarajan K, Bennett A, Agostini P, Naidu B. Is preoperative physiotherapy/pulmonary rehabilitation beneficial in lung resection patients? Interact Cardiovasc Thorac Surg. 2011;13:300–2.

Newth CJ, Venkataraman S, Willson DF, Meert KL, Harrison R, Dean JM, Pollack M, Zimmerman J, Anand KJ, Carcillo JA, Nicholson CE. Weaning and extubation readiness in pediatric patients. Pediatr Crit Care Med. 2009;10:1–11.

Nzegwu NI, Mack T, DellaVentura R, Dunphy L, Koval N, Levit O, Bhandari V. Systematic use of the RAM nasal cannula in the Yale-New Haven Children's Hospital Neonatal Intensive Care Unit: a quality improvement project. J Matern Fetal Neonatal Med. 2015;28:718–21.

O'Callaghan C. Targeting drug delivery to the lungs by inhalation. Mediators Inflamm. 1994;3:S31–3.

Pasquina P, Tramer MR, Walder B. Prophylactic respiratory physiotherapy after cardiac surgery: systematic review. BMJ (Clinical Research Ed). 2003;327:1379.

Pediatric Acute Lung Injury Consensus Conference Group. Pediatric acute respiratory distress syndrome: consensus recommendations from the Pediatric Acute Lung Injury Consensus Conference. Pediatr Crit Care Med. 2015;16:428–39.

Pelosi P, Jaber S. Noninvasive respiratory support in the perioperative period. Curr Opin Anaesthesiol. 2010;23:233–8.

Petkar KC, Chavhan SS, Agatonovik-Kustrin S, Sawant KK. Nanostructured materials in drug and gene delivery: a review of the state of the art. Crit Rev Ther Drug Carrier Syst. 2011;28:101–64.

Quasney MW, Lopez-Fernandez YM, Santschi M, Watson RS. The outcomes of children with pediatric acute respiratory distress syndrome: proceedings from the Pediatric Acute Lung Injury Consensus Conference. Pediatr Crit Care Med. 2015;16:S118–31.

Randolph AG, Wypij D, Venkataraman ST, Hanson JH, Gedeit RG, Meert KL, Luckett PM, Forbes P, Lilley M, Thompson J, Cheifetz IM, Hibberd P, Wetzel R, Cox PN, Arnold JH. Effect of mechanical ventilator weaning protocols on respiratory outcomes in infants and children: a randomized controlled trial. JAMA. 2002;288:2561–8.

Rastogi R, Sultana Y, Ali A, Aqil M. Particulate and vesicular drug carriers in the management of tuberculosis. Curr Drug Deliv. 2006;3:121–8.

Rimensberger PC, Cheifetz IM. Ventilatory support in children with pediatric acute respiratory distress syndrome: proceedings from the Pediatric Acute Lung Injury Consensus Conference. Pediatr Crit Care Med. 2015;16:S51–60.

Rothaar RC, Epstein SK. Extubation failure: magnitude of the problem, impact on outcomes, and prevention. Curr Opin Crit Care. 2003;9:59–66.

Saikia B, Kumar N, Sreenivas V. Prediction of extubation failure in newborns, infants and children: brief report of a prospective (blinded) cohort study at a tertiary care paediatric centre in India. SpringerPlus. 2015;4:827.

Sapru A, Flori H, Quasney MW, Dahmer MK. Pathobiology of acute respiratory distress syndrome. Pediatr Crit Care Med. 2015;16:S6–22.

Schindler MB. Prediction of ventilation weaning outcome: children are not little adults. Crit Care. 2005;9:651–2.

Seguin J, Albright B, Vertullo L, Lai P, Dancea A, Bernier PL, Tchervenkov CI, Calaritis C, Drullinsky D, Gottesman R, Zappitelli M. Extent, risk factors, and outcome of fluid overload after pediatric heart surgery*. Crit Care Med. 2014;42:2591–9.

Sinitsky L, Walls D, Nadel S, Inwald DP. Fluid overload at 48 hours is associated with respiratory morbidity but not mortality in a general PICU: retrospective cohort study. Pediatr Crit Care Med. 2015;16:205–9.

Squires AJ, Hyndman M. Prevention of nasal injuries secondary to NCPAP application in the ELBW infant. Neonatal Netw: NN. 2009;28:13–27.

Stream AR, Bull TM. Experiences with treprostinil in the treatment of pulmonary arterial hypertension. Ther Adv Respir Dis. 2012;6:269–76.

Sunder RA, Haile DT, Farrell PT, Sharma A. Pediatric airway management: current practices and future directions. Paediatr Anaesth. 2012;22:1008–15.

Tamburro RF, Kneyber MC. Pulmonary specific ancillary treatment for pediatric acute respiratory distress syndrome: proceedings from the Pediatric Acute Lung Injury Consensus Conference. Pediatr Crit Care Med. 2015;16:S61–72.

Thiagarajan RR, Bratton SL, Martin LD, Brogan TV, Taylor D. Predictors of successful extubation in children. Am J Respir Crit Care Med. 1999;160:1562–6.

Tobin MJ, Jubran A. Variable performance of weaning-predictor tests: role of Bayes' theorem and spectrum and test-referral bias. Intensive Care Med. 2006;32:2002–12.

Tripp HF, Bolton JW. Phrenic nerve injury following cardiac surgery: a review. J Card Surg. 1998;13:218–23.

Valentine SL, Nadkarni VM, Curley MA. Nonpulmonary treatments for pediatric acute respiratory distress syndrome: proceedings from the Pediatric Acute Lung Injury Consensus Conference. Pediatr Crit Care Med. 2015;16:S73–85.

Villar J, Perez-Mendez L, Lopez J, Belda J, Blanco J, Saralegui I, Suarez-Sipmann F, Lopez J, Lubillo S, Kacmarek RM. An early PEEP/FIO2 trial identifies different degrees of lung injury in patients with acute respiratory distress syndrome. Am J Respir Crit Care Med. 2007;176:795–804.

Walker RW, Ellwood J. The management of difficult intubation in children. Paediatr Anaesth. 2009;19 Suppl 1:77–87.

Wielenga JM, van den Hoogen A, van Zanten HA, Helder O, Bol B, Blackwood B. Protocolized versus non-protocolized weaning for reducing the duration of invasive mechanical ventilation in newborn infants. Cochrane Database Syst Rev. 2016;3:CD011106.

Wilkinson D, Andersen C, O'Donnell CP, De Paoli AG, Manley BJ. High flow nasal cannula for respiratory support in preterm infants. Cochrane Database Syst Rev. 2016;2:CD006405.

Wood M. Pharmacokinetic drug interactions in anaesthetic practice. Clin Pharmacokinet. 1991;21:285–307.

Wratney AT, Benjamin Jr DK, Slonim AD, He J, Hamel DS, Cheifetz IM. The endotracheal tube air leak test does not predict extubation outcome in critically ill pediatric patients. Pediatr Crit Care Med. 2008;9:490–6.

Yang KL, Tobin MJ. A prospective study of indexes predicting the outcome of trials of weaning from mechanical ventilation. N Engl J Med. 1991;324:1445–50.

Yoder BA, Stoddard RA, Li M, King J, Dirnberger DR, Abbasi S. Heated, humidified high-flow nasal cannula versus nasal CPAP for respiratory support in neonates. Pediatrics. 2013;131:e1482–90.

Zarbock A, Mueller E, Netzer S, Gabriel A, Feindt P, Kindgen-Milles D. Prophylactic nasal continuous positive airway pressure following cardiac surgery protects from postoperative pulmonary complications: a prospective, randomized, controlled trial in 500 patients. Chest. 2009;135:1252–9.

Chapter 36
Cardiac Anesthesia in Infants and Children: Postoperative Bleeding and Coagulation Management

Pablo Motta and Antonio Pérez Ferrer

Introduction

Clinical monitoring for intraoperative bleeding starts as soon as heparin is reversed by surgical inspection of the operative site. Once the chest is closed, monitoring the chest tube output (CTO) is of paramount importance. Acceptable CTO is less than 1–2 mL/kg/h even though it could be higher in the first 2 h (3–4 mL/kg/h). Bleeding should be prevented and addressed early to avoid the use of blood products. Increasing literature shows that allogeneic blood transfusions are associated with thrombosis, acute renal failure (ARF), transfusion-related immunomodulation (TRIM), transfusion-related acute lung injury (TRALI), and transfusion-associated circulatory overload (TACO), worsening postoperative outcomes. In addition to reoperation, bleeding complications in cardiac surgery are associated with postoperative stroke, mechanical ventilation, ICU stay, 30-day mortality, and hospital cost (Thiele and Raphael 2014; Christensen et al. 2009, 2012; Guay and Rivard 1996; Guzzetta et al. 2015; Hayashi et al. 2011).

P. Motta (✉)
Department of Pediatric Cardiac Anesthesia,
Texas Children's Hospital – Baylor College of Medicine, Houston, TX, USA
e-mail: pxmotta@texaschildrens.org

A.P. Ferrer
Department of Anesthesiology, La Paz University Hospital, Madrid, Spain
e-mail: antonioperezferrer@gmail.com

© Springer International Publishing Switzerland 2017
A. Dabbagh et al. (eds.), *Congenital Heart Disease in Pediatric
and Adult Patients*, DOI 10.1007/978-3-319-44691-2_36

Table 36.1 Risk factors for postoperative bleeding

Preoperative factors		
Age	Neonates Prematures Low birth weight	Undeveloped coagulation system and calcium hemostasis
Comorbidities	Acquired coagulopathies	Dilution and trauma post CPB Renal or hepatic insufficiency
	Congenital coagulopathies	von Willebrand disease
Medications	Antiplatelets agents	Aspirin <ADP-receptor antagonist <GPIIb/GPIIIa inhibitor
	Anticoagulants	LMWH Direct factor X inhibitors Thrombin inhibitors vitamin-K antagonist
Intraoperative factors		
Procedure related	Neonatal repairs	Norwood, ASO Truncus repair TAPVR
	Single-ventricle palliation	Glenn Shunt Fontan
	Aortic reconstruction	Multiple suture lines
	Redo surgery	Numerous adhesions
	ECMO/VAD	
CPB related	Hemodilution	Major effect in infants
	Hypothermia	DHCA
	Coagulation derangements	Hyperfibrinolysis Residual heparin Protamine overdose

CPB cardiopulmonary bypass, *LMWH* low molecular weight heparin, *ASO* arterial switch operation, *TAPVR* total anomalous pulmonary venous return, *ECMO* extracorporeal membrane oxygenation, *VAD* ventricular assist device, *DHCA* deep hypothermia circulatory arrest

Risk Factors for Postoperative Bleeding

There are several preoperative risk factors for postoperative bleeding pediatric cardiac surgery that can be classified as specific to the patient, to congenital heart disease, and those related to the surgical procedure and cardiopulmonary bypass (CPB) (Table 36.1).

Preoperative Risk Factors

Age is inversely related with the risk of bleeding. Neonates and particularly premature babies are the highest-risk group for postoperative bleeding. Neonates do not a have a completely developed coagulation system at birth, but there is a balance between the low levels of endogenous procoagulants and anticoagulant systems (Arnold 2014). In addition neonates do not regulate calcium hemostasis well, which is essential in the coagulation process (Jain et al. 2010). Traditional coagulation testing such as prothrombin time (PT), thrombin time (TT), and activated partial thromboplastin time (APTT) are prolonged in neonates (Long et al. 2011). Refer to Chap. 10 for extensive discussion regarding preoperative testing.

Comorbidities like congenital coagulopathies (e.g., von Willebrand disease) or acquired coagulopathies secondary to diabetes and liver or kidney dysfunction also increase the bleeding risk.

Single-ventricle patient in the pre-Fontan stage has coagulation anomalies characterized by lower levels of protein C, protein S, antithrombin III, and factors II, V, VII, and X and longer prothrombin times probably due to chronic passive congestion of the liver. These factor anomalies tend to correct post-Fontan surgery probably due to improvement in systemic oxygenation and overall perfusion (Cheung et al. 2005). Independent from the primary lesion, cyanotic heart disease is associated with secondary erythrocytosis as a compensatory mechanism for hypoxemia. This compensatory increase in the red cell mass reduces the plasma volume with the consecutive reduction in coagulating factors, fibrinogen, and platelet count increasing the postoperative bleeding risk. The effect on the coagulation is directly related to the amount of hypoxia and polycythemia (Zabala and Guzzetta 2015). Cyanotic patients with multiple aortopulmonary collateral vessels have an increased venous return to the heart affecting surgical visualization and increasing postoperative bleeding due to poor surgical hemostasis (Donmez and Yurdakok 2014).

Antiplatelet agent and anticoagulants are commonly used in pediatric patients with congenital heart disease and have been implicated in increasing surgical bleeding. Of the antiplatelets, aspirin has the lower risk of bleeding, ADP-receptor antagonist has an intermediate risk, and the GPIIb/GPIIIa receptor antagonists have the highest risk. Aspirin causes an irreversible inhibition of the platelet cyclo-oxygenase 1 (COX1) which is responsible of formation thromboxane A_2 essential for platelet activation and aggregation. Aspirin duration of action is related to the platelet turnover (about 10 days) because the inhibition is not reversible. About 10 % of the platelet COX1 activity recovers per day due to platelet turnover, and only 20 % of the platelet COX1 activity is needed to achieve a normal hemostasis (Awtry and Loscalzo 2000). ADP-receptor antagonist such as clopidogrel affects the geometry of the platelets making them spherical and unable to aggregate (Wijeyeratne and Heptinstall 2011). GPIIb/GPIIIa receptor antagonists are used infrequently in pediatrics, but they will also increase the risk of bleeding due to the profound capacity to prevent platelet aggregation, thrombus formation, and distal thromboembolism. Alternatively early withdrawal of aspirin and/or clopidogrel is not feasible in shunt-dependent patients at life-threatening risk for thrombosis. Similarly in emergency cases like heart transplant with harvesting or left ventricular assist device (VAD), patient undergoes surgery under full anti-aggregation and anticoagulation. Preoperatively the platelet count in these patients is normal since the production is not affected. Platelet functional studies such as PFA-100 and multiplate platelet aggregometer, which are described at length in Chap. 10, can detect platelet inhibition but are not used routinely in the preoperative period. Platelet aggregation studies showed conflicting data in terms of predicting not postoperative blood loss and more research is needed (Hofer et al. 2011; Orlov et al. 2014). Recently in adults undergoing heart surgery, low platelet activity predicted 30-day mortality bringing up the question when to discontinue the antiplatelet agents (Kuliczkowski et al. 2016).

Anticoagulants are another group of medications strongly associated with postoperative bleeding. Unfractioned heparin (UH), which is a mixture of polymers of sulfated glycosaminoglycans (molecular weight 5–30 kd), potentiates the anticoagulant effects of antithrombin III. Heparin has a short half-life since is it cleared from the circulation by endothelial cells (saturable mechanism) and by kidney excretion. Due to the extensive metabolism, UH is administered as a bolus and followed by an infusion. Target APTT is 1.5–2.5 normal values. Heparin is usually stopped 6 h before surgery, and residual effect can be checked by the activated clotting time (ACT) in the operating room. Normal ACT values are 80–160 s. Heparin concentration measurement in pediatrics has not correlated well with antifactor Xa activity and is not commonly used to detect residual UH effect (Gruenwald et al. 2000).

Low molecular weight heparin (LMWH) is a depolymerized molecule with an average weight of 5 kd which its effect is mediated by the inhibition of factor Xa. Due to lack of monitoring needed, longer half-life and predictable effect LMWH have gained popularity in the pediatric population. LMWH should be held 12 h before surgery, and if needed its residual effect can be checked by the antifactor Xa levels (0.5–1.0 U/mL therapeutic, 0.1–0.3 U/mL prophylactic).

Direct factor X inhibitors have limited indications in pediatrics, and its use has been restricted to heparin-induced thrombocytopenia. Due to its long half-life and lack of an antidote, these drugs are not ideal to be used in the preoperative period (Young 2008).

Vitamin-K antagonists like Coumadin inhibits the production of vitamin-K-dependent coagulation factors (II, VII, IX, and X). In addition Coumadin also inhibits the production of physiologic anticoagulant proteins C and S. Its effect is monitored by the international normalized ratio (INR). Therapeutic INR values depend on the indication (INR 2–3 thromboembolism, INR 2.5–3.5 mechanical valve). Vitamin-K antagonist's long half-life makes it impractical for the perioperative period and is usually held for 3–5 days and transitioned to UH. If emergency cardiac surgery is needed in a patient on Coumadin, its effect can be reversed with prothrombin complex concentrate (PCC) which is going to be later in the chapter.

Intraoperative Risk Factors

The intraoperative risk factors for bleeding are related to the procedure and to the cardiopulmonary bypass. Complex procedures by RACHS-1 score such as neonatal repairs (e.g., Norwood, arterial switch, truncus repair, and total anomalous pulmonary vein repair), single-ventricle palliation (Glenn Shunt and Fontan), redo surgeries, and aortic surgeries are the highest risk for perioperative bleeding (Guay and Rivard 1996; Guzzetta et al. 2015). Duration of surgery has been related with postoperative bleeding measured by chest tube output and ROTEM trace abnormalities (Hayashi et al. 2011).

Table 36.2 Priming volume hemodilution effect by weight

Flow (ml/min)	Weight (kg)	CPB circuit	Priming volume (ml)	Hemodilution (%)
0–500	0–6	3/16" art ¼" ven	~350 ml	70–137
500–1000	<6–7	¼" art and ven	~450 ml	76–88
1000–2000	7–15	¼" art 3/8″ ven	~650 ml	54–111
2000–3000	15–18	¼" art 3/8″ ven	~850 ml	59–70
3000–4000	18–25	¼" or 3/8″ art, 3/8" ven	~1200 ml	64–83

Ultimately high risks for postoperative bleeding are patients on mechanical circulation with either extracorporeal membrane oxygenator (ECMO) or ventricular assist device (VAD). ECMO patients are kept fully anticoagulated on UH infusion to avoid thrombosis triggered by the contact of patients' blood with ECMO circuit. In addition to coagulation activation, there is a dilutional effect on coagulation factors due to the ECMO prime. The target values for anticoagulation while on ECMO are ACT of 180–220 s, antifactor Xa levels of 0.3–0.7 IU/mL, and/or APTTs of 1.5–2.5 times the normal. Currently most of the ECMO circuits are heparin coated decreasing the amount of UH needed. Low levels of anticoagulation could lead into ECMO circuit thrombosis, but on the other hand excessive anticoagulation could lead to bleeding. Neurological injury due central nervous system (CNS) bleeding is the most feared complication of ECMO and frequent cause of withdrawing support.

VAD patients do not need full intravenous anticoagulation, but they are still at risk from thrombosis and emboli from the device, cannulas, and valves (e.g., Berlin Heart). Most institutions follow the Edmonton triple antithrombotic protocol entailing aspirin, dipyridamole, and either warfarin ≥12 months or enoxaparin <12 months. During the ECMO wean or VAD harvesting coagulation point of care (POC), testing is crucial to minimize the bleeding risk and conduct a coagulation goal-directed therapy (Annich and Adachi 2013; Esper et al. 2014; Seibel et al. 2008).

Cardiopulmonary bypass (CPB) causes massive physiologic changes in children characterized by hemodilution, coagulation activation, and hyperfibrinolysis (Sniecinski and Chandler 2011). The hemodilution effect is inversely proportional to size, neonates and infants being the ones affected the most (Table 36.2). The artificial surface of the CPB circuit activates platelets and the kallikrein-kinin system promoting thrombosis (Fig. 36.1). Heparin use even though effective to avoid circuit thrombosis and thrombin formation does not inhibit completely platelet and coagulation activation. During the CPB run, there is also platelet sequestration, downregulation of GPIIb/GPIIIa receptor, and destruction due to thrombogenic bypass circuit surfaces. Due to these facts platelet function and fibrinogen concentration are affected the most post CPB in pediatric cardiac surgery (up to 50 % of baseline values). An early study by Miller et al. showed that platelets and cryoprecipitate (rich in fibrinogen) restore hemostasis in the initial post CPB period (Miller et al. 1997, 2000). Infant CPB is conducted under some degree of hypothermia for most

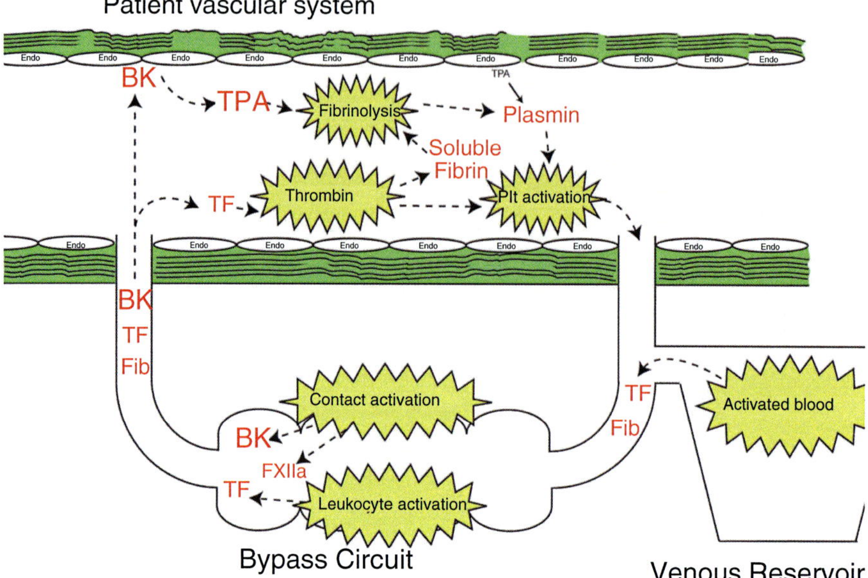

Fig. 36.1 Summary of hemostatic activation mechanisms on cardiopulmonary bypass (*CPB*). *BK* bradykinin, *FXIIa* activated factor XII, *TF* tissue factor, *TPA* tissue plasminogen activator, *Plt* platelets, *Fib* fibrin degradation products, *Endo* endothelium. Details provided in text (Published with permission from Wolters Kluwer Health, Inc. Sniecinski and Chandler 2011)

procedures and in some cases (e.g., aortic reconstruction – Norwood) under deep hypothermia circulatory arrest (DHCA). Mossad et al. showed that when comparing with adult cardiac surgery, pediatric patients have a higher incidence of DHCA use and blood transfusion requirements in the perioperative period (Mossad et al. 2007). Coagulation and inflammation activation is caused by the stress caused by the trauma of the circulating blood components with the artificial surface of the CPB circuit. Due to immaturity of coagulation and immune system, this activation is more profound in neonates and infants. Modulation of the stress response with intravenous steroid is common practice even though there is doubtful evidence for its use. Steroid will decrease the inflammatory mediators interleukin-1, interleukin-6, interleukin-8, tumor necrosis factor, leukotrienes, and endotoxin, but its effects on coagulation and postoperative bleeding are not well defined (Augoustides 2012). The priming solution varies with patient size and weight. Usually prime solution for patients <18 kg includes packed red blood cells (PRBC), crystalloids (e.g., PlasmaLyte), colloid (e.g., albumin), and/or fresh frozen plasma (FFP), trying to keep the solution as physiological as possible. In addition to the prime solution heparin, buffer solution (e.g., sodium bicarbonate), mannitol, and steroids are added. The use of FFP for CPB prime is debatable. Traditionally FFP is added to blood prime in patients <18 kg, but there is no evidence that this practice will improve outcomes and decrease postoperative bleeding. Desborough et al. in a

Cochrane database of systematic reviews showed that in patients without coagulopathy, the addition of FFP did not improve the outcome (Desborough et al. 2015). Miao et al. showed that adding FFP to the CPB in a population of cyanotic patient (6 months–3 years) undergoing cardiac surgery did not decrease postoperative bleeding. Preoperative fibrinogen was an independent predictor of postoperative blood loss (Miao et al. 2014).

Pathophysiology of Postoperative Bleeding

Cardiac surgery exposes the subendothelium, which is rich in thromboplastin, triggering platelet activation and aggregation binding to the von Willebrand factor and collagen forming the initial vascular plug. The coagulation system through the factors IX (FIXa) and factor X (FXa) is activated by the binding of the wound tissue factor (TF) to active factor VII (FVIIa) transforming prothrombin to thrombin. The activated platelets, factors V, VIII, and XI, work as catalyst accelerating the coagulation process. Next the clot stabilizes with fibrinogen and factor XIII. Finally, once the clot is formed and stable, the fibrinolytic system avoids further thrombus formation (Fig. 36.2).

Uncontrolled surgical bleeding can lead to coagulation activation by exposure of the subendothelium, coagulation factor loss, and thrombocytopenia. Blood product replacement should be balanced (e.g., packed red blood cells, coagulation factors, fibrinogen, and platelets) and POC targeted. Isolated PRBC replacement further dilutes coagulation factors, fibrinogen, and platelets perpetuating the vicious circle of coagulopathy and further bleeding. Hypothermia, acidosis, low-ionized calcium, and hyperfibrinolysis should also be tackled since they are major contributors of maintaining the postoperative bleeding cycle. CPB rewarming strategies are crucial since infants are prone to hypothermia due to widespread use of hypothermia and DHCA in pediatric cardiac surgery. Neonates and infants due to limited fat stores, inability to shiver, and larger ratio of body surface area to weight are especially susceptible to hypothermia. Hypothermia affects coagulation factors and platelet function perpetrating postoperative bleeding. Furthermore uncorrected hypothermia will increase oxygen consumption causing metabolic acidosis impairing hemostasis even further. Hypocalcemia is common in infants due to sarcoplasmic reticulum underdevelopment and reduced calcium storages. Furthermore massive use of citrated blood product will decrease ionized calcium even further (Kozek-Langenecker 2014). Residual heparin effect due to reheparinization and/or excess protamine has also been associated to postoperative bleeding. Lastly hyperfibrinolysis in pediatric cardiac surgery is a potential cause of postoperative bleeding. Miller et al. were the first group to described hyperfibrinolysis using thromboelastogram (TEG) in the post-protamine period. In his series hyperfibrinolysis was uncommon (2 out 32 patients, 6.25 %) and only present in the bigger patients (>8 kg cohort) (Miller et al. 1997, 2000).

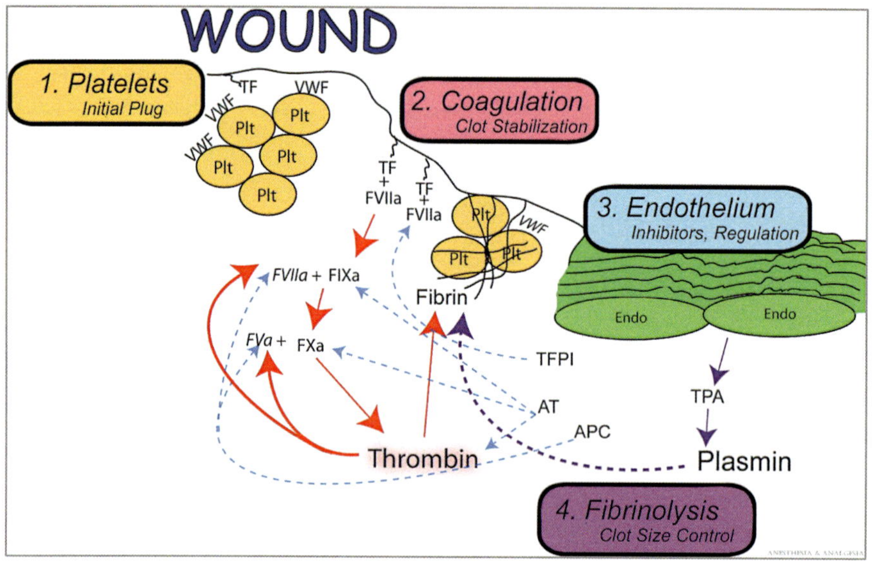

Fig. 36.2 Normal hemostasis. (*1*) Initial plug formation begins with von Willebrand factor (VWF) binding to collagen in the wound and platelets (Plt) adhering to VWF. (*2*) Coagulation is initiated by small amounts of active factor VII (FVIIa) in blood binding to the exposed tissue factor (TF) in the wound, leading to activation of factor IX (FIXa) and factor X (FXa), which in turn initiates the conversion of prothrombin to thrombin. Thrombin creates a positive feedback loop by activating factors VIII (FVIIIa) and V (FVa), which increases FIXa and FXa's conversion of prothrombin to thrombin. This local burst of thrombin production at the wound site converts soluble fibrinogen into a fibrin mesh that stabilizes the initial plug. (*3*) Clot formation away from the site of injury is prevented by antithrombin (AT), which destroys thrombin and FXa, FIXa, and FXIa, activated protein C (APC), which destroys FVIIIa and FVa, and tissue factor pathway inhibitor (TFPI), which destroys TF-VIIa complexes. (*4*) Additionally, the endothelium (Endo) secretes tissue plasminogen activator (TPA), which binds to fibrin and converts plasminogen to plasmin, which in turn lyses the fibrin. Once a stable clot is formed and the wounded tissue is no longer exposed, the regulatory proteins and fibrinolytic proteins prevent further thrombus formation (Published with permission from Wolters Kluwer Health, Inc. Sniecinski and Chandler 2011)

Point of Care Testing and Algorithms in Postoperative Bleeding

A detailed description of the value of POC in postoperative bleeding is available in Chap. 10. The value of ROTEM, TEG, and traditional preoperative testing in predicting bleeding after pediatric cardiac surgery is under investigation. POC algorithms have been used for the stepwise approach of postoperative bleeding which is also presented in Chap. 10. The aim of POC algorithms is a targeted treatment of postoperative bleeding minimizing blood transfusion while improving surgical outcomes. Romlin et al. demonstrated that ROTEM could be used early during the rewarming period of CPB before hemoconcentration accelerating the analysis by running the HEPTEM/FIBTEM receiving information of clot firmness after just 10 min (Romlin et al. 2013). The same Swedish group studied a pediatric cardiac

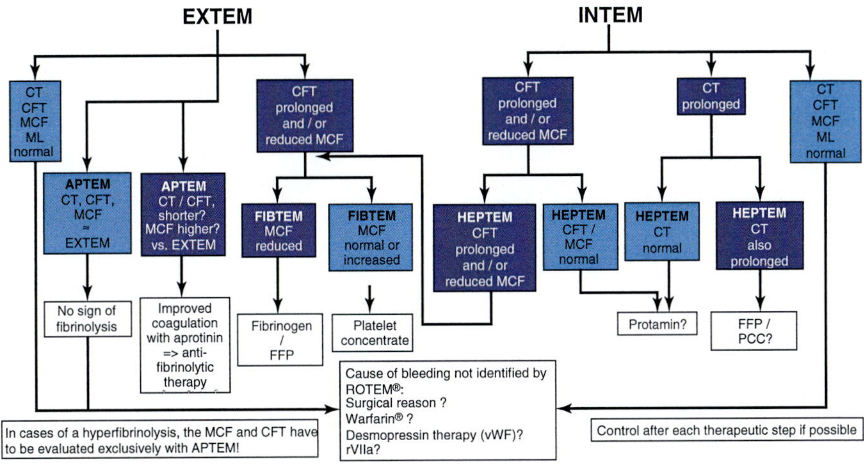

Fig. 36.3 Differential diagnostic and therapeutic ROTEM® algorithm used in the Clinic Cologne–Merheim (Vorweg et al. 2001) and reproduced in ROTEM promotional material (Calatzis et al. 2013)

surgery population using TEG as POC testing showing decreased transfusion rate of PRBC and FFP while receiving more platelets and fibrinogen (Romlin et al. 2011). Other studies like the one by Lee et al. could not show that ROTEM predicted chest tube output after cardiac surgery (Lee et al. 2012).

Currently at Texas Children's in high-risk patients, we use ROTEM as POC running HEPTEM and FIBTEM upon rewarming of CPB following Romlin et al.'s approach. The more prevailing finding is the decrease of maximum clot firmness (MCF) in both tests (HEPTEM MCF <50 mm, FIBTEM <9 mm). We utilize a modified version of the Clinic Cologne–Merheim algorithm (Vorweg et al. 2001) (Fig. 36.3) (See section "Case Vignette"). Espinosa et al. showed that ROTEM and TEG parameters correlated well with post CPB hemostasis changes and plasma fibrinogen and helped to guide fibrinogen replacement (Espinosa et al. 2014). Nakayama in pediatric cardiac surgical population validated the use of thromboelastometry-based algorithm reducing postoperative bleeding and decreasing the intensive care unit stay versus conventional treatment (ACT and platelet count transfusion guided) (Nakayama et al. 2015).

Prophylaxis

Preoperative Optimization

It is important in the preoperative visit to review all active medications and its indications. As detailed before, antiplatelet agents should be discontinued 5–7 days before surgery unless the risk of thrombosis is extremely high (e.g., shunt-dependent lesion with low SaO_2). LMWH treatment can be continued in the preoperative period, but the last dose should be given subcutaneously 8–12 h before elective surgery. Vitamin-K antagonist should be stopped after overlapping treatment with UH as an inpatient and reaching a target APTT 1.5–2.5 normal values. Residual Coumadin effect should be ruled out on the day of surgery with a normalized INR value. It usually takes 3–5 days to normalize the INR after stopping Coumadin (Society of Thoracic Surgeons Blood Conservation Guideline Task F et al. 2007; Kozek-Langenecker et al. 2013).

Herbal medications use is not as prevalent in children as in adults with a reported use of 3.5 % vs. 16 %, respectively. Many of the herbal supplements such as garlic, ginkgo biloba, *Panax ginseng*, and/or ginger that can affect coagulation and should be stopped a week before surgery (Kaufman et al. 2002; Everett et al. 2005).

Cyanotic heart disease patients and specially those with hematocrit >65 % are admitted to the hospital before surgery for preoperative hydration and to avoid triggering hyperviscosity syndrome with prolonged preoperative fasting. Intraoperative acute red cell reduction by replacing equal volume with plasma or albumin has shown to increase cardiac output and cerebral blood flow. In addition platelet function and hemostasis will improve within a few hours of phlebotomy. Sahoo et al. showed that hemodilution to a hematocrit of 45 % in patients with cyanotic heart disease undergoing Blalock–Taussig (BT) shunt decreases postoperative blood loss and increases shunt patency (Sahoo et al. 2007).

Intraoperative

General Measures

Control of surgical bleeding is crucial to stop triggering the coagulation cascade by the tissue factor and to avoid consumption coagulopathy. Furthermore the persistent factors of bleeding should be corrected, for example, hypothermia, acidosis, electrolyte disturbance, and erythrocytosis. Even how rewarming is conducted is very important to avoid the temperature after-drop after weaning of CPB with core hypothermia. Saleh et al. showed that decreasing the temperature gradient between the heater–cooler unit and the patient core temperature to only 3 °C improved the hemodynamics, lowered the inotropic requirement, improved the hemostasis, and decreased the ICU stay (Saleh and Barr 2005).

During CPB heparin anticoagulation is used to decrease coagulation activation and to avoid thrombosis of the bypass circuit. The benefits of the use of heparin concentration-based systems (Hepcon HMS; Medtronic, Minneapolis, MN) to titrate heparin effect are still debated in cardiac surgery. Guzzetta et al. showed that a heparin concentration-based system protocol in infants (<6 months) was associated with reduced activation of the hemostatic system decreasing postoperative blood loss and avoiding blood transfusion (Guzzetta et al. 2008). In an adult population, Ichikawa et al. showed that residual UH by Hepcon did not correlate with postoperative bleeding after cardiac surgery (Ichikawa et al. 2014). Protamine binds ionically to UH to reverse its effect.

The adequate dosing of protamine is crucial because the incomplete reversal of UH will affect the patient hemostasis. On the other hand, excess protamine can lead to hypercoagulable state due to its inhibition of serine proteases debilitating the clot strength and clot kinetics and decreasing platelet aggregation. Again the use of Hepcon monitoring for protamine titration is still controversial. Gautam et al. recommended calculating protamine dosing with patient-estimated blood volume instead of dosing to the combined blood volume (pump+patient blood volume) to avoid prolongation of the initiation of the clotting time due to excess protamine (Gautam et al. 2013). Other strategies used to decrease the CPB activation of inflammatory and coagulation pathways are to limit cardiotomy suction, improve CPB circuit biocompatibility, supplement antithrombin III, and prophylactic use of antifibrinolytics.

Prophylactic Agents

Antifibrinolytics (Table 36.3)

The lysine analogs tranexamic acid (TXA) and ε-aminocaproic acid (EACA) are the two current commercially available antibrinolytics in the United States. Current guidelines recommend the intraoperative use of antibrinolytics to reduce perioperative bleeding in high-, medium-, and low-risk cardiovascular surgery. Comparative studies in children with cyanotic heart disease undergoing corrective surgery between TXA and EACA showed no difference in terms of reducing postoperative blood loss, as well as blood and blood product use (Chauhan et al. 2004; Martin

Table 36.3 Antifibrinolytics

Drug	Mechanism of action	Pharmacokinetics	Therapeutic concentration/dose	Adverse effects
Tranexamic acid	Inhibits the degradation of fibrinogen	*Protein binding* 3% V_d, 0.39 L/kg *Half-life*, 2 h *Excretion* renal via glomerular filtration (95% of unchanged)	20 mcg/mL *Bolus dose* 6.4 mg/kg *Infusion* between 2.0 and 3.1 mg/kg/h (decrease infusion with increase weight)	Seizures Thrombosis

ε-Aminocaproic acid	Inhibits the degradation of fibrinogen	*Protein binding*
		 V_d, 0.42 L/kg
		 Half-life, 77 min
		 Excretion renal via glomerular filtration
			50–130 mg/l
			 Pediatric
			   Bolus 75 mg/kg over 10 min
			   Infusion 75 mg/kg
			   Pump prime 250 μg per 1 ml of prime
			 Neonates
			   Bolus 40 mg/kg
			   Infusion of 30 mg/kg^{-1}/h
			   Pump prime 0.1 mg per 1 ml of prime
				Thrombosis

et al. 2011a). In addition, in newborn surgery, EACA and TXA have been equally effective to prevent postoperative bleeding (Martin et al. 2011b).

The mechanism of action of lysine analogs is to bind competitively to the lysine-binding site on plasminogen, which inhibits the attachment of plasmin to fibrin, impeding the degradation of fibrin and fibrinolysis.

Large differences have been reported in the pharmacokinetics of antifibrinolytics between adults and children undergoing cardiac surgery on CPB especially in neonates due to their lack of renal and liver maturation. In addition neonates suffer a massive hemodilution effect (50–100 % of their blood volume), diluting the coagulation factors as well as the antifibrinolytic drug (Nilsson 1980; Ririe et al. 2002).

The pharmacokinetics of TXA is characterized by low protein binding (3 %) and low volume of distribution (0.39 L/kg). The elimination half-life is 2 h and is eliminated unchanged by urinary excretion primarily via glomerular filtration. The therapeutic drug concentration for fibrinolysis inhibition is 10–20 mcg/mL.

Traditionally dosing schemes derived from adult studies recommended 100 mg/kg over 15 min followed by a continuous infusion of 10 mg/kg/h, and 100 mg/kg was injected into the pump reservoir. Following concerns of increases in seizure activity, the TXA dosing has been decreased to 30 mg/kg load, 15 mg/kg/h infusion, and 2 mg/kg in the CPB prime (Murkin et al. 2010). Recent pharmacokinetic studies suggested lower weight-adjusted dose to achieve a therapeutic concentration of 20 mcg/kg. The recommended TXA bolus dose is 6.4 mg/kg followed by a continuous infusion between 2.0 and 3.1 mg/kg/h (infusion rate decreases with increasing weight) (Grassin-Delyle et al. 2013).

High-dose TXA regimens in older patients undergoing CPB with open-chamber cardiac surgery have been associated with clinical seizures in susceptible patients. The proposed mechanisms for the seizures include decreased blood flow and inhibition of γ-aminobutyric acid A (GABA-A) receptors. The GABA-A receptors hyperpolarize the brain by increasing the chloride conductance through the receptor. TXA blocking the GABA-A receptor lowers the depolarization threshold and enhances excitotoxicity (Eaton et al. 2015).

The EACA has similar pharmacokinetics to TXA with no protein binding, volume of distribution (0.42 L/kg), and an elimination half-life of 77 min.

More than 80 % is eliminated unchanged in the urine by glomerular filtration.

The therapeutic drug concentration for fibrinolysis inhibition is 50–130 mg/L.

Established EACA dosing in pediatric cardiovascular surgery is 100 mg/kg IV bolus followed by 100 mg/kg infusion and 100 mg/kg added to the pump prime. However a recent study showed that EACA clearance is reduced in neonates undergoing elective cardiac surgery due to the decreased glomerular filtration rate compared with older patients. For this reason the loading dose and infusion dose need to be decreased to about 50 % of dose required in children and adults. Currently simulation studies recommend a priming dose of 0.1 mg EACA per 1 ml of blood prime, an IV loading dose of 40 mg/kg, with an infusion of 30 mg/kg/h. Using this dosing regimen maintained a steady state concentration of 100 mg/L needed to prevent fibrinolysis.

All antifibrinolytic therapy increases the risk of thrombosis either with the use of TXA or EACA so its administration is usually stopped once surgery is finished unless a pattern of hyperfibrinolysis is identified in the POC testing.

The serine protease inhibitor aprotinin is the most effective antifibrinolytic, but it was withdrawn from the US market due to safety concerns. Fergusson et al. in a multicentric randomized trail (BART study) comparing TXA, EACA, and aprotinin in high-risk cardiac surgery demonstrated that, even though it was the most effective drug to decrease the risk of massive bleeding, aprotinin increased the risk of mortality by 2.1 %. The mortality is due to increase risk of cardiac death (cardiogenic shock, right ventricular failure, congestive heart failure, or myocardial infarction). In other studies aprotinin has been linked with acute renal failure (Fergusson et al. 2008).

Treatment

The treatment of postoperative bleeding should be multimodal. One hand should address the blood loss with PRBC replacement, but the other hand ought to treat the coagulation disorder guided by POC testing. Massive blood transfusion is defined by the replacement of one or more circulating blood volumes. The estimated blood volume (EBV) decreases with age (Table 36.4). It is important in pediatric to calculate the maximal allowable blood loss (MABL):

$$MABL = \left(starting\,Hct - lowest\,acceptable\,Hct \right) / starting\,Hct \times EBV$$

The specific coagulation problem should be identified and addressed.

Abnormal Clot Generation

Abnormal clot generation is considered when the clotting time (CT) is prolonged in EXTEM (>90 s) and INTEM (>240 s).

Table 36.4 Estimated blood volume by age

Age	Estimated blood volume (ml/kg)
Premature infant	90–100
Term infant – 3 months	80–90
Children >3 months	70

Table 36.5 Kcentra composition

Ingredient	Kcentra 500 units
Total protein	120–280 mg
Factor II	380–800 units
Factor VII	200–500 units
Factor IX	400–620 units
Factor X	500–1020 units
Protein C	420–820 units
Protein S	240–680 units
Heparin	8–40 units
Antithrombin III	4–30 units
Human albumin	40–80 mg
Sodium chloride	60–120 mg
Sodium citrate	40–80 mg
HCl	Small amounts
NaOH	Small amounts

Prothrombin Complex Concentrates (PCCs)

Prothrombin complex concentrates (PCCs) are the component of choice to treat abnormal clot generation and for reversal of oral anticoagulation before emergent cardiac surgery. PCCs are vitamin-K-dependent coagulation factors. In the United States the PCC available is Kcentra® (CSL Behring LLC, Kankakee, IL 60901) in which components are detailed in Table 36.5. The initial dose should be adjusted to the patients with INR. If the starting INR is between 2 and 4, the Kcentra® initial dose should be 25 IU/kg but not to exceed 2500. For INRs between 4 and 6, the initial dose should be 35 U/kg, and for INRs >6 IU/kg the initial dose should be 50 IU/kg. There is very limited published information in pediatrics with Kcentra®. Beaty et al. just published the initial experience at our center with Kcentra® (Beaty et al. 2016; Demeyere et al. 2010). Thromboembolic events have been reported with the repeated use of PCC.

Activated Factor VII

Activated factor VII (factor VIIa) is usually considered for patients with intractable bleeding after pediatric cardiac surgery once other treatments have been used and failed. Okonta et al. reviewed the published experience with factor VIIa, which shows that it is effective in decreasing postoperative bleeding once other measures have failed. The recommended starting dose is 90 μg/kg; repeated doses might be given at 2-h interval (maximum of two doses). Thrombosis is the principal complication that has been reported with an incidence 4.2 %. Patients on ECMO are at the highest risk for thrombosis. Thrombosis of the ECMO circuit has been reported. Lastly Kcentra® contains 200–500 units of factor VII so the use of factor VIIa should be avoided in these cases (Okonta et al. 2012; Guzzetta et al. 2012).

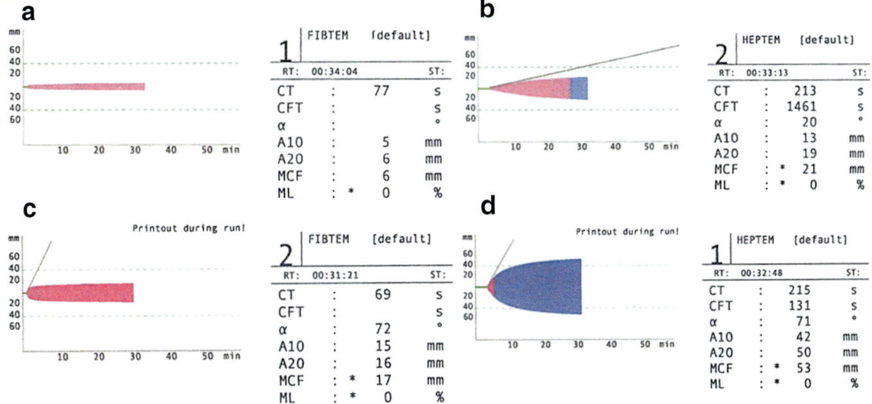

Fig. 36.4 (**a, b**) ROTEM tracing shows a decreased MCF in FIBTEM (<7–12 mm) and/or decreased MCF in the HEPTEM (<50 mm). (**c, d**) The ROTEM tracing showed a FIBTEM MCF >17 mm and HEPTEM MCF >53 mm after the patient received 10 ml/kg of platelets and 70 ml/kg of fibrinogen concentrate (RiaSTAPTM, CSL Behring LLC, Kankakee, IL)

Abnormal Clot Stability

Abnormal clot stability is suspected when the ROTEM maximum lysis (ML) >15 % of maximum clot firmness (MCF) in EXTEM (Fig. 36.4). Comparing EXTEM with APTEM, results can be used to diagnose hyperfibrinolysis. If the APTEM results improve the EXTEM, one hyperfibrinolysis should be considered.

Antifibrinolytics

Antifibrinolytics are the agents of choice to treat hyperfibrinolysis diagnosed by a pattern of abnormal clot stability on EXTEM. In high-risk cardiovascular surgery, antifibrinolytics are used as a prophylactic agent as described above. If they have not been used prophylactically and an ML >15 % of MCF in EXTEM, either EACA or TXA should be started.

Clot Firmness

The clot firmness is affected when there is decreased concentration of fibrinogen, factor XIII, and/or platelets. The ROTEM tracing shows a decreased MCF in FIBTEM (<7–12 mm) and/or decreased MCF in the HEPTEM/EXTEM/INTEM (<50 mm). Since fibrinogen is an intravascular component and there is no tissue reservoir, is first coagulation factor to drop after uncontrolled bleeding. There are two ways of replacing fibrinogen.

Fibrinogen Concentrate

Fibrinogen concentrate is obtained from human plasma by pasteurization and sterile filtration achieving a complete virus inactivation, which precludes viral disease transmission. Another advantage of fibrinogen concentrates in pediatric patients is the small volume required for its reconstitution avoiding volume overload complications (e.g., TACO or TRALI) and dilution of platelets and/or PRBC. Galas et al. showed that fibrinogen concentrate is as effective as cryoprecipitate in postoperative bleeding after pediatric cardiac surgery (Galas et al. 2014). RiaSTAP® (CSL Behring LLC Kankakee, IL 60901) is commercially available in the United States. The recommended dose if the fibrinogen level is known is:

$$\text{Dose}\left(\text{mg}\,/\,\text{kg}\right) = \left[\text{Target Fib}\left(\text{mg}\,/\,\text{dL}\right) - \text{measured Fib}\left(\text{mg}\,/\,\text{dL}\right)\right] \\ /1.7\left(\text{mg}\,/\,\text{dL per mg}\,/\,\text{kg}\right)$$

If the plasma concentration of fibrinogen is unknown, the starting dose is 70 mg/kg body weight.

Cryoprecipitate

Cryoprecipitate is the cold-insoluble white precipitate that forms when a unit of FFP is thawed at 1–6 °C and is kept at room air with a very short half-life of 4 h. A unit of cryoprecipitate (5–15 ml) contains fibrinogen (150–250 mg), factor VIII (80–150 UI), von Willebrand factor (40–70 % plasma concentration), factor XIII (30 % of original plasma concentration), and fibronectin (30–60 mg). In a cardiac surgery population, patients who received cryoprecipitate associated with FFP experience less bleeding than patients treated with FFP alone. Cryoprecipitate use is associated with increased 5-year mortality in cardiac surgery, but it may be related to the severity of the bleeding itself not the cryoprecipitate. The dose used is variable. In our center we start with 1 unit every 5 kg in neonates and infants. Re-dosing is based on fibrinogen levels and/or FIBTEM tracing.

Since the availability of fibrinogen concentrates, cryoprecipitate is the second-line treatment of postoperative bleeding due to hypofibrinogenemia due to concerns of transmission blood-borne pathogen, TACO, and TRALI (Nascimento et al. 2014; Gorlinger et al. 2013).

Platelets

Platelets are prepared from the platelet-rich plasma component by apheresis. The platelets come from either a single or random donor platelets. Platelets have a short shelf life of only 4 days since they are stored at room temperature (20–24 °C) with continuous agitation to avoid aggregation. Due to this issue, platelets have the highest rate of bacterial contamination. Although irradiation is used to kill viable lymphocytes, compatibility between recipients and donors is recommended in infants and children. Platelets transfusion is indicated when POC testing shows a decreased MCF in the HEPTEM/EXTEM/INTEM (<50 mm) with normal MCF in FIBTEM. Platelet count after cardiac surgery is an unreliable trigger for transfusion since platelets tend to clump in the post-hypothermic CPB period. In infants and neonates, we dose 1 unit every 5 kg of body weight. Platelet administration is not devoid of complications, and adult studies have shown association between platelet transfusion and TRALI and ischemic events.

Fresh Frozen Plasma

Fresh frozen plasma (FFP) is prepared from the platelet-rich plasma component of whole blood or by apheresis and contains anti-ABO antibodies, and it is stored at –18 °C or cooler. Factors V and VIII activity diminishes after 24 h. The freezing process kills the leukocytes, and further irradiation is not needed. FFP is thawed in a water bath at 30–37 °C for approximately 20–30 min before transfusion. Similarly to PRBC patients can only receive plasma with anti-ABO antibodies that will not react with the patient's ABO surface antigens. Currently FFP is used if individual components are not available for prolonged CT in EXTEM (>90 s) and INTEM (>240 s) and oral anticoagulant reversal. Starting dose is 5–10 mL/kg, but oftentimes higher doses are needed to achieve hemostasis. FFP volumes >15 mL/kg are associated with TACO, TRALI, sepsis, and nosocomial infections (Khan et al. 2007; Sarani et al. 2008).

Packed Red Blood Cells

Packed red blood cells are necessary to increase the blood's oxygen-carrying capacity and therefore increase end-organ perfusion. The threshold for transfusion depends on age, weight, physiology (cyanotic vs. acyanotic), ongoing blood loss, and adequacy of oxygenation/perfusion. In general PRBC transfusion is indicated if hemoglobin concentration is <7 g/dL; however the threshold for transfusion can be higher in the premature, cyanosis, or chronic conditions (Guzzetta 2011). The physiologic nadir for hemoglobin occurs at approximately 2–3 months of age. The use of somatic and cerebral oximetry can guide transfusion in critical patients. Leukocyte reduction used to decrease febrile nonhemolytic transfusion reactions, alloimmunization of recipients to HLA antigens, and transmission of cytomegalovirus (CMV) even though the evidence is inconclusive (Simancas-Racines et al. 2015). PRBC are stored at 1–6 °C in the anticoagulant/preservative solution citrate, phosphate, dextrose, adenine-formula 1 (CPDA-1). The hematocrit on PRBC is 65–80 % with a shelf life of 35 days. Irradiation is used to prevent transfusion-associated graft-versus-host disease in immunocompromised patients or transplant candidates but decreases shelf life (28 days). The target hematocrit on bypass is a debatable issue.

No difference in outcomes has been seen between hematocrit of 25 and 35 % during CPB for pediatric congenital heart surgery in terms of blood product use, psychomotor development, and imaging (Newburger et al. 2008). Before going on, CPB is important to calculate the predicted hematocrit change (Δ Htc), and the PRBC need to achieve a desired hematocrit on CBP with the following formulas:

$$\Delta Htc = Htc_{pt} \times Pt_{BV} / Pt_{BV} + CPB_{PB}$$

$$PRBC(mL) = \left[Htc_{CPB} \times (Pt_{BV} + CPB_{PB}) - (Pt_{BV} \times Htc_{pt}) \right] / 60\%$$

Where Pt_{BV} is patient blood volume, CBP_{PB} is priming volume, PRBC is packed red blood cells, Htc_{pt} is patient hematocrit, and Htc_{CPB} is the hematocrit on the prime.

Adverse Effects (Table 36.6)

Transfusion-related acute lung injury (TRALI) is characterized by non-cardiogenic pulmonary edema and severe hypoxia. The treatment is symptomatic with supporting measures including mechanical ventilation.

TRALI is the most common transfusion-related cause of death. There is a two-hit hypothesis for TRALI. First is transfused neutrophils activating the endothelial cell in the lung, followed by the second hit which is overwhelming inflammatory response, capillary leakage, and pulmonary edema. Transfusion circulatory overload (TACO) is the second leading cause of transfusion-related death. TACO is considered as acute pulmonary edema during or shortly after

Table 36.6 Transfusion complications

Metabolic	Hypocalcemia and hypomagnesemia (e.g., citrate toxicity)
	Hyperkalemia secondary to PRBC leakage: worse in old (>7 days) and irradiated blood
	Hypothermia
	Acidosis due to PRBC shift to anaerobic metabolism increasing lactic acid
	Shifts in the oxygen–hemoglobin dissociation curve
Infectious	Decreased by screening tests but not zero due to false-negative screen
	Hepatitis A, B, and C
	HIV
	Human T lymphotropic virus I and II
Immune mediated	Incompatibility: clerical error while checking blood products
	Graft-versus-host disease is caused by lymphocytes contained in a transfused blood component proliferate and causes host tissue destruction
	Hemolytic transfusion reactions
	Febrile nonhemolytic transfusion reactions
	Allergic reactions
	Transfusion-related acute lung injury
	Post-transfusion purpura
	Transfusion-related immunomodulation
	Alloimmunization

transfusion and is associated with symptoms and signs of congestive cardiac failure. TACO is associated with elevated B-type natriuretic peptide due to chamber distension (Toy et al. 2012; Iyengar et al. 2013).

Outcome

Guzzetta et al. showed that neonates who bleed more (upper quartile) post cardiac surgery on CPB had a statistically significant increased risk of postoperative dialysis and ECMO support (Guzzetta 2011). In addition neonates who had higher incidence of postoperative bleeding had longer hospital stay were at a higher risk for in-hospital mortality. Wolf et al. demonstrated that early postoperative bleeding was independently associated with an increased mortality, postoperative mechanical ventilation, and intensive care unit stay in infants after cardiac surgery (Wolf et al. 2014).

Case Vignette

Six-month-old boy (6.5 kg/66 cm) with past medical history of dextrocardia, double-inlet left ventricle, ventricular septal defect, subpulmonic stenosis, and right ventricular hypoplasia. He was palliated as a newborn with a modified right BT shunt (3.5 mm), and he was receiving aspirin until the day of surgery. In addition to his cardiac condition, the patient carries sickle cell trait with a hemoglobin (Hb) S of 39 %.

Currently the patient is experiencing desaturation (SaO_2 low 70s) due to outgrowth of the BT shunt and is scheduled for bidirectional cavo-pulmonary shunt (Glenn shunt) and pulmonary valve oversaw on CPB. The CPB prime volume for this size patient is 350 ml, and the estimated patient's blood volume is ~500 ml. To avoid a sickle cell crisis while in surgery due to the elevated Hb S (39 %), an exchange transfusion was planned on starting CPB (Table 36.7). The total prime volume ~900 ml was set to match the circuit prime volume and the patient's estimated blood volume.

Due to a complex anatomy, the repair was long with a CPB duration of 294 min and a cross clamp time of 146 min. In addition to the prime blood products, two additional units of PRBC and one unit of FFP were administered during CPB. The patient has several risk factors for postoperative bleeding including size, weight, cyanotic heart disease with single-ventricle physiology, aspirin until day of surgery, Glenn shunt surgery, long cardiopulmonary bypass, and a complete exchange transfusion. POC testing with ROTEM was used showing a decreased MCF in the FIBTEM y HEPTEM (Fig. 36.4a, b). This POC testing finding was consistent with the clinical scenario in which the patient due to the complete exchange transfusion the platelets were removed from the circulation and the fibrinogen was remarkably

Table 36.7 CPB prime for exchange transfusion

PRBC	595 ml
FFP	335 ml
Heparin	3500 U
NaHCO$_3$	20 mEq
CaCl$_2$	500 mg
EACA	420 mg

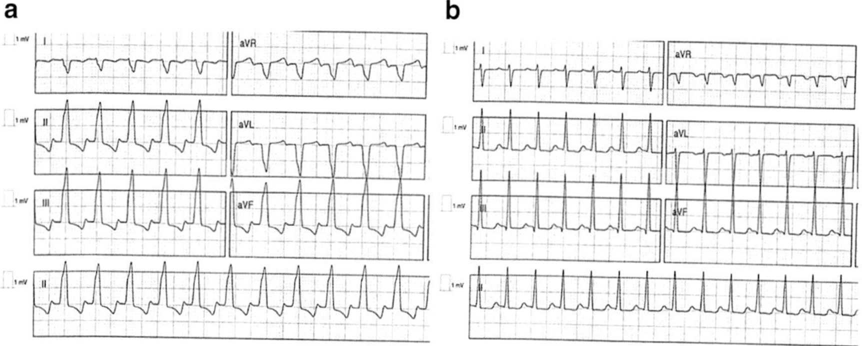

Fig. 36.5 (**a**) EKG trace showing a wide complex tachycardia secondary to hyperkalemia (K = 6.5 mEq/L) due to the multiple PRBC use. (**b**) EKG trace normalized after the potassium dropped to 5.2 mEq/L due to 15 min PRBC washing and increasing ionized Ca to 1.3 mEq/L

hemodiluted. Following our institutional POC, ROTEM-guided transfusion protocol recommended the administration of platelets and fibrinogen (Fig. 36.4). Once the aorta was unclamped, the EKG showed a wide complex tachycardia probably secondary to hyperkalemia (K = 6.5 mEq/L) due to the multiple PRBC use (Fig. 36.5a). After 15 min of washing the PRBC and increasing the ionized Ca to 1.3 mEq/L, the potassium dropped to 5.2 mEq/L and the EKG normalized (Fig. 36.5b). There was still profuse bleeding from the suture lines once the patient was weaned off CPB, and heparin was reversed with protamine achieving a baseline ACT. The patient received 10 ml/kg of platelets and 70 ml/kg of fibrinogen concentrate (RiaSTAPTM, CSL Behring LLC, Kankakee, IL) with remarkable clinical response. The ROTEM tracing showed a FIBTEM MCF >17 mm and HEPTEM MCF >53 mm (Fig. 36.4c, d). The patient was admitted to the ICU and weaned off the ventilator the next day. He did not present with any further bleeding problems.

References

Annich G, Adachi I. Anticoagulation for pediatric mechanical circulatory support. Pediatr Crit Care Med. 2013;14:S37–42.

Arnold PD. Coagulation and the surgical neonate. Paediatr Anaesth. 2014;24:89–97.

Augoustides JG. The inflammatory response to cardiac surgery with cardiopulmonary bypass: should steroid prophylaxis be routine? J Cardiothorac Vasc Anesth. 2012;26:952–8.

Awtry EH, Loscalzo J. Aspirin. Circulation. 2000;101:1206–18.

Beaty RS, Moffett BS, Mahoney Jr DH, Yee DL, Lee-Kim YJ. Use of 4-factor prothrombin concentrate (kcentra) in hospitalized pediatric patients. Ann Pharmacother. 2016;50:70–1.

Calatzis A, Spannagl M, Vorweg M (2013) ROTEM Analysis Targeted Treatment of Acute Haemostatic Disorders. ROTEM Promotional Analysis booklet.

Chauhan S, Das SN, Bisoi A, Kale S, Kiran U. Comparison of epsilon aminocaproic acid and tranexamic acid in pediatric cardiac surgery. J Cardiothorac Vasc Anesth. 2004;18:141–3.

Cheung EW, Chay GW, Ma ES, Cheung YF. Systemic oxygen saturation and coagulation factor abnormalities before and after the fontan procedure. Am J Cardiol. 2005;96:1571–5.

Christensen MC, Dziewior F, Kempel A, von Heymann C. Increased chest tube drainage is independently associated with adverse outcome after cardiac surgery. J Cardiothorac Vasc Anesth. 2012;26:46–51.

Christensen MC, Krapf S, Kempel A, von Heymann C. Costs of excessive postoperative hemorrhage in cardiac surgery. J Thorac Cardiovasc Surg. 2009;138:687–93.

Demeyere R, Gillardin S, Arnout J, Strengers PF. Comparison of fresh frozen plasma and prothrombin complex concentrate for the reversal of oral anticoagulants in patients undergoing cardiopulmonary bypass surgery: a randomized study. Vox Sang. 2010;99:251–60.

Desborough M, Sandu R, Brunskill SJ, Doree C, Trivella M, Montedori A, Abraha I, Stanworth S. Fresh frozen plasma for cardiovascular surgery. Cochrane Database Syst Rev. 2015;7:CD007614.

Donmez A, Yurdakok O. Cardiopulmonary bypass in infants. J Cardiothorac Vasc Anesth. 2014;28:778–88.

Eaton MP, Alfieris GM, Sweeney DM, Angona RE, Cholette JM, Venuto C, Anderson B. Pharmacokinetics of epsilon-aminocaproic acid in neonates undergoing cardiac surgery with cardiopulmonary bypass. Anesthesiology. 2015;122:1002–9.

Esper SA, Levy JH, Waters JH, Welsby IJ. Extracorporeal membrane oxygenation in the adult: a review of anticoagulation monitoring and transfusion. Anesth Analg. 2014;118:731–43.

Espinosa A, Stenseth R, Videm V, Pleym H. Comparison of three point-of-care testing devices to detect hemostatic changes in adult elective cardiac surgery: a prospective observational study. BMC Anesthesiol. 2014;14:80.

Everett LL, Birmingham PK, Williams GD, Brenn BR, Shapiro JH. Herbal and homeopathic medication use in pediatric surgical patients. Paediatr Anaesth. 2005;15:455–60.

Fergusson DA, Hebert PC, Mazer CD, Fremes S, MacAdams C, Murkin JM, Teoh K, Duke PC, Arellano R, Blajchman MA, Bussieres JS, Cote D, Karski J, Martineau R, Robblee JA, Rodger M, Wells G, Clinch J, Pretorius R, Investigators B. A comparison of aprotinin and lysine analogues in high-risk cardiac surgery. N Engl J Med. 2008;358:2319–31.

Galas FR, de Almeida JP, Fukushima JT, Vincent JL, Osawa EA, Zeferino S, Camara L, Guimaraes VA, Jatene MB, Hajjar LA. Hemostatic effects of fibrinogen concentrate compared with cryoprecipitate in children after cardiac surgery: a randomized pilot trial. J Thorac Cardiovasc Surg. 2014;148:1647–55.

Gautam NK, Schmitz ML, Harrison D, Zabala LM, Killebrew P, Belcher RH, Prodhan P, McKamie W, Norvell DC. Impact of protamine dose on activated clotting time and thromboelastography in infants and small children undergoing cardiopulmonary bypass. Paediatr Anaesth. 2013;23:233–41.

Gorlinger K, Shore-Lesserson L, Dirkmann D, Hanke AA, Rahe-Meyer N, Tanaka KA. Management of hemorrhage in cardiothoracic surgery. J Cardiothorac Vasc Anesth. 2013;27:S20–34.

Grassin-Delyle S, Couturier R, Abe E, Alvarez JC, Devillier P, Urien S. A practical tranexamic acid dosing scheme based on population pharmacokinetics in children undergoing cardiac surgery. Anesthesiology. 2013;118:853–62.

Gruenwald C, de Souza V, Chan AK, Andrew M. Whole blood heparin concentrations do not correlate with plasma antifactor Xa heparin concentrations in pediatric patients undergoing cardiopulmonary bypass. Perfusion. 2000;15:203–9.

Guay J, Rivard GE. Mediastinal bleeding after cardiopulmonary bypass in pediatric patients. Ann Thorac Surg. 1996;62:1955–60.

Guzzetta NA, Allen NN, Wilson EC, Foster GS, Ehrlich AC, Miller BE. Excessive postoperative bleeding and outcomes in neonates undergoing cardiopulmonary bypass. Anesth Analg. 2015;120:405–10.

Guzzetta NA, Bajaj T, Fazlollah T, Szlam F, Wilson E, Kaiser A, Tosone SR, Miller BE. A comparison of heparin management strategies in infants undergoing cardiopulmonary bypass. Anesth Analg. 2008;106:419–25, table of contents.

Guzzetta NA. Benefits and risks of red blood cell transfusion in pediatric patients undergoing cardiac surgery. Paediatr Anaesth. 2011;21:504–11.

Guzzetta NA, Russell IA, Williams GD. Review of the off-label use of recombinant activated factor VII in pediatric cardiac surgery patients. Anesth Analg. 2012;115:364–78.

Hayashi T, Sakurai Y, Fukuda K, Yada K, Ogiwara K, Matsumoto T, Yoshizawa H, Takahashi Y, Yoshikawa Y, Hayata Y, Taniguchi S, Shima M. Correlations between global clotting function tests, duration of operation, and postoperative chest tube drainage in pediatric cardiac surgery. Paediatr Anaesth. 2011;21:865–71.

Hofer A, Kozek-Langenecker S, Schaden E, Panholzer M, Gombotz H. Point-of-care assessment of platelet aggregation in paediatric open heart surgery. Br J Anaesth. 2011;107:587–92.

Ichikawa J, Kodaka M, Nishiyama K, Hirasaki Y, Ozaki M, Komori M. Reappearance of circulating heparin in whole blood heparin concentration-based management does not correlate with postoperative bleeding after cardiac surgery. J Cardiothorac Vasc Anesth. 2014;28:1003–7.

Iyengar A, Scipione CN, Sheth P, Ohye RG, Riegger L, Bove EL, Devaney EJ, Hirsch-Romano JC. Association of complications with blood transfusions in pediatric cardiac surgery patients. Ann Thorac Surg. 2013;96:910–6.

Jain A, Agarwal R, Sankar MJ, Deorari A, Paul VK. Hypocalcemia in the newborn. Indian J Pediatr. 2010;77:1123–8.

Kaufman DW, Kelly JP, Rosenberg L, Anderson TE, Mitchell AA. Recent patterns of medication use in the ambulatory adult population of the United States: the Slone survey. JAMA. 2002;287:337–44.

Khan H, Belsher J, Yilmaz M, Afessa B, Winters JL, Moore SB, Hubmayr RD, Gajic O. Fresh-frozen plasma and platelet transfusions are associated with development of acute lung injury in critically ill medical patients. Chest. 2007;131:1308–14.

Kozek-Langenecker SA, Afshari A, Albaladejo P, Santullano CA, De Robertis E, Filipescu DC, Fries D, Gorlinger K, Haas T, Imberger G, Jacob M, Lance M, Llau J, Mallett S, Meier J, Rahe-Meyer N, Samama CM, Smith A, Solomon C, Van der Linden P, Wikkelso AJ, Wouters P, Wyffels P. Management of severe perioperative bleeding: guidelines from the European Society of Anaesthesiology. Eur J Anaesthesiol. 2013;30:270–382.

Kozek-Langenecker SA. Coagulation and transfusion in the postoperative bleeding patient. Curr Opin Crit Care. 2014;20:460–6.

Kuliczkowski W, Sliwka J, Kaczmarski J, Zysko D, Zembala M, Steter D, Zembala M, Gierlotka M, Kim MH, Serebruany V. Low platelet activity predicts 30 days mortality in patients undergoing heart surgery. Blood Coagul Fibrinolysis. 2016;27:199–204.

Lee GC, Kicza AM, Liu KY, Nyman CB, Kaufman RM, Body SC. Does rotational thromboelastometry (ROTEM) improve prediction of bleeding after cardiac surgery? Anesth Analg. 2012;115:499–506.

Long E, Pitfield AF, Kissoon N. Anticoagulation therapy: indications, monitoring, and complications. Pediatr Emerg Care. 2011;27:55–61; quiz 62–54.

Martin K, Breuer T, Gertler R, Hapfelmeier A, Schreiber C, Lange R, Hess J, Wiesner G. Tranexamic acid versus varepsilon-aminocaproic acid: efficacy and safety in paediatric cardiac surgery. Eur J Cardiothorac Surg. 2011a;39:892–7.

Martin K, Gertler R, Sterner A, MacGuill M, Schreiber C, Horer J, Vogt M, Tassani P, Wiesner G. Comparison of blood-sparing efficacy of epsilon-aminocaproic acid and tranexamic acid in newborns undergoing cardiac surgery. Thorac Cardiovasc Surg. 2011b;59:276–80.

Miao X, Liu J, Zhao M, Cui Y, Feng Z, Zhao J, Long C, Li S, Yan F, Wang X, Hu S. The influence of cardiopulmonary bypass priming without FFP on postoperative coagulation and recovery in pediatric patients with cyanotic congenital heart disease. Eur J Pediatr. 2014;173:1437–43.

Miller BE, Guzzetta NA, Tosone SR, Levy JH. Rapid evaluation of coagulopathies after cardiopulmonary bypass in children using modified thromboelastography. Anesth Analg. 2000;90:1324–30.

Miller BE, Mochizuki T, Levy JH, Bailey JM, Tosone SR, Tam VK, Kanter KR. Predicting and treating coagulopathies after cardiopulmonary bypass in children. Anesth Analg. 1997;85:1196–202.

Mossad EB, Machado S, Apostolakis J. Bleeding following deep hypothermia and circulatory arrest in children. Semin Cardiothorac Vasc Anesth. 2007;11:34–46.

Murkin JM, Falter F, Granton J, Young B, Burt C, Chu M. High-dose tranexamic acid is associated with nonischemic clinical seizures in cardiac surgical patients. Anesth Analg. 2010;110:350–3.

Nakayama Y, Nakajima Y, Tanaka KA, Sessler DI, Maeda S, Iida J, Ogawa S, Mizobe T. Thromboelastometry-guided intraoperative haemostatic management reduces bleeding and red cell transfusion after paediatric cardiac surgery. Br J Anaesth. 2015;114:91–102.

Nascimento B, Goodnough LT, Levy JH. Cryoprecipitate therapy. Br J Anaesth. 2014;113:922–34.

Newburger JW, Jonas RA, Soul J, Kussman BD, Bellinger DC, Laussen PC, Robertson R, Mayer Jr JE, del Nido PJ, Bacha EA, Forbess JM, Pigula F, Roth SJ, Visconti KJ, du Plessis AJ, Farrell DM, McGrath E, Rappaport LA, Wypij D. Randomized trial of hematocrit 25% versus 35% during hypothermic cardiopulmonary bypass in infant heart surgery. J Thorac Cardiovasc Surg. 2008;135:347–54, 354 e341-344.

Nilsson IM. Clinical pharmacology of aminocaproic and tranexamic acids. J Clin Pathol Suppl (R Coll Pathol). 1980;14:41–7.

Okonta KE, Edwin F, Falase B. Is recombinant activated factor VII effective in the treatment of excessive bleeding after paediatric cardiac surgery? Interact Cardiovasc Thorac Surg. 2012;15:690–4.

Orlov D, McCluskey SA, Selby R, Yip P, Pendergrast J, Karkouti K. Platelet dysfunction as measured by a point-of-care monitor is an independent predictor of high blood loss in cardiac surgery. Anesth Analg. 2014;118:257–63.

Ririe DG, James RL, O'Brien JJ, Lin YA, Bennett J, Barclay D, Hines MH, Butterworth JF. The pharmacokinetics of epsilon-aminocaproic acid in children undergoing surgical repair of congenital heart defects. Anesth Analg. 2002;94:44–9, table of contents.

Romlin BS, Wahlander H, Berggren H, Synnergren M, Baghaei F, Nilsson K, Jeppsson A. Intraoperative thromboelastometry is associated with reduced transfusion prevalence in pediatric cardiac surgery. Anesth Analg. 2011;112:30–6.

Romlin BS, Wahlander H, Synnergren M, Baghaei F, Jeppsson A. Earlier detection of coagulopathy with thromboelastometry during pediatric cardiac surgery: a prospective observational study. Paediatr Anaesth. 2013;23:222–7.

Sahoo TK, Chauhan S, Sahu M, Bisoi A, Kiran U. Effects of hemodilution on outcome after modified Blalock-Taussig shunt operation in children with cyanotic congenital heart disease. J Cardiothorac Vasc Anesth. 2007;21:179–83.

Saleh M, Barr TM. The impact of slow rewarming on inotropy, tissue metabolism, and "after drop" of body temperature in pediatric patients. J Extra Corpor Technol. 2005;37:173–9.

Sarani B, Dunkman WJ, Dean L, Sonnad S, Rohrbach JI, Gracias VH. Transfusion of fresh frozen plasma in critically ill surgical patients is associated with an increased risk of infection. Crit Care Med. 2008;36:1114–8.

Seibel K, Berdat P, Boillat C, Wagner B, Zachariou Z, Kessler U. Hemostasis management in pediatric mechanical circulatory support. Ann Thorac Surg. 2008;85:1453–6.

Simancas-Racines D, Osorio D, Martí-Carvajal AJ, Arevalo-Rodriguez I. Leukoreduction for the prevention of adverse reactions from allogeneic blood transfusion. Cochrane Database Syst Rev. 2015;12:CD009745.

Sniecinski RM, Chandler WL. Activation of the hemostatic system during cardiopulmonary bypass. Anesth Analg. 2011;113:1319–33.

Society of Thoracic Surgeons Blood Conservation Guideline Task F, Ferraris VA, Ferraris SP, Saha SP, Hessel 2nd EA, Haan CK, Royston BD, Bridges CR, Higgins RS, Despotis G, Brown JR, Society of Cardiovascular Anesthesiologists Special Task Force on Blood T, Spiess BD, Shore-Lesserson L, Stafford-Smith M, Mazer CD, Bennett-Guerrero E, Hill SE, Body S. Perioperative blood transfusion and blood conservation in cardiac surgery: the Society of Thoracic Surgeons and The Society of Cardiovascular Anesthesiologists clinical practice guideline. Ann Thorac Surg. 2007;83:S27–86.

Thiele RH, Raphael J. A 2014 update on coagulation management for cardiopulmonary bypass. Semin Cardiothorac Vasc Anesth. 2014;18:177–89.

Toy P, Gajic O, Bacchetti P, Looney MR, Gropper MA, Hubmayr R, Lowell CA, Norris PJ, Murphy EL, Weiskopf RB, Wilson G, Koenigsberg M, Lee D, Schuller R, Wu P, Grimes B, Gandhi MJ, Winters JL, Mair D, Hirschler N, Sanchez Rosen R, Matthay MA, Group TS. Transfusion-related acute lung injury: incidence and risk factors. Blood. 2012;119:1757–67.

Vorweg M, Hartmann B, Knuttgen D, Jahn MC, Doehn M. Management of fulminant fibrinolysis during abdominal aortic surgery. J Cardiothorac Vasc Anesth. 2001;15:764–7.

Wijeyeratne YD, Heptinstall S. Anti-platelet therapy: ADP receptor antagonists. Br J Clin Pharmacol. 2011;72:647–57.

Wolf MJ, Maher KO, Kanter KR, Kogon BE, Guzzetta NA, Mahle WT. Early postoperative bleeding is independently associated with increased surgical mortality in infants after cardiopulmonary bypass. J Thorac Cardiovasc Surg. 2014;148:631–6 e631.

Young G. New anticoagulants in children. Hematology Am Soc Hematol Educ Program. 2008;2008:245–50.

Zabala LM, Guzzetta NA. Cyanotic congenital heart disease (CCHD): focus on hypoxemia, secondary erythrocytosis, and coagulation alterations. Paediatr Anaesth. 2015;25:981–9.

Chapter 37
Postoperative Central Nervous System Management in Patients with Congenital Heart Disease

Ali Dabbagh and Michael A.E. Ramsay

The Impact of CNS Outcome in Pediatric Cardiac Surgery

The mortality rate of neonates and pediatrics with congenital heart diseases has decreased during the last decades due to advanced techniques of care especially the perioperative surgical, anesthetic, and intensive care. However, emerging concern has increased regarding neurologic and neurodevelopmental outcome of these patients, with broad list of etiologies and multifactorial risk factors. Different studies have quoted different results for the rate of neurologic injuries: even as high as 70% in some studies (Mahle et al. 2002; Galli et al. 2004; McQuillen et al. 2007; Block et al. 2010; Hirsch et al. 2012; Gaynor et al. 2015; van Tilborg et al. 2016).

Growing evidence suggests that congenital heart disease is by itself a risk factor for increased chance of neurologic injuries: brain injuries are found in about one-third of those full-term neonates who have underlying congenital heart disease. Neonates and infants with congenital heart disease are much more vulnerable to global hypoxic–ischemic insult and white matter injuries including periventricular leukomalacia (PVL). Besides the innate vulnerability of the developing brain to any insult, there are a multitude of perioperative risk factors and perioperative events that increase the chance of brain injuries in this patient population and are discussed in the next section (Mahle et al. 2002; Galli et al. 2004; Miller et al. 2004, 2007; McQuillen et al. 2007; Beca et al. 2009; Block et al. 2010).

A. Dabbagh, MD, FCA (✉)
Cardiac Anesthesiology Department, Anesthesiology Research Center,
Shahid Beheshti University of Medical Sciences, Tehran, Iran
e-mail: alidabbagh@yahoo.com; alidabbagh@sbmu.ac.ir

M.A.E. Ramsay, MD, FRCA
Texas A&M Health Science Center, Baylor University Medical Center
and Baylor Research Institute, Dallas, TX, USA
e-mail: michaera@BaylorHealth.edu

© Springer International Publishing Switzerland 2017
A. Dabbagh et al. (eds.), *Congenital Heart Disease in Pediatric and Adult Patients*, DOI 10.1007/978-3-319-44691-2_37

Risk Factors for CNS Injury in Neonates and Infants Undergoing Cardiac Surgery

Neonates and infants undergoing cardiac surgery are at increased risk of CNS injury before the operation; in fact, many studies have demonstrated inherent genetic and/ or developmental risk factors in association with congenital heart disease (Markowitz et al. 2007; Albers et al. 2010).

Besides, the perioperative period imposes an extra burden on these patients which affects the outcome. Here we discuss these risk factors in brief; a number of them could be modifiable; however, regarding the others, we have limited options.

Many studies have been performed to assess the weight of different risk factors on occurrence of CNS injuries in patients with congenital heart disease undergoing surgery, including both a relatively great number of primary studies and an acceptable number of reviews. We could categorize these risk factors based on a time-based schedule (Markowitz et al. 2007; Williams and Ramamoorthy 2007; Massaro et al. 2008; Nelson et al. 2008; Albers et al. 2010; Sterken et al. 2015):

- Preoperative risk factors (from the fetal period up to the time of operation)
- Intraoperative risk factors (i.e., throughout the time of operation)
- Postoperative risk factors (i.e., during postoperative period which is after termination of surgery and patient transfer to cardiac ICU)

Preoperative Risk Factors for CNS Injuries in Neonates and Children

The main *preoperative risk* factors are summarized in Table 37.1. The majority of these risk factors are not modifiable when the patient undergoes the perioperative care for congenital cardiac surgery; however, some are modifiable, and the others should be recognized in order to manage or at least estimate the risk of the patient in perioperative period (Hsia and Gruber 2006; McQuillen et al. 2007; Lee et al. 2008; Massaro et al. 2008; Albers et al. 2010).

Intraoperative Risk Factors for CNS Injuries in Neonates and Children

The main *intraoperative risk* factors could be mainly categorized under cardiopulmonary bypass (CPB)-related factors which are summarized in Table 37.2; however, intraoperative risk factors are not just limited to this table (Shen et al. 2003; Hsia and Gruber 2006; Lee et al. 2008; Massaro et al. 2008; Albers et al. 2010; Kaltman et al. 2010; Dabbagh et al. 2012).

Table 37.1 *Preoperative* risk factors affecting CNS outcome in neonatal and pediatric congenital heart surgery

Risk factor	Relationship with CNS disorders
Genetic risk factors	Genetic syndromes have a very worse effect on CNS outcome; among them, these are the main ones: trisomy 21, DiGeorge syndrome, conotruncal anomalies, VACTERL, and velocardiofacial syndrome (Atallah et al. 2007; Gaynor et al. 2007; Lee et al. 2008; Kaltman et al. 2010; Chung et al. 2015) Most of the above genetic syndromes have a common syndrome: 22q11 chromosome deletion (Goldmuntz 2005) In neonates with 22q11.2 deletion syndrome, the chance for congenital heart disease is about 80 % (Momma 2010) Carotti et al. have described a number of conotruncal anomalies associated with 22q11 deletion syndrome: "tetralogy of Fallot, pulmonary atresia with ventricular septal defect, truncus arteriosus, interrupted aortic arch, isolated anomalies of the aortic arch, and ventricular septal defect" which are usually associated with other "anomalies of the aortic arch, pulmonary arteries, infundibular septum, and semilunar valves" (Carotti et al. 2008) Other genetic syndromes that are associated with developmental delay in children with congenital heart disease are Alagille, CHARGE, Down, Jacobsen, Noonan, Turner, and Williams (Marino et al. 2012) Genetic vulnerability, genetic predisposition, and perioperative genomics affect CNS outcome in patients undergoing congenital heart surgery; e.g., *APO-E allele polymorphism* is associated with increased chance of CNS disorders (Gaynor et al. 2003, 2007; Marino et al. 2012)

Impaired development of CNS in utero	Antenatal administration of the following could help prevent in utero CNS injuries especially for protection of oligodendrocytes:
	    Free radical scavengers including vitamin E
	    Anti-inflammatory and/or anti-cytokine agents to decrease chance of fetal/maternal inflammation
	    Antibiotics to decrease chance of infection
	(Volpe 2001; Rezaie and Dean 2002; Lee et al. 2008; Licht et al. 2009)

Congenital structural CNS malformations and/or acquired CNS disorders or injuries in utero or during the perioperative period	There is increased chance of congenital structural CNS disorders in patients with CHD; *cerebral dysgenesis* has a wide spectrum from microdysgenesis to major anatomical congenital defects like corpus callosum agenesis, white matter injury, microcephaly, and incomplete opercularization; also, "hypotonia, seizures, feeding difficulties, and brain imaging abnormalities like stroke, hemorrhage, or periventricular leukomalacia" are among the lesions in these patients (Newburger and Bellinger 2006; Licht et al. 2009; Rollins and Newburger 2014)
Antenatal hemodynamic instability and/or preoperative hemodynamic instability including preoperative hypoxia or severe acidosis	Before birth, impaired fetal blood flow and the resulting decrease in brain oxygen delivery are the main sources of brain insults (Licht et al. 2009; Kaltman et al. 2010) After birth, decreased or impaired oxygen delivery to brain results in injuries to the CNS especially the white matter or those regions communicating different parts of the brain (Kaltman et al. 2010) Cardiac arrest and cardiopulmonary resuscitation are both associated with increased risk of worse neurologic and/or neurodevelopmental outcome, either before birth or during the preoperative period (Marino et al. 2012; Rollins and Newburger 2014)

(continued)

Table 37.1 (continued)

Risk factor	Relationship with CNS disorders
Preoperative hyperthermia	Even mild degrees of hyperthermia in ischemic CNS regions could have considerable and significant impacts on CNS status; these deleterious effects should especially be avoided in patients undergoing DHCA; CNS tissue is highly sensitive to ischemia, and temperature changes especially during pre-bypass period and early post-bypass (Shum-Tim et al. 1998; Nussmeier 2005; Shamsuddin et al. 2015; Hu et al. 2016)
Preoperative hypoglycemia	Tight control of blood glucose is controversial; however, hypoglycemia should be avoided (Hirsch et al. 2012)
Prematurity	Congenital heart disease patients with prematurity (<37 weeks, especially those weighing less than 1500 g at birth) are at high risk for developmental delays and/or disorders (Marino et al. 2012; Rollins and Newburger 2014); currently, despite great improvements in care of the neonates in NICUs, about 5–10 % of premature neonates have major motor deficits, while more than 50 % have significant impairments in behavioral, cognitive, or sensory fields (Khalil et al. 2014; Back 2015; Li et al. 2015)
Low birth weight	LBW is an important risk factor because it could be the result of many other independent risk factors including "prematurity, associated genetic syndromes, placental insufficiency, and intrauterine growth restriction" (Gaynor et al. 2007; Lee et al. 2008)
Perinatal asphyxia and/or cardiorespiratory problems in perinatal period	Increase the chance of perinatal hypoxic–ischemic insult to the brain (Gaynor et al. 2007; Lee et al. 2008)
Trauma during birth	Increases the chance for cerebral hemorrhage and/or hypoxic–ischemic insults, which could be possibly a potential source for CNS injuries (Kelly et al. 2014; Li et al. 2015)
Age at the time of surgery	Early corrective surgery vs. late correction is still controversial; early correction is in favor of improved cardiac; also, CNS plasticity in neonates could possibly compensate for the effects of CPB; on the other hand, later correction might be in favor of improved CNS outcome and preventing untoward effects of CPB on CNS; controversy still exists (Kaltman et al. 2010; Barron 2013)
Preoperative treatments	Treatments like balloon atrial septostomy is associated with increased risk of stroke in preoperative period; though some studies have not confirmed this (McQuillen et al. 2006; Lee et al. 2008; Beca et al. 2009)
Underlying cardiac lesion	Some specific preoperative cardiac disorders are associated with increased risk of postoperative CNS lesions, e.g., single ventricle anatomy, d-transposition of the great arteries, and tetralogy of Fallot (Mahle et al. 2002; Bellinger et al. 2011, 2015a, b; Goldberg et al. 2014; Dehaes et al. 2015)
Mechanical support/ heart transplantation	Patients receiving mechanical support both in preoperative period or during postoperative care (either as extracorporeal membrane oxygenation or ventricular assist devices) are at risk of hemodynamic instability; besides, they are at increased risk of thromboembolic events; on the other hand, patients with heart transplantation are at increased risk for worse CNS outcome (Massaro et al. 2008; Marino et al. 2012; Rollins and Newburger 2014)

Table 37.2 *Intraoperative* and *cardiopulmonary bypass (CPB)*-related factors affecting CNS outcome in neonatal and pediatric congenital heart surgery

Potential risks	How to prevent or compensate
Gaseous microemboli	Using arterial filters (at least 40 μ; smaller 20 μ filters are superior); using microporous hollow fiber oxygenators; debubbling the oxygenator before CPB with extreme accuracy and vigilance
Macroemboli and particles (especially clots); low levels of antithrombin III	Ensuring enough dose of heparin for anticoagulation before establishment of CPB; using fresh frozen plasma (FFP) in prime volume to compensate for lower levels of antithrombin III, which is common especially in neonates and infants less than 6 months of age; possibly, antithrombin III supplementation is much more efficacious than FFP (Codispoti et al. 2001; Kaltman et al. 2010)
Inflammation due to CPB circuit	A number of anti-inflammatory strategies have been suggested in many studies, in order to be used during CPB; these include steroids (especially methylprednisolone), heparin-coated circuits, leukocyte filtration strategies, using ischemic preconditioning models for the brain, institution of modified ultrafiltration, etc.; none have been proved as a definite therapy (Shen et al. 2003; Ungerleider and Shen 2003; Lee et al. 2008; Kaltman et al. 2010)
Potential episodes of systemic hypotension or hypoperfusion during CPB	Appropriate monitoring; administering more flow during CPB than "full-flow bypass" (Shamsuddin et al. 2015)
Hemodilution during CPB	Avoiding extreme hemodilution during CPB with different methods like priming part of the circuit with RBCs, managing cardioplegia, and using minimum volume circuits; it has been recommended to adjust hematocrit levels with CPB temperature (in Celsius); however, strong evidence recommends strict avoidance of hematocrit levels below 24 % (Ungerleider and Shen 2003; Durandy 2010; Kaltman et al. 2010; Hirsch et al. 2012)
DHCA (deep hypothermic circulatory arrest)	DHCA is a real risk especially when prolonged more than 45 min; administering antegrade cerebral perfusion or regional low flow cerebral perfusion (Gaynor et al. 2007; Kaltman et al. 2010) Alternative neuroprotective strategies like antegrade cerebral perfusion (ACP) have been used for CNS preservation; however, regional cerebral perfusion (RCP) has not been much in favor of improved outcomes (Fraser and Andropoulos 2008; Nelson et al. 2008; Ohye et al. 2009; Kaltman et al. 2010) At least 20 min of cooling should be allowed in order to have appropriate cerebral cooling before DHCA (Hsia and Gruber 2006) Using packed ice around the head during DHCA (Hsia and Gruber 2006; O'Neill et al. 2012)
Rate and duration of core cooling	
pH management during core cooling	Most clinicians have shifted to pH-stat strategy especially when using DHCA (Hsia and Gruber 2006; Abdul Aziz and Meduoye 2010)
Air trapping and air emboli after cardiac chambers are opened	Preventing air ejection into the arterial system after removal of aortic cross clamp by the surgeon; if air bubbling occurs, reestablishment of CPB and other measures like hyperbaric oxygen therapy could be useful

(continued)

Table 37.2 (continued)

Potential risks	How to prevent or compensate
Impaired cerebral perfusion; hemodynamic perturbations of cerebral blood flow (CBF)	Ensuring adequate cerebral perfusion pressure (CPP) and cerebral blood flow (CBF) during CPB; preventing hypotension during CPB; avoiding hemoglobin drop; checking CPB circuit for proper and appropriate size of arterial and venous cannulae; sufficient setting of the CPB reservoir and venous cannulae to ensure venous drainage (Dehaes et al. 2015)
Oxidative stress of the CNS	Antioxidative measurements; normoxic management and avoidance of hyperoxia and controlled reoxygenation during CPB especially in cyanotic patients; monitoring with F(2)-isoprostanes (F(2)-IsoPs), neuron-specific enolase (NSE), S-100 beta, C-reactive protein (Arneson and Roberts 2007; Kaltman et al. 2010; Morita 2012; Cardenas-Rodriguez et al. 2013; Kochanek et al. 2013; Caputo et al. 2014)
Anesthetic drugs	There is great amount of concern in favor of anesthetic neurotoxicity in animal models of developing brain; however, clinically there is still controversy without decisive results, and those studies performed in human have failed to confirm these studies in human pediatric and neonatal anesthesia (McCann and Soriano 2012; Vutskits 2012; Zhou and Ma 2014; Hansen 2015)

Postoperative Risk Factors for CNS Injuries in Neonates and Children

During the *postoperative* period, a number of events go on. First of all, the aftermath of surgical trauma, with all its inflammatory events, affects different organs including CNS. Second, factors like "impaired autoregulation, unstable hemodynamics, hyperthermia after cardiopulmonary bypass, pain, and vanished effects of anesthetic drugs leading to arousal after anesthesia" superimpose the potential underlying factors which may lead to unwanted CNS complications. The main *postoperative risk factors* are categorized in Table 37.3 (Hsia and Gruber 2006; Lee et al. 2008; Massaro et al. 2008; Albers et al. 2010; Kaltman et al. 2010).

Classification of CNS Deficits

The risk of neurologic injuries and adverse neurodevelopmental outcomes is higher in neonates and infants with congenital heart disease (Sherlock et al. 2009). In these patients, CNS deficits are categorized under three main classes:

- Neurologic deficits
- Neurocognitive and neurodevelopmental disorders
- White matter injuries (WMI) including periventricular leukomalacia (PVL)

Table 37.3 *Postoperative* risk factors affecting CNS outcome in neonatal and pediatric congenital heart surgery

Risk factor	How to prevent or compensate
Impaired CNS autoregulation	Hemodynamic stability and prevention of hypotension; ensuring adequate CNS oxygen delivery; prevention of low hematocrit levels; ensuring adequate ventilation and oxygenation
Clinical seizure and/or electroencephalographic (EEG) seizure (i.e., nonconvulsive seizure)	Continuous EEG monitoring; especially for patients at risk of seizure or with underlying CNS disorders; if seizure starts from frontal lobe, a worse "Psychomotor Developmental Index" is predicted in patients under 1 year
Postoperative hyperthermia	Even mild degrees of hyperthermia in ischemic CNS regions could have considerable and significant impacts on CNS status; these deleterious effects should especially be avoided in patients undergoing DHCA; CNS tissue is highly sensitive to ischemia and temperature changes especially during pre-bypass period and early post-bypass (Shum-Tim et al. 1998; Nussmeier 2005; Shamsuddin et al. 2015; Hu et al. 2016)
Postoperative arterial and/or venous desaturation	Optimizing oxygenation, ventilation, hemodynamics, and hematocrit level prevents systemic desaturation; residual shunts or single ventricle anatomy affect significantly the level of postoperative saturation; systemic venous desaturation is an important indicator of decreased systemic oxygen delivery; postoperative monitoring with both "cerebral NIRS" and "somatic NIRS" could be a useful guide to foresee this event
Single ventricle anatomy	Increases the risk of arterial hypoxemia; also, there is increased chance for systemic emboli; all are potential risk factors for postoperative CNS injuries; respiratory maneuvers, preventing hyperventilation and hypocapnia and stable hemodynamics, could help decrease the risk; also, cerebral and somatic NIRS could be of use (Dehaes et al. 2015). Goldberg et al. demonstrated impaired neurodevelopmental state in children with single right ventricle anatomy at 3 years of age (Goldberg et al. 2014)
Increased intracranial pressure (ICP)	Increased ICP leads to decreased cerebral perfusion pressure; head elevation and other maneuvers for prevention of ICP increase should be used
Low cardiac output state (LCOS)	LCOS is predicted to occur 6–18 h after surgery and occurs in 25 % of infants and neonates undergoing congenital heart surgery; residual defects like hypoplastic left heart syndrome are associated with increased chance of LCOS and hemodynamic support with pharmacologic agents (including but not limited to milrinone, dobutamine, and levosimendan) could be used to treat LCOS
Role of oxidative stress on CNS injury and refractory seizure	Antioxidative measurements; normoxic management and avoidance of hyperoxia during CPB especially in cyanotic patients; monitoring with F(2)-isoprostanes (F(2)-IsoPs), neuron-specific enolase (NSE), S-100 beta, C-reactive protein (Morita 2012; Cardenas-Rodriguez et al. 2013; Kochanek et al. 2013)
ICU length of stay	Increased ICU stay associated with higher chance of intelligent quotient (IQ) drop (Newburger et al. 2003; Newburger and Bellinger 2006; Marino et al. 2012; Rollins and Newburger 2014)

(continued)

Table 37.3 (continued)

Risk factor	How to prevent or compensate
Mechanical support/ heart transplantation	Patients receiving mechanical support both in preoperative period or during postoperative care (either as extracorporeal membrane oxygenation or ventricular assist devices) are at risk of hemodynamic instability; besides, they are at increased risk of thromboembolic events; on the other hand, patients with heart transplantation are at increased risk for worse CNS outcome (Massaro et al. 2008; Marino et al. 2012; Rollins and Newburger 2014)

Neurologic Deficits

Neurologic injuries are a common finding in neonates and infants with underlying congenital heart diseases; also, these lesions are among the most important perioperative complications in these patients. The following are among the most common neurologic disorders in these patients (Kinney et al. 2005; Chen et al. 2009; Sherlock et al. 2009; Block et al. 2010; Gaynor et al. 2015):

- White matter injuries (including periventricular leukomalacia or diffuse white matter gliosis)
- Stroke with a 10 % prevalence; half occurring preoperatively (Chen et al. 2009)
- Seizures
- Intraventricular hemorrhage (IVH)
- Visual disturbances
- Gray matter lesions
- Focal neurologic injuries

Neonatal stroke and periventricular leukomalacia (PVL) are the two most significant lesions in patients undergoing congenital heart surgery (Sherlock et al. 2009); however, seizures, either convulsive or nonconvulsive, are among the most serious neurologic complications after congenital heart surgery in neonates and infants; nonconvulsive seizure presenting only as EEG seizure activity is much more common than convulsive seizures in this patient population (Abend et al. 2013).

Neonatal Seizure

Neonatal seizure still remains a great challenge and a clinical dilemma; among the main reasons for this fact, the following could be mentioned:

- Ambiguous presentations.
- Failure of immediate detection.
- Paucity of evidence-based management protocols, especially regarding the standard treatment.
- Poor outcomes.

- Adverse neurodevelopmental outcome and epilepsy are the main considerations as the aftermath of neonatal seizure in the long term, mandating careful follow-up for neonatal seizure patients.

The incidence of neonatal seizure is the highest among all age groups: 1.5–3 per 1000 live births (Silverstein and Jensen 2007; Jensen 2009).

Etiology Among a long list of etiologic factors, these four classes remain the main etiologies for neonatal seizure in 80–85 % of patients (Silverstein and Jensen 2007; Jensen 2009; Kang and Kadam 2015):

- Hypoxic–ischemic encephalopathy (HIE)
- Hemorrhagic events
- Metabolic disorders
- Infectious processes

Among all the above, hypoxic–ischemic encephalopathy (HIE) is the etiology of neonatal seizure in about two-thirds of patients (Jensen 2009).

However, these different etiologies lead to different severities of the disease and diverse outcome; some of the seizures with non-HIE etiologies have good outcomes, while the outcome in HIE is much worse. So, underlying mechanism in neonatal seizure remains a crucial issue in diagnosis and treatment of neonatal seizure (Kang and Kadam 2015).

Risk factors for seizure in neonatal and pediatric patients undergoing cardiac surgery are diverse and heterogeneous; however, the main risk factors in this specific patient population include:

- DHCA
- Longer duration of circulatory arrest
- Asphyxia at birth
- Respiratory distress
- A complication due to use of extracorporeal membrane oxygenation (ECMO)
- Some of the underlying cardiac anomalies like VSD (Helmers et al. 1997; Jensen 2009)

Diagnosis In diagnosis of neonatal seizure, the availability of both amplitude-integrated EEG (aEEG) and standard EEG are very decisive; unless we use aEEG in NICU, a considerable part of patients with neonatal seizure would be undetected (Boylan et al. 2015; Kang and Kadam 2015). aEEG is a bedside tool for neurophysiologic assessment; uses fewer channels than standard EEG; so, aEEG is much easier, both regarding its use and interpretation and could help earlier diagnosis much more than conventional EEG; however standard EEG is more sensitive for diagnosis of seizure. However, it is not a mandatory that aEEG be interpreted by a neurologist. Of course, standard EEG remains the decisive method of diagnosis for neurophysiologic assessments. A full discussion on CNS monitoring tools including EEG could be found in Chap. 9 "CNS Monitoring." For long-term brain imaging and follow-up studies, MR images are one of the best available options; long-term outcome differs based on the underlying etiology; hence, long-term follow-up is a basic rule.

Treatment Though a considerable number of studies have been done to determine the best therapeutic protocol for neonatal seizures, satisfactory evidence is still lacking; however, phenobarbital is considered as the drug of choice; however, its efficacy and the pharmacologic profile of the drug is still the subject of some studies. The final word in selection of the best available anticonvulsant therapeutic protocol is to be said (Hellstrom-Westas et al. 2015; Kang and Kadam 2015).

Neurocognitive and Neurodevelopmental Disorders

Congenital heart disease increases the risk of neurodevelopmental performance including the scores on intelligence, alertness, executive functions, attention and memory, and possibly the daily life care and school function (Sterken et al. 2015). Since neurodevelopmental and neurocognitive aspects of care are of great concern, clinicians have tried to improve this aspect of postoperative outcome; however, difficulties in daily functioning and academic achievements in such patients still remains a problem (Gaynor et al. 2015).

Neurocognitive disorders are categorized under a common framework in DSM-5. Generally, the main characteristic of neurocognitive disorders is "a decline from a previously attained level of cognitive function" and includes "delirium, mild cognitive impairment and dementia" (Hsia and Gruber 2006; Snookes et al. 2010; Sachdev et al. 2014; Simpson 2014). Based on DSM-5 classification, there are six neurocognitive domains:

1. Perceptual motor function: visual perception, visuoconstructional reasoning, and perceptual motor coordination
2. Language: object naming, word finding, fluency, grammar and syntax, and receptive language
3. Learning and memory: free recall, cued recall, recognition memory, semantic and autobiographical long-term memory, and implicit learning
4. Social cognition: recognition of emotions, theory of mind, and insight
5. Complex attention: sustained attention, divided attention, selective attention, and processing speed
6. Executive function: planning, decision making, wording memory, responding to feedback, and inhibition flexibility

For assessment of cognitive function, both clinical neurodevelopmental testing and follow-up MRIs are of great importance; these two remain the main surrogate outcome measures in the aftermath of congenital heart surgeries (Kaltman et al. 2010). For example, there is a specific type of brain injury seen in pediatric patients undergoing congenital heart surgery described by Soul et al.; they found subtle hemorrhagic events, demonstrated in brain MRI as "foci of hemosiderin"; in their study, these lesions were found in postoperative brain MRI, and they described them as small hemorrhagic lesions with the etiology being different from the etiology of hypoxic–ischemic lesions or periventricular leukomalacia. These subtle hemorrhagic foci could be detected by exact MRI studies during serial assessments; also, they have an adverse impact on neurodevelopmental outcome of the children undergoing congenital heart surgery (Soul et al. 2009; Albers et al. 2010).

White Matter Injuries (WMI) Including Periventricular Leukomalacia (PVL)

During recent years, the improved quality of care in NICUs has led to improvements in outcome in some aspects of white matter injuries (WMI); however, there are still areas which are not much well managed. For a better understanding, let's first review the current classification for WMI based on the many of studies performed in this area, both on animal and human samples (Segovia et al. 2008; Buser et al. 2010; Back et al. 2012; Dean et al. 2013; Back 2014, 2015; Back and Miller 2014; McClendon et al. 2014; van Tilborg et al. 2016).

WMI occurs in two forms:

- Selective death of premyelinating oligodendrocytes is more common and involves widespread lesions which are often detected in autopsies and yield to microscopic cysts; however, they are not very well defined by MRI; this type of lesions leads to widespread renewal of premyelinating oligodendrocytes; then leading to reactive gliosis, the final outcome is arrest in maturation of premyelinating oligodendrocytes.
- The other form is widespread "pan-cellular death and necrosis" resulting in cystic PVL and larger lesions compared with the first group; this type of lesion leads to glial and axonal loss.

Both of these lesions lead to "myelination failure" which is discussed more in the next paragraphs.

Definition of PVL Necrosis in deep white matter, which is presented as multifocal symmetrical necrosis areas, often known as cystic PVL or cPVL; the process of necrosis involves premyelinating oligodendrocytes; these necrotic areas are often adjacent to the external angles of the lateral ventricles (Rezaie and Dean 2002; Back 2014; McClendon et al. 2014).

Etiology (Including Predisposing Factors and Mechanisms of Injury)

Risk Factors These are among the mostly reported risk factors for PVL (Herzog et al. 2015; Shang et al. 2015):

- Prematurity
- Preterm infants
- Gestational age of ≤ 32 weeks
- Perinatal infections (especially chorioamnionitis)

- Perinatal hypoxia and/or respiratory distress
- Low-birth-weight infants
- Maternal obesity
- Preterm premature rupture of the membranes (PROM)

Also, there seems to be a negative correlation between gestational age and birth weight (Shang et al. 2015). Resch et al. in a cohort study found "respiratory distress syndrome, preterm premature rupture of the membranes, and chorioamnionitis" as the most common clinical findings associated with PVL (Resch et al. 2015). Chorioamnionitis has been proposed as a risk factor for PVL in many studies, mainly due to its inflammatory effects; however, some controversy exists (Wu and Colford 2000; Chau et al. 2014; Herzog et al. 2015).

Mechanism of Injury Decreased perfusion of the periventricular areas during systemic hypotension and inflammatory responses during the perinatal period has been proposed as the two main mechanisms of injury for PVL; in infants with PVL, higher serum levels of interleukin-1 beta (IL-1β) and tumor necrosis factor-alpha (TNF-α) have been demonstrated, which are accompanied by other proinflammatory mechanisms leading to white matter damage in PVL, while antenatal steroid might suppress the prevalence of PVL (Canterino et al. 2001; du Plessis and Volpe 2002; Rezaie and Dean 2002; Kohelet et al. 2006; Tsukimori et al. 2007; Hagberg et al. 2015; van Tilborg et al. 2016). New insights to inflammatory mechanisms of PVL are in the way: Vontell et al. demonstrated increased expression of glial toll-like receptor 3 (TLR3) protein in infants with PVL which could result in impaired development in preterm infants (Vontell et al. 2013, 2015).

However, the most probable pathologic mechanism of PVL is that etiologic insults result in "acute death in premyelinating oligodendrocytes"; this insult is potentially by microglial activation and liberation of "reactive oxygen and nitrogen species"; these oligodendrocytes should normally be changed to myelinating cells; finally, their failure in normal growth leads to a pathologic process associated with "rapid regeneration of premature oligodendrocytes" which happens during a crucial period of neural circuitry development. Immature neurons are more resistant to cellular death; however, even after the mildest insults in premature neurons, extensive interference and disruption is seen in the maturation process of their dendritic synapses and dendritic latticework; the final result of these insults is impaired cerebral growth and development in neonatal brain and thereafter (Haynes et al. 2003; Back 2014, 2015; Back and Miller 2014; McClendon et al. 2014; van Tilborg et al. 2016).

Prevalence

In neonates with congenital heart disease, PVL is a frequent finding even before they undergo cardiac surgery (Miller et al. 2007), and more than 50% of these patients demonstrate mild ischemic CNS lesions in brain MRI during the postoperative period, often in the form of PVL (Mahle et al. 2002). Also, Galli et al. found that more than 50 % of neonates undergoing cardiac surgery had PVL after surgery; however, in their study, PVL occurred rarely after in older infants after cardiac surgery (Galli et al. 2004).

Clinical Presentation of PVL

PVL has been demonstrated as a risk factor for the following abnormalities with different frequencies (Gurses et al. 1999; Kohelet et al. 2006; Glass et al. 2008; van Haastert et al. 2008; Resch et al. 2015; Shang et al. 2015; van Tilborg et al. 2016):

- Visual impairment
- Auditory disorders
- Sensory disorders
- Gross motor function
- Convulsive or nonconvulsive seizure (not a frequent comorbidity; maximum in 25 % of PVL patients)
- Mental retardation
- Language impediments
- Cognitive impairment
- Psychological disturbances (like autism spectrum disorders, ADHD, and other psychological disturbances)
- Abnormal gait patterns
- Intraventricular hemorrhage

Infants with PVL are at increased risk of seizure; also, it has been demonstrated that in infants with PVL, the following risk factors are significant independent predictors of seizures (Kohelet et al. 2006):

- Decreasing gestational age
- Intraventricular hemorrhage
- Posthemorrhagic hydrocephalus
- Sepsis
- Necrotizing enterocolitis

Diagnosis

Besides the clinical findings, especially in long-term follow-up terms, the diagnosis was commonly confirmed using cerebral ultrasonography; however, recent studies have shown MR images of significantly greater diagnostic value which could detect lesions not detected by cerebral ultrasonography; neuroimaging methods and their biomarkers are not only used as diagnostic and prognostic markers but also they are used as efficient tools for follow-up assessments, long-term outcome assessment, and evaluation of neuroprotective measures (Panigrahy et al. 2012; Kwon et al. 2014; Englander et al. 2015; Van't Hooft et al. 2015).

Treatment

Currently, no well-defined treatment for PVL is available; however, the current research in the field of "molecular mechanisms underlying impeded oligodendrocyte maturation" may help us discover novel therapies; till then, recognition of at-risk patients, prevention of additional injuries, and rehabilitation for the aftermath of the disease remain the mainstay (van Tilborg et al. 2016).

Postoperative Delirium in Pediatric Patients Postoperative delirium after pediatric cardiac surgery is a challenging issue.

Based on DSM-5 criteria, delirium is "characterized by disturbance in attention that makes it difficult for the individual to direct, sustain and shift their focus" (Joshi et al. 2012). According to Sachdev et al., these are the main diagnostic features of delirium based on DSM-5 criteria (Sachdev et al. 2014):

1. Disturbance in attention or awareness.
2. Time course of the disturbance is short, hours to a few days, with fluctuation during the daily time course.
3. Added by a cognition disturbance like "memory deficit, disorientation, language, visuospatial ability, or perception."
4. Numbers 1 and 3 are not better explained in the context of any other neurocognitive disorder.
5. Clinical and/or paraclinical findings demonstrate that the disturbance is directly due to physiological results of another underlying medical and/or substance-induced disorder.

Currently, due to paucity of evidence, at times our practice in this issue is some extrapolations from adult cardiac surgery to pediatric cardiac surgery, and the practice is based on consensus than pure evidence; for example, it is recommended not to use benzodiazepines for treatment of postoperative delirium after pediatric cardiac surgery just because studies in adult cardiac surgery have demonstrated these drugs as potentially deliriogenic.

Keeping the above sentences in mind, general consensus is in favor of pharmacological treatments for postoperative pediatric delirium, just in cases that non-pharmacological treatments go unsuccessful, with the aim to prevent the child from potential self-hazards, discomforting, or endangering himself/herself; since if a child is delirious, he/she will interfere with the treatment process; on the other hand, a well-treated child helps the treatment team to open "appropriate environment" for the parents to take part in the process of care; also, if a delirious child is untreated, the risk of unplanned events decreases: events like unplanned endotracheal extubation or loss of intravenous lines, arterial line, or central line (Malarbi et al. 2011).

Clinical Assessment and Monitoring of Delirium in Pediatric Cardiac Surgery

It is necessary to perform repeated and specific methods for screening of delirium; this approach mandates validated delirium scoring systems developed for pediatric age groups, including (Daoud et al. 2014; Baron et al. 2015):

- pCAM-ICU: the Pediatric Confusion Assessment Method for the Intensive Care Unit (for ages ≥5 years)
- PAED Scale: the Pediatric Anesthesia Emergence Delirium Scale (for ages 1–17 years)
- CAP-D: the Cornell Assessment of Pediatric Delirium, which is a modification of the PAED designed for detection of hypoactive delirium
- CAP-D(R): the revised Cornell Assessment of Pediatric Delirium

Treatment of Postoperative Delirium

Pediatric delirium when recognized responds well to therapy, including both pharmacologic and non-pharmacologic treatments; once the pharmacologic treatment is tailored appropriately, it improves the course of treatment (Schieveld et al. 2007; Madden et al. 2011; Hipp and Ely 2012).

A detailed discussion on pharmacotherapy of postoperative delirium after pediatric cardiac surgery is presented in Chap. 4 of this book; also, Table 4.20 provides a list of drugs used for treatment of pediatric ICU delirium; however, the principles of treatment in hyperactive delirium include the following key items:

- There are some anesthetic drugs with delirium preventing effects when given as premedication or as analgesic during anesthesia, including clonidine (4 µg/kg), propofol, ketamine, halothane, dexmedetomidine, gabapentin, midazolam, magnesium, hydroxyzine, dexamethasone, or opioids (e.g., fentanyl); these agents decrease the chance and/or severity of postoperative delirium in children undergoing general anesthesia; so, especial attention to pain management and also using sedative background medication especially with alpha-2 agonist activity have an important role in prevention of postoperative pediatric delirium (Dahmani et al. 2010, 2014; Costi et al. 2014; Lambert et al. 2014; van Hoff et al. 2015).
- Some anesthetic agents may provoke delirium after general anesthesia; among volatile agents, sevoflurane could increase the chance of delirium especially when the patient is not premedicated (Messieha 2013).
- Pharmacologic treatment, when started, should be continued until full treatment and should be tapered off; abruptly "cutting the off" is dangerous.
- Intravenous haloperidol and oral risperidone are the main drugs used for pharmacologic treatment; risperidone has less adverse events than haloperidol; risperidone has no intravenous form, while in ICU, intravenous forms are at times the preferred choice; atypical antipsychotics like quetiapine are used as off-label pharmacological agents for adult delirium; however, there are limited data for

their application in pediatric delirium; the median daily dose of quetiapine is about 1.3 mg/kg/day with a median treatment duration of 12 days (Warshaw and Mechlin 2009; Madden et al. 2011; McPheeters et al. 2011; Joyce et al. 2015).

- Delirium scoring during pharmacologic treatment is critical and should be done at least 3 times a day; at least one of the scoring systems named in the previous paragraphs should be used as a routine assessment tool; when any of these tools is chosen, monitoring the level of sedation/agitation, assessment of patient behavior regarding psychometric performance, and the clinical opinion of the caregivers should be among the main considerations (Schieveld et al. 2009; van Dijk et al. 2012; Daoud et al. 2014).
- The main complications of pharmacologic therapy include extrapyramidal symptom (including dystonia, akathisia, hyperpyrexia, etc.) and lengthening of QTc interval which might lead to lethal torsade de pointes (Brahmbhatt and Whitgob 2016).

CNS Monitoring

A full chapter of this book deals with CNS monitoring, and the interested audiences could study about it in Chap. 9.

References

Abdul Aziz KA, Meduoye A. Is pH-stat or alpha-stat the best technique to follow in patients undergoing deep hypothermic circulatory arrest? Interact Cardiovasc Thorac Surg. 2010;10:271–82.

Abend NS, Dlugos DJ, Clancy RR. A review of long-term EEG monitoring in critically ill children with hypoxic-ischemic encephalopathy, congenital heart disease, ECMO, and stroke. J Clin Neurophysiol. 2013;30:134–42.

Albers EL, Bichell DP, McLaughlin B. New approaches to neuroprotection in infant heart surgery. Pediatr Res. 2010;68:1–9.

Arneson KO, Roberts 2nd LJ. Measurement of products of docosahexaenoic acid peroxidation, neuroprostanes, and neurofurans. Methods Enzymol. 2007;433:127–43.

Atallah J, Joffe AR, Robertson CM, Leonard N, Blakley PM, Nettel-Aguirre A, Sauve RS, Ross DB, Rebeyka IM. Two-year general and neurodevelopmental outcome after neonatal complex cardiac surgery in patients with deletion 22q11.2: a comparative study. J Thorac Cardiovasc Surg. 2007;134:772–9.

Back SA. Cerebral white and gray matter injury in newborns: new insights into pathophysiology and management. Clin Perinatol. 2014;41:1–24.

Back SA. Brain injury in the preterm infant: new horizons for pathogenesis and prevention. Pediatr Neurol. 2015;53:185–92.

Back SA, Miller SP. Brain injury in premature neonates: a primary cerebral dysmaturation disorder? Ann Neurol. 2014;75:469–86.

Back SA, Riddle A, Dean J, Hohimer AR. The instrumented fetal sheep as a model of cerebral white matter injury in the premature infant. Neurotherapeutics. 2012;9:359–70.

Baron R, Binder A, Biniek R, Braune S, Buerkle H, Dall P, Demirakca S, Eckardt R, Eggers V, Eichler I, Fietze I, Freys S, Frund A, Garten L, Gohrbandt B, Harth I, Hartl W, Heppner HJ, Horter J, Huth R, Janssens U, Jungk C, Kaeuper KM, Kessler P, Kleinschmidt S, Kochanek M,

Kumpf M, Meiser A, Mueller A, Orth M, Putensen C, Roth B, Schaefer M, Schaefers R, Schellongowski P, Schindler M, Schmitt R, Scholz J, Schroeder S, Schwarzmann G, Spies C, Stingele R, Tonner P, Trieschmann U, Tryba M, Wappler F, Waydhas C, Weiss B, Weisshaar G. Evidence and consensus based guideline for the management of delirium, analgesia, and sedation in intensive care medicine. Revision 2015 (DAS-Guideline 2015) – short version. Ger Med Sci. 2015;13:Doc19. e-journal.

Barron DJ. Tetralogy of Fallot: controversies in early management. World J Pediatr Congenit Heart Surg. 2013;4:186–91.

Beca J, Gunn J, Coleman L, Hope A, Whelan LC, Gentles T, Inder T, Hunt R, Shekerdemian L. Pre-operative brain injury in newborn infants with transposition of the great arteries occurs at rates similar to other complex congenital heart disease and is not related to balloon atrial septostomy. J Am Coll Cardiol. 2009;53:1807–11.

Bellinger DC, Rivkin MJ, DeMaso D, Robertson RL, Stopp C, Dunbar-Masterson C, Wypij D, Newburger JW. Adolescents with tetralogy of Fallot: neuropsychological assessment and structural brain imaging. Cardiol Young. 2015a;25:338–47.

Bellinger DC, Watson CG, Rivkin MJ, Robertson RL, Roberts AE, Stopp C, Dunbar-Masterson C, Bernson D, DeMaso DR, Wypij D, Newburger JW. Neuropsychological status and structural brain imaging in adolescents with single ventricle who underwent the fontan procedure. J Am Heart Assoc. 2015b;4:pii: e002302.

Bellinger DC, Wypij D, Rivkin MJ, DeMaso DR, Robertson Jr RL, Dunbar-Masterson C, Rappaport LA, Wernovsky G, Jonas RA, Newburger JW. Adolescents with d-transposition of the great arteries corrected with the arterial switch procedure: neuropsychological assessment and structural brain imaging. Circulation. 2011;124:1361–9.

Block AJ, McQuillen PS, Chau V, Glass H, Poskitt KJ, Barkovich AJ, Esch M, Soulikias W, Azakie A, Campbell A, Miller SP. Clinically silent preoperative brain injuries do not worsen with surgery in neonates with congenital heart disease. J Thorac Cardiovasc Surg. 2010;140:550–7.

Boylan GB, Kharoshankaya L, Wusthoff CJ. Seizures and hypothermia: importance of electroencephalographic monitoring and considerations for treatment. Semin Fetal Neonatal Med. 2015;20:103–8.

Brahmbhatt K, Whitgob E. Diagnosis and management of delirium in critically ill infants: case report and review. Pediatrics. 2016;137:1–5.

Buser JR, Segovia KN, Dean JM, Nelson K, Beardsley D, Gong X, Luo NL, Ren J, Wan Y, Riddle A, McClure MM, Ji X, Derrick M, Hohimer AR, Back SA, Tan S. Timing of appearance of late oligodendrocyte progenitors coincides with enhanced susceptibility of preterm rabbit cerebral white matter to hypoxia-ischemia. J Cereb Blood Flow Metab. 2010;30:1053–65.

Canterino JC, Verma U, Visintainer PF, Elimian A, Klein SA, Tejani N. Antenatal steroids and neonatal periventricular leukomalacia. Obstet Gynecol. 2001;97:135–9.

Caputo M, Mokhtari A, Miceli A, Ghorbel MT, Angelini GD, Parry AJ, Suleiman SM. Controlled reoxygenation during cardiopulmonary bypass decreases markers of organ damage, inflammation, and oxidative stress in single-ventricle patients undergoing pediatric heart surgery. J Thorac Cardiovasc Surg. 2014;148:792–801.e798; discussion 800–791.

Cardenas-Rodriguez N, Huerta-Gertrudis B, Rivera-Espinosa L, Montesinos-Correa H, Bandala C, Carmona-Aparicio L, Coballase-Urrutia E. Role of oxidative stress in refractory epilepsy: evidence in patients and experimental models. Int J Mol Sci. 2013;14:1455–76.

Carotti A, Digilio MC, Piacentini G, Saffirio C, Di Donato RM, Marino B. Cardiac defects and results of cardiac surgery in 22q11.2 deletion syndrome. Dev Disabil Res Rev. 2008;14:35–42.

Chau V, McFadden DE, Poskitt KJ, Miller SP. Chorioamnionitis in the pathogenesis of brain injury in preterm infants. Clin Perinatol. 2014;41:83–103.

Chen J, Zimmerman RA, Jarvik GP, Nord AS, Clancy RR, Wernovsky G, Montenegro LM, Hartman DM, Nicolson SC, Spray TL, Gaynor JW, Ichord R. Perioperative stroke in infants undergoing open heart operations for congenital heart disease. Ann Thorac Surg. 2009;88:823–9.

Chung JH, Cai J, Suskin BG, Zhang Z, Coleman K, Morrow BE. Whole-genome sequencing and integrative genomic analysis approach on two 22q11.2 deletion syndrome family trios for genotype to phenotype correlations. Hum Mutat. 2015;36:797–807.

Codispoti M, Ludlam CA, Simpson D, Mankad PS. Individualized heparin and protamine management in infants and children undergoing cardiac operations. Ann Thorac Surg. 2001;71:922–7; discussion 927–928.

Costi D, Cyna AM, Ahmed S, Stephens K, Strickland P, Ellwood J, Larsson JN, Chooi C, Burgoyne LL, Middleton P. Effects of sevoflurane versus other general anaesthesia on emergence agitation in children. Cochrane Database Syst Rev. 2014;9:Cd007084.

Dabbagh A, Rajaei S, Bahadori Monfared A, Keramatinia AA, Omidi K. Cardiopulmonary bypass, inflammation and how to defy it: focus on pharmacological interventions. Iran J Pharm Res. 2012;11:705–14.

Dahmani S, Delivet H, Hilly J. Emergence delirium in children: an update. Curr Opin Anaesthesiol. 2014;27:309–15.

Dahmani S, Stany I, Brasher C, Lejeune C, Bruneau B, Wood C, Nivoche Y, Constant I, Murat I. Pharmacological prevention of sevoflurane- and desflurane-related emergence agitation in children: a meta-analysis of published studies. Br J Anaesth. 2010;104:216–23.

Daoud A, Duff JP, Joffe AR. Diagnostic accuracy of delirium diagnosis in pediatric intensive care: a systematic review. Crit Care. 2014;18:489.

Dean JM, McClendon E, Hansen K, Azimi-Zonooz A, Chen K, Riddle A, Gong X, Sharifnia E, Hagen M, Ahmad T, Leigland LA, Hohimer AR, Kroenke CD, Back SA. Prenatal cerebral ischemia disrupts MRI-defined cortical microstructure through disturbances in neuronal arborization. Sci Transl Med. 2013;5:168ra167.

Dehaes M, Cheng HH, Buckley EM, Lin PY, Ferradal S, Williams K, Vyas R, Hagan K, Wigmore D, McDavitt E, Soul JS, Franceschini MA, Newburger JW, Ellen Grant P. Perioperative cerebral hemodynamics and oxygen metabolism in neonates with single-ventricle physiology. Biomed Opt Express. 2015;6:4749–67.

du Plessis AJ, Volpe JJ. Perinatal brain injury in the preterm and term newborn. Curr Opin Neurol. 2002;15:151–7.

Durandy Y. Perfusionist strategies for blood conservation in pediatric cardiac surgery. World J Cardiol. 2010;2:27–33.

Englander ZA, Sun J, Laura C, Mikati MA, Kurtzberg J, Song AW. Brain structural connectivity increases concurrent with functional improvement: evidence from diffusion tensor MRI in children with cerebral palsy during therapy. NeuroImage Clin. 2015;7:315–24.

Fraser Jr CD, Andropoulos DB. Principles of antegrade cerebral perfusion during arch reconstruction in newborns/infants. Semin Thorac Cardiovasc Surg Pediatr Card Surg Annu. 2008;2008:61–8.

Galli KK, Zimmerman RA, Jarvik GP, Wernovsky G, Kuypers MK, Clancy RR, Montenegro LM, Mahle WT, Newman MF, Saunders AM, Nicolson SC, Spray TL, Gaynor JW. Periventricular leukomalacia is common after neonatal cardiac surgery. J Thorac Cardiovasc Surg. 2004;127:692–704.

Gaynor JW, Gerdes M, Zackai EH, Bernbaum J, Wernovsky G, Clancy RR, Newman MF, Saunders AM, Heagerty PJ, D'Agostino JA, McDonald-McGinn D, Nicolson SC, Spray TL, Jarvik GP. Apolipoprotein E genotype and neurodevelopmental sequelae of infant cardiac surgery. J Thorac Cardiovasc Surg. 2003;126:1736–45.

Gaynor JW, Stopp C, Wypij D, Andropoulos DB, Atallah J, Atz AM, Beca J, Donofrio MT, Duncan K, Ghanayem NS, Goldberg CS, Hovels-Gurich H, Ichida F, Jacobs JP, Justo R, Latal B, Li JS, Mahle WT, McQuillen PS, Menon SC, Pemberton VL, Pike NA, Pizarro C, Shekerdemian LS, Synnes A, Williams I, Bellinger DC, Newburger JW. Neurodevelopmental outcomes after cardiac surgery in infancy. Pediatrics. 2015;135:816–25.

Gaynor JW, Wernovsky G, Jarvik GP, Bernbaum J, Gerdes M, Zackai E, Nord AS, Clancy RR, Nicolson SC, Spray TL. Patient characteristics are important determinants of neurodevelopmental outcome at one year of age after neonatal and infant cardiac surgery. J Thorac Cardiovasc Surg. 2007;133:1344–53, 1353.e1341-1343.

Glass HC, Fujimoto S, Ceppi-Cozzio C, Bartha AI, Vigneron DB, Barkovich AJ, Glidden DV, Ferriero DM, Miller SP. White-matter injury is associated with impaired gaze in premature infants. Pediatr Neurol. 2008;38:10–5.

Goldberg CS, Lu M, Sleeper LA, Mahle WT, Gaynor JW, Williams IA, Mussatto KA, Ohye RG, Graham EM, Frank DU, Jacobs JP, Krawczeski C, Lambert L, Lewis A, Pemberton VL, Sananes R, Sood E, Wechsler SB, Bellinger DC, Newburger JW. Factors associated with neurodevelopment for children with single ventricle lesions. J Pediatr. 2014;165:490–6.e498.

Goldmuntz E. DiGeorge syndrome: new insights. Clin Perinatol. 2005;32:963–78, ix-x.

Gurses C, Gross DW, Andermann F, Bastos A, Dubeau F, Calay M, Eraksoy M, Bezci S, Andermann E, Melanson D. Periventricular leukomalacia and epilepsy: incidence and seizure pattern. Neurology. 1999;52:341–5.

Hagberg H, Mallard C, Ferriero DM, Vannucci SJ, Levison SW, Vexler ZS, Gressens P. The role of inflammation in perinatal brain injury. Nat Rev Neurol. 2015;11:192–208.

Hansen TG. Anesthesia-related neurotoxicity and the developing animal brain is not a significant problem in children. Paediatr Anaesth. 2015;25:65–72.

Haynes RL, Folkerth RD, Keefe RJ, Sung I, Swzeda LI, Rosenberg PA, Volpe JJ, Kinney HC. Nitrosative and oxidative injury to premyelinating oligodendrocytes in periventricular leukomalacia. J Neuropathol Exp Neurol. 2003;62:441–50.

Hellstrom-Westas L, Boylan G, Agren J. Systematic review of neonatal seizure management strategies provides guidance on anti-epileptic treatment. Acta Paediatr. 2015;104:123–9 (Oslo, Norway: 1992).

Helmers SL, Wypij D, Constantinou JE, Newburger JW, Hickey PR, Carrazana EJ, Barlow JK, Kuban KC, Holmes GL. Perioperative electroencephalographic seizures in infants undergoing repair of complex congenital cardiac defects. Electroencephalogr Clin Neurophysiol. 1997;102:27–36.

Herzog M, Cerar LK, Srsen TP, Verdenik I, Lucovnik M. Impact of risk factors other than prematurity on periventricular leukomalacia. A population-based matched case control study. Eur J Obstet Gynecol Reprod Biol. 2015;187:57–9.

Hipp DM, Ely EW. Pharmacological and nonpharmacological management of delirium in critically ill patients. Neurotherapeutics. 2012;9:158–75.

Hirsch JC, Jacobs ML, Andropoulos D, Austin EH, Jacobs JP, Licht DJ, Pigula F, Tweddell JS, Gaynor JW. Protecting the infant brain during cardiac surgery: a systematic review. Ann Thorac Surg. 2012;94:1365–73; discussion 1373.

Hsia TY, Gruber PJ. Factors influencing neurologic outcome after neonatal cardiopulmonary bypass: what we can and cannot control. Ann Thorac Surg. 2006;81:S2381–8.

Hu Z, Xu L, Zhu Z, Seal R, McQuillan PM. Effects of hypothermic cardiopulmonary bypass on internal jugular bulb venous oxygen saturation, cerebral oxygen saturation, and bispectral index in pediatric patients undergoing cardiac surgery: a prospective study. Medicine. 2016;95:e2483.

Jensen FE. Neonatal seizures: an update on mechanisms and management. Clin Perinatol. 2009;36:881–900, vii.

Joshi A, Krishnamurthy VB, Purichia H, Hollar-Wilt L, Bixler E, Rapp M. "What's in a name?" Delirium by any other name would be as deadly. A review of the nature of delirium consultations. J Psychiatr Pract. 2012;18:413–8.

Joyce C, Witcher R, Herrup E, Kaur S, Mendez-Rico E, Silver G, Greenwald BM, Traube C. Evaluation of the safety of quetiapine in treating delirium in critically ill children: a retrospective review. J Child Adolesc Psychopharmacol. 2015;25:666–70.

Kaltman JR, Andropoulos DB, Checchia PA, Gaynor JW, Hoffman TM, Laussen PC, Ohye RG, Pearson GD, Pigula F, Tweddell J, Wernovsky G, Del Nido P. Report of the pediatric heart network and national heart, lung, and blood institute working group on the perioperative management of congenital heart disease. Circulation. 2010;121:2766–72.

Kang SK, Kadam SD. Neonatal seizures: impact on neurodevelopmental outcomes. Front Pediatr. 2015;3:101.

Kelly P, Hayman R, Shekerdemian LS, Reed P, Hope A, Gunn J, Coleman L, Beca J. Subdural hemorrhage and hypoxia in infants with congenital heart disease. Pediatrics. 2014;134:e773–81.

Khalil A, Suff N, Thilaganathan B, Hurrell A, Cooper D, Carvalho JS. Brain abnormalities and neurodevelopmental delay in congenital heart disease: systematic review and meta-analysis. Ultrasound Obstet Gynecol. 2014;43:14–24.

Kinney HC, Panigrahy A, Newburger JW, Jonas RA, Sleeper LA. Hypoxic-ischemic brain injury in infants with congenital heart disease dying after cardiac surgery. Acta Neuropathol. 2005;110:563–78.

Kochanek PM, Berger RP, Fink EL, Au AK, Bayir H, Bell MJ, Dixon CE, Clark RS. The potential for bio-mediators and biomarkers in pediatric traumatic brain injury and neurocritical care. Front Neurol. 2013;4:40.

Kohelet D, Shochat R, Lusky A, Reichman B. Risk factors for seizures in very low birthweight infants with periventricular leukomalacia. J Child Neurol. 2006;21:965–70.

Kwon SH, Vasung L, Ment LR, Huppi PS. The role of neuroimaging in predicting neurodevelopmental outcomes of preterm neonates. Clin Perinatol. 2014;41:257–83.

Lambert P, Cyna AM, Knight N, Middleton P. Clonidine premedication for postoperative analgesia in children. Cochrane Database Syst Rev. 2014;1:Cd009633.

Lee JK, Blaine Easley R, Brady KM. Neurocognitive monitoring and care during pediatric cardiopulmonary bypass-current and future directions. Curr Cardiol Rev. 2008;4:123–39.

Li Y, Yin S, Fang J, Hua Y, Wang C, Mu D, Zhou K. Neurodevelopmental delay with critical congenital heart disease is mainly from prenatal injury not infant cardiac surgery: current evidence based on a meta-analysis of functional magnetic resonance imaging. Ultrasound Obstet Gynecol. 2015;45:639–48.

Licht DJ, Shera DM, Clancy RR, Wernovsky G, Montenegro LM, Nicolson SC, Zimmerman RA, Spray TL, Gaynor JW, Vossough A. Brain maturation is delayed in infants with complex congenital heart defects. J Thorac Cardiovasc Surg. 2009;137:529–36; discussion 536–527.

Madden K, Turkel S, Jacobson J, Epstein D, Moromisato DY. Recurrent delirium after surgery for congenital heart disease in an infant. Pediatr Crit Care Med. 2011;12:e413–5.

Mahle WT, Tavani F, Zimmerman RA, Nicolson SC, Galli KK, Gaynor JW, Clancy RR, Montenegro LM, Spray TL, Chiavacci RM, Wernovsky G, Kurth CD. An MRI study of neurological injury before and after congenital heart surgery. Circulation. 2002;106:I109–14.

Malarbi S, Stargatt R, Howard K, Davidson A. Characterizing the behavior of children emerging with delirium from general anesthesia. Paediatr Anaesth. 2011;21:942–50.

Marino BS, Lipkin PH, Newburger JW, Peacock G, Gerdes M, Gaynor JW, Mussatto KA, Uzark K, Goldberg CS, Johnson Jr WH, Li J, Smith SE, Bellinger DC, Mahle WT. Neurodevelopmental outcomes in children with congenital heart disease: evaluation and management: a scientific statement from the American Heart Association. Circulation. 2012;126:1143–72.

Markowitz SD, Ichord RN, Wernovsky G, Gaynor JW, Nicolson SC. Surrogate markers for neurological outcome in children after deep hypothermic circulatory arrest. Semin Cardiothorac Vasc Anesth. 2007;11:59–65.

Massaro AN, El-Dib M, Glass P, Aly H. Factors associated with adverse neurodevelopmental outcomes in infants with congenital heart disease. Brain Dev. 2008;30:437–46.

McCann ME, Soriano SG. General anesthetics in pediatric anesthesia: influences on the developing brain. Curr Drug Targets. 2012;13:944–51.

McClendon E, Chen K, Gong X, Sharifnia E, Hagen M, Cai V, Shaver DC, Riddle A, Dean JM, Gunn AJ, Mohr C, Kaplan JS, Rossi DJ, Kroenke CD, Hohimer AR, Back SA. Prenatal cerebral ischemia triggers dysmaturation of caudate projection neurons. Ann Neurol. 2014;75:508–24.

McPheeters ML, Warren Z, Sathe N, Bruzek JL, Krishnaswami S, Jerome RN, Veenstra-Vanderweele J. A systematic review of medical treatments for children with autism spectrum disorders. Pediatrics. 2011;127:e1312–21.

McQuillen PS, Barkovich AJ, Hamrick SE, Perez M, Ward P, Glidden DV, Azakie A, Karl T, Miller SP. Temporal and anatomic risk profile of brain injury with neonatal repair of congenital heart defects. Stroke. 2007;38:736–41.

McQuillen PS, Hamrick SE, Perez MJ, Barkovich AJ, Glidden DV, Karl TR, Teitel D, Miller SP. Balloon atrial septostomy is associated with preoperative stroke in neonates with transposition of the great arteries. Circulation. 2006;113:280–5.

Messieha Z. Prevention of sevoflurane delirium and agitation with propofol. Anesth Prog. 2013;60:67–71.

Miller SP, McQuillen PS, Hamrick S, Xu D, Glidden DV, Charlton N, Karl T, Azakie A, Ferriero DM, Barkovich AJ, Vigneron DB. Abnormal brain development in newborns with congenital heart disease. N Engl J Med. 2007;357:1928–38.

Miller SP, McQuillen PS, Vigneron DB, Glidden DV, Barkovich AJ, Ferriero DM, Hamrick SE, Azakie A, Karl TR. Preoperative brain injury in newborns with transposition of the great arteries. Ann Thorac Surg. 2004;77:1698–706.

Momma K. Cardiovascular anomalies associated with chromosome 22q11.2 deletion syndrome. Am J Cardiol. 2010;105:1617–24.

Morita K. Surgical reoxygenation injury of the myocardium in cyanotic patients: clinical relevance and therapeutic strategies by normoxic management during cardiopulmonary bypass. Gen Thorac Cardiovasc Surg. 2012;60:549–56.

Nelson DP, Andropoulos DB, Fraser Jr CD. Perioperative neuroprotective strategies. Semin Thorac Cardiovasc Surg Pediatr Card Surg Annu. 2008;2008:49–56.

Newburger JW, Bellinger DC. Brain injury in congenital heart disease. Circulation. 2006;113:183–5.

Newburger JW, Wypij D, Bellinger DC, du Plessis AJ, Kuban KC, Rappaport LA, Almirall D, Wessel DL, Jonas RA, Wernovsky G. Length of stay after infant heart surgery is related to cognitive outcome at age 8 years. J Pediatr. 2003;143:67–73.

Nussmeier NA. Management of temperature during and after cardiac surgery. Tex Heart Inst J. 2005;32:472–6.

O'Neill B, Bilal H, Mahmood S, Waterworth P. Is it worth packing the head with ice in patients undergoing deep hypothermic circulatory arrest? Interact Cardiovasc Thorac Surg. 2012;15:696–701.

Ohye RG, Goldberg CS, Donohue J, Hirsch JC, Gaies M, Jacobs ML, Gurney JG. The quest to optimize neurodevelopmental outcomes in neonatal arch reconstruction: the perfusion techniques we use and why we believe in them. J Thorac Cardiovasc Surg. 2009;137:803–6.

Panigrahy A, Wisnowski JL, Furtado A, Lepore N, Paquette L, Bluml S. Neuroimaging biomarkers of preterm brain injury: toward developing the preterm connectome. Pediatr Radiol. 2012;42 Suppl 1:S33–61.

Resch B, Resch E, Maurer-Fellbaum U, Pichler-Stachl E, Riccabona M, Hofer N, Urlesberger B. The whole spectrum of cystic periventricular leukomalacia of the preterm infant: results from a large consecutive case series. Childs Nerv Syst. 2015;31:1527–32.

Rezaie P, Dean A. Periventricular leukomalacia, inflammation and white matter lesions within the developing nervous system. Neuropathology. 2002;22:106–32.

Rollins CK, Newburger JW. Cardiology patient page. Neurodevelopmental outcomes in congenital heart disease. Circulation. 2014;130:e124–6.

Sachdev PS, Blacker D, Blazer DG, Ganguli M, Jeste DV, Paulsen JS, Petersen RC. Classifying neurocognitive disorders: the DSM-5 approach. Nat Rev Neurol. 2014;10:634–42.

Schieveld JN, Leroy PL, van Os J, Nicolai J, Vos GD, Leentjens AF. Pediatric delirium in critical illness: phenomenology, clinical correlates and treatment response in 40 cases in the pediatric intensive care unit. Intensive Care Med. 2007;33:1033–40.

Schieveld JN, van der Valk JA, Smeets I, Berghmans E, Wassenberg R, Leroy PL, Vos GD, van Os J. Diagnostic considerations regarding pediatric delirium: a review and a proposal for an algorithm for pediatric intensive care units. Intensive Care Med. 2009;35:1843–9.

Segovia KN, McClure M, Moravec M, Luo NL, Wan Y, Gong X, Riddle A, Craig A, Struve J, Sherman LS, Back SA. Arrested oligodendrocyte lineage maturation in chronic perinatal white matter injury. Ann Neurol. 2008;63:520–30.

Shamsuddin AM, Nikman AM, Ali S, Zain MR, Wong AR, Corno AF. Normothermia for pediatric and congenital heart surgery: an expanded horizon. Front Pediatr. 2015;3:23.

Shang Q, Ma CY, Lv N, Lv ZL, Yan YB, Wu ZR, Li JJ, Duan JL, Zhu CL. Clinical study of cerebral palsy in 408 children with periventricular leukomalacia. Exp Ther Med. 2015;9:1336–44.

Shen I, Giacomuzzi C, Ungerleider RM. Current strategies for optimizing the use of cardiopulmonary bypass in neonates and infants. Ann Thorac Surg. 2003;75:S729–34.

Sherlock RL, McQuillen PS, Miller SP, aCCENT. Preventing brain injury in newborns with congenital heart disease: brain imaging and innovative trial designs. Stroke. 2009;40:327–32.

Shum-Tim D, Nagashima M, Shinoka T, Bucerius J, Nollert G, Lidov HG, du Plessis A, Laussen PC, Jonas RA. Postischemic hyperthermia exacerbates neurologic injury after deep hypothermic circulatory arrest. J Thorac Cardiovasc Surg. 1998;116:780–92.

Silverstein FS, Jensen FE. Neonatal seizures. Ann Neurol. 2007;62:112–20.

Simpson JR. DSM-5 and neurocognitive disorders. J Am Acad Psychiatry Law. 2014;42:159–64.

Snookes SH, Gunn JK, Eldridge BJ, Donath SM, Hunt RW, Galea MP, Shekerdemian L. A systematic review of motor and cognitive outcomes after early surgery for congenital heart disease. Pediatrics. 2010;125:e818–27.

Soul JS, Robertson RL, Wypij D, Bellinger DC, Visconti KJ, du Plessis AJ, Kussman BD, Scoppettuolo LA, Pigula F, Jonas RA, Newburger JW. Subtle hemorrhagic brain injury is associated with neurodevelopmental impairment in infants with repaired congenital heart disease. J Thorac Cardiovasc Surg. 2009;138:374–81.

Sterken C, Lemiere J, Vanhorebeek I, Van den Berghe G, Mesotten D. Neurocognition after paediatric heart surgery: a systematic review and meta-analysis. Open Heart. 2015;2:e000255.

Tsukimori K, Komatsu H, Yoshimura T, Hikino S, Hara T, Wake N, Nakano H. Increased inflammatory markers are associated with early periventricular leukomalacia. Dev Med Child Neurol. 2007;49:587–90.

Ungerleider RM, Shen I. Optimizing response of the neonate and infant to cardiopulmonary bypass. Semin Thorac Cardiovasc Surg Pediatr Card Surg Annu. 2003;6:140–6.

Van't Hooft J, van der Lee JH, Opmeer BC, Aarnoudse-Moens CS, Leenders AG, Mol BW, de Haan TR. Predicting developmental outcomes in premature infants by term equivalent MRI: systematic review and meta-analysis. Syst Rev. 2015;4:71.

van Dijk M, Knoester H, van Beusekom BS, Ista E. Screening pediatric delirium with an adapted version of the Sophia Observation withdrawal Symptoms scale (SOS). Intensive Care Med. 2012;38:531–2.

van Haastert IC, de Vries LS, Eijsermans MJ, Jongmans MJ, Helders PJ, Gorter JW. Gross motor functional abilities in preterm-born children with cerebral palsy due to periventricular leukomalacia. Dev Med Child Neurol. 2008;50:684–9.

van Hoff SL, O'Neill ES, Cohen LC, Collins BA. Does a prophylactic dose of propofol reduce emergence agitation in children receiving anesthesia? A systematic review and meta-analysis. Paediatr Anaesth. 2015;25:668–76.

van Tilborg E, Heijnen CJ, Benders MJ, van Bel F, Fleiss B, Gressens P, Nijboer CH. Impaired oligodendrocyte maturation in preterm infants: potential therapeutic targets. Prog Neurobiol. 2016;136:28–49.

Volpe JJ. Neurobiology of periventricular leukomalacia in the premature infant. Pediatr Res. 2001;50:553–62.

Vontell R, Supramaniam V, Thornton C, Wyatt-Ashmead J, Mallard C, Gressens P, Rutherford M, Hagberg H. Toll-like receptor 3 expression in glia and neurons alters in response to white matter injury in preterm infants. Dev Neurosci. 2013;35:130–9.

Vontell R, Supramaniam V, Wyatt-Ashmead J, Gressens P, Rutherford M, Hagberg H, Thornton C. Cellular mechanisms of toll-like receptor-3 activation in the thalamus are associated with white matter injury in the developing brain. J Neuropathol Exp Neurol. 2015;74:273–85.

Vutskits L. Anesthetic-related neurotoxicity and the developing brain: shall we change practice? Paediatr Drugs. 2012;14:13–21.

Warshaw G, Mechlin M. Prevention and management of postoperative delirium. Int Anesthesiol Clin. 2009;47:137–49.

Williams GD, Ramamoorthy C. Brain monitoring and protection during pediatric cardiac surgery. Semin Cardiothorac Vasc Anesth. 2007;11:23–33.

Wu YW, Colford Jr JM. Chorioamnionitis as a risk factor for cerebral palsy: a meta-analysis. JAMA. 2000;284:1417–24.

Zhou Z, Ma D. Anaesthetics-induced neurotoxicity in developing brain: an update on preclinical evidence. Brain Sci. 2014;4:136–49.

Chapter 38
Perioperative Management Endocrine Problems in Pediatric Cardiac Surgical Patients

Mahin Hashemipour, Elham Hashemi Dehkordi, Neda Mostofizadeh, Fahimeh Soheilipour, Mahmoud Ghasemi, Ali Mazaheri, and Noushin Rostampour

Part 1: Perioperative management of patients on steroids requiring surgery
Part 2: Perioperative management of hypothyroid and hyperthyroid patients
Part 3: Pituitary gland in perioperative period
Part 4: Perioperative management in diabetic patients
Part 5: Perioperative management in patients with parathyroid disorders
Part 6: Perioperative management in patients with metabolic disorders

M. Hashemipour, MD
Endocrine and Metabolism Research Center, Isfahan University of Medical Sciences, Isfahan, Iran
e-mail: e_hashemi@med.mui.ac.ir

E.H. Dehkordi, MD • N. Mostofizadeh, MD (✉)
Child Growth and Development Research Center, Isfahan University of Medical Sciences, Isfahan, Iran
e-mail: hashemielham@ymail.com; nmostofizadeh@yahoo.com; nmostofizadeh@med.mui.ac.ir

F. Soheilipour, MD
Minimally Invasive Surgery Research Center, Iran University of Medical Sciences, Tehran, Iran
e-mail: fsoheilipour@yahoo.com; Soheilipour.f@iums.ac.ir

M. Ghasemi, MD
Pediatric Department, Kermanshah University of Medical Sciences, Kermanshah, Iran
e-mail: mghasemi51@ymail.com; mahmoud.ghasemi@kums.ac.ir

A. Mazaheri, MD
Pediatric Department, Lorestan University of Medical Sciences, Lorestan, Iran
e-mail: alimazaherimed@yahoo.com

N. Rostampour, MD
Pediatric Department, Shahrekord University of Medical Sciences, Shahrekord, Iran
e-mail: rostampour_n@yahoo.com; Rostampour@skums.ac.ir

© Springer International Publishing Switzerland 2017
A. Dabbagh et al. (eds.), *Congenital Heart Disease in Pediatric and Adult Patients*, DOI 10.1007/978-3-319-44691-2_38

Perioperative Management of Patients on Steroids Requiring Surgery

Acute physical or emotional stresses are the most important activators of the hypo-thalamic–pituitary–adrenal (HPA) axis (Antoni 1986; Aguilera 1994; Thomason et al. 1999). Surgery is one the most potent activators of the axis. The degree of activeness depends on factors such as type of the surgery and the anesthetic agents used during the procedure (Chernow et al. 1987; Jabbour 2001; Bromberg et al. 1991).

The level of cortisol changed during both major and minor surgeries. It fell initially after premedication and rose rapidly during surgery. Its rising trend continued after surgery, i.e., during reversal of anesthesia, extubation, and recovery period mainly in response to pain. The pattern of response was similar in minor surgeries but the peak values are smaller than major surgeries (Udelsman et al. 1987; Shaw and Mandell 1999; Raff et al. 1987).

The peak values occur immediately (4–6 h) after surgery and fell to reach its baseline value after 24 h (Shaw and Mandell 1999).

When to Suspect an Impaired HPA Axis?

The exact time period it takes for a patient to become adrenally suppressed while treated with glucocorticoids, and the time it takes to recover adrenal function after discontinuation of steroids, is not known. It depends on dose, time of day, and the duration of previous glucocorticoid therapy (Graber et al. 1965; Westerhof et al. 1972; Cooper and Stewart 2003).

Following group of patients classified in this group are:

1. Patients receiving glucocorticoid with a dose similar to the physiologic range for 1–2 months
2. Patients receiving prednisone with a dose of 5–20 mg daily or an equivalent dose of another steroid for more than 3 weeks (Westerhof et al. 1972; Cooper and Stewart 2003)
3. Patients receiving prednisone or its equivalent in doses higher than 20 mg daily for more than 3 weeks (Udelsman et al. 1987)
4. Patients receiving glucocorticoids and has clinical Cushing's syndrome

Treatment strategy for this group of patients, according to our suggestion, is additional perioperative glucocorticoid coverage during perioperative period in accordance with the magnitude of the stress.

Patients with Non-suppressed HPA Axis

Following group of patients classified in this group are:

1. Patients who have received any dose of glucocorticoid for less than 3 weeks (Axelrod 2003)

2. Patients who have received morning doses of prednisone with a dose of less than 5 mg daily or its equivalent including *methylprednisolone* (4 mg daily), *dexamethasone* (0.5 mg daily), or *hydrocortisone* (20 mg daily) for any duration of use (Larochelle et al. 1993; Harter et al. 1963)
3. Patients who have received *prednisone* with a dose of less than 10 mg daily or its equivalent every other day (Fauci 1978; Ackerman and Nolan 1968; Marik and Varon 2008)

Suggested treatment for this group of patients is to receiving a maintenance dose of their normal daily dose of glucocorticoids during perioperative period.

This group of patients does not need to be evaluated for HPA axis suppression, because the test could not accurately predict development of adrenal crisis postoperatively (Kehlet and Binder 1973a, b; Christy 1988). It is recommended to monitor these patients for any evidence of hemodynamic instability perioperatively (Kehlet and Binder 1973b; Christy 1988).

Patients with Uncertain Status of HPA Axis

There are two approaches for this group of patients. The first approach is perioperative administration of glucocorticoids. The second one which is recommended for those patients who have enough time is to measure morning serum cortisol level or evaluate the responsiveness of the adrenal to ACTH stimulation before surgery.

Other Groups of Patients

Patients Using Inhaled Steroids

This group of patients does not need any additional perioperative glucocorticoid treatment except in cases with Cushingoid clinical manifestation or signs or symptoms of adrenal insufficiency perioperatively.

Using inhaled glucocorticoids could have suppressive effect on the HPA axis in patients receiving the following dose of the inhaled steroids:

1. Inhaled glucocorticoid with daily doses greater than 0.8 mg (Lipworth 1999)
2. Fluticasone with a daily dose of 0.75 mg (Glowniak and Loriaux 1997)
3. Beclomethasone, triamcinolone, or budesonide with a daily dose of 1.5 mg

Patients Using Topical Steroids

The potency or dose of topical steroid which could induce secondary adrenal suppression is not determined clearly. Some factors such as application to a large surface area of the skin or highly permeable areas, use of high-potency glucocorticoid as little as 2 g/day for 2 or more weeks, long-term use, occlusive dressings, poor skin integrity, liver failure, and young age could increase the risk of adrenal suppression (Shapiro et al. 1990).

Patients Using Intra-articular and Spinal Glucocorticoid Injections

For patients who have received three or more intra-articular or spinal glucocorticoid injections during the last 3 months before surgery or those with Cushingoid appearance, HPA axis evaluation is recommended (Dahl 2006; Reeback et al. 1980).

Guidelines for Dosing Glucocorticoids in the Perioperative Period

The required dose of glucocorticoids will be determined according to the three main factors including the preoperative dose and the duration of glucocorticoid use as well as the anticipated duration of surgery (Friedman et al. 1995).

Surgical Procedures

The consensus conference for congenital adrenal hyperplasia is recommended in the following protocol for surgical procedures with duration of 30–45 min (Wood et al. 1997):

- 0–3 years: hydrocortisone 25-mg IV
- 3–12 years: hydrocortisone 50-mg IV
- 12 years and older: hydrocortisone 100-mg IV

The initial bolus dose with mentioned dosage is followed at a constant rate over a 24-h period. Considering the clinical improvement of the patient, the stress doses of hydrocortisone are tapered rapidly by 50 % reducing of the dose, daily.

For surgeries with duration longer than 30–45 min, the suggested protocol is as follows (Coursin and Wood 2002):

1. Before induction of anesthesia: rapid intravenous injection of hydrocortisone with a dose of 25 mg/m^2.
2. During surgery: an approximately 50-mg/m^2 dose of hydrocortisone as a constant intravenous infusion.
3. For the first 24 h after surgery: an approximately 25- to 50-mg/m^2 dose of hydrocortisone as a constant intravenous infusion for patients unable to take oral hydrocortisone postoperatively.
4. 24 h after surgery: hydrocortisone replacement therapy with the same dose is continued for three to four times by constant IV infusion or orally. In cases with significant hypotension or electrolyte abnormalities, an additional hydrocortisone may be needed. The stress dosing is continued until the patient becomes stable hemodynamically and afebrile and can tolerate oral intake of glucocorticoids.

5. For switching the intravenous administration to oral form, the intravenous dose is reduced, and triple dose oral hydrocortisone replacement therapy with a dose of 30–50 mg/m^2 daily is initiated.

   The dose of oral hydrocortisone replacement therapy could be gradually reduced to reach to its maintenance levels in a 5-day period.

   The maintenance dose for patients with primary and secondary adrenal insufficiency is 10–15 mg/m^2 and 6–8 mg/m^2 daily, respectively.

6. For patients with mineralocorticoid deficiency, fludrocortisone at maintenance doses is initiated as soon as patient can tolerate oral fluids.

7. An alternative approach which is followed by some centers is continuous infusion of hydrocortisone with a daily dose of 100 mg/m^2 after the initial bolus dose mentioned above.

Pituitary Gland in Perioperative Period

Pituitary gland as the "master gland" has an important role in the secretion of five groups of hormones that some of them directly regulate the secretion of other endocrine glands and some others have an important role in preventing water and electrolyte imbalance. In perioperative period, it is very important to diagnose any degree of deficient secretion of adrenocorticotropic hormone (ACTH), thyroid-stimulating hormone (TSH), and antidiuretic hormone (ADH) from ether anterior or posterior pituitary gland. It may cause central adrenal insufficiency (AI), central hypothyroidism and central diabetes insipidus (DI). In apposite, deficient secretion of FSH, LH, prolactin, and GH has less effect in perioperative management of children although GH has an important role in glucose homeostasis, providing euglycemic state especially in neonatal period and early infancy (Demirbilek et al. 2014; Kelly et al. 2008).

Central Adrenal Insufficiency

Its signs and symptoms include fatigue, weakness, arthralgia, myalgia, and hypoglycemia. It does not include volume depletion, salt wasting, and hyperkalemia; that is because of mineralocorticoid deficiency, but dilutional hyponatremia is not uncommon in this situation because cortisol deficiency – even without aldosterone deficiency – may cause free water retention. The diagnosis of central adrenal in suffice the same as primary form of this life-threatening situation is very important in perioperative management of children as an adult patient. It must be tested by measuring serum cortisol level at 8:00 AM. The values below 3 µg/dL are suggestive of cortisol deficiency, and values above 18 µg/dL are indicative of cortisol and ACTH sufficiency. For cortisol values persistently between these two numbers (3 and 18 µg/dL), it is recommended to have an ACTH reserve test that is discussed with more details in other parts of this chapter. It is very important to know that partial ACTH deficiency may be with few or no significant signs or symptoms, and so, in all patients with suspected pituitary insufficiency, the adequacy of hypothalamic–pituitary–adrenal axis should be evaluated biochemically. The appropriate treatment of central AI, the same as primary form, is very important and lifesaving in perioperative management of children. It will be discussed in different parts of this chapter.

Central Hypothyroidism

Central hypothyroidism is defined by low or low normal free T4 with normal or minimally increased TSH values. It may have different degrees of weight gain, fatigue, constipation, cold intolerance, dry skin, and bradycardia. When the diagnosis is established by laboratory, it is recommended to start levothyroxine before anesthesia and surgery to minimize perioperative problems such as delayed recovery of anesthesia, neuropsychiatric disturbances, and ileus and electrolyte abnormalities.

The initial dose is the same as primary hypothyroidism, but in dose adjustment, it is important to know that TSH values were normal from the first time and through the course of treatment, so we must consider free T4 values to adjust the levothyroxine dosage.

The second important point in this area is that glucocorticoid replacement therapy is essential before levothyroxine if there is a concomitant adrenal insufficiency as a part of hypopituitarism. It is because of the effect of thyroid hormones in increasing cortisol metabolism and consequently precipitating adrenal crisis.

Central Diabetes Insipidus (DI)

Childhood central DI, due to deficient secretion of ADH, is caused by familial or congenital disorders, head trauma, neurosurgery, central nervous system tumors in hypothalamus or pituitary region especially craniopharyngiomas, infiltrative disorders, hypoxic encephalopathy, and anorexia nervosa. But the most common causes are cranial tumors, Langerhans cell histiocytosis, and idiopathic conditions. The diagnosis is made by the presence of polyuria (urine output exceeding 2 li/m²/day) and polydipsia with elevated or high normal serum sodium concentration and urine-specific gravity less than 1005.

In children with central DI, before inducing anesthesia, it is important to be sure about being patient in euvolemic and normonatremic state. When the thirst mechanism is intact and in adult patients who are completely conscious, replacement of the water loses usually is done by oral intake. But in young children and in those who are unable to drink fluids by themselves, the same as in unconscious patient, hypernatremia may occur. On the other hand, overtreatment of pediatric patient with cent DI may cause the more dangerous risk of water intoxication. So, management of these children in perioperative period is frequently complicated by the risk of hyper- or hyponatremia and over- or underhydration.

Some physicians prefer not to replace ADH and elevate total fluid intake of these children to about twice maintenance amount that is 3 li/m^2/day for minimizing the risk of hyponatremic encephalopathy and water intoxication.

Some other endocrinologists prefer to manage DI children in perioperative period with intermittent intramuscular vasopressin injection instead of using long-acting intranasal dDAVP.

Another group suggests treating these patients in perioperative management using continuous low-dose IV infusion of aqueous vasopressin with fluid restriction. The infusion rate should be started with minimal dosage and titrated upward to the desired effect that is urine output less than 2 ml/kg/h.

As we know, frequent monitoring of serum sodium concentration, urine volume, and urine-specific gravity is the most important part in all of these protocols.

In Conclusion

For any suspected patient to have pituitary insufficiency, the adequacy of different pituitary axis should be tested before surgery to rule out life-threatening ACTH deficiency or other important involvements such as central DI or central hypothyroidism.

Perioperative Management of Diabetes Mellitus in Children

Introduction

Diabetes mellitus (DM) is well defined as a syndrome determined by inconsistent fasting or postprandial hyperglycemia that is caused by complete or relative insulin deficiency and its metabolic consequences, which include agitated metabolism of protein and fat. Results achieved from different researches about diabetes mellitus were the result of the combination of the fault of insulin secretion and its activity in the target organs.

Typical lab data: urinary glucose and ketone loss; arbitrary serum glucose >200 mg/dL, fasting serum glucose >126 mg/dL with 2-h intervening value >200 mg/dL on oral glucose tolerance test.

In the United States, both types (type I and type II) of diabetes mellitus in children were increased; therefore the management of these patients is becoming very complicated. Anesthesiologists when making an appropriate management plan for DM disease in children must be carefully considered about pathophysiology, attitude of regimen, control of sugar in diet, surgery intendancy, and anticipated postoperative care. Because of complexity and variability of current diabetes treatment options, the preoperative plan should be made in consultation with a pediatric endocrinologist.

Perioperative management of glucose concentration revolves among several key objectives that are briefly mentioned on the title listed in below:

1. Reduction of comprehensive patient morbidity and mortality
2. Avoidance of severe hyperglycemia or hypoglycemia
3. Maintenance of physiological electrolyte and fluid balance
4. Impediment of ketoacidosis
5. Preparation of certain glycemic target levels less than 180 mg/dl in the critical patients and less than 140 mg/dl in the stable patients

In patients who used insulin, frequent glucose monitoring should be utilized to guarantee that glucose values are in normal ranges. Patients should be monitoring the blood glucose contents watchfully including before and after meals as well as before sleeping. In addition, finger stick glucose monitoring should be completed every 4–6 h in any patient who is nil per os (NPO), with supplemental insulin used to correct hyperglycemias' back to normal values.

Preoperative care should be given for children with type I or type II diabetes treated with insulin.

- When shown any general anesthesia in the patients must be accepted by personnel's of the hospital., Should be planned as the first case in each day and To avoid ketoacidosis, even in the diet of patients, should be insulin taken by any persons that shown this disease.

Patients may initially receive an intravenous (IV) infusion without dextrose for minor surgery or procedures (lasting for less than 2 h) if treated with basal/bolus insulin regimen or continuous subcutaneous insulin infusion (CSII).

They should initially receive an IV infusion with dextrose for major surgery or procedures (lasting for at least 2 h) or if treated with NPH insulin.

Careful glucose monitoring was required before the procedures to detect hypoglycemia and hyperglycemia.

Anesthetist should manage the time of presurgical food and fluid limitations.

In the treated patients, the required specific adjustment of the insulin panel are made depending on the type of surgery (major or minor), the patient's insulin regimen, and the time of the surgical daily method (morning or afternoon).

Intraoperative Care

Blood glucose monitoring should be taken at least hourly during and immediately after general anesthesia:

- In major surgery (lasting for at least 2 h) or patients treated with NPH insulin, an IV injection with dextrose should be used to prevent hypoglycemia risk in any child's treatment.
- If treated with basal/bolus insulin regimen or CSII, an IV injection should be used initially without dextrose during minor surgery or other methods (lasting for less than 2 h).

- Insulin and dextrose infusion should be adjusted to maintain suitable blood glucose in the range of 5–10 mmol/L (90–180 mg/dl).
- If there is an unexpected acute drop in blood pressure, normal saline (NS) (0.9 %NaCl) or Ringer's lactate must be infused rapidly. In this circumstance, potassium-containing fluids must *not* be infused rapidly.

Postoperative Care

- Once the child is able to return to oral nutrition, they pick up usual diabetic treatment regimen in the daily meals by specific attentions. Give short- or rapid-acting insulin (based on the child's usual insulin: carbohydrate ratio and correction factor), if needed, to decrease hyperglycemia or to match food intake.

For Emergency Surgery

- The endocrinologists and the consultant should be contacted about all patients with diabetes who require emergency surgery.
- In preparation for emergency surgery, the child should first be appraised clinically and biochemically. In these methods, blood gas including glucose and ketones test, U&E tests, FBE, and other pre-op bloods should be examined and registered in the documents of patients.
- If ketoacidosis is observed, treatment according to the *DKA protocol* (BSPED Recommended Guideline 2015) (developed by researchers in last years ago) should be started immediately, and the patient's circulating volume and electrolytes should be stabilized before the surgery operation.
- When DKA is detected, initial insulin injection rates are 0.1 U/kg/h and 0.05 U/kg/h in a child under 2 years.
- Insulin injection rate should be continued until ketones have washed and acidosis has improved.
- Once ketones have cleared and acidosis has been corrected, the insulin infusion rates may be decreased, and the dextrose level of IV fluids should be adjusted as appropriate to maintain BGLs between 5 and 10 mmol/L (90–180 mg/dl). Maintenance insulin injection rates once ketosis/acidosis has fully cleared are usually in the range of 0.02–0.03 U/kg/h; therefore, the endocrinologists will advise this protocol for use in patients and high-risk children.
- If there is no signal of ketoacidosis observed, the child should be fasted and commenced on intravenous dextrose/saline (start with 0.45 % NaCl+5 % dextrose+20 mmol/L KCl) with continuous IV insulin infusion. The insulin infusion is made up by the addition of 50 units of regular insulin (Actrapid HM or Humulin R) to 49.5 ml 0.9 % NaCl (1 unit/ml solution).
- The insulin infusion may be carried as a sideline with the maintenance fluids via a three-way tap, provided a syringe pump is used. The parents of patients should be ensuring that the insulin is clearly labeled and achieved from creditable companies in the entire world.

- Initial rate of the insulin infusion should be 0.02–0.03 U/kg/h (note that this maintenance rate is much lower than the rate required in treating DKA). It should be started with the deal of 0.02 U/kg/h if BGL is <10.0 mmol/L (180 mg/dl) and 0.03 U/kg/h if BGL >10.0 mmol/L.
- If the patient is usually controlled with insulin pump therapy, subcutaneous insulin with the pump should be discontinued half an hour after IV insulin, and intravenous fluid infusion should be started.
- BGLs should be monitored and measured hourly in the time of insulin infusion.
- BGLs should be kept in the ranges of 5.0 and 10.0 mmol/L (90–180 mg/dl).
- If two continuance hourly BGLs are above 10.0 mmol/L (180 mg/dl), the rate of insulin infusion should be enhanced in the ranges of 0.005–0.01 U/kg/h (in order to carry out this assay, we must first attempt it on lab animals and then infuse it in humans specifically in patients).

If any BGL is >15.0 mmol/L (270 mg/dl), check if blood ketones were tested by Optium™ meter as recommended by manufacturers.

- If any BGL is <5.0 mmol/L (90 mg/dl), the insulin rate can be reduced by the same enhancement of infusion (0.005–0.01 U/kg/h) to prevent the hypoglycemia. If the insulin rate is already at 0.02 U/kg/h, the increase in the dextrose level of intravenous fluids can be up to 10 %.
- With regard to subcutaneous insulin injection in the post-op period should be discussed for any child by the diabetes team. This problem may vary depending on the patient's usual uptake insulin regimen and their ability to tolerate oral diet. This action is possible to recommence CSII in the postoperative period even if the patient is being kept nil by mouth; this should be done by the endocrinology team, because they know well what time it is suitable for recommend rates and settings on an individual basis.
- Sometimes in rare cases, the patients are unable to eat food/enteral nutrition for long duration postoperatively (age >2 days), it may be possible to reduce the frequency of BGL testing once a stable state has been reached in the post-op period. Endocrinologists will recommend the best program for any patients.

Children with diabetes mellitus need to help and care, and usually, their parents are the best information about their disease.

Perioperative Management in Patients with Metabolic Disorders

Introduction

Inborn errors of metabolism are a group of genetic disorders that result from deficiency of an enzyme or its cofactor (Sutton, accessed July 7, 2014). The presence of these disorders could influence and complicate the management of surgery (Hines and

Marschall 2012). Clinical manifestations have a wide variety, from clinically asymptomatic to severe presentation.

Hypoglycemia

One of the most important issues that should be noticed in patients suffering from metabolic disorders is the increase in the risk of hypoglycemia during stressful conditions. So, regular fasting prior to surgery in these patients should be adjusted on the basis of patient's history and fasting tolerance. In short or minor procedures, surgery could be performed at noon or later after receiving glucose. In most situations, patients should receive fluid containing 10 % glucose at a rate of 2500 ml/m^2/day, and if needed, the rate of infusion must be changed to achieve fixed blood glucose level.

Maintaining blood glucose >4 mmol/L (70 mg/dl) has been recommended (Hoffmann et al. 2010).

Phenylketonuria

Phenylketonuria (PKU) is a disorder of amino acid metabolism on which phenylalanine accumulates as a consequence of phenylalanine hydroxylase deficiency (Nyhan 2005). Some of the presentations of PKU having an impact on the management of anesthesia are mental retardation, seizure, and friable skin. Those suffering from this disorder are susceptible to pressure damage due to their friable skin. Associated vitamin B12 deficiency may be seen in patients on strict diets (Hines and Marschall 2012).

Preoperative Management

Adequacy of dietary therapy should be evaluated before the surgery by checking levels of phenylalanine and vitamin B12 within 72 h of elective procedures. Patients with high plasma level of phenylalanine are at risk of seizure and abnormal neurological and/or emotional behaviors. Low phenylalanine level is associated with liver dysfunction, hypoglycemia, and abnormal neurological and psychological activity. In the case of abnormal levels, elective operation may be postponed (Dal and Celiker 2004). In patients with B12 deficiency, nitrous oxide can cause myeloneuropathy and B12 deficiency and hence should be avoided (Dal and Celiker 2004; Hines and Marschall 2012). It has been mentioned that more sensitivity of PKU patients to narcotics and respiratory depression following narcotic drugs might be a trigger for seizure during the postanesthetic period (Dal and Celiker 2004; Hines and Marschall 2012).

Propionic and Methylmalonic Acidemia

Methylmalonic and propionic academia are autosomal recessive disorders, due to methylmalonyl-coA mutase and propionyl-coA carboxylase deficiency, respectively. Increasing protein catabolism during perioperative period could raise the probability of acidosis. Information about the management of these patients during surgery is limited, but there are some recommendations to minimize catabolism.

Preoperative Management

In emergency operations and major procedures (>30 min), plasma ammonia, pH, and blood gases should be checked. If serum ammonia is above 100 µmol/L, PH <7.3, or base deficit >10 mmol/L or when the patient condition is not well, specialist consultation should be arranged and elective surgery should be canceled. Make sure that the child is well 48 h before the elective surgery.

Otherwise, postpone the operation. It is important that the last metabolic investigation must have taken place less than 3 months prior to elective surgery (Baumgartner et al. 2014). It has been suggested that elective surgery should be delayed 4 weeks after the recent infection (Harker et al. 2000). Stop feeds based on minimal requirement for surgery and start carbohydrate-containing fluids or 10% glucose parenterally with appropriate electrolyte.

In B12 responsive patients, administer hydroxocobalamin in dose of 1 mg parenterally, 1 day before and on the day of surgery. L-Carnitine is another essential drug that should be given to these patients in the amount of 100 mg/kg/day (max 12 g for adults). The mentioned management should be maintained during the procedure. Intravenous lipid infusion (1–2 g/kg/day) is also helpful in longer operations (Harker et al. 2000; Karagoz et al. 2006).

Nitrous oxide in methylmalonic acidemia may be avoided because it could result in methylmalonic acidemia following the inhibition of cobalamin coenzymes. It is believed that some muscle relaxants including atracurium, cisatracurium, succinylcholine, and mivacurium should be avoided in propionic academia because their metabolites contain odd-chain organic molecules. Because a small portion of fat in propofol is metabolized to propionic acid, this medication is not safe in propionic academia (Harker et al. 2000). Sensitivity to central nervous depressant effects of volatile anesthetics and narcotics has been observed in hypotonic and lethargic patients with propionic acidemia. Another important complication in propionic acidemia is airway problems; these complications could be minimized by delaying tracheal extubation until muscle strength is regained (Harker et al. 2000; Karagoz et al. 2006).

Postoperative Management

Start feeding when the patient is metabolically stable; after tolerating food, discontinue IV infusion. In the case of delayed or complicated recovery, ammonia, blood gases, and electrolytes should be evaluated. Antiemetic drugs including ondansetron could help patients but metoclopramide should be avoided. L-Carnitine and glucose infusion should be continued. Adding intralipid is helpful in some cases (1–2 g/kg/day). After regaining full recovery and normal metabolic state, discharge is recommended (Baumgartner et al. 2014).

Maple Syrup Urine Disease

Maple syrup urine disease (MSUD) is a disorder of branched-chain amino acid that results from defective carboxylation of these amino acids. Surgery and anesthesia introduce a number of problems in these patients. MSUD patients are at risk of hypoglycemia, cerebral edema, ketoacidosis, and neurological decline during perioperative period (Fuentes-Garcia and Falcon-Arana 2009; Hines and Marschall 2012).

Preoperative Management

Blood ammonia, PH, electrolyte, and plasma amino acid concentration as well as urine ketone should be checked before the operation (Hoffmann et al. 2010). Poor feeding could increase leucine concentration in plasma, so correction of dehydration prior to surgery is important (Fuentes-Garcia and Falcon-Arana 2009). Administration of glucose is a good way to reduce catabolism (Hoffmann et al. 2010). One of the lethal factors in these patients is overhydration; therefore, a conservative fluid management should be used in order to reduce the risk of brain edema (Kahraman et al. 1996; Fuentes-Garcia and Falcon-Arana 2009). For selecting anesthetic technique, it should be kept in mind that these patients are susceptible to convulse. Administration of ketamin in MSUD patients with seizure is controversial (Kahraman et al. 1996).

Urea Cycle Defects

Urea cycle is a pathway detoxified ammonia to urea. Involvement of the enzymes in this pathway is called urea cycle disorder (Kliegman et al. 2015).

The preoperative approach in urea cycle defects is similar to organic academia, but in these patients, hyperammonemia should be avoided and monitored carefully (Hoffmann et al. 2010).

Preoperative Management

Intravenous arginine is indicated to patients receiving citrulline or arginine medication. The previous usual dose should be used and added to 2.5 g of arginine to 50 cc 10 % glucose administrated via syringe pump. Use the IV mixture of benzoate-phenylacetate for patients receiving either of these drugs and diluted the same way described for arginine. These drugs could be started in postoperative period in the case of short procedures, but it is recommended to administer intraoperatively in long operations and hyperammonemia states and if there is high probability of catabolism (Hoffmann et al. 2010).

Fatty Acid Oxidation Defects

Acute breakdown of muscle following anesthesia is a problem in patient with fatty acid oxidation disorder especially in carnitine palmitoyl transferase II deficiency and long-chain hydroxyacyl-coA dehydrogenase deficiency. Renal failure may be seen in these patients due to myoglobinuria. The avoidance of fasting and the administration of IV glucose and water are the best strategies to prevent complication of surgery and anesthesia. Start with 10 % glucose or higher if myoglobinuria is present. In some situations, insulin should be considered to maintain euglycemia (Hoffmann et al. 2010).

Homocystinuria

Homocystinuria is a rare metabolic disease due to the defect of transsulfuration of precursors of cystine. High plasma homocystine has atherogenic and thrombophilic activity. Employing pyridoxine or betaine in perioperative period decreases the risk of thromboembolism by lowering homocystine concentration. Appropriate preoperative hydration and dextran infusion are suggested to prevent vein thrombosis (Hines and Marschall 2012).

Mucopolysaccharidosis

Mucopolysaccharidosis (MPS) are a group of metabolic disorders in which glycosaminoglycan is stored in tissues, and they are classified in seven types (I, II, III, IV, VI, VII, IX) (Nyhan 2005; Gurumurthy et al. 2014). These disorders have some characteristics influencing the anesthesia management including instability of atlantoaxial joint, kyphoscoliosis, probability of cardiopulmonary involvement, and cord compression. Because of the difficulty of anesthesia in these patients, general anesthesia should be performed only in centers familiar with these diseases and by an experienced team (Hoffmann et al. 2010; Hendriksz et al. 2015). Cervical instability has high risk of anesthesia which is more prominent in Morquio (MPS IV) but also seen in MPS I and VI (Hoffmann et al. 2010).

Preoperative Management

A careful history of anesthesia problems should be taken and complete physical examination should be done. It is necessary to be aware of cardiopulmonary and cervical spine conditions. Determine blood pressure, EKG, and echocardiogram for all patients, evaluate pulmonary function test in case of kyphoscoliosis, and reevaluate recent X-ray of the chest. If patient is suspected to cord compression, spine MRI should be performed. Airway management and intubation are other major problems in MPS patients. They may be required smaller tubes than predicted for age. Macroglossia, micrognathia, and neck instability exacerbate these problems (Hoffmann et al. 2010).

Postoperative Management

Postoperative airway obstruction may be seen in these patients, so postoperative care is also important. In order to reduce this problem, intraoperative corticosteroids may be needed before extubation. Waiting until the complete reversal effect of myorelaxants is recommended; another helpful way is the assignment of a nasopharyngeal airway (Braunlin et al. 2011; Ziyaeifard et al. 2014).

References

Ackerman GL, Nolan CM. Adrenocortical responsiveness after alternate-day corticosteroid therapy. N Engl J Med. 1968;278:405–9.

Adlerberth A, Stenström G, Hasselgren P. The selective beta 1-blocking agent metoprolol compared with antithyroid drug and thyroxine as preoperative treatment of patients with hyperthyroidism. Results from a prospective, randomized study. Ann Surg. 1987;205:182.

Aguilera G. Regulation of pituitary ACTH secretion during chronic stress. Front Neuroendocrinol. 1994;15:321–50.

Antoni FA. Hypothalamic control of adrenocorticotropin secretion: advances since the discovery of 41-residue corticotropin-releasing factor. Endocr Rev. 1986;7:351–78.

Axelrod L. Perioperative management of patients treated with glucocorticoids. Endocrinol Metab Clin North Am. 2003;32:367–83.

Ayuk J, Gittoes NJ. How should hypomagnesaemia be investigated and treated? Clin Endocrinol (Oxf). 2011;75:743–6.

Bardin CW. Current therapy in endocrinology and metabolism. 3rd ed. Toronto: B.C. Decker; 1988.

Baumgartner MR, Hörster F, et al. Proposed guidelines for the diagnosis and management of methylmalonic and propionic acidemia. Orphanet J Rare Dis. 2014;9:130.

Bennett-Guerrero E, Kramer DC, Schwinn DA. Effect of chronic and acute thyroid hormone reduction on perioperative outcome. Anesth Analg. 1997;85:30–6.

Bhalla P, Eaton FE, Coulter JB, Amegavie FL, Sills JA, Abernethy LJ. Lesson of the week: hyponatraemic seizures and excessive intake of hypotonic fluids in young children. BMJ. 1999;319:1554–7.

Braunlin EA, Harmatz PR, Scarpa M, Furlanetto B, Kampmann C, Loehr JP, Ponder KP, Roberts WC, Rosenfeld HM, Giugliani R. Cardiac disease in patients with mucopolysaccharidosis: presentation, diagnosis and management. J Inherit Metab Dis. 2011;34:1183–97.

Brent GA, Hershman JM. Thyroxine therapy in patients with severe nonthyroidal illnesses and low serum thyroxine concentration*. J Clin Endocrinol Metab. 1986;63:1–8.

Bromberg JS, Alfrey EJ, Barker CF, Chavin KD, Dafoe DC, Holland T, Naji A, Perloff LJ, Zellers LA, Grossman RA. Adrenal suppression and steroid supplementation in renal transplant recipients. Transplantation. 1991;51:385–95.

Burg FD, Gellis SS, Kagan BM, Ingelfinger JR, Wald ER. Gellis & Kagan's current pediatric therapy 14. Philadelphia: Saunders; 1993.

Canaris GJ, Manowitz NR, Mayor G, Ridgway EC. The Colorado thyroid disease prevalence study. Arch Intern Med. 2000;160:526–34.

Chaudhary H, Bhakhri BK, Datta V. Central diabetes insipidus in newborns: unique challenges in management. Pediatr Endocrinol Rev. 2011;9:476–8.

Chernow B, Alexander HR, Smallridge RC, Thompson WR, Cook D, Beardsley D, Fink MP, Lake CR, Fletcher JR. Hormonal responses to graded surgical stress. Arch Intern Med. 1987;147: 1273–8.

Cho YH, Tchan M, Roy B, Halliday R, Wilson M, Dutt S, Siew S, Munns C, Howard N. Recombinant parathyroid hormone therapy for severe neonatal hypoparathyroidism. J Pediatr. 2012;160:345–8.

Christy NP. Corticosteroid withdrawal. In: Bardin CW, editor. Current therapy in endocrinology and metabolism-3. 3rd ed. Toronto: B.C. Decker; 1988. p. 113.

Cooper MS, Gittoes NJ. Diagnosis and management of hypocalcaemia. BMJ. 2008;336:1298–302.

Cooper MS, Stewart PM. Corticosteroid insufficiency in acutely ill patients. N Engl J Med. 2003;348:727–34.

Coursin DB, Wood KE. Corticosteroid supplementation for adrenal insufficiency. JAMA. 2002;287:236–40.

Crowley Jr WF, Ridgway EC, Bough EW, Francis GS, Daniels GH, Kourides IA, Myers GS, Maloof F. Noninvasive evaluation of cardiac function in hypothyroidism: response to gradual thyroxine replacement. N Engl J Med. 1977;296:1–6.

Dahl R. Systemic side effects of inhaled corticosteroids in patients with asthma. Respir Med. 2006;100:1307–17.

Dal D, Celiker V. Anesthetic management of a strabismus patient with phenylketonuria. Peadiatr Anaesth. 2004;14:697–702.

De Sanctis V, Soliman A, Yassin M, Garofalo P. Cortisol levels in central adrenal insufficiency: light and shade. Pediatr Endocrinol Rev. 2015;12:283–9.

Demirbilek H, Tahir S, Baran RT, Sherif M, Shah P, Ozbek MN, Hatipoglu N, Baran A, Arya VB, Hussain K. Familial isolated growth hormone deficiency due to a novel homozygous missense mutation in the growth hormone releasing hormone receptor gene: clinical presentation with hypoglycemia. J Clin Endocrinol Metab. 2014;99:E2730–4.

Fauci AS. Alternate-day corticosteroid therapy. Am J Med. 1978;64:729–31.

Feek CM, Sawers JSA, Irvine WJ, Beckett GJ, Ratcliffe WA, Toft AD. Combination of potassium iodide and propranolol in preparation of patients with Graves' disease for thyroid surgery. N Engl J Med. 1980;302:883–5.

Fish LH, Schwartz HL, Cavanaugh J, Steffes MW, Bantle JP, Oppenheimer JH. Replacement dose, metabolism, and bioavailability of levothyroxine in the treatment of hypothyroidism. N Engl J Med. 1987;316:764–70.

Fommei E, Iervasi G. The role of thyroid hormone in blood pressure homeostasis: evidence from short-term hypothyroidism in humans. J Clin Endocrinol Metab. 2002;87:1996–2000.

Fredlund BO, Olsson SB. Long QT interval and ventricular tachycardia of "torsade de pointe" type in hypothyroidism. Acta Med Scand. 1983;213:231–5.

Friedman RJ, Schiff CF, Bromberg JS. Use of supplemental steroids in patients having orthopaedic operations. J Bone Joint Surg. 1995;77:1801–6.

Frost L, Vestergaard P, Mosekilde L. Hyperthyroidism and risk of atrial fibrillation or flutter: a population-based study. Arch Intern Med. 2004;164:1675–8.

Fuentes-Garcia D, Falcon-Arana L. Perioperative management of a patient with maple syrup urine disease. Br J Anaesth. 2009;102:144–5.

Gallo S, Comeau K, Vanstone C, Agellon S, Sharma A, Jones G, L'Abbe M, Khamessan A, Rodd C, Weiler H. Effect of different dosages of oral vitamin D supplementation on vitamin D status in healthy, breastfed infants: a randomized trial. JAMA. 2013;309:1785–92.

Garcia M, Fernandez A, Moreno JC. Central hypothyroidism in children. Endocr Dev. 2014;26:79–107.

Gardiner L. Royal Children's Hospital, Melbourne, 1870–1970: a history. Melbourne: Royal Children's Hospital; 1970.

Geffner DL, Hershman JM. β-adrenergic blockade for the treatment of hyperthyroidism. Am J Med. 1992;93:61–8.

Glowniak JV, Loriaux DL. A double-blind study of perioperative steroid requirements in secondary adrenal insufficiency. Surgery. 1997;121:123–9.

Graber AL, Ney RL, Nicholson WE, Island DP, Liddle GW. Natural history of pituitary-adrenal recovery following long-term suppression with corticosteroids 1. J Clin Endocrinol Metab. 1965;25:11–6.

Graettinger JS, Muenster JJ, Checchia CS, Grissom RL, Campbell JA. A correlation of clinical and hemodynamic studies in patients with hypothyroidism. J Clin Invest. 1958;37:502.

Green S, Ng J. Hypothyroidism and anaemia. Biomed Pharmacother. 1985;40:326–31.

Gurumurthy TS, et al. Management of an anticipated difficult airway in Hurler's syndrome. J Anaesthesiol Clin Pharmacol. 2014;30:558–61.

Ham PB, Cunningham AJ, Mentzer CJ, Ahmad A, Young LS, Abuzeid AM. Traumatic panhypopituitarism resulting in acute adrenal crisis. J Trauma Acute Care Surg. 2015;79:484–9.

Harker HE, Emhardt JD, Hainline BE. Propionic acidemia in a four-month-old male: a case study and anesthetic implications. Anesth Analg. 2000;91:309–11.

Harter JG, Reddy WJ, Thorn GW. Studies on an intermittent corticosteroid dosage regimen. N Engl J Med. 1963;269:591–6.

Haug R. Recovery of the hypothalmic-pituitary adrenal (HPA) axis in patients with rheumatic diseases receiving low-dose prednisone: La Rochelle GE, La Rochelle AG, Ratner RE, et al. Am J Med. 1993;95:258. J Oral Maxillofac Surg. 1994;52:203.

Hays MT, Nielsen KR. Human thyroxine absorption: age effects and methodological analyses. Thyroid. 1994;4:55–64.

Hendriksz CJ, Berger KI, Giugliani R, Harmatz P, Kampmann C, Mackenzie WG, Raiman J, Villarreal MS, Savarirayan R. International guidelines for the management and treatment of Morquio A syndrome. Am J Med Genet A. 2015;167:11–25.

Hines RL, Marschall K. Stoelting's anesthesia and co-existing disease. Philadelphia: Elsevier; 2012.

Hoffmann GF, Zschocke J, Nyhan WL. Inherited metabolic diseases: a clinical approach. Heidelberg: Springer; 2010.

Hollowell JG, Staehling NW, Flanders WD, Hannon WH, Gunter EW, Spencer CA, Braverman LE. Serum TSH, T4, and thyroid antibodies in the United States population (1988 to 1994): National Health and Nutrition Examination Survey (NHANES III). J Clin Endocrinol Metab. 2002;87:489–99.

Jabbour SA. Steroids and the surgical patient. Med Clin North Am. 2001;85:1311–7.

Kahraman S, Ercan M, Akkuş O, Erçelen O, Erdem K, Coşkun T. Anesthesia management in maple syrup urine disease. Anaesthesia. 1996;51:575–8.

Karagoz AH, Uzümcügil F, Celebi N, Canbay O, Ozgen S. Anesthetic management of a 2-year-old male with propionic acidemia. Paediatr Anaesth. 2006;16(12):1290–1291.

Kehlet H, Binder C. Adrenocortical function and clinical course during and after surgery in unsupplemented glucocorticoid-treated patients. Br J Anaesth. 1973a;45:1043–8.

Kehlet H, Binder C. Value of an ACTH test in assessing hypothalamic-pituitary-adrenocortical function in glucocorticoid-treated patients. BMJ. 1973b;2:147–9.

Kelly A, Tang R, Becker S, Stanley CA. Poor specificity of low growth hormone and cortisol levels during fasting hypoglycemia for the diagnoses of growth hormone deficiency and adrenal insufficiency. Pediatrics. 2008;122:e522–8.

Kliegman RM, Nelson WE. Nelson textbook of pediatrics. Philadelphia: Saunders Elsevier; 2011.

Kliegman RM, Behrman RE, Nelson WE. Nelson textbook of pediatrics. Philadelphia: Elsevier; 2015.

Kreisman SH, Hennessey JV. Consistent reversible elevations of serum creatinine levels in severe hypothyroidism. Arch Intern Med. 1999;159:79–82.

Kumar R. Vitamin D and calcium transport. Kidney Int. 1991;40:1177–89.

Ladenson PW, Goldenheim PD, Ridgway EC. Prediction and reversal of blunted ventilatory responsiveness in patients with hypothyroidism. Am J Med. 1988;84:877–83.

Ladenson PW, Levin AA, Ridgway EC, Daniels GH. Complications of surgery in hypothyroid patients. Am J Med. 1984;77:261–6.

Laroche CM, Cairns T, Moxham J, Green M. Hypothyroidism presenting with respiratory muscle weakness. Am Rev Respir Dis. 1988;138:472–4.

Lipworth BJ. Systemic adverse effects of inhaled corticosteroid therapy: a systematic review and meta-analysis. Arch Intern Med. 1999;159:941–55.

Loughead JL, Mimouni F, Tsang RC. Serum ionized calcium concentrations in normal neonates. Am J Dis Child. 1988;142:516–8.

Ma NS, Fink C, Geffner ME, Borchert M. Evolving central hypothyroidism in children with optic nerve hypoplasia. J Pediatr Endocrinol Metab. 2010;23:53–8.

Manfredi E, ZAANE B, Gerdes VE, Brandjes DP, Squizzato A. Hypothyroidism and acquired von Willebrand's syndrome: a systematic review. Haemophilia. 2008;14:423–33.

Marik PE, Varon J. Requirement of perioperative stress doses of corticosteroids: a systematic review of the literature. Arch Surg. 2008;143:1222–6.

Marx SJ. Hyperparathyroid and hypoparathyroid disorders. N Engl J Med. 2000;343:1863–75.

Meneghini LF. Perioperative management of diabetes: translating evidence into practice. Cleve Clin J Med. 2009;76 Suppl 4:S53–9.

Meyer T, Ruppert V, Karatolios K, Maisch B. Hereditary long QT syndrome due to autoimmune hypoparathyroidism in autoimmune polyendocrinopathy-candidiasis-ectodermal dystrophy syndrome. J Electrocardiol. 2007;40:504–9.

Misra M, Pacaud D, Petryk A, Collett-Solberg PF, Kappy M. Vitamin D deficiency in children and its management: review of current knowledge and recommendations. Pediatrics. 2008;122:398–417.

Newfield RS. Recombinant PTH for initial management of neonatal hypocalcemia. N Engl J Med. 2007;356:1687–8.

Nyhan WL, Ozand PT. Atlas of metabolic diseases. 2nd ed. London: Chapman &Hall; 2005.

Ooi HL, Maguire AM, Ambler GR. Desmopressin administration in children with central diabetes insipidus: a retrospective review. J Pediatr Endocrinol Metab. 2013;26:1047–52.

Park YJ, Yoon JW, Kim KI, Lee YJ, Kim KW, Choi SH, Lim S, Choi DJ, Park K-H, Choh JH. Subclinical hypothyroidism might increase the risk of transient atrial fibrillation after coronary artery bypass grafting. Ann Thorac Surg. 2009;87:1846–52.

Raff H, Norton AJ, Flemma RJ, Findling JW. Inhibition of the adrenocorticotropin response to surgery in humans: interaction between dexamethasone and fentanyl*. J Clin Endocrinol Metab. 1987;65:295–8.

Reeback J, Chakraborty J, English J, Gibson T, Marks V. Plasma steroid levels after intra-articular injection of prednisolone acetate in patients with rheumatoid arthritis. Ann Rheum Dis. 1980;39:22–4.

Rehman HU, Mohammed K. Perioperative management of diabetic patients. Curr Surg. 2003;60:607–11.

Reichel H, Koeffler HP, Norman AW. The role of the vitamin D endocrine system in health and disease. N Engl J Med. 1989;320:980–91.

Reifschneider K, Auble BA, Rose SR. Update of endocrine dysfunction following pediatric traumatic brain injury. J Clin Med. 2015;4:1536–60.

Rhodes ET, Ferrari LR, Wolfsdorf JI. Perioperative management of pediatric surgical patients with diabetes mellitus. Anesth Analg. 2005;101:986–99, table of contents.

Rhodes ET, Gong C, Edge JA, Wolfsdorf JI, Hanas R. ISPAD Clinical Practice Consensus Guidelines 2014. Management of children and adolescents with diabetes requiring surgery. Pediatr Diabetes. 2014;15 Suppl 20:224–31.

Robson WL, Leung AK. Hyponatremia in children treated with desmopressin. Arch Pediatr Adolesc Med. 1998;152:930–1.

Ross AC, Manson JE, Abrams SA, Aloia JF, Brannon PM, Clinton SK, Durazo-Arvizu RA, Gallagher JC, Gallo RL, Jones G, Kovacs CS, Mayne ST, Rosen CJ, Shapses SA. The 2011 report on dietary reference intakes for calcium and vitamin D from the Institute of Medicine: what clinicians need to know. J Clin Endocrinol Metab. 2011;96:53–8.

Schlegel A. Metyrapone stimulation test to diagnose central adrenal insufficiency. Lancet Diabetes Endocrinol. 2015;3:407.

Schrier RW. Body water homeostasis: clinical disorders of urinary dilution and concentration. J Am Soc Nephrol. 2006;17:1820–32.

Shafer R, Prentiss R, Bond J. Gastrointestinal transit in thyroid disease. Gastroenterology. 1984;86:852–5.

Shapiro R, Carroll PB, Tzakis AG, Cemaj S, Lopatin WB, Nakazato P. Adrenal reserve in renal transplant recipients with cyclosporine, azathioprine, and prednisone immunosuppression. Transplantation. 1990;49:1011–2.

Shaw M, Mandell BF. Perioperative management of selected problems in patients with rheumatic diseases. Rheum Dis Clin North Am. 1999;25:623–38.

Sherman SI, Ladenson PW. Percutaneous transluminal coronary angioplasty in hypothyroidism. Am J Med. 1991;90:367–70.

Siafakas N, Salesiotou V, Filaditaki V, Tzanakis N, Thalassinos N, Bouros D. Respiratory muscle strength in hypothyroidism. Chest. 1992;102:189–94.

Silva PP, Bhatnagar S, Herman SD, Zafonte R, Klibanski A, Miller KK, Tritos NA. Predictors of hypopituitarism in patients with traumatic brain injury. J Neurotrauma. 2015;32:1789–95.

Sperling MA. Pediatric endocrinology. Philadelphia: Elsevier Science Health Science; 2014.

Squizzato A, Romualdi E, Buller H, Gerdes V. Thyroid dysfunction and effects on coagulation and fibrinolysis: a systematic review. J Clin Endocrinol Metab. 2007;92:2415–20.

Stathatos N, Wartofsky L. Perioperative management of patients with hypothyroidism. Endocrinol Metab Clin North Am. 2003;32:503–18.

Stockigt J. Guidelines for diagnosis and monitoring of thyroid disease: nonthyroidal illness. Clin Chem. 1996;42:188–92.

Sudhakaran S, Surani SR. Guidelines for perioperative management of the diabetic patient. Surg Res Pract. 2015;2015:284063.

Sutton V. Inborn errors of metabolism: classification.http://www.uptodate.com. Accesed 7 Jul 2014.

Taddei S, Caraccio N, Virdis A, Dardano A, Versari D, Ghiadoni L, Salvetti A, Ferrannini E, Monzani F. Impaired endothelium-dependent vasodilatation in subclinical hypothyroidism: beneficial effect of levothyroxine therapy. J Clin Endocrinol Metab. 2003;88:3731–7.

Thakker RV. Hypocalcemia: pathogenesis, differential diagnosis and management. Am Soc Bone Min Res. 2006;35:213.

Thomas TC, Smith JM, White PC, Adhikari S. Transient neonatal hypocalcemia: presentation and outcomes. Pediatrics. 2012;129:e1461–7.

Thomason J, Girdler N, Kendall-Taylor P, Wastell H, Weddel A, Seymour R. An investigation into the need for supplementary steroids in organ transplant patients undergoing gingival surgery. J Clin Periodontol. 1999;26:577–82.

Tripathi M, Karwasra RK, Parshad S. Effect of preoperative vitamin D deficiency on postoperative hypocalcemia after thyroid surgery. Thyroid Res. 2014;7:8.

Tunbridge W, Evered D, Hall R, Appleton D, Brewis M, Clark F, Evans JG, Young E, Bird T, Smith P. The spectrum of thyroid disease in a community: the Whickham survey. Clin Endocrinol (Oxf). 1977;7:481–93.

Udelsman R, Norton JA, Jelenich SE, Goldstein DS, Linehan WM, Loriaux DL, Chrousos GP. Responses of the hypothalamic-pituitary-adrenal and renin-angiotensin axes and the sympathetic system during controlled surgical and anesthetic stress. J Clin Endocrinol Metab. 1987;64:986–94.

Urbano FL. Signs of hypocalcemia: Chvostek's and Trousseau's signs. Hosp Physician. 2000;36: 43–5.

Vanderpump M, Tunbrldge W, French J, Appleton D, Bates D, Clark F, Evans JG, Hasan D, Rodgers H, Tunbridge F. The incidence of thyroid disorders in the community: a twenty-year follow-up of the Whickham Survey. Clin Endocrinol (Oxf). 1995;43:55–68.

Vickers P, Garg K, Arya R, Godha U, Mathur P, Jain S. The role of selective beta 1-blocker in the preoperative preparation of thyrotoxicosis: a comparative study with propranolol. Int Surg. 1989;75:179–83.

Walsh JP, Bremner AP, Feddema P, Leedman PJ, Brown SJ, O'Leary P. Thyrotropin and thyroid antibodies as predictors of hypothyroidism: a 13-year, longitudinal study of a community-based cohort using current immunoassay techniques. J Clin Endocrinol Metab. 2010;95:1095–104.

Wassner AJ, Cohen LE, Hechter E, Dauber A. Isolated central hypothyroidism in young siblings as a manifestation of PROP1 deficiency: clinical impact of whole exome sequencing. Horm Res Paediatr. 2013;79:379–86.

Weinberg AD, Brennan MD, Gorman CA, Marsh HM, O'Fallon WM. Outcome of anesthesia and surgery in hypothyroid patients. Arch Intern Med. 1983;143:893–7.

Werner SC, Ingbar SH, Braverman LE, Utiger RD. Werner & Ingbar's the thyroid: a fundamental and clinical text. Philadelphia: Lippincott Williams & Wilkins; 2000.

Westerhof L, Van Ditmars M, Der Kinderen P, Thijssen J, Schwarz F. Recovery of adrenocortical function during long-term treatment with corticosteroids. BMJ. 1972;2:195–7.

Wise-Faberowski L, Soriano SG, Ferrari L, McManus ML, Wolfsdorf JI, Majzoub J, Scott RM, Truog R, Rockoff MA. Perioperative management of diabetes insipidus in children [corrected]. J Neurosurg Anesthesiol. 2004;16:14–9.

Woeber KA. Thyrotoxicosis and the heart. N Engl J Med. 1992;327:94–8.

Wood AJ, Lamberts SW, Bruining HA, de Jong FH. Corticosteroid therapy in severe illness. N Engl J Med. 1997;337:1285–92.

Ziyaeifard M, Azarfarin R, Ferasatkish R, Dashti M. Management of difficult airway with laryngeal mask in a child with mucopolysaccharidosis and mitral regurgitation: a case report. Res Cardiovasc Med. 2014;3:e174561.

Chapter 39
Perioperative Pain Management in Patients with Congenital Heart Disease

Evelyn C. Monico and Zoel Augusto Quiñónez

Introduction

Two areas regarding the care of children with heart disease that are underappreciated in the literature are the development and management of chronic postoperative pain as well as the use of neuraxial and regional techniques in patients with congenital heart disease. Given the surprisingly high prevalence, and the inadequate treatment, of persistent pain after surgery in children, it is of benefit to the anesthesiologist to understand its presentation and trajectory. This may allow for its recognition in the perioperative setting and referral for proper management.

Likewise, the benefit of regional anesthetic techniques seems to be underappreciated in children with congenital heart disease (Gottlieb and Andropoulos 2013; Ing and Twite 2015). With advancement and availability of ultrasound making regional anesthetic techniques safer and more accessible, superficial and deep peripheral nerve or plexus blocks are options for these patients, particularly for those patients that may not tolerate general anesthesia. Here, we present several techniques that may be beneficial in the care of children with heart disease.

Chronic Postsurgical Pain

Persistent or chronic postsurgical pain occurs in approximately 20 % of all children having major surgery. Postsurgical pain, defined as pain that persists beyond the expected time of healing, may last months to years past the time of surgery, leading

E.C. Monico, MD (✉) • Z.A. Quiñónez, MD
Texas Children's Hospital, Baylor College of Medicine,
6621 Fannin Street, Suite A3300, Houston, TX 77030, USA
e-mail: ecmonico@texaschildrens.org; zoel.quinonez@bcm.edu;
zaquinon@texaschildrens.org

© Springer International Publishing Switzerland 2017
A. Dabbagh et al. (eds.), *Congenital Heart Disease in Pediatric and Adult Patients*, DOI 10.1007/978-3-319-44691-2_39

to a decline in health-related quality-of-life measures (HRQOL) and greater activity limitations (Merskey and Bogduk 1994; Rabbitts et al. 2015a). In a study of 60 children, 10–18 years of age, undergoing spine and chest wall surgery, children followed two distinct trajectories. Early recovery was characterized by decreasing pain from 2 weeks to 4 months, and a late recovery trajectory was characterized by increasing pain from admission to 2 weeks after surgery, followed by decreasing pain to 4 months and 1 year after surgery (Rabbitts et al. 2015b). After controlling for sex and age, presurgical parental pain catastrophizing strongly predicted a late recovery trajectory. Surprisingly, the child's own pain catastrophizing and baseline pain did not predict the child's recovery trajectory.

Neuropathic pain from direct surgical nerve injury is believed to account for the vast majority of persistent postsurgical pain, but there are patient-specific characteristics that may also determine why only some patients with surgical nerve injury go on to develop chronic postsurgical pain. Among these patient characteristics are genetic factors, preexisting pain, pain memories, age, and gender (Kehlet et al. 2006).

The synaptic plasticity of neurons at the spinal cord level, particularly those in the dorsal horn, are currently thought to be at the root of how acute surgical pain becomes chronic continuous or chronic intermittent postsurgical pain. These neurons are responsible for amplifying the initial nociceptive surgical stimulus both temporally and regionally at the periphery (Fig. 39.1) (Kehlet et al. 2006). This phenomenon has been termed central sensitization, and it starts with the activation of high-threshold peripheral nociceptors by a noxious stimulus and the simultaneous activation of the inflammatory cascade at the periphery, which in turn influence neurons (Kehlet et al. 2006). These two separate processes lead to changes in intracellular kinases and proteins in dorsal horn second-order neurons, thus fundamentally changing gene transcription and ultimately resulting in a reduction of inhibitory neurotransmitters and an increase in excitatory transmitters. This change in the balance of neuronal excitability occurs almost immediately and last several days. Neurons that were normally not activated by painful stimulus suddenly become responsive to non-painful, i.e., normal, sensory stimuli, even in areas beyond the original injury site.

Fig. 39.1 Sites and mechanisms responsible for chronic postsurgical neuropathic pain: (*1*) Denervated Schwann cells and infiltrating macrophages distal to nerve injury produce local and systemic chemicals that drive pain signaling. (*2*) Neuroma at site of injury is a source of ectopic spontaneous excitability in sensory fibers. (*3*) Changes in gene expression in dorsal root ganglion alter excitability, responsiveness, transmission, and survival of sensory neurons. (*4*) Dorsal horn is a site of altered activity and gene expression, producing central sensitization, loss of inhibitory interneurons, and microglial activation, which together amplify sensory flow. (*5*) Brainstem descending controls modulate transmission in spinal cord. (*6*) Limbic system and hypothalamus contribute to altered mood, behavior, and autonomic reflexes. (*7*) Sensation of pain generated in the cortex (past experiences, cultural inputs, and expectations converge to determine what patient feels). (*8*) Genomic DNA predispose (or not) patient to chronic pain and affect their reaction to treatment (Taken from Kehlet and colleagues (2006))

Pain After Sternotomy

Persistent postsurgical pain is a well-established entity in the adult pain literature, but in children, it has only recently been recognized as an important consequence of surgery. We know from adult studies that the prevalence of persistent pain after sternotomy ranges from 20 to 50 % (Eisenberg et al. 2001; Meyerson et al. 2001;

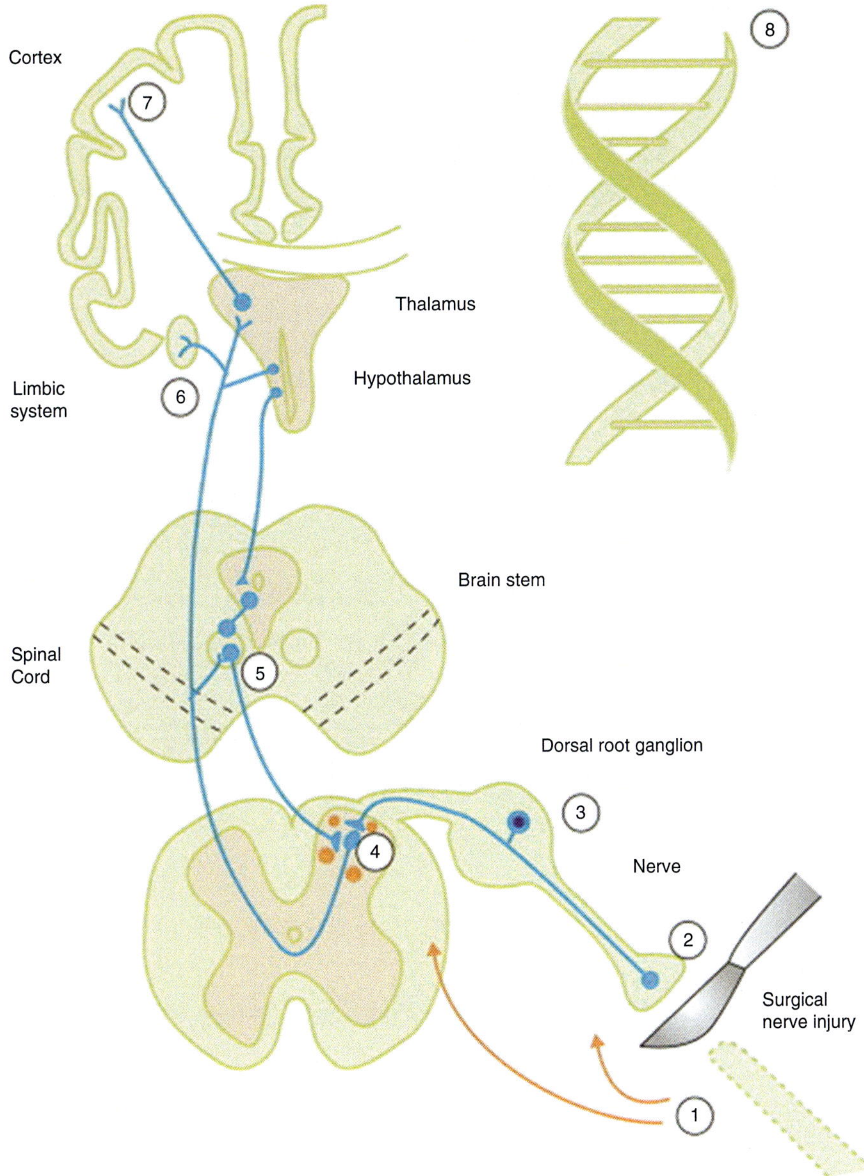

Bruce et al. 2003; Lahtinen et al. 2006; van Gulik et al. 2011; Rodriguez-Aldrete et al. 2015). In adults, chronic pain after sternotomy most closely presents like neuropathic pain, although in some cases, it is mixed with inflammatory or nociceptive pain. This observation is consistent with what we know about chronic postsurgical pain, which is that it is more common after surgeries where surgical nerve injury is most likely to occur (Kehlet et al. 2006).

Children commonly undergo cardiac surgery that requires sternotomy for repair of lesions that include, but are not limited to, Tetralogy of Fallot, transposition of the great arteries, and hypoplastic left heart syndrome. Most recently, Lauridsen and colleagues (2014) studied 121 children ages 0–12 that required median sternotomy. They found that 4 years after cardiac surgery, roughly 20 % of these children had recent or persistent pain. In 24 out of the 26 children with pain reports, pain could be provoked by physical activity, and 12 out of the 26 children reported a pain intensity ≥ 4 on a numerical rating scale (Lauridsen et al. 2014). Based on these children's reported pain characteristics, post-sternotomy pain appears to have a neuropathic component. Redo sternotomy, a known risk factor in adults for persistent postsurgical pain, did not prove in this study to be a risk factor for the development of persistent post-sternotomy pain, though there was a trend toward a higher pain prevalence in children with more than one sternotomy (van Gulik et al. 2011). Thus far, surgical technique (mini-sternotomy versus full-sternotomy) for atrial septal defect repair has failed to show a significant difference in immediate postoperative pain scores and development of chronic pain (Laussen et al. 2000).

Pain After Thoracotomy

Thoracotomies are one of the most painful surgical procedures in children, having a higher analgesic requirement than other incisions (Shima et al. 1996; Gerner 2008). Chronic post-thoracotomy pain (CPTP), defined as persistent or recurring incisional pain for at least 2 months after thoracotomy, is rarely studied in children (Merskey 1999). Chou and colleagues (2014) recently reported a prevalence of chronic pain in a predominantly male population of 51 subjects who had their first thoracotomy at a median 5.7 years of age to be 1.96 % (0.00–10.4 % CI) (Chou et al. 2014). The results from this retrospective cross-sectional study, which mostly looked at children with a single nonelective thoracotomy, stand in contrast to CPTP prevalence data in adults, which has been quoted to be as high as 50 %. These results are also different from previous pediatric studies that estimate CPTP in adults who were 20 years status post-thoracotomy for coarctation repair between age of zero and 25 years old as 16 % (Matsunaga et al. 1990; Pluijms et al. 2006; Kristensen et al. 2010). It is possible that in children increased CNS plasticity accompanies the synaptic abundance and may allow for a reduced period of recovery, but prospective studies are needed (Johnston 2009).

In the immediate postoperative period, pain after thoracotomy can hinder respiratory dynamics by promoting splinting and delay mobilization. The postoperative course can be particularly rocky after posterolateral thoracotomies that do not employ a muscle-sparing technique, as the serratus anterior and latissimus dorsi muscles are compromised resulting in more postoperative nerve impairment0 (Ponn et al. 1992; Benedetti et al. 1998). Pediatric or adult data do not strongly support a surgical technique as being advantageous in preventing CPTP, but it is understood that minimizing muscle injury and rib retraction is likely to preserve intercostal nerves. It is generally desirable to minimize opioids in most cases since opioids can further compromise the patient's respiratory function and trigger opioid-related side effects like nausea and constipation. Institutions today typically treat the immediate postoperative pain from thoracotomy with thoracic epidural analgesia (TEA), patient-controlled analgesia (PCA), paravertebral catheters, intercostal nerve catheters, or a combination of these (TEA plus PCA). Due to evidence of equivalent analgesia with a more favorable side-effect profile, ultrasound-guided thoracic paravertebral blocks are increasingly challenging the long-held gold standard TEA. Several small pediatric retrospective studies exist comparing different analgesic modalities in the immediate postoperative period, but these studies are often too small and with too brief follow-up periods to definitively show superiority of one analgesic technique over another, particularly as it pertains to the development of chronic postsurgical pain (Gonzalez et al. 2015). This is a controversy that extends into adult literature. In a Cochrane Database Systematic Review from 2012 where 250 adults were included as participants, regional anesthesia for thoracotomy to prevent chronic pain at 6 months had an odds ratio of 0.33 (95 % CI 0.20 to 0.56), and paravertebral block for breast cancer surgery to prevent chronic postsurgical pain at 5–6 months had an odds ratio of 0.37 (95 % CI 0.14 to 0.94) (Andreae and Andreae 2012). Another important controversy that adult studies have tackled has been the question of preoperative versus postoperative TEA for thoracotomies. While there seems to be no difference in their incidence of CPTP, preoperative TEA seems to perform as a better analgesic for acute postoperative pain (Andreae and Andreae 2012). The methodology of many of the included studies was intermediate, and the inclusion of children in further studies is needed to generalize this data to the pediatric population. There are currently no pediatric studies supporting the use of gabapentinoids, antidepressants, ketamine, local anesthetic infiltration, or cryoanalgesia to prevent CPTP.

Management of CPTP and Post-sternotomy Pain

For post-sternotomy and post-thoracotomy pain, ruling out secondary pain due to wound dehiscence, broken sternal wires causing tissue injury, or a localized infection precedes the diagnosis of a primary pain syndrome. The etiology of CPTP is both neuropathic, from iatrogenic intercostal nerve injury, and myofascial in origin (Gerner 2008; Steegers et al. 2008; Wildgaard et al. 2009). In adult patients, there seems to be some association between poorly controlled pain and the appearance of neuropathic features in the acute postoperative period with the eventual development of CPTP, but this has not been fully studied in the pediatric population (Searle et al. 2009). Sensory deficits and paresthesias, particularly allodynia, defined as pain elicited by a non-painful stimulus such as clothes or light touch, are frequently encountered along the thoracotomy scar and along the territory of intercostal nerves (Merskey and Bogduk 1994). Patients with a greater component of neuropathic pain can suffer with severe pain that can be continuous or paroxysmal and that interferes with sleep, school, sports, and activities of daily living. To make the diagnosis of neuropathic pain, there must be pain in a dermatomal distribution, partial or complete sensory loss in all or part of the painful area, and the presence of disease or injury preceding pain (Kehlet et al. 2006). Initial management of CPTP is usually conservative and starts with an anti-neuropathic agent such as gabapentinoids (gabapentin or pregabalin), serotonin-norepinephrine reuptake inhibitors, or a tricyclic antidepressant like amitriptyline dosed based on the child's weight. If pain persists and medical therapy fails to relieve the neuropathic symptoms, an intercostal nerve injection, a paravertebral single injection or catheter, pulsed radiofrequency of the dorsal root ganglion, or intercostal radiofrequency ablation can be considered, but pediatric data is lacking (Fishman et al. 2010). One could consider trigger point injections or botox injections into the intercostal muscles to address the myofascial component of the pain (Fishman et al. 2010). There is currently no supportive evidence in children for minimally invasive pain therapies, such as nerve blocks, and the evaluation of a child with CPTP should include a referral to an interdisciplinary pediatric pain clinic to investigate the physiologic and psychosocial contributors of pain chronicity (Cohen et al. 2008).

The concepts in management for post-sternotomy pain are similar to those of CPTP. Given that much of post-sternotomy pain has a neuropathic quality, anti-neuropathic agents (gabapentinoids, serotonin-norepinephrine reuptake inhibitors, tricyclic antidepressant) are potential therapies once secondary pain has been ruled out. Referral to an interdisciplinary pediatric pain clinic should also be considered for assessment and management of chronic post-sternotomy pain.

Useful Regional Techniques in Patients with Congenital Heart Disease

For children with congenital heart disease undergoing noncardiac surgery, regional anesthesia may provide the benefit of analgesia while minimizing the respiratory depressant effects of opiate analgesics (Harnik et al. 1986). The following are neuraxial and regional techniques that may be useful alone or in combination with general anesthesia for the care of patients with congenital heart disease.

Neuraxial Blocks

Spinal and epidural blocks have been used for adults and children undergoing cardiac surgery, and it has been a standard in at least one center (Hammer et al. 2000; Peterson et al. 2000; Steven and McGowan 2000; Weiner et al. 2012). And although the risk of epidural hematoma seems exceptionally low, the potentially devastating neurologic injury that may occur in patients undergoing systemic anticoagulation dissuades practitioners from utilizing neuraxial techniques (Chaney 2009; Weiner et al. 2012). This may be of greater concern for cyanotic patients with increased risk for epidural collateral vessels, increased central venous pressures, and coagulopathy (Steven and McGowan 2000).

Nonetheless, neuraxial blocks have benefits for children with congenital heart disease undergoing noncardiac surgery, including thoracolumbar and lower extremity procedures (Hardacker and Tolley 2004). Intrathecal blocks, as well as caudal, thoracic, or lumbar epidural blocks, are useful in a variety of thoracolumbar procedures, and placement of an epidural catheter allows for continuous postoperative pain control (Hardacker and Tolley 2004; Ivani and Mosseti 2009).

Both spinal and epidural anesthesia in combination with general anesthesia have been shown to mitigate the stress response to cardiothoracic surgery better than systemic opiates, which may improve patient outcomes (Anand et al. 1990; Anand and Hickey 1992; Wolf et al. 1998). This includes attenuating hemodynamic changes, mitigating immunologic and metabolic derangements, and moderating platelet activation. The improved respiratory mechanics seen after thoracotomy, along with the decreased need for narcotics, can also facilitate extubation (Slinger et al. 1995). Reports of successful and safe use of these techniques for women with congenital heart disease in the peripartum period seem to indicate their safety in high-risk patients with single-ventricle physiology and pulmonary hypertension (Fong et al. 1990; Peng et al. 1997; Lockhart et al. 1999; Maxwell et al. 2013).

Only minor, if any, self-resolving hemodynamic changes have been seen with neuraxial techniques, including high spinal anesthesia, in children with congenital heart disease, and they are typically not observed in those less than 8 years old (Murat et al. 1987; Hammer et al. 2000; Finkel et al. 2003; Kachko et al. 2012; Shenkman et al. 2012). Neuraxial anesthesia can therefore likely be performed with less of a concern for hemodynamic changes in these younger children.

While neurologic injury has been reported even after uneventful epidural block placement, neurologic injury is rare, with only 9 transient neurologic injuries in 37,543 epidural blocks, including caudal epidural blocks, reviewed in French, British, and American pediatric databases (Meyer et al. 2012).

Peripheral Block Techniques

Given the concern for devastating neurologic injuries, even after uneventful placement of thoracic epidural catheters, safety has driven use of regional anesthetic techniques with a lower risk profile. Additionally, in patients in whom neuraxial anesthesia is contraindicated, or those undergoing unilateral or ambulatory procedures, alternative truncal blocks from which patients may recover more quickly may be preferred (Oliver and Oliver 2013). The following are chest and abdominal blocks that avoid the neuraxial space.

Paravertebral Blocks

The paravertebral nerve blocks (PVNB) were described as early as 1919, but its use in children is more recent (Giesecke et al. 1988; Lönnqvist 1992). Like epidural and spinal anesthesia, paravertebral nerve blocks have been shown to attenuate the sympathetic and hormonal response to surgery (Giesecke et al. 1988). Generally used for thoracic and abdominal surgeries, PVNB have been shown to be effective in the management of intraoperative and postoperative pain associated with thoracic and abdominal procedures in children, and they possibly reduce the odds of developing chronic postoperative pain, although more prospective studies are needed, particularly in children (Lönnqvist 1992; Karmakar et al. 1996; Shah et al. 1997; Richardson and Lönnqvist 1998; Andreae and Andreae 2013; Qi et al. 2014). Recently, a study by Hall Burton and Boretsky (2014) suggests that there may be no difference in efficacy between bilateral PVNB and thoracic epidurals for minimally invasive thoracoscopic NUSS procedures (Hall Burton and Boretsky 2014).

Several techniques for the placement of paravertebral blocks have been described, initially using a landmark-based technique and subsequently incorporating the use of nerve stimulation and ultrasound (Lönnqvist 1992; Ben-Ari et al. 2009; O Riain et al. 2010). The traditional parasagittal approach, though, poses difficulty in visualizing the block needle using ultrasound in smaller children (Boretsky et al. 2013). We, thus, advocate the use of the lateral in-line approach to the paravertebral space first described in children by Boretsky and colleagues, which accounts for the limitations of the traditional approaches in this population (Fig. 39.2) (Boretsky et al. 2013). Even with a landmark-based, blind approach, Lönnqvist (1992) demonstrated a reliably unilateral spread of contrast spanning four to six adjacent ribs in 7-month to 8-year-old children after a single contrast injection, in contrast to adults where injections at multiple levels are sometimes required (Boretsky 2014).

Given the limited reported experience with thoracic paravertebral blocks in children, complication rates are difficult to ascertain, but currently, no permanent neurologic injury has been reported with thoracic paravertebral blocks in children (Naja and Lönnqvist 2001; Polaner et al. 2012). Additionally, rates of dural and

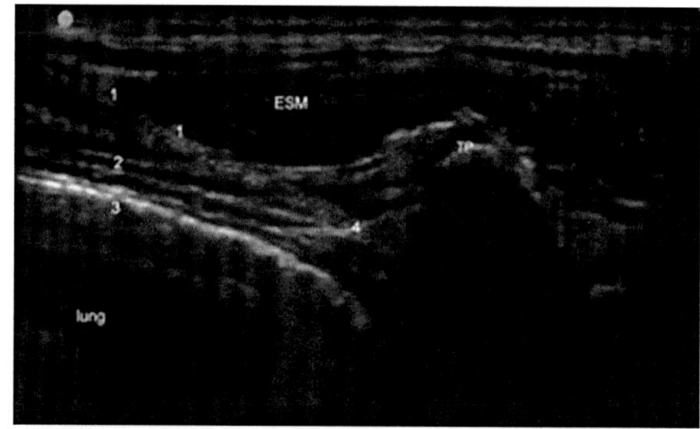

Fig. 39.2 Ultrasound anatomy of PVNB. Internal intercostal membrane (*IICM*) seen connecting the edge of the internal intercostal muscle to the lower edge of the TP. (*1*) Tuohy needle. (*2*) Intercostal muscles. (*3*) Parietal pleura. (*4*) IICM; *TP* transverse process, *ESM* erector spinae muscle

vascular puncture appear to be lower with PVNB (0 and 0 %) than with thoracic epidural (1.3 and 2.3 %), even when bilateral paravertebral nerve blocks are performed, and complication rates appear to be lower than those of adults undergoing PVNB (Naja and Lönnqvist 2001).

The added benefit of more hemodynamic stability with PVNB than with thoracic epidural blocks (less hypotension and requiring less volume and vasopressor therapy to maintain target hemodynamics) may be of benefit to those with congenital heart disease (Richardson et al. 1999; Pintaric et al. 2011). This may be due to PVNB providing a unilateral sympathetic block as opposed to the bilateral blockade with thoracic epidural (Casati et al. 2006).

In addition to surgeries requiring thoracotomy, such as aortic coarctation and vascular ring repair, we have successfully used thoracic PVNB, in combination with general anesthesia, for placement or replacement of abdominal pacemakers in children and adults. But they would likely be of benefit for many thoracic and abdominal procedures where providers wish to minimize the systemic effects of narcotics and avoid the risk of a sympathectomy from a neuraxial technique.

Pecs Blocks/Serratus Plane Block

The Pecs and serratus plane blocks provide anesthesia and analgesia to the ipsilateral hemithorax and are now more commonly used for breast surgeries and other thoracic procedures. The Pecs 1 block was initially described by Blanco (2011) and involved putting local anesthetic in the interfacial plane between the pectoralis major and pectoralis minor muscles (Blanco 2011). This block was designed to provide sensory blockade to the pectoralis major muscle and the overlying skin via the medial and lateral pectoral nerves, as well as intercostal nerves (Blanco 2011; Blanco et al. 2012).

Designed to have improved local anesthetic spread to the lateral branches of the intercostal nerves and to address serratus pain after chest expander placement, Blanco and colleagues (2012) then described the Pecs 2 block (Blanco et al. 2012; Blanco 2014). After injection of local anesthetic between the pectoralis minor and serratus anterior muscles, they provided radiographic evidence of local anesthetic spread to the long thoracic nerve (supplies the serratus anterior muscle) and as far down as the T8 dermatomal level. In an effort to make the block easier to perform and to improve its safety, Blanco and colleagues (2013) then described the serratus plane block, performed farther laterally than the Pecs 2 block, but designed for similar local anesthetic spread (Blanco et al. 2013). Rather than deposit local anesthetic between interfacial planes between the pectoralis minor and serratus anterior, it is deposited either above or below the serratus anterior muscle at the midaxillary line (Fig. 39.3).

In this last study, a wide area of sensory blockade was seen to reliably extend along the anterior hemithorax, the axilla, and the posterior hemithorax from the T2 to at least T6 when injected below the serratus anterior and T2 to at least T8 when injected above the serratus anterior. Injecting above the serratus anterior muscle was associated with a longer duration of intercostal nerve paresthesia as well (752 min versus 386 min) (Blanco et al. 2013).

The only randomized control trial comparing general anesthesia alone to general anesthesia plus Pecs 1/Pecs 2 blocks demonstrated improved pain control, a decreased need for intraoperative and postoperative opiates, lower postoperative nausea and vomiting scores, faster discharge from the postanesthesia recovery unit and the hospital, as well as lower sedation scores for those receiving regional anesthesia (Bashandy and Abbas 2015). Of note, these were women without congenital cardiac disease undergoing a modified radical mastectomy.

In patients with congenital heart disease, this series of blocks may have utility for those undergoing thoracic or axillary procedures, such as pacemaker placement in

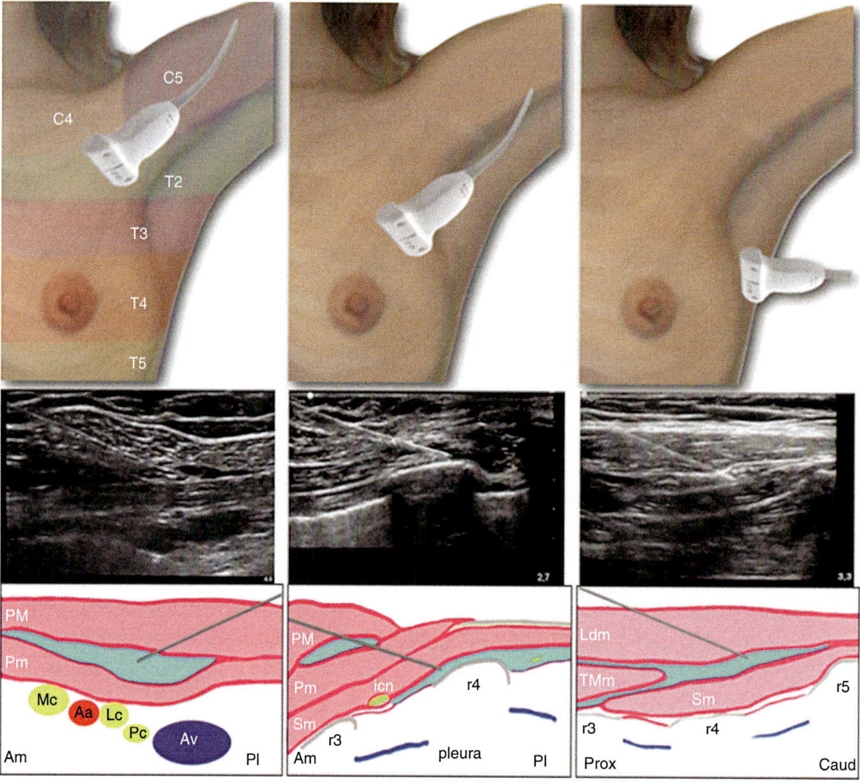

Fig. 39.3 Ultrasound probe position, ultrasound image of needle, and diagram for Pecs 1 (*left*), Pecs 2* (*middle*), and serratus plane (*right*) blocks. *Needle shown between pectoralis minor and serratus anterior muscles in the ultrasound image, but local anesthetic shown under the serratus anterior muscle in the diagram. Blanco and colleagues have clarified that injection above or below muscle is acceptable for the Pecs 2 block. *PM* pectoralis major, *Pm* pectoralis minor, *Ldm* latissimus dorsi, *Tmm* Teres major, *Sm* serratus muscle, *Icn* intercostal nerve, *Lc* lateral cord, *Pc* posterior cord, *Mc* medial cord of the brachial plexus, *Aa* axillary artery, *Av* axillary vein, together with the ribs, three (*r3*), four (*r4*), and rib five (*r5*), *Am* orientation anteromedial, *PI* posterolateral, *Prox* proximal, *Caud* caudal (Taken from Blanco and colleagues (2013))

older children, as well as vascular access (Fujiwara et al. 2014). For procedures extending from the axilla to the upper arm, such as vascular access, supplementing with a supraclavicular brachial plexus block may be of benefit (Purcell and Wu 2014; Tan and Quek 2015).

At our institution, we have used Pecs 1 alone as well as in combination with a Pecs 2 block, as described by Bashandy and colleagues (2015), in combination with general anesthesia, with good analgesic effect for pacemaker placements and pacemaker generator changes confined to the chest (Bashandy and Abbas 2015).

No complications have been reported, but large studies have yet to be conducted, and given that the first of these blocks was described in 2011, there is limited experience on which to base complication rates associated with Pecs and serratus plane blocks.

Transversus Abdominis Plane (TAP) Block

Depositing local anesthetic in the interfacial plane between the internal oblique and transversus abdominis muscles constitutes a TAP block. This block was traditionally performed using a landmark technique at the lumbar triangle of Petit, through which thoracic nerve segments below T9 enter (Figs. 39.4 and 39.5) (Rozen et al. 2008). Ultrasound has allowed more precise deposition of local anesthetic in different portions of the interfascial plane (Fig. 39.6). While Støving and colleagues (2015) demonstrated heterogeneity in the abdominal paresthesia created by an ultrasound-guided TAP block, they also confirmed that the block reliably affects only the lower thoracic and lumbar dermatomes ipsilaterally (Støving et al. 2015).

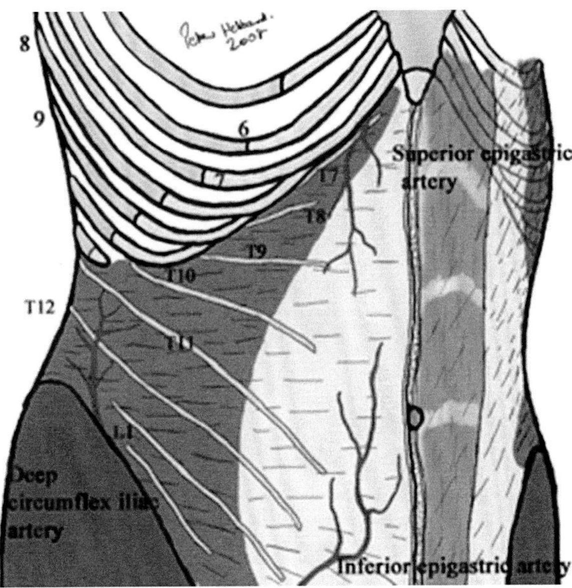

Fig. 39.4 Distribution of nerves in the transversus abdominis plane (Taken from Mai et al. (2012))

Fig. 39.5 Surface anatomy relevant to the TAP Block. (**a**) Anatomy of the TOP. (**b**) Needle insertion into the TOP. (**c**) Injection of local anesthetic into the TAP. *TOP* lumbar triangle of Petit; *LD* latissimus dorsi muscle, *EO* external oblique muscle (Taken from McDonnell and colleagues (2007))

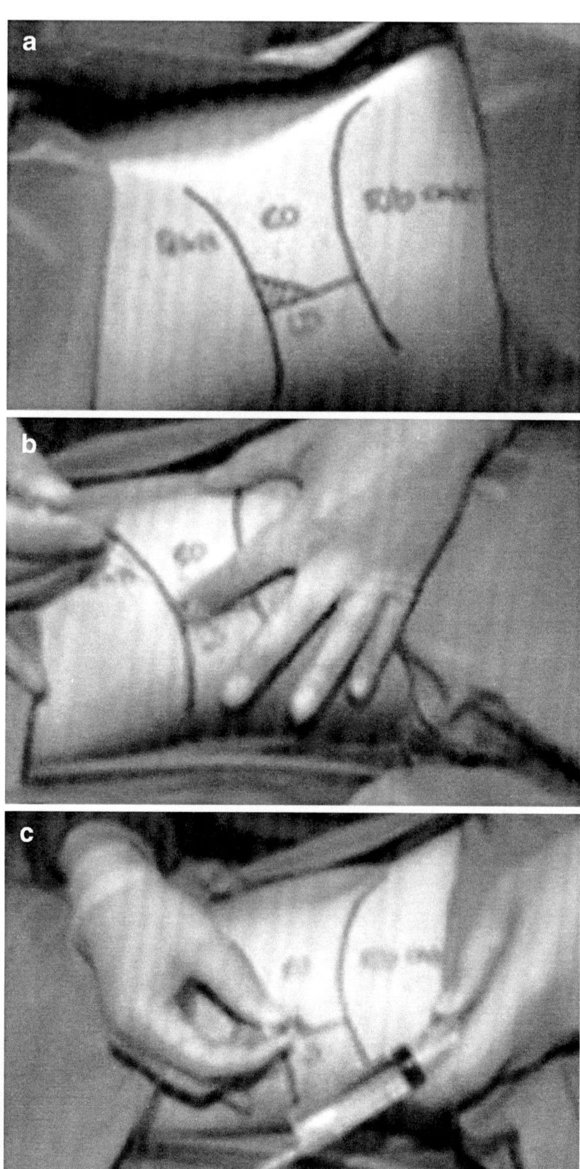

This finding is supported by studies that show no benefit to TAP blocks when the surgical site is outside of this effective area in many or all of the studied patients (Lorenzo et al. 2014; Faasse et al. 2015; Lapmahapaisan et al. 2015). Moreover, Rozen and colleagues (2008) suggested that TAP blocks would likely only be useful for lower abdominal surgery after their anatomic examination of the abdominal innervation of the thoracolumbar nerves (Rozen et al. 2008). Several studies and

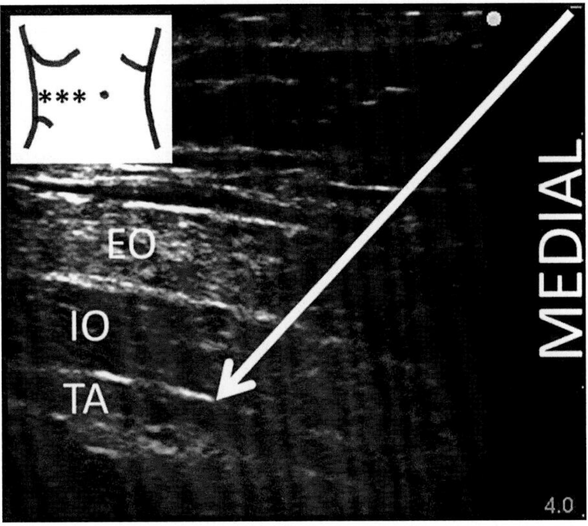

Fig. 39.6 In-line TAP block approach. *** position of ultrasound probe for in-line approach. *Arrow* path of the needle from medial to lateral. *EO* external oblique muscle, *IO* internal oblique muscle, *TA* transversus abdominis muscle (Taken from Steffel and colleagues (2016))

reviews have shown decreased opiate use, improved pain scores, and decreased PONV after placement of a TAP block for lower abdominal and midline procedures (McDonnell et al. 2007; Bryskin et al. 2015; Suresh et al. 2015; Hamill et al. 2016).

At our institution, TAP blocks have been used, in combination with general anesthesia, with good analgesic results for patients with congenital heart disease undergoing laparoscopic or open gastrostomy tube placement, and in combination with a femoral nerve block for one unstable and awake patient requiring Impella® (Abiomed; Danvers, MA) left ventricular assist device placement via femoral arterial approach. It is important to note that TAP blocks only provide analgesia or anesthesia to the abdominal wall, and patients may require supplemental analgesics for visceral pain associate with surgery. This was highlighted by Bryskin and colleagues (2015), where patients receiving a TAP block, compared to caudal epidural block, for bilateral ureteral implant surgery using a low transverse incision had higher pain scores in the recovery unit and had higher requirement for a bladder antispasmotic (oxybutynin) but required less cumulative opiates over the first 24 h after surgery (Bryskin et al. 2015).

Complications are rare for TAP blocks, but care must be taken to avoid entering the peritoneal space, particularly because of the proximity of vital organs (McDonnell et al. 2007; Farooq and Carey 2008; Long et al. 2014; Bryskin et al. 2015; Faasse et al. 2015; Lapmahapaisan et al. 2015).

In summary, perioperative physicians should understand how to recognize persistent pain after surgery related to thoracotomy or sternotomy. These children may require referral to a specialized pain provider for care. There is evidence for the use of regional anesthetic techniques in the prevention of chronic pain, but larger randomized control trials are needed. Regional techniques, though, help improve pain scores and decrease the side effects related to systemic opioids. Additionally, they may be particularly useful in unstable children who may not tolerate general anesthesia, intubation, and positive pressure ventilation.

References

Anand KJ, Hansen DD, Hickey PR. Hormonal-metabolic stress responses in neonates undergoing cardiac surgery. Anesthesiology. 1990;73:661–70.

Anand KJ, Hickey PR. Halothane-morphine compared with high-dose sufentanil for anesthesia and postoperative analgesia in neonatal cardiac surgery. N Engl J Med. 1992;326:1–9.

Andreae MH, Andreae DA. Local anaesthetics and regional anaesthesia for preventing chronic pain after surgery. Cochrane Database Syst Rev. 2012;10:CD007105.

Andreae MH, Andreae DA. Regional anaesthesia to prevent chronic pain after surgery: a Cochrane systematic review and meta-analysis. Br J Anaesth. 2013;111:711–20.

Bashandy GM, Abbas DN. Pectoral nerves I and II blocks in multimodal analgesia for breast cancer surgery: a randomized clinical trial. Reg Anesth Pain Med. 2015;40:68–74.

Ben-Ari A, Moreno M, Chelly JE, Bigeleisen PE. Ultrasound-guided paravertebral block using an intercostal approach. Anesth Analg. 2009;109:1691–4.

Benedetti F, Vighetti S, Ricco C, Amanzio M, Bergamasco L, Casadio C, Cianci R, Giobbe R, Oliaro A, Bergamasco B, Maggi G. Neurophysiologic assessment of nerve impairment in posterolateral and muscle-sparing thoracotomy. J Thorac Cardiovasc Surg. 1998;115: 841–7.

Blanco R. The 'pecs block': a novel technique for providing analgesia after breast surgery. Anaesthesia. 2011;66:847–8.

Blanco R. A reply. Anaesthesia. 2014;69:1173–4.

Blanco R, Fajardo M, Parras Maldonado T. Ultrasound description of Pecs II (modified Pecs I): a novel approach to breast surgery. Rev Esp Anestesiol Reanim. 2012;59:470–5.

Blanco R, Parras T, McDonnell JG, Prats-Galino A. Serratus plane block: a novel ultrasound-guided thoracic wall nerve block. Anaesthesia. 2013;68:1107–13.

Boretsky K, Visoiu M, Bigeleisen P. Ultrasound-guided approach to the paravertebral space for catheter insertion in infants and children. Paediatr Anaesth. 2013;23:1193–8.

Boretsky KR. Regional anesthesia in pediatrics: marching forward. Curr Opin Anaesthesiol. 2014;27:556–60.

Bruce J, Drury N, Poobalan SA, Jeffrey RR, Smith SWC, Chambers AW. The prevalence of chronic chest and leg pain following cardiac surgery: a historical cohort study. Pain. 2003;104:265–73.

Bryskin RB, Londergan B, Wheatley R, Heng R, Lewis M, Barraza M, Mercer E, Ye G. Transversus abdominis plane block versus caudal epidural for lower abdominal surgery in children: a double-blinded randomized controlled trial. Anesth Analg. 2015;121:471–8.

Casati A, Alessandrini P, Nuzzi M, Tosi M, Iotti E, Ampollini L, Bobbio A, Rossini E, Fanelli G. A prospective, randomized, blinded comparison between continuous thoracic paravertebral and epidural infusion of 0.2% ropivacaine after lung resection surgery. Eur J Anaesthesiol. 2006;23:999–1004.

Chaney MA. Thoracic epidural anaesthesia in cardiac surgery – the current standing. Ann Card Anaesth. 2009;12:1–3.

Chou J, Chan C-w, Chalkiadis GA. Post-thoracotomy pain in children and adolescence: a retrospective cross-sectional study. Pain Med. 2014;15:452–9.

Cohen LL, Lemanek K, Blount RL, Dahlquist LM, Lim CS, Palermo TM, McKenna KD, Weiss KE. Evidence-based assessment of pediatric pain. J Pediatr Psychol. 2008;33:939–55; discussion 956–937.

Eisenberg E, Pultorak Y, Pud D, Bar-El Y. Prevalence and characteristics of post coronary artery bypass graft surgery pain (PCP). Pain. 2001;92:11–7.

Faasse MA, Lindgren BW, Frainey BT, Marcus CR, Szczodry DM, Glaser AP, Suresh S, Gong EM. Perioperative effects of caudal and transversus abdominis plane (TAP) blocks for children undergoing urologic robot-assisted laparoscopic surgery. J Pediatr Urol. 2015;11:121. e121-127.

Farooq M, Carey M. A case of liver trauma with a blunt regional anesthesia needle while performing transversus abdominis plane block. Reg Anesth Pain Med. 2008;33:274–5.

Finkel JC, Boltz MG, Conran AM. Haemodynamic changes during high spinal anaesthesia in children having open heart surgery. Paediatr Anaesth. 2003;13:48–52.

Fishman S, Ballantyne J, Rathmell JP, Bonica J. Bonica's management of pain. 4th ed. Baltimore: Lippincott Williams & Wilkins; 2010.

Fong J, Druzin M, Gimbel AA, Fisher J. Epidural anacsthcsia for labour and caesarean section in a parturient with a single ventricle and transposition of the great arteries. Can J Anaesth. 1990;37:680–4.

Fujiwara A, Komasawa N, Minami T. Pectoral nerves (PECS) and intercostal nerve block for cardiac resynchronization therapy device implantation. Springerplus. 2014;3:409.

Gerner P. Postthoracotomy pain management problems. Anesthesiol Clin. 2008;26:355–67, vii.

Giesecke K, Hamberger B, Järnberg PO, Klingstedt C. Paravertebral block during cholecystectomy: effects on circulatory and hormonal responses. Br J Anaesth. 1988;61:652–6.

Gonzalez KW, Dalton BG, Millspaugh DL, Thomas PG, St Peter SD. Epidural versus patient-controlled analgesia after pediatric thoracotomy for malignancy: a preliminary review. Eur J Pediatr Surg. 2015;26:340–3.

Gottlieb EA, Andropoulos DB. Anesthesia for the patient with congenital heart disease presenting for noncardiac surgery. Curr Opin Anaesthesiol. 2013;26:318–26.

Hall Burton DM, Boretsky KR. A comparison of paravertebral nerve block catheters and thoracic epidural catheters for postoperative analgesia following the Nuss procedure for pectus excavatum repair. Paediatr Anaesth. 2014;24:516–20.

Hamill JK, Rahiri J-L, Liley A, Hill AG. Rectus sheath and transversus abdominis plane blocks in children: a systematic review and meta-analysis of randomized trials. Paediatr Anaesth. 2016;26:363–71.

Hammer GB, Ngo K, Macario A. A retrospective examination of regional plus general anesthesia in children undergoing open heart surgery. Anesth Analg. 2000;90:1020–4.

Hardacker DM, Tolley JA. Postoperative neuraxial pain relief in the pediatric patient. Semin Pediatr Surg. 2004;13:203–9.

Harnik EV, Hoy GR, Potolicchio S, Stewart DR, Siegelman RE. Spinal anesthesia in premature infants recovering from respiratory distress syndrome. Anesthesiology. 1986;64:95–9.

Ing RJ, Twite MD. The year in review: anesthesia for congenital heart disease 2014. Semin Cardiothorac Vasc Anesth. 2015;19:12–20.

Ivani G, Mosseti V. Pediatric regional anesthesia. Minerva Anestesiol. 2009;75:577–83.

Johnston MV. Plasticity in the developing brain: implications for rehabilitation. Dev Disabil Res Rev. 2009;15:94–101.

Kachko L, Birk E, Simhi E, Tzeitlin E, Freud E, Katz J. Spinal anesthesia for noncardiac surgery in infants with congenital heart diseases. Paediatr Anaesth. 2012;22:647–53.

Karmakar MK, Booker PD, Franks R, Pozzi M. Continuous extrapleural paravertebral infusion of bupivacaine for post-thoracotomy analgesia in young infants. Br J Anaesth. 1996;76:811–5.

Kehlet H, Jensen TS, Woolf CJ. Persistent postsurgical pain: risk factors and prevention. Lancet. 2006;367:1618–25.

Kristensen AD, Pedersen TAL, Hjortdal VE, Jensen TS, Nikolajsen L. Chronic pain in adults after thoracotomy in childhood or youth. Br J Anaesth. 2010;104:75–9.

Lahtinen P, Kokki H, Hynynen M. Pain after cardiac surgery: a prospective cohort study of 1-year incidence and intensity. Anesthesiology. 2006;105:794–800.

Lapmahapaisan S, Tantemsapya N, Aroonpruksakul N, Maisat W, Suraseranivongse S. Efficacy of surgical transversus abdominis plane block for postoperative pain relief following abdominal surgery in pediatric patients. Paediatr Anaesth. 2015;25:614–20.

Lauridsen MH, Kristensen AD, Hjortdal VE, Jensen TS, Nikolajsen L. Chronic pain in children after cardiac surgery via sternotomy. Cardiol Young. 2014;24:893–9.

Laussen PC, Bichell DP, McGowan FX, Zurakowski D, DeMaso DR, del Nido PJ. Postoperative recovery in children after minimum versus full-length sternotomy. Ann Thorac Surg. 2000;69:591–6.

Lockhart EM, Penning DH, Olufolabi AJ, Bell EA, Booth JV, Kern FH. SvO2 monitoring during spinal anesthesia and cesarean section in a parturient with severe cyanotic congenital heart disease. Anesthesiology. 1999;90:1213–5.

Long JB, Birmingham PK, De Oliveira GS, Schaldenbrand KM, Suresh S. Transversus abdominis plane block in children: a multicenter safety analysis of 1994 cases from the PRAN (Pediatric Regional Anesthesia Network) database. Anesth Analg. 2014;119:395–9.

Lönnqvist PA. Continuous paravertebral block in children. Initial experience. Anaesthesia. 1992;47:607–9.

Lorenzo AJ, Lynch J, Matava C, El-Beheiry H, Hayes J. Ultrasound guided transversus abdominis plane vs surgeon administered intraoperative regional field infiltration with bupivacaine for early postoperative pain control in children undergoing open pyeloplasty. J Urol. 2014;192:207–13.

Mai CL, Young MJ, Quraishi SA. Clinical implications of the transversus abdominis plane block in pediatric anesthesia. Paediatr Anaesth. 2012;22(9):831–40.

Matsunaga M, Dan K, Manabe FY, Hara F, Shono S, Shirakusa T. Residual pain of 90 thoracotomy patients with malignancy and non-malignancy. Pain. 1990;41 Suppl 5:s148.

Maxwell BG, El-Sayed YY, Riley ET, Carvalho B. Peripartum outcomes and anaesthetic management of parturients with moderate to complex congenital heart disease or pulmonary hypertension*. Anaesthesia. 2013;68:52–9.

McDonnell JG, O'Donnell B, Curley G, Heffernan A, Power C, Laffey JG. The analgesic efficacy of transversus abdominis plane block after abdominal surgery: a prospective randomized controlled trial. Anesth Analg. 2007;104:193–7.

Merskey H. Comments on Woolf et al. Pain 77(1998):227–9. Re: mechanisms and the classification of pain. Pain. 1999;82:319–20.

Merskey H, Bogduk N. Classification of chronic pain: descriptions of chronic pain syndromes and definitions of pain terms. 2nd ed. Seattle: IASP Press; 1994.

Meyer MJ, Krane EJ, Goldschneider KR, Klein NJ. Case report: neurological complications associated with epidural analgesia in children: a report of 4 cases of ambiguous etiologies. Anesth Analg. 2012;115:1365–70.

Meyerson J, Thelin S, Gordh T, Karlsten R. The incidence of chronic post-sternotomy pain after cardiac surgery – a prospective study. Acta Anaesthesiol Scand. 2001;45:940–4.

Murat I, Delleur MM, Esteve C, Egu JF, Raynaud P, Saint-Maurice C. Continuous extradural anaesthesia in children. Clinical and haemodynamic implications. Br J Anaesth. 1987;59:1441–50.

Naja Z, Lönnqvist PA. Somatic paravertebral nerve blockade. Incidence of failed block and complications. Anaesthesia. 2001;56:1184–8.

O Riain SC, Donnell BO, Cuffe T, Harmon DC, Fraher JP, Shorten G. Thoracic paravertebral block using real-time ultrasound guidance. Anesth Analg. 2010;110:248–51.

Oliver J-A, Oliver L-A. Beyond the caudal: truncal blocks an alternative option for analgesia in pediatric surgical patients. Curr Opin Anaesthesiol. 2013;26:644–51.

Peng TC, Chuah EC, Tan PP. Epidural anesthesia for emergency caesarean section in a patient with single ventricle and aortic stenosis. Acta Anaesthesiol Sin. 1997;35:39–44.

Peterson KL, DeCampli WM, Pike NA, Robbins RC, Reitz BA. A report of two hundred twenty cases of regional anesthesia in pediatric cardiac surgery. Anesth Analg. 2000;90:1014–9.

Pintaric TS, Potocnik I, Hadzic A, Stupnik T, Pintaric M, Novak Jankovic V. Comparison of continuous thoracic epidural with paravertebral block on perioperative analgesia and hemodynamic stability in patients having open lung surgery. Reg Anesth Pain Med. 2011;36:256–60.

Pluijms WA, Steegers MAH, Verhagen AFTM, Scheffer GJ, Wilder-Smith OHG. Chronic post-thoracotomy pain: a retrospective study. Acta Anaesthesiol Scand. 2006;50:804–8.

Polaner DM, Taenzer AH, Walker BJ, Bosenberg A, Krane EJ, Suresh S, Wolf C, Martin LD. Pediatric Regional Anesthesia Network (PRAN): a multi-institutional study of the use and incidence of complications of pediatric regional anesthesia. Anesth Analg. 2012;115:1353–64.

Ponn RB, Ferneini A, D'Agostino RS, Toole AL, Stern H. Comparison of late pulmonary function after posterolateral and muscle-sparing thoracotomy. Ann Thorac Surg. 1992;53:675–9.

Purcell N, Wu D. Novel use of the PECS II block for upper limb fistula surgery. Anaesthesia. 2014;69:1294.

Qi J, Du B, Gurnaney H, Lu P, Zuo Y. A prospective randomized observer-blinded study to assess postoperative analgesia provided by an ultrasound-guided bilateral thoracic paravertebral block for children undergoing the Nuss procedure. Reg Anesth Pain Med. 2014;39:208–13.

Rabbitts JA, Palermo TM, Zhou C, Mangione-Smith R. Pain and health-related quality of life after pediatric inpatient surgery. J Pain. 2015a;16:1334–41.

Rabbitts JA, Zhou C, Groenewald CB, Durkin L, Palermo TM. Trajectories of postsurgical pain in children: risk factors and impact of late pain recovery on long-term health outcomes after major surgery. Pain. 2015b;156:2383–9.

Richardson J, Lönnqvist PA. Thoracic paravertebral block. Br J Anaesth. 1998;81:230–8.

Richardson J, Sabanathan S, Jones J, Shah RD, Cheema S, Mearns AJ. A prospective, randomized comparison of preoperative and continuous balanced epidural or paravertebral bupivacaine on post-thoracotomy pain, pulmonary function and stress responses. Br J Anaesth. 1999;83:387–92.

Rodriguez-Aldrete D, Candiotti KA, Janakiraman R, Rodriguez-Blanco YF. Trends and New evidence in the management of acute and chronic post-thoracotomy pain-an overview of the literature from 2005 to 2015. J Cardiothorac Vasc Anesth. 2015;30:762–72.

Rozen WM, Tran TMN, Ashton MW, Barrington MJ, Ivanusic JJ, Taylor GI. Refining the course of the thoracolumbar nerves: a new understanding of the innervation of the anterior abdominal wall. Clin Anat. 2008;21:325–33.

Searle RD, Simpson MP, Simpson KH, Milton R, Bennett MI. Can chronic neuropathic pain following thoracic surgery be predicted during the postoperative period? Interact Cardiovasc Thorac Surg. 2009;9:999–1002.

Shah R, Sabanathan S, Richardson J, Mearns A, Bembridge J. Continuous paravertebral block for post thoracotomy analgesia in children. J Cardiovasc Surg (Torino). 1997;38:543–6.

Shenkman Z, Johnson VM, Zurakowski D, Arnon S, Sethna NF. Hemodynamic changes during spinal anesthesia in premature infants with congenital heart disease undergoing inguinal hernia correction. Paediatr Anaesth. 2012;22:865–70.

Shima T, Momose K, Tokutomi S, Satoh K, Hashimoto Y. Postoperative analgesic requirements after various operations. Masui. 1996;45:370–3.

Slinger P, Shennib H, Wilson S. Postthoracotomy pulmonary function: a comparison of epidural versus intravenous meperidine infusions. J Cardiothorac Vasc Anesth. 1995;9:128–34.

Steegers MAH, Snik DM, Verhagen AF, van der Drift MA, Wilder-Smith OHG. Only half of the chronic pain after thoracic surgery shows a neuropathic component. J Pain. 2008;9:955–61.

Steven JM, McGowan FX. Neuraxial blockade for pediatric cardiac surgery: lessons yet to be learned. Anesth Analg. 2000;90:1011–3.

Støving K, Rothe C, Rosenstock CV, Aasvang EK, Lundstrøm LH, Lange KHW. Cutaneous sensory block area, muscle-relaxing effect, and block duration of the transversus abdominis plane block: a randomized, blinded, and placebo-controlled study in healthy volunteers. Reg Anesth Pain Med. 2015;40:355–62.

Steffel L, Kim TE, Howard SK, Ly DP, Kou A, King R, Mariano ER. Comparative Effectiveness of Two Ultrasound-Guided Regional Block Techniques for Surgical Anesthesia in Open Unilateral Inguinal Hernia Repair. J Ultrasound Med. 2016;35(1):177–82.

Suresh S, Taylor LJ, De Oliveira GS. Dose effect of local anesthetics on analgesic outcomes for the transversus abdominis plane (TAP) block in children: a randomized, double-blinded, clinical trial. Paediatr Anaesth. 2015;25:506–10.

Tan YR, Quek KHY. Tackling the axillary blind spot with PECS II. Anaesthesia. 2015;70:230–1.

van Gulik L, Janssen LI, Ahlers SJGM, Bruins P, Driessen AHG, van Boven WJ, van Dongen EPA, Knibbe CAJ. Risk factors for chronic thoracic pain after cardiac surgery via sternotomy. Eur J Cardiothorac Surg. 2011;40:1309–13.

Weiner MM, Rosenblatt MA, Mittnacht AJC. Neuraxial anesthesia and timing of heparin administration in patients undergoing surgery for congenital heart disease using cardiopulmonary bypass. J Cardiothorac Vasc Anesth. 2012;26:581–4.

Wildgaard K, Ravn J, Kehlet H. Chronic post-thoracotomy pain: a critical review of pathogenic mechanisms and strategies for prevention. Eur J Cardiothorac Surg. 2009;36:170–80.

Wolf AR, Doyle E, Thomas E. Modifying infant stress responses to major surgery: spinal vs extradural vs opioid analgesia. Paediatr Anaesth. 1998;8:305–11.

Chapter 40
Postoperative Renal Management, Fluid/Electrolyte Management and Acid–Base Disorders

Felice Eugenio Agrò, Marialuisa Vennari, and Alessandro Centonze

Introduction

Maintaining electrolyte, acid–base and fluid balance is the final goal of any clinical treatment in the setting of cardiac surgery and in particular with the complex clinic of congenital heart diseases. In these cases, the preservation of fluid, ionic, osmolar and acid–base balance is the sum of complex clinic evaluations and actions, taking into account the kind of surgery, the alterations due to anaesthesia, the effects of cardiopulmonary bypass, patient's comorbidities and his own response to surgical stress. The complexity of clinical management is increased by the strict interconnection existing between electrolytes, acid–base system and fluid distributions: any change in one of them is responsible of modification of both the remainders. Moreover, the balance of each system is physiologically maintained through modification in the balance of the remainders. The character actor of these regulator mechanisms is the kidney: any alteration in renal function modifies the multifaceted homeostasis of the 'milieu intérieur' of the human body. The role played by kidneys is an additional problem in the clinical management of cardiac surgery patients, considering that renal impairment is one of the most frequent complications. In clinical practice, clinicians are often faced with much uncertainty that should be in part overcome through an adequate knowledge of human physiology.

F.E. Agrò, MD (✉) • M. Vennari, MD • A. Centonze, MD
Anesthesia, Intensive Care and Pain Management Department,
University School of Medicine Campus Bio-Medico of Rome,
Via A. Del Portillo 200, 00128 Rome, Italy
e-mail: f.agro@unicampus.it; m.vennari@unicampus.it; a.centonze@unicampus.it

© Springer International Publishing Switzerland 2017
A. Dabbagh et al. (eds.), *Congenital Heart Disease in Pediatric
and Adult Patients*, DOI 10.1007/978-3-319-44691-2_40

Physiology: From Birth to Adults

Fluid Balance and Distribution

In adults the total body water (TBW) represents the 60 % of the body weight. It is mainly distributed in the intracellular space (ICS = 55 % of body water) and the extracellular space (ECS = 45 %). The ECS is divided into three additional compartments:

- The intravascular space (IVS, plasma = 15 % of ECS)
- The interstitial space (ISS = 45 % of ECS)
- The transcellular space (TCS = 40 % of ECS) (Agrò and Vennari 2013) (Fig. 40.1)

The TCS is a functional compartment represented by the amount of fluid and electrolytes continually exchanged (in and out) by cells with the ISS and by the IVS with the ISS. Other fluids composing the ECS are secretions, ocular fluid and cerebrospinal fluid (Agrò and Vennari 2013).

The TBW represents about 90 % of total body weight in neonates. It decreases significantly during the first 6 months of life and reaches adult levels after 1 year of age. The ECS constitutes the main part of TBW and decreases in parallel from 40 % in term newborns to adult levels after 1 year of age (Suempelmann et al. 2013). The ECS expansion in neonates is mainly due to higher ISS fluid than adults. This becomes relevant as neonates have difficulty mobilizing fluid and electrolyte excess, potentially leading to pulmonary or peripheral oedema (Sulemanji and Vakili 2013). The composition of the ECS fluid and plasma is similar in neonates, children and adults, but dehydration occurs more rapidly in children because they need more fluids (Suempelmann et al. 2013) (Table 40.1).

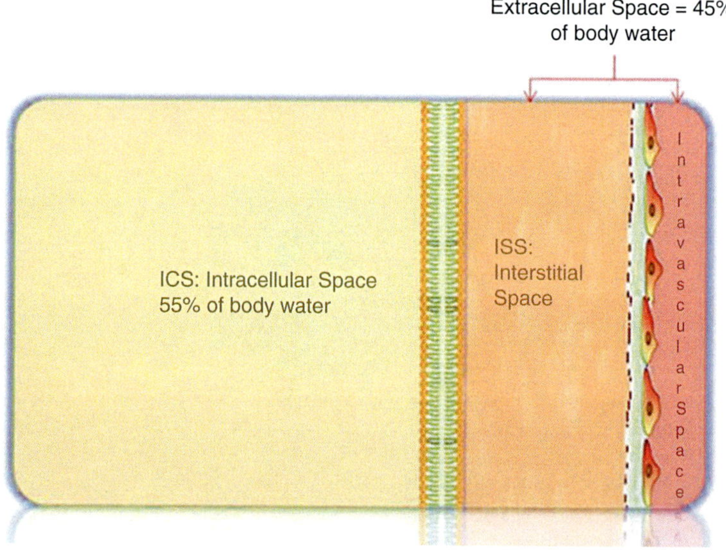

Fig. 40.1 Body water distribution (From Agrò and Vennari 2013, pp 1–26)

Soon after birth, kidneys eliminate sodium and water excess in the ECS determining a redistribution of body water and the early postnatal weight loss (a decrease in 5–10 % of body weight). The site where most of the sodium exchange is done is in the distal tube (O'Brien and Walker 2014).

Expansion of the ECS by excessive administration of sodium and water, particularly before the postnatal diuresis has occurred, has an adverse effect on outcomes, especially in extremely low birth weight infants (Bell et al. 1980; Stephens et al. 2008). A Cochrane review of randomized controlled studies comparing liberal to restricted water (and sodium) intake in preterm neonates showed a significant increase in postnatal weight gain, in the risk of patent ductus arteriosus (PDA) and necrotizing enterocolitis, with an increased incidence of bronchopulmonary dysplasia, intracranial haemorrhage and death (Bell and Acarregui 2008). A retrospective chart review of 204 premature neonates (gestational age < 32 weeks) suggested that restricted water intake in the first 3 days of life (constant calorie intake) was protective for the development of PDA, with a statistical significance observed for analysis accorded for gestational age and severity of illness (Stephens et al. 2008). A randomized controlled trial in preterm newborns (gestational age <30 weeks) showed that early sodium supplementation (4 mmol/kg/day) was associated with delayed postnatal diuresis, delayed reduction in ECS water and increased oxygen requirement at 1 month (Hartnoll et al. 2000a, b). Moreover, excessive sodium administration may result in fluid retention, oedema and hypernatraemia, even in term neonates.

The ICS water does not vary much during infancy, from 30 % at birth to 40 % in adult (Friis-Hansen 1961). In adults, insensible water losses (IWL) consist mostly of water lost via evaporation through the skin (2/3) or respiratory tract (1/3). In neonates, IWL from the skin depend on gestational age: the more preterm the infant, the greater the transepidermal water loss. This is due to a higher body surface area/weight ratio and to a thin and fragile skin, poorly keratinized, especially in preterm neonates (Modi 2005). IWL may increase using a radiant warmer or phototherapy, determining a significant effect on fluid balance. In extreme preterm infants, IWL may exceed renal water losses. Evaporation of water from the skin is associated with cooling due to the effect of the latent heat of evaporation. Difficulty in keeping a baby warm may be a sign of excessive IWL. IWL may be reduced by nursing preterm infants <2 weeks of age in a heated humidified incubator (>80 % humidity). However, if the baby is taken out of the incubator (for instance, for surgery) or if the incubator is left open for procedures, this protection will be lost. IWL decrease as preterm neo-

Table 40.1 Composition of the ECS fluid, plasma and ICS fluid

Properties	Plasma	ISS fluid	ICS fluid
Colloid osmotic pressure (mmHg)	25	4	–
Osmolality (mOsmol/kg)	280	280	280
pH	7.4	7.4	7.2
Na^+ (mmol/l)	142	143	10
K^+ (mmol/l)	4	4	155
Cl^- (mmol/l)	103	115	8
Ca^{2+} (mmol/l)	2.5	1.3	<0.001

nates mature, and ambient humidity may be gradually decreased with time. In ventilated babies, humidification reduces IWL from the lungs. It is also required for babies receiving nasal CPAP or nasal 'high flow' therapy. Postextubation, respiratory IWL may be high if a neonate receives unhumidified O_2 via nasal cannulas. IWL cannot be measured but should be estimated to allow for appropriate fluid prescription. IWL can be estimated using the following formula (Jansen et al. 2012):

$$IWL = fluid\,intake - urine\,output + weight\,loss\left(or - weight\,gain\right).$$

Fluid and Solute Movements

Fluid and electrolyte balance is both an external balance between the body and its environment and an internal balance between the ECS and ICS, and between the IVS and ISS. This balance is based on specific chemical and physical properties of body fluids, such as ionic composition, pH, protein content, osmotic pressure, osmolarity and colloid osmotic pressure, leading water and solutes to move across the compartments (Agrò and Vennari 2013). Body compartments are surrounded by a semipermeable membrane through which fluids and solutes selectively pass according to the properties of the fluids (Musso et al. 2004). Moreover, water and solute movement between the IVS and ISS is regulated by the capillary endothelium and the overlying capillary endothelial glycocalyx, which together form the endothelial glycocalyx layer (EGL). The glycocalyx consists of glycoproteins and proteoglycans containing glycosaminoglycans attached to the endoluminal surface of the capillary endothelium. It is a dynamic structure continuously degraded and resynthetized, impermeable to large molecules (>70 kDa), and probably it is the main responsible for the oncotic gradient across IVS and ISS. Albumin is contained within the EGL, and normal plasma albumin levels are required to assure EGL functions (Young 2012). Furthermore, glycocalyx prevents the endothelial adhesion of inflammatory cells, reducing the risks of an increased endothelial permeability. A glycocalyx damage leads larger molecules to pass from the IVS into the ISS, reducing the IVS–ISS oncotic gradient and increasing the ISS volume with tissue oedema. Various conditions associated to cardiac surgery may potentially destroy glycocalyx: hemodilution, ischaemia and reperfusion damage and inflammation (Young 2012).

Electrolyte Balance

Ionic balance is based on the principle of the 'electric neutrality': the sum of cations must be the same of the sum of anions. In other words, the net sum of the electric charge in the body fluids is zero. Ionic composition of ICS and ECS is

Fig. 40.2 Gamble gram. Electric neutrality principle: the sum of plasmatic cations is equivalent to the sum of plasmatic anions (Modified from Agrò et al. 2014)

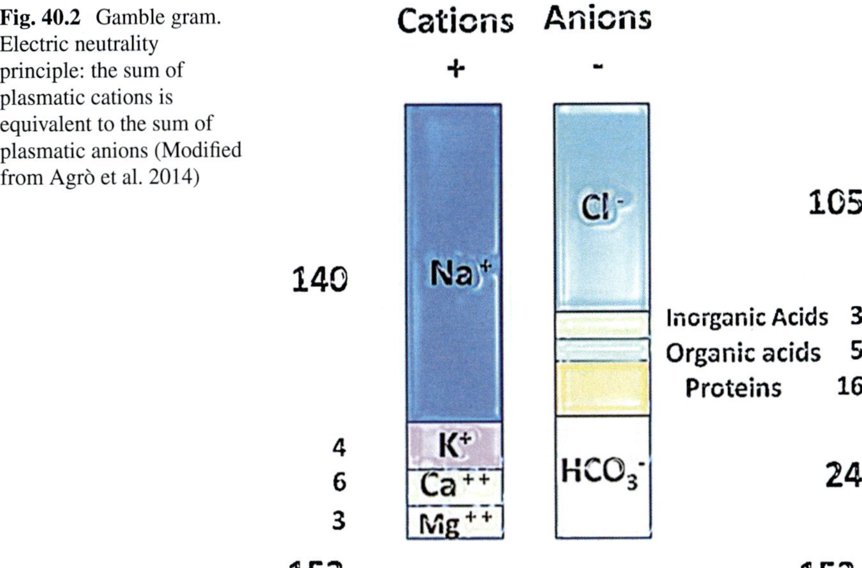

different, and further differences exist in the ECS between the IVS and the ISS (Table 40.1). In clinical practice, the only value directly measurable is the plasmatic concentration of each ion. Generally, this value is considered as a reference to evaluate the presence of electrolyte alterations. The relationship between the ionic plasmatic composition and the neutrality principle is expressed by Gamble gram (Fig. 40.2). Examining the Gamble gram is immediately evident that the sum of cations ($Na^+ + K^+ + Ca^{++} + Mg^{++}$ + others) is 154 mEq/L and is the same of anions (Cl^- + bicarbonate + proteins + phosphates + sulphates + organic acids). Na^+ and K^+ represent the 94 % of all IVS cations, while Cl^- and bicarbonate represent the 84 % of all anions. Na^+, K^+, Ca^{++} and Mg^{++} are electrolytes generally measured through laboratory exams, while bicarbonate is only calculated using Henderson–Hasselbalch equation when arterial blood sample is performed (Gamble 1947).

Sodium

Sodium is the most highly represented cation in the ECS and it has a key hemodynamic role: it is the main determinant of ECS volume, contributes to renin–angiotensin–aldosterone system (RAAS) activation and regulates ADH secretion. Sodium concentration determines body fluid osmolarity. Changes in sodium plasma level are responsible for modification in fluid movement across the body space, determining ICS and ECS volume variation. The normal sodium concentration in plasma and the ISS is about 142 mEq/L, and it is higher than the ICS concentration (10 mEq/L)

(Agrò and Vennari 2013). Neonates are susceptible to sodium disorders, and both sodium content and water amount administered through IV fluids should be considered carefully. Aldosterone secretion is slow to be reduced in the face of a sodium load, for instance, from isotonic fluid boluses, intravenous flushes and drugs, and may result in hypernatraemia or sodium retention with oedema formation. It is recommended that neonates are given sodium-free fluids until after the postnatal diuresis to allow for contraction of the ECS volume (O'Brien and Walker 2014), but inadequate sodium intake thereafter will result in hyponatraemia (Hartnoll et al. 2000a, b). This is particularly important in preterm neonates as the renin–angiotensin–aldosterone system (RAAS) is less active, causing a limited ability to retain sodium in the distal renal tubule. Inadequate sodium intake is associated with severe hyponatraemia and poor long-term neurological outcomes in preterm neonates (Baraton et al. 2009).

Potassium

Potassium is the main cation of the ICS. It plays a central role in determining the resting cell membrane potential, especially for excitable cells such as myocytes. Therefore, it influences the transmission of impulses along the cardiac pacemakers (potentially predisposing to arrhythmias) and the contraction of myocardial cells. It is also involved in a variety of metabolic processes, including energy production and the synthesis of nucleic acids and proteins (Agrò and Vennari 2013). The kidney plays an important role in maintaining potassium balance in the body. Potassium is freely filtered by the glomerulus and reabsorption occurs in the proximal tubules. There is some reabsorption in the ascending loop, but the final urinary concentration is determined by the secretion in the distal tubule. In premature neonates, hyperkalaemia is usually evident due the immaturity of the distal tubules. The peritubular and luminal permeability to potassium may also contribute to the physiologic positive balance. A major determinant of potassium balance is cellular metabolism. There is a shift of potassium from the ISS to the ECS immediately after the birth in preterm infants (Lorenz et al. 1997). Once the kidney adapts to the extrauterine environment, the increased diuresis facilitates potassium excretion and the regulation of serum potassium levels.

Calcium

Calcium balance in the body is maintained by a well-coordinated mechanism between the gastrointestinal tract, bone and kidneys. The kidneys regulate calcium reabsorption throughout the nephron via various active and passive processes. Calcium is involved in endocrine, exocrine and neurocrine secretion, coagulation activation, muscle contraction (it has a great inotropic effect), potential membrane depolarization, cell growth and enzymatic regulation and in the metabolism of other electrolytes (especially potassium and magnesium). Calcium may circulate in the plasma bound to albumin and free from proteins. Free calcium may be ionized (physiologically active) or nonionized (chelated with inorganic anions such as sulphate, citrate and phosphate). The amounts of the three forms are altered by many factors, such as pH, plasma protein levels (hypoalbuminaemia reduces total calcium, but not free fraction) and percentage of anions associated with ionized calcium (blood products contain citrate) (Agrò and Vennari 2013). Although there is a strong correlation between serum total calcium levels and serum-ionized calcium, total calcium can be a poor predictor of calcium status especially in neonates. Low levels of calcium are common in premature infants, but seldom results in tetany or decreased cardiac contractility (Venkataraman et al. 1985). Calcium levels tend to stabilize and reach childhood levels by the first week of life (Sulemanji and Vakili 2013).

Phosphorus

Phosphorus is similarly and concordantly regulated with calcium. It has an important role in bone structure and various metabolic processes. The normal plasma phosphorus level is maintained through a balance between intestinal absorption versus renal excretion. Renal excretion is the primary mechanism by which phosphorus is regulated in the body. Parathyroid hormone (PTH) is the most potent hormone that controls urinary excretion of phosphorus. Elevation in phosphorus levels induce the secretion of PTH, which in turn leads to the secretion of phosphorus via the kidneys. Excess phosphorus develops a complex with calcium resulting in a decrease in the production of calcitriol, thereby reducing calcium absorption in the gut (Agrò and Vennari 2013).

Magnesium

Magnesium is the physiological antagonist of calcium. It plays a crucial role in neuromuscular stimulation and modulation of excitable cell activity (membrane-stabilizing activity); it also acts as a cofactor of several enzymes involved in the metabolism of three major categories of nutrients: carbohydrates, lipids and proteins (Agrò and Vennari 2013).

Chloride

Chloride is the most important anion of the ECS. Together with sodium, it determines the ECS volume, and it plays a crucial role in acid–base balance (SID approach). It is also responsible for the resting potential of the membrane and action potential, and plasma osmotic pressure (Agrò and Vennari 2013).

Bicarbonate

Bicarbonate is the main buffer system of the blood. It plays a critical role in maintaining acid–base balance. Two-thirds of the CO_2 in the human body is metabolized as bicarbonate, through the action of carbonic anhydrase. The equilibrium between CO_2 and bicarbonate leads to the elimination of volatile acid. The bicarbonate buffer system is described by the following equilibrium reaction:

$$CO_2 + H_2O \leftrightarrow H_2CO_3 \leftrightarrow HCO_3^- + H^+$$

When there is an increased concentration of H^+, the system reacts by shifting the reaction equilibrium to the left (towards the production of CO_2); while when the concentration of H^+ is reduced, the system moves to the right, resulting in the production of H^+. The bicarbonate buffer system works 'in concert' with several organs. Bicarbonate has a normal plasma concentration of about 24 mmol/L (Agrò and Vennari 2013).

Acid–Base Balance

The acid–base balance is regulated by a combination of the respiratory, buffer and renal systems. The buffer system constitutes the bicarbonate–carbonic acid buffer, haemoglobin–oxyhaemoglobin buffer, protein buffer and the phosphorus buffer mechanisms. The buffer systems are adapted to serve as the primary mechanism for maintaining acid–base balance in the newborns (Sulemanji and Vakili 2013). With low serum bicarbonate levels and ongoing physiologic demands, the premature infants have a tendency to acidosis. It is known that administration of bicarbonate gives little benefit in comparison of risks, including intraventricular haemorrhage, deteriorating cardiac function and the worsening of intracellular acidosis (Aschner and Poland 2008). However, if strictly needed, bicarbonate should be administered at a very slow rate in order to minimize fluctuations in cerebral hemodynamics (Berg et al. 2010). Term neonates, with the exception of those having congenital complications, usually have a stable physiologic transition from foetal life to extra-uterine surrounding. Cardiovascular, respiratory and cerebral hemodynamic mechanisms are in equilibrium with each other and generally result in a balanced acid–base homeostasis. The acid–base balance is maintained closely by complex interactions between the respiratory system and the kidneys. The acceptable values in term infants compared to preterm infants (o28 weeks) are as follows: pH > 7.30 (>7.28), $PaCO_2$ 40–50 (40–50), bicarbonate (HCO_3) 20–24 (18–24) and PaO_2 50–70 (50–65). The respiratory effort in the term infants is almost always stable with marginal predisposition to respiratory acidosis. At the same time, the buffer systems and tubular handling of the term infant kidney are also mature to handle any non-respiratory-induced acidosis within 72 h following birth (Malan et al.

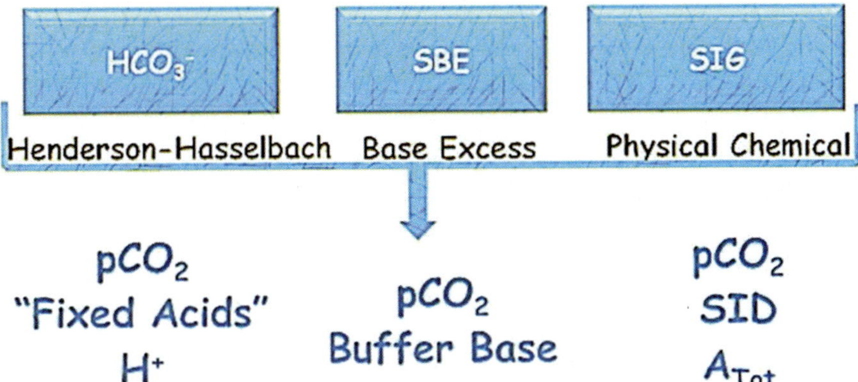

Fig. 40.3 The three possible approaches to acid–base balance system description. Some factors (i.e. pCO₂) are considered by all the approaches (Modified from Agrò and Vennari 2013, pp 1–26)

1965). Classically, there have been three different clinical approaches to acid–base physiology and management:

- The descriptive approach
- The semi-quantitative approach
- The quantitative approach

The first is mainly founded on Henderson–Hasselbalch equation, the second on base excess (BE) and the third on strong ion difference (SID) (Fig. 40.3). They use distinct variables derived from a set of master equations that can be transferred from one approach to the other two (Agrò and Vennari 2013; Kellum 2005):

- $\mathrm{pH} = \mathrm{pKa} + \log\left(\left[\mathrm{HCO_3^-}\right] / \left[\mathrm{pCO_2}\right]\right)$

- $\mathrm{BE} = \left(\mathrm{HCO_3^-} - 24.4 + \left[2.3 \times \mathrm{Hb} + 7.7\right] \times \left[\mathrm{pH} - 7.4\right]\right) \times \left(1 - 0.023 \times \mathrm{Hb}\right)$

- $\mathrm{pH} = \mathrm{pK1} + \log\left\{\mathrm{SID^+} - \left[\mathrm{ATOT} / \left(1 + 10\mathrm{p}^{\mathrm{Ka-pH}}\right)\right]\right\} / \mathrm{pCO_2}$

Renal Physiology

Renal function is related to the maturation and size of the nephrons, which have the ability to filter the blood and to collect the filtrate. At birth, the kidneys are still undeveloped with reduced ability in reabsorption. Thus, newborns cannot concentrate urine as effectively as adults, and they are unable to excrete large salt loads. After 1 month, the kidneys reach about 60 % of their maturation, but the reabsorptive capacity remains lower than in adults. In the first 2 years, the maturity and function of the kidneys increase greatly and reach adult levels (Suempelmann et al. 2013; Bissonnette Bruno 2011).

Renal Blood Flow

Renal blood flow (RBF) changes throughout the years from newborns to adults. It is influenced by the ratio of renal/systemic vascular resistance and the cardiac output (CO). RBF is only about 3–7 % of the CO in the foetus (Rudolph and Heymann 1968). After the birth, it is improved consequentially to a reduction in renal vascular resistances and an increase in CO. In the first week of life, RBF is only the 10 % of CO. In the neonate, the relation between RBF and kidney weight, body weight and surface area is lower than the adult (Sulemanji and Vakili 2013). From childhood to adults, a combination of increased renal perfusion pressure and decreased renal vascular resistance leads to an improvement of RBF up to 25 % of CO (Musso et al. 2004). The clearance of p-aminohippurate has traditionally been used to measure the effective renal plasma flow (ERPF). The ERPF has been reported as:

- <20 mL/min/1.73 m^2 in the premature infant
- 45 mL/min/1.73 m^2 by 35 weeks of gestation
- 83 mL/min/1.73 m^2 in term infants (Musso et al. 2004)

It progressively increases to reach 300 mL/min/1.73 m^2 by toddler age and finally reaches adult rate of 650 mL/min/1.73 m^2 by 2 years of age. This increase is associated with a proportionally higher flow to the outer cortical region. At any age, ERPF may be modified by renal flow autoregulation. However, autoregulation is less efficient in infants, especially at lower baseline values as in newborns (Musso et al. 2004).

Glomerular Filtration Rate

The determinants of glomerular filtration rate (GFR) are:

- Starling forces across the capillary wall
- Permeability of the glomerular wall
- Total surface area of the capillaries
- RBF (Fig. 40.4)

GFR is established during intrauterine life, but it is insignificant because the kidneys do not primarily function as a water- and fluid-regulating organ. After birth it significantly increases, as the kidney assumes its role in fluid, water and electrolyte balances (Yared 2004). In the newborn, GFR is about 40 mL/min/1.73 m^2 and it reaches 66 mL/min/1.73 m^2 by 2 weeks of age. Adult levels of 100–125 mL/min/1.73 m^2 are reached at around 2 years of age (Schwartz et al. 1987). In addition, maximal urine concentration capacity of the term infants (700 mOsm) does not reach adult levels (1400 mOsm) until 6–12 months of age (Rudolph and Heymann 1968). In very low birth weight (VLBW) infants, the increase in GFR is generally reduced than normal weight infants, reaching normal levels later in childhood. Neonates, especially premature, have a limited ability to handle fluid loads:

$$P_f = P_c - (P_B + \pi_p)$$

$$P_f = 60 - (18 + 32) = 10 \text{ mmHg}$$

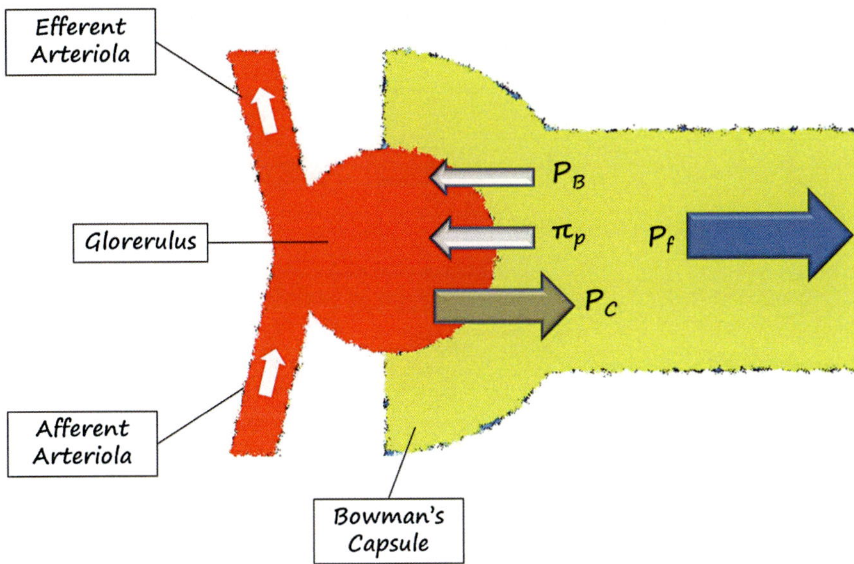

Fig. 40.4 Determinant of glomerular filtration. *Pf* filtration pressure, *Pc* hydrostatic pressure in the capillary (glomerulus), *πp* colloid osmotic pressure in Bowman's capsule, *PB* hydrostatic pressure in Bowman's capsule

variations in GFR are clinically relevant because they affect fluid and electrolyte homeostasis as well as excretion of drugs (Iacobelli et al. 2007).

A variety of mechanisms are involved in GFR regulation. First of all, macula densa cells of the tubuloglomerular system regulate GFR according to the rate of distal tubular flow and the chloride concentration of the tubular fluid: a high chloride concentration is interpreted as an elevated GFR, while a low chloride concentration as a low GFR. Macula densa cells regulate the afferent arteriole and glomerular capillary tone leading to an adjustment in the GFR (Koeppen and Stanton 2004) (Fig. 40.5). The myogenic reflex regulates GFR based on renal perfusion pressure. Decreased perfusion pressure leads to a dilation of the afferent arteriole and vasoconstriction of the efferent arteriole (Koeppen and Stanton 2004) (Fig. 40.5).

Renal perfusion pressure is firstly compromised in many clinical settings such as cardiac dysfunction, hypovolaemia or septic shock. In any case (normal, reduced or increased intravascular volume), GFR is maintained by an increase in the filtration fraction in the context of diminished CO and RBF. The myogenic reflex is initially adequate, but as cardiac function continues to deteriorate, it no longer can maintain

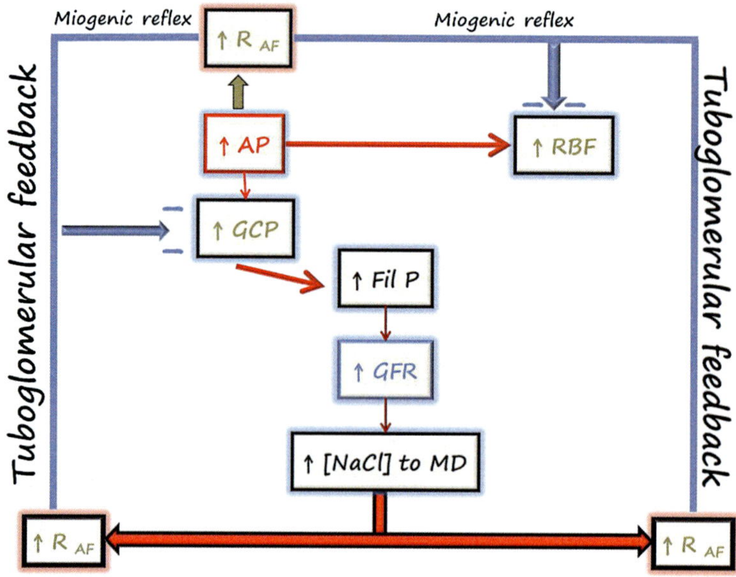

Fig. 40.5 The tubuloglomerular system and the myogenic reflex

an acceptable GFR. As a consequence, GFR decreases secondary to diminished renal perfusion leading to accumulation of water and solutes via multiple sodium-retaining systems. Water- and salt-retaining mechanisms are used by kidneys to restore CO and arterial pressure. Depending on the nature and degree of CO reduction, the retention may lead to a vicious cycle of worsening oedema and congestion. However, a drastic RBF decrease may overwhelm the kidney's ability to autoregulate, resulting in a dramatic GFR diminution. When a mild to moderate reduction of renal perfusion develops, GFR may be maintained via various mechanisms that act on the afferent (vasodilator prostaglandins) and efferent (angiotensin II) arteriolar systems. However, any aggravation of this system by exogenous factors (ACE inhibitors and/or NSAIDs) may produce an important fall in the GFR (Ricci et al. 2011a).

The renin–angiotensin–aldosterone system (RAAS) is activated by secretion of norepinephrine in the peripheral vessels. The RAAS action determines intrarenal vasoconstriction and subsequently diminished RBF with increased sodium retention (DiBona and Sawin 1991, 1995; DiBona and Kopp 1997) (Fig. 40.6). The RAAS is responsible for regulating blood pressure, RBF, fluid and electrolyte balance. Renin is the key component of the system. It is produced in the kidney by the juxtaglomerular cells. The mechanism controlling release of renin is well established by late gestation. Hypotension, haemorrhage, furosemide, ACE inhibitors, prostaglandins, vasopressin and atrial natriuretic peptide are all known factors that influence renin secretion. Renin triggers the formation of angiotensin I (ATI) which subsequently gets converted to angiotensin II (ATII) by angiotensin-converting enzyme (ACE). ATII, through plasma membrane receptors ATI and ATII, increases systemic blood pressure determining a vasoconstriction of small vessels with an increase in

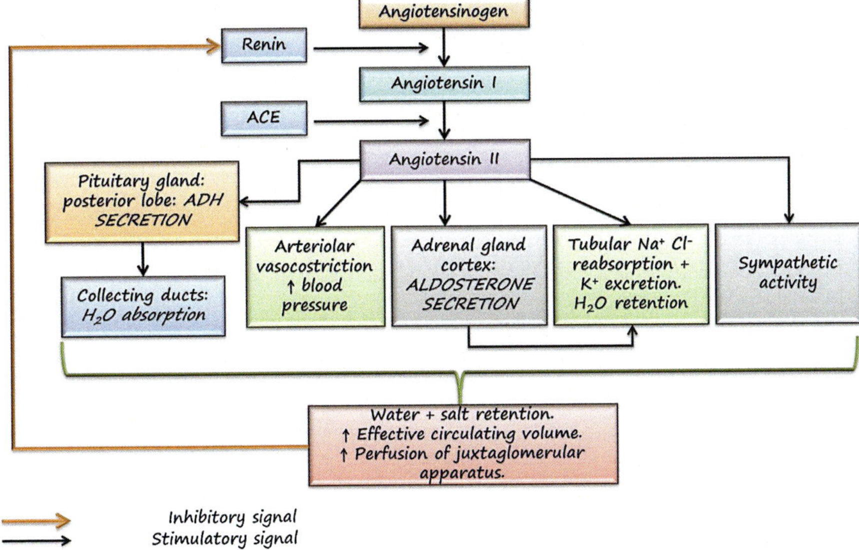

Fig. 40.6 Renin–angiotensin–aldosterone system: hypovolaemia reduces perfusion of juxtaglomerular apparatus, with renin release. Circulating renin converts angiotensinogen to angiotensin I, subsequently angiotensin-converting enzyme (ACE) acts on angiotensin I converting it to angiotensin II. This hormone increases NSS activity, increases reabsorption of Na and water by kidneys directly and through aldosterone action and determines vasoconstriction and ADH secretion (Modified from Agrò and Vennari 2013, pp 71–92)

peripheral resistances. Furthermore, ATII can increase CO through increasing myocardial contractility (Sulemanji and Vakili 2013). ATII has an autocrine effect: it is the primary vasoconstrictor of the renal vessels, modulating reabsorption of sodium and water by kidneys (Kobori et al. 2007). ATII renal action is greatest on the efferent arteriole than afferent, leading to an increase in the filtration fraction with retention of water and sodium (Ichikawa et al. 1984). Moreover, the release of ATII leads to the production and secretion of aldosterone by the zona glomerulosa of the adrenal gland. Aldosterone acts on the mineral corticoid receptors of the kidney, heart, brain, colon and vessel walls. Aldosterone effect on kidney determines sodium retention, which eventually leads to retention of water (Garty 1992).

Components of RAAS are present during early gestation, but their activity and function are somewhat different than adults. RAAS is active in the kidney prior of foetal urine production. This may suggest a role in regulating growth and development of the nephron. At birth, plasma renin activity is increased and continues to stay elevated through infancy. It begins to decline to adult levels by 6–9 years of age (Stalker et al. 1967). Both ATI and ATII receptor expression increase exponentially after birth (Tufro-McReddie et al. 1993), contributing to vasoconstriction of the neonatal kidney. Likewise, there is augmented production of renin, AT and ACE in the postnatal kidney. These effects are counteracted by the postnatal increase in prostaglandins, nitric oxide and kinins which promote vasodilatation and contribute to the maturational increase in RBF (Carey et al. 2000). When CO is reduced, prolonged sodium retention persists with subsequent accumulation of extracellular water. Moreover, a clinical study showed a severe reduction of GFR in young rats VS a mild reduction in adults, when renal perfusion pressure is decreased by 30% (Yared and Yoshioka 1988). Micropuncture experiments revealed that the young rats had decreased glomerular capillary pressure due to incompetence of the ATII-mediated vasoconstriction effects: the young rats may not be able to activate ATII, and the immature efferent arteriole may not respond to ATII the same way as in adults. This is not due to receptor and angiotensin availability but instead to immature post-receptor processes (Yared and Yoshioka 1988).

Aldosterone is one component through which angiotensin regulates sodium reabsorption, influencing fluid and electrolyte balance. The foetal response to secrete aldosterone is less than that seen in adults due to the relative insensitivity of the adrenal gland (Robillard et al. 1982). It is well known that infants with poor cardiac function secondary to congenital heart disease are at risk for acute kidney injury. Mechanoreceptors in the aortic arch, left ventricle and renal afferent arterioles sense systemic arterial pressure and regulate IVS volume. Arterial underfilling activates the sympathetic nervous system with an increase in myocardial contractility, heart rate and peripheral and renal vasoconstriction. Stimulation of the RAAS also contributes to systemic vasoconstriction as well as vasoconstriction of the efferent and afferent arterioles mediated by AT II. Sympathetic stimulation and ATII increase sodium transport in the proximal tubule and deliver less sodium to the distal tubule. This leads to persistent aldosterone-mediated sodium retention in the collecting duct (Fig. 40.7). Moreover RAAS activation can have deleterious effects on the heart. In fact, aldosterone increases myocardial collagen deposition, fibrosis, inflammation and remodelling of the heart and blood vessels (Schrier et al. 2010). ATII additionally contributes to left ventricular hypertrophy as well as remodelling (Booz and Baker 1996).

The antidiuretic hormone (ADH) is secreted from the posterior pituitary in response to severe arterial underfilling leading to osmolarity modification. Stimulation of ADH receptors leads to the expression of aquaporin-2 water channels on the apical surface of the collecting duct, resulting in an increase of water reabsorption restoring osmolarity and volume of IVS (Fig. 40.7). The persistent activation of these adaptive mechanisms leads to fluid overload, worsening heart failure and decreased renal perfusion (Funayama et al. 2004; Pedersen et al. 2003).

The atrial natriuretic peptide (ANP) increases GFR by constriction of efferent arteriole and dilatation of the afferent arteriole (Marin-Grez et al. 1986). ANP also acts on sympathetic renal effect: it may reverse sympathetic-induced afferent vasoconstriction and potentiate efferent arteriolar vasoconstriction. These effects may suggest a role of ANP in maintaining GFR in heart failure patients, in which ANP values are elevated and renal perfusion pressure is reduced. In addition, ANP counteracts the effects of ATII on the proximal tubule in regard to sodium and water retention: it promotes natriuresis by inhibiting tubular sodium reabsorption (Harris et al. 1987). Moreover, ANP inhibits renin secretion and reduces aldosterone secretion by the zona glomerulosa of the adrenal cortex. It also counteracts maladaptive cardiac hypertrophy and remodelling mechanisms.

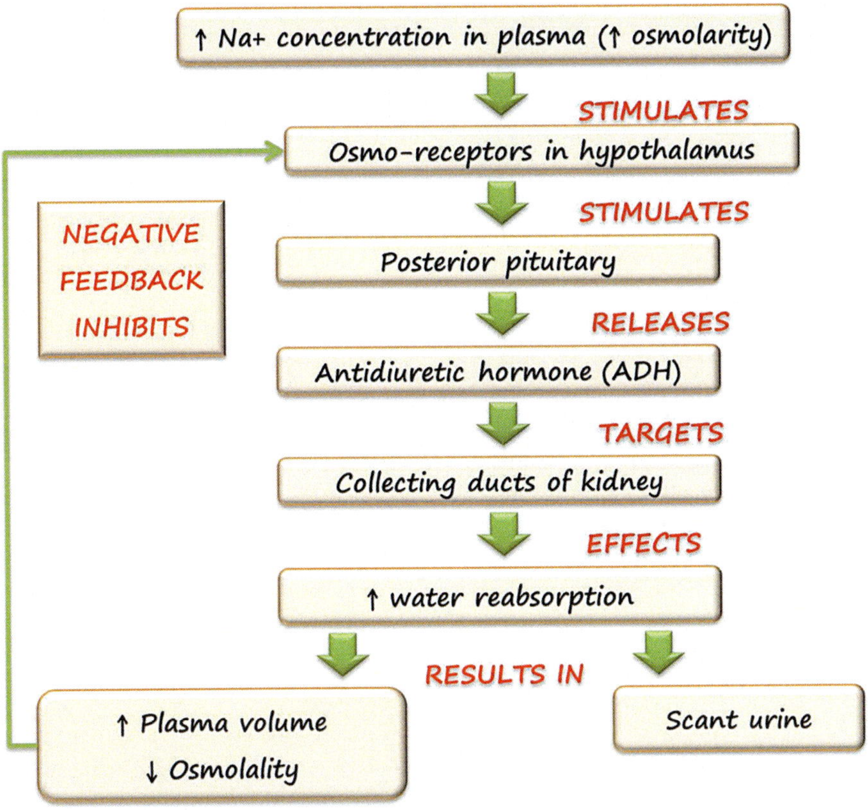

Fig. 40.7 Mechanism of ADH secretion: when fluid volume decreases, plasma sodium concentration and plasmatic osmolarity increases, leading to hypothalamic osmoreceptor stimulation. The hypothalamus will then stimulate the posterior pituitary gland that releases antidiuretic hormone. ADH will make renal distal tubules able to reabsorb water into the IVS in order to maintain homeostasis of fluid balance. ADH secretion is more sensible to plasmatic osmolarity than circulating blood (Modified from Agrò and Vennari 2013, pp 71–92)

The brain natriuretic peptide (BNP) is produced mostly in the ventricular myocardium and has similar action respect with ANP. ANP and BNP react to the effects of the RAAS and sympathetic activation seen in acute cardiac dysfunction. Studies have shown that BNP secretion increase after a left ventricular dysfunction (Wei et al. 1993). BNP's effect is similar to those of ANP.

Prostaglandins are potent renal vasodilators produced by arachidonic acid in many cells throughout the body. The major action of prostaglandins is to modulate the actions of vasoconstrictors.

Nitric oxide is an endothelium-derived gas synthesized from the amino acid L-arginine by nitric oxide synthase. It diffuses across the endothelial membrane and enters vascular smooth muscle cells, inducing vasodilatation. In the kidneys, the afferent arteriole is more sensitive than the efferent arteriole to the vasodilator effects of NO. The main action of NO is to modulate the action of angiotensin.

Urine Concentration and Sodium Excretion Fraction

The ability to maintain a negative water and sodium balance through a high sodium excretion is inversely proportional to the infant's maturity. As a result, this process results in a greater loss and lasts longer in premature infants.

After the postnatal diuresis, the neonate grows rapidly. Renal function is ideally adapted to cope with a liquid (milk) diet with relatively low sodium content. Sodium is required for growth and is retained avidly in the distal tubules under the influence of the renin–angiotensin–aldosterone system (RAAS). Although the kidney has a full complement of nephrons from around 35 weeks' gestation, the renal tubules are short, and there is limited ability to concentrate the urine (Haycock 2005). High volumes of dilute urine are therefore produced (urinary osmolarity 300 mOsmol*kg^{-1}) at a rate of around 2–3 mL*kg^{-1}*h^{-1} (45–50 mL*kg^{-1}*day^{-1}). Neonates are also able to produce more dilute urine in the face of a high water load (provided ADH levels are not elevated), but they have limited ability to concentrate the urine and so become dehydrated easily (Bell and Acarregui 2008). Growth of the kidney is associated with increasing complexity and length of the renal tubules and increasing ability to concentrate the urine, so that by a year of age, infants are able to vary the concentration of urine between 50 and 1400 mOsmol/kg, as in adults (Haycock 2005).

Fractional excretion of sodium (FE Na) is highest during the first 10 days of life and decreases to below 0.4 % by 1 month of age which is comparable to adults. FE Na may increase secondary to hypoxia, respiratory distress, hyperbilirubinaemia, increased fluid or salt intake and diuretic administration (Jose et al. 1994). The major regulators of FE Na are the renin–angiotensin–aldosterone system, atrial natriuretic peptides, prostaglandins and catecholamines (Nafday 2005). It is the balance between these factors that compensates for the immaturity of the nephron in order to maintain systemic homeostasis.

Acute Kidney Injury After Congenital Heart Disease Surgery

Congenital heart disease surgery is one of the most common causes of renal failure. In fact, adult and paediatric cardiac surgery is complicated in 30–40 % of cases by acute kidney injury (AKI), and it is associated with adverse outcomes, including diminished quality of life, prolonged intensive care and hospital stays and increased long-term mortality, particularly in patients who require dialysis. Furthermore, even minor degrees of postoperative AKI caused a significant increase in mortality and morbidity.

Epidemiology of AKI

The incidence of AKI after cardiac surgery in both paediatric and adult patients may be widely variable because of the shortage of standardized definitions. It has been shown that AKI has an incidence of 7.2–48 % with a mortality of 14–80 % (Kuitunen et al.

2006) in adult postoperative cardiac patients, depending on the definition used and the population analysed. Moreover, AKI is the strongest independent risk factor for mortality (Lassnigg et al. 2004), following adult cardiac surgery. In paediatric patients, the incidence of AKI after congenital heart surgery varies in a wide range between 3 and 61 % with mortality from 20 to 79 % (Picca et al. 1995; Aydin et al. 2012). Price et al. (Price et al. 2008) linked a worsening in renal function (increase in Scr>0.3 mg/dL) with acute decompensate heart failure. They found an incidence of worsening renal function in 48 % of patient with acute decompensated heart failure, and it was related with in-hospital death or requirement for mechanical circulatory support.

Aetiology and Pathogenesis of AKI Post-Cardiac Surgery

A lot of factors are essential in the development of AKI after cardiac surgery. In fact, the pathogenesis is related to the complex interaction between tubular, vascular and inflammatory factors. It is well known as, both in child and adult patients, AKI after cardiac surgery mainly caused by acute tubular necrosis (ATN). Microscopically, ischaemia (e.g. as a result of CPB, low cardiac output, circulatory arrest) produces an ATP depletion that activates oxidative and cell death mechanism, with a loss of brush borders and disruption of cell polarity and cytoskeleton. These lead to cell apoptosis and, gradually, to a desquamation of tubule cells into the lumen, causing a cast obstruction. Moreover, the ischemic insult modifies the renal blood flow, causing hypoperfusion of the outer medulla. In this manner, the microvasculature becomes both a 'source of' and a 'target for' the inflammatory injury present in the ischemic kidney (Devarajan 2006). Injured endothelia and tubule cells are part of an inflammatory response which involve the systemic inflammatory response syndrome (SIRS) existing during and after CPB. Furthermore, these events may be exacerbating during reperfusion (see later). It is important to consider that, according to a low mean arterial pressure and high renovascular resistance, normal infants have a lower GFR, making the infant kidney weaker in than adult patients. Several factors may contribute to the failure of this mechanism in congenital heart disease paediatric patients than adults. Hypoxaemia, resulting from preoperative cyanosis or postoperative pulmonary impairment, reduces RBF and GFR, inducing hypotension, hypervolaemia and activation of the RAAS.

Frequently, patients need intubation and mechanical ventilation both in pre- and postoperative phase. Positive pressure ventilation impairs renal function because of it decreases the venous return and consequently the cardiac output, with an increase in renal sympathetic nervous activity and serum vasopressin levels.

Hypothermia, induced in operation theatre, causes renal vasoconstriction and a decrease in GFR.

As previously described, the angiotensin II activity plays a central role in the maintenance of GFR, because of causing vasoconstriction of post-glomerular, efferent arteriole. Prostaglandin synthase inhibitors, such as indomethacin, used in patient with patent ductus arteriosus, may blunt the vasodilatation of afferent arterioles needed to maintain adequate perfusion of the newborn kidney. Moreover,

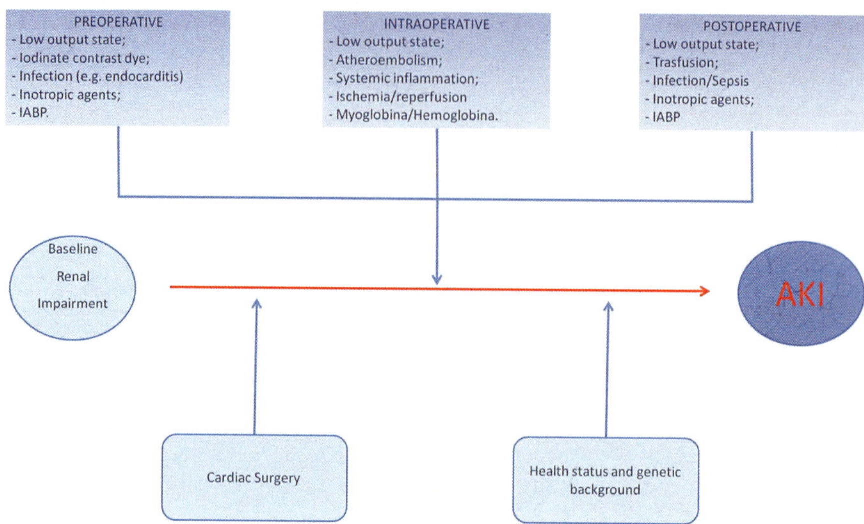

Fig. 40.8 Main risk factors of post-cardiac surgery AKI

compared with adults, paediatric patients are more sensitive to the use of inhibitors of ACE inhibitors. The use of nephrotoxic drug or contrast in pre- and postoperative phase may induce directly tubular injury (Picca et al. 2008).

Postoperatively, sepsis may contribute to renal damage, because it induces an inflammatory response that leads to a production of vasoactive mediators that may worsen GFR and precipitate a heart failure.

All these mechanisms contribute to cell death, resulting in necrosis and/or apoptosis and even in patient death. A recent case–control study has been conducted to identify independent risk factors for AKI and dialysis. Among them are preoperative use of mechanical ventilation, milrinone, or gentamicin, intraoperative milrinone or furosemide, duration of anaesthesia, multiple cross clamps and transfusion of blood products (Chiravuri et al. 2011). As mentioned before, a lot of studies show that preoperative state of the congenital heart disease patient may also influence the development and the prognosis of AKI. Preoperative conditions favouring AKI are central venous hypertension, systolic arterial hypotension, pump failure or low cardiac output syndrome, use of inotropic and vasopressor drugs, high-risk complex operation, cyanotic cardiac disease and circulatory arrest (Pedersen 2012). Several of the risk factors are mutually related to each other, and identification of independent risk factors is dependent on the specific variables (Fig. 40.8). One of most important factors that may affect renal function, however, remains CPB.

CPB and Ultrafiltration

Historically, CPB was associated with a multiorgan dysfunction that may result in increase in morbidity and mortality in patients who underwent cardiac surgery, particularly in the smallest neonates after repair of complex congenital heart defects.

This is due to hemodilution and hypothermia, often in association with tissue ischaemia. Moreover, CPB may increase TBW, which participate to organ dysfunction and tissue oedema. Nowadays, improvements in the technology of CPB and use of ultrafiltration have significantly reduced morbidity after cardiac surgery.

Physiopathology

It is well known that patients undergoing cardiac surgery without CPB have preserved renal function and a milder systemic inflammatory response as compared to those requiring CPB (Ascione et al. 1999). This evidence is particularly strong in younger patients (especially neonates), as a result of their small body surface area. Two are the underlying causes of renal impairment: the hemodynamic changes during CPB and the activation of immune response. First, there is an association between CPB duration and the risk of AKI in infants (Picca et al. 1995). The non-pulsatile flow modifies the arterial resistance, with subsequent alteration in organ perfusion. This suboptimal perfusion may not compensate kidney oxygen consumption, resulting in ischaemia and initial organ damage. Reperfusion may worsen ischaemia, inducing cell death and inflammation, resulting in tissue damage and eventually organ dysfunction. Moreover, ischaemia and alteration in blood flow activate the RAAS, leading to fluid accumulation and initial fluid retention. The mechanic and ischemic insult produced by CPB cause also a systemic inflammatory response. First of all, blood components are exposed to the foreign surface of the CPB circuit. Per se, this can cause an inflammatory response (Abu-Omar and Ratnatunga 2006; Asimakopoulos 2001). In fact, an activation of the complement system and a secretion of various proinflammatory cytokines such as IL-8, IL-10 and TNF-α have been found in patients who underwent CPB (Abu-Omar and Ratnatunga 2006; Asimakopoulos 2001). Furthermore, the production of proinflammatory mediators is stimulated by renal ischaemia. Particularly, the activation of the complement system plays a central role: it may cause a direct injury to the renal tubular epithelial cells and may promote secretion of cytokines, which worsen the epithelial damage. The oxygen-free radicals released from the ischemic tissue may contribute to end-organ damage. Finally, CPB increases the activation of neutrophils, monocytes and endothelial cells which have also been implicated in the development of kidney injury.

Ultrafiltration

One of the most important findings after CPB is a fluid overload (FO), which typically is more prominent in neonates (Berdat et al. 2004). Haemodilution, as a result of the large circuit priming volumes, may be associated with vital organ dysfunction and tissue oedema (Apostolakis et al. 2010). Moreover, a large volume and blood component shifts have been demonstrated in patients with congenital heart disease undergoing surgery with CPB, due to the inflammatory response and the production of vasoactive mediators that increase capillary permeability (Rosner and Okusa

2006). Miniaturization of CPB circuit (Merkle et al. 2004) and the use of intraoperative ultrafiltration are improvements that could have a significant impact on the prevention of AKI during CPB. Ultrafiltration (also known as haemoconcentration) is a variety of membrane filtrations in which water and low molecular weight solutes are removed from plasma, throughout a semipermeable membrane, by a transmembrane pressure gradient (a process known as solvent drag), so that the composition of the ultrafiltrate is related to the pore size of the haemofilter. The first application of ultrafiltration for the CPB was during rewarming, the so-called conventional ultrafiltration (CUF). With this technique, the ultrafilter (UF) of the perfusate is performed, while the patient is still being assisted by the lung–heart machine and the haemoconcentrator is connected to the recirculation line between the oxygenator and the venous reservoir. The volume of the venous reservoir of the bypass circuit restricts the volume of filtrate that can be removed during CUF, providing only a limited ability to remove excess water and reverse hemodilution (Cooper et al. 2011). For this reasons, Naik and colleagues (Naik et al. 1991a, b) introduced an ultrafiltration technique after separation from CPB, which they termed modified ultrafiltration (MUF). The difference is that blood is removed from the arterial cannulas and passed through a haemoconcentrator. Blood remaining in the venous reservoir is ultrafiltrated, haemoconcentrated and then returned to the right atrium (so-called arteriovenous MUF). A roller pump maintains a flow rate of approximately 200 mL/min with a filtration rate of 150 mL/min. Typically, the duration of ultrafiltration is approximately 20–30 min, but has a high institutional variability. Haemoconcentration is carried out until a haematocrit value of 40 % is achieved or no blood remains in the bypass circuit. A similar process, called veno-venous MUF, has been used too. Blood is withdrawn from the right atrium and returned to the right atrium. No direct comparisons of the effectiveness of arteriovenous MUF and veno-venous MUF have been performed. Various advantages are associated with the use of MUF. In a lot of studies, it has been demonstrated that MOF decreases FO, postoperative blood loss and blood product use (Naik et al. 1991b); improve left ventricular systolic function, with an increase in arterial blood pressure (Naik and Elliott 1993); improve alveolar–arterial oxygen gradient and lung compliance and decrease the frequency of pulmonary hypertensive episodes (Davies et al. 1998); decrease the duration of postoperative ventilation (Koutlas et al. 1997); and decrease the incidence of pleural effusions after cavopulmonary connection and the Fontan procedure (Koutlas et al. 1997). It has not been well elucidated the mechanism by which MUF causes these beneficial effects. Initially, the benefit appeared to be caused simply by removing FO decreasing tissue oedema. Subsequent studies showed a large amount in the ultrafiltrate of inflammatory mediators and vasoactive substances, including IL-6, IL-8, and IL-10, TNF-α and endothelin 1 (Elliott 1999), so that early removal of the mediators may decrease the inflammatory cascade (Bando et al. 1998). As mentioned, CUF and MUF are two different processes, not competing, but can be complementary techniques with potentially additive positive effects. Filtration during CPB (CUF) may be used to remove inflammatory mediators and vasoactive substances, whereas MUF is performed after CPB to reverse haemodilution and decrease tissue oedema. Nowadays, the improvement in technology (small circuits, decrease use of haemodilution, less use of hypothermia and circulatory arrest) may change the indication for ultrafiltration during CPB.

Clinical Pictures

Classification and Diagnosis

Historically, the diagnosis of AKI was based on a rising serum creatinine (SCr) or a reduction in the urine output. However, these two parameters are delayed and unreliable measure in the acute setting (Bellomo et al. 2004a): age, gender, lean muscle mass, muscle metabolism and hydration status influence SCr, making its plasma levels variable. Moreover, a reduction of about 50 % of renal function is needed to measure a modification of SCr. At lower GFR rates, the amount of tubular Cr secretion results in overestimation of renal function. Finally, during acute changes in GFR, SCr does not accurately depict kidney function until steady-state equilibrium has been reached, which may require several days. Nevertheless, nowadays the absolute value of or a change in SCr remains the most widely used method for the diagnosis of AKI; in fact, there are more than 30 definitions of AKI in the current literature based on it. This lack of standardized definition has resulted in the reported incidence of AKI ranging from 1 to 25 % and a mortality ranging from 7 to 80 %, if aetiology is based on a primary renal disease or if it is part of a multiorgan dysfunction syndrome (MODS). We are given below of the most commonly used definition in the literature (Table 40.2).

RIFLE Classification System

In 2004 an interdisciplinary collaboration, the Acute Dialysis Quality Initiative (www.adqi.net) group, has defined the range of acute renal dysfunction using the so-called RIFLE classification system. It classifies three grades of increasing severity of acute renal dysfunction and two outcomes (Bellomo et al. 2004b):

- Risk (R) – 1.5-fold increases in SCr, greater than 25 % decrease in GFR, or urine output of less than 0.5 ml/kg/h for 6 h
- Injury (I) – twofold increase in SCr, greater than 50 % decrease in GFR, or urine output of less than 0.5 ml/kg/h for 12 h
- Failure (F) – threefold increase in Scr (>4 mg/dl), greater than 75 % decrease in GFR, or urine output of less than 0.3 ml/kg/h for 24 h or anuria for 12 h

Table 40.2 Definition of AKI by AKIN classification, RIFLE and pRIFLE scoring system

AKIN		RIFLE				pRIFLE		
Stage	SCr	Class	Urine output	SCr or GFR	Class	Urine output	eCrCl	
I	Increase>0.3 mg/dL or >150–200 % from baseline	Risk	<0.5 mL/kg/h × 8 h	SCr increase 150 % or GFR decrease by 25 % from baseline	Risk	<0.5 mL/kg/h × 8 h	Decrease by 25 %	
II	Increase>200–300 % from baseline	Injury	<0.5 mL/kg/h × 16 h	SCr increase 200 % or GFR decrease by 50 % from baseline	Injury	<0.5 mL/kg/h × 16 h	Decrease by 50 %	
III	Increase>300 % from baseline or SCr>4 mg/dL with an acute raise at least 0.5 mg/dL	Fail	<0.3 mL/kg/h × 24 h or Anuric × 12 h	SCr increase 300 % or SCr>4 mg/dL with an acute increase of 0.5 mg/dL or GFR decrease by 75 % from baseline	Fail	<0.3 mL/kg/h × 24 h or anuric × 12 h	Decrease by 75 % or<35 mL/min/1.73 m^2	
		Loss	Failure>4 weeks		Loss	Failure>4 weeks		
		ESRD	Failure>3 mouths		ESRD	Failure>3 mouths		

- Loss (L) – persistent acute renal failure defined as the need for renal replacement therapy for greater than 4 weeks
- End-stage renal disease (E) – need for renal replacement therapy for more than 3 months (Bellomo et al. 2004b)

The three severity grades are defined on the basis of the changes in SCr and/or GFR from baseline value and/or urine output where the worst of each criterion is used. The two outcome criteria, loss and end-stage renal disease, are defined by the duration of loss of kidney function. There is a reasonable correlation between stage of AKI based on RIFLE criteria and mortality. The criteria have been validated as predictive of mortality in studies on different adult patient populations, including cardiac surgical patients (Ricci et al. 2008a).

pRIFLE Classification System

In 2007, a modified paediatric version of the RIFLE classification system, pRIFLE, was proposed to classify AKI in paediatrics, and then it has also been developed and validated (Akcan-Arikan et al. 1997). It uses the same stages of acute kidney injury as the RIFLE criteria, but the SCr, GFR and urine output are inferior. pRIFLE criteria have been found to be predictive of outcomes, specifically mortality (Plotz et al. 2008), and it has been validated by various single-centre studies.

AKIN Classification System

In 2007, the Acute Kidney Injury Network (AKIN) developed a later version of the RIFLE classification: the new system classifies AKI into stages I–III on the basis of small (>/0.3 mg/dL) increases in serum creatinine levels or oliguria in 48 h (Mehta et al. 2007). Instead of RIFLE classification, the AKIN introduce some modifications:

- AKI is defined by the decrease of renal function in about 48 h, defined as an increase in absolute SCr of at least 0.3 mg/dL, or defined by a percentage increase in SCr $\geq 50\%$ (1.5× first value) or by a decrease in the urine output (documented oliguria <0.5 mL/kg/h for more than 6 h); stage 1 corresponds to the risk class, but it also considers an absolute increase in SCr ≥ 0.3 mg/dL.
- Stages 2 and 3 define the injury and failure classes, respectively; stage 3 also considers patients needing renal replacement therapy, independently of the stage (defined by SCr and/or UO).
- A correct state of hydration and the exclusion of renal obstruction are necessary for the diagnosis of AKI.
- The AKIN classification only does not consider either the GFR or baseline SCr; it requires at least two values of SCr obtained within a period of 48 h.
- The two outcome classes (loss of kidney function and end-stage kidney disease) were removed from the classification.

Difference Between RIFLE, pRIFLE and AKIN Classification

The AKIN classification allows only the identification of more AKI patients, despite not exhibiting a better prognostic acuity in terms of in-hospital mortality. Moreover, it theoretically improves the RIFLE criteria sensitivity and specificity, although the advantages of the RIFLE modifications have not been proven (Lopes et al. 2008; Conlon et al. 1994).

The Multi-societal Database Committee for Pediatric and Congenital Heart Disease Classification

In 2008, the Multi-societal Database Committee for Pediatric and Congenital Heart Disease developed consensus definitions used by the STS Congenital Heart Surgery Database – the largest database on paediatric and congenital cardiac operations in the world – for renal dysfunction and renal failure requiring dialysis (Welke et al. 2008). Renal dysfunction was defined as oliguria with sustained urine output < 0.5 cc/ kg per h for 24 h and/or a rise in creatinine > 1.5 times upper limits of normal for age, without the need for dialysis (including peritoneal dialysis and/or haemodialysis) or haemofiltration. Renal failure requiring dialysis was defined as oliguria with sustained urine output < 0.5 cc/kg per h for 24 h and/or a rise in creatinine > 1.5 times upper limits of normal for age, with the need for dialysis (including peritoneal dialysis and/or haemodialysis) or haemofiltration (Welke et al. 2008).

Lab Findings: New Biomarkers

Novel biomarkers for AKI have been developed in recent years, with potentially high sensitivity and specificity. These include plasma biomarkers (NGAL and cystatin C) and urine biomarkers (NGAL, IL-18, KIM-1 and L-FABP). Measurement should be technically easy with good reproducibility. So, it should be easier determining the timing of the initial insult, even in the absence of typical clinical signs, assessing the duration of AKI and correlating with both prognosis and response to treatment. Based on the differential expression of the biomarkers, it is also likely that the AKI panels will help distinguish between the various types and aetiologies of AKI and should enable early intervention.

Among the new markers, urine NGAL, IL-18 and serum cystatin C appear to perform best for the early diagnosis of AKI.

Neutrophil Gelatinase-Associated Lipocalin (NGAL)

Human NGAL is a small protein (around 25 KDalton) normally bound to gelatinase from neutrophils, involved in innate immunity. It is also present at very low levels, in several human tissues such as kidney, lungs, stomach and colon.

Many studies found that in case of acute kidney injury, after an ischemic or nephrotoxic injury, NGAL gene is upregulated and the protein is secreted very quickly into the blood (Mishra et al. 2003). Because its small dimension, it is rapidly excreted, so it is easily and early detected in the urine. In patients who developed AKI, urinary NGAL levels increase within 2 h and peak at 6 h. These features have led many authors to consider NGAL as a biomarker of ischemic AKI (Mishra et al. 2005; Haase-Fielitz et al. 2009). However, it was found that NGAL is most sensitive and specific in relatively uncomplicated patients with AKI (Haase et al. 2009) and also its dosage can be affected by several variables, such as pre-existing renal disease and systemic or urinary tract infections (Picca et al. 1995).

Interleukin 18

IL-18 is a proinflammatory cytokine involved in cell-mediated immunity following infection with microbial products such as lipopolysaccharide. It was found that urinary level of IL-18 increases in ischemic AKI, but it is not influenced by nephrotoxins, chronic renal diseases or urinary tract infections. In cardiac surgery patients who developed AKI, urinary IL-18 was induced within 6 h and peaked at 12 h after CPB. So it can be used as marker of injured tubules. Urinary levels of NGAL and IL-18 have been proven to represent early, predictive, sequential AKI biomarkers in children undergoing cardiopulmonary bypass (Parikh et al. 2004).

Cystatin C

Cystatin C is a small protein normally produced by nucleated cells. It is a potent inhibitor of lysosomal proteinases and probably the most important cysteine proteinases inhibitor. It is removed from the bloodstream by glomerular filtration, and it is reabsorbed and catabolized but is not secreted by the tubules. If kidney function and GFR decline, the blood levels of cystatin C rise. Since the blood levels of cystatin C are not influenced by age, gender or muscle mass, it was found that serum levels of cystatin C are a more precise test of kidney function than SCr in patients with chronic kidney disease (Dharnidharka et al. 2002). Some studies showed that cystatin C can be considered a good predictor for renal replacement therapy need (Herget-Rosenthal et al. 2004a) and it might be predictive of AKI in intensive care setting (Herget-Rosenthal et al. 2004b). In a recent study in paediatric post-CPB patients, cystatin C levels at 12 h after CPB were strong independent predictors of AKI (Krawczeski et al. 2010).

The importance of the new biomarkers for AKI has been recently shown by Haase et al., confirming that an increase in the levels of these molecules is strongly related to an increased length of hospital stay, even in patients with normal creatinine value (Haase et al. 2011).

Treatment Course

Fluid Management

During the perioperative period, patients with chronic heart decompensation require a great amount of fluid. As a consequence, fluid management became of utmost importance: the volume needed should be administered to maintain perfusion, but FO should be avoided. Fluid intake calculation should take into account all sources of fluid, including intravenous crystalloid, parental nutrition, drug infusion, fluid bolus. Fluid management is a challenging task: in the past, a positive fluid balance was associated with a clinical benefit; nowadays, there are increasing evidences that positive fluid balances in the order of 5–10% of body weight are associated with worsening organ dysfunction in the critically ill and with worse postoperative outcomes after surgery. In clinical practice, fluid management after congenital heart disease surgery is more complicated considering the risk of prerenal AKI in case of excessive fluid restriction and the risk of kidney damages related to fluid and sodium overload and the effect of acidosis and hyperchloraemia on renal flow. As a consequence, the amount and the kind of infused fluid play a crucial role in determining or worsening a renal dysfunction.

Fluid Overload

Fluid overload, deriving from the inability or impossibility to optimize endovascular filling, has been clearly identified as an independent risk of mortality, length of mechanical ventilation and hospital stay (Ricci et al. 2011a). Particularly, because of an increased TBW amount and the highest possibility of interstitial fluid spill over, smallest patients and newborns are the most delicate patients, especially when inflammatory conditions are present, such as post CPB. So, the prevailing consensus is to avoid a hypervolaemic state in the immediate postoperative period as an FO is considered a risk factor for multiorgan dysfunction. Different factors contribute to the development of FO. CPB leads to haemodilution and increased capillary permeability, both of which promote extravasation of fluid into the ECS. Moreover, postoperative administration of fluid and blood product worsens the third-space accumulation of water. Subsequently, increasing oedema leads to the raising of the intra-abdominal pressure, decreasing renal perfusion. When combined with postoperative myocardial dysfunction, there is also a stimulus FO via the RAAS. Given the acute nature of CPB-mediated kidney injury and the observation that most patients have normal renal function prior to surgery, these patients may be ideal candidates for aggressive postoperative goal-directed protocols aimed at avoiding FO and optimizing tissue perfusion.

Goal-Directed Fluid Therapy

Adequate fluid resuscitation is essential to restore cardiac output, systemic blood pressure and renal perfusion in patients with shock secondary to low cardiac output, but fluid responsiveness of cardiac output is dependent both on the volume of the central venous reservoirs and venous tone. When managing fluid resuscitation, the best strategy may be to ensure a sufficient preload to generate adequate cardiac output rather than simply responding to hypotension. Goal-directed therapy (GDT) allows physicians to the treatment of hypotension, including volume expansion with boluses of crystalloid or colloid, or the use of inotropes, only to patients who need them, in order to assure sufficient DO_2 to fulfil the metabolic requirement of the particular patients. This approach may help to determine when fluid resuscitation can safely be stopped, avoiding FO (Agrò and Vennari 2014). Defined haemodynamic variables are necessary to evaluate volume status and to test fluid responsiveness. Filling pressure, central venous pressure (CVP), pulmonary capillary wedge pressure (PCWP) and mean arterial pressure (MAP) are the most commonly used and known parameters to evaluate fluid replacement in cardiosurgical ICU (Kastrup et al. 2007). Despite being easily achieved and their values simply interpreted, they have limited predictive value as indicators of fluid responsiveness due to the different underlying cardiac compliance and value competence (Osman et al. 2007). Many studies have shown that CVP does not adequately reflect preload and fails to predict fluid responsiveness (Agrò and Vennari 2014; Kastrup et al. 2007). In one study PCWP was found to adequately predict fluid responsiveness in 19 patients who have undergone CABG (Bennett-Guerrero et al. 2002). Other studies found a significant CVP and PCWP increase after a fluid challenge, but they do not correlate to an increase in stroke volume (Wiesenack et al. 2001). Moreover, pressure parameters are altered by intra-abdominal pressure variation, modification of cardiac compliance, pulmonary resistance, and cardiac pathologies (Marik et al. 2008). As a result they are not very reliable and useful in cardiac surgery patient who present at less one of these conditions. More recently, the use of respiratory variation of arterial pressure, such as pulse pressure variation (PPV), stroke volume variation (SVV) and continuous cardiac index (CI) to predict fluid responsiveness, has shown some interesting data in both operating room and intensive care units (Teboul and Monnet 2009). Both high PPV and SVV are indicators of hypovolaemia, indicate fluid responsiveness and correlate to the CI increase after fluid challenge administration (Habicher et al. 2011). This evidence was confirmed in a study on off-pump CABG patients, in which both SVV and PPV strongly correlated to CI improvement after a fluid challenge, with respect to filling pressure (Habicher et al. 2011). As a consequence, dynamic parameters such as PPV and SVV are able to adequately distinguish fluid responder and fluid nonresponder patients and are suitable to guide fluid management in the perioperative period of cardiac surgery, with respect to filling pressure. Unfortunately, these dynamic indices, robust and reliable under specific conditions (mechanical ventilation, closed chest, sinus rhythm, low tidal volume ventilation, absence of right ventricular failure), have not been validated during open-chest settings.

The esophageal Doppler (ED) estimations might be more reliable, even if biased by the need of a learning curve. It allows measurement such as left ventricular end-diastolic area (LVEDA) and the blood velocity at the level of the descending aorta. The flow time in the descending aorta, corrected for HR (FTc normally 330–360 ms), corresponds to the SV. At lower velocities, hypovolaemia should be suspected. FTc correlates with LVEDA (Agrò and Vennari 2014). ED requires shorter operator training than other systems and does not require calibration, but it is difficult to use in awake patients and in a prolonged monitoring, and finally its results may be operator dependent. GDT using ED was shown to improve patient outcomes (Agrò and Vennari 2014).

In the last years, new devices, assessing dynamic and volumetric parameters, have been developed. They are PICCO system and PiCCO$_2$, PULSION Medical Systems, Munich, Germany; FloTrac, Edwards Lifesciences; and LiDCOrapid, LiDCO, London, UK. These devices use trans-pulmonary thermodilution and/or pulse wave analysis. When the methodologies are used in combination, the validity of pulse pressure analysis depends on periodic recalibration through thermodilution (Agrò and Vennari 2014; Reuter et al. 2010). These systems require invasive arterial lines and a central venous catheter, but they are less invasive than PAC. All these systems have to be compared to the Swan–Ganz or pulmonary artery catheter (PAC), which remains the gold standard, despite its limits. In fact, many clinical trials showed that PAC is not suitable for GDT in the routine perioperative setting. Its use is further discouraged by the invasiveness of the procedure, which exposes patients to complications. In addition, PAC cannot be used without adequate training and experience. Finally, its performance mainly refers to filling pressure values (PVC, PCWP), which have been found to be not so effective in clinical practice. Consequently, its fame in the literature and in clinics has decreased over the years (Agrò and Vennari 2014). Low cardiac output should be managed with a multimodal monitoring and treatment tailored to the single patient and clinical picture trying to obtain the best balance between fluids, inotropes and vasopressors during the whole intra- and postoperative phase.

The maintaining of an adequate cardiac output with no FO is the first goal of perioperative fluid management in cardiac heart surgery, avoiding primary, secondary and iatrogenic renal dysfunction.

Type of Fluid Solution

In 2001, a survey of paediatric anaesthetists suggested that the choice of fluids for plasma volume expansion in infants and children varied by geographical location, with semi-synthetic colloids commonly used and albumin mainly used for neonates (Soderlind et al. 2001). Recently, the evidence about which fluid to use are changed, suggesting caution regarding the use of albumin, the use of semi-synthetic colloids and excessive volumes of intravenous crystalloid in perioperative or critically ill patient (Myburgh and Mythen 2013). At the state of the art, crystalloids are suggested for continuous losses (perspiratio insensibilis and urinary output), while colloids are suggested for temporary losses (IVS loss, such as due to haemorrhage) (Agrò et al. 2013a).

Colloids

Colloids are distributed in the IVS, with a larger increase in plasma volume because they contain oncotic particles. They have a longer duration of action, with smaller volumes needed for a specific target volume expansion than crystalloids (Agrò et al. 2013a). If endothelial permeability is intact, colloids are retained in the IVS, with a subsequent increase of the plasma oncotic pressure and the diffusion of fluids from the ISS to the IVS (Agrò and Vennari 2014). Colloids have a 'contest volume effect': in hypovolaemic patients, they have a volume effect>90% of the volume infused; in normovolaemic patients, two-thirds of the infused volume shifts to the ISS within minutes. Consequently, they should be used only in hypovolaemia, even when there is capillary membrane damage. In fact, in this case, hypovolaemia is connected to the shift into the ISS of protein-rich fluids, with a plasma COP reduction. Colloids that are able to increase COP are needed: their use may reduce ISS overload.

In 2006, Verheij et al. (2006a) showed that following cardiac surgery, volume expansion and cardiac output were significantly higher after colloid infusion than after the administration of crystalloids. He found colloids were approximately five times as efficient in expanding the IVS volume with respect to saline 0.9%. Ley et al. (1990) compared fluid replacement with crystalloids or colloids in patients undergoing coronary artery bypass or valve substitution. Patients treated with HES showed a reduced length of ICU stay than patients treated with normal saline solution. In addition, they required less fluid infusion after surgery and showed better haemodynamic performance than the crystalloid group (Agrò et al. 2013a).

Despite this evidence, colloids have been associated with coagulopathy, and platelet dysfunction, predisposing cardiac surgery patients to postoperative bleeding (in particular when high MW molecules and CPB are involved) and to anaphylaxis (especially gelatins), may cause tubular damage with renal dysfunction (Agrò et al. 2013a). All colloids can induce kidney injury. The anatomic feature of colloid-induced renal damage is an *osmotic nephrosis-like lesion.* The most likely mechanism of renal dysfunction is a tubular obstruction caused by hyperoncotic urine formation with the storage of colloidal molecules filtered by the glomeruli. This mechanism is further impaired by a condition of dehydration. Another suggested mechanism is an increase in plasma oncotic pressure, with secondary renal macromolecules accumulation. Adequate hydration using crystalloids may prevent this injury (Agrò et al. 2013b). The proposed risk factors for colloid-related kidney dysfunction are age (older patients have a higher risk), hypovolaemia, previous kidney alterations (chronic or acute injury due to other causes) and other comorbidities (such as diabetes and others conditions causing direct or indirect renal alterations). Other risk factors are the type of colloid administered (higher MMW and MS) and the total amount infused per kg of body weight (Agrò et al. 2013b). Clinical evidences of the renal effects of colloid use (especially hydroxyethyl starches) are not uniform, and there is still intense debate as to whether there is truly a critical creatinine level for their administration. Up to some years ago, the use of low MMW and low MS hydroxyethyl starches (HES) was thought to be relatively safe on renal function with respect to other colloids. More recently many issues have been relieved by literature. Initially the administration of the newest-generation HES was suggested to reduce the risk of short-term and long-term renal injury (Agrò et al. 2013b; Mitra and Khandelwal 2009). In a study on brain-dead kidney donors, Blasco et al. (2008) compared HES 130/0.4 and HES 200/0.62. At 1 month and 1 year post-administration, they found better effects on renal function (lower serum creatinine) with HES 130/0.4 than with HES 200/0.62 (Feng et al. 2006). The use of fourth-generation HES seems to cause much less harm than older-generation HES, even in patients with previous renal impairment. The infusion of 500 mL of HES 6%/130/0.4 did not cause any kidney damage in volunteers showing mild-to-severe renal dysfunction (Agrò et al. 2013b; Jungheinrich et al. 2002). In a review comprising 34 studies (2607 patients), HES was compared with other fluids. According to other studies, the results evidenced an increased risk of acute renal dysfunction, of long-term renal damage and mortality with HES (even third- and fourth-generation HES), especially in patients with sepsis (Agrò et al. 2013b; Perner et al. 2012; Myburgh et al. 2012). On the basis of these evidences, HES use (included modern HES) has been restricted in Europe, with specific reference to patient with renal dysfunction or undergoing dialysis. Their use remains justified in case of severe hypovolaemic shock. According to the recent literature, the newest-generation HES seems to be the better colloidal solutions with respect to kidney oncotic damage while assuring an adequate volume replacement. However, the influence of HES on kidney function remains controversial, and large studies are still needed to evaluate the incidence of acute kidney injury with HES in patients without sepsis, directly applying the RIFLE criteria, by precisely measuring the GFR and urine output together with creatinine and NGAL (Young 2012; Agrò et al. 2013b). The need for studies with a specific subset of patients (i.e. cardiac surgery patients) is crucial in the perioperative management of population with a high risk of AKI, such as congenital heart disease patients, considering colloid use is largely diffused in the intra- and postoperative setting (i.e. CBP priming).

Crystalloids

Crystalloids are mainly distributed in the ISS, with less effectiveness in maintaining plasma volume, because they do not contain oncotic particles (Agrò and Vennari 2014). Their duration of action is short, with large volume needed for a specific target volume expansion (Rackow et al. 1983). Their infusion dilutes plasma proteins, thus reducing the COP. Consequently, there is a diffusion of fluids from the IVS to the ISS. This fluid shift increases when vascular permeability is altered, increasing interstitial oedema. A relationship between the administration of high fluid volumes and increased mortality has been reported in cardiac surgery patients (Pradeep et al. 2010). According to the literature, the use of crystalloids for volume stabilization in patients with circulatory shock is related to a higher risk of altered lung function because of pulmonary oedema (fluid overload, referred to as 'Da Nang lung' based on the large number of cases in the Vietnam war) (Agrò et al. 2013a). In particular, the use of crystalloids seems to be less appropriate in patients with reduced myocardial function. Animal studies on acute normovolaemic haemo-dilution with Ringer's lactate vs. HES demonstrated that HES group presented a significant increase in cardiac output. Moreover, the microscopic study of left ventricular wall revealed the destruction of myofilaments, and mucosal gastric pH was significantly reduced (index of hypoperfusion) in the Ringer's lactate group (Otsuki et al. 2007). CBP with crystalloids has also been associated with postoperative myocardial oedema and cerebral dysfunction with respect to colloids (Iriz et al. 2005). On the other hand, Ringer's solutions were found to not increase pulmonary water volume with respect to dextran 70, after CABG procedures, with no difference on PO_2/FIO_2 (Karanko et al. 1987). Similar results were found in a more recent study comparing 0.9 % saline, 4 % gelatin, 6 % HES 200/0.5 and 5 % albumin in a sample of major vascular surgery: no difference was found in PaO_2/FIO_2 ratio and in pulmonary leak index among the groups (Verheij et al. 2006b). When evaluating the effect of different types of fluid replacement therapies, one of most important factors that have to be taken into account is the electrolytic composition. For many years, many clinicians have preferred 'balanced salt solutions' such as Hartmann's or Ringer's lactate in anaesthetic practice. Normal saline contains a higher than physiological concentration of sodium and chloride ions, which may result in hyperchloraemic acidosis and adverse effects on renal or immune function (Myburgh and Mythen 2013), leading to increased vascular tone and a reduction in GFR. So, plasma-adapted and plasma-balanced solutions have a lower risk of AKI, even in cardiac patients, as well as bleeding risk and inflammation response (Agrò et al. 2013a). An observational study of patients in an adult ICU where there was a change from high chloride-containing solutions (0.9 % saline, gelatin, albumin in saline) to restricted chloride-containing solutions (PlasmaLyte, Hartmann's, chloride-poor 20 % albumin) suggested the low chloride-containing solutions were associated with less acute kidney injury and need renal replacement therapy (Yunos et al. 2012). Similarly, review of a large database of adults undergoing open abdominal surgery showed fewer major complications (blood transfusion, acid–base disturbance, postoperative infection and renal impairment) and improved mortality in those who received a balanced salt solution (PlasmaLyte) compared with 0.9 % saline (Shaw et al. 2012).

Concerns Regarding Paediatric Patients

According to Holliday and Segar (1957), for half a century, the administration of hypotonic fluids with 5 % glucose added was considered the gold standard for maintenance fluid therapy in children. Recently, many authors have found the wide use of such fluids causing serious complications, such as hyponatraemia or hyperglycaemia, and, more rarely, resulting in permanent neurological consequences or death (Duke and Molyneux 2003).

Two main factors lead to the development of perioperative hyponatraemia: the stress-induced ADH secretion, which decreases the body's ability to excrete free water, and the use of hypotonic solutions as a source of free water. Infants are particularly susceptible to hyponatraemia-related complications, because they have a reduced Na-K-ATPase activity and their brain size/cranial vault ratio is higher (Ayus et al. 2008). Severe hyponatraemia may become a very dangerous condition, leading to a shift of water from ISS into neuronal cells, with subsequent increase in brain volume, leading to cerebral oedema, brainstem herniation and death. All of these sequels can be avoided by the use of balanced electrolyte solutions containing both a physiological osmolarity and electrolyte composition with metabolic anions (acetate, lactate or malate) as bicarbonate precursors for acid–base stabilization (Sumpelmann et al. 2010). Infants have higher metabolic requirements than adults, potentially leading to perioperative lipolysis and hypoglycaemia. Hypoglycaemia can result in cerebral metabolism and blood flow alterations (Sieber and Traystman 1992) and subsequently in long-lasting neurodevelopment impairment, if unrecognized or undertreated. Administering a 5 % dextrose solution in the perioperative period can prevent hypoglycaemia, although these solutions often cause hyperglycaemia because of stress-induced insulin resistance (Welborn et al. 1986). Hyperglycaemias may damage the brain, because of increased lactate levels, leading to intracellular acidosis that compromises cellular functions (Bailey et al. 2010). The literature suggests the use of isotonic solutions with a reduced dextrose (i.e., 1–2.5 %) concentration to avoid the above-mentioned consequences of hypoglycaemia/lipolysis and hyperglycaemia in children (Sumpelmann et al. 2011).

Parental Nutrition

In the postoperative phase, one of the major factors affecting fluid balance is parental nutrition (Ricci et al. 2011a). In most cases, more than 60 % of total postoperative fluid administered result from parental nutrition. Undernutrition is a serious risk for patients with chronic heart diseases (CHD), both in the pre- and postoperative phase. Postoperatively, surgical stress causes a great amount of energy wasting. Moreover, undernutrition can be exacerbated further by fluid restriction and AKI occurrence (Zappitelli et al. 2008). Inadequate nutrition provision might be associated with decreased patient survival rate in CHD patient, even if there are no studies that confirm it.

Monitoring Daily Fluid Balance

Daily fluid balance should be accurately monitored in postoperative care, avoiding a positive fluid balance. Alternatively, fluid balance might be monitored by daily measurement of patient's weight. An interesting recent weight-based determination of FO status in PICU patients requiring RRT showed that weight-based definition of FO is useful in defining FO at CRRT initiation and is associated with increased mortality in a broad paediatric critically ill patient population (Selewski et al. 2011). Many studies in other critically ill paediatric patient populations with acute renal failure have recently demonstrated that nonsurviving patients have greater degrees of FO at the initiation of RRT, even when corrected for their severity of illness (Ricci et al. 2011a). The prevention of FO is thus an important clinical goal for critically ill patients.

Pharmacologic Management of Fluid Overload

Conventional treatment of FO in the ICU involves the use of diuretics. In the recent years, novel evidence regarding newer agents is available, which may serve as primary or adjunct agents in achieving negative fluid balance.

Dopamine

Historically, low-dose or 'renal-dose' dopamine (1–3 mcg/kg/min) was used as medical management of AKI, in the attempt to increase renal blood flow and enhance urine output, throughout the stimulation of D-1 renal receptor. However, multiple studies and meta-analyses have demonstrated that renal-dose dopamine is ineffective in AKI in adult patients (Lauschke et al. 2006).

Loop Diuretics

Loop diuretics are the most used in the critically ill patients, and furosemide is by far the most popular one. It can be administered both in continuous infusion and in bolus. Compared with bolus administration, the continuous infusion has been demonstrated to be generally more advantageous: it results in an almost comparable urinary output with a much lower dose, less hourly fluctuations and less urinary wasting in sodium and chloride (Luciani et al. 1997; Singh et al. 1992). Furosemide use is associated with side effects, the major of which are electrolyte disturbance (hypokalaemia and hyponatraemia), metabolic alkalosis with hypochloraemia and diuretic resistance. In particular, the last effect consists in an absolute or relative inefficiency of diuretic standard dosing. It derives from heart failure per se (inability to reach the optimal peak intraluminal levels of drug), hypoalbuminaemia (that causes less intravascular bindings of the diuretics and less delivery to the proximal tubular cells), hyponatraemia (hyperaldosteronism, vasopressin production and less free water excretion), and the so-called braking effect (decreased responsiveness to diuretics due to histological modifications of loop and tubular cells). Few strategies have been developed to overcome diuretic resistance: use of continuous infusion, increase dosage of loop diuretics, use of combined therapy to block sodium reabsorption, correction of electrolyte balance, metabolic derangements and excessive vascular depletion. Not infrequently, diuretics may be associated with adverse outcome: in the adult population, their use does not prevent the occurrence of AKI, and sometimes it has been associated with increased mortality rates (Mehta et al. 2002). However, it has been shown that furosemide use has a protective effect on 60-day mortality, except when adjusted for fluid balance, suggesting that the benefit of furosemide in critically ill patients is derived from the reduction in fluid balance (Wiedemann et al. 2006).

Nesiritide

Nesiritide is a recombinant form of human BNP, with effects on the regulation of fluid balance and vascular resistance. As mentioned before, there are two most important natriuretic peptides in cardiac setting: atrial natriuretic peptide (ANP) and brain natriuretic peptide (BNP). ANP, synthesized and mostly stored in the atria, causes diuresis, natriuresis and vasorelaxation and inhibits the release and action of aldosterone, than ADH. Brain natriuretic peptide (BNP) is a hormone secreted in the ventricles, in response to ventricular wall stretch caused by hypertrophy or volume overload. It promotes natriuresis and diuresis and induces vasodilatation and antagonizes the effect of antidiuretic hormone and aldosterone throughout dedicated receptors in the vascular endothelium, myocardium and kidneys, antagonizing the effect.

In congenital heart surgery patients, an increase in early postoperative BNP levels has been reported, particularly after repair of tetralogy of Fallot, intracardiac left-to-right shunts and extracardiac Fontan completion (Costello et al. 2004). Moreover, increasing in BNP levels has been associated with increased CPB times and increased aortic cross clamp times (Costello et al. 2005). The mechanism by which CPB impairs the biological activity of the natriuretic hormone system is not known. Decreased biological activity and poor responsiveness of the natriuretic hormone system might play a role in the development of fluid retention after CPB (Costello et al. 2005).

Nesiritide works on several sites. In the heart, it has a lusitropic effect, acting on intracellular substrates to reduce cytosolic calcium, so causing myocytes relaxation. In the kidney, it increases GFR, and consequently diuresis, by afferent arteriolar vasodilatation and efferent arteriolar vasoconstriction. Indirectly, it augments diuresis inhibiting the effects of the sympathetic nervous system and angiotensin II on proximal tubular sodium absorption, blunting aldosterone production and inhibiting the effect of vasopressin at the medullary collecting duct (Costello-Boerrigter et al. 2003). All these physiological effects lead to the therapeutic benefits of venous, arterial and coronary vasodilatation with a decrease in excessive preload and afterload, resulting in increased cardiac output. So, nesiritide has a therapeutic benefit in adults with congestive heart failure (CHF) and is currently approved for use in acute congestive heart failure (Aronson and Burger 2002). Similarly, it can have positive effect on low cardiac output syndrome (LCOS). Data suggest that, as well as increasing urine output, it may decrease pulmonary vascular resistance and central venous filling pressure, having a favourable trend in cardiac index and systemic vascular resistance (Hiramatsu et al. 1998). It is also associated with improved fluid balance when associated to routine inotropes and diuretic therapy (Mahle et al. 2005). Moreover, preliminary data propose that the infusion of nesiritide has favourable renal and haemodynamic effects after CPB in adults (Hayashi et al. 2003) and children on extracorporeal membrane oxygenation (Smith et al. 2005) and with CHF (Feingold and Law 2004), even if there are limited studies in children thus far (Moffett et al. 2006).

At least, caution regarding the use of nesiritide in adults as a sole diuretic agent has recently been advised.

Fenoldopam

Fenoldopam is a selective D-1 receptor partial agonist, registered as antihypertensive agent. It promotes the relaxation of vascular smooth muscle, particularly the renal and splanchnic arteries. In the kidney, it increases RBF, tubular sodium excretion and urine output, by blunting aldosterone. It is rapidly titratable, with an elimination half-life of less than 10 min. Several reports suggest that fenoldopam infusions provide renal protection after CPB and during critical illness in adults (Halpenny et al. 2001). Regarding paediatric postoperative cardiac population, data available are limited and do not confirm the adults' results (Ricci et al. 2008b). It is possible that neonatal kidneys are relatively resistant to D-1 receptor stimulation, due to differences in receptor density and affinity and in coupling to intracellular second messengers: neonates might require higher fenoldopam doses to achieve significant clinical effects (about 10 times the adult dose) (Ricci et al. 2011b).

Renal Replacement Therapy

In patients with acute renal failure, starting renal replacement therapy (RRT) may be due to different clinical settings. In 2007, the Prospective Pediatric Continuous Renal Replacement Therapy Registry Group (ppCRRT) showed that the main reasons that induce physicians to start RRT in paediatric patients are fluid overload and electrolyte imbalance (Symons et al. 2007). Other causes can be the increase of uraemia, the need to eliminate toxins and the presence of metabolic imbalance. Regarding the choice of RRT modality, intermittent haemodialysis (IHD), peritoneal dialysis or continuous renal replacement therapy (CRRT) are based on several factors such as:

- Physicians' preferences and expertise
- Patient needs
- Goal of the therapy
- Availability of equipment
- Cost

Most used criteria to start RRT are presented in Table 40.3. Recent indications suggest a wider use of RRT in paediatric and adult patients with AKI than in past years (Picca et al. 2008). This is particularly important especially when the fluid balance cannot be properly controlled with diuretic therapy. In these patients, the early use of RRT prevents or limits FO, allowing adequate nutritional support without worsening the accumulation of fluids. FO is associated with increased mortality in patients receiving CRRT (Bagshaw et al. 2009). It is suggested that RRT should be started within the first 48 h of ICU admission in critically ill AKI patients (Ricci et al. 2011a). Although there are no specific recommendations for RRT in patients without AKI, there is a wide consensus that RRT can improve the prognosis of patients with multiple organ failure (MOF). Goldstein et al. (2005) suggested that

Table 40.3 Conventional criteria for initiation CRRT

Indication	Description
Anuria	Negligible urine output for 6 h
Severe oliguria	Urine output < 200 mL/12 h
Hyperkalaemia	$K^+ > 6.5$ mmol/L
Severe metabolic acidosis	pH < 7.2 despite normal or low CO_2 in arterial blood
Volume overload	Especially pulmonary oedema unresponsive to diuretics
Pronounced azotaemia	Urea concentration > 30 mmol/L or creatinine concentration > 300 μmol/L
Complication of uraemia	For example, encephalopathy, neuropathy, pericarditis

the benefit received from the RRT is due to the prevention of FO. They reported that prognosis of patients with MOF was significantly better for patients with less than 20 % of FO versus greater than 20 % of FO at CRRT initiation. However, regarding the time of starting RRT, international recommendations are not very clear. In this field, the term 'early' or 'late' are both related to the time from ICU admission to CRRT start or to the severity of metabolic alterations present at CRRT initiation (Bellomo et al. 2012).

In 2007, Palevsky reviewed 11 studies from 1961 to 2006 evaluating the timing of initiation of RRT based on the blood urea nitrogen (BUN) level. In the studies analysed, the cut-off BUN value for early initiation ranged from <60 to 150 mg/dL and for late initiation ranged from >60 to 200 mg/dL (Palevsky 2007). In Liu's report of the Project to Improve Care in Acute Renal Disease (PICARD) study (Liu et al. 2006), a better prognosis was found when RRT was started with a BUN <73 mg/dL ($P < .0001$) and when CRRT was the initial RRT modality ($P < .0001$).

In the literature, there are no data regarding the timing of initiation of RRT based on a BUN level in paediatric patients. Instead, in the last decade, FO was recognized as an independent predictor of mortality in paediatric patients with AKI. In 2001, Goldstein et al. analysed the outcome of children receiving CVVH (Goldstein et al. 2001). They reported a formula to calculate the percentage of FO:

$$FO = \left(\text{fluid intakes} - \text{fluid losses} / \text{body weigh at PICU admission}\right) \times 100$$

Patients with less FO at the time of CRRT initiation had a better outcome. Similarly, an interesting recent weight-based determination of FO status in PICU patients requiring CRRT reported that weight-based determination of FO is related to increased mortality in a broad critically ill patients (Selewski et al. 2011). In 2009, Hayes et al. showed an OR death of 6.1 when FO was >20 % upon initiation of CRRT (Hayes et al. 2009). They also reported a better outcome when CRRT was started with <20 % FO, in terms of shorter need of ventilatory support, shorter PICU stay, and increased renal recovery rate. Most recently, Sutherland et al. reviewed the ppCRRT Registry data: FO was found to be associated with the mortality in paediatric patients receiving CRRT (Sutherland et al. 2010). Patients with <10 % FO upon initiation of CRRT had a significantly lower mortality rate compared to patients with an FO between 10 and 20 % and FO > 20 %. The multivariate regression analysis revealed a 3 % increase in mortality for each 1 % increase in FO present at CRRT start.

Regarding the timing of discontinuation of CRRT, even in this field, the indications are not clear. At the state of the art, there have been no precise recommendations to determine when to discontinue RRT. Usually, RRT is discontinued after renal function has recovered, the electrolytes and metabolic balance have normalized, and the urine output is enough to maintain a negative fluid balance. In 2009, Uchino et al. (2009) reviewed the current practice for the discontinuation of CRRT in 54 adult centres in 23 countries. They concluded that a urinary volume of >436 mL/d without diuretics or >2330 mL/d with diuretic therapy may be used as a threshold to stop RRT. If confirmed, these data may be a valid indication in the future.

In paediatric patients, two dialysis modalities are most frequently used: peritoneal dialysis and continuous renal replacement therapy.

Peritoneal Dialysis

Peritoneal dialysis (PD) is an RRT using patient's peritoneum as a semipermeable dialysis membrane. Fluid is introduced through a permanent catheter in the abdomen and flushed out either every night while the patient sleeps (automatic peritoneal dialysis) or during the day (continuous ambulatory peritoneal dialysis). The peritoneal membrane is vascularized. Solutes move thanks to a concentration gradient between the blood and the dialysis solution. This process called diffusion is also dependent on the molecular size of the solute and the effective surface area and permeability of the peritoneal membrane. Ultrafiltration of water across the peritoneal membrane occurs primarily due to the osmotic gradient generated by the glucose concentration in the dialysis fluid. This technique presents the main advantage to be easy to use, it does not need vascular access (often complicated in infants), and it is generally better tolerated than haemodialysis in haemodynamically unstable patients. However, peritoneal dialysis can be complicated by obstruction of the peritoneal dialysis catheter. Drainage from the peritoneal dialysis can be disrupted due to catheter kinking, fibrin clots or omental wrapping. Furthermore, it was observed that PD is less efficient than haemodialysis in restoring water, electrolytic and metabolic balance. This is true, especially with regard to water removal, with direct consequence on fluid balance. Given these limitations, the early application of PD in order to achieve the prevention and treatment of FO is presently accepted (Alkan et al. 2006). PD also presents limited efficiency in depurative function (Ricci et al. 2008c). In particular it does not provide adequate removal of molecules, and it is not the optimum choice in cases of patients with severe life-threatening hyperkalaemia who require rapid reduction of serum potassium. Another important limitation of PD is that in case of haemodynamic instability, the application of high dialysate volumes is difficult, because changes in atrial conformation, mean pulmonary artery and systemic pressure have been observed (Dittrich et al. 2000). Because high dialysate volumes may not be tolerated in critically ill infants, a PD prescription of 10 mL/kg, previously defined as 'low-volume PD', is commonly used during neonatal RRT (Morelli et al. 2007). In a recent study, the role of prophylactic peritoneal dialysis has been evaluated. It was shown that patients in the PD group had a greater negative fluid balance and decreased levels of IL-6 and IL-8, suggesting removal of inflammatory cytokines by PD. Moreover, these patients had lower inotropic needs, despite typical concerns for negative haemodynamic effects. Finally, the results were statistically significant for decreased duration of mechanical ventilation in the PD group (Sasser et al. 2014).

Continuous Renal Replacement Therapy

CRRT is one of the techniques of extracorporeal dialysis. The use of extracorporeal dialysis is recently increasing, according to the explained limitations of PD, especially in critical post heart surgery patients (Jander et al. 2007) (Table 40.4).

Extracorporeal dialysis can be used with several modalities, such as intermittent haemodialysis, continuous haemofiltration or haemodiafiltration. The choice is influenced by many factors, including the goals of dialysis, the advantages and disadvantages of each modality, and institutional resources. Intermittent haemodialysis may be not well tolerated from paediatric patients, especially in those with haemodynamic instability (Flynn 2002), because of its rapid rate of solute clearance (Sadowski et al. 1994).

CRRT is an extracorporeal blood purification therapy used in case of acute or chronic kidney disease intended to replace the lost function of kidneys, aimed at being applied for 24 h a day (Ronco and Bellomo 1996). CRRT provides slow and balanced fluid removal that even unstable patients – those with shock or severe

Table 40.4 Differences between PD and CRRT

	Advantages	Disadvantages
CRRT	Better haemodynamic stability Fewer cardiac arrhythmias Improved nutritional support Better pulmonary gas exchange Better fluid control Better biochemical control	Greater vascular access problems Higher risk of systemic bleeding Long-term immobilization of patient More filter problems (ruptures, clotting) Greater cost
PD	Easy to perform Does not require vascular access Does not require heparinization	Risk of peritonitis Catheter problems (obstruction, kinking, fibrin clots, omental wrapping) Difficult to optimize ultrafiltration Does not provide efficient removal of water Both ultrafiltration and solute clearance are slow

fluid overload – can more easily tolerate. Both adult and paediatric patients can undergo CRRT therapy, and it can be adapted quickly to meet changing needs. However, there are special considerations to take into account when prescribing therapy to smaller patients. The use of CRRT requires a central double-lumen veno-venous haemodialysis catheter. Having functional vascular access is critical for the success of all modalities of renal replacement therapy. Normally, a 7 French double-lumen haemodialysis catheter is wide enough in diameter to achieve adequate blood flows for dialysis while minimizing risk of clots in the extracorporeal circuit. Typical locations for placement include the internal jugular, subclavian or femoral veins. In the past, the preferred site for haemodialysis catheter was considered the subclavian vein, but recently it was observed that subclavian access increases the risk for subclavian stenosis and may compromise placement of an AV fistula in the future. So internal jugular vein is generally considered the best access (Ronco and Ricci 2015). The femoral vein is not ideal because increased abdominal pressure could affect blood flow rates. Femoral access is also the most difficult to keep sterile.

One of the main problems that occur with the use of CRRT is the formation of clots in the extracorporeal circuit that necessitate the discontinuation of treatment and the replacement of the entire extracorporeal circuit. Activation of the clotting cascade is due to the contact between circulating blood and artificial surfaces. Repeated changes of the haemofilter result in loss of blood for the patient. This is the reason why anticoagulation remains an area of intense research regarding the use of RRT. Both heparin and citrate are used as anticoagulation, and both have been shown to achieve comparable filter survival (Brophy et al. 2005). However, despite small doses of heparin are used, the anticoagulant effect, especially in critically ill patients, can be significant. Regarding citrate, patients with liver dysfunction may develop citrate toxicity, and then citrate presents a hepatic metabolism.

Normally, the initial blood flow setting ranges from 4 to 5 mL/kg/min. Recommended dialysate or replacement fluid rate is typically 2000–3000 mL/1.73 m²/h. Ultrafiltration rates typically start at 1–2 mL/kg/h.

Regarding the best CRRT modality to support AKI in paediatric patients, it was recently shown in vitro that haemofiltration and haemodialysis have the same purification performance at the low blood flow typically used in paediatric patients (Parakininkas and Greenbaum 2004). Even if CVVH at low blood flows used in paediatric patients may result in an excessive haemoconcentration and formation of clots, however haemofiltration is considered to have a better clearance capacity of medium- and small-weight solutes than haemodialysis. For this reason, finally, CVVH is preferred to CVVHD RRT of paediatric patients. During the treatment, a careful monitoring should be applied, because – even if the continuous therapy has less impact on haemodynamic than intermittent one – still small changes in blood flow rate can cause significant changes in the haemodynamic one. Also the formation of clots and the consequent need to change the circuit can result in the loss of blood that in paediatric patients may be significant. Furthermore, it is important to continuously monitor electrolyte balance, because at the initiation of CRRT, many dangerous electrolyte disturbances may occur.

Finally, ECMO is a commonly utilized technique to support post cardiosurgical respiratory and cardiac failure. The use of CRRT circuits to ECMO, in series, has been recently reported as an effective solution for renal dysfunction treatment during CRRT (Ricci et al. 2011a).

Electrolyte Management

Sodium

In the cardiac surgery patient, sodium overload is the most common alteration due to fluid administration and to the surgical stress response (increased level of aldosterone and cortisol). In this case, it is accompanied by hypervolaemia and fluid overload, with interstitial oedema (Young 2012). Hypernatraemia may be also due to a loss of hypotonic fluids. Renal losses may be caused by furosemide use, osmotic diuresis (severe hyperglycaemia, uraemia, mannitol overdose), pre-existing renal diseases and the development of ATN (polyuric phase). In these cases, sodium losses are associated to water losses, with a reduction of IVS fluid and the presence of signs and symptoms of hypovolaemia (Agrò and Vennari 2013). Less frequently, hypernatremia may be due to a loss of free body water (hypernatremia due to sodium concentration). In this case, EVS volume is preserved. The most frequent cause of normovolaemic hypernatremia is the lack of an adequate restoration of perspiratio insensibilis, especially when it is increased (i.e. patients with fever).

In the postoperative period, many cardiac surgery patients may present a reduction of sodium plasma levels, due to a shift of water from ICS to IVS rather than a reduction in total body sodium. The shift is caused by hyperglycaemia (diluting hyponatremia) triggered by the surgical stress response, by the reduction in insulin production and insulin resistance and by an overload in the bypass pump priming (Young 2012). A similar mechanism may be triggered by mannitol overdose. In these cases, hyponatremia is accompanied by hypertonicity (plasma osmolarity > 300 mOsm/L) (Agrò and Vennari 2013). Other causes responsible for hyponatremia in the ICU cardiac surgery patient are associated to a reduction of plasma osmolarity (true hyponatremia). In this case, IVS volume may be normal-increased or reduced (Agrò and Vennari 2013).

Advanced heart failure, severe hypovolaemia and hepatic complications with ascites alter ADH release and the kidneys' capacity to dilute urines, leading to hyponatremia with IVS volume reduction and interstitial oedema development.

The use of diuretics (especially if inappropriate), and the development of SIADH due to cerebral complications or prolonged mechanical ventilation, may cause normo-hypervolaemic hyponatremia without oedema.

Hyponatremia with hypovolaemia may be due to cerebral salt wasting (cerebral complications), hypokalaemia, renal losses and extra-renal losses. The most frequent cause of renal losses in the cardiac surgery patient is diuretics use and the development of ATN. Possible extra-renal losses are PONV, gastric suction and diarrhoea (i.e. related to enteral nutrition in long-stay patient). In the critic patient, frequent causes of hypovolaemic hyponatremia are third-space syndromes.

Potassium

Maintaining adequate potassium levels is crucial for bypass pump separation and to prevent postoperative dysrhythmias. In the perioperative setting, many factors may affect potassium plasma levels in different directions. Generally, factors determining a reduction of potassium levels are predominant; as a consequence, potassium loss must be adequately prevented and managed (Young 2012).

Hyperkalaemia may be the consequence of an increase in total potassium body stores or of a shift of potassium from the ICS to the ECS (Agrò and Vennari 2013).

In the cardiac surgery patient, an increase in potassium is commonly due to ICS shift caused by acidaemia, hypoinsulinaemia and haemolysis and to potassium i.v. load due to cardioplegia (Young 2012).

In case of postoperative ATN, hyperkalaemia often reflects a reduced renal excretion of potassium due to reduced tubular secretion, rather than a reduced glomerular filtration. Adrenal dysfunction (due to disease or drugs), with reduced aldosterone production, can lead to potassium retention (Agrò and Vennari 2013). Muscular weakness, up to paralysis, is one of the main manifestations of hyperkalaemia. Cardiac signs are increased automaticity and repolarization of the myocardium, leading to ECG alterations and arrhythmias. Mild hyperkalaemia may appear with T waves and a prolonged P-R interval; severe hyperkalaemia may cause a wide QRS complex, asystole or ventricular fibrillation (Agrò and Vennari 2013).

The management of hyperkalaemia includes heart protection and facilitating in ICS redistribution of potassium. Rapid-effect therapies are the administration of calcium gluconate, insulin with glucose (considering patient glycaemia) and correction of acidaemia through bicarbonate administration or hyperventilation. In acute and severe cases (often associated to AKI and development of postoperative complication such as sepsis), CRRT may be indicated considering other electrolytes and acid–base status. Additional therapies are resin exchange, diuretics, aldosterone agonists and β-adrenergic agonists. They act long term, and their use is suitable in long-stay ICU patients who have developed a chronic condition determining hyperkalaemia (Agrò and Vennari 2013).

Cardiac surgery patient often presents hypokalaemia, which may be caused by an absolute deficiency of total body potassium stores or by an abnormal shift of potassium from the ECS to the ICS (despite a normal total potassium) (Agrò and Vennari 2013).

In the perioperative setting, a reduction in potassium level is due to augmented catecholamine production with increase skeletal uptake, diuresis caused by hypothermia, furosemide and mannitol use during CPB, and increased cortisol and aldosterone levels due to surgical stress. Other causes may be gastrointestinal loss or renal losses due to diuretic or the development of acute renal damage. Hypokalaemia is always associated to metabolic alkalosis (Agrò and Vennari 2013).

Calcium

Hypocalcaemia is frequent during the intraoperative period. Hypocalcaemia refers to free ionized calcium levels in the plasma. It develops when calcium concentrations are low, but plasma protein levels are normal. As a consequence, it is necessary to know if the calcium value measured is the total plasma value (in this case, it should be adjusted for albumin value) or the ionized fraction (Agrò and Vennari 2013).

In the cardiac surgery patients, hypocalcaemia is generally limited, and it is caused by citrate use, haemodilution, increase of albumin-binding fraction and hypomagnesaemia. In these cases, hypocalcaemia is treated in order to normalize calcium level and to uptake its effects on myocardium (protection and inotropism) and vessels (vasopressor) (Young 2012). In the ICU setting, the most frequent cause of hypocalcaemia is hypoalbuminaemia. Other causes are the development of post-operative renal dysfunctions, hyperventilation, blood transfusion (citrate chelation) and septic complications (the pathogenesis of the mechanisms correlating sepsis and hypocalcaemia is not fully understood) (Young 2012).

Magnesium

Hypomagnesaemia is frequent in the postoperative period after cardiac surgery. It may be triggered by hyperaldosteronism (heart failure, stress response), by calcium alteration (hypercalcemia) and by the use of drugs such as diuretics or adrenergic drugs (Agrò and Vennari 2013). The effects of magnesium deficits are neuromuscular excitability disorders (related to the concurrent development of hypercalcaemia), such as involuntary contraction of the facial muscles, cramps, tetany and arrhythmias, or other symptoms mainly related to metabolism, such as morning fatigue. Hypomagnesaemia may lead to hypertension, coronary vasoconstriction and arrhythmias (Young 2012; Kimura et al. 1989; Booth et al. 2003). It may also be characterized by an alteration of consciousness, as demonstrated by confusion, hallucinations and epilepsy.

Magnesium supplementation has been demonstrated to reduce the reperfusion injury, by blocking calcium ingress in myocardial cells and acting as a free radical scavenger (Young 2012; Garcia et al. 1998). In fact, in animal studies, magnesium use has been related with a reduction of infarct size. The timing of administration appears to be very important: no effects have been found when administration is realized early after the reperfusion (Young 2012;

Ravn et al. 1999; Herzog et al. 1995). Literature also demonstrated that after CABG, magnesium supplementation reduces the risk of postoperative arrhythmias, improves the short-term neurological function and may have a significant opioid-sparing effect (Young 2012; England et al. 1992).

Magnesium inhibits platelets function with a prolongation of bleeding time at 24 h after cardiac surgery. However, a correlation of this effect with an increase of postoperative blood losses is not clear (Young 2012; Gries et al. 1999). On the other side, a recent study demonstrated reduced postoperative bleeding and transfusional need after CABG, in patient receiving magnesium (Young 2012; Dabbagh et al. 2010).

Hypermagnesaemia is less frequent in cardiac surgery patient. The most common and probable cause is kidney failure. Haemolysis, hypocalcaemia, adrenal insufficiency, diabetic ketoacidosis, lithium intoxication and hyperparathyroidism are other predisposing conditions. Hypermagnesaemia is characterized by weakness, hypocalcaemia, nausea and vomiting, hypotension, breathing symptoms and arrhythmias up to asystole (Agrò and Vennari 2013).

In severe cases, the first line in hypomagnesaemia management is the administration of calcium gluconate, since calcium is the natural antagonist of magnesium. Subsequently, according to renal function, diuretics or dialysis are needed (Agrò and Vennari 2013).

Basis of Pathophysiology Acid–Base Balance in the Postoperative ICU Setting of Cardiac Surgery

Maintaining acid–base balance during and after cardiac surgery is essential for the success of the surgery, especially for procedure requiring prolonged bypass time. As an example, cardiac surgery patients are at high risk for developing arrhythmias: the presence of a neutral pH is necessary to obtain a response to pharmacological and electric treatments. At the same time, acid–base status is considered as an index of adequate perfusion of tissue (i.e. lactate increase, adequate renal compensation) and may modify blood flux distribution. Moreover, pH and pCO_2 variation may influence Hb-curve dissociation reducing Hb saturation (acidosis, pCO_2 increases) or reducing Hb capacity to transfer O_2 to tissue (alkalosis, pCO_2 decreases) (Agrò et al. 2013a). Literature demonstrated in experimental and clinical studies the influence of pH on vascular tone resulting in possible blood flux redistribution and blood pressure alteration (Celotto et al. 2008). Both modification of ECS pH (pHe) and ICS pH (pHi) may cause these alterations, through many proposed mechanisms: neurotransmitters release, prostanoids, purines, smooth cells hyperpolarization, NO, changes in intracellular calcium concentration (Franco-Cereceda et al. 1993; Ishizaka and Kuo 1996). Moreover, acid–base balance alterations have been related to modification of endothelium activity, with different effects according to the type of considered vessel (Celotto et al. 2008).

On the other hand, cardiac surgery is responsible for profound alteration in acid–base system. At the base of this modification, there are different mechanisms, causing an impact on acid–base balance in opposite directions (Dobell et al. 1960; Gibbon et al. 1950). These mechanisms depend on (Young 2012; Ito et al. 1957; Litwin et al. 1959):

- Type of oxygenator and the type of blood flow during the CPB
- CPB duration
- Kind and duration of postoperative mechanical ventilation
- Hypotension in the postoperative setting (need for inotropes and/or vasoactive drugs, bleeding)
- Kind of fluid used for priming and for liquid management (balanced vs. unbalanced)
- Temperature modifications (hypothermia reduces buffer system dissociation, determining a 'natural alkaline shift', while CO_2 becomes more soluble and pCO_2 is decreased)
- Haemolysis

Metabolic Acidosis

The more frequent alteration of acid–base equilibrium in cardiac patients is metabolic acidosis (Young 2012). It is thought to be due to pre-existing respiratory alkalosis, increased lactate levels, hypoxia and hypoperfusion (Dobell et al. 1960; Ito et al. 1957). Acidosis induces systemic vasodilatation (included coronary) and pulmonary vasoconstriction (Young 2012). Although vasodilatation may have a positive effect, such as an increase in coronary blood flow, its consequence may be detrimental in patient presenting a cardiac dysfunction after the surgery (Celotto et al. 2008; Clancy and Gonzalez 1975; Ely et al. 1982). Moreover, acidosis reduces the responsiveness to catecholamines, decreasing pharmacological effectiveness of the treatment of postoperative haemodynamic instability and further precipitating patients' conditions. Pulmonary vasoconstriction may increase pulmonary resistance and decompensate the haemodynamic and respiratory status of cardiac surgery patients (Celotto et al. 2008).

In ICU patients, there often is a hyperchloraemic acidosis caused by i.v. fluid infusion, especially when large amounts are needed and unbalanced nor plasma-adapted solutions are used (Young 2012; Morgan 2005).

A severe and prolonged reduction of diuresis and the development of postoperative AKI (especially ATN) may also be the cause of metabolic acidosis due to altered chloride levels and bicarbonate excretion and reduced lactate and other not volatile acids' clearance, especially in patients with pre-existing or precipitating renal dysfunction (Beers 2009).

In complicated, long-stay ICU patient, the need for enteral nutrition, gastric aspiration and the development of gastrointestinal dysfunction such as diarrhoea may be other causes of metabolic acidosis with normal AG (Beers 2009).

According to the management of all acid–base alteration, the treatment of metabolic acidosis is to eliminate the underlying cause or causes. As a consequence, an adequate integration between ABG information, patient clinic, patient anamnesis and therapy in course is fundamental.

The use of i.v. bicarbonate is generally indicated when acidaemia (especially severe acidaemia) is developing. Sodium bicarbonate use may be more useful in some cases and even deleterious in some others.

When acidaemia is the consequence of a loss of bicarbonate or inorganic acids (AG normal, Cl^- increased, HCO_3^- reduced), the use of i.v. bicarbonate is considered appropriate to restore plasma levels. When acidaemia is due to organic nonmeasurable acids (more frequently lactic acidosis), the use of bicarbonate is controversial: it may be helpful to avoid deleterious consequence of acidity (i.e. protein denaturation), but may cause other deleterious mechanisms (Young 2012; Beers 2009).

Bicarbonate reacts with H^+ producing H_2CO_3 and finally CO_2 that is eliminated through the lungs. In patients under mechanical ventilation, clinicians may modify ventilator parameters in order to optimize the clearance of pCO_2. In patients with spontaneous breathing and in those with pulmonary complication (i.e. postoperative pneumonia, pleural effusion in case of cardiac insufficiency, pulmonary oedema), increasing VCO_2 may be difficult even when using invasive and non-invasive ventilation. As a consequence, pCO_2 retentions with respiratory acidosis may develop aggravating the patient status. The overproduction of CO_2 may aggravate intracellular acidosis because the infused bicarbonate does not pass across the cellular membrane, while the obtained CO_2 freely pass. It reacts with endocellular water finally producing H^+ (Young 2012; Beers 2009).

Sodium bicarbonate administration may depress cardiac function, worsening the haemodynamic status of postoperative ICU patient, especially when there has just been a cause of cardiac failure.

Considering that bicarbonate is administered with sodium too, the development of hypernatremia and hyperosmolarity is possible, especially when large amounts of sodium bicarbonate are used (Young 2012; Beers 2009). Finally, the administration of exogenous bicarbonate reduces free ionized Ca^{2+} and K^+ levels that may be deleterious in patients with hypokalaemic acidosis (generally due to renal loss of salts) (Young 2012; Beers 2009).

In mechanical ventilated patient, hyperventilation may be used without bicarbonate administration in order to compensate metabolic acidosis. The consequence is the induction of a respiratory alkalosis that may reduce the hepatic clearance of lactate with a reduction of portal flux, potentially generating liver hypoxia and increase of lactate production (Young 2012; Beers 2009).

In case of postoperative AKI, the use of CRRT should be precociously considered (Young 2012; Beers 2009).

In any case, bicarbonate is generally used when (Young 2012; Beers 2009):

- pH < 7.2; bicarbonate is < 12 mEq/L.
- Hyperkalaemia develops with difficulties to control its value with other treatments.

- Acidosis is symptomatic.
- Patient is waiting for CRRT.

Sodium bicarbonate amount (bicarbonate deficit) may be calculated according to bicarbonate value (Beers 2009)

$$HCO_3^- \ deficit = 0.4 \ body \ weight \times \left(goal \ HCO_3^- - measured \ HCO_3^- \right)$$

or BE (Beers 2009)

$$HCO_3^- \ deficit = BE \left(mEq \, / \, L \right) \times body \ weight \, / \, 4.$$

Metabolic Alkalosis

Metabolic alkalosis is less frequent with respect to metabolic acidosis in cardiac surgery patients. Generally, it is due to a predominance of bicarbonate levels caused by retention, loss (renal and gastrointestinal), intracellular H^+ shift and/or alkali administration (Beers 2009).

In ICU setting metabolic alkalosis is generally caused by acid losses and may be due to secondary hyperaldosteronism caused by hypovolaemia, heart failure, renal artery stenosis (polivasculopatic patients), cirrhosis (patients with hepatic diseases) or renal impairment, HCl and KCl losses due to PONV (especially when high dose of opioid is needed) or gastric suction. Hypokalaemia and hypomagnesaemia are other causes of metabolic alkalosis because K^+ and Mg^{2+} renal reabsorption is realized through H^+ exchange (Young 2012; Beers 2009). However, the most frequent cause of metabolic alkalosis in postoperative ICU patients is the use of diuretics (especially furosemide in continuous infusion). Furosemide may lead to metabolic alkalosis through different mechanisms: hyperaldosteronism due to hypovolaemia, Cl^- losses and hypokalaemia (Young 2012; Beers 2009).

Other causes of metabolic alkalosis are due to bicarbonate retention overload, such as post-hypercapnic persistent elevation of bicarbonate, generally associated to K^+, Cl^- and volume depletion, lactate or ketoacidosis conversion to bicarbonate (augmented after bicarbonate administration for acidosis) and $NaHCO_3$ loading (Young 2012; Beers 2009).

A cause of metabolic alkalosis may be the administration of some kind of antibiotics such as carbenicillin, penicillin and ticarcillin. It should be considered in ICU patients (generally complicated, long-stay patients) with a prolonged therapy with them or with a recent story of protracted use (Young 2012; Beers 2009).

When a metabolic alkalosis persists during the time, it indicates an increased renal reabsorption of bicarbonates. The more frequent stimuli for bicarbonate reabsorption are hypovolaemia (GFR reduction) and hypokalaemia. In fact, in case of hypovolaemia, the kidney increases Na^+ (and water) reabsorption to restore IVS volume. Sodium is reabsorbed as NaCl or $NaHCO_3$. Maintaining IVS volume is more vital than correct alkalaemia; as a consequence, $NaHCO_3$ will be reabsorbed till IVS volume is restored. This mechanism is present only if hypovolaemia is caused by acid fluid losses (vomitus, gastric suction, diuretics). Hypokalaemia leads to a shift of H^+ from ECS to ICS, with stimulus (intracellular acidosis) to H^+ secretion and HCO_3 reabsorption in tubular cells. Frequently two or more causes of metabolic alkalosis may coexist: for example, the use of diuretic may cause hypovolaemia and hypokalaemia (Young 2012; Beers 2009; Narins and Gardner 1981).

The treatment of metabolic alkalosis depends on the cause. Metabolic alkalosis involving Cl^- losses responds to administration of fluid containing NaCl. Generally 0.9 % saline solution is used. In order to avoid other electrolytic disorders, the infusion of a balanced solution may be suggested. It is recommendable to start the infusion at a rate of 50–100 mL/h and to subsequently increase the rate, according to the estimated and measured losses (Young 2012; Beers 2009).

When metabolic alkalosis is not Cl^- responsive, the correction of K^+ and Mg^{2+} levels is needed. According to Stewart's approach, K^+ deficit should be replaced using KCl. In fact in case of hypokalaemia, the deficit is manly in the ICS: the administered K^+ moves into cells, while Cl^- remains in ECS reducing SID (and SBE), with an acidifying effect (Young 2012; Beers 2009).

The correction of volume and Cl^- and/or K^+ depletion lead to K^+/H^+ exchange, restoring H^+ plasma levels and reducing Na^+ (and consequently HCO_3^-) reabsorption.

Respiratory Acidosis and Alkalosis

Respiratory acidosis is due to CO_2 accumulation caused by a reduced elimination or an increased production.

A reduction in CO_2 elimination is caused by hypoventilation. Frequent causes of hypoventilation in cardiac surgery in the ICU settings may be caused by sedation effects (during weaning from MV and in the immediate postextubation period), neuromuscular blocker effects (fast-track protocols or long-stay patients with protracted curarization), postoperative pain and the development of complications such as cerebral complications or abdominal complications (ascites, abdominal distension), cardiac failure with pulmonary oedema or/and pleural effusion, pneumothorax (post central line positioning or MV related), pneumonia (VAP) and atelectasis. Other causes of hypoventilation may be due to patient's comorbidity such as COPD, OSAS and restrictive pulmonary diseases. These diseases may cause chronic acidosis that may be associated to acute causes (Young 2012; Beers 2009).

Frequent causes of CO_2 overproduction may be hypovolaemia, sepsis and an inadequate artificial nutrition (long-stay patient) with an excess of calories. On the other hand, malnutrition may cause muscular weakness (Young 2012; Beers 2009).

Finally it is fundamental to remember the detrimental effect of a prolonged MV on respiratory muscles and its effects during MV weaning attempts and the role of oxygen administration resulting in hyperoxaemia and subsequent hypoventilation (Young 2012; Beers 2009).

Treatment is based on the management of the underlying cause and the increase of alveolar ventilation.

Respiratory alkalosis is caused by an increase of alveolar ventilation. Many stimuli may lead to hyperventilation as a physiologic response: hypoxemia, hypotension, severe anaemia and metabolic acidosis. These causes are often present in the cardiac surgery patient in the ICU setting, especially in complicated cases (Young 2012; Beers 2009).

Other causes leading to respiratory alkalosis are fever and sepsis, pain (insufficient analgesic administration), anxiety and agitation (postoperative delirium, central complication), COPD and pulmonary embolism (Young 2012; Beers 2009).

Finally the most frequent cause of respiratory alkalosis in the ICU patients is iatrogenic: mechanical ventilation. It may be the cause of pseudo-respiratory alkalosis: in cases of hypoperfusion–hypoxemia, the underlying metabolic acidosis is masked by a CO_2 elimination over the normal rate and due to the mechanical control of alveolar ventilation. This alteration may be detected studying the arterial–venous difference in pCO_2, pH and the other ABG markers of metabolic acidosis such as AG and SID (Young 2012; Beers 2009).

A Practical Approach to…

A practical approach to the management of main modification in fluids, electrolytes and acid–base balances should consider that they are interconnected by three principles:

- The electric neutrality principle
- The iso-osmolarity principle
- The neutrality principle

As a consequence, modification in each one of the balances determines modification on both the other two. Clinical scenarios are further complicated by the role of the kidney in modulating each of the three principles.

Fluid Management

1. Postoperative salt and water should be titrated to each patient's individual requirements.
2. Control volaemia using CVP and wedge pressure. The ideal value for atrial pressures is 15 mmHg. CVP may reach 18 mmHg and wedge pressure 20 mmHg in case of:

   - Hypotrophy
   - Hypocontractility
   - Partial obstruction of ventricular outflow
   - Pulmonary hypertension

During post-op with significant right atrium dilation, such as anomalous pulmonary vein drainage, the right atrium is overly complacent, and CVP oscillates between 5 and 10 mmHg. In surgery with atriopulmonary anastomosis, in the immediate postoperative care, CVP should remain between 18 and 20 mmHg (Joao and Faria Junior 2003).

3. The volume of crystalloids offered during the first 24 h may be as follows:

- 40% of basic needs in the form of glucose solution with calcium, for surgery involving CPB
- 60% for surgery without CPB (Joao and Faria Junior 2003)

4. Acute fluid loss (bleeding/drain losses) within the first 12 h post-op should be replaced with equal volumes of fluid (crystalloid/colloid/fresh whole blood).

5. Avoid excessive volume replacement in response to hypotension or low atrial pressures, because it may be associated with significant increase in total body water particularly in the presence of capillary leak syndrome. Fluid overload may lead to excess lung water and exacerbate pulmonary hypertension, hypoxaemia, V/Q mismatch and cardiac failure. A possible strategy guiding filling is represented in Fig. 40.9.

6. The choice of replacement fluid should be guided by the haematocrit and the lesion. Patients with a persisting cyanotic lesion will require a higher Hb than those with a non-cyanotic lesion. The following values may be useful:

- Acyanotic heart diseases: Hb 10, Ht 30–35%
- Cyanotic heart diseases: Hb 15, Ht 40–45%
- Blalock–Taussig: Hb 13–14, Ht 40%, in order to avoid obstructing the shunt (Cruz et al. 2015)

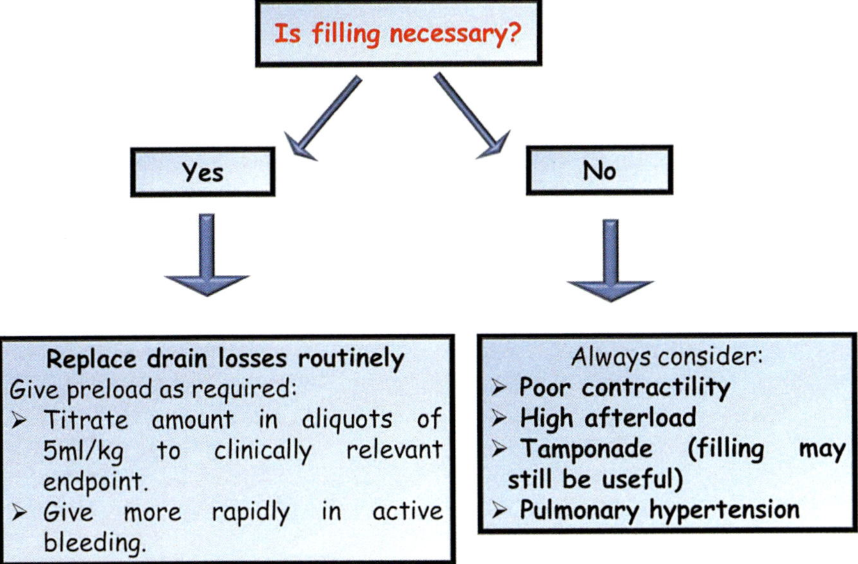

Fig. 40.9 A suitable filling strategy

7. Consider that fluid administration may modify acid–base status:

   - Delusional acidosis
   - Hyperchloraemic acidosis (reduces renal perfusion and GFR potentially deteriorating renal function)
   - Role of metabolizable anions

Renal Management

1. Hourly urine output should be measured in all patients, preferably by urinary catheter initially. A urine output ≥ 1 mL/kg/h should be maintained.
2. The overall balance to aim for should be determined by their clinical status.
3. If:

   - Diuresis < 1 mL/kg/h.
   - Hematuria arises.
   - Potassium > 5 mEq/L.
   - Creatinine > 1 mg/dL.

   Renal insufficiency may possibly develop.
4. If after the correction of volaemia (Fig. 40.9) oliguria persists, furosemide is indicated at a dosage of 1 m/kg up to a maximum of 6 mg/kg/day in an attempt to stimulate diuresis (Cruz et al. 2015).
5. Nesiretide, fenoldopam and dopamine may be used related to patient's individual clinical status.
6. If after stimulation and restricted hydration (including all drugs and infusions, but not boluses of volume expanders/blood products) hypervolaemia remains and urea and creatinine levels are increased, it may indicate RRT. The modality, type and settings have been indicated in Sect. 40.7.

Acid–Base Disorders Management

Eight clinical issues should be solved:

1. pH (acidosis or alkalosis?)
2. pCO_2 (same or opposite direction with respect to pH?)
3. HCO_3^- (same or opposite direction with respect to pH?)
   The answers to these questions may be found using a graphic tool (Fig. 40.10).
4. Is there compensation according to Boston rules?
   Boston rules and their interpretation are presented in Table 40.5.
5. Is there an anion gap (AG)? (Fig. 40.11)

$$AG = \left(Na^+ + K^+\right) - \left(Cl^- + HCO_3^-\right) = 8 - 16$$

AG evaluation is presented in Fig. 40.11.

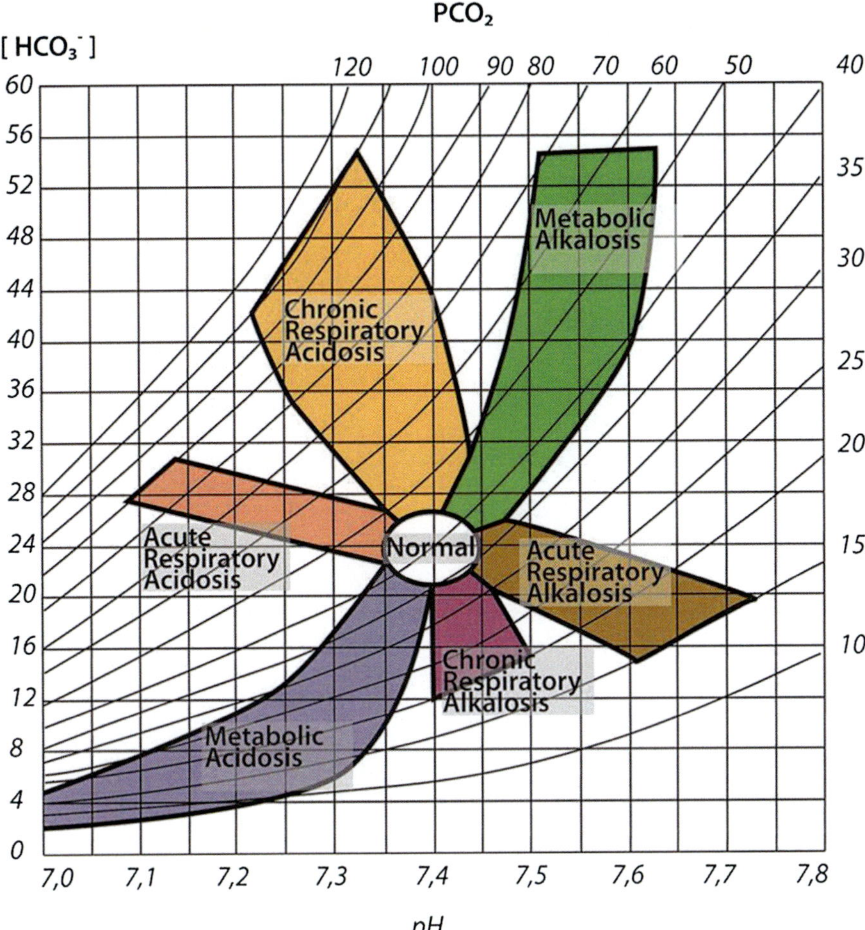

Fig. 40.10 A graphic tool to rapidly identify acid–base patient disorders knowing pH, [HCO$_3^-$] and pCO$_2$

6. If AG is increased, evaluate Delta Gap. It could reveal the presence of more than one acid–base (Fig. 40.12):

$$\text{Delta gap} = \left(\text{Measured AG} - \text{Normal AG}\right) / \left(\text{Normal HCO}_3^- - \text{Measured HCO}_3^-\right)$$
$$= \left(\text{Measured AG} - 12\right) / \left(24 - \text{measured HCO}_{3-}\right) = \Delta AG / \Delta HCO_3^-.$$

7. What is the SID (strong ion difference) value?

$$SID = \left(\left[Na^+\right] + \left[K^+\right] + \left[Ca^{2+}\right] + \left[Mg^{2+}\right]\right)$$
$$- \left(\left[Cl^-\right] + \left[A^-\right] + \left[SO_4^{2-}\right]\right) = 38 - 42$$

Table 40.5 Boston rules

pH	Disorder	HCO$_3$	PCO$_2$	Compensation evaluation	Comment
≤7.38 acidosis	Metabolic	≤24 mEq/L	↓ 1.5 mmHg for each 1 mEq/L of HCO$_3$ ↓	pCO$_2$ value higher	Respiratory acidosis
				pCo$_2$ value lower	Respiratory alkalosis
	Respiratory	↑ 1 mEq/L (acute), ↑ 4 mEq/L (chronic) for each 10 mmHg of pCO$_2$ ↑	≥40 mmHg	HCO$_3$ value higher	Metabolic alkalosis
				HCO$_3$ value lower	No time for compensation or metabolic acidosis
≥7.42 alkalosis	Metabolic	≥24 mEq/L	↑0.7 mmHg for each 1 mEq/L of HCO$_3$↑	pCO$_2$ value higher	Respiratory acidosis
				pCo$_2$ value lower	Respiratory alkalosis
	Respiratory	↓ 1 mEq/L (acute), ↓ 4 mEq/L (chronic) for each 10 mmHg of pCO$_2$ ↓	≤40 mmHg	HCO$_3$ value higher	No time for compensation or metabolic alkalosis
				HCO$_3$ value lower	Metabolic acidosis

From Agrò and Vennari (2013)

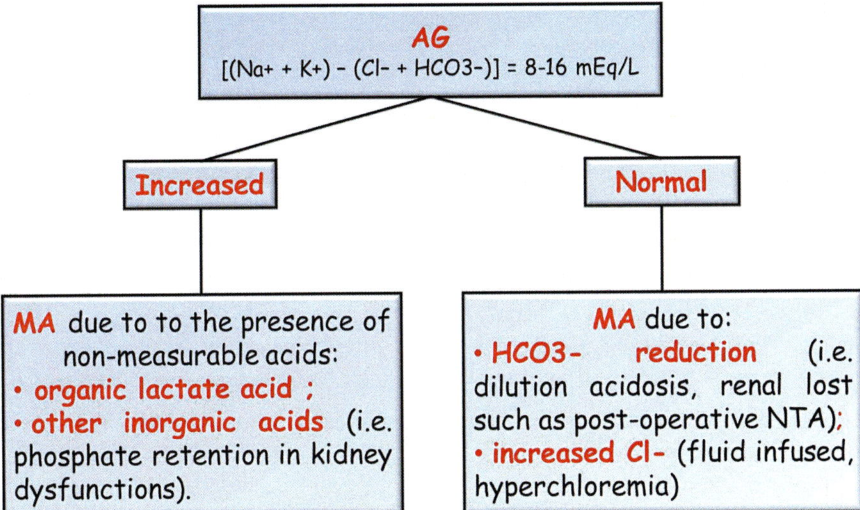

Fig. 40.11 Evaluation of anion gap. MA, metabolic acidosis

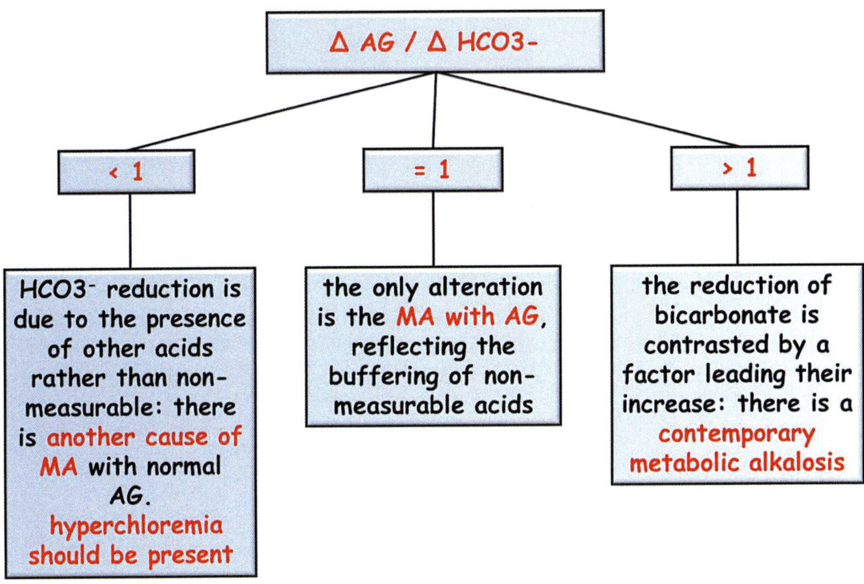

Fig. 40.12 Evaluation of delta gap. MA, metabolic acidosis

Table 40.6 Metabolic disorders according to SID

Metabolic acidosis	↓ SID RTA, TPN, normal saline, anion exchange resins, diarrhoea and loss of pancreatic secretions	↓ SID Ketoacidosis, lactic acidosis, salicylate, methanol
Metabolic alkalosis	↑ SID Loss of Cl⁻: vomitus, gastric drainage, diuretics, posthypercapnia, villous adenoma with diarrhoea, mineralocorticoid excess, Cushing's, Liddle's, Bartter's, liquorice; sodium excess; Ringer's, TPN, transfusions	↓ A_{tot} Hypoalbuminaemia (nephrotic syndrome, cirrhosis)

From Agrò and Vennari (2013)

SID variation according to metabolic disorders is presented in Table 40.6.

8. Electrolytes

Consider the values of main electrolytes are crucial. As evidenced by SID acid–base, status alteration is always accompanied by electrolyte alteration and vice versa. Examples are:

- Hyperkalaemia induced by acidosis (both metabolic and respiratory)
- Hypochloraemia in metabolic alkalosis
- Hyperchloraemia in metabolic acidosis

The role of chloride levels (mainly modified during fluid administration) is crucial in acid–base status because of its inverse relation with bicarbonate.

Bibliography

Abu-Omar Y, Ratnatunga C. Cardiopulmonary bypass and renal injury. Perfusion. 2006;21: 209–13.

Agrò FE, Vennari M. Physiology of body fluid compartments and body fluid movements. In: Agrò FE, editor. Body fluid management – from physiology to therapy. 1st ed. Milan: Springer; 2013.

Agrò FE, Vennari M. Clinical treatment: the right fluid in the right quantity. In: Agrò FE, editor. Body fluid management – from physiology to therapy. 1st ed. Milan: Springer; 2014.

Agrò FE, Fries D, Vennari M. Cardiac surgery. In: Agrò FE, editor. Body fluid management – from physiology to therapy. 1st ed. Milan: Springer; 2013a.

Agrò FE, Fries D, Benedetto M. How to maintain and restore the balance: colloids. In: Agrò FE, editor. Body fluid management – from physiology to therapy. 1st ed. Milan: Springer; 2013b.

Agrò FE, Vennari M, Benedetto M. Fluid management and electrolyte balance. In: Dabbag A, Esmalian F, Aranky SF, editors. Postoperative critical care for cardiac surgical patients. Berlin/ Heidelberg: Springer; 2014. p. 313–83.

Akcan-Arikan A, Zappitelli M, Loftis LL, et al. Modified RIFLE criteria in critically ill children with acute kidney injury. Kidney Int. 1997;71:1028–35.

Alkan T, Akcevin A, Turkoglu H, et al. Postoperative prophylactic peritoneal dialysis in neonates and infants after complex congenital cardiac surgery. ASAIO J. 2006;52:693–7.

Apostolakis EE, Koletsis EN, Baikoussis NG, et al. Strategies to prevent intraoperative lung injury during cardiopulmonary bypass. J Cardiothorac Surg. 2010;5:1.

Aronson D, Burger AJ. Intravenous nesiritide (human B-type natriuretic peptide) reduces plasma endothelin-1 levels in patients with decompensated congestive heart failure. Am J Cardiol. 2002;90:435–8.

Aschner JL, Poland RL. Sodium bicarbonate: basically useless therapy. Pediatrics. 2008;122: 831–5.

Ascione R, Lloyd CT, Underwood MJ, et al. On-pump versus off-pump coronary revascularization: evaluation of renal function. Ann Thorac Surg. 1999;68:493–8.

Asimakopoulos G. Systemic inflammation and cardiac surgery: an update. Perfusion. 2001;16: 353–60.

Aydin SI, Seiden HS, Blaufox AD, Parnell VA, Choudhury T, Punnoose A, Schneider J. Acute kidney injury after surgery for congenital heart disease. Ann Thorac Surg. 2012;94: 1589–95.

Ayus JC, Achinger SG, Arieff A. Brain cell volume regulation in hyponatremia: role of sex, age, vasopressin, and hypoxia. Am J Physiol Renal Physiol. 2008;295:F619–24.

Bagshaw SM, Uchino S, Bellomo R, et al. Timing of renal replacement therapy and clinical outcomes in critically ill patients with severe acute kidney injury. J Crit Care. 2009;24:129–40.

Bailey AG, McNaull PP, Jooste E, Tuchman JB. Perioperative crystalloid and colloid fluid management in children: where are we and how did we get here? Anesth Analg. 2010;110:375–90.

Bando K, Turrentine MW, Vijay P, et al. Effect of modified ultrafiltration in high-risk patients undergoing operations for congenital heart disease. Ann Thorac Surg. 1998;66:821–7. discussion 8.

Baraton L, Ancel PY, Flamant C, et al. Impact of changes in serum sodium levels on 2-year neurologic outcomes for very preterm neonates. Pediatrics. 2009;124:e655–61.

Beers M. Acid–base regulation and disorders. In: Beers M, editor. The Merck manual XVIII. Merck Edition. NJ, USA. 2009.

Bell EF, Acarregui MJ. Restricted versus liberal water intake for preventing morbidity and mortality in preterm infants. Cochrane Database Syst Rev. 2008;(1):CD000503.

Bell EF, Warburton D, Stonestreet BS. Effect of fluid administration on the development of symptomatic patent ductus arteriosus and congestive heart failure in premature infants. N Engl J Med. 1980;302:598–604.

Bellomo R, Kellum JA, Ronco C. Defining acute renal failure: physiological principles. Intensive Care Med. 2004a;30:33–7.

Bellomo R, Ronco C, Kellum JA, et al. Acute renal failure – definition, outcome measures, animal models, fluid therapy and information technology needs: the Second International Consensus Conference of the Acute Dialysis Quality Initiative (ADQI) Group. Crit Care. 2004b;8:R204–12.

Bellomo R, Kellum JA, Ronco C. Acute kidney injury. Lancet. 2012;380:756–66.

Bennett-Guerrero E, Kahn RA, Moskowitz DM, et al. Comparison of arterial systolic pressure variation with other clinical parameters to predict the response to fluid challenges during cardiac surgery. Mt Sinai J Med. 2002;69:96–100.

Berdat PA, Eichenberger E, Ebell J, et al. Elimination of proinflammatory cytokines in pediatric cardiac surgery: analysis of ultrafiltration method and filter type. J Thorac Cardiovasc Surg. 2004;127:1688–96.

Berg CS, Barnette AR, Myers BJ, et al. Sodium bicarbonate administration and outcome in preterm infants. J Pediatr. 2010;157:684–7.

Bissonnette Bruno. Pediatric anesthesia: basic principles – state of the art – future. Shelton: People's Medical Publishing House – USA; 2011.

Blasco V, Leone M, Antonini F, et al. Comparison of the novel hydroxyethylstarch 130/0.4 and hydroxyethylstarch 200/0.6 in brain-dead donor resuscitation on renal function after transplantation. Br J Anaesth. 2008;100:504–8.

Booth JV, Phillips-Bute B, McCants CB, et al. Low serum magnesium level predicts major adverse cardiac events after coronary artery bypass graft surgery. Am Heart J. 2003;145:1108–13.

Booz GW, Baker KM. Role of type 1 and type 2 angiotensin receptors in angiotensin II-induced cardiomyocyte hypertrophy. Hypertension. 1996;28:635–40.

Brophy PD, Somers MJ, Baum MA, et al. Multi-centre evaluation of anticoagulation in patients receiving continuous renal replacement therapy (CRRT). Nephrol Dial Transplant. 2005;20:1416–21.

Carey RM, Wang ZQ, Siragy HM. Role of the angiotensin type 2 receptor in the regulation of blood pressure and renal function. Hypertension. 2000;35:155–63.

Celotto AC, Capellini VK, Baldo CF, et al. Effects of acid–base imbalance on vascular reactivity. Braz J Med Biol Res. 2008;41:439–45.

Chiravuri SD, Riegger LQ, Christensen R, et al. Factors associated with acute kidney injury or failure in children undergoing cardiopulmonary bypass: a case-controlled study. Paediatr Anaesth. 2011;21:880–6.

Clancy RL, Gonzalez NC. Effect of respiratory and metabolic acidosis on coronary vascular resistance (38528). Proc Soc Exp Biol Med. 1975;148:307–11.

Conlon PJ, Stafford-Smith M, White WD, et al. Acute renal failure following cardiac surgery. Nephrol Dial Transplant. 1994;14:1158–62.

Cooper DS, Charpie JR, Flores FX, et al. Acute kidney injury and critical cardiac disease. World J Pediatr Congenit Heart Surg. 2011;2:411–23.

Costello JM, Backer CL, Checchia PA, et al. Alterations in the natriuretic hormone system related to cardiopulmonary bypass in infants with congestive heart failure. Pediatr Cardiol. 2004;25:347–53.

Costello JM, Backer CL, Checchia PA, et al. Effect of cardiopulmonary bypass and surgical intervention on the natriuretic hormone system in children. J Thorac Cardiovasc Surg. 2005;130:822–9.

Costello-Boerrigter LC, Boerrigter G, Burnett Jr JC. Revisiting salt and water retention: new diuretics, aquaretics, and natriuretics. Med Clin North Am. 2003;87:475–91.

Cruz I, Stuart B, Caldeira D, et al. Controlled pericardiocentesis in patients with cardiac tamponade complicating aortic dissection: experience of a centre without cardiothoracic surgery. Eur Heart J Acute Cardiovasc Care. 2015;4:124–8.

Dabbagh A, Rajaei S, Shamsolahrar MH. The effect of intravenous magnesium sulfate on acute postoperative bleeding in elective coronary artery bypass surgery. J Perianesth Nurs. 2010;25:290–5.

Davies MJ, Nguyen K, Gaynor JW, et al. Modified ultrafiltration improves left ventricular systolic function in infants after cardiopulmonary bypass. J Thorac Cardiovasc Surg. 1998;115:361–9. discussion 9–70.

Devarajan P. Update on mechanisms of ischemic acute kidney injury. J Am Soc Nephrol. 2006;17:1503–20.

Dharnidharka VR, Kwon C, Stevens G. Serum cystatin C is superior to serum creatinine as a marker of kidney function: a meta-analysis. Am J Kidney Dis. 2002;40:221–6.

DiBona GF, Kopp UC. Neural control of renal function. Physiol Rev. 1997;77:75–197.

DiBona GF, Sawin LL. Role of renal nerves in sodium retention of cirrhosis and congestive heart failure. Am J Physiol. 1991;260:R298–305.

DiBona GF, Sawin LL. Increased renal nerve activity in cardiac failure: arterial vs. cardiac baroreflex impairment. Am J Physiol. 1995;268:R112–6.

Dittrich S, Vogel M, Dahnert I, et al. Acute hemodynamic effects of post cardiotomy peritoneal dialysis in neonates and infants. Intensive Care Med. 2000;26:101–4.

Dobell AR, Gutelius JR, Murphy DR. Acidosis following respiratory alkalosis in thoracic operations with and without heart-lung bypass. J Thorac Cardiovasc Surg. 1960;39:312–7.

Duke T, Molyneux EM. Intravenous fluids for seriously ill children: time to reconsider. Lancet. 2003;362:1320–3.

Elliott M. Modified ultrafiltration and open heart surgery in children. Paediatr Anaesth. 1999;9:1–5.

Ely SW, Sawyer DC, Scott JB. Local vasoactivity of oxygen and carbon dioxide in the right coronary circulation of the dog and pig. J Physiol. 1982;332:427–39.

England MR, Gordon G, Salem M, Chernow B. Magnesium administration and dysrhythmias after cardiac surgery. A placebo-controlled, double-blind, randomized trial. JAMA. 1992;268:2395–402.

Feingold B, Law YM. Nesiritide use in pediatric patients with congestive heart failure. J Heart Lung Transplant. 2004;23:1455–9.

Feng X, Yan W, Liu X, et al. Effects of hydroxyethyl starch 130/0.4 on pulmonary capillary leakage and cytokines production and NF-kappaB activation in CLP-induced sepsis in rats. J Surg Res. 2006;135:129–36.

Flynn JT. Choice of dialysis modality for management of pediatric acute renal failure. Pediatr Nephrol. 2002;17:61–9.

Franco-Cereceda A, Kallner G, Lundberg JM. Capsazepine-sensitive release of calcitonin gene-related peptide from C-fibre afferents in the guinea-pig heart by low pH and lactic acid. Eur J Pharmacol. 1993;238:311–6.

Friis-Hansen B. Body water compartments in children: changes during growth and related changes in body composition. Pediatrics. 1961;28:169–81.

Funayama H, Nakamura T, Saito T, et al. Urinary excretion of aquaporin-2 water channel exaggerated dependent upon vasopressin in congestive heart failure. Kidney Int. 2004;66:1387–92.

Gamble J. Chemical anatomy, physiology and pathology of extracellular fluid. Cambridge: Harvard University Press; 1947.

Garcia LA, Dejong SC, Martin SM, et al. Magnesium reduces free radicals in an in vivo coronary occlusion-reperfusion model. J Am Coll Cardiol. 1998;32:536–9.

Garty H. Regulation of Na+ permeability by aldosterone. Semin Nephrol. 1992;12:24–9.

Gibbon Jr JH, Allbritten Jr FF, Stayman Jr JW, Judd JM. A clinical study of respiratory exchange during prolonged operations with an open thorax. Ann Surg. 1950;132:611–25.

Goldstein SL, Currier H, Graf C, et al. Outcome in children receiving continuous venovenous hemofiltration. Pediatrics. 2001;107:1309–12.

Goldstein SL, Somers MJ, Baum MA, et al. Pediatric patients with multi-organ dysfunction syndrome receiving continuous renal replacement therapy. Kidney Int. 2005;67:653–8.

Gries A, Bode C, Gross S, et al. The effect of intravenously administered magnesium on platelet function in patients after cardiac surgery. Anesth Analg. 1999;88:1213–9.

Haase M, Bellomo R, Devarajan P, et al. Accuracy of neutrophil gelatinase-associated lipocalin (NGAL) in diagnosis and prognosis in acute kidney injury: a systematic review and meta-analysis. Am J Kidney Dis. 2009;54:1012–24.

Haase M, Devarajan P, Haase-Fielitz A, et al. The outcome of neutrophil gelatinase-associated lipocalin-positive subclinical acute kidney injury: a multicenter pooled analysis of prospective studies. J Am Coll Cardiol. 2011;57:1752–61.

Haase-Fielitz A, Bellomo R, Devarajan P, et al. Novel and conventional serum biomarkers predicting acute kidney injury in adult cardiac surgery--a prospective cohort study. Crit Care Med. 2009;37:553–60.

Habicher M, Perrino Jr A, Spies CD, et al. Contemporary fluid management in cardiac anesthesia. J Cardiothorac Vasc Anesth. 2011;25:1141–53.

Halpenny M, Lakshmi S, O'Donnell A, et al. Fenoldopam: renal and splanchnic effects in patients undergoing coronary artery bypass grafting. Anaesthesia. 2001;56:953–60.

Harris PJ, Thomas D, Morgan TO. Atrial natriuretic peptide inhibits angiotensin-stimulated proximal tubular sodium and water reabsorption. Nature. 1987;326:697–8.

Hartnoll G, Betremieux P, Modi N. Randomised controlled trial of postnatal sodium supplementation on body composition in 25 to 30 week gestational age infants. Arch Dis Child Fetal Neonatal Ed. 2000a;282:F24–8.

Hartnoll G, Betremieux P, Modi N. Randomised controlled trial of postnatal sodium supplementation on oxygen dependency and body weight in 25–30 week gestational age infants. Arch Dis Child Fetal Neonatal Ed. 2000b;82:F19–23.

Hayashi Y, Ohtani M, Hiraishi T, et al. Synthetic human alpha-atrial natriuretic peptide infusion in management after open heart operations. ASAIO J. 2003;49:320–4.

Haycock G. Disorders of the kidney and urinary tract. In: Rennie J, editor. Roberton's text-book of neonatology. 4th ed. Edinburgh: Elsevier Churchill Livingstone; 2005. p. 929–44.

Hayes LW, Oster RA, Tofil NM, Tolwani AJ. Outcomes of critically ill children requiring continuous renal replacement therapy. J Crit Care. 2009;24:394–400.

Herget-Rosenthal S, Poppen D, Husing J, et al. Prognostic value of tubular proteinuria and enzymuria in nonoliguric acute tubular necrosis. Clin Chem. 2004a;50:552–8.

Herget-Rosenthal S, Marggraf G, Husing J, et al. Early detection of acute renal failure by serum cystatin C. Kidney Int. 2004b;66:1115–22.

Herzog WR, Schlossberg ML, MacMurdy KS, et al. Timing of magnesium therapy affects experimental infarct size. Circulation. 1995;92:2622–6.

Hiramatsu T, Imai Y, Takanashi Y, et al. Hemodynamic effects of human atrial natriuretic peptide after modified Fontan procedure. Ann Thorac Surg. 1998;65:761–4.

Holliday MA, Segar WE. The maintenance need for water in parenteral fluid therapy. Pediatrics. 1957;19:823–32.

Iacobelli S, Loprieno S, Bonsante F, et al. Renal function in early childhood in very low birthweight infants. Am J Perinatol. 2007;24:587–92.

Ichikawa I, Pfeffer JM, Pfeffer MA, et al. Role of angiotensin II in the altered renal function of congestive heart failure. Circ Res. 1984;55:669–75.

Iriz E, Kolbakir F, Akar H, et al. Comparison of hydroxyethyl starch and ringer lactate as a prime solution regarding S-100beta protein levels and informative cognitive tests in cerebral injury. Ann Thorac Surg. 2005;79:666–71.

Ishizaka H, Kuo L. Acidosis-induced coronary arteriolar dilation is mediated by ATP-sensitive potassium channels in vascular smooth muscle. Circ Res. 1996;78:50–7.

Ito I, Faulkner WR, Kolff WJ. Metabolic acidosis and its correction in patients undergoing open-heart operation; experimental basis and clinical results. Cleve Clin Q. 1957;24:193–203.

Jander A, Tkaczyk M, Pagowska-Klimek I, et al. Continuous veno-venous hemodiafiltration in children after cardiac surgery. Eur J Cardiothorac Surg. 2007;31:1022–8.

Jansen LA, Safavi A, Lin Y. Preclosure fluid resuscitation influences outcome in gastroschisis. Am J Perinatol. 2012;29:307–12.

Joao PR, Faria Junior F. Immediate post-operative care following cardiac surgery. J Pediatr (Rio J). 2003;79 Suppl 2:S213–22.

Jose PA, Fildes RD, Gomez RA, et al. Neonatal renal function and physiology. Curr Opin Pediatr. 1994;6:172–7.

Jungheinrich C, Scharpf R, Wargenau M, et al. The pharmacokinetics and tolerability of an intravenous infusion of the new hydroxyethyl starch 130/0.4 (6%, 500 mL) in mild-to-severe renal impairment. Anesth Analg. 2002;95:544–51, table of contents.

Karanko MS, Klossner JA, Laaksonen VO. Restoration of volume by crystalloid versus colloid after coronary artery bypass: hemodynamics, lung water, oxygenation, and outcome. Crit Care Med. 1987;15:559–66.

Kastrup M, Markewitz A, Spies C, et al. Current practice of hemodynamic monitoring and vasopressor and inotropic therapy in post-operative cardiac surgery patients in Germany: results from a postal survey. Acta Anaesthesiol Scand. 2007;51:347–58.

Kellum JA. Clinical review: reunification of acid–base physiology. Crit Care. 2005;9:500–7.

Kimura T, Yasue H, Sakaino N, et al. Effects of magnesium on the tone of isolated human coronary arteries. Comparison with diltiazem and nitroglycerin. Circulation. 1989;79:1118–24.

Kobori H, Nangaku M, Navar LG, et al. The intrarenal renin-angiotensin system: from physiology to the pathobiology of hypertension and kidney disease. Pharmacol Rev. 2007;59:251–87.

Koeppen BM, Stanton BA. The renal system. In: Berne RM, editor. Physiology. 5th ed. New York: Elsevier; 2004.

Koutlas TC, Gaynor JW, Nicolson SC, et al. Modified ultrafiltration reduces postoperative morbidity after cavopulmonary connection. Ann Thorac Surg. 1997;64:37–42. discussion 3.

Krawczeski CD, Vandevoorde RG, Kathman T, et al. Serum cystatin C is an early predictive biomarker of acute kidney injury after pediatric cardiopulmonary bypass. Clin J Am Soc Nephrol. 2010;5:1552–7.

Kuitunen A, Vento A, Suojaranta-Ylinen R, et al. Acute renal failure after cardiac surgery: evaluation of the RIFLE classification. Ann Thorac Surg. 2006;81:542–6.

Lassnigg A, Schmidlin D, Mouhieddine M, et al. Minimal changes of serum creatinine predict prognosis in patients after cardiothoracic surgery: a prospective cohort study. J Am Soc Nephrol. 2004;15:1597–605.

Lauschke A, Teichgraber UK, Frei U, Eckardt KU. 'Low-dose' dopamine worsens renal perfusion in patients with acute renal failure. Kidney Int. 2006;69:1669–74.

Ley SJ, Miller K, Skov P, Preisig P. Crystalloid versus colloid fluid therapy after cardiac surgery. Heart Lung. 1990;19:31–40.

Litwin MS, Panico FG, Rubini C, et al. Acidosis and lacticacidemia in extracorporeal circulation: the significance of perfusion flow rate and the relation to preperfusion respiratory alkalosis. Ann Surg. 1959;149:188–99.

Liu KD, Himmelfarb J, Paganini E, et al. Timing of initiation of dialysis in critically ill patients with acute kidney injury. Clin J Am Soc Nephrol. 2006;1:915–9.

Lopes JA, Fernandes P, Jorge S, et al. Acute kidney injury in intensive care unit patients: a comparison between the RIFLE and the Acute Kidney Injury Network classifications. Crit Care. 2008;12:R110.

Lorenz JM, Kleinman LI, Markarian K. Potassium metabolism in extremely low birth weight infants in the first week of life. J Pediatr. 1997;131:81–6.

Luciani GB, Nichani S, Chang AC, et al. Continuous versus intermittent furosemide infusion in critically ill infants after open heart operations. Ann Thorac Surg. 1997;64:1133–9.

Mahle WT, Cuadrado AR, Kirshbom PM, et al. Nesiritide in infants and children with congestive heart failure. Pediatr Crit Care Med. 2005;6:543–6.

Malan AF, Evans A, Heese HD. Serial acid–base determinations in normal premature and full-term infants during the first 72 hours of life. Arch Dis Child. 1965;40:645–50.

Marik PE, Baram M, Vahid B. Does central venous pressure predict fluid responsiveness? A systematic review of the literature and the tale of seven mares. Chest. 2008;134:172–8.

Marin-Grez M, Fleming JT, Steinhausen M. Atrial natriuretic peptide causes pre-glomerular vasodilatation and post-glomerular vasoconstriction in rat kidney. Nature. 1986;324:473–6.

Mehta RL, Pascual MT, Soroko S, Chertow GM. Diuretics, mortality, and nonrecovery of renal function in acute renal failure. JAMA. 2002;288:2547–53.

Mehta RL, Kellum JA, Shah SV, et al. Acute Kidney Injury Network: report of an initiative to improve outcomes in acute kidney injury. Crit Care. 2007;11:R31.

Merkle F, Boettcher W, Schulz F, et al. Perfusion technique for nonhaemic cardiopulmonary bypass prime in neonates and infants under 6 kg body weight. Perfusion. 2004;19:229–37.

Mishra J, Ma Q, Prada A, et al. Identification of neutrophil gelatinase-associated lipocalin as a novel early urinary biomarker for ischemic renal injury. J Am Soc Nephrol. 2003;14:2534–43.

Mishra J, Dent C, Tarabishi R, et al. Neutrophil gelatinase-associated lipocalin (NGAL) as a biomarker for acute renal injury after cardiac surgery. Lancet. 2005;365:1231–8.

Mitra S, Khandelwal P. Are all colloids same? How to select the right colloid? Indian J Anaesth. 2009;53:592–607.

Modi N. Fluid and electrolyte balance. In: Rennie J, editor. Roberton's textbook of neonatology. 4th ed. Edinburgh: Churchill Livingstone; 2005. p. 335–54.

Moffett BS, Jefferies JL, Price JF, et al. Administration of a large nesiritide bolus dose in a pediatric patient: case report and review of nesiritide use in pediatrics. Pharmacotherapy. 2006;26: 277–80.

Morelli S, Ricci Z, Di Chiara L, et al. Renal replacement therapy in neonates with congenital heart disease. Contrib Nephrol. 2007;156:428–33.

Morgan TJ. The meaning of acid–base abnormalities in the intensive care unit: part III -- effects of fluid administration. Crit Care. 2005;9:204–11.

Musso CG, Ghezzi L, Ferraris J. Renal physiology in newborns and old people: similar characteristics but different mechanisms. Int Urol Nephrol. 2004;36:273–6.

Myburgh JA, Mythen MG. Resuscitation fluids. N Engl J Med. 2013;69:2462–3.

Myburgh JA, Finfer S, Bellomo R, et al. Hydroxyethyl starch or saline for fluid resuscitation in intensive care. N Engl J Med. 2012;367:1901–11.

Nafday S. Renal disease. In: MacDonald MG, Mullett MD, Seshia MMK, editors. Avery's neonatology-pathophysiology and the management of the newborn. 6th ed. Philadelphia: Lippincott; 2005. p. 981–1056.

Naik SK, Elliott MJ. Ultrafiltration and paediatric cardiopulmonary bypass. Perfusion. 1993;8: 101–12.

Naik SK, Knight A, Elliott MJ. A successful modification of ultrafiltration for cardiopulmonary bypass in children. Perfusion. 1991a;6:41–50.

Naik SK, Knight A, Elliott M. A prospective randomized study of a modified technique of ultrafiltration during pediatric open-heart surgery. Circulation. 1991b;84:III422–31.

Narins RG, Gardner LB. Simple acid–base disturbances. Med Clin North Am. 1981;65:321–46.

O'Brien F, Walker IA. Fluid homeostasis in the neonate. Paediatr Anaesth. 2014;24:49–59.

Osman D, Ridel C, Ray P, et al. Cardiac filling pressures are not appropriate to predict hemodynamic response to volume challenge. Crit Care Med. 2007;35:64–8.

Otsuki DA, Fantoni DT, Margarido CB, et al. Hydroxyethyl starch is superior to lactated Ringer as a replacement fluid in a pig model of acute normovolaemic haemodilution. Br J Anaesth. 2007;98:29–37.

Palevsky PM. Clinical review: timing and dose of continuous renal replacement therapy in acute kidney injury. Crit Care. 2007;11:232.

Parakininkas D, Greenbaum LA. Comparison of solute clearance in three modes of continuous renal replacement therapy. Pediatr Crit Care Med. 2004;5:269–74.

Parikh CR, Jani A, Melnikov VY, et al. Urinary interleukin-18 is a marker of human acute tubular necrosis. Am J Kidney Dis. 2004;43:405–14.

Pedersen K. Acute kidney injury in children undergoing surgery for congenital heart disease. Eur J Pediatr Surg. 2012;22:426–33.

Pedersen RS, Bentzen H, Bech JN, et al. Urinary aquaporin-2 in healthy humans and patients with liver cirrhosis and chronic heart failure during baseline conditions and after acute water load. Kidney Int. 2003;63:1417–25.

Perner A, Haase N, Guttormsen AB, et al. Hydroxyethyl starch 130/0.42 versus Ringer's acetate in severe sepsis. N Engl J Med. 2012;367:124–34.

Picca S, Principato F, Mazzera E, et al. Risks of acute renal failure after cardiopulmonary bypass surgery in children: a retrospective 10-year case–control study. Nephrol Dial Transplant. 1995;10:630–6.

Picca S, Ricci Z, Picardo S. Acute kidney injury in an infant after cardiopulmonary bypass. Semin Nephrol. 2008;28:470–6.

Plotz FB, Bouma AB, van Wijk JA, et al. Pediatric acute kidney injury in the ICU: an independent evaluation of pRIFLE criteria. Intensive Care Med. 2008;34:1713–7.

Pradeep A, Rajagopalam S, Kolli HK, et al. High volumes of intravenous fluid during cardiac surgery are associated with increased mortality. HSR Proc Intensive Care Cardiovasc Anesth. 2010;2:287–96.

Price JF, Mott AR, Dickerson HA, et al. Worsening renal function in children hospitalized with decompensated heart failure: evidence for a pediatric cardiorenal syndrome? Pediatr Crit Care Med. 2008;9:279–84.

Rackow EC, Falk JL, Fein IA, et al. Fluid resuscitation in circulatory shock: a comparison of the cardiorespiratory effects of albumin, hetastarch, and saline solutions in patients with hypovolemic and septic shock. Crit Care Med. 1983;11:839–50.

Ravn HB, Moeldrup U, Brookes CI, et al. Intravenous magnesium reduces infarct size after ischemia/reperfusion injury combined with a thrombogenic lesion in the left anterior descending artery. Arterioscler Thromb Vasc Biol. 1999;19:569–74.

Reuter DA, Huang C, Edrich T, et al. Cardiac output monitoring using indicator-dilution techniques: basics, limits, and perspectives. Anesth Analg. 2010;110:799–811.

Ricci Z, Cruz D, Ronco C. The RIFLE criteria and mortality in acute kidney injury: a systematic review. Kidney Int. 2008a;73:538–46.

Ricci Z, Stazi GV, Di Chiara L, et al. Fenoldopam in newborn patients undergoing cardiopulmonary bypass: controlled clinical trial. Interact Cardiovasc Thorac Surg. 2008b;7: 1049–53.

Ricci Z, Morelli S, Ronco C, et al. Inotropic support and peritoneal dialysis adequacy in neonates after cardiac surgery. Interact Cardiovasc Thorac Surg. 2008c;7:116–20.

Ricci Z, Iacoella C, Cogo P. Fluid management in critically ill pediatric patients with congenital heart disease. Minerva Pediatr. 2011a;63:399–410.

Ricci Z, Luciano R, Favia I, et al. High-dose fenoldopam reduces postoperative neutrophil gelatinase-associated lipocaline and cystatin C levels in pediatric cardiac surgery. Crit Care. 2011b;15:R160.

Robillard JE, Gomez RA, VanOrden D, et al. Comparison of the adrenal and renal responses to angiotensin II fetal lambs and adult sheep. Circ Res. 1982;50:140–7.

Ronco C, Bellomo R. Basic mechanisms and definitions for continuous renal replacement therapies. Int J Artif Organs. 1996;19:95–9.

Ronco C, Ricci Z. Pediatric continuous renal replacement: 20 years later. Intensive Care Med. 2015;41(6):985–93.

Rosner MH, Okusa MD. Acute kidney injury associated with cardiac surgery. Clin J Am Soc Nephrol. 2006;1:19–32.

Rudolph AM, Heymann MA. The fetal circulation. Annu Rev Med. 1968;19:195–206.

Sadowski RH, Harmon WE, Jabs K. Acute hemodialysis of infants weighing less than five kilograms. Kidney Int. 1994;45:903–6.

Sasser WC, Dabal RJ, Askenazi DJ, et al. Prophylactic peritoneal dialysis following cardiopulmonary bypass in children is associated with decreased inflammation and improved clinical outcomes. Congenit Heart Dis. 2014;9:106–15.

Schrier RW, Masoumi A, Elhassan E. Aldosterone: role in edematous disorders, hypertension, chronic renal failure, and metabolic syndrome. Clin J Am Soc Nephrol. 2010;5:1132–40.

Schwartz GJ, Brion LP, Spitzer A. The use of plasma creatinine concentration for estimating glomerular filtration rate in infants, children, and adolescents. Pediatr Clin North Am. 1987;34: 571–90.

Selewski DT, Cornell TT, Lombel RM, et al. Weight-based determination of fluid overload status and mortality in pediatric intensive care unit patients requiring continuous renal replacement therapy. Intensive Care Med. 2011;37:1166–73.

Shaw AD, Bagshaw SM, Goldstein SL, et al. Major complications, mortality, and resource utilization after open abdominal surgery: 0.9% saline compared to Plasma-Lyte. Ann Surg. 2012;255:821–9.

Sieber FE, Traystman RJ. Special issues: glucose and the brain. Crit Care Med. 1992;20:104–14.

Singh NC, Kissoon N, al Mofada S, et al. Comparison of continuous versus intermittent furosemide administration in postoperative pediatric cardiac patients. Crit Care Med. 1992;20: 17–21.

Smith T, Rosen DA, Russo P, et al. Nesiritide during extracorporeal membrane oxygenation. Paediatr Anaesth. 2005;15:152–7.

Soderlind M, Salvignol G, Izard P, et al. Use of albumin, blood transfusion and intraoperative glucose by APA and ADARPEF members: a postal survey. Paediatr Anaesth. 2001;11:685–9.

Stalker HP, Holland NH, Kotchen JM, et al. Plasma renin activity in healthy children. J Pediatr. 1967;89:256–8.

Stephens BE, Gargus RA, Walden RV. Fluid regimens in the first week of life may increase risk of patent ductus arteriosus in extremely low birth weight infants. J Perinatol. 2008;28:123–8.

Suempelmann R, Vennari M, Agrò FE. Fluid management in pediatric patients. In: Agrò FE, editor. Body fluid management – from physiology to therapy. Milan: Springer; 2013.

Sulemanji M, Vakili K. Neonatal renal physiology. Semin Pediatr Surg. 2013;22:195–8.

Sumpelmann R, Mader T, Eich C, et al. A novel isotonic-balanced electrolyte solution with 1% glucose for intraoperative fluid therapy in children: results of a prospective multicentre observational post-authorization safety study (PASS). Paediatr Anaesth. 2010;20:977–81.

Sumpelmann R, Becke K, Crean P, et al. European consensus statement for intraoperative fluid therapy in children. Eur J Anaesthesiol. 2011;28:637–9.

Sutherland SM, Zappitelli M, Alexander SR, et al. Fluid overload and mortality in children receiving continuous renal replacement therapy: the prospective pediatric continuous renal replacement therapy registry. Am J Kidney Dis. 2010;55:316–25.

Symons JM, Chua AN, Somers MJ, et al. Demographic characteristics of pediatric continuous renal replacement therapy: a report of the prospective pediatric continuous renal replacement therapy registry. Clin J Am Soc Nephrol. 2007;2:732–8.

Teboul JL, Monnet X. Detecting volume responsiveness and unresponsiveness in intensive care unit patients: two different problems, only one solution. Crit Care. 2009;13:175.

Tufro-McReddie A, Harrison JK, Everett AD, et al. Ontogeny of type 1 angiotensin II receptor gene expression in the rat. J Clin Invest. 1993;91:530–7.

Uchino S, Bellomo R, Morimatsu H, et al. Discontinuation of continuous renal replacement therapy: a post hoc analysis of a prospective multicenter observational study. Crit Care Med. 2009;37:2576–82.

Venkataraman PS, Blick KE, Fry HD, et al. Postnatal changes in calcium-regulating hormones in very-low-birth-weight infants. Effect of early neonatal hypocalcemia and intravenous calcium infusion on serum parathyroid hormone and calcitonin homeostasis. Am J Dis Child. 1985;139:913–6.

Verheij J, van Lingen A, Beishuizen A, et al. Cardiac response is greater for colloid than saline fluid loading after cardiac or vascular surgery. Intensive Care Med. 2006a;32:1030–8.

Verheij J, van Lingen A, Raijmakers PG, et al. Effect of fluid loading with saline or colloids on pulmonary permeability, oedema and lung injury score after cardiac and major vascular surgery. Br J Anaesth. 2006b;96:21–30.

Wei CM, Kao PC, Lin JT, et al. Circulating beta-atrial natriuretic factor in congestive heart failure in humans. Circulation. 1993;88:1016–20.

Welborn LG, McGill WA, Hannallah RS, et al. Perioperative blood glucose concentrations in pediatric outpatients. Anesthesiology. 1986;65:543–7.

Welke KF, Dearani JA, Ghanayem NS, et al. Renal complications associated with the treatment of patients with congenital cardiac disease: consensus definitions from the Multi-Societal Database Committee for Pediatric and Congenital Heart Disease. Cardiol Young. 2008;18 Suppl 2:222–5.

Wiedemann HP, Wheeler AP, Bernard GR, et al. Comparison of two fluid-management strategies in acute lung injury. N Engl J Med. 2006;354:2564–75.

Wiesenack C, Prasser C, Keyl C, Rodig G. Assessment of intrathoracic blood volume as an indicator of cardiac preload: single transpulmonary thermodilution technique versus assessment of pressure preload parameters derived from a pulmonary artery catheter. J Cardiothorac Vasc Anesth. 2001;15:584–8.

Yared II A. Postnatal development of glomerular filtration. In: Polin RA, Fox WW, editors. Fetal and neonatal physiology. 2nd ed. Philadelphia: W.B. Saunders Co; 2004. p. 1588–92.

Yared A, Yoshioka T. Uncoupling of the autoregulation of renal blood flow and glomerular filtration rate in immature rats: role of the renin-angiotensin system. Kidney Int. 1988;33:414.

Young R. Perioperative fluid and electrolyte management in cardiac surgery: a review. J Extra Corpor Technol. 2012;44:P20–6.

Yunos NM, Bellomo R, Hegarty C, et al. Association between a chloride-liberal vs chloride-restrictive intravenous fluid administration strategy and kidney injury in critically ill adults. JAMA. 2012;308:1566–72.

Zappitelli M, Goldstein SL, Symons JM, et al. Protein and calorie prescription for children and young adults receiving continuous renal replacement therapy: a report from the Prospective Pediatric Continuous Renal Replacement Therapy Registry Group. Crit Care Med. 2008;36:3239–45.

Part VI
Anesthesia and Critical Care Outside the
Cardiac Operating Room

Chapter 41
Congenital Cardiac Intensive Care and Management of Cardiac Arrest

Pooja Nawathe

Background

Congenital heart disease (CHD) is the most common congenital anomaly with a worldwide prevalence of 9 per 1000 live births (van der Linde et al. 2011). Congenital heart disease incidence has remained stable (Hoffman and Kaplan 2002), but longevity has improved. Since the advent of neonatal repair of complex lesions in the 1970s, an estimated 85 % of patients survive into adult life. Over 90 % of infants born with congenital heart anomalies can now expect to reach adulthood (Khairy et al. 2010), and it is anticipated that almost 1 in 150 young adults in the next decade will have some form of CHD (Khairy et al. 2008).

Adults with congenital heart disease remain at risk for frequent hospitalizations (Somerville 1997). In a study by O'Leary et al. (2013) from 1998 to 2010, adult admission volume was 87.8 % higher during the second half of the study period compared with the first half, while pediatric admissions only grew by 32.8 %. While many neonatal to childhood operations are viewed as "corrective" in terms of reestablishing normal physiology, the need for reoperation or other interventions later in life are quite common.

Congenital Cardiac Critical Care is an evolving multidisciplinary field with the congenital heart disease specialist (pediatric and adult), congenital cardiac surgeon, perfusionist, pediatric and adult congenital cardiac nurses, advanced nurse practitioners, respiratory therapists, child life therapist, and family members. Optimal care of the neonate, infant, adolescent, and adult with CHD requires an understanding of complex congenital cardiac anomalies, cardiopulmonary interactions, transitional circulation of the neonate, cardiopulmonary bypass (CPB) effects, airway management, multiorgan system management, and mechanical ventilation.

P. Nawathe, MD, FAAP
Congenital Heart Program, Cedars-Sinai Heart Institute,
127 S. SanVicente Blvd, Suite A3409, Los Angeles, CA 90048, USA
e-mail: Pooja.Nawathe@csmc.edu

© Springer International Publishing Switzerland 2017
A. Dabbagh et al. (eds.), *Congenital Heart Disease in Pediatric and Adult Patients*, DOI 10.1007/978-3-319-44691-2_41

Cardiovascular Physiology and Shock

Circulatory dysfunction occurs when the cardiovascular system is unable to deliver oxygen and nutrients to the tissues at a rate that fulfills their metabolic demands (demand >supply). This causes many of the compensatory mechanisms to be activated. When this cardiovascular failure occurs acutely, shock ensues. When chronic cardiovascular failure exists, supply cannot meet necessary increases in demand, congestive heart failure occurs. This leads to compensatory mechanisms functioning at or near their maximum for substance delivery.

Oxygen extraction ratio (O_2Er)
$O_2ER = SaO_2 - SmvO_2/SaO_2$
SaO_2, arterial O_2 saturation; $SmvO_2$, mixed venous O_2 saturation; oxygen extraction
   ratios based on mixed venous oximetry
25 % normal
30–40 % increased
40–50 % impending shock
>50–60 % shock, elevated lactate levels
Normal O_2 extraction ratios for central venous oximetry
Right atrium 25 %
Jugular vein 35 %, superior vena cava 30 %, inferior vena cava 20 %

Pulmonary Vascular Resistance (PVR) and Pulmonary Blood Flow (PBF) Regulation

Thorough understanding of the pharmacologic and ventilator management of PVR is crucial for the management of CHD patients. Medical conditions, created in the OR and ICU, increase reactivity and resistance of the PVR and may be significantly risky if not done with appropriate knowledge and skills. CPB, endotracheal suctioning, decreasing lung volumes (pneumothoraces, surgically retracting, intrabdominal hypertension, pleural and peritoneal collections), alveolar hypoxia, and hypoventilation can alter PVR.

Hypoventilation with associated acidosis and hypercapnia increases PVR. Hyperventilation to a pH of >7.50 reliably decreases PVR. Hyperventilation is not a preferred long-term measure to decrease PVR as it decreases cerebral blood flow.

Heart Disease and Cerebral Function

In children, complications of cardiac surgery are one of the major sources of neurodevelopmental sequelae of CHD. The most prominent of the acute complications are focal and generalized seizures, intracranial hemorrhage, and spinal cord infarction. Cerebral palsy, gait disorders, seizures, and learning disorders are the chronic problems.

Pharmacology

The following two tables summarize the various catecholamine end organ receptors with physiologic actions.

Epidemiology, Prevention, and Outcome of In-Hospital Cardiopulmonary Arrest in CHD Patients

In 1999, Rhodes et al. (1999) showed that the outcome of cardiac arrest in infants after congenital heart surgery was better than that for pediatric intensive care unit populations as a whole. Univentricular physiology did not increase the risk of death after cardiac arrest. Infants with more hemodynamic compromise before the arrest as demonstrated with lower mean arterial blood pressure and higher inotropic support were less likely to survive.

Diagnosis of Cardiac Arrest

For the child who suffers a cardiac arrest in the OR, electronic monitoring will generally alert the anesthesiologist to an actual or impending cardiac arrest. The electrocardiogram (ECG) may indicate nonperfusing rhythms such as ventricular fibrillation and asystole, end-tidal carbon dioxide (ETCO$_2$) may decrease precipitously reflecting a decrease in cardiac output as a result of a decreased delivery of carbon dioxide (CO$_2$) to the lungs, and a pulse oximeter may lose its regular waveform in the absence of pulsatile blood flow. Granting the importance of these monitors, the diagnosis of cardiopulmonary arrest still rests on the absence of a pulse in a major artery (e.g., carotid, femoral, or brachial artery) as determined by palpation in the presence of unconsciousness and apnea.

Mechanics of Cardiopulmonary Resuscitation

Management proceeds along the well-known airway, breathing, circulation (ABC) algorithm with the exception that the child with ventricular fibrillation or pulseless ventricular tachycardia should receive electrical defibrillation without delay. Airway access in children with ventricular fibrillation or pulseless ventricular tachycardia should be performed secondarily. CPR should be continued without interruption until a shock can be delivered.

Airway

Before tracheal intubation, the child's airway can usually be managed effectively with bag-valve-mask (BVM) ventilation with proper head positioning and jaw thrust. Although tracheal intubation ensures optimal control of the airway for effective ventilation, multiple attempts at tracheal intubation by an inexperienced operator may seriously compromise the airway and increases the cumulative duration of "no-flow" (i.e., no CPR) time.

In the child without an artificial airway, the use of BVM devices may result in a significant risk of gastric inflation, followed by pulmonary aspiration of gastric contents. Abdominal distention (gastric and bowel) can significantly compromise oxygenation; therefore, the stomach should be vented when excessive gastric inflation occurs. One study found a 28 % incidence of pulmonary aspiration in a series of failed resuscitations (Lawes and Baskett 1987). For this reason as well as for the risk of barotrauma and volutrauma, excessive inflation pressures should be avoided. However, effective bilateral ventilation is best judged by visualizing bilateral chest excursions and listening to the quality of the breath sounds rather than setting a preset maximal inflation pressure.

Tracheal intubation should be performed as soon as appropriate personnel and equipment are available. The $ETCO_2$ is a valuable method of confirming the correct placement of the tracheal tube. In the absence of capnography, a disposable colorimetric $ETCO_2$ device serves the same purpose. However, it is important to appreciate that $ETCO_2$ measurements are meaningful only in the presence of effective pulmonary circulation, such that a lack of color change may reflect either improper placement of the tube or a lack of pulmonary blood flow resulting from ineffective chest compressions or a massive pulmonary embolism. It is also essential to use the proper size colorimetric device for the child's weight because the adult size may not detect the presence of CO_2 and may lead the user to misdiagnose a successful intubation.

Breathing

In the inpatient environment, equipment necessary to ventilate the lungs emergently should be readily available. Because the equipment provided for emergency ventilatory support may differ from standard equipment, depending on the location within a hospital, the anesthesiologist needs to be familiar with all of the equipment in the hospital in which he or she practices. Anesthesiologists are skilled providers of ventilatory support, but in the context of a cardiac arrest, must return to the basics and remember that *if there is no chest movement, there is no ventilation*. If no chest movement occurs during BVM ventilation despite an apparently good seal between the mask and the child's face, the underlying cause, be it upper airway obstruction, whether anatomic or presence of a foreign body, bilateral tension pneumothoraces, or severe bronchospasm must be considered.

Table 41.1a Endogenous receptors of the sympathetic nervous system and their activation effects

Location	Type of receptor	Effects of simulation
Heart		
Sinus node	β_1	Increase in heart rate
Atrioventricular node	β_1	Increase in heart rate
Coronary circulation	α	Vasoconstriction
Coronary circulation	DA	Vasodilation
Peripheral vasculature		
Pulmonary	α	Vasoconstriction
Renal	DA	Vasodilation
Mesenteric and splanchnic	DA, β_1	Vasodilation
Skin	α	Vasoconstriction
Skeletal muscle	β_1	Vasodilation
Nonvascular		
Bronchial tree	β_2	Bronchodilation
Renal tubule	DA	Diuresis

Overventilation is common during CPR, resulting in greater mean intrathoracic pressures than required, which decreases venous return and reduces cardiac output (Aufderheide et al. 2004). In cardiopulmonary arrest, less than normal minute ventilation may be appropriate, because cardiac output and delivery of CO_2 to the lungs are diminished. If an artificial airway is not in place for single person rescue, two breaths should be given for each 30 chest compressions. If an artificial airway is not in place for two person rescue, two breaths should be given after each 15 chest compressions. Once an artificial airway is in place, a ventilator rate of 8–10 per minute *without* pausing during rapid chest compressions should be used (Tables 41.1a and 41.1b).

Circulation

During cardiac arrest, chest compressions provide the sole perfusion to a child's vital organs; therefore, optimal performance of CPR is critical. Key elements to providing quality chest compressions include (1) ensuring an adequate rate (100 compressions per minute), (2) ensuring adequate chest wall depression (one third to half of the anteroposterior chest diameter), (3) releasing completely between compressions to allow full chest wall recoil, (4) minimizing interruptions in chest compressions, and (5) ensuring that the child is on a sufficiently hard surface to allow effective chest compressions (ECC Committee, Subcommittees and Task Forces of the American Heart Association 2005). In short, push hard and push fast, release completely, and do not interrupt compressions unnecessarily. Incomplete recoil during CPR is associated with higher intrathoracic pressures and significantly decreased venous return, and coronary and cerebral perfusion (Berg et al. 2010).

Table 41.1b Physiological effects of different agents

Drug	Receptor					Effects					
	α	β_1	β_2	DA	Na^+/K^+ ATPase	CO	Contractility	SVR	MAP	PCWP	HR
Dopamine	++	++	+	++		↑↑	↑	↑↔↓	↑↔	↑↔	↑
Dobutamine	+	+++	+			↑↑	↑↔	↓	↓↔	↔	↑↔
Isoproterenol		+++	+++			↑↑	↔	↓↓	↓	↓	↑↑
Milrinone						↑↑	↑	↓↓	↓↔	↑↔	↑↔
Epinephrine	+++	+++	+++			↑↑	↑↔	↑↔↓	↑↔	↑↔	↔/↑/↑↑
Norepinephrine	+++	+				↑↔↓	↑	↑↑↑	↑↑	↑↔	↑/↑↑
Nitroprusside						↑	↔	↓↓	↓	↓	↑↔
Nitroglycerin						↑	↔	↓	↓	↓↔	↑↔
Enalapril						↑	↔	↓	↓	↓↔	↑↔
Digoxin					+++	↑	↑				

ATPase adenosine triphosphatase, *DA* dopamine, *CO* cardiac output, *SVR* systemic vascular resistance, *HR* heart rate, *MAP* mean arterial pressure, *PCWP* pulmonary capillary wedge pressure

If a child is small enough (e.g., younger than 6 months) that the person providing chest compressions can comfortably encircle the chest with his or her hands, chest compressions should be performed using the circumferential technique, with thumbs depressing the sternum and the fingers supporting the infant's back and circumferentially squeezing the thorax. In larger infants, the sternum can be compressed using two fingers, and in the child, either one or two hands can be used, depending on the size of the child and of the rescuer (Berg et al. 2010). Whichever method is used, focused attention must remain on delivering effective compressions with *minimal interruptions* (Kleinman et al. 2010). In all cases other than circumferential CPR, a backboard must be used. Properly delivered chest compressions are tiring to the provider, and providers should rotate approximately every 2 min to prevent compressor fatigue and deterioration in the quality and rate of chest compressions (Berg et al. 2010).

Mechanisms of Blood Flow

External chest compressions provide cardiac output through two mechanisms: the cardiac pump mechanism and the thoracic pump mechanism. By the cardiac pump mechanism of blood flow, blood is squeezed from the heart by compression of the heart between the sternum and the vertebral column, exiting the heart only anterograde because of the closure of the atrioventricular valves. Between compressions, ventricular pressure decreases below atrial pressure, allowing the atrioventricular valves to open and the ventricles to fill. This sequence of events resembles the normal cardiac cycle. Although the cardiac pump is likely not the dominant blood flow mechanism during most closed-chest CPR, specific clinical situations have been identified in which the cardiac pump mechanism is more prominent. For example, a smaller, more compliant chest may allow for more direct cardiac compression. Increasing the applied force during chest compressions also increases the likelihood of direct cardiac compression.

Several observations do not support the cardiac pump as the primary mechanism of blood flow during CPR. Angiographic studies show that blood passes from the vena cava through the right heart into the pulmonary artery and from the pulmonary veins through the left heart into the aorta during a single chest compression (Niemann et al. 1981; Cohen et al. 1982). Echocardiographic studies show that the atrioventricular valves are open during blood ejection (Niemann et al. 1981; Werner et al. 1981; Rich et al. 1981). Without the closure of the atrioventricular valves during chest compression, the cardiac pump mechanisms cannot account for forward movement of blood during CPR.

In 1976, Criley and colleagues (1976) made the dramatic observation that several patients who developed ventricular fibrillation during cardiac catheterization produced enough blood flow to maintain consciousness by repetitive coughing (Criley et al. 1976). The production of blood flow by increasing thoracic pressure without direct cardiac compression describes the thoracic pump mechanism, in which the heart is a passive conduit for blood flow. The intrathoracic pressure is greater than the extrathoracic pressure during the compression phase of CPR, at which time blood flows out of the thorax, with venous valves preventing excessive retrograde blood flow. Experimental and clinical data support both mechanisms of blood flow during CPR in human infants.

Rate and Duty Cycle

The recommended rate of chest compressions for all patients is 100 per minute, with great care taken to minimize interruptions in chest compressions and to ensure adequate compression depth (Kleinman et al. 2010). This rate represents a compromise that attempts to maximize contributions from both the thoracic pump and cardiac pump mechanism of blood flow.

Duty cycle is defined as the percent of the compression–relaxation cycle that is devoted to compression. If blood flow is generated by direct cardiac compression, then primarily the force of compression determines the stroke volume. Prolonging the compression (increasing the duty cycle) beyond the time necessary for full ventricular ejection should have no additional effect on stroke volume. Increasing the rate of compressions should increase cardiac output, because a fixed volume of blood is ejected with each cardiac compression. In contrast, if blood flow is produced by the thoracic pump mechanism, the volume of blood that is ejected comes from a large reservoir of blood contained within the capacitance vessels in the chest. With the thoracic pump mechanism, flow is enhanced by increasing either the force of compression or the duty cycle but is not affected by changes in compression rate over a wide range of rates, given a set duty cycle (Chandra et al. 1990).

Different animal models yield conflicting results as to the optimal compression rate and duty cycle. However, a rate of compression during conventional CPR of 100 per minute satisfies both those who prefer the faster rates and those who support a longer duty cycle. This is true because it is easier to produce a longer duty cycle when compressions are administered at a faster rate (Maier et al. 1984; Ornato et al. 1988).

Defibrillation and Cardioversion

In children with ventricular fibrillation or pulseless ventricular tachycardia, the immediate management should be defibrillation, without delay to secure an airway.

Electric Countershock

Electric countershock, or defibrillation, is the treatment of choice for ventricular fibrillation and pulseless ventricular tachycardia. Defibrillation should not be delayed to secure an airway, because the likelihood of restoring an organized rhythm decreases with increased duration of fibrillation. Ventricular fibrillation is terminated by simultaneous depolarization and sustained contraction of a critical mass of myocardium (Zipes et al. 1975), allowing the return of spontaneous, coordinated cardiac contractions, assuming the myocardium is well oxygenated and the acid–base status is relatively normal. Drug treatment may be required as an adjunct to defibrillation, but by itself cannot be relied on to terminate ventricular fibrillation.

An older generation of defibrillator that is still present in many hospitals delivers energy in a monophasic damped sinusoidal waveform. This type of instrument delivers a single, unidirectional current with a gradual decrease to zero current. By contrast, the newer generation of biphasic defibrillator delivers a current in a positive direction for a set period, followed by a reversal in current. Biphasic defibrillators are more effective than monophasic defibrillators in terminating ventricular fibrillation in adults; therefore, their use is recommended where possible. If available, use of pediatric attenuator pads or a pediatric mode on the AED should be used in children 1–8 years of age, but if unavailable (and a standard defibrillator is similarly unavailable), an unmodified AED should be used.

In the majority of adult cases, energy levels of 100–200 J are successful when shocks are delivered with minimal delay (Weaver et al. 1982; Campbell et al. 1977). The goal of defibrillation is to deliver a minimum of electrical energy to a critical mass of ventricular muscle while avoiding excessive current that could further damage the heart. The most reliable predictor of success of defibrillation is the duration of fibrillation before the first countershock (Kerber and Sarnat 1979). Acidosis and hypoxemia also decrease the success of defibrillation (Kerber and Sarnat 1979).

Practical Aspects of Defibrillation in Children

Correct paddle size and position are critical to the success of defibrillation. The largest paddle size appropriate for the child should be used because a larger size reduces the density of current flow, which in turn reduces myocardial damage. In general, adult paddles should be used in children weighing more than 10 kg, and infant paddles should be used in infants weighing less than 10 kg. Paddle force is important as well. If the entire paddle does not rest *firmly* on the chest wall, a current of increased density will be delivered to a small contact point. Paddles should be positioned on the chest wall so that the bulk of myocardium lies directly between them. One paddle is placed to the right of the upper sternum below the clavicle; the other is positioned just caudad and to the left of the left nipple. For children with dextrocardia, the position of the paddles should be a mirror image. An alternative approach is to place one paddle anteriorly over the left precordium and the other paddle posteriorly between the scapulae.

The interface between the paddle and chest wall can be gel pads, electrode cream, or electrode paste. The electrode cream produces less impedance than the paste. *Electric current follows the path of least resistance, so care should be taken that the interface material from one paddle does not touch that of the other paddle. This is especially important in infants, in whom the distance between paddles is small.* If the gel is continuous between paddles, a short circuit is created, and an insufficient amount of current will traverse the heart. The use of bare metal paddles increases the risk of arcing and worsens cutaneous burns from defibrillation. The use of self-adhesive pads is preferable when feasible.

In an oxygen (O_2)-enriched atmosphere, sparking from poorly applied defibrillator paddles can cause a fire. Therefore, any sources of free-flowing O_2 should be removed to a distance of at least 1 m from the child. These potentially hazardous O_2 sources include nasal cannula O_2, "blow-by" O_2, and nebulizers powered by O_2. By contrast, O_2 in a closed circuit may remain on the child. For example, it is not necessary to disconnect the ventilator from the child's tracheal tube (if a ventilator is disconnected, the fresh gas flow should be turned off because large volumes of O_2 flow through disconnected ventilators).

For the first defibrillation attempt, 2 J/kg of delivered energy should be administered. After shock delivery, CPR should resume immediately with chest compressions for five duty cycles (2 min). If one shock fails to eliminate ventricular fibrillation, the incremental benefit of another immediate shock is small. Resumption of CPR is likely to confer a greater benefit than another shock. CPR may provide coronary perfusion, increasing the likelihood of defibrillation with a subsequent shock. It is important to minimize the time between chest compressions and shock delivery and between shock delivery and resumption of postshock compressions (Kleinman et al. 2010). Approximately 2 min of CPR should be delivered before a second attempt at defibrillation at twice the original energy level (4 J/kg) (Kleinman et al. 2010).

If ventricular fibrillation or pulseless ventricular tachycardia persists beyond the second defibrillation attempt, standard doses of epinephrine should be administered (with subsequent doses every 3–5 min during persistent cardiac arrest). After 2 min of chest compressions, defibrillation should be attempted again, followed by administration of amiodarone (5 mg/kg) or lidocaine (1 mg/kg) with subsequent defibrillation attempts. It is not necessary to increase the energy level on each successive shock during defibrillation after the second dose. However, successful defibrillation has been reported with currents in excess of 4 J/kg without adverse sequelae, up to a maximum dose not exceeding 10 J/kg or the adult level, whichever is less (Kleinman et al. 2010). This sometimes occurs when a fixed energy level, adult automated external defibrillator (AED) is used in a small child.

Open-Chest Defibrillation

If the chest is already open in the OR or easily opened as in a fresh postoperative cardiac patient, ventricular fibrillation should be treated with open-chest defibrillation, using internal paddles applied directly to the heart. These should have a diameter of 6 cm for adults, 4 cm for children, and 2 cm for infants. Handles should be insulated. Saline-soaked pads or gauzes should be placed between the paddles and the heart. One electrode is placed behind the left ventricle and the other over the right ventricle on the anterior surface of the heart. The energy level used should begin at 5 J in infants and 20 J in adults.

Automated External Defibrillation

The use of AEDs is now a standard therapy in out-of-hospital resuscitation of adults (Berg et al. 2010; Weaver et al. 1982). AEDs are now deemed appropriate for use in children older than 1 year. If available, the use of pediatric attenuator pads or a pediatric mode on the AED should be used in children 1–8 years of age, but if unavailable (and a standard defibrillator is similarly unavailable), an unmodified AED should be used.

Transcutaneous Cardiac Pacing

In the absence of in situ pacing wires or an indwelling transvenous or esophageal pacing catheter, transcutaneous cardiac pacing (TCP) is the preferred method for temporary electrical cardiac pacing in children with asystole or severe bradycardia. TCP is indicated for children whose primary problem is impulse formation or conduction, with preserved myocardial function. It is most effective in those with sinus bradycardia or high-grade atrioventricular block, with slow ventricular response but adequate stroke volume. TCP is not indicated for children during prolonged arrest, because in this situation, it usually results in electrical but not mechanical cardiac capture, and its use may delay or interfere with other resuscitative efforts.

To set up pacing, one electrode is placed anteriorly at the left sternal border and the other posteriorly just below the left scapula. Smaller electrodes are available for infants and children, but adult-sized electrodes can be used in children weighing more than 15 kg. ECG leads should be connected to the pacemaker, the demand or asynchronous mode selected, and an age-appropriate heart rate used. The stimulus output should be set at zero when the pacemaker is turned on and then increased gradually until electrical capture is identified on the monitor. After electrical capture is achieved, whether an effective arterial pulse is generated must be determined. If not, additional resuscitative efforts should be initiated.

The most serious complication of TCP is the induction of a ventricular arrhythmia. Fortunately, this is rare and may be prevented by pacing only in the demand mode. Mild transient erythema beneath the electrodes is common. Skeletal muscle contraction can be minimized by using large electrodes, a 40-ms pulse duration, and the smallest stimulus required for capture. If defibrillation or cardioversion is necessary, a distance of 2–3 cm must be allowed between the electrode and paddles to prevent arcing of the current.

Vascular Access and Monitoring During Cardiopulmonary Resuscitation

Vascular Access and Fluid Administration

One of the key aspects of successful CPR is early establishment of a route for administration of fluids and medications. If intravenous access cannot be established rapidly, the intraosseous or endotracheal route should be used.

Endotracheal Medication Administration

In the absence of other vascular access, medications including lidocaine, atropine, naloxone, and epinephrine (mnemonic LANE) can be administered via the endotracheal tube (Ward 1983; Johnston 1992). The use of ionized medications such as sodium bicarbonate or calcium chloride is not recommended by this route. The peak concentration of epinephrine or lidocaine administered via the endotracheal route may be less compared with the intraosseous route. For example, the peak drug concentration of epinephrine after endotracheal administration was only 10 % of that after intravenous administration in anesthetized dogs. The recommended dose for epinephrine via the endotracheal tube is ten times the intravenous or intraosseous dose or 0.1 mg/kg for bradycardia or pulseless arrest.

The volume and the diluent in which the medications are administered through an endotracheal tube may be important. When large volumes of fluid are used, pulmonary surfactant may be altered or destroyed, resulting in atelectasis. The total volume of fluid delivered into the trachea with each drug administered should not exceed 10 mL in children and 5 mL in infants and neonates (Greenberg et al. 1981). However, administering an adequate volume of a drug is important to reach a large area of mucosal surface beyond the tip of the endotracheal tube for absorption. Absorption into the systemic circulation may be further enhanced by deep intrapulmonary administration by passing a catheter beyond the tip of the tracheal tube deep into the bronchial tree. The risk associated with the endotracheal route of drug administration is the formation of an intrapulmonary depot of drug, which may prolong the drugs' effect. This could theoretically result in postresuscitation hypertension and tachycardia or the recurrence of fibrillation after normal circulation is restored.

Monitoring During Cardiopulmonary Resuscitation

A basic clinical examination is vital during cardiac arrest. The chest is carefully observed for adequacy of bilateral chest expansion with artificial ventilation and for equal and normal breath sounds. In addition, the depth of compression and the position of the rescuer's hands should be constantly reevaluated in performing chest compressions by palpation of a major artery. Palpation is essential in establishing the absence of a pulse and in assessing the adequacy of blood flow during chest compressions. Palpating the peripheral pulses may be inaccurate, especially during intense vasoconstriction associated with the use of epinephrine.

An indwelling arterial catheter, when available, is a valuable monitor in assessing the arterial blood pressure. Specific attention should be paid to diastolic blood pressure as it relates directly to adequacy of coronary perfusion during CPR. In addition, arterial access allows for frequent blood sampling, particularly for measurement of arterial pH and blood gases. Pulse oximetry can be used during CPR to determine the O_2 saturation and may be of value in assessing the adequacy of cardiac output, as reflected in the plethysmograph. The ECG can suggest metabolic imbalances and diagnose electrical disturbances.

The $ETCO_2$ monitor provides important information during the course of resuscitation. Leading resuscitation organizations strongly recommend the use of capnography to confirm correct placement of the endotracheal tube, to monitor the quality of CPR, and to provide an early indicator of ROSC (Deakin et al. 2010). Because the generation of exhaled CO_2 depends on pulmonary blood flow, it can provide a useful indicator of the adequacy of cardiac output generated by chest compressions. As the cardiac output increases, the $ETCO_2$ increases and the difference between end-tidal and arterial CO_2 becomes smaller (Tang et al. 1991). In animal models, $ETCO_2$ during CPR correlates with coronary perfusion pressure and with ROSC (Sanders et al. 1989; von Planta et al. 1989). A reduced $ETCO_2$ may occur transiently in the presence of adequate chest compressions after administration of epinephrine owing to an increase in intrapulmonary shunting. The International Liaison Committee on Resuscitation (ILCOR) in its international consensus (2010) acknowledges the fact that low values of ETCO2 are associated with low probability of survival, and the committee believes however that there are insufficient data to support or refute a specific cut-off of ETCO2 as a prognostic indicator of outcome during adult cardiac arrest. Touma and Davies (2013) did a systematic review studying the prognostic value of end-tidal carbon dioxide during cardiac arrest. The ability of ETCO2 cut-off values to reliably predict the outcome of resuscitation with high accuracy is not established. ETCO2 monitoring may be considered to evaluate quality of chest compressions, but there is no pediatric evidence that ETCO2 monitoring improves outcomes from cardiac arrest (de Caen et al. 2015).

Temperature should be monitored during and after CPR. The resuscitation of the child with hypothermia as the cause of cardiac arrest must be continued until the child's core temperature exceeds 95 °F (35 °C). A glass bulb thermometer measures the temperature to very low values. Repeated measurements of core body temperature should be made at several sites (rectal, bladder, esophageal, axillary, or tympanic membrane) where possible, to avoid misleading temperature readings from a single site, because local body temperature may vary with changes in regional blood flow during CPR. Hyperthermia should be aggressively treated in the peri-arrest period, because postarrest hyperthermia is associated with worse outcomes in children (Hickey et al. 2000). Evidence suggests a benefit to induced hypothermia after resuscitation from cardiac arrest in adults (Hypothermia After Cardiac Arrest Study Group 2002; Bernard et al. 2002) and after perinatal hypoxic or ischemic injury (Shankaran et al. 2002). The data available to support the use of hypothermia in infants and children after cardiac arrest is from case series and retrospective studies. In the recently published Therapeutic Hypothermia After Pediatric Cardiac Arrest (THAPCA) study, therapeutic hypothermia, as compared with therapeutic normothermia, did not confer a significant benefit with respect to survival with good functional outcome at 1 year (Moler et al. 2015).

Medications Used During Cardiopulmonary Resuscitation

α- and β-Adrenergic Agonists

In 1963, only 3 years after the original description of closed-chest CPR, Redding and Pearson (1963) demonstrated that early administration of epinephrine in a canine model of cardiac arrest improved the success rate of CPR. They also demonstrated that the increase in aortic diastolic pressure with the administration of α-adrenergic agonists was responsible for the improved success of resuscitation. They theorized that vasopressors such as epinephrine were of value because the drug increased peripheral vascular tone and, hence, coronary perfusion pressure. The relative importance of α- and β-adrenergic agonist actions during resuscitation has been widely investigated. In a canine model of cardiac arrest, only 27 % of dogs that received a pure β-adrenergic receptor agonist along with an α-adrenergic antagonist were resuscitated successfully, compared with 100 % of dogs that received a pure α-adrenergic agonist and a β-adrenergic antagonist. Other investigators have demonstrated that the α-adrenergic effects of epinephrine resulted in intense vasoconstriction of the resistance vessels of all organs of the body, except those supplying the heart and brain (Michael et al. 1984). Because of the widespread vasoconstriction in nonvital organs, adequate perfusion pressure and thus blood flow to the heart and brain can be achieved despite the fact that cardiac output is very low during CPR (Michael et al. 1984; Koehler and Michael 1985; Schleien et al. 1986).

The increase in aortic diastolic pressure associated with epinephrine administration during CPR is critical for maintaining coronary blood flow and enhancing the success of resuscitation (Niemann et al. 1985; Sanders et al. 1984). Even though the contractile state of the myocardium is increased by the use of β-adrenergic agonists in the spontaneously beating heart, β-adrenergic agonists may actually decrease myocardial blood flow by increasing intramyocardial wall pressure and vascular resistance during CPR (Downey et al. 1979). By its inotropic and chronotropic effects, β-adrenergic stimulation increases myocardial O_2 demand, which, when superimposed on low coronary blood flow, increases the risk of ischemic injury.

Any medication that causes systemic arterial vasoconstriction can be used to increase aortic diastolic pressure and resuscitate the heart. For example, pure α-adrenergic agonists can be used in place of epinephrine during CPR. Phenylephrine and methoxamine, two α-adrenergic agonists, have been used in animal models of CPR with success equal to that of epinephrine. Their use results in a greater O_2 supply to demand ratio in the ischemic heart and at least a theoretical advantage over the combined α- and β-adrenergic agonist effects of epinephrine. These agonists, as well as other classes of vasopressors such as vasopressin, have been used successfully for resuscitation.

The merits of using a pure α-adrenergic agonist during CPR have been questioned by some investigators. Although the inotropic and chronotropic effects of β-adrenergic agonists may have deleterious hemodynamic effects during CPR for ventricular fibrillation, increases in both heart rate and contractility will increase cardiac output when spontaneous coordinated ventricular contractions are achieved.

Epinephrine

Epinephrine (adrenaline) is an endogenous catecholamine with potent α- and β-adrenergic stimulating properties. The α-adrenergic action increases systemic and pulmonary vascular resistance, increasing both systolic and diastolic blood pressure. The increase in diastolic blood pressure directly increases coronary perfusion pressure, thereby increasing coronary blood flow and increasing the likelihood of ROSC (Niemann et al. 1985; Sanders et al. 1984). The β-adrenergic effect increases myocardial contractility and heart rate and relaxes smooth muscle in the skeletal muscle vascular bed and bronchi. Epinephrine also increases the vigor and intensity of ventricular fibrillation, increasing the likelihood of successful defibrillation (Otto and Yakaitis 1984).

Larger than necessary doses of epinephrine may be deleterious. Epinephrine may worsen myocardial ischemic injury secondary to increased O_2 demand and may result in postresuscitative tachyarrhythmias, hypertension, and pulmonary edema. Epinephrine causes hypoxemia and an increase in alveolar dead space ventilation by redistributing pulmonary blood flow (Tang et al. 1991; von Planta et al. 1993). Prolonged peripheral vasoconstriction by excessive doses of epinephrine may delay or impair reperfusion of systemic organs, particularly the kidneys and the gastrointestinal tract.

Routine use of large-dose epinephrine in in-hospital pediatric cardiac arrest should be *avoided*. A randomized, controlled trial in 2003 compared high-dose with standard-dose epinephrine for children with in-hospital cardiac arrest refractory to initial standard-dose epinephrine. Survival was reduced at 24 h, with a trend toward decreased survival to hospital discharge in the children who received large doses of epinephrine (Perondi et al. 2004). Despite these data, large doses of epinephrine may be considered in special cases (e.g., β-blocker overdose), particularly when diastolic blood pressure remains low despite excellent chest compression and several standard doses of epinephrine.

Vasopressin

Vasopressin is a long-acting endogenous hormone that causes vasoconstriction (V1 receptor) and reabsorption of water in the renal tubule (V2 receptor). In experimental models of cardiac arrest, vasopressin increases blood flow to the heart and brain and improves long-term survival compared with epinephrine (Lindner et al. 1995; Prengel et al. 1996). In a randomized trial comparing the efficacy of epinephrine to vasopressin in shock-resistant out-of-hospital ventricular fibrillation in adults, vasopressin produced a greater rate of ROSC (Lindner et al. 1997). In a study of in-hospital adult cardiac arrest, vasopressin produced a rate of survival to hospital discharge similar to that of epinephrine (Babbs et al. 2001). In a recent meta-analysis of vasopressin for cardiac arrest (Mentzelopoulos et al. 2012), vasopressin use in the resuscitation of cardiac arrest patients is not associated with any overall benefit or harm.

In a pediatric porcine model of prolonged ventricular fibrillation, the use of vasopressin and epinephrine in combination resulted in greater left ventricular blood flow than either vasopressor alone, and both vasopressin alone and vasopressin plus epinephrine resulted in superior cerebral blood flow than epinephrine alone (Wenzel et al. 2002). By contrast, in a pediatric porcine model of *asphyxial* cardiac arrest, ROSC was more likely in piglets treated with epinephrine than in those treated with vasopressin (Voelckel et al. 2000). Pediatric (Mann et al. 2002; Matok et al. 2007; Gil-Anton et al. 2010) case series and reports suggested that vasopressin (Mann et al. 2002) or its long-acting analog, terlipressin (Matok et al. 2007; Gil-Anton et al. 2010), may be effective in refractory cardiac arrest. In a 2009 National Registry of Cardiopulmonary Resuscitation (NRCPR) review, vasopressin was associated with reduced ROSC and a trend toward reduced 24-h and discharge survival. There is insufficient evidence to make a recommendation for its routine use during cardiac arrest (Kleinman et al. 2010).

Atropine

Atropine, a parasympatholytic agent, blocks cholinergic stimulation of the muscarinic receptors in the heart, increasing the sinus rate and shortening atrioventricular node conduction time. Atropine may activate latent ectopic pacemakers. Atropine has little effect on systemic vascular resistance, myocardial perfusion pressure, or contractility (Brown and Laiken 2011).

Atropine is indicated for the treatment of asystole, pulseless electrical activity, bradycardia associated with hypotension, second- and third-degree heart block, and slow idioventricular rhythms. Atropine is particularly effective in clinical conditions associated with excessive parasympathetic tone. *However, for children with asystole or symptomatic bradycardia associated with severe hypotension, epinephrine is the medication of choice and atropine should be regarded as a second-line drug.*

A dose of 0.02 mg/kg with no minimum dose may be considered when atropine is used as a premedication for emergency intubation. This new recommendation applies to the use of atropine as a premedication for infants and children during emergency intubation (de Caen et al. 2015). Although a minimum dose of 0.1 mg has been entrenched in the literature, it is not evidence-based (Dauchot and Gravenstein 1971; Kottmeier and Gravenstein 1968). The increase in heart rate after intravenous atropine (20 μg/kg) in infants and children may be attenuated compared with that in adults (Dauchot and Gravenstein 1971). Atropine may be given by any route, including intravenous, intraosseous, endotracheal, intramuscular, and subcutaneous. After intravenous administration, its onset of action is within 30 s, and its peak effect occurs in 1–2 min. The recommended adult dose is 0.5 mg every 3–5 min until the desired heart rate is obtained, up to a maximum of 3 mg.

Sodium Bicarbonate

The routine use of sodium bicarbonate during CPR remains controversial, and it remains American Heart Association Class Indeterminate. Acidosis may depress myocardial function, prolong diastolic depolarization, depress spontaneous cardiac activity, decrease the electrical threshold for ventricular fibrillation, and reduce the cardiac response to catecholamines (Huang et al. 1995; Burchfield et al. 1993; Pannier and Leusen 1968). Acidosis also vasodilates systemic vessels and attenuates the vasoconstrictive response of peripheral vessels to catecholamines (Wood et al. 1963), which is the opposite of the desired vascular effect during CPR. In children with a reactive pulmonary vascular bed, acidosis causes pulmonary hypertension. Therefore, correction of even mild acidosis may be helpful in resuscitating children with increased pulmonary vascular resistance. Additionally, the presence of severe acidosis may increase the threshold for myocardial stimulation in a child with an artificial cardiac pacemaker (Dohrmann and Goldschlager 1985). Other situations in which administration of bicarbonate is indicated include tricyclic antidepressant overdose, hyperkalemia, hypermagnesemia, or sodium channel blocker poisoning.

Potentially deleterious effects of bicarbonate administration include metabolic alkalosis, hypercapnia, hypernatremia, and hyperosmolality. In a 2004 multicenter cohort study of in-hospital pediatric cardiac arrest, the use of sodium bicarbonate was associated with increased mortality (Meert et al. 2009). Alkalosis causes a leftward shift of the oxyhemoglobin dissociation curve and thus impairs the release of O_2 from hemoglobin to tissues at a time when O_2 delivery may already be reduced (Bishop and Weisfeldt 1976). Alkalosis also can result in hypokalemia by enhancing potassium influx into cells and in ionic hypocalcemia by increasing protein binding of ionized calcium. The marked hypercapnic acidosis that occurs during CPR in the venous circulation, including the coronary sinus, may be exacerbated by the administration of bicarbonate (Grundler et al. 1986). Myocardial acidosis during cardiac arrest is associated with decreased myocardial contractility (Pannier and Leusen

1968). Hypernatremia and hyperosmolality may decrease tissue perfusion by increasing interstitial edema in microvascular beds.

Paradoxical intracellular acidosis after bicarbonate administration can occur with the rapid entry of CO_2 into cells with a slow egress of hydrogen ions out of cells; however, in neonatal rabbits recovering from hypoxic acidosis, bicarbonate administration increased both arterial pH and intracellular brain pH as measured by nuclear magnetic resonance spectroscopy (Sessler et al. 1987; Cohen et al. 1990). Likewise, in rats, intracellular brain adenosine triphosphate concentration did not change during severe intracellular acidosis in the brain produced by extreme hypercapnia (Cohen et al. 1990). In a separate animal study, bicarbonate slowed the rate of decrease of both arterial and cerebral pH during prolonged CPR, suggesting that the blood–brain pH gradient is maintained during CPR (Eleff et al. 1995). Given the potentially deleterious effects of bicarbonate administration, its use should be *limited to cases in which there is a specific indication*, as discussed earlier.

Calcium

Calcium administration during CPR should be restricted to cases with a specific indication for calcium (e.g., hypocalcemia, hyperkalemia, hypermagnesemia, and calcium channel blocker overdose). These restrictions are based on the possibility that exogenously administered calcium may worsen ischemia–reperfusion injury. Intracellular calcium overload occurs during cerebral ischemia by the influx of calcium through voltage-dependent and agonist-dependent (e.g., *N*-methyl-D-aspartate [NMDA]) calcium channels. Calcium plays an important role in the process of cell death in many organs, possibly by activation of intracellular enzymes such as nitric oxide synthase, phospholipase A and C, and others (Morley et al. 1994).

The calcium ion is essential in myocardial excitation–contraction coupling, in increasing ventricular contractility, and in enhancing ventricular automaticity during asystole. Ionized hypocalcemia is associated with decreased ventricular performance and the peripheral blunting of the hemodynamic response to catecholamines (Bristow et al. 1977; Urban et al. 1988). Severe ionized hypocalcemia has been documented in adults suffering from out-of-hospital cardiac arrest (Urban et al. 1988) and in animals during prolonged CPR (Cairns et al. 1991). Thus, children at risk for ionized hypocalcemia should be identified and treated as expeditiously as possible. Both total and ionized hypocalcemia may occur in children with either chronic or acute disease. Ionized hypocalcemia also occurs during massive or rapid transfusion of blood products (particularly whole blood and fresh frozen plasma) because citrate and other preservatives in stored blood products rapidly bind calcium. Because of this effect, ionized hypocalcemia is a known cause of cardiac arrest in the OR and should be treated immediately with calcium chloride or calcium gluconate (see Chap. 10). The magnitude of hypocalcemia in this setting depends on the rate and volume of blood products administered and the hepatic and renal function of the child. Administration of fresh frozen plasma at a rate in excess of 1 mL/kg/min significantly decreases the ionized calcium concentration in anesthetized children (Cote et al. 1988).

The pediatric dose of calcium chloride for resuscitation is 20 mg/kg with a maximum dose of 2 g. Calcium gluconate is as effective as calcium chloride in increasing the ionized calcium concentration (Heining et al. 1984; Cote et al. 1987). The dose of calcium gluconate should be three times that of calcium chloride (milligram per kilogram) (i.e., 20 mg/kg calcium chloride is equivalent to 60 mg/kg calcium gluconate), with a maximum dose of 2 g in children. Calcium should be given slowly through a large-bore, free-flowing intravenous cannula, or preferably a central venous line. When administered too rapidly, calcium may cause bradycardia, heart block, or ventricular standstill. Severe tissue necrosis occurs when calcium infiltrates into subcutaneous tissue. Calcium administration is not recommended for pediatric cardiopulmonary arrest in the absence of documented hypocalcemia, calcium channel blocker overdose, hypermagnesemia, or hyperkalemia (class III, level of evidence [LOE] B). Routine calcium administration in cardiac arrest provides no benefit and may be harmful (Dohrmann and Goldschlager 1985; Srinivasan et al. 2008).

Glucose

The administration of glucose during CPR should be restricted to children with documented hypoglycemia because of the possible detrimental effects of hyperglycemia on the brain during or after ischemia. The mechanism by which hyperglycemia exacerbates ischemic neurologic injury may be due to an increased production of lactic acid in the brain by anaerobic metabolism. During ischemia under normoglycemic conditions, brain lactate concentration reaches a plateau. In a hyperglycemic milieu, however, brain lactate concentration continues to increase for the duration of the ischemic period (Siesjo 1984).

Clinical studies have shown a direct correlation between the initial post-cardiac arrest serum glucose concentration and poor neurologic outcome (Pulsinelli et al. 1983; Longstreth and Inui 1984; Ashwal et al. 1990; Longstreth et al. 1986), although the greater glucose concentration may be a marker rather than a cause of more severe brain injury (Longstreth and Inui 1984). However, given the likelihood of additional ischemic and hypoxic events in the postresuscitation period, it seems prudent to maintain serum glucose concentrations within the normal range. Additional studies are needed to determine if the benefit from tight control of serum glucose after cardiac arrest outweighs the risk of iatrogenic hypoglycemia. Some groups of children, including preterm infants and debilitated children with small endogenous glycogen stores, are more prone to developing hypoglycemia during and after a physiologic stress such as surgery. Bedside monitoring of the serum glucose concentration is critical during and after a cardiac arrest and allows for the opportunity to administer glucose before the critical point of small substrate delivery has been reached. The dose of glucose generally needed to correct hypoglycemia is 0.5 g/kg given as 5 mL/kg of 10 % dextrose in infants or

1 mL/kg of 50 % dextrose in an older child. The osmolarity of 50 % dextrose is approximately 2700 mOsm/L and has been associated with intraventricular hemorrhage in neonates and infants; therefore, the more dilute concentration is recommended in infants.

Amiodarone

The role of amiodarone was established for cardiac arrest after a series of studies showed it to be more effective than lidocaine in the management of refractory tachyarrhythmias in adults. Compared with lidocaine, amiodarone results in an increased rate of survival to hospital admission in patients with shock-resistant out-of-hospital ventricular fibrillation (Sarkozy and Dorian 2003).

Early reports on the use of oral amiodarone in children were favorable (Coumel et al. 1983; Pickoff et al. 1983; Coumel and Fidelle 1980). Recent data on amiodarone use in children are limited to case reports and descriptive case series. Nevertheless, it is now used widely for serious pediatric arrhythmias in the nonresuscitation environment and appears to be effective and have an acceptable short-term safety profile.

The pharmacology of amiodarone is complex and may explain the wide range of its usefulness. It is primarily classified as a Vaughn-Williams class III agent that blocks the adenosine triphosphate–sensitive outward potassium channels causing prolongation of the action potential and refractory period; however, this effect requires intracellular accumulation. On intravenous loading, the antiarrhythmic effects are primarily due to noncompetitive α- and β-adrenergic receptor blockade, calcium channel blockade, and effects on inward sodium current causing a decrease in anterograde conduction across the atrioventricular node and an increase in the effective atrioventricular refractory period. The α-adrenergic blockade leads to vasodilation, which may increase coronary blood flow. It is poorly absorbed orally, requiring intravenous loading in urgent situations. The full antiarrhythmic impact requires a loading period of up to 1–3 weeks to achieve intracellular levels and full potassium channel blocking effects.

Hypotension is commonly reported with intravenous administration and may limit the rate at which the drug can be given; however, the development of hypotension is less common with the newer, aqueous formulation (Somberg et al. 2002). The overall hemodynamic impact of intravenous administration will depend on the balance of its effect on rate control, myocardial performance, and vasodilation. Dosage recommendations for children are based on limited clinical studies. The dose is extrapolated from data on adults, 5 mg/kg intravenously for life-threatening arrhythmias. This dose can be repeated if necessary to control the arrhythmia. Intravenous loading doses are followed by a continuous infusion of 10–20 mg/kg/day if there is a risk of arrhythmia recurrence. The ideal rate of bolus administration is unclear; in adults, once diluted, it is given as an intravenous push. It is best administered over 20–60 min to avoid profound vasodilation. We recommend slow intravenous push

(2–3 min) for pulseless ventricular tachycardia or ventricular fibrillation until the arrhythmia is controlled and then a slower bolus (up to 10 min) for the remainder of the dose. An alternative dosing regimen for children is 1 mg/kg intravenous push every 5 min up to 5 mg/kg. The use of the small aliquot bolus technique may be particularly appropriate for infants younger than 12 months of age.

Amiodarone-induced torsades de pointes has been described (Silvetti et al. 2001). The use of amiodarone should be avoided in combination with other drugs that prolong the QT interval, as well as in the setting of hypomagnesemia and other electrolyte abnormalities that predispose to torsades de pointes. Severe bradycardia and heart block have also been described, especially in the postoperative period, and ventricular pacing wires are recommended in this setting. Both amiodarone and inhalation anesthetic agents prolong the QT interval; however, no specific data exist to evaluate the use of amiodarone for ventricular arrhythmias in children receiving inhalation anesthetics. It would seem prudent to be especially vigilant for this adverse effect in this circumstance.

Noncardiac adverse effects are often seen, especially with chronic dosing (Jafari-Fesharaki and Scheinman 1998). The most serious of these has been the development of interstitial pneumonitis seen most commonly in patients with preexisting lung disease (Jessurun et al. 1998). The incidence in children is unknown. Rarely, an acute illness similar to acute respiratory distress syndrome illness has been reported in both infants and adults at the initiation of treatment (Birmingham 1998). The lung disease may remit with early discontinuation of the drug. Hypothyroidism, hepatotoxicity, photosensitivity, and corneal opacities are also common side effects with chronic use (Jafari-Fesharaki and Scheinman 1998).

The 2005 and 2010 PALS guidelines recommended administering amiodarone in preference to lidocaine for the management of ventricular fibrillation or pulseless ventricular tachycardia. Valdes et al. in a pediatric observational study, showed improved ROSC with the use of lidocaine as compared with amiodarone (Valdes et al. 2014). There was no association between lidocaine or amiodarone use and survival to hospital discharge. Hence, the 2015 Pediatric Cardiac Arrest Algorithm (de Caen et al. 2015) reflects the change in recommendation to use either lidocaine or amiodarone for refractory ventricular fibrillation or pulseless VT.

Lidocaine

Lidocaine is a class IB antiarrhythmic that decreases automaticity of pacemaker tissue that prevents or terminates ventricular arrhythmias as a result of accelerated ectopic foci. Lidocaine abolishes reentrant ventricular arrhythmias by decreasing the action potential duration and the conduction time of Purkinje fibers and increases the effective refractory period of Purkinje fibers, reducing the nonuniformity of contraction. Lidocaine has no effect on atrioventricular nodal conduction time, so it is ineffective in the treatment of atrial or atrioventricular junctional arrhythmias. In healthy adults, no change in heart rate or blood pressure occurs with lidocaine administration. In patients with cardiac disease, there may be a slight decrease in ventricular function when a lidocaine bolus is administered intravenously.

In children with normal cardiac and hepatic function, an initial intravenous bolus of 1 mg/kg of lidocaine is given, followed by a continuous intravenous infusion at a rate of 20–50 µg/kg/min. If the arrhythmia recurs, a second intravenous bolus at the same dose can be given. In children with severely decreased cardiac output, a bolus of no greater than 0.75 mg/kg is administered, followed by an infusion at the rate of 10–20 µg/kg/min. In children with hepatic disease, dosages should be decreased by 50 %. Children with renal insufficiency have normal lidocaine pharmacokinetics; however, toxic metabolites may accumulate in children receiving infusions over a long period. In children with hypoproteinemia, the dose of lidocaine also should be lowered, because of the increase in free fraction of the drug.

Toxic effects of lidocaine occur when the serum concentration exceeds 7–8 µg/mL and include seizures, psychosis, drowsiness, paresthesias, disorientation, agitation, tinnitus, muscle spasms, and respiratory arrest. The treatment of choice for lidocaine-induced seizures is a benzodiazepine (midazolam or lorazepam) or a barbiturate (e.g., phenobarbital; chronic therapy also increases the hepatic metabolism of lidocaine) (Greenblatt et al. 1976). Conversion of second-degree heart block to complete heart block has been described (Lichstein et al. 1973), as has severe sinus bradycardia.

Special Cardiac Arrest Situations

Perioperative Cardiac Arrest

The incidence, causes, and risk factors associated with anesthesia- and operative-related cardiac arrest have been evaluated by the Pediatric Perioperative Cardiac Arrest Registry (Bhananker et al. 2007; Geiduschek 1998). Cardiovascular causes of cardiac arrest were the most common (41 % of all arrests), with hypovolemia from blood loss and hyperkalemia from transfusion of stored blood as the most common identifiable cardiovascular causes. Among respiratory causes of arrest (27 %), airway obstruction from laryngospasm was the most common cause. Vascular injury incurred during placement of central venous catheters was the most common equipment-related cause of arrest. The cause of arrest varied by phase of anesthesia care.

Cardiac arrest in the OR should have the greatest potential for a successful outcome, because it is a witnessed arrest with virtually instantaneous availability of skilled personnel, monitoring equipment, resuscitative equipment, and drugs. Whenever a cardiac arrest occurs in the OR, the circumstances causing the arrest should be rapidly determined. The circumstances of the arrest may provide a clue as to the cause, such as hyperkalemia after succinylcholine administration or rapid blood transfusion, hypocalcemia during a rapid infusion of fresh frozen plasma or large blood transfusion, or a sudden fall in $ETCO_2$ indicating air, blood clot, or tumor embolism. A bradyarrhythmia always must be assumed to be first resulting from hypoxemia; second, caused by anesthetic overdose (real or relative); and third, possibly related to a vagal reflex caused by surgical or airway manipulation. Administering 100% O_2 and ensuring adequate ventilation is always the first maneuver, regardless of the cause of the bradycardia. In reflex-induced bradycardia, atropine may be the first drug of choice, but in extreme cases of bradycardia, whatever the mechanism, epinephrine should be used. Hypotension and a low cardiac output state must be rapidly corrected by appropriate administration of intravenous fluids, vasopressors, and adequate chest compressions to circulate drugs to have the needed clinical effect. Once chest compressions are required, the standard American Heart Association recommendations for CPR generally apply and this includes the frequent administration of epinephrine.

Hyperkalemia

A child with a hyperkalemic cardiac arrest may be identified by history, by the progression of ECG changes leading up to the arrest, or by initial laboratory results. A high index of suspicion must be maintained for hyperkalemia as a cause of cardiac arrest because it requires specific therapy. Along with the usual resuscitation algorithms, immediate therapy to antagonize the effects of an increased serum potassium level is necessary. Calcium gluconate or calcium chloride will antagonize the effects of hyperkalemia at the myocardial cell membrane, increasing the threshold for fibrillation. Sodium bicarbonate and hyperventilation will increase the serum pH and shift potassium from the extracellular to the intracellular compartment; insulin (with concomitant dextrose) will also cause potassium to shift intracellularly (0.1 unit/kg of insulin with 0.5 g/kg of dextrose; 2 mL/kg of dextrose 25%). The serum potassium concentration must be monitored frequently during this treatment, preferably by point-of-care testing modalities. Because these therapies shift potassium intracellularly, therapy to remove potassium from the body (furosemide, hemodialysis, sodium polystyrene sulfonate) also may be indicated.

References

Ashwal S, et al. Prognostic implications of hyperglycemia and reduced cerebral blood flow in childhood near-drowning. Neurology. 1990;40(5):820–3.

Aufderheide TP, et al. Hyperventilation-induced hypotension during cardiopulmonary resuscitation. Circulation. 2004;109(16):1960–5.

Babbs CF, et al. Use of pressors in the treatment of cardiac arrest. Ann Emerg Med. 2001;37(4 Suppl):S152–62.

Berg MD, et al. Part 13: pediatric basic life support: 2010 American Heart Association guidelines for cardiopulmonary resuscitation and emergency cardiovascular care. Circulation. 2010;122(18 Suppl 3):S862–75.

Bernard SA, et al. Treatment of comatose survivors of out-of-hospital cardiac arrest with induced hypothermia. N Engl J Med. 2002;346(8):557–63.

Bhananker SM, et al. Anesthesia-related cardiac arrest in children: update from the Pediatric Perioperative Cardiac Arrest Registry. Anesth Analg. 2007;105(2):344–50.

Birmingham WP. More on an infant with acute pulmonary toxicity during amiodarone therapy. Am J Cardiol. 1998;81(9):1171.

Bishop RL, Weisfeldt ML. Sodium bicarbonate administration during cardiac arrest. Effect on arterial pH PCO2, and osmolality. JAMA. 1976;235(5):506–9.

Bristow MR, et al. Ionized calcium and the heart. Elucidation of in vivo concentration-response relationships in the open-chest dog. Circ Res. 1977;41(4):565–74.

Brown JH, Laiken N. Muscarinic receptor agonists and antagonists. In: Brunton LL, Chabner BA, Knollmann BC, editors. Goodman & Gilman's the pharmacological basis of therapeutics. New York: McGraw-Hill; 2011.

Burchfield DJ, et al. Effects of graded doses of epinephrine during asphxia-induced bradycardia in newborn lambs. Resuscitation. 1993;25(3):235–44.

Cairns CB, et al. Ionized hypocalcemia during prolonged cardiac arrest and closed-chest CPR in a canine model. Ann Emerg Med. 1991;20(11):1178–82.

Campbell NP, et al. Transthoracic ventricular defibrillation in adults. Br Med J. 1977;2(6099): 1379–81.

Chandra NC, et al. Observations of hemodynamics during human cardiopulmonary resuscitation. Crit Care Med. 1990;18(9):929–34.

Cohen JM, et al. Timing of pulmonary and systemic blood flow during intermittent high intrathoracic pressure cardiopulmonary resuscitation in the dog. Am J Cardiol. 1982;49(8):1883–9.

Cohen Y, et al. Stability of brain intracellular lactate and 31P-metabolite levels at reduced intracellular pH during prolonged hypercapnia in rats. J Cereb Blood Flow Metab. 1990;10(2):277–84.

Cote CJ, et al. Calcium chloride versus calcium gluconate: comparison of ionization and cardiovascular effects in children and dogs. Anesthesiology. 1987;66(4):465–70.

Cote CJ, et al. Ionized hypocalcemia after fresh frozen plasma administration to thermally injured children: effects of infusion rate, duration, and treatment with calcium chloride. Anesth Analg. 1988;67(2):152–60.

Coumel P, Fidelle J. Amiodarone in the treatment of cardiac arrhythmias in children: one hundred thirty-five cases. Am Heart J. 1980;100(6 Pt 2):1063–9.

Coumel P, Lucet V, Do Ngoc D. The use of amiodarone in children. Pacing Clin Electrophysiol. 1983;6(5 Pt 1):930–9.

Criley JM, Blaufuss AH, Kissel GL. Cough-induced cardiac compression. Self-administered from of cardiopulmonary resuscitation. JAMA. 1976;236(11):1246–50.

Dauchot P, Gravenstein JS. Effects of atropine on the electrocardiogram in different age groups. Clin Pharmacol Ther. 1971;12(2):274–80.

de Caen AR, et al. Part 12: pediatric advanced life support: 2015 American Heart Association guidelines update for cardiopulmonary resuscitation and emergency cardiovascular care. Circulation. 2015;132(18 Suppl 2):S526–42.

Deakin CD, et al. Part 8: advanced life support: 2010 International consensus on cardiopulmonary resuscitation and emergency cardiovascular care science with treatment recommendations. Resuscitation. 2010;81 Suppl 1:e93–174.

Dohrmann ML, Goldschlager NF. Myocardial stimulation threshold in patients with cardiac pacemakers: effect of physiologic variables, pharmacologic agents, and lead electrodes. Cardiol Clin. 1985;3(4):527–37.

Downey JM, Chagrasulis RW, Hemphill V. Quantitative study of intramyocardial compression in the fibrillating heart. Am J Physiol. 1979;237(2):H191–6.

ECC Committee, Subcommittees and Task Forces of the American Heart Association. 2005 American Heart Association guidelines for cardiopulmonary resuscitation and emergency cardiovascular care. Circulation. 2005;112(24 Suppl):Iv1–203.

Eleff SM, et al. Acidemia and brain pH during prolonged cardiopulmonary resuscitation in dogs. Stroke. 1995;26(6):1028–34.

Geiduschek JM. Registry offers insight on preventing cardiac arrest in children. Soc Am Anesth. 1998;62:6–18.

Gil-Anton J, et al. Pediatric cardiac arrest refractory to advanced life support: is there a role for terlipressin? Pediatr Crit Care Med. 2010;11(1):139–41.

Greenberg MI, Roberts JR, Baskin SI. Use of endotracheally administered epinephrine in a pediatric patient. Am J Dis Child. 1981;135(8):767–8.

Greenblatt DJ, Gross PL, Bolognini V. Pharmacotherapy of cardiopulmonary arrest. Am J Hosp Pharm. 1976;33(6):579–83.

Grundler W, Weil MH, Rackow EC. Arteriovenous carbon dioxide and pH gradients during cardiac arrest. Circulation. 1986;74(5):1071–4.

Heining MP, Band DM, Linton RA. Choice of calcium salt. A comparison of the effects of calcium chloride and gluconate on plasma ionized calcium. Anaesthesia. 1984;39(11):1079–82.

Hickey RW, et al. Hypothermia and hyperthermia in children after resuscitation from cardiac arrest. Pediatrics. 2000;106(1 Pt 1):118–22.

Hoffman JI, Kaplan S. The incidence of congenital heart disease. J Am Coll Cardiol. 2002;39(12):1890–900.

Huang YG, et al. Cardiovascular responses to graded doses of three catecholamines during lactic and hydrochloric acidosis in dogs. Br J Anaesth. 1995;74(5):583–90.

Hypothermia After Cardiac Arrest Study Group. Mild therapeutic hypothermia to improve the neurologic outcome after cardiac arrest. N Engl J Med. 2002;346(8):549–56.

Jafari-Fesharaki M, Scheinman MM. Adverse effects of amiodarone. Pacing Clin Electrophysiol. 1998;21(1 Pt 1):108–20.

Jessurun GA, Boersma WG, Crijns HJ. Amiodarone-induced pulmonary toxicity. Predisposing factors, clinical symptoms and treatment. Drug Saf. 1998;18(5):339–44.

Johnston C. Endotracheal drug delivery. Pediatr Emerg Care. 1992;8(2):94–7.

Kerber RE, Sarnat W. Factors influencing the success of ventricular defibrillation in man. Circulation. 1979;60(2):226–30.

Khairy P, et al. Multicenter research in adult congenital heart disease. Int J Cardiol. 2008;129(2):155–9.

Khairy P, et al. Changing mortality in congenital heart disease. J Am Coll Cardiol. 2010;56(14):1149–57.

Kleinman ME, et al. Part 14: pediatric advanced life support: 2010 American Heart Association guidelines for cardiopulmonary resuscitation and emergency cardiovascular care. Circulation. 2010;122(18 Suppl 3):S876–908.

Koehler RC, Michael JR. Cardiopulmonary resuscitation, brain blood flow, and neurologic recovery. Crit Care Clin. 1985;1(2):205–22.

Kottmeier CA, Gravenstein JS. The parasympathomimetic activity of atropine and atropine methylbromide. Anesthesiology. 1968;29(6):1125–33.

Lawes EG, Baskett PJ. Pulmonary aspiration during unsuccessful cardiopulmonary resuscitation. Intensive Care Med. 1987;13(6):379–82.

Lichstein E, Chadda KD, Gupta PK. Atrioventricular block with lidocaine therapy. Am J Cardiol. 1973;31(2):277–81.

Lindner KH, et al. Vasopressin improves vital organ blood flow during closed-chest cardiopulmonary resuscitation in pigs. Circulation. 1995;91(1):215–21.

Lindner KH, et al. Randomised comparison of epinephrine and vasopressin in patients with out-of-hospital ventricular fibrillation. Lancet. 1997;349(9051):535–7.

Longstreth Jr WT, Inui TS. High blood glucose level on hospital admission and poor neurological recovery after cardiac arrest. Ann Neurol. 1984;15(1):59–63.

Longstreth Jr WT, et al. Neurologic outcome and blood glucose levels during out-of-hospital cardiopulmonary resuscitation. Neurology. 1986;36(9):1186–91.

Maier GW, et al. The physiology of external cardiac massage: high-impulse cardiopulmonary resuscitation. Circulation. 1984;70(1):86–101.

Mann K, Berg RA, Nadkarni V. Beneficial effects of vasopressin in prolonged pediatric cardiac arrest: a case series. Resuscitation. 2002;52(2):149–56.

Matok I, et al. Beneficial effects of terlipressin in prolonged pediatric cardiopulmonary resuscitation: a case series. Crit Care Med. 2007;35(4):1161–4.

Meert KL, et al. Multicenter cohort study of in-hospital pediatric cardiac arrest. Pediatr Crit Care Med. 2009;10(5):544–53.

Mentzelopoulos SD, et al. Vasopressin for cardiac arrest: meta-analysis of randomized controlled trials. Resuscitation. 2012;83(1):32–9.

Michael JR, et al. Mechanisms by which epinephrine augments cerebral and myocardial perfusion during cardiopulmonary resuscitation in dogs. Circulation. 1984;69(4):822–35.

Moler FW, et al. Therapeutic hypothermia after out-of-hospital cardiac arrest in children. N Engl J Med. 2015;372(20):1898–908.

Morley P, Hogan MJ, Hakim AM. Calcium-mediated mechanisms of ischemic injury and protection. Brain Pathol. 1994;4(1):37–47.

Niemann JT, et al. Pressure-synchronized cineangiography during experimental cardiopulmonary resuscitation. Circulation. 1981;64(5):985–91.

Niemann JT, et al. Predictive indices of successful cardiac resuscitation after prolonged arrest and experimental cardiopulmonary resuscitation. Ann Emerg Med. 1985;14(6):521–8.

O'Leary JM, et al. The changing demographics of congenital heart disease hospitalizations in the United States, 1998 through 2010. JAMA. 2013;309(10):984–6.

Ornato JP, et al. Effect of cardiopulmonary resuscitation compression rate on end-tidal carbon dioxide concentration and arterial pressure in man. Crit Care Med. 1988;16(3):241–5.

Otto CW, Yakaitis RW. The role of epinephrine in CPR: a reappraisal. Ann Emerg Med. 1984;13(9 Pt 2):840–3.

Pannier JL, Leusen I. Contraction characteristics of papillary muscle during changes in acid-base composition of the bathing-fluid. Arch Int Physiol Biochim. 1968;76(4):624–34.

Perondi MB, et al. A comparison of high-dose and standard-dose epinephrine in children with cardiac arrest. N Engl J Med. 2004;350(17):1722–30.

Pickoff AS, et al. Use of amiodarone in the therapy of primary ventricular arrhythmias in children. Dev Pharmacol Ther. 1983;6(2):73–82.

Prengel AW, Lindner KH, Keller A. Cerebral oxygenation during cardiopulmonary resuscitation with epinephrine and vasopressin in pigs. Stroke. 1996;27(7):1241–8.

Pulsinelli WA, et al. Increased damage after ischemic stroke in patients with hyperglycemia with or without established diabetes mellitus. Am J Med. 1983;74(4):540–4.

Redding JS, Pearson JW. Evaluation of drugs for cardiac resuscitation. Anesthesiology. 1963;24:203–7.

Rhodes JF, et al. Cardiac arrest in infants after congenital heart surgery. Circulation. 1999;100 Suppl 2:II-194–9.

Rich S, Wix HL, Shapiro EP. Clinical assessment of heart chamber size and valve motion during cardiopulmonary resuscitation by two-dimensional echocardiography. Am Heart J. 1981;102(3 Pt 1):368–73.

Sanders AB, Ewy GA, Taft TV. Prognostic and therapeutic importance of the aortic diastolic pressure in resuscitation from cardiac arrest. Crit Care Med. 1984;12(10):871–3.

Sanders AB, et al. End-tidal carbon dioxide monitoring during cardiopulmonary resuscitation. A prognostic indicator for survival. JAMA. 1989;262(10):1347–51.

Sarkozy A, Dorian P. Strategies for reversing shock-resistant ventricular fibrillation. Curr Opin Crit Care. 2003;9(3):189–93.

Schleien CL, et al. Effect of epinephrine on cerebral and myocardial perfusion in an infant animal preparation of cardiopulmonary resuscitation. Circulation. 1986;73(4):809–17.

Sessler D, et al. Effects of bicarbonate on arterial and brain intracellular pH in neonatal rabbits recovering from hypoxic lactic acidosis. J Pediatr. 1987;111(6 Pt 1):817–23.

Shankaran S, et al. Whole-body hypothermia for neonatal encephalopathy: animal observations as a basis for a randomized, controlled pilot study in term infants. Pediatrics. 2002;110(2 Pt 1):377–85.

Siesjo BK. Cerebral circulation and metabolism. J Neurosurg. 1984;60(5):883–908.

Silvetti MS, et al. Amiodarone-induced torsade de pointes in a child with dilated cardiomyopathy. Ital Heart J. 2001;2(3):231–6.

Somberg JC, et al. Intravenous lidocaine versus intravenous amiodarone (in a new aqueous formulation) for incessant ventricular tachycardia. Am J Cardiol. 2002;90(8):853–9.

Somerville J. Management of adults with congenital heart disease: an increasing problem. Annu Rev Med. 1997;48:283–93.

Srinivasan V, et al. Calcium use during in-hospital pediatric cardiopulmonary resuscitation: a report from the National Registry of Cardiopulmonary Resuscitation. Pediatrics. 2008;121(5): e1144–51.

Tang W, et al. Pulmonary ventilation/perfusion defects induced by epinephrine during cardiopulmonary resuscitation. Circulation. 1991;84(5):2101–7.

Touma O, Davies M. The prognostic value of end tidal carbon dioxide during cardiac arrest: a systematic review. Resuscitation. 2013;84(11):1470–9.

Urban P, et al. Cardiac arrest and blood ionized calcium levels. Ann Intern Med. 1988;109(2): 110–3.

Valdes SO, et al. Outcomes associated with amiodarone and lidocaine in the treatment of in-hospital pediatric cardiac arrest with pulseless ventricular tachycardia or ventricular fibrillation. Resuscitation. 2014;85(3):381–6.

van der Linde D, et al. Birth prevalence of congenital heart disease worldwide: a systematic review and meta-analysis. J Am Coll Cardiol. 2011;58(21):2241–7.

Voelckel WG, et al. Comparison of epinephrine and vasopressin in a pediatric porcine model of asphyxial cardiac arrest. Crit Care Med. 2000;28(12):3777–83.

von Planta M, et al. End tidal carbon dioxide as an haemodynamic determinant of cardiopulmonary resuscitation in the rat. Cardiovasc Res. 1989;23(4):364–8.

von Planta I, et al. Coronary perfusion pressure, end-tidal CO_2 and adrenergic agents in haemodynamic stable rats. Resuscitation. 1993;25(3):203–17.

Ward Jr JT. Endotracheal drug therapy. Am J Emerg Med. 1983;1(1):71–82.

Weaver WD, et al. Ventricular defibrillation – a comparative trial using 175-J and 320-J shocks. N Engl J Med. 1982;307(18):1101–6.

Wenzel V, et al. The use of arginine vasopressin during cardiopulmonary resuscitation. An analysis of experimental and clinical experience and a view of the future. Anaesthesist. 2002;51(3): 191–202.

Werner JA, et al. Visualization of cardiac valve motion in man during external chest compression using two-dimensional echocardiography. Implications regarding the mechanism of blood flow. Circulation. 1981;63(6):1417–21.

Wood WB, Manley Jr ES, Woodbury RA. The effects of CO_2-induced respiratory acidosis on the depressor and pressor components of the dog's blood pressure response to epinephrine. J Pharmacol Exp Ther. 1963;139:238–47.

Zipes DP, et al. Termination of ventricular fibrillation in dogs by depolarizing a critical amount of myocardium. Am J Cardiol. 1975;36(1):37–44.

Chapter 42
Pediatric Cardiac Surgery in Emerging Countries

William Novick and Marcelo Cardarelli

The Burden of Congenital Heart Disease in the World and in Emerging Nations in Particular

The infant mortality rate (IMR) of a country, defined as the number of infants dying before reaching 1 year of age for every 1000 children born alive during the same year, is a commonly used indicator to reflect the health status of a population.

While nearly 70 countries have managed to achieve single-digit IMRs, close to 124 emerging countries continue to have IMRs in the two and even three digits.

Countries making an epidemiological transition by conquering the prevailing and preventable causes of infant mortality through simple measures, such as sanitation and vaccines, must still struggle in order to achieve single-digit IMRs. Many factors contribute to a persistently high neonatal and infant mortality rates, and root causes are compounded and assorted, but a significant contributor to the infant death toll is the uniform incidence of birth defects across geographical, socioeconomic, and political borders (Gilboa et al. 2010).

Globally, close to 2 % of all neonatal deaths can be attributed to cardiac malformations (Rao 2007); therefore, new public health approaches and strategies must be developed to deal with the devastating effects of congenital heart disease (CHD).

W. Novick, MD (✉)
International Child Health, University of Tennessee Health Science Center, Memphis, TN, USA

William Novick Global Cardiac Alliance, Memphis, TN, USA
e-mail: bill.novick@cardiac-alliance.org

M. Cardarelli, MD, MPH
William Novick Global Cardiac Alliance, Memphis, TN, USA
e-mail: marcelo.cardarelli@cardiac-alliance.org

Inova Children Hospital, Fairfax, VA, USA

© Springer International Publishing Switzerland 2017
A. Dabbagh et al. (eds.), *Congenital Heart Disease in Pediatric and Adult Patients*, DOI 10.1007/978-3-319-44691-2_42

Using publicly available data (2013a, b), we calculated the yearly incidence of severe/moderate congenital heart disease for 180 countries. Based on 2009–2010 population data, the incidence of CHD was estimated by multiplying the number of live births times the prevailing rate of CHD among newborns.

Since mild forms of CHD rarely require interventions in the first year of life, hence, not affecting the infant mortality rate of a nation, they were excluded from our calculations.

Based on a published review of 62 publications on the incidence of CHD, we adopted for our calculations a very conservative incidence rate of six moderate/severe CHD cases per 1000 children born alive (Hoffman and Kaplan 2002). As a result, we have calculated an incidence of 809,936 children born with moderate or severe forms of CHD and requiring surgical treatment or catheterization every year.

With a global burden of 810,000 new cases every year, the questions then become how many of those new patients do receive the proper intervention/surgery, and it is here where the numbers are less clear.

We accessed the list of self-registered pediatric cardiac surgeons on the Cardio-Thoracic Surgery Network (CTSNet) as a proxy for the availability of pediatric cardiology/pediatric cardiac surgery services in any given country. The Cardio-Thoracic Surgery Network (CTSNet) is a not-for-profit organization jointly overseen by the Society of Thoracic Surgeons, the American Association for Thoracic Surgery, and the European Association for Cardio-Thoracic Surgery (EACTS) as well as numerous cardiothoracic surgery organizations from around the world (http://www.ctsnet.org). The number of cardiothoracic surgeons that list themselves as practicing in the pediatric subspecialty amounts to 3,200 around the world, a number that no doubt would become significantly smaller if we were to subject every self-listed pediatric cardiac surgeon to some stricter account of formal training experience and exclusive dedication. The second issue regarding the true number of available surgeons is given by the uneven geographic distribution of those specialists able to perform surgical procedures or manage treatment in these newborns.

While the calculated ratio of new patients born with CHD per congenital heart surgeon is 200/1 at the global level, the inequities are profound and dramatically different among continents. We found the most homogeneous distribution of surgeons in Europe where that ratio is close to 55 newborns with CHD/year per listed surgeon. Meanwhile, the American continent as a whole has a ratio of 91 newborns with CHD per listed surgeon, but with significant disproportions in the ratios between North American continent and the rest. While the United States and Canada have a low ratio (41 children born with CHD per listed surgeon), Latin America and the Caribbean have significantly higher ones (193 newborns with CHD per listed surgeon). Yet, the most dramatic shortage of pediatric heart surgeons can be seen in Asia and Africa with ratios of CHD newborns to surgeon of 486 and 1069, respectively. Oceania, on the other hand, has ratios comparable to those of developed nations (45 CHD newborns/year per listed surgeon).

Using a conservative estimate of 60 newborn children with CHD/surgeon ratio as a measure that may convey the ability of health services to deal with a modern approach with the burden of this disease, we could speculate that only 30 countries are providing appropriate care to all their patients. This represents appropriate diagnosis treatment for 68,827 patients born every year with moderate to severe CHD out of 809,000. Estimates of as low as 1.5 % of children born outside of industrialized countries receive needed surgery (Leon-Wyss et al. 2009). Clearly a substantial shortage of physicians, healthcare professionals, facilities, and budgets are dedicated to the management of this significant problem.

Shortages and Solutions

Human Resources

It is clear that one of the most significant shortages to solve the problem of children and adults with CHD in emerging countries is the human factor. Unlike infrastructure (hospitals, operating room, intensive care units, monitors, etc.) or supplies (oxygenators, sutures, sterile supplies), human resources require a significant time investment, besides the cost, never shorter than 5–10 years. Upon the decision of a government, a Ministry of Health or a local foundation to act upon the lack of congenital heart surgery services, given allocated resources, a building project may require anywhere between 1 and 3 years. Disposables, medications, sterile supplies, and instruments can be obtained, given enough economic resources, almost immediately. Human shortages (nurses, anesthesiologists, intensive care physicians, surgeons), on the other hand, are a very expensive item, it is in short supply, and it requires anywhere from 4 to 10 years of tertiary education to build.

No amount of economic resources can speed up the process of knowledge accumulation and expertise gathering that these professionals need to transit before becoming proficient at the management of CHD, and it is only with long-term planning that any society can satisfy its healthcare need in this and many other complex areas.

Because of this reason, the diagnosis and treatment of CHD in children and adults in emerging countries currently depends heavily on the support of international charity organizations and the use of alternative training pathways to achieve self-sufficient centers.

Developing a Sustainable Congenital Heart Center in an Emerging Country

Models of Assistance

The options available to either improve pediatric cardiac services at an existing site or to engage in the development of a new program are numerous and should be tailored to the desires and capabilities of the local stakeholders (Dearani et al. 2010).

Regardless of which model is decided upon, all participants must be fully vested in a long-term commitment.

Over the years we have employed four distinctive models of assistance, all having great benefits as well as drawbacks.

Education abroad Sending personnel abroad for education and training to centers of excellence for brief or extended periods of time has been used for years as a mechanism to initiate or improve a local program in pediatric cardiac care. The benefits of such a model are obvious. The trainees are exposed to centers practicing pediatric cardiac care in well-equipped institutions that have had many years to establish their programs. Typically teams at these sites have matured into cohesive units which function seamlessly. Sending young inexperienced personnel into such situations can and does lead to excitement about returning home to provide similar services. However without adequate leadership support at home, administrative commitment, and appropriate financing, this excitement rapidly disappears upon returning home to the realities of working in a low- to middle-income country (LMIC) health system. Language and cultural differences may interfere with optimizing the benefits that such an opportunity can present. In a number of Western countries, visits to centers of excellence may be observational only secondary to medicolegal issues and licensing. In the United States, direct patient care is unlikely unless the visitor has passed appropriate standardized tests and is in the position to be licensed locally. Such a program requires considerable time and financial expense (Novick et al. 2008). It is important that the personnel chosen to receive this opportunity be sufficiently mature and knowledgeable to reap the benefits. We usually recommend that at least two individuals make these visits abroad to provide support to each other during the visit and to serve as the core for change upon return home. We have used this model to provide education to groups of physicians, nurses, and technicians from a number of countries (Croatia, Bosnia, Kazakhstan, Nepal, Ukraine).

Experienced physician returns to lead program Individual senior physicians who have a desire to return home or simply a desire to assist a country in need after they have created a successful program abroad can have a major impact on program development in LMICs. The obstacles of adequate financing and political and governmental support still remain, but having an experienced senior-level leader to advocate for and direct program development is extremely beneficial to overall program sustainability and success. We have employed this model in Honduras and Nicaragua.

Visiting team of specialists The model most frequently used today is when a team of pediatric cardiac specialists visits a particular institution for a varying number of trips per year for an extended period of time. The composition of the visiting team is critical for success at every level. A visiting team must be cognizant that the receiving team will view them both positively and skeptically and realize that all aspects of the visit will be reviewed. Cultural, religious, and political differences may be present, and the visiting team must respect these differences if the success of the program is to be complete. Our teams are typically comprised of senior-level pediatric cardiac specialists including surgeon, anesthesiologist, cardiologist, intensivist, ICU nurses and nurse practitioners, respiratory therapist, and when needed a biomedical engineer. Visits including travel time are usually limited to 2 weeks and local holiday and weekend work schedules adhered to. Depending upon local infrastructure and personnel, 1–3 children receive operations daily and a similar number of catheterizations depending upon the need.

The key difference between these trips and those commonly referred to as "surgical safari" is the frequency of trips annually (3–6) and the number of years committed to developing pediatric cardiac services (5–7). We have used this model in 34 countries and helped to develop independently functioning pediatric cardiac units in 53 different institutions. Not all programs have been successful, and we have canceled 12 programs after the first 1–3 trips secondary to a variety of factors we deemed unacceptable.

One-year program We developed a unique program assistance scheme whereby we embed a team of specialists' in-country on a near continuous basis for 12 consecutive months. The team consists of a surgeon, anesthesiologist, perfusionist, intensivist, and 2–4 ICU nurses/practitioners. The surgical component spends 1 month on-site, departs for 1–2 weeks, and returns for a month on a continuous type schedule for 12 consecutive months. The ICU team arrives with the surgical team, and a portion of this team remains during the absence of the surgical team. Such a schedule allows for 41–42 weeks of surgical coverage and education, and the ICU team spends 48 weeks on-site with breaks for holidays only. The purpose of this program is to provide immediate coverage for neonates and complex cases on a nearly continuous basis to countries with a population and birthrate that can provide sufficient clinical work. The result is a rapid expansion of services and a concentrated period of education and training. We have used this program in two countries to date, Iraq and Libya. Such a program is covered by both volunteers and dedicated full-time staff from the charity.

The decision of which model to use is dependent upon the local stakeholders needs for clinical and educational services in addition to the financial support provided by the visiting and local teams. The philosophical and financial support by the hospital administration and Ministry of Health of the respective regions/countries is critical to program growth and eventual sustainability.

A Success Story

The cardiac unit at the Zaitcev Institute for General and Urgent Surgery serves both adults and children, draws from a population close to 2.9 million, and has the financial support of the Ukrainian National Academy of Medical Sciences. It has a

Table 42.1 A summary of pediatric assistance program

	Period A	Period B	p
Total number of RACHS-1 classifiable cases	154	767	
RACHS-1 classifiable patients/year (95 % CI)	19.3 (14.3–4.2)	95.9 (63.2–128.6)	*<0.0001*
Median age, year	7	1.3	

single-plane cardiac catheterization laboratory, one dedicated operating room and an eight-bed cardiac surgical intensive care unit (CSICU) with no separation of care between adults and children.

Our pediatric assistance program was launched in May 2008, and it consisted of visiting international teams every approximately 3 months for 2-week periods, and it has been focused into five main areas:

- On-site surgical and interventional activity with side-by-side training of the local team
- Education (on-site lectures, quality assessment conferences, morbidity and mortality conferences)
- Biomedical engineering support (donation of equipment and supplies, continuous engineering support)
- Development of a teamwork culture with nurse empowerment and a horizontal hierarchy
- Data collection

Using the Risk Adjustment for Congenital Heart Surgery (RACHS-1) model of risk stratification (Jenkins et al. 2002) and reviewing patient data and demographics for 7 years before our involvement (Period A – year 2000–2008) and 7 years since our assistance program was implemented (period B – 2008–2015), we show an increase in annual volume of cases and a trend toward treatment at a younger age (Table 42.1).

In Chart 42.1 we can clearly visualize the increment in case complexity with a significant decreased in mortality (66.7–11.7 %) for category RACHS-3 cases ($p=0.05$).

Analysis of the Five Main Areas of Program Assistance

On-Site Surgical and Interventional Activity

The principal purpose of an assistance program is not to perform, but to teach by working side-by-side with the local teams, while performing. There is no theoretical or classroom-style teaching stronger than hands-on exercise. The establishment of a patient discussion conference is the first step in accomplishing this goal. All patients selected for intervention/surgery during the 2-week visit periods are open for discussion, and relevant information is equally shared. We believe it is during this process

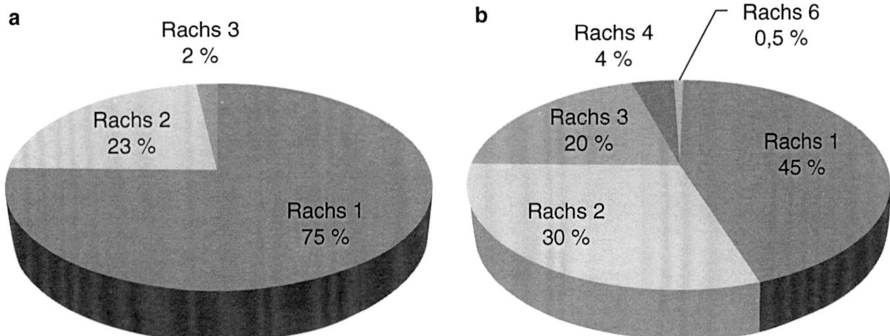

Chart 42.1 (**a**): Period A (before program assistance). (**b**): Period B (after program assistance)

of sharing the information available and the experiences of the most senior leaders of our teams that the hosting team benefits the most. While in occidental societies, we believe that the opportunity to openly discuss and question the decision-making process is fundamental for the good outcome of the patients and is not an exercise commonly carried out in other cultures. The agreement to question leadership and decisions is a learned habit that promotes good leadership skills while fostering change, keystones to the development of modern cardiac surgery centers.

Equally important is the shared experience in the operating room or catheterization suite. Our programmatic approach to the sharing/educating experience permits the transition of leadership roles over a variable period of time, from the visiting to the local team. Our expectations are that while at the beginning of the program assistance implementation, the visiting team (us) will lead and partake in most if not all of the interventions/surgeries, and over time the local surgeon(s) and interventional cardiologist will share a larger proportion of responsibility in the decision making and the actual doing of the procedure. Using the Kharkiv experience, the proportion of locally led surgeries during international assistance trips significantly increased from 0 % in 2008 to 76.2 % in 2010, finalizing with 100 % locally led surgeries in 2015. Likewise, surgical milestones made by the local team with international team assistance include first times as primary surgeon for a tetralogy of Fallot full repair (2009), complete AV canal repair (2011), and the arterial switch operation (2012). Since 2010, a second local pediatric heart surgeon has also begun training as lead surgeon.

It is important to consider that the volume and complexity of cases is kept up during the periods when we are not visiting and assisting, demonstrating a solid movement toward self-sustainability.

Education

The role of formal education should not be underestimated. Fundamental concepts must be mastered in the safe environment a classroom provides before put to practice. We believe the introduction of nurses and perfusionist to the most updated concepts to be of essential importance. Constant improvement, a concept ligated to high-reliability organizations (HROs) (organizations such as airlines and nuclear power plants that cannot afford the occurrence of even a single unwanted event) depends greatly on education and insight. Using this concept to develop a cardiac surgery center implies a trend toward zero tolerance for mishaps. Unwanted events are to be avoided by planning ahead rather than coping with them by relying on multiple safety mechanisms.

At the core of high-reliability organizations (HROs) are five key concepts, which we believe are essential for any improvement initiative to succeed (Hines et al. 2008):

Sensitivity to operations: Preserving constant awareness by leaders and staff of the state of the systems and processes that affect patient care. This awareness is the key to noting risks and preventing them.

Reluctance to simplify: Simple processes are good, but simplistic explanations for why things work or fail are risky. Avoiding overly simple explanations of failure (unqualified staff, inadequate training, communication failure, etc.) is essential in order to understand the true reasons patients are placed at risk.

Preoccupation with failure: When near misses occur, these are viewed as evidence of systems that should be improved to reduce potential harm to patients. Rather than viewing near misses as proof that the system has effective safeguards, they are viewed as symptomatic of areas in need of more attention.

Deference to expertise: If leaders and supervisors are not willing to listen and respond to the insights of the staff who knows how processes really work and the risks patients really face, you will not have a culture in which high reliability is possible.

Resilience: Leaders and staff need to be trained and prepared to know how to respond when system failures do occur.

These thought processes should be implemented from the beginning and kept in play as case mix complexity grows and a new personnel is incorporated.

Biomedical Engineering Support

Pediatric cardiac care is heavily reliant upon equipment in order to safely carry out the procedures and care of children during and after intervention. The level of technological sophistication that has been achieved in today's equipment provides us with safeguards previously unavailable. However these features also come with significant costs, which few LMIC can afford. Moreover, although much of the improvement in hardware was healthcare professional driven, it is not essential in order to provide safe cardiac care to children. Adequate equipment which has been refurbished and certified for human use can be acquired at a fraction of the cost of the new one, and in many cases as developed country hospitals upgrade their equipment one can obtain the replaced equipment for shipping costs alone.

Our approach has been to provide critical pieces of needed equipment which has been refurbished but which is not so outdated that replacement parts or entire pieces cannot be found readily. The equipment is tested before it is shipped from the United States, and an experienced biomedical engineer travels with the team's first trip into each country annually. Repairs are made on this first trip; equipment in need of replacement is identified and sought for between trips. We have used point-of-care testing as a means to bypass local laboratory deficiencies or inefficiencies. We routinely bring two handheld point-of-care devices and supply of necessary cartridges on all trips where we are knowledgeable of local laboratory shortcomings.

A Different Way of Doing Business

There are many issues confronting a team from a developed country visiting a center in an LMIC, which directly impact the decision to operate, subsequent patient care, and utilization of resources. Children in North America and Europe are now operated on mostly as newborns and infants, and it is unusual to provide a primary operation on someone in late childhood or adolescence. The consequences of chronic congenital heart disease are apparent, and given the paucity of resources available for extended or sophisticated care, special approaches need to be adopted to care safely for these children.

Chronic, pulmonary hypertension and polycythemia are just a few of the consequences of chronic congenital heart disease which the clinician faces and can impact results if approached as a child in a developed country. Pulmonary hypertension secondary to untreated L-to-R shunts is extremely common, and nitric oxide and extracorporeal membrane oxygenation devices are basically nonexistent. We have modified our ventricular septal defect patch closure allowing for R-to-L shunting postoperatively should pulmonary hypertensive crises develop (Novick et al. 2005). Moreover due to the ubiquitous presence of sildenafil, all patients demonstrating bidirectional shunting prior to operation are treated for periods of days prior to operation and continued in the immediate postoperative period for periods of 1 week to 3 months.

Malnutrition is common and infectious complications are more common after surgery than in the developed world (Jenkins et al. 2014). To minimize postoperative nosocomial pneumonia, we pursue a program of fast-track recovery in every child operated upon. Just over 70 % of the children we operate on are extubated in the first 4 h after arrival in the ICU (Shekerdemian et al. 2000). Our protocol for pain management in the immediate postoperative period of acetaminophen and ibuprofen helps us to facilitate early extubation with a very low rate of re-intubation.

Children requiring pulmonary ventricle to pulmonary artery valve conduits have few options in LMICs. The cost of a commercial valve conduit can be prohibitive unless funded by the government or donated by the visiting team. We have adopted the use of a number of unique materials to provide these children with options to commercial valve conduits including autologous pericardium, PTFE large-sized conduits, and more recently de-cellularized intestinal submucosa scaffolding (Gilbert et al. 2011).

Development of a Teamwork Culture with Nurse Empowerment and a Horizontal Hierarchy

In our experience, when we start the process of developing a new assistance program in emerging countries, the more resisted changes to introduce are those that are viewed as a traumatic change in culture. This phenomenon is particularly evident in health center located in countries where the decision-making authority is traditional and pyramidal. By this we mean, from top to bottom, from older to younger, from doctors to nurses, and from surgeon to everyone else in the group.

One of the pillars of our philosophy rests in the horizontalization of hierarchy. Our organization functions by allowing individuals to challenge and discuss any and all the options in the daily management of patients, independently of degrees, roles, and age and based solely in experience. We try to convey and implement, when possible, a similar approach to problems in those programs under our assistance.

This philosophy of horizontal hierarchy is not limited to bedside clinical issues. We actually manage our organization in a similar way. While there are fixed roles and responsibilities within our organization, any and all issues are open for discussion, and while a decision-making structure is in place, all voices are heard before making final decisions.

The empowerment of bedside nurses, operating room technicians, perfusionists, respiratory techs, etc. can be extremely helpful in the process of creating a culture where patient safety is paramount.

Data Collection

The collection of data on interventions is an important building block in the development of any pediatric cardiac program. Program growth and improvement cannot be measured unless data is gathered on each patient and analyzed on a quarterly/annual basis. We encourage all our affiliate programs to develop a local in-house database and to subscribe to one of the many international databases. We have maintained a comprehensive database on all operations performed during all our visits and have nearly 8,000 primary operations archived to date.

There are a number of database registries available for use through the Society of Thoracic Surgery, the European Congenital Heart Surgeons Association, and The Asian Society for Cardiovascular and Thoracic Surgery. We, and others, have noted reluctance over the years for new programs to share their data with international registries secondary to reluctance to disclose surgical or interventional results that fall below international standards. As such we embarked on an effort to create a database and registry with Boston Children's Hospital and the University of Geneva in 2007 which allows enrollment of programs only located in LMICs.

This initiative is the International Quality Improvement Collaborative (IQIC) in pediatric cardiac surgery in developing countries and now has more than 30 institutions participating throughout the world. The IQIC is unique in that in addition to routine reporting of results of the group and individual institutions, it routinely provides webinars. The webinars are structured to improve specific aspects of the care of children with cardiac interventions. The first publication from the IQIC analyzed the results of the webinars on surgical site infections. To date this service is provided without cost to the participants.

Data Monitoring

Although not a systemic part of our program assistance methodology, we believe real-time data monitoring is as important as data acquisition for the development of a solid cardiac surgery program. Outcomes data, once entered in our database, must be brought to life by some type of data monitoring system that provides a current and dynamic view of the outcomes as they happen. This type of data management (data acquisition followed by data visualization) avoids the perils of looking retrospectively to the data and making the adjustments a year or 6 months after we realize a trend toward declining clinical outcomes has been occurring.

We favor the use of software such as the Variable Life-Adjusted Display (VLAD) currently used by the Society for Cardiothoracic Surgery in Great Britain and Ireland (Novick et al. 2008) to assess and to present to the public the mortality of their cardiac surgery centers. This program, which was provided free of charge to us by the University College of London Operational Research Unit (Clinical Operational Research Unit 2016), allows for real-time monitoring of binary variables based on an observed/expected calculation.

Figure 42.1 shows data on the eight common outcomes quality measures (Jacobs et al. 2012) in 2709 of our surgeries carried out in 10 LMICs between January 2008 and June 2013. The difference in trends is self-evident. While our observed outcomes are better than expected (above the horizontal line) for five important quality measures (surgery for chylothorax, diaphragm plication, mediastinitis, need for a permanent pacemaker, and sepsis), we were trending below the expected results on two critical variables (take-back for bleeding and reoperation/revision during the same admission) (Cardarelli et al. 2014).

The visualization of the available data in our database allowed for a detailed analysis, utilizing the same software, of the countries where these two outcomes were lagging. For instance, after assigning an expected incidence of 0.031 % to the *take-back for bleeding* events, we realized that our bleeding issues were not generalized but rather limited to five of the ten countries we were operating in Fig. 42.2.

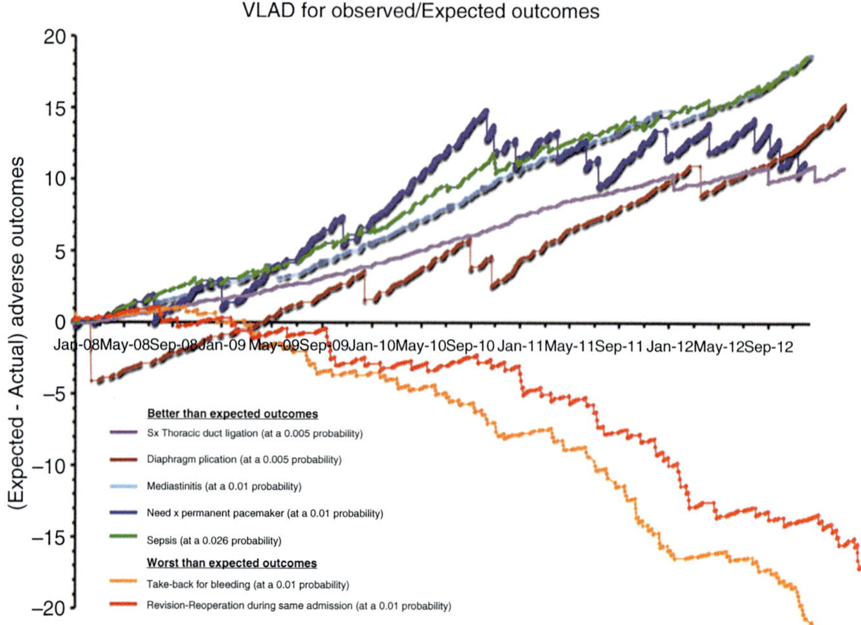

Fig. 42.1 Shows visualization of data collected on eight common quality measures over a 4-year period (Jan 2008–Sept 2012). Lines below the expected horizon (*horizontal line*) demonstrate worst than expected complications in the areas of take-back for bleeding and unexpected reoperation/revision during the same hospitalization

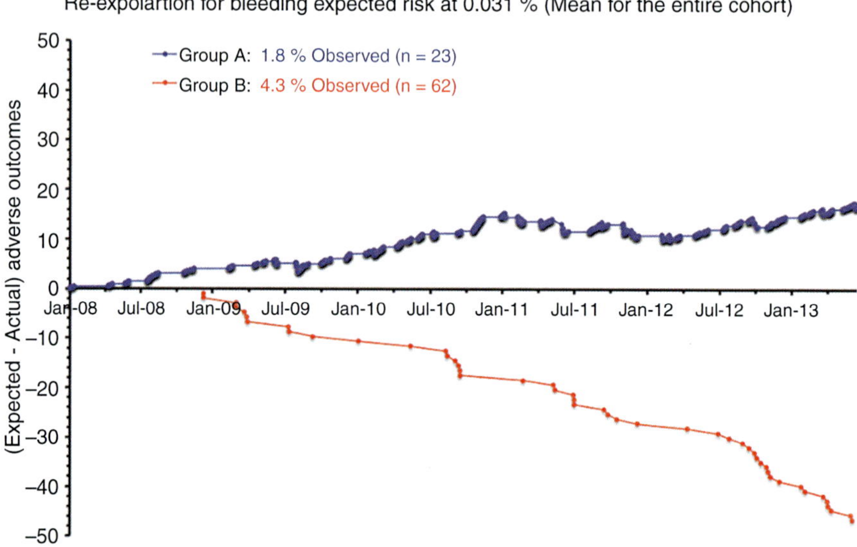

Fig. 42.2 Countries in *Group A* had a better than expected frequency of surgical bleeding with an overall 1.8 % rate. Meanwhile, countries in *Group B* performed worse than expected with a take-back rate for bleeding of 4.3 %

The main advantage of the use of this type of tools is the real-time visualization of a problem since this graph can be actualized as soon as data on a new patient is added in the software-running score sheet.

Summary

Despite enormous scientific progress in many areas of medicine and public health, even today, a significant proportion of children born with congenital heart disease in Asia, Africa, and Latin America do not receive proper diagnosis or treatment.

The human toll has never been calculated, and the economic burden of this unsatisfied demand for services is overwhelming but never before has been properly addressed. While in the short term, this problem is unlikely to be solved; well-planned surgical/educational humanitarian campaigns combined with adequate locally budgeted resources and a sustainable plan may, in the long term, create the conditions by which most children born with heart defects in the developing world could be diagnosed and treated in time to have a full and productive life.

References

2013a. http://www.who.int/en. In.

2013b. http://www.worldbank.org/. In.

Cardarelli M, Molloy F, Novick W. 2014. Use of variable-adjusted display to benchmark pediatric cardiac surgery morbidity among emerging countries. In: 22nd annual meeting of Asian Society for Cardiovascular and Thoracic Surgery Istanbul, Turkey.

Clinical Operational Research Unit C. 2016. www.ucl.ac.uk/operational-research.

Dearani JA, Neirotti R, Kohnke EJ, Sinha KK, Cabalka AK, Barnes RD, Jacobs JP, Stellin G, Tchervenkov CI, Cushing JC. Improving pediatric cardiac surgical care in developing countries: matching resources to needs. Semin Thorac Cardiovasc Surg Pediatr Card Surg Annu. 2010;13:35–43.

Gilbert CL, Gnanapragasam J, Benhaggen R, Novick WM. Novel use of extracellular matrix graft for creation of pulmonary valved conduit. World J Pediatr Congenit Heart Surg. 2011;2:495–501.

Gilboa SM, Salemi JL, Nembhard WN, Fixler DE, Correa A. Mortality resulting from congenital heart disease among children and adults in the United States, 1999 to 2006. Circulation. 2010;122:2254–63.

Hines S, Luna K, Lofthus J, et al. Becoming a high reliability organization: operational advice for hospital leaders. (Prepared by the Lewin Group under Contract No. 290-04-0011.) AHRQ Publication No 08-0022. Rockville: Agency for Healthcare Research and Quality April; 2008.

Hoffman JI, Kaplan S. The incidence of congenital heart disease. J Am Coll Cardiol. 2002;39: 1890–900.

Jacobs JP, Jacobs ML, Austin 3rd EH, Mavroudis C, Pasquali SK, Lacour-Gayet FG, Tchervenkov CI, Walters 3rd H, Bacha EA, Nido PJ, Fraser CD, Gaynor JW, Hirsch JC, Morales DL, Pourmoghadam KK, Tweddell JS, Prager RL, Mayer JE. Quality measures for congenital and pediatric cardiac surgery. World J Pediatr Congenit Heart Surgery. 2012;3:32–47.

Jenkins KJ, Castaneda AR, Cherian KM, Couser CA, Dale EK, Gauvreau K, Hickey PA, Koch Kupiec J, Morrow DF, Novick WM, Rangel SJ, Zheleva B, Christenson JT. Reducing mortality and infections after congenital heart surgery in the developing world. Pediatrics. 2014;134: e1422–30.

Jenkins KJ, Gauvreau K, Newburger JW, Spray TL, Moller JH, Iezzoni LI. Consensus-based method for risk adjustment for surgery for congenital heart disease. J Thorac Cardiovasc Surg. 2002;123:110–8.

Leon-Wyss JR, Veshti A, Veras O, Gaitan GA, O'Connell M, Mack RA, Calvimontes G, Garcia F, Hidalgo A, Reyes A, Castaneda AR. Pediatric cardiac surgery: a challenge and outcome analysis of the Guatemala effort. Semin Thorac Cardiovasc Surg Pediatr Card Surg Annu. 2009:8–11. doi:10.1053/j.pcsu.2009.01.003.

Novick WM, Sandoval N, Lazorhysynets VV, Castillo V, Baskevitch A, Mo X, Reid RW, Marinovic B, Di Sessa TG. Flap valve double patch closure of ventricular septal defects in children with increased pulmonary vascular resistance. Ann Thorac Surg. 2005;79:21–8. discussion 21–28.

Novick WM, Stidham GL, Karl TR, Arnold R, Anic D, Rao SO, Baum VC, Fenton KE, Di Sessa TG. Paediatric cardiac assistance in developing and transitional countries: the impact of a fourteen year effort. Cardiol Young. 2008;18:316–23.

Rao SG. Pediatric cardiac surgery in developing countries. Pediatr Cardiol. 2007;28:144–8.

Shekerdemian LS, Penny DJ, Novick W. Early extubation after surgical repair of tetralogy of Fallot. Cardiol Young. 2000;10:636–7.

Index

© Springer International Publishing Switzerland 2017

A. Dabbagh et al. (eds.), *Congenital Heart Disease in Pediatric
and Adult Patients*, DOI 10.1007/978-3-319-44691-2